**Essential Revision Notes
for the European Exam in Core Cardiology**

Essential Revision Notes for the European Exam in Core Cardiology

Second Edition

EDITED BY

Daniel X Augustine
Consultant Cardiologist, Royal United Hospitals Bath NHS Foundation Trust, UK;
Honorary Professor, University of Bath, UK

John Graby
Cardiology Specialist Registrar, Royal United Hospitals Bath NHS Foundation Trust, UK

Ali Khavandi
Consultant Cardiologist, Royal United Hospitals Bath NHS Foundation Trust, UK

Sri Raveen Kandan
Consultant Cardiologist, Royal United Hospitals Bath NHS Foundation Trust, UK

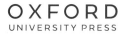

Great Clarendon Street, Oxford, OX2 6DP,
United Kingdom

Oxford University Press is a department of the University of Oxford.
It furthers the University's objective of excellence in research, scholarship,
and education by publishing worldwide. Oxford is a registered trade mark of
Oxford University Press in the UK and in certain other countries

© Oxford University Press 2025

The moral rights of the authors have been asserted

First Edition published in 2014
Second Edition published in 2025

All rights reserved. No part of this publication may be reproduced, stored in
a retrieval system, or transmitted, in any form or by any means, without the
prior permission in writing of Oxford University Press, or as expressly permitted
by law, by licence or under terms agreed with the appropriate reprographics
rights organization. Enquiries concerning reproduction outside the scope of the
above should be sent to the Rights Department, Oxford University Press, at the
address above

You must not circulate this work in any other form
and you must impose this same condition on any acquirer

Published in the United States of America by Oxford University Press
198 Madison Avenue, New York, NY 10016, United States of America

British Library Cataloguing in Publication Data

Data available

Library of Congress Control Number: 2024942014

ISBN 978–0–19–879546–9

DOI: 10.1093/med/9780198795469.001.0001

Printed in the UK by
Bell & Bain Ltd., Glasgow

Oxford University Press makes no representation, express or implied, that the
drug dosages in this book are correct. Readers must therefore always check
the product information and clinical procedures with the most up-to-date
published product information and data sheets provided by the manufacturers
and the most recent codes of conduct and safety regulations. The authors and
the publishers do not accept responsibility or legal liability for any errors in the
text or for the misuse or misapplication of material in this work. Except where
otherwise stated, drug dosages and recommendations are for the non-pregnant
adult who is not breast-feeding

The manufacturer's authorised representative in the EU for product safety is
Oxford University Press España S.A. of El Parque Empresarial San Fernando de
Henares, Avenida de Castilla, 2 – 28830 Madrid (www.oup.es/en or product.
safety@oup.com). OUP España S.A. also acts as importer into Spain of
products made by the manufacturer.

Huge thanks for the support of my wife, Ellie and my junior A team—Josh, Zach, Luke & Yasmin. Dan Augustine

For Ellen and Huw, and my parents for all the opportunities they provided. John Graby

*For my father, who taught me to give my best in everything that I do; and my mother, whose selflessness and sacrifice created endless opportunities for our family.
Sri Raveen Kandan*

Preface

The European Exam in Core Cardiology (EECC) is led by the European Society of Cardiology, in conjunction with the European Union of Medical Specialists and the national cardiac societies. It is designed to assess core cardiology knowledge and is part of an assessment strategy for current specialist trainees in cardiology, our future leaders in cardiology.

Essential revision notes for the European Exam in Core Cardiology is the first text book of its kind, aimed to help cardiology trainees prepare for the EECC. The book is based upon the ESC Core Curriculum syllabus (2020) and written by cardiology trainees with experience in the exam as well as established consultants throughout Europe, from a variety of specialties. Falling between a reference textbook and pocket handbook, Essential revision notes for the EECC is a practical, contemporary, concise yet comprehensive cardiology textbook.

Since initiation in 2018, this project has not been without hurdles. The book was restructured in 2020 following the new syllabus launch and since then updated ESC guidelines have been incorporated into the book. There was a hiatus during the COVID-19 pandemic and following ease of restrictions, publishing houses have understandably taken time to reintegrate to allow onward publication. Despite all of this, the contributors to the book have been outstanding and the Editors would like to extend their sincere gratitude to all of our contributors.

We hope this revision aid helps cardiology trainees throughout Europe, our future cardiology leaders.

Acknowledgements

The editors would like to thank the OUP team for their help during the drafting and processing of the book. A special thanks in particular goes to James Oates for his support and advice during the whole project.

We would like to thank the following colleagues for contributing images:

Dr Kevin Carson, Consultant Cardiologist, Royal United Hospitals Bath NHS Foundation Trust, UK

Dr Edward Duncan, University Hospitals Bristol and Weston NHS Foundation Trust, UK

Dr Thomas W Johnson, University Hospitals Bristol and Weston NHS Foundation Trust, UK

Dr David Little, Consultant Radiologist, Royal United Hospitals Bath NHS Foundation Trust, UK

Dr Nathan Manghat, University Hospitals Bristol and Weston NHS Foundation Trust, UK

Contents

List of Contributors xv
Levels of evidence xxi
List of abbreviations xxiii

1 IMAGING 1

1.1 Echocardiography 3
Luigi P. Badano, Elena Surkova, Denisa Muraru, Chiara Palermo, and Patriza Aruta

1.2 Cardiac magnetic resonance imaging 65
Theo Karamitsos and Chrysovalantou Nikolaidou

1.3 Cardiac computed tomography 91
Jonathan Rodrigues, Benjamin Hudson, Oliver Gosling, and Kate Liang

1.4 Nuclear techniques 107
Nik Sabharwal and Katharine Thomas

2 CORONARY ARTERY DISEASE 121

2.1 Acute coronary syndrome 123
Mark Mariathas, and Florence Mouy

2.2 Chronic coronary syndrome 147
Phillip Freeman and Majd Protty

2.3 Cardiac catheterization 165
Daniel McKenzie and Paul Brady

3 VALVULAR HEART DISEASE 195

3.1 Epidemiology 197
Sarah Hudson and Daniel X Augustine

3.2 Aortic valve disease 199
Sarah Hudson and Daniel X Augustine

3.3 Mitral valve disease 211
Sarah Hudson and Daniel X Augustine

3.4 Tricuspid valve disease 223
Sarah Hudson and Daniel X Augustine

3.5 Pulmonary valve disease 229
Sarah Hudson and Daniel X Augustine

3.6 Mixed and multi-valvular disease 233
Shaun Robinson

3.7 Prosthetic valves 243
Sarah Hudson and Daniel X Augustine

3.8 Infective endocarditis 249
Bernard Prendergast, James Harrison, and James Tomlinson

4 RHYTHM DISORDERS 271

4.1 The electrocardiogram 273
S M Afzal Sohaib and Mark Elliott

4.2 Transient loss consciousness 303
Boon Lim and Katharine Thomas

4.3 Bradycardia and pacemakers 317
Richard Bond and Howell Williams

4.4 Supraventricular tachycardia 335
Richard Bond, Howell Williams, Christopher N. Floyd, and Alexander Carpenter

4.5 Atrial fibrillation 355
Kim Rajappan and Dan Raine

4.6 Atrial flutter 369
Kim Rajappan and Dan Raine

4.7 Ventricular arrhythmia 375
Richard Bond and Howell Williams

4.8 Cardiac ion channel dysfunction 383
Richard Bond, Howell Williams, Victoria McKay, and Stewart Brown

4.9 Implantable cardioverter defibrillator 391
Richard Bond and Howell Williams

4.10 Cardiac resynchronization therapy and His bundle pacing 409
Richard Bond and Howell Williams

5 HEART FAILURE 417

5.1 Heart failure syndromes 419
Abdul Hameed, Andrew Clark, Christopher N Floyd, and Alexander Carpenter

5.2 Cardiomyopathies 461
Angus Nightingale, Eva Sammut, Victoria McKay, Stewart Brown, and Rhian Richardson

5.3 Pericardial disease 499
Nav Masani and Abbas Zaidi

5.4 Cardiac tumours 517
Arjun Ghosh

5.5 Cardio-oncology 527
Arjun Ghosh

6 ACUTE CARDIOVASCULAR CARE 537

6.1 Acute cardiovascular care 539
Ben Gibbison and Ursula McHugh

6.2 Cardiac arrest and resuscitation 567
Richard Bond and Ahmed Merghani

6.3 Sudden cardiac death 573
Richard Bond and Ahmed Merghani

7 PREVENTION, REHABILITATION AND SPORT 585

7.1 Sports cardiology 587
Joyee Basu, Jamie O'Driscoll, and Daniel X Augustine

7.2 Primary prevention 617
Scott Murray and David Murphy

7.3 Arterial hypertension 629
Tim Fairbairn and James Redfern

7.4 Dyslipidaemia 643
Scott Murray, David Murphy, Christopher N. Floyd, and Alexander Carpenter

7.5 Diabetes 665
Mimi Z. Chen and Konstantinos Gkastaris

7.6 Cardiac rehabilitation 679
Dimitra Nikoletou

8 CARDIAC PATIENTS IN OTHER SETTINGS 691

8.1 Aortic disease 693
David Wilson

8.2 Trauma to the aorta or heart 723
David Wilson

8.3 Peripheral artery disease 727
Marcus Brooks and Fjalar Elvarsson

8.4 Thromboembolic disease 743
Jay Suntharalingam and James Harper

8.5 Pulmonary hypertension 759
Gerry Coghlan, Hossam Fayed, and Ruta Virsinskaite

8.6 Adult congenital heart disease 775
Ali Khavandi, Graham Stuart and Victoria North

8.7 Cardiovascular disease in pregnancy 813
Stephanie Curtis and Yasmin Ismail

9 CARDIOLOGICAL CONSULTATION 835

9.1 The patient undergoing non-cardiac surgery 837
James Rosengarten, Hiten Patel, and Thomas White

9.2 The patient with neurological symptoms 857
James Choulerton, Helen Sims, Oliver Watkinson, and Laura Pannell

9.3 The patient with chronic kidney disease 869
Diana Vassallo and Dimitrios Poulikakos

9.4 The patient with pulmonary disease 885
Patrick Murphy and Georgios Kaltsakas

9.5 The patient with rheumatic disorders 901
John D. Pauling and Lesley-Anne Bissell

9.6 The patient with erectile dysfunction 923
Greg Shaw, Piotr Pawel Swiniarski, and David Ralph

10 GENETICS AND CLINICAL PHARMACOLOGY 929

10.1 Genetics 931
Victoria McKay and Stewart Brown

10.2 Clinical pharmacology 943
Christopher N. Floyd and Alexander Carpenter

Index 947

Contributors

Joanna Abramik
Cardiology Specialist Registrar, University Hospitals Bristol and Weston NHS Foundation Trust, Bristol, UK

Patriza Aruta
Policlinico University Hospitals "G. Rodolico-San Marco," Division of Cardiology San Marco Hospital, Catania, Italy

Daniel X Augustine
Consultant Cardiologist, Royal United Hospitals Bath NHS Foundation Trust, UK; Honorary Professor, University of Bath, Bath, UK

Luigi P. Badano
Professor of Cardiovascular Medicine, University of Milano-Bicocca, Milan, Italy

Joyee Basu
Cardiology Specialist Registrar, John Radcliffe Hospital, Oxford, UK

Lesley-Anne Bissell
Consultant Rheumatologist & Honorary Senior Lecturer, Leeds Teaching Hospitals NHS Trust and University of Leeds, Leeds, UK

Richard Baker
Consultant Cardiologist, Musgrove Park Hospital, Somerset NHS Foundation Trust, Taunton, UK

Richard Bond
Consultant Cardiologist and Electrophysiologist, Gloucestershire Royal Hospital NHS Foundation Trust, Gloucester, UK

Paul Brady
Cardiology Specialist Registrar, Bristol Heart Institute, University Hospitals Bristol NHS Foundation Trust & Severn Deanery, UK

Marcus Brooks
Consultant Vascular Surgeon, North Bristol NHS Trust, Bristol, UK

Stewart Brown
Cardiology Specialist Registrar & Research Fellow, Musgrove Park Hospital, Somerset NHS Foundation Trust & Severn Deanery, UK

Alexander Carpenter
Cardiology Specialist Registrar and MRC Clinical Research Training Fellow, Bristol Heart Institute, University Hospitals Bristol NHS Foundation Trust & Severn Deanery, UK

Mimi Z. Chen
Consultant Endocrinologist & Honorary Senior Lecturer, St. George's University Hospitals NHS Foundation Trust & St. George's, University of London, London, UK

James Choulerton
Consultant Stroke Physician, Royal United Hospital Bath NHS Foundation Trust, Bath, UK

Andrew Clark
Professor of Cardiology, Hull York Medical School, Hull, UK

Gerry Coghlan
Consultant Cardiologist, Royal Free Hospital, London, UK

Stephanie Curtis
Consultant Cardiologist, University Hospitals Bristol and Weston NHS Foundation Trust, UK

Mark Elliott
Cardiology Specialist Registrar, North East Thames Deanery, UK

Fjalar Elvarsson
Consultant Vascular Surgeon, Västmanland Hospital, Västerås, Sweden

Tim Fairbairn
Consultant Cardiologist, Liverpool Heart and Chest Hospital, Liverpool, UK

Hossam Fayed
Structural Heart Fellow, Kings College Hospital, London and Hon. Clinical Lecturer, Institute of Cardiovascular Science, University College London, London, UK

Christopher N. Floyd
Visiting Senior Lecturer in Clinical Pharmacology & Therapeutics, King's College London, London, UK

Phillip Freeman
Interventional Cardiologist and Cardiac MRI, Aalborg University Hospital, Aalborg, Denmark

Arjun K. Ghosh
Consultant Cardiologist, Cardio-Oncology services at Barts Heart Centre, St Bartholomew's Hospital and University College London Hospital, London, UK

Ben Gibbison
Associate Professor in Cardiac Anaesthesia and Intensive Care, University of Bristol, Bristol, UK

Konstantinos Gkastaris
Consultant in Diabetes and Endocrinology, St. Luke's Hospital, Panorama, Thessaloniki, Greece

Oliver Gosling
Consultant Cardiologist, Cardiology Department, Musgrove Park Hospital, Taunton, UK

Abdul Hameed
Consultant Cardiologist and Honorary Senior Lecturer, Sheffield Teaching Hospitals Trust and Hull University Teaching Hospitals NHS Trust, UK

James Harper
Consultant Respiratory Physician, Royal United Hospitals Bath NHS Foundation Trust, Bath, UK

James Harrison
Department of Cardiology, Guy's and St. Thomas' NHS Foundation Trust, London, UK

Benjamin J. Hudson
Consultant Radiologist, Royal United Hospitals Bath NHS Foundation Trust, Bath, UK

Sarah Hudson
Consultant Cardiologist, Wye Valley NHS Trust, Hereford, UK

Georgios Kaltsakas
Consultant Respiratory Physician and Honorary Senior Lecturer, Guy's and St Thomas' NHS Foundation Trust & King's College London, London, UK

Theo Karamitsos
Division of Cardiovascular Medicine, Radcliffe Department of Medicine, John Radcliffe Hospital, Oxford, UK

Ali Khavandi
Consultant Cardiologist, Royal United Hospitals Bath NHS Foundation Trust, UK

Kate Liang
Cardiology Specialist Registrar, Bristol Heart Institute, University Hospitals Bristol and Weston NHS Trust, Bristol, UK

Boon Lim
Consultant Cardiologist, Hammersmith Hospital, Imperial College Healthcare NHS Trust, London, UK

Mark Mariathas
Consultant Cardiologist, Bristol Heart Institute, University Hospitals Bristol NHS Foundation Trust, UK

Nav Masani
Consultant Cardiologist, Cardiff & Vale University Health Board, Cardiff, UK

Ursula McHugh
Consultant Anaesthetist, St James's Hospital, Dublin, Ireland

Victoria McKay
Consultant in Cardiovascular Clinical Genetics, Liverpool Centre for Genomic Medicine & Liverpool Heart and Chest NHS FT, Liverpool, UK

Daniel McKenzie
Consultant Cardiologist, Royal United Hospitals Bath NHS Foundation Trust, Bath, UK

Ahmed Merghani
Consultant Cardiologist and Electrophysiologist, University Hospital of Northern British Columbia, Prince George, Canada

Florence Mouy
Cardiology Specialist Registrar, Royal United Hospitals Bath NHS Foundation Trust, Bath UK

Denisa Muraru
Cardiologist, University of Milano-Bicocca, Istituto Auxologico Italiano, IRCCS, San Luca Hospital, Milan, Italy

David Murphy
Cardiology Specialist Registrar & Research Fellow, Royal United Hospitals Bath NHS Foundation Trust & Severn Deanery, UK

Patrick B Murphy
Consultant in Sleep, Ventilation and Respiratory Medicine, Reader in Respiratory Medicine, King's College London, London, UK

Scott Murray
Consultant Cardiologist & Honorary Senior Lecturer, Wirral University Teaching Hospital & Liverpool Centre for Cardiovascular Science, Liverpool, UK

Angus Nightingale
Consultant Cardiologist, Bristol Heart Institute, University Hospitals Bristol NHS Foundation Trust, Bristol, UK

Chrysovalantou Nikolaidou
Oxford Centre for Clinical Magnetic Resonance Research, University of Oxford, UK

Dimitra Nikoletou
Associate Professor in Exercise Rehabilitation, St George's University of London, London, UK

Victoria North
Consultant Cardiologist (Congenital Heart Disease), Bristol Heart Institute, University Hospitals Bristol NHS Foundation Trust, Bristol, UK

Jamie O'Driscoll
Reader in Cardiovascular Physiology, School of Psychology and Life Sciences, Canterbury Christ Church University

Chiara Palermo
Cardiac Sonographer, University of Padua, Azienda Ospedale-Università Padova, Padua, Italy

Katherine Thomas
Clinical Research Fellow, University of Oxford, Oxford, UK

Laura Pannell
Cardiology Research Fellow and Specialist Registrar, Bristol Heart Institute, University Hospitals Bristol NHS Foundation Trust, Bristol, UK

Hiten Patel
Cardiologist, Eastbourne District General Hospital, UK

John D. Pauling
Consultant Rheumatologist and Senior Lecturer, North Bristol NHS Trust, Bristol, UK; Translational Health Sciences, Bristol Medical School, University of Bristol, Bristol, UK

Dimitrios Poulikakos
Consultant Renal Physician Salford Royal NHS Foundation Trust & Honorary Senior Lecturer, Salford Royal NHS Foundation Trust & University of Manchester, Manchester, UK

Bernard Prendergast
Consultant Cardiologist, St Thomas' Hospital and Cleveland Clinic London, London, UK

Majd Protty
WCAT Clinical Lecturer in Interventional Cardiology, Cardiff University, UK

Dan Raine
Consultant Cardiologist and Electrophysiologist, Norfolk and Norwich University Hospital, Norwich, UK

Kim Rajappan
Consultant Cardiologist and Electrophysiologist, John Radcliffe Hospital, Oxford University Hospitals NHS Foundation Trust, Oxford, UK

David Ralph
Consultant Urologist at University College London and Medical Director of St Peter's Andrology Centre, London, UK

James Redfern
Consultant Cardiologist, Countess of Chester Hospital, UK

Rhian Richardson
Specialty Doctor in Cardiology, Royal United Hospital Bath NHS Foundation Trust, Bath, UK

Shaun Robinson
Consultant Clinical Scientist, Imperial College Healthcare NHS Trust, London, UK

Jonathan Rodrigues
Consultant Cardiothoracic Radiologist, Royal United Hospitals NHS Foundation Trust, Honorary Senior Lecturer, Department of Health, University of Bath, Chief Medical Officer and Co-Founder, Heart & Lung Imaging LTD

James Rosengarten
Consultant Cardiologist, East Kent Hospitals University NHS Foundation Trust, UK

Nikant Sabharwal
Consultant Cardiologist, John Radcliffe Hospital, Oxford University Hospitals NHS Foundation Trust, Oxford, UK

Eva Sammut
Consultant Cardiologist, Bristol Heart Institute, University Hospitals Bristol NHS Foundation Trust, Bristol, UK

Greg Shaw
Lead for Robotic Urology & Professor of Urology, University College London Hospitals NHS Foundation Trust & University College London, UK

Helen Sims
Geriatric and Stroke Specialist Registrar, North Bristol NHS Trust & Severn Deanery, UK

S M Afzal Sohaib
Consultant Cardiologist (Electrophysiology & Devices), St Bartholomew's Hospital, London, & King George Hospital, Essex, UK

Graham Stuart
Consultant Cardiologist (Congenital Heart Disease) & Honorary Associate Professor in Sports and Exercise Cardiology, Bristol Heart Institute & Bristol Royal Hospital for Children, University Hospitals Bristol NHS Foundation Trust & University of Bristol, Bristol, UK

Jay Suntharalingam
Consultant Respiratory Physician, Royal United Hospitals Bath NHS Foundation Trust, Bath, UK; Honorary Professor, Department for Health, University of Bath, Bath, UK

Elena Surkova
Honorary Consultant Cardiologist, Royal Brompton and Harefield Hospitals, Guy's and St Thomas' NHS Foundation Trust, London, UK

Piotr Pawel Swiniarski
Lecturer, Department of Urology and Andrology, Ludwik Rydygier Medical College NCU in Bydgoszcz, Poland & Nicolaus Copernicus University in Torun, Poland

James Tomlinson
Cardiology Specialist Registrar, Royal United Hospitals Bath NHS Foundation Trust, Bath, UK

Katharine Thomas
Clinical Research Fellow, University of Oxford, Oxford, UK

Diana Vassallo
Consultant in Nephrology and General Medicine, Department of Medicine, Mater Dei Hospital, Msida, Malta

Ruta Virsinskaite
Clinical Research Fellow in Pulmonary Hypertension, National Pulmonary Hypertension Service, Royal Free London NHS Foundation Trust, London, UK

Oliver Watkinson
Consultant Cardiologist, Royal United Hospitals Bath NHS Foundation Trust, Bath, UK

Thomas White
Cardiology Specialist Registrar, Royal United Hospital Bath NHS Foundation Trust & Severn Deanery, UK

Howell Williams
Cardiology Specialist Registrar, Bristol Heart Institute, University Hospitals Bristol and Weston NHS Foundation Trust & Severn Deanery, UK

David Wilson
Consultant Cardiologist, Worcestershire Acute Hospitals NHS Trust, UK

Abbas Zaidi
Consultant Cardiologist, Cardiff & Vale University Health Board, Cardiff, UK

Levels of evidence

This revision book has been written to reflect the latest European Society of Cardiology (ESC) guidelines and evidence, whilst aligning with the 2020 ESC Core Curriculum. As such, when presented, evidence is graded in line with ESC assessment of recommendation and level of evidence, as presented in table form below.

Table 1 ESC graded classes of recommendation

	Definition	Wording to use
Class I	Evidence and/or general agreement that a given treatment or procedure is beneficial, useful, effective.	Is recommended or is indicated
Class II	Conflicting evidence and/or a divergence of opinion about the usefulness/efficacy of the given treatment or procedure.	
Class IIa	Weight of evidence/opinion is in favour of usefulness/efficacy.	Should be considered
Class IIb	Usefulness/efficacy is less well established by evidence/opinion.	May be considered
Class III	Evidence or general agreement that the given treatment or procedure is not useful/effective, and in some cases may be harmful.	Is not recommended

Table 2 ESC graded level of evidence

Level of evidence A	Data derived from multiple randomized clinical trials or meta-analyses.
Level of evidence B	Data derived from a single randomized clinical trial or large non-randomized studies.
Level of evidence C	Consensus of opinion of the experts and/or small studies, retrospective studies, registries.

List of abbreviations

6MWT	6 minute walk test	APS	anti-phospholipid syndrome
99mTc-PYP	Technetium99m-pyrophosphate	AR	aortic regurgitation
		ARB	angiotensin II receptor blockers
AAA	abdominal aortic aneurysm		
AADs	anti-arrhythmic drugs	ARD	autoimmune rheumatic disease
AAV	ANCA-associated systemic vasculitis		
		ARNI	angiotensin receptor and neprilysin inhibitor
ABI	ankle-brachial index		
ACE	angiotensin converting enzyme	ARR	absolute risk reduction
		ARVC	arrhythmogenic right ventricular cardiomyopathy
ACEi	angiotensin converting enzyme inhibitor		
		AnkS	ankylosing spondylitis
ACHD	adult congenital heart disease	AS	aortic stenosis
aCL	anticardiolipin antibodies	ASA	American Society of Anesthesiologists
ACPA	anto-citrullinated protein antibodies		
		ASCVD	atherosclerotic cardiovascular disease
ACR	albumin creatinine ratio		
ACS	acute coronary syndrome	ASD	atrial septal defect
ADA	American Diabetes Association	ASOT	anti-streptolysin-O titre
		ASV	adaptive servo-ventilation
AHI	apnoea-hypopnoea index	AT	atrial tachycardia
AF	atrial fibrillation	AtriTP	adenosine triphosphate
AFL	atrial flutter	ATP	anti-tachycardia pacing
AH	atrio-Hisian	AUC	area under curve
AHRE	atrial high rate episodes	AV	atrioventricular
AIDS	acquired immunodeficiency syndrome	AVA	aortic valve area
		AVM	arteriovenous malformation
ALCAPA	left coronary artery from pulmonary artery	AVN	atrioventricular node
		AVNRT	atrioventricular nodal re-entrant tachycardia
ALS	advanced life support		
ALT	alanine transaminase	AVRT	atrioventricular re-entrant tachycardia
AMI	acute myocardial infarction		
ANCA	anti-neutrophil cytoplasm antibodies	AVSD	atrioventricular septal defect
anti-β2GPI	anti-beta2-glycoprotein I	BAV	bicuspid aortic valve
Ao	aorta	BB	beta blocker
AP	accessory pathway	BBB	bundle branch block
Apo- (A or B)	Apolipoprotein	BCT	broad complex tachycardia

BiPAP	bilevel positive airway pressure	CPET	cardio pulmonary exercise test
BMS	bare metal stent	CPPD	calcium pyrophosphate dehydrate
BMI	body mass index		
BNP	b-type natriuretic peptide	CPR	cardiopulmonary resuscitation
BP	blood pressure		
BPPV	benign paroxysmal positional vertigo	CPVT	catecholaminergic polymorphic ventricular tachycardia
BT	Blalock–Taussig		
Ca2+	calcium	CrCl	creatinine clearance
CABG	coronary artery bypass graft	CRP	c reactive protein
CACS	coronary artery calcium score	CRT	cardiac resynchronization therapy
CAD	coronary artery disease	CRT-P/D	cardiac resynchronization therapy pacemaker/ defibrillator
CAM	cancer associated myositis		
CAPS	catastrophic antiphospholipid syndrome		
		CS	coronary sinus
CAT	COPD assessment tool	CSA	central sleep apnoea
CAV	chronic allograft vasculopathy	CSM	carotid sinus massage
		CSR	Cheyne–Stokes respiration
CCB	calcium channel blocker	CSS	carotid sinus syndrome
CI	cardiac index	CT	computerized tomography/ computed tomography
CCF	congestive cardiac failure		
ccTGA	congenitally corrected transposition of the great arteries	CTA	computed tomography angiography
		CTD	connective tissue disease
CCU	coronary care unit	CTI	cavotricuspid isthmus
CFAE	complex fractionated atrial electrogram	cTnI	cardiac troponin I
		cTnT	cardiac troponin T
CHB	complete heart block	CTPA	computed tomography pulmonary angiogram
CHD	coronary heart disease		
CHF	congestive heart failure	CV	cardiovascular
CHG	comparative genomic hybridization	CVA	cerebrovascular accident
		CVD	cardiovascular disease
CIED	cardiovascular implantable electronic device	CVE	cardiovascular event
		CVP	central venous pressure
CIMT	carotid intimal media thickness	CW	continuous wave
CK	creatinine kinase	CXR	chest X-ray
CKD	chronic kidney disease	DA	ductus arteriosus
CL	clearance	DASH	dietary approaches to stop hypertension
CLI	critical limb ischaemia		
Cmax	maximum plasma concentration	DBP	diastolic blood pressure
		DC	direct current
CMR	cardiac magnetic resonance imaging	DCCT	Diabetes Control and Complications Trial
CO	cardiac output	DCCV	direct current cardioversion
CoA	coarctation of the aorta	DCI	diving decompression illness
COPD	chronic obstructive pulmonary disease	DCM	dilated cardiomyopathy
		dcSSc	diffuse cutaneous systemic sclerosis
CPAP	continuous positive airway pressure		
		DES	drug eluting stent

DFT	defibrillation threshold	**FFR**	fractional flow reserve
Dm	dermatomyositis	**FH**	familial hypercholesterolaemia
DM	diabetes mellitus		
DMARD	disease modifying antirheumatic drug	**FISH**	fluorescent in-situ hybridization
DMD	Duchenne muscular dystrophy	**FMD**	flow-mediated dilatation
DNA	deoxyribonucleic acid	**FPG**	fasting plasma glucose
DNAR	do not attempt resuscitation	**FO**	foramen ovale
DOAC	direct oral anticoagulant	**FVC**	forced vital capacity
DPP-4	dipeptidyl peptidase-4	**GAD**	glutamic acid decarboxylase
DSM	defibrillation safety margin	**GCA**	giant cell arteritis
DVLA	Driver and Vehicle Licensing Agency	**GCS**	Glasgow coma scale
		GDM	gestational diabetes mellitus
DVT	deep vein thrombosis	**GI**	gastrointestinal
EAM	electro-anatomic mapping	**GOLD**	global initiative on obstructive lung disease
ECG	electrocardiogram		
ECMO	extracorporeal membrane oxygenation	**GP**	general population
		GPA	granulomatosis with polyangiitis
ECV	extracellular volume		
ED	erectile dysfunction	**GRACE**	Global Registry of Acute Coronary Events
EDS	Ehlers–Danlos syndrome		
EDTA	ethylenediaminetetraacetic acid	**HB**	His bundle
		HbA1c	glycated haemoglobin A1c
EEG	electroencephalogram	**HCM**	hypertrophic cardiomyopathy
EF	ejection fraction		
eGFR	estimated glomerular filtration rate	**HCN**	hyperpolarization-activated cyclic nucleotide-gated
EGPA	eosinophilic granulomatosis with polyangiitis	**HD**	heart disease
		HDL	high-density lipoprotein
EHRA	European Heart Rhythm Association	**HDL-C**	high-density lipoprotein cholesterol
EMG	electromyography	**HF**	heart failure
EP	electrophysiology	**HFmrEF**	heart failure with mid-range ejection fraction
EPA	eicosapentaenoic acid		
EPS	electrophysiology study	**HFpEF**	heart failure with preserved ejection fraction
ER	early repolarization		
ESC	European Society of Cardiology	**HFrEF**	heart failure with reduced ejection fraction
ESKD	end-stage kidney disease	**H-ISDN**	hydralazine and isosorbide dinitrate
ESR	estimated sediment rate		
ESRF	end-stage renal failure	**HIV**	human immunodeficiency virus
EU	European Union		
EULAR	European League Against Rheumatism	**HLA-B27**	Human leukocyte antigen B27
F	bioavailability	**HLHS**	hypoplastic left heart syndrome
FCH	familial combined hyperlipidaemia		
		HR	heart rate
FDG	18F-fluorodeoxyglucose	**HRA**	high right atrium
FEV1	forced expiratory volume in one second	**HRT**	hormone replacement therapy
FFAs	free fatty acids	**HSP**	Henoch–Schönlein purpura

IBD	inflammatory bowel disease	Lp(a)	lipoprotein a
IBM	inclusion body myositis	LPA	left pulmonary artery
ICD	implantable cardiac defibrillator	LQTS	long QT syndrome
		LSCD	left cardiac sympathetic denervation
ID	iron deficiency		
IDL	intermediate low density lipoprotein	LV	left ventricle
		LVAD	left ventricular assist device
IFCC	International Federation of Clinical Chemistry	LVEDP	left ventricular end-diastolic pressure
IFG	impaired fasting glucose	LVEF	left ventricular ejection fraction
IGT	impaired glucose tolerance		
IHD	ischaemic heart disease	LVH	left ventricular hypertrophy
IL-6	interleukin 6	LVNC	left ventricular non-compaction
ILD	interstitial lung disease		
ILR	implantable loop recorders	LVOT	left ventricular outflow tract
INR	international normalized ratio	LVSD	left ventricular systolic dysfunction
IR	insulin resistance	mAbs	monoclonal antibodies
IAS	intra-atrial septum	MACE	major adverse cardiovascular event
ITU	intensive therapy unit		
i.v.	intravenous	MAP	mean aortic pressure
IVC	inferior vena cava	MAPCAs	major aortopulmonary collateral arteries
IVIG	intravenous immunoglobulin		
IwFR	instantaneous wave-free ratio	MAT	multi-focal atrial tachycardia
		MCS	mechanical circulatory support
JBS	Joint British Societies		
JVP	jugular venous pressure	MD	myotonic dystrophy
K+	potassium	MDT	multi-disciplinary team
KD	Kawasaki's disease	MEC	minimum effective concentration
KDOQI	Kidney Disease Outcomes Quality Initiative		
		MELAS	mitochondrial encephalopathy with lactic acidosis and stroke-like episodes
Kg	kilogram		
LA	left atrium		
LAC	lupus anticoagulant		
LACS	lacunar syndrome	MERRF	myoclonic epilepsy with ragged red fibres
LAD	left axis deviation		
LADA	latent auto-immune diabetes in adults	MetS	metabolic syndrome
		Mg2+	magnesium
LBBB	left bundle branch block	MIx	mechanical index
LDL	low-density lipoprotein	MI	myocardial infarction
LDL-C	low-density lipoprotein cholesterol	MMAS	Massachusetts Male Aging Study
LDLR	low-density lipoprotein receptor	mMRC-D	modified Medical Research Council dyspnoea score
LFT	liver function test	MODY	mature-onset diabetes of the young
LGE	late gadolinium enhancement		
LI-SWT	low-intensity extracorporeal shock wave therapy	MPA	main pulmonary artery
		MPA	microscopic polyangiitis
LMWH	low molecular weight heparin	MR	mitral regurgitation
		MRIA	magnetic resonance imaging angiography
LOC	loss of consciousness		

MRA	mineralocorticoid receptor antagonist	**PAD**	peripheral artery disease
MRI	magnetic resonance imaging	**PAF**	paroxysmal atrial fibrillation
MS	Marfan's syndrome	**PAH**	pulmonary arterial hypertension
MSD	myositis spectrum disease	**PAI-1**	plasminogen activator inhibitor-1
MTC	maximum tolerated concentration	**PAN**	polyarteritis nodosa
MUFA	monounsaturated fatty acids	**PAP**	pulmonary artery pressure
MV	mitral valve	**PAPVD**	partial anomalous pulmonary venous drainage
Na+	sodium		
NAC	N-acetyl cysteine	**PCI**	percutaneous coronary intervention
NAM	necrotizing autoimmune myositis	**PCR**	protein creatinine ratio
NCEP ATP	National Cholesterol Education Program Adult Treatment Panel	**PCSK9**	proprotein convertase subtilisin/kexin type 9
		PCWP	pulmonary capillary wedge pressure
NDCC	non dihydropyridine calcium channel blockers	**PD**	pharmacodynamics
NICE	National Institute for Health and Care Excellence	**PDA**	patent ductus arteriosus
		PDE5i	phosphodiesterase type 5 inhibitor
NIV	non-invasive ventilation	**PE**	pulmonary embolism
NO	nitric oxide	**PEA**	pulseless electrical activity
NOAC	non-vitamin K antagonist oral anticoagulants	**PET**	positron emission tomography
NP	natriuretic peptides	**PFO**	patent foramen ovale
NRT	nicotine replacement therapy	**PH**	pulmonary hypertension
NSAID	non-steroidal anti-inflammatory drug	**PHT**	pressure half-time
NSTEMI	non ST-elevation myocardial infarction	**PISA**	proximal isovelocity surface area
NSVT	non-sustained ventricular tachycardia	**PJRT**	persistent junctional reciprocating tachycardia
nT-pro BNP	N-terminal pro B-type natriuretic peptide	**PK**	pharmacokinetics
		PM	polymyositis
NYHA	New York Heart Association	**PMT**	pacemaker-mediated tachycardia
OAC	oral anticoagulants		
OGTT	oral glucose tolerance test	**PNES**	psychogenic non-epileptic seizures
OH	orthostatic hypotension		
OHS	obesity hypoventilation syndrome	**POCS**	posterior circulation stroke
		POTS	postural orthostatic tachycardia syndrome
OMT	optimal medical therapy		
OR	odds ratio	**PPAR-a**	proliferator-activated receptor-a
OSA	obstructive sleep apnoea		
OSAHS	obstructive sleep apnoea/ hypopnoea syndrome	**PPG**	photoplethysmography
		PPM	permanent pacemaker
P	pacemaker	**PR**	pulmonary regurgitation
PA	pulmonary artery	**PS**	pulmonary stenosis
PaCO2	partial pressure of carbon dioxide	**PsA**	psoriatic arthritis
		PSG	polysomnography
PACS	partial anterior circulation stroke	**pSS**	primary Sjögren's syndrome
		PSV	primary systemic vasculitides

PT	prothrombin time	SNP	single nucleotide polymorphisms
PTH	parathyroid hormone		
PUFA	polyunsaturated fatty acids	SNRT	sinus node recovery time
PV	pulmonary vein	SpA	spondyloarthropathy
PVi	plasma viscosity	SPECT	single-photon emission computed tomography
PVARP	post-ventricular atrial refractory period	SQTS	short QT syndrome
PVC	premature ventricular complex	SR	sinus rhythm
		SRP	signal recognition peptide
PVD	peripheral vascular disease	SSc	systemic sclerosis
PVI	pulmonary vein isolation	STE	speckle-tracing 2-dimensional echocardiography
PVR	pulmonary vascular resistance	STEMI	ST elevation myocardial infarction
PW	pulsed wave		
QTc	corrected QT	SUDS	sudden unexplained death syndrome
RA	rheumatoid arthritis		
RA	right atrium	SV	stroke volume
RAAS	renin angiotensin aldosterone system	SVA	systemic venous atrium
		SVC	superior vena cava
RAD	right axis deviation	SVR	systemic vascular resistance
RAS	reflex anoxic seizures	SVT	supraventricular tachycardia
RAS	renin angiotensin system	T1	Thallium-201
RBBB	right bundle branch block	T1/2	half-life
RCT	randomized controlled trial	T1DM	type 1 diabetes mellitus
REM	rapid eye movement	T2DM	type 2 diabetes mellitus
RF	rheumatoid factor	TACS	total anterior circulation stroke
RHD	rheumatic heart disease		
RNA	ribonucleic acid	TAK	Takayasu's arteritis
ROSC	return of spontaneous circulation	TAPVD	Total anomalous pulmonary venous drainage
RP	relapsing polychondritis	TAVI	transcatheter aortic valve implantation
RPA	right pulmonary artery		
RR	relative risk	TC	total cholesterol
RRT	renal replacement therapy	TCPC	total cavopulmonary connection
RRR	relative risk reduction		
RUPV	right upper pulmonary vein	TDI	tissue doppler imaging
RV	right ventricle	TG	triglycerides
RVH	right ventricular hypertrophy	TGA	transposition of the great arteries
RVOT	right ventricular outflow tract		
SA	sino-atrial	TIA	transient ischaemic attack
SADS	sudden arrhythmic death syndrome	TLOC	transient loss of consciousness
SBP	systolic blood pressure	tmax	time to maximum plasma concentration
SCD	sudden cardiac death		
SCORE	Systematic Coronary Risk Evaluation	TOE	trans-oesophageal echocardiogram
SGLT2	sodium-glucose co-transporter-2	ToF	tetralogy of Fallot
		tPA	tissue plasminogen activator
S-ICD	subcutaneous implantable cardioverter-defibrillator	TR	tricuspid regurgitation
		TRV	tricuspid valve velocity
SLE	systemic lupus erythematous	TSH	thyroid stimulating hormone

TTE	transthoracic echocardiogram	**VED**	vacuum-erection devices
TTR	transthyretin	**VEGF**	vascular endothelial growth factor
TV	tricuspid valve		
TVR	tricuspid valve repair/replacement	**VF**	ventricular fibrillation
		VLDL	very low-density lipoprotein
UFH	unfractionated heparin	**VSD**	ventricular septal defect
UK	United Kingdom	**VT**	ventricular tachycardia
UKPDS	UK Prospective Diabetes Study	**VTE**	venous thromboembolism
		VUS	variants of unknown significance
V	volume of distribution		
VA	ventriculoarterial	**WES**	whole exome sequencing
VC	valved conduit	**WGS**	whole genome sequencing
VC	vena contracta	**WHO**	World Health Organization
VE	ventricular ectopic	**WPW**	Wolff–Parkinson–White

CHAPTER 1

IMAGING

1.1 Echocardiography

Luigi P. Badano, Elena Surkova, Denisa Muraru, Chiara Palermo, and Patriza Aruta

TABLE OF CONTENTS

1.1.1 Techniques 3
 M-mode 3
 Two-dimensional (2D) mode 4
 Three-dimensional (3D) mode 7
 Doppler imaging (blood flow, tissue) 9
 Deformation imaging (speckle-tracking and Doppler-based strain analysis) 12
 Contrast echocardiography 12
 Stress-echo modalities (exercise and/or pharmacological echo) 14
 Transoesophageal echocardiography 15
1.1.2 Global LV and RV systolic and diastolic function 16
 Global LV systolic function 16
 LV diastolic function 16
 Global RV systolic function 17
 RV diastolic function 23
 Regional LV function: Ischaemia 23
1.1.3 LV mass, scaling for body size, and hypertrophy 24
1.1.4 Cardiac chambers anatomy, size, function 27
 Left ventricle 27
 Right ventricle 28
 RV volumetric analysis 29
 Left atrium 30
 Right atrium 32
1.1.5 Primary and secondary cardiomyopathies (dilated, hypertrophic, restrictive, arrhythmogenic) 33
 Dilated cardiomyopathy 33
 Hypertrophic cardiomyopathy 33
 Arrhythmogenic RV cardiomyopathy 35
 LV myocardial non-compaction 36
1.1.6 Valvular morphology and function 37
 Aortic stenosis 37
 Low-flow, low-gradient AS 37
 Pulmonary stenosis 38
 Mitral stenosis 38
 Tricuspid stenosis 40
 Mitral regurgitation 41
 Tricuspid regurgitation 45
 Aortic regurgitation 47
 Pulmonary regurgitation 50
1.1.7 Prosthetic valves 51
1.1.8 Endocarditis 51
1.1.9 Pericardial disease 52
 Pericardial effusion 52
 Cardiac tamponade 53
 Constrictive pericarditis 53
 Pericardial cyst 54
 Congenital absence of pericardium (total or partial) 54
1.1.10 Cardiac masses 54
1.1.11 Congenital heart disease 55
 Atrial septal defect (ASD) 55
 Coronary sinus defect (or unroofed coronary sinus) 56
 Sinus venosus defect 56
 Ventricular septal defect (VSD) 57
 Patent Ductus Arteriosus (PDA) 57
 Aortic coarctation 57
1.1.12 Pulmonary hypertension 58
1.1.13 Non-invasive haemodynamics 58
1.1.14 Liver congestion and venous flow, respiratory changes of the vena cava 60
 Pathology to anticipate and to screen for in emergency echocardiography 64
1.1.15 Aortic root assessment 64

1.1.1 Techniques

M-mode

M-Mode is produced by the transmission and reception of an ultrasound signal along a single line. As a result it:

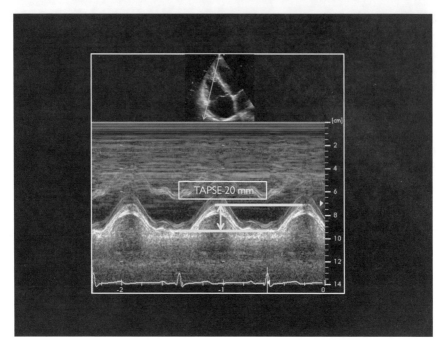

Figure 1.1.1 Measurement of TAPSE using M-mode.

- has high temporal resolution
- allows precise measurements of time intervals and timing of events
- is routinely used to obtain certain parameters: tricuspid / mitral annular plane systolic excursion (TAPSE/MAPSE) for right/left ventricular (RV/LV) longitudinal function assessment (Figure 1.1.1); movement/contraction patterns and respiratory shift of interventricular septum (IVS)

Tips for correct use
- Ensure correct orientation of the ultrasound beam (e.g. perpendicular to IVS to avoid oblique measurements).
- Anatomical M-mode allows manual orientation of the ultrasound bean which can help overcome misalignment during live acquisition (Figure 1.1.2).
- Increase the sweep speed to 100 mm/s for precise measurement of timing of events.

Two-dimensional (2D) mode
- The ultrasound beam sweeps across a sector scan of variable width. The reflected ultrasounds generate electrical signals in the crystals, which are used to produce a 2D image on the screen.
- It is the main conventional echocardiographic mode used to assess morphology and function of cardiac chambers, valves, vessels and pericardium in clinical cardiology.
- Standard 2D views include:
    - Parasternal long-axis view (Figure 1.1.3 A)
    - RV inflow view (Figure 1.1.3 B)
    - RV outflow view

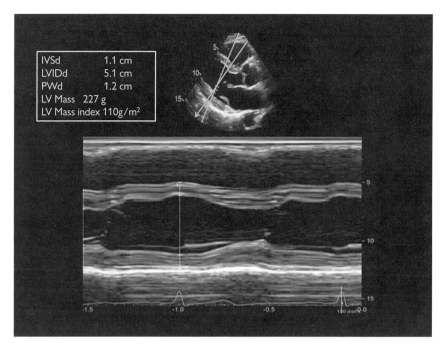

Figure 1.1.2 Measurement of LV mass using anatomical M-mode (green line).

- Parasternal short-axis view at mitral valve (MV) level (Figure 1.1.3 C)
- Parasternal short-axis view at papillary muscle level (Figure 1.1.3 D)
- Parasternal short-axis view at level of the apex of left ventricle (LV)
- Parasternal short-axis view at great vessels level (Figure 1.1.3 E)
- Apical 4-chamber (4Ch) view (Figure 1.1.3 F)
- Apical RV-focused 4Ch view (Figure 1.1.3 G)
- Apical 5-chamber (5Ch) view (Figure 1.1.3 H)
- Apical 2-chamber (2Ch) view (Figure 1.1.3 I)
- Apical 3-chamber (3Ch) view (Figure 1.1.3 J)
- Subcostal view (4Ch view (Figure 1.1.3 K); interatrial septum view; inferior vena cava (IVC) long-axis view; subcostal short-axis view)
- Suprasternal view (Figure 1.1.3 L).

Tips for correct use

- Optimize the image before acquisition by adjusting depth, sector width, gain settings, time gain compensation, and focus position.
- Include the structure/s of interest within the sector scan.
- Obtain a clear visualization of endocardium and record loops at the required temporal resolution (frame rate).
- Ensure that the apical views are acquired from the lowest position of the transducer on the chest to avoid foreshortening of the cardiac chambers.
- Acquire images at particular respiratory phases to minimize heart–lung interactions if needed.

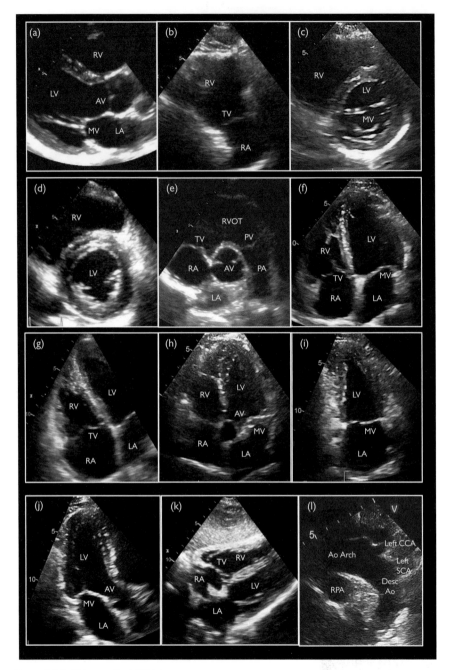

Figure 1.1.3 Main standard 2DE views.

(A) Parasternal long-axis view; (B) RV inflow view; (C) Parasternal short-axis view at MV level; (D) Parasternal short-axis view at papillary muscle level; (E) Parasternal short-axis view at great vessels level; (F) Apical 4Ch view; (G) Apical RV-focused 4Ch view; (H) Apical 5Ch view; (I) Apical 2Ch view; (J) Apical 3Ch view; (K) Subcostal 4Ch view; (L) Suprasternal view.

Abbreviations: Ao—aorta/aortic; AV—aortic valve; CCA—common carotid artery; LA—left atrium; LV—left ventricle; MV—mitral valve; PV—pulmonary valve; RA—right atrium; RPA—right pulmonary artery; RV—right ventricle; RVOT—RV outflow tract; SCA—subclavian artery; TV—tricuspid valve.

Three-dimensional (3D) mode

3D echocardiography provides *real-time single-beat* and *ECG gated multi-beat pyramidal data set acquisitions* containing the cardiac structures.

The main advantages are to allow:

- The display images of cardiac structures in motion from any perspective by cropping and volume rendering the data set (Figure 1.1.4);
- Quantitative assessment of cardiac structures (Figure 1.1.5);
- Multi-slice display of cardiac chambers allowing assessment of regional wall motion and morphology (Figure 1.1.6);
- Direct volumetric analysis of all cardiac chambers without geometrical assumptions about their shape/morphology

Main limitations:

- Temporal resolution / spatial resolution trade-off
- Highly dependent on image quality
- Multi-beat acquisition requires regular heart rhythm and adequate patient breath-holding

Tips for correct use

- Optimize the image before acquisition by adjusting depth, sector width, gain settings
- Position the structure of interest in the middle of the sector
- Keep the sector as narrow as possible, with minimal depth to increase temporal resolution.

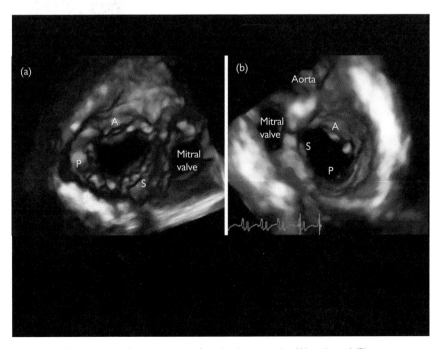

Figure 1.1.4 *En-face* view of tricuspid valve from both ventricular (A) and atrial (B) prospective.
Abbreviations: A—anterior, P—posterior, and S—septal leaflets of tricuspid valve.

8   1.1 Echocardiography

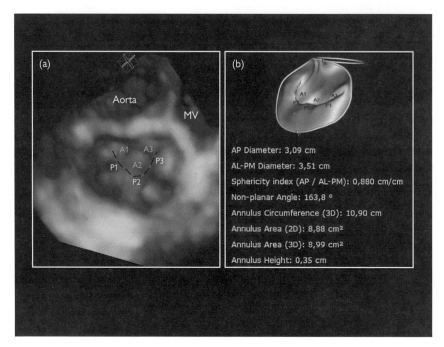

Figure 1.1.5 3DE assessment of complex MV prolapse. (A) *En-face* view of the MV from atrial prospective showing the location and extent of the prolapsing segments of posterior MV leaflet. (B) Surface rendering of the MV providing an automated quantitative analysis of valve morphology and geometry useful for surgical planning.

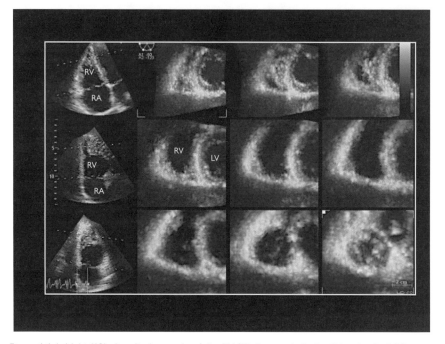

Figure 1.1.6 Multi (12)-slice display mode of the RV 3D data set including 3 longitudinal (0°, 60°, and 120°), and 9 transversal equidistant tomographic views between the apex and the base enabling RV regional wall motion analysis.

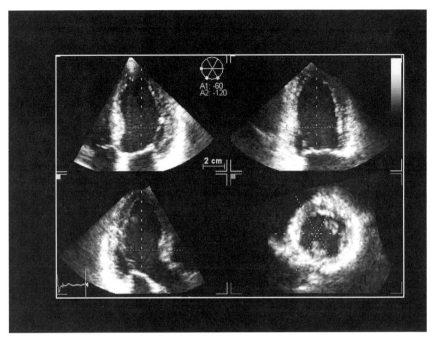

Figure 1.1.7 Three-plane acquisition mode allowing simultaneous acquisition of 3 longitudinal (0°, 60°, and 120°) and one short-axis LV views.

- Ensure that all parts of the structure of interest are included in the acquired volume
- Ensure that the ECG tracing is stable and of good quality with a well-defined R wave

A 3D probe can also allow simultaneous acquisition of 2D images in two or three planes—Simultaneous *multi-plane acquisition mode* (Figure 1.1.7).

Doppler imaging (blood flow, tissue)

Doppler imaging allows evaluation of the direction and velocity of blood flow or tissue motion based on the Doppler shift between the sent and the received signal.

Blood flow Doppler enables assessment of:

- Valve function (calculation of valve gradient, valve functional area, and effective regurgitant orifice area) (Figures 1.1.8–1.1.9)
- Haemodynamic parameters (calculation of stroke volume (SV), cardiac output (CO) (Figure 1.1.9), intracardiac pressures, flow resistance, and the detection of intracardiac shunts)
- LV filling pressure and diastolic function
- Coronary flow reserve.

Modalities

- Pulsed-wave (PW) Doppler: this is used to measure localized low velocity flow within the sample volume (e.g. normal LV/RV inflow and outflow, flow in pulmonary and hepatic veins)

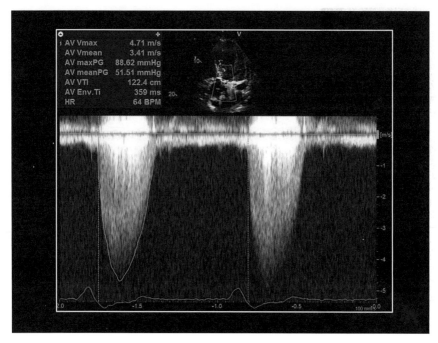

Figure 1.1.8 CW Doppler of aortic flow in a patient with severe aortic stenosis.

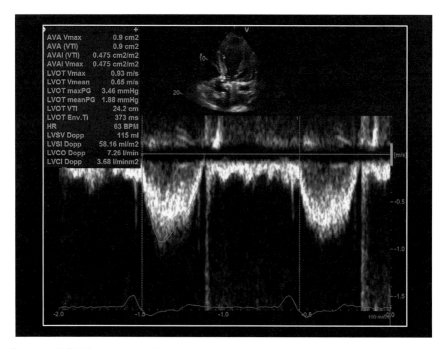

Figure 1.1.9 PW Doppler of LVOT flow of the same patient as in Figure 1.1.5. Functional aortic valve area (AVA) was assessed by continuity equation (see section 1.3.6). LV stroke volume (LVSV) and cardiac output (LVCO) were calculated using LVOT diameter, velocity-time integral (VTI) and heart rate (see section 1.3.13).

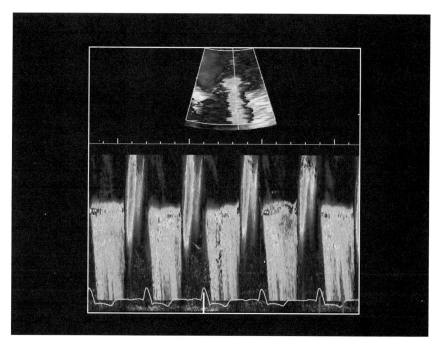

Figure 1.1.10 Colour M-mode showing holosystolic regurgitant flow in a patient with severe mitral regurgitation.

- Continuous-wave (CW) Doppler: this is used to assess high flow velocities (e.g. valvular stenosis and regurgitation, shunts)
- Colour-flow Doppler: this is used to visually assess direction and turbulence of the flow. Colour M-mode also allows analysis of flow timing (Figure 1.1.10)

Tissue Doppler Imaging (TDI) measures tissue velocities along the ultrasound beam. It is routinely used for assessment of:

- LV filling pressures
- Longitudinal component of RV systolic function (Figure 1.1.11)

Modalities
- PW spectral tissue Doppler (Figure 1.1.11 A)
- Colour tissue Doppler (Figure 1.1.11 B)

Tips for correct use
- Ensure there is alignment of the ultrasound beam along the direction of flow/tissue displacement and correct positioning of control volume
- Use high acquisition frame rate to get high temporal resolution
- Maximize spectral displays to precisely trace and measure maximal velocities
- Increase the sweep speed to 100 mm/s
- Use correct colour scale and baseline shifting when required (e.g. measurement of proximal isovelocity surface area (PISA))
- Average over five cardiac cycles in atrial fibrillation

1.1 Echocardiography

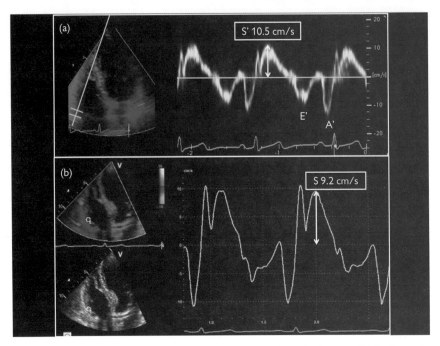

Figure 1.1.11 Tissue Doppler in assessment of RV longitudinal systolic function. (A) Peak systolic velocity of the lateral tricuspid annulus by tissue PW Doppler (S') and (B) mean myocardial velocities by colour tissue Doppler (S).

Deformation imaging (speckle-tracking and Doppler-based strain analysis)

- During the cardiac cycle, the LV follows a complex pattern of movements including twisting and rotation (both clock- and counter clockwise)
- During systole the ventricular myocardium undergoes shortening in the longitudinal and circumferential planes and thickening in the radial plane
- Strain is defined as the fractional change in length of a myocardial segment relative to its resting length in longitudinal, circumferential, and radial direction and is expressed as a percentage
- Strain rate is the rate of strain deformation and is usually expressed in 1/s
- Myocardial deformation imaging can be performed using either colour TDI, grey scale 2D images (Figure 1.1.12) or 3D data sets (Figure 1.1.13). 2D speckle tracking longitudinal strain is the most frequently used parameter

  Indications for 2D speckle tracking echocardiography include:

- Differential diagnosis of cardiomyopathies and detection of sub-clinical LV dysfunction
- Monitoring cardiotoxicity during chemotherapy
- A marker of LV function in heart failure with preserved ejection fraction

Contrast echocardiography

- A technique based on the use of agitated saline solution or specific contrast agents containing microbubbles to enhance the signal of blood.
- Agitated saline contrast:
    - Agitated saline solution (with or without blood) produces large bubbles filled with air that cannot cross the pulmonary capillaries when injected in a peripheral vein.

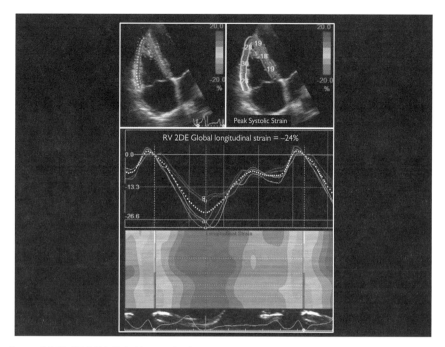

Figure 1.1.12 2DE RV Global longitudinal strain.

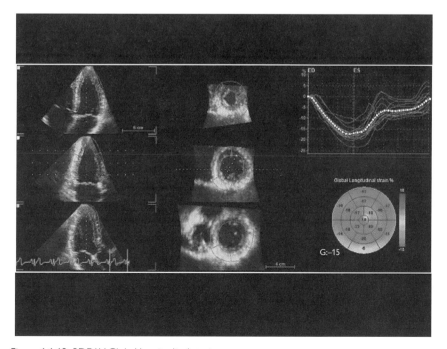

Figure 1.1.13 3DE LV Global longitudinal strain.

Table 1.1.1 Contrast agents used in echocardiography

	Sonovue	Optison	Luminity
Mean bubble size	2.0–8.0 μm	3.0–4.5 μm	1.1–2.5 μm
Outer shell	Predominantly phospholipid	Human albumin	Predominantly phospholipid
Inner gas	Sulphur hexafluoride	Perfluoropropane	Perfluoropropane
Storage	No special precautions	at 2–8 °C	at 2–8 °C
Reported side effects	Headache; nausea; chest pain; injection site reaction; paraesthaesia; vasodilation	Headache; nausea and/or vomiting; warm sensation or flushing; dizziness	Headache; flushing; back pain

- ■ This type of contrast is mainly used to detect right to left shunts and the persistent left superior vena cava.
- Microbubble contrast (Table 1.1.1):
  - ■ Is homogeneous and small in size.
  - ■ They oscillate when exposed to ultrasound and produce harmonic signals at multiple frequencies. This signal is used to opacify the blood pool and improve the visualization of the blood–tissue interface
  - ■ Consists of an outer shell and incapsulated inner gas
  - ■ Has a diameter < 8 μm allowing passage through the pulmonary capillaries. Therefore, their injection into a peripheral vein allows pronounced contrast enhancement of both right and left cardiac chambers even in the absence of shunts
  - ■ Remain entirely intravascular at all times
  - ■ Have high echogenicity
  - ■ Interact with ultrasound in three ways depending on the mechanical index (MI):
    - very low power (MI < 0.1) does not affect microbubbles and so there is no signal
    - high power (MI > 0.5, such as standard 2D echo using MI of 1.0–1.4). This level would destroy the outer shells
    - intermediate power (MI 0.1–0.5) causes bubbles to resonate which leads to generation of signal. *Most commonly used for contrast echocardiography.*

Indications and contraindications for left heart contrast agents are listed in Table 1.1.2.

Stress-echo modalities (exercise and/or pharmacological echo)

A stress echo can be achieved using both physiological (exercising on a treadmill or stationery bicycle) or pharmacological methods (most frequently achieved by using an infusion of dobutamine).

Specific indications for a stress echocardiography include:

- Diagnosis of an ischaemic heart disease
- Prognosis and risk stratification in patients with established coronary artery disease
- Pre-operative risk assessment in non-cardiac surgery
- Evaluation for possible cardiac aetiology of exertional dyspnoea
- Evaluation after coronary revascularization
- Evaluation of certain valve diseases

Table 1.1.2 Indications and contraindications for left heart contrast agents

Indications	Contraindications
• Cavity opacification (ventricular volumes and function, wall motion abnormalities at rest and during stress) • Detection of thrombus/mass • LV apical pathology (apical hypertrophic cardiomyopathy; LV non-compaction; apical thrombi, pseudoaneurysm) • Doppler signal enhancement (tricuspid regurgitation)	• Known hypersensitivity to contrast agent or constituent chemical • Known hypersensitivity to blood/albumin (for Optison only) • Right-to-left or bidirectional intracardiac shunts • 30 min close monitoring for patients with severe pulmonary hypertension or unstable cardiovascular conditions may be considered

Transoesophageal echocardiography

Due to close proximity of oesophagus to the aorta and heart, TOE allows the use of higher frequency transducers to provide higher quality images of cardiac structures and vessels, including those which are very difficult to visualize using transthoracic echocardiography (TTE) (e.g. left atrial appendage, pulmonary veins, superior vena cava)

TOE is particularly useful in the following situations:

- search for a potential source of cardiac embolism
- infective endocarditis
- aortic dissection or aneurysm
- mitral regurgitation (Figure 1.1.14)

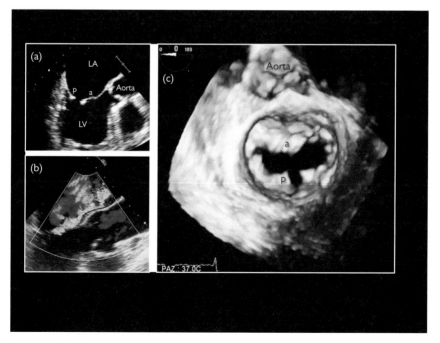

Figure 1.1.14 TOE in a patient with cleft of posterior leaflet of the MV. (A and B) Mid-oesophageal long-axis views showing severe mitral regurgitation with highly eccentric regurgitant jet in colour Doppler. (C) *En-face* view of MV obtained by transoesophageal 3DE clearly demonstrating cleft of posterior MV leaflet.
Abbreviations: a—anterior MV leaflet; LA—left atrium; p—posterior MV leaflet.

- suspected structural or non-structural valve prosthesis dysfunction
- monitoring/guiding intracardiac transcatheter procedures
- monitoring left ventricular function in those undergoing high risk non cardiac surgery
- perioperative monitoring of cardiac surgery procedures

1.1.2 Global LV and RV systolic and diastolic function

Global LV systolic function

- The most commonly used parameter of global LV function is LV ejection fraction (EF). This is calculated from end-diastolic (EDV) and end-systolic (ESV) LV volumes using the formula:

$$EF = (EDV - ESV)/EDV$$

- LV volumes can be obtained by either 2DE (Figure 1.1.15) or 3DE (Figure 1.1.16)
- Strengths and limitations of methods for assessment of LV systolic function are described in Table 1.1.3. Table 1.1.4 provides the reference values for parameters of LV size and function.

LV diastolic function

The integrated approach of LV diastolic function assessment includes:

- 2DE/3DE: assessment of LV geometry and function (EF), left atrial (LA) maximal volume

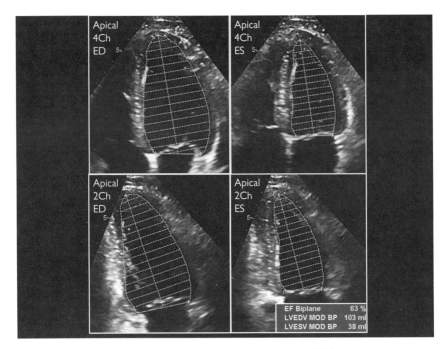

Figure 1.1.15 Left ventricular volumes and function assessment using 2DE.
For correct use of Simpson's algorithm it is necessary to (i) acquire LV focused apical 4Ch and 2Ch views; (ii) trace LV endocardium at end-diastole (ED) (the first frame after mitral valve closure or the frame with the largest LV dimensions/volume) and end-systole (ES) (the frame after aortic valve closure or the frame with the smallest LV dimensions/volume) in both views; (iii) include papillary muscles and trabeculations into cavity. Compare the LV length in both apical 4Ch and 2Ch views to avoid foreshortening.

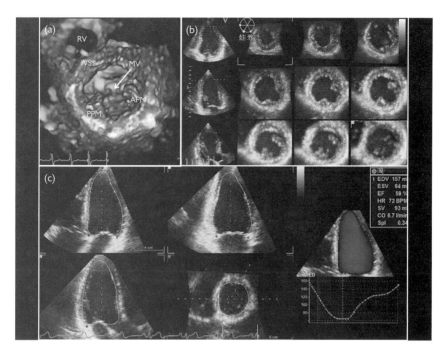

Figure 1.1.16 Left ventricular assessment using 3DE.
3D data set was obtained from the apical 4-chamber view using full-volume multi-beat acquisition with minimal depth and sector angle encompassing the entire LV. (A) Volume rendering display of the LV allowing visualization of morphology and spatial relationships of adjacent structures. (B) Multi (12)-slice display for morphological and functional analysis at different regional levels. (C) Three longitudinal views (4Ch, 2Ch, 3Ch, and the adjustable short-axis view) are used to visualize the accuracy of the semi-automated endocardial tracking. The time-volume curve demonstrates the change in LV volume during the cardiac cycle. LV volumes, EF and LV shape analysis (3D sphericity index, SpI) are extracted from the endocardial 3D surface reconstruction.
Additional abbreviations: APM—anterior papillary muscle; PPM—posterior papillary muscle.

- PW Doppler echocardiography: assessment of mitral inflow and pulmonary to derive pulmonary artery pressures (PAP)
- PW TDI: assessment of early and late diastolic mitral annular velocities

Figure 1.1.17 demonstrates the recommended algorithm for diagnosis of LV diastolic dysfunction.

Global RV systolic function

- RV systolic dysfunction is an independent predictor of cardiovascular morbidity and mortality
- RVEF is possible only using 3DE
- Conventional 2D/M-mode echocardiography provides a number of echocardiographic parameters for clinical use:
  1. **RV fractional area change (FAC)** (Figure 1.1.18) is calculated using the following formula: RV FAC = (RV EDA – RV ESA)/RV EDA, where EDA and ESA are the areas of RV cavity in the RV-focused apical 4Ch view obtained at end-diastole and end-systole, respectively.

Advantages	Limitations	Tips for correct use
Reflects both longitudinal and radial components of RV contraction Established prognostic value Correlates with RV EF	Requires good endocardial border delineation Neglects the contribution of RV outflow tract (RVOT) to overall systolic function Fair inter-observer reproducibility	Use RV-focused 4Ch view Adjust depth and gain settings to optimize image quality Avoid tracing pitfalls

Table 1.1.3 Echocardiographic parameters of LV systolic function.

Parameter	Method/Technique	Advantages	Limitations
EF (%)	**2DE biplane disc summation (Simpson's algorithm)**	Relatively easy to perform Corrects for shape distortions visible in apical 4Ch and 2Ch views Established prognostic values Correlates with LV EF by cardiac magnetic resonance (CMR)	Requires good endocardial border delineation in apical 4Ch and 2Ch planes Based on geometrical assumptions Blind to shape distortions not visualized in apical 4Ch and 2Ch planes Underestimates volumes in apical foreshortening
	2DE area–length method	Relatively easy to perform Partial correction for shape distortion	Heavily based on geometrical assumptions Underestimates volumes in apical foreshortening Limited published data in normal population
	3DE	Does not rely on geometrical assumptions Unaffected by apical foreshortening More accurate and reproducible than 2DE Validated against CMR Established prognostic value	Requires post processing and experience Dependent on good acoustic window and image quality Lower temporal resolution Requires regular heart rhythm and patient's cooperation
Global longitudinal strain (GLS) (%)	**Peak value of 2D longitudinal speckle tracking derived strain**	Angle independent Established prognostic value	Requires good image quality in apical 4Ch, 3Ch, and 2Ch planes Represents only longitudinal component of LV systolic function Vendor dependent

Table 1.1.4 Reference values for LV volumes and systolic function

Parameter	Abnormality threshold	
	Male	Female
2DE EDV index (ml/m²)	> 74	> 61
2DE ESV index (ml/m²)	> 31	> 24
3DE EDV index (ml/m²)*	> 79	> 71
3DE ESV index (ml/m²)*	> 32	> 28
LV EF (%)**	< 52	< 54
2DE GLS (%)	–20 (the lower absolute value of strain is likely to be abnormal)	

* LV volumes measured with 3DE are usually larger than those calculated with 2DE and cannot be used interchangeably.
** LV EF of 51–41% in male and 53–41% in female patients are considered as mildly abnormal; 30–40% moderately abnormal and < 30% severely abnormal.

2. **Tricuspid annular plane systolic excursion (TAPSE)** is obtained from the apical 4Ch view by positioning the M-mode cursor at the lateral part of tricuspid annulus and measuring the excursion distance on the M-mode tracing (Figure 1.1.1).

Advantages	Limitations	Tips for correct use
Easy to obtain Less dependent on image quality Established prognostic value	Reflects only the longitudinal function Neglects the contribution of the IVS and the RVOT Angle dependency Unreliable after procedures that affect the overall heart motion (e.g. cardiac surgery)	Align the scan line along the direction of the tricuspid annulus displacement

3. **S-wave velocities of the lateral tricuspid annulus by TDI** can be obtained with PW (S') and colour tissue Doppler (S) (Figure 1.1.11). They are not identical, as the former reflects peak myocardial velocities, whereas the latter represents mean myocardial velocities, which are usually lower.

Advantages	Limitations	Tips for correct use
S'-wave velocity: Easy to perform Reproducible Validated against RV EF Established prognostic value S-wave velocity: Allows multisite sampling on the same beat	Angle dependent Not fully representative of RV global function, particularly after cardiac surgery Requires postprocessing (for S-wave velocity)	Ensure sufficient image quality of RV free wall Align the scan line along the direction of the tricuspid lateral annulus displacement (for S'-wave velocity)

4. **PW Doppler-derived RV myocardial performance index (RIMP, Tei index)** A non-geometric index of global ventricular function. RIMP is calculated as the ratio between the total RV isovolumic time (isovolumic contraction + isovolumic relaxation) and the RV ejection time (Figure 1.1.19) using the following formula: RIMP = (TCO − ET)/ET.

TCO is the time interval between tricuspid valve closure and opening time and ET is transpulmonary ejection time.

Advantages	Limitations	Tips for correct use
Established prognostic value	Requires matching for R-R intervals when measurements are performed on separate recordings Unreliable when RA pressure is elevated Limited use in normal RV	Use only in regular heart rate Use a sweep speed of 100 mm/s to increase the accuracy of time measurements Avoid in patients with elevated RA pressure

5. **TDI-derived RIMP** allows to measure isovolumic and ejection time intervals in the same cardiac cycle from myocardial velocities of the lateral tricuspid annulus (Figure 1.1.20): RIMP = (IVRT + IVCT)/ET, where IVRT is isovolumic relaxation time, IVCT is isovolumic contraction time, and ET is ejection time.
6. **3DE-derived RV EF** is the only parameter providing direct assessment of true global RV pump function from EDV and ESV measurements (Figure 1.1.21). It is accurate, reproducible and correlates well with cardiac magnetic resonance (CMR).

Normal values of RV systolic function parameters are presented in Table 1.1.5.

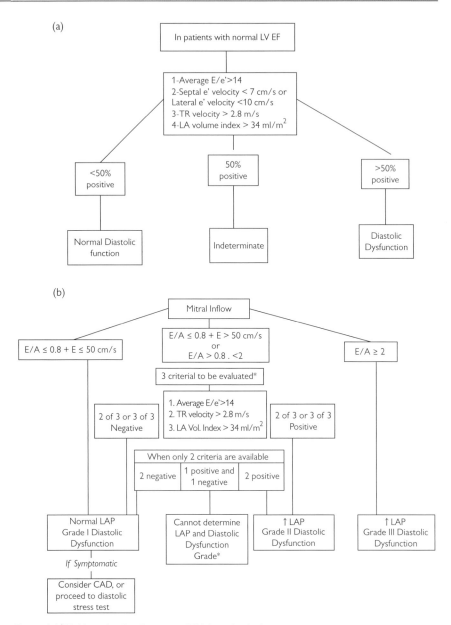

Figure 1.1.17 Algorithm for diagnosis of LV diastolic dysfunction.
Reproduced from Nagueh SF, Smiseth OA, Appleton CP, et al. Recommendations for the Evaluation of Left Ventricular Diastolic Function by Echocardiography: An Update from the American Society of Echocardiography and the European Association of Cardiovascular Imaging. J Am Soc Echocardiogr. 2016 Apr;29(4):277–314. doi: 10.1016/j.echo.2016.01.011 with permission from Elsevier.

(A) Algorithm for diagnosis of LV diastolic dysfunction in subjects with normal LVEF. (B) Algorithm for estimation of LV filling pressures and grading LV diastolic function in patients with depressed LVEFs and patients with myocardial disease and normal LVEF after consideration of clinical and other 2D data.

1.1.2 Global LV and RV systolic and diastolic function

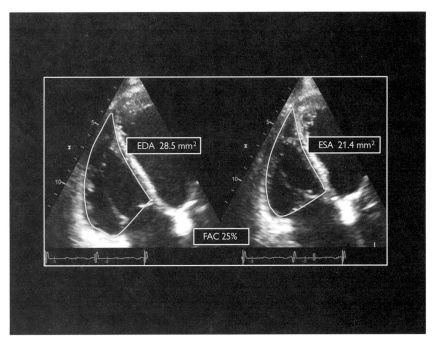

Figure 1.1.18 Measurement of fractional area change.

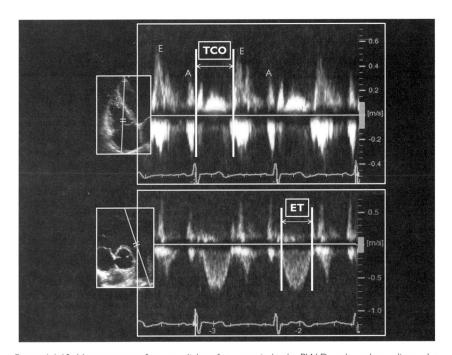

Figure 1.1.19 Measurement of myocardial performance index by PW Doppler echocardiography.

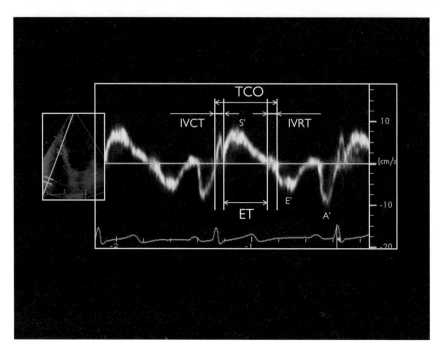

Figure 1.1.20 Measurement of myocardial performance index by PW TDI.

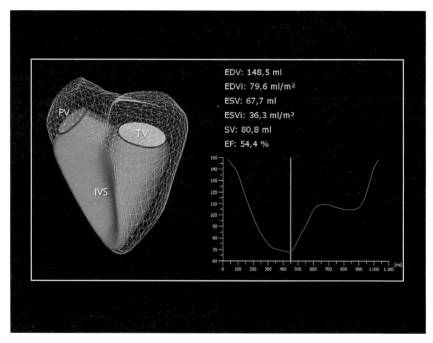

Figure 1.1.21 3DE volumetric analysis of RV volumes and ejection fraction.

Table 1.1.5 Normal values for echocardiographic parameters of RV systolic function

Parameter	Normal values (mean ± SD)	Abnormality threshold
FAC (%)	49 ± 7	< 35
TAPSE (mm)	24 ± 3.5	< 17
Pulsed Tissue Doppler S' wave (cm/sec)	14.1 ± 2.3	< 9.5
Colour Tissue Doppler S wave (cm/sec)	9.7 ± 1.85	< 6.0
Pulsed Doppler RIMP	0.26 ± 0.085	> 0.43
Tissue Doppler RIMP	0.38 ± 0.08	> 0.54
3D RV EF (%)	58 ± 6.5	< 45

RV diastolic function

Evaluation of RV diastolic function is rarely considered as part of routine echo examination. The assessment includes evaluation of:

- RV inflow by PW Doppler sampling at the tips of the tricuspid valve leaflets
- TDI velocities of the tricuspid annulus at RV free wall
- RA maximal volume
- IVC/hepatic veins

All parameters are preload-dependent.

Grading of RV diastolic dysfunction

- tricuspid E/A < 0.8—impaired relaxation;
- tricuspid E/A of 0.8 to 2.1 and E/e' > 6 and/or diastolic flow predominance in the hepatic veins—pseudonormal filling;
- tricuspid E/A > 2.1 and deceleration time < 120 ms—restrictive filling.

Regional LV function: Ischaemia

- Visual assessment of endocardial excursion and wall thickening is used for evaluation of regional LV wall motion by echocardiography
- The LV is divided into 16 segments (6 basal, 6 mid, and 4 apical; Figure 1.1.22), which reflect coronary perfusion territories (Figure 1.1.23).
- The 17-segment model (containing additional apical segment—'apical cap') should be used for myocardial perfusion studies or for comparison with other imaging modalities.
- Thickening of each segment should be analysed individually in multiple views (apical, parasternal long- and short-axis).

For regional wall motion assessment, scoring systems can be used (Table 1.1.6).

- Hibernating myocardium is viable myocardium supplied by coronary branches that have critical stenosis. It can be diagnosed using low-dose dobutamine stress echocardiography. A biphasic response (augmentation of segments' thickening at low-dose dobutamine followed by segmental function deterioration at higher doses) has the highest specificity for diagnosing this condition.
- Myocardial stunning is the reversible dysfunction of acutely ischaemic segments after reestablishment of myocardial reperfusion. In contrast to hibernating myocardium, stunned myocardium is not accounted for by tissue damage or reduced blood flow and function recovers spontaneously.

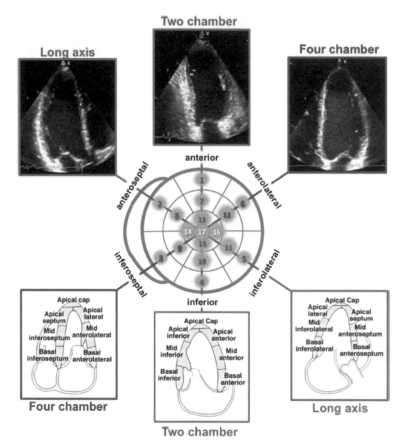

Figure 1.1.22 LV segmentation. Orientation of apical four-chamber, apical two-chamber, and apical long-axis views in relation to the bull's-eye display of the LV segments (centre). Top panels show actual images, and bottom panels schematically depict the LV wall segments in each view.

Reproduced from Lang RM, Badano LP, Mor-Avi V, et al. Recommendations for cardiac chamber quantification by echocardiography in adults: an update from the American Society of Echocardiography and the European Association of Cardiovascular Imaging. J Am Soc Echocardiogr. 2015 Jan;28(1):1–39.e14. doi: 10.1016/j.echo.2014.10.003 with permission from Elsevier.

- Regional wall motion abnormalities may also occur in the absence of coronary artery disease; for example in cardiomyopathies, left bundle branch block, RV pressure, or volume overload, post cardiac surgery.

1.1.3 LV mass, scaling for body size, and hypertrophy

- Several algorithms have been introduced for LV mass assessment using M-mode, 2DE, and 3DE. All measurements should be obtained at end-diastole.
  1. **Linear measurements** (M-mode or 2D-guided) (Figure 1.1.2) are performed from parasternal long- or short-axis view using Cube formula:

$$\text{LV mass} = 0.8\,(1.04([\text{LVIDd} + \text{PWd} + \text{IVSd}]^3 - [\text{LVIDd}]^3)) + 0.6 \text{ g},$$

where LVIDd—LV internal diameter in diastole; PWd—LV posterior wall thickness in diastole; IVSd—IVS thickness in diastole.

1.1.3 LV mass, scaling for body size, and hypertrophy

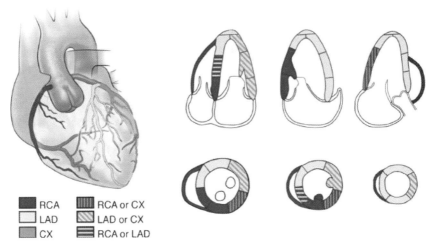

- RCA
- LAD
- CX
- RCA or CX
- LAD or CX
- RCA or LAD

Figure 1.1.23 Typical distributions of the right coronary artery (RCA), the left anterior descending coronary artery (LAD), and the circumflex coronary artery (CX). The arterial distribution varies among patients. Some segments have variable coronary perfusion.

Reproduced from Lang RM, Badano LP, Mor-Avi V, et al. Recommendations for cardiac chamber quantification by echocardiography in adults: an update from the American Society of Echocardiography and the European Association of Cardiovascular Imaging. J Am Soc Echocardiogr. 2015 Jan;28(1):1–39.e14. doi: 10.1016/j.echo.2014.10.003 with permission from Elsevier.

Advantages	Limitations	Tips for correct use
Fast and easy to use Established prognostic value A lot of published data Fairly accurate in normally shaped LV	Based on geometric assumption (assumes that LV has ellipsoid shape with symmetric distribution of hypertrophy) Requires alignment of ultrasound beam perpendicular to LV long axis Since linear measurements are cubed, even small measurement errors have an impact on accuracy	Measurements should be obtained perpendicular to the LV long axis (use anatomical M-mode if necessary) Measurement should be performed at the level of the tips of mitral valve leaflets

Table 1.1.6 Scoring to assess wall motion of the LV

Wall motion pattern	Thickening during systole	Score*	Clinical scenarios
Normal/Hyperkinetic	Normal or increased (usually > 30% increase compared to diastolic wall thickness)	1	Normal
Hypokinetic	Reduced (10–30% thickening compared to diastolic wall thickness)	2	Ischaemia, hibernation, stunning
Akinetic	Absent or negligible thickening (< 10% thickening compared to diastolic wall thickness)	3	Scar, ischaemia, hibernation, stunning
Dyskinetic	Systolic thinning or stretching	4	Scar, aneurysm

*Wall motion score index is the sum of individual segment scores divided by the number of interpretable segments.

2. **2D-based methods** include *Truncated ellipsoid formula* (LV mass is calculated using several diameters obtained from apical 4Ch view) and *Area–length formula* (LV mass is calculated using the epicardial and endocardial cross-sectional LV areas in short-axis view at the level of papillary muscles).

Advantages	Limitations	Tips for correct use
Partial correction for shape distortions Less dependent on geometrical assumptions than the linear measurements	Good epi- and endocardial definition is required Higher measurement variability Limited normative and prognostic data	Attention should be paid to correct orientation of parasternal short-axis view (no oblique planes)

3. **3DE** allows for direct measurement of LV mass from 3D data set (Figure 1.1.24).

Advantages	Limitations
No geometrical assumptions about LV cavity shape and hypertrophy distribution Higher accuracy Higher inter-measurement and test/retest reproducibility	Dependent on image quality Epicardium may be difficult to visualize, particularly at the apex Limited normative and prognostic data

The following considerations about LV mass assessment should be taken into account:

- LV mass varies according to age, gender, body size, ethnicity
- Indexing to BSA is currently recommended

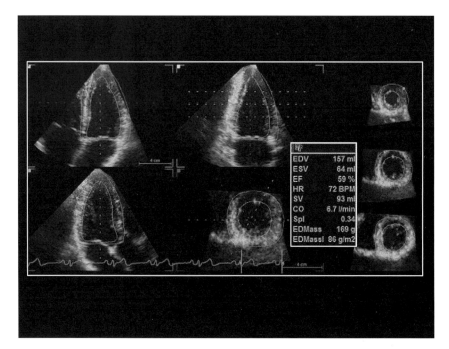

Figure 1.1.24 Measurement of LV mass by 3DE.

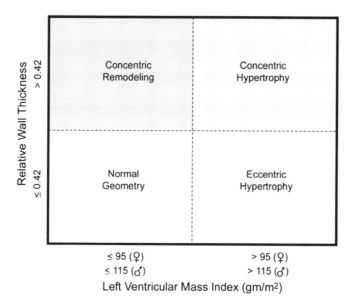

Figure 1.1.25 Assessment of RWT and LV mass index to establish geometry. Patients with normal LV mass can have either concentric remodelling (normal LV mass with increased RWT > 0.42) or normal geometry (RWT ≤ 0.42) and normal LV mass. Patients with increased LV mass can have either concentric (RWT > 0.42) or eccentric (RWT ≤ 0.42) hypertrophy. These LV mass measurements are based on linear measurements.

Reproduced from Lang RM, Badano LP, Mor-Avi V, et al. Recommendations for cardiac chamber quantification by echocardiography in adults: an update from the American Society of Echocardiography and the European Association of Cardiovascular Imaging. J Am Soc Echocardiogr. 2015 Jan;28(1):1-39.e14. doi: 10.1016/j.echo.2014.10.003 with permission from Elsevier.

- In normally shaped LV, both M-mode and 2DE formulas can be used
- In abnormally shaped ventricles or in patients with asymmetric or localized hypertrophy, 3D echo is more accurate method for LV mass assessment
- Reference upper limits for linear measurements: 95 g/m² in women and 115 g/m² in men; for 2D measurements: 88 g/m² in women and 102 g/m² in men

The relative wall thickness (RWT = (2 × posterior wall thickness)/(LV internal diameter at end-diastole) permits further categorization of LV hypertrophy and remodelling (Figure 1.1.25. Reproduction of Figure 6, Comparison of RWT. from Lang et al. J Am Soc Echocardiogr 2015;28:1–39.)

1.1.4 Cardiac chambers anatomy, size, function

Left ventricle

- **Linear measurements** (M-mode tracing or 2D-guided linear measurements) should be obtained from the parasternal long axis view at end-diastole and end-systole

Advantages	Limitations	Tips for correct use
Fast and easy to use A lot of published data High temporal resolution (especially, for M-mode)	Requires alignment of ultrasound beam perpendicular to the LV long axis Single dimension, i.e. representative only in normally shaped LV	Measurements should be obtained perpendicular to the LV long axis (use anatomical M-mode if necessary) (Figure 1.1.2) Measurements should be performed at the level of the tips of mitral valve leaflets

Table 1.1.7 Reference values for LV internal diameters

Parameter	Male	Female
End-diastolic diameter (mm)	42.0–58.4	37.8–52.2
End-systolic diameter (mm)	25.0–39.8	21.6–34.8

Table 1.1.7 provides the reference values for LV internal diameters.
Volumetric measurements (see Tables 1.1.3 and 1.1.4)

- LV volumes should be used to report LV size
- Clinical and prognostic significance of LV volumes has been demonstrated in numerous cardiovascular disorders.
- EDV and ESV can be assessed by 2DE (using either biplane discs' summation algorithm or area–length method) (Figure 1.1.15) or 3DE (Figure 1.1.16).
- LV volumes obtained from linear measurements (Teichholz or Quinones methods) are inaccurate and currently are not recommended for LV volumetric analysis.
- LV volumes measured by 3DE have been reported to be more accurate than those calculated by 2DE (when compared to CMR) and more reproducible
- LV EDV and ESV vary according to gender and body size, consequently the indexing of volumes to BSA is recommended.

Right ventricle

- Care should be taken to obtain the true RV-focused 4Ch image with the LV apex at the centre of the scanning sector, while displaying the largest basal RV diameter and thus avoiding foreshortening.
- Normal values for RV 2D linear and area dimensions are listed in Table 1.1.8.

Table 1.1.8 Normal values for the RV size parameters

Parameter	Normal values (mean±SD) Male	Normal values (mean±SD) Female	Abnormality threshold Male	Abnormality threshold Female
RV basal diameter (mm)	33 ± 4		> 41	
RV mid diameter (mm)	27 ± 4		> 35	
RV longitudinal diameter	71 ± 6		> 83	
RVOT proximal diameter (mm)	28 ± 3.5		> 35	
RVOT distal diameter (mm)	22 ± 2.5		> 27	
RV EDA (cm^2)	17 ± 3.5	14 ± 3	> 24	> 20
RV EDA indexed to BSA (cm^2/m^2)	8.8 ± 1.9	8.0 ± 1.75	> 12.6	> 11.5
RV ESA (cm^2)	9 ± 3	7 ± 2	> 15	> 11
RV ESA indexed to BSA (cm^2/m^2)	4.7 ± 1.35	4.0 ± 1.2	> 7.4	> 6.4
3D EDV indexed to BSA (ml/m^2)	61 ± 13	53 ± 10.5	> 87	> 74
3D ESV indexed to BSA (ml/m^2)	27 ± 8.5	22 ± 7	> 44	> 36

1.1.4 Cardiac chambers anatomy, size, function   29

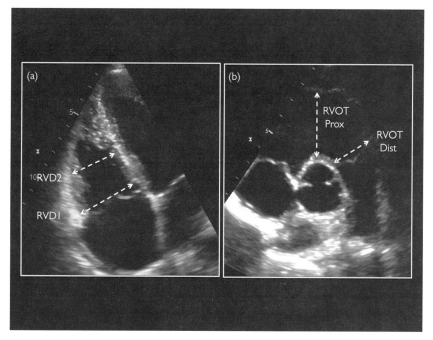

Figure 1.1.26 RV linear measurements. (A) RV basal (RVD1) and mid diameters (RVD2) should be obtained at end-diastole from RV-focused 4Ch view. (B) RVOT proximal (RVOT Prox) diameter should be measured at end-diastole from parasternal short-axis view from the anterior RV wall to the aortic valve (or to the interventricular septal-aortic junction in parasternal long-axis view); RVOT distal diameter (RVOT Dist) should be measured just proximal to the pulmonary valve.

Linear measurements should be obtained at end-diastole from different echocardiographic views. The following RV diameters are recommended in current guidelines (Figure 1.1.26):

- RV basal diameter
- RV mid diameter
- RVOT proximal diameter
- RVOT distal diameter

RV diameters may vary significantly with minor rotation or tilting the transducer and should be performed in standard recommended views.

Area measurements include RV EDA and ESA obtained by manual tracing of the RV endocardial border in RV-focused apical 4Ch view (Figure 1.1.18).

- Ensure that the entire RV including the apex and the free wall is encompassed in the imaging sector during both systole and diastole.
- Include trabeculae in the RV cavity.

RV volumetric analysis

- 3DE RV volumes and EF closely correlate (but slightly underestimate) RV volumes measured by CMR.
- Limitations for 3D RV imaging include:
    - high dependence on image quality
    - i-ncomplete visualization in case of severe dilation
    - need for regular heart rate.

Left atrium

Internal linear dimensions

- LA anteroposterior diameter can be measured by M-mode tracings (Figure 1.1.27 A) or 2D-guided measurement (Figure 1.1.27 B).
- Acquired at end-systole in parasternal long axis view at the level of the aortic sinuses.

Advantages	Limitations	Tips for correct use
Fast and easy to use A lot of published data Reproducible, high temporal resolution (for M-mode measurements)	Single dimension only; not representative of actual LA size (i.e. in LA dilatation) May be affected by dilated aortic root	Measurements should be obtained perpendicular to the aortic root long axis (use anatomical M-mode if necessary) Measure from leading edge to leading edge

Area measurement

- More representative of actual LA size than anteroposterior diameter only.
- LA area should be measured in apical 4Ch view at LV end-systole by tracing the LA inner border. Exclude the area between the MV annulus and the leaflets, and the inlet of pulmonary veins (Figure 1.1.28 A).
- When measuring it is important to obtain a dedicated 4Ch view to avoid LA foreshortening.

Normal values of LA diameter and area are listed in Table 1.1.9.

2DE-derived LA maximal volume

- 2D volumetric measurements are based on tracings of the blood–tissue interface on apical 4Ch and 2Ch views (Figure 1.1.28 A and B, respectively).

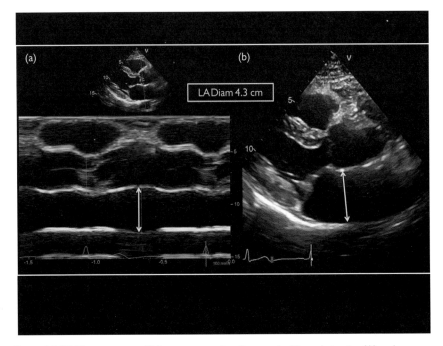

Figure 1.1.27 Measurement of LA anteroposterior diameter by M-mode tracing (A) and 2D-guided measurement (B).

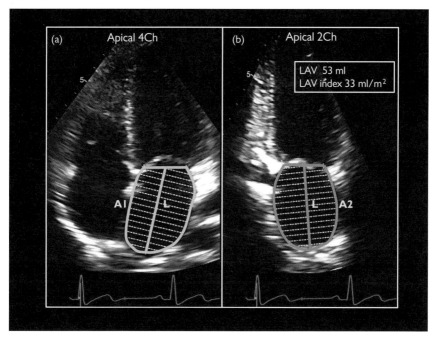

Figure 1.1.28 Measurements of LA area (A) and LA volume (A and B) by 2DE. LA volume was calculated utilizing two currently recommended methods:

1. Method of discs, applying the following equation: $\pi/4(h) \sum(D1)(D2)$, where h is the height of the discs and D1 and D2 are orthogonal minor and major transverse axes of each disc.

2. Area-length method, applying the following equation: $8/3\pi \cdot [(A1 \cdot A2)/L]$, where A1 and A2 are the LA areas measured in the apical 4Ch and 2Ch views and L is the shortest of the two long axes.

Algorithms used:

- Biplane method of discs (Simpson's algorithm);
- Area–length method.

Note, that area–length method provides slightly larger LA volume than method of discs.

Advantages	Limitations	Tips for correct use
Relatively easy to use A lot of published data Prognostic significance More representative of actual LA size than diameters/areas	Based on geometrical assumption (elliptical shape of LA) May be affected by LA foreshortening Inaccurate in irregular LA shape	Dedicated, non-shortened LA views should be used Endocardial tracing should exclude atrial appendage and pulmonary veins Connect MV leaflet insertions on the annulus with straight line

Table 1.1.9 Normal values for LA linear and area measurements

Parameter	Male	Female
Anteroposterior diameter (cm)	2.7–3.8	3.0–4.0
Anteroposterior diameter index (cm/m²)	1.5–2.3	1.5–2.3
LA area index (cm²/m²)	9.3 ± 1.7	8.9 ± 1.5

1.1 Echocardiography

Table 1.1.10 Reference values and severity partition cut-off values for 2DE-derived LA volume

	Normal	Mildly abnormal	Moderately abnormal	Severely abnormal
LA volume index (ml/m^2)	16–34	35–41	42–48	> 48

Reference values for 2DE-derived LA volume are listed in Table 1.1.10.
3DE assessment of LA volumes and function (Figure 1.1.29)

- Limited availability of normative data 3DE and so not recommended for routine use, yet.

Recommendations for LA size measurements

- LA volume measured by biplane methods is the preferred parameter;
- LA dimensions and volumes should be indexed to BSA;
- The upper limit of normality for 2DE LA volume is 34 ml/m^2 for both genders.

Right atrium

- Most commonly performed from a dedicated apical 4Ch view at end-systole (frame just prior to tricuspid valve opening)
- Trace the RA blood–tissue interface and exclude the area between tricuspid annulus and leaflets (Figure 1.1.30).
- The normal ranges for 2DE RA volume are 25 ± 7 ml/m^2 in men and 21 ± 6 ml/m^2 in women.

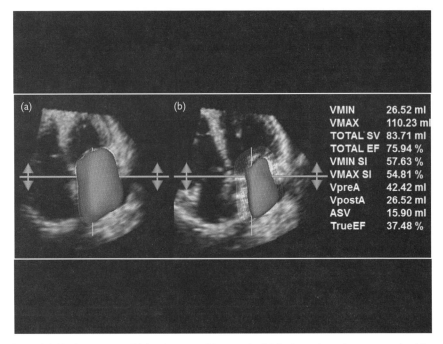

Figure 1.1.29 Assessment of LA volumes and function by 3DE. Green beutels represent the LA volume in real time. (A) Maximal LA volume (VMAX); (B) minimal LA volume (VMIN) with white cage showing the maximal LA volume.

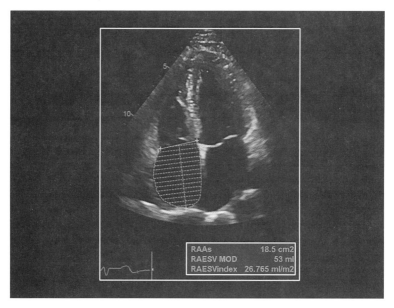

Figure 1.1.30 Measurement of RA area (RAAs) and end-systolic volume by method of discs (RAESV MOD).

1.1.5 Primary and secondary cardiomyopathies (dilated, hypertrophic, restrictive, arrhythmogenic)

Dilated cardiomyopathy

The main diagnostic findings are:

- Dilatation of the LV cavity (LV EDV index > 112 ml/m^2)
- Thinning of LV walls
- EF < 45%

Associated echocardiographic findings are:

- spherical shape of the LV
- LV systolic dyssynchrony
- LV diastolic dysfunction
- presence of wall motion abnormalities even with normal coronary arteries
- presence of thrombi
- dilatation of the atria/RV
- functional mitral regurgitation (MR)
- pulmonary hypertension

Hypertrophic cardiomyopathy

The following echo parameters should be assessed and reported in patients with HCM:

- Presence, extent (maximal wall thickness), and distribution of LV hypertrophy
- LV global systolic function and regional wall motion
- Presence of dynamic LV obstruction at rest and with Valsalva manoeuvre or exercise

- RV hypertrophy
- LA volume (LA 2D parasternal diameter if using HCM risk calculator)
- LV diastolic function (LV relaxation and filling pressures)
- Systolic PAP
- MV and papillary muscle evaluation
    - presence of systolic anterior motion of leaflets and/or chordae
    - direction, mechanism, and severity of MR.

Diagnosis

- Wall thickness ≥ 15 mm in one or more LV myocardial segments which cannot be explained solely by loading conditions
- In first-degree relatives of patients with unequivocal disease (LVH ≥ 15 mm), the clinical diagnosis of HCM should be suspected ad further investigated if there is unexplained increased LV wall thickness ≥ 13 mm in one or more LV myocardial segments.
- Measurement of the maximum diastolic wall thickness is recommended, using 2D short-axis views in all LV segments, from base to apex is recommended.

Asymmetrical septal hypertrophy

- ratio of IVS / posterior LV wall thickness > 1.3 in normotensive patients or > 1.5 in patients with arterial hypertension is a frequent (but non-specific) finding in HCM.

LVOT (or mid-cavity) obstruction

- Peak pressure gradient ≥ 30 mmHg at rest or during physiological provocation (Valsalva manoeuvre, standing, or exercise).
- A gradient of ≥ 50 mmHg is usually considered a threshold for haemodynamically significant LVOT obstruction.
- Echocardiographic reports should describe the site of obstruction and the peak gradient.
- In symptomatic patients with a resting or provoked peak LVOT gradient < 50 mmHg, assessment during exercise in the standing, sitting, or semi-supine position is recommended to detect provocable LVOT obstruction and exercise-induced MR.
- Other morphological features that contribute to LVOT obstruction include
    - papillary muscle abnormalities (hypertrophy, anterior and internal displacement, direct insertion into the anterior mitral valve leaflet)
    - mitral leaflet abnormalities such as elongation or accessory tissue.

Systolic anterior motion of the MV leaflets

- Approximately one-third of HCM patients have resting systolic anterior motion of the MV leaflets that is related to the LVOT obstruction
- One-third of patients have latent obstruction only during Valsalva manoeuvre.
- It is important to consider systolic anterior motion-related MR if eccentric posteriorly directed MR jet is noted.
- MR is usually more severe and frequent in obstructive HCM.

In patients undergoing septal myectomy, perioperative TOE is recommended to:

- confirm the mechanism of LVOT obstruction.
- guide the surgical strategy.
- assess post-surgical complications.
- detect residual LVOT obstruction.

Differential diagnosis between HCM and hypertensive heart disease is described in Table 1.1.11.

Table 1.1.11 Differential diagnosis between HCM and hypertensive heart disease

Echocardiographic finding	HCM	Arterial hypertension
LV hypertrophy	Severe, frequently asymmetric	Moderate, concentric. or mildly asymmetric
IVS/posterior wall thickness	> 1.3 (> 1.5 in patients with arterial hypertension)	< 1.3 (< 1.5)
LVOT obstruction	Frequent	Rare
LV diastolic function	Impaired	May be normal

Arrhythmogenic RV cardiomyopathy

- Arrhythmogenic RV cardiomyopathy (ARVC) is an inherited disorder characterized by fatty or fibro-fatty replacement of the RV myocardium, resulting in ventricular arrhythmias, RV dilatation, and slowly progressive RV dysfunction.
- Diagnostic criteria include electrocardiographic, echocardiographic, and CMR findings.

The following 2DE parameters are included as diagnostic criteria in current clinical guidelines and should be carefully evaluated in all patients with (suspected) ARVC:

Major 2DE criteria

Regional RV akinesia, dyskinesia, or aneurysm (Figure 1.1.31) and one of the following measured at end-diastole:

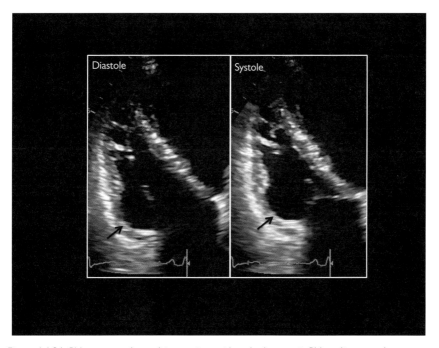

Figure 1.1.31 RV aneurysm (arrow) in a patient with arrhythmogenic RV cardiomyopathy.

- RVOT diameter in parasternal long-axis view ≥ 32 mm (≥ 19 mm/m^2), or
- RVOT diameter in parasternal short-axis view (RVOT prox diameter in Figure 1.1.25B) ≥ 36 mm (≥ 21 mm/m^2), or
- FAC ≤ 33% (Figure 1.1.18).

Minor 2DE criteria

Regional RV akinesia or dyskinesia and one of the following measured at end-diastole:

- RVOT diameter in parasternal long-axis view 29 to 32 mm (PLAX/BSA ≥ 16 to < 19 mm/m^2), or
- RVOT diameter in parasternal short-axis view 32 to 36 mm (PSAX/BSA ≥ 18 to < 21 mm/m^2), or
- FAC 33–40%.

LV myocardial non-compaction

LV myocardial non-compaction is related to the absence of involution of LV trabeculae during the embryogenic process.

Echocardiographic diagnostic findings include:

- Multiple trabeculations with deep endomyocardial recesses (Figure 1.1.32)
- Two-layer myocardial structure with a thin compacted and a thick non-compacted layers;
- Colour Doppler evidence of perfused intertrabecular recesses (Figure 1.1.32 C)
- Systolic thickness of noncompacted vs compacted layer ratio > 2
- LV function can be either preserved or decreased

Contrast echocardiography with contrast agents may improve the accuracy of the diagnosis.

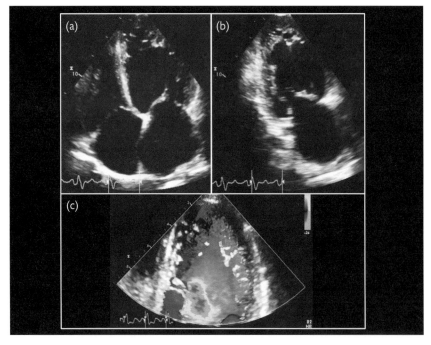

Figure 1.1.32 Increased LV trabeculation and thick non-compacted layer in a patient with LV myocardial non-compaction seen in apical 4Ch view (A), 2Ch view (B), and colour Doppler (C).

1.1.6 Valvular morphology and function

Aortic stenosis

Three main haemodynamic parameters are recommended for the echocardiographic evaluation of AS severity:

A) AS peak jet velocity (Figure 1.1.8):
- Should be obtained from multiple views (apical 5Ch, 3Ch views, right parasternal view) using CW Doppler.
- Align the ultrasound beam along the direction of aortic flow to avoid underestimation of peak velocities and gradients.
- A dedicated small dual-crystal CW Doppler transducer (Pedof) is recommended.
- A peak velocity of ≤ 2.5 m/s is consistent with aortic sclerosis.
- Peak velocity of ≥ 4 m/s is consistent with severe aortic stenosis.

B) Mean aortic transvalvular pressure gradient (Figure 1.1.8):
- The mean gradient is obtained by tracing the spectral Doppler of the aortic flow in CW and calculated by averaging the instantaneous gradients over the ejection period.
- Misalignment of the beam with the direction of the jet is the most common source of gradient underestimation.
- A mean gradient of ≥ 40 mmHg is consistent with severe aortic stenosis.

C) Aortic valve area (AVA) by continuity equation (Figures 1.1.8 and 1.1.9):
- AVA is calculated by continuity equation:

$$AVA = CSA_{LVOT} \cdot VTI_{LVOT} / VTI_{AV},$$

where CSA_{LVOT}—cross-sectional area of LVOT (CSA = π (LVOT diameter^2/4), VTI_{LVOT} and VTI_{AV}—velocity time integral of flow through LVOT and aortic valve, respectively.

- LVOT diameter should be measured in a parasternal long-axis view from the inner edge to inner edge of the LVOT at the point of insertion of aortic cusps, in mid-systole.
- The assumption of a circular LVOT shape is one limitation of the continuity equation. Due to its elliptical shape in majority of patients, LVOT area may be underestimated and as consequence AVA will be underestimated.
- Direct LVOT planimetry by 3DE or computed tomography should be considered when there is discrepancy between valve area and gradients.
- VTI_{LVOT} should be assessed by tracing of PW Doppler LVOT flow from the apical 5Ch or 3Ch view. The PW Doppler sample volume should be positioned just proximal to the aortic valve.
- The role of indexing of AVA by BSA is controversial. It is important in children, adolescents, and small adults with:
  - BSA < 1.5 m^2;
  - Body mass index < 22 kg/m^2;
  - Height < 135 cm.
- In obese patients AVA indexing by BSA is not recommended, as the AVA does not increase with excess body weight and it may overestimate the severity of the stenosis.

Recommendations for grading of AS severity are listed in Table 1.1.12.

Low-flow, low-gradient AS

Suspected when the discrepancy between AVA and aortic transvalvular pressure gradient occurs (AVA < 1 cm^2, however the peak velocity < 4 m/s and the mean pressure gradient < 40 mmHg).

Table 1.1.12 Assessment of aortic stenosis severity by echocardiography

Parameter	Mild	Moderate	Severe
Peak velocity (m/s)	2.6–2.9	3.0–3.9	≥ 4
Mean gradient (mmHg)	< 20	20–40	> 40
AVA (cm^2)	> 1.5	1.0–1.5	< 1.0
AVA index (cm^2/m^2)	> 0.85	0.60–0.85	< 0.60
LVOT/Aortic valve velocity ratio	> 0.50	0.25–0.50	< 0.25

Types:

- Low-flow, low-gradient AS with reduced LV EF (when LV EF < 50%, and SV index < 35 ml/m^2);
- Low-flow, low-gradient AS with preserved LV EF ('paradoxical' low-flow, low-gradient AS). It may occur in patients with small, hypertrophied LV resulting in SV index < 35 ml/m^2 despite normal EF.

Low-dose dobutamine stress echocardiography is indicated in low-flow, low-gradient AS to distinguish between pseudo severe and true severe AS:

- An increase in effective AVA > 1.0 cm^2 suggests pseudo severe AS;
- An increase in AS jet velocity > 4 m/s and a mean gradient > 30–40 mmHg provided that AVA does not exceed 1.0 cm^2 suggests true severe AS.
- Absence of contractile reserve (failure to increase SV by > 20%) makes the diagnosis difficult. Additionally, it predicts poor long-term outcome and high surgical mortality.

Pulmonary stenosis

Quantitative assessment of pulmonary stenosis severity is based mainly on the transpulmonary peak velocity and pressure gradient (Table 1.1.13).

Mitral stenosis

Assessment of MS severity

Mitral valve area < 1.0 cm^2 is consistent with severe mitral stenosis.

There are several techniques used to assess mitral stenosis severity:

A) 2D planimetry (Figure 1.1.33 B)
   a. It is less dependent on flow, heart rate, chamber compliance, or concomitant MR than Doppler methods.
   b. Planimetry should be performed at the level of the MV leaflet tips with the smallest opening orifice.

Table 1.1.13 Grading of pulmonary stenosis severity

	Mild	Moderate	Severe
Peak velocity (m/s)	< 3	3–4	> 4
Peak gradient (mmHg)	< 36	36–64	> 64

1.1.6 Valvular morphology and function   39

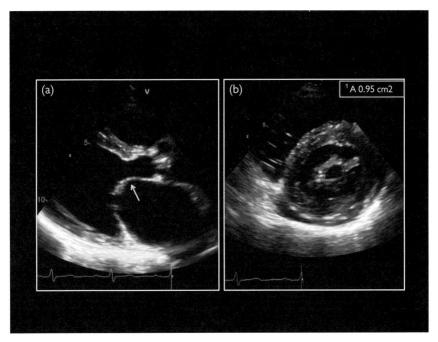

Figure 1.1.33 Doming of anterior mitral valve leaflet (arrow, A) and 'fish-mouth' appearance of mitral valve (B) in a patient with rheumatic mitral stenosis.

  c. Tracing is made at the black–white interface from at least three cardiac cycles in sinus rhythm and five cardiac cycles in atrial fibrillation.
B) 3DE planimetry
  a. Overcomes important limitations of 2DE planimetry, e.g. avoids oblique short-axis views; enables correct positioning of the cut plane in relation to MV orifice location and opening direction thus increasing accuracy of measurement (Figure 1.1.34).
C) Pressure half-time (PHT)
  a. This is the time interval between the maximal trans-mitral pressure gradient and the time point at which this gradient attains the half of its maximal value.
  b. Mitral valve area is calculated by the following formula: $MVA(cm^2) = 220/PHT(ms)$. This method should be used in conjunction with other methods to assess mitral valve severity
D) Continuity equation
  a. This relies on the law of volume conservation. MV area can be calculated by the following formula:

$$MVA = CSA_{LVOT} \times VTI_{LVOT} / VTI_{MV},$$

where CSA_{LVOT}—cross-sectional area of LVOT, VTI_{LVOT} and VTI_{MV}—velocity time integral of flow though LVOT and MV, respectively. This method is more prone to error measurements and cannot be used in the presence of more than mild aortic or mitral regurgitation. Furthermore, it estimates functional MV area which is not the same as anatomic valve area.

E) Trans-mitral diastolic pressure gradient
  a. Mean pressure gradient is calculated by averaging the instantaneous gradients over the diastolic flow period.

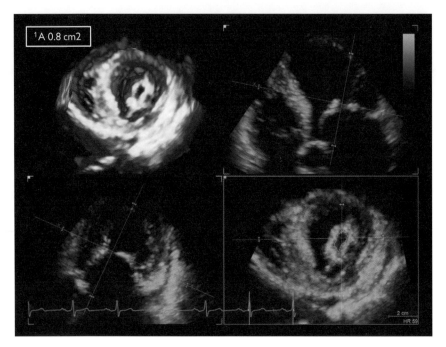

Figure 1.1.34 3DE planimetry of mitral valve area.

b. Pressure gradient depends on flow rate, heart rate, chamber compliance, and concomitant MR.
c. A mean gradient of > 10 mmHg is consistent with severe mitral stenosis.

Recommendations for grading of mitral stenosis severity are listed in Table 1.1.14.

Tricuspid stenosis

Increased transvalvular gradients are frequently associated with TR and high transvalvular flow.

Assessment of tricuspid stenosis severity

A) Valve anatomy (thickening and limited mobility of the leaflets, presence of calcification)
B) Pressure gradient is the most reliable method to assess the severity of tricuspid stenosis. Due to respiratory variations of tricuspid inflow care should be taken to measure gradients in end expiration (or average through respiratory cycle).

Table 1.1.14 Assessment of mitral stenosis severity by echocardiography

Parameter	Mild	Moderate	Severe
Specific findings			
Mitral valve area (cm^2)	> 1.5	1.0–1.5	< 1.0
Supportive findings			
Mean gradient (at heart rate 60–80 per sec) (mmHg)	< 5	5–10	> 10
Pulmonary artery pressure (mmHg)	< 30	30–50	> 50

Table 1.1.15 Findings consistent with haemodynamically significant tricuspid stenosis

Mean pressure gradient	≥ 5 mmHg
Velocity time interval	> 60 cm
PHT	≥ 190 ms
Tricuspid valve area (continuity equation)	≤ 1 cm^2

C) PHT and tricuspid valve area assessed by continuity equitation have limited use due to load dependence, difficulties in precise assessment of RVOT diameter and the frequent presence of concomitant severe TR.
D) 3DE is the only method allowing direct planimetry of the tricuspid orifice. Limited validation data are currently available for this technique.
E) Important supportive findings in severe tricuspid stenosis are the RA enlargement and IVC dilatation.

Recommendations for grading of mitral stenosis severity are listed in Table 1.1.15.

Mitral regurgitation

Assessment of MV morphology

- 2D TTE and TOE are widely used to assess the MV anatomy and the mechanism of MR.
- Assessment should be performed from multiple views allowing to visualize MV in different planes (Figure 1.1.3 A, C, F, H, I, J).
- 3DE significantly improves the understanding of the MV morphology.
- 3DE allows the display of the *en face* view of the valve both from atrial and ventricular perspectives
- 3DE enables precise anatomical and functional analysis. This modality is clinically valuable particularly in cases with complex MV prolapse (Figure 1.1.5).

Assessment of MR severity

A) Colour Doppler imaging of the regurgitant jet is the most common way to detect MR and visually estimate its severity.

Advantages	Limitations	Tips for correct use
Easy to use Evaluation of the spatial orientation of MR jet Good screening test for differentiation between mild vs. severe MR	Does not provide accurate quantitative assessment of the severity of MR	Optimize colour gain and scale Evaluate in multiple (at least in two orthogonal) views Use only for detecting of MR, proceed with quantitative approach if more than a small central MR jet is observed

B) Vena contracta (VC) is the area of the regurgitant jet as it leaves the regurgitant orifice.
   - Width reflects the regurgitant orifice area: an important criteria of MR severity.
   - VC measurements are based on the assumption that the regurgitant orifice is circular. While it may be true in organic MR, in functional MR it can be more oval shaped (elongated along the mitral coaptation line).

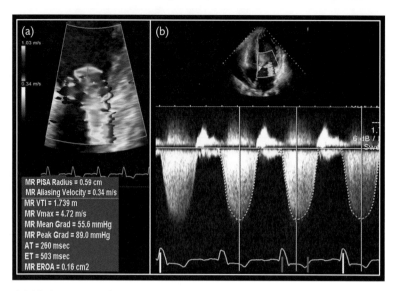

Figure 1.1.35 Assessment of severity of MR by PISA method. (A) Measurement of PISA radius. (B) Tracing of MR signal in CW Doppler.

C) PISA method (Figure 1.1.35)
- Flow converges towards a restrictive orifice, remaining laminar and forming isovelocity surfaces that approximate hemispheres.
- The isovelocity surface should be equal to the flow through regurgitant orifice PISA method allows to calculate regurgitant volume (R Vol) and effective regurgitant orifice area (EROA) using the following formulas:

Advantages	Limitations	Tips for correct use
Relatively easy and fast Can be used in eccentric jet Not affected by other valve regurgitation	Based on the assumption that regurgitant orifice is circular Affected by systolic changes in regurgitant flow Small errors lead to large mistakes due to small absolute values of VC Not applicable in multiple jets	Measure in two orthogonal planes Optimize colour gain/scale (40–70 cm/s) Zoom the selected zone Reduce the colour sector size and depth to maximize frame rate Measure VC immediately distal to the regurgitant orifice, perpendicular to the direction of the jet

$$EROA = (2\pi\, r^2 \times V_a) / \text{Peak velocity}_{MR},$$
$$R\, Vol = EROA \times VTI_{MR},$$

Where: r—PISA radius, V_a—aliasing velocity, Peak velocity$_{MR}$—peak velocity of regurgitant jet, VTI_{MR}—velocity time integral of regurgitant jet.

Advantages	Limitations	Tips for correct use
Quantitative assessment of valve lesion severity (EROA) and volume overload (R Vol) Can be used in eccentric jet Not affected by the aetiology of MR or other valve regurgitation Flow convergence at 50 cm/s alerts to significant MR	Based on the assumption that PISA is a hemisphere PISA shape affected by the aliasing velocity, by systolic changes in regurgitant flow, and by adjacent structures Small errors in PISA radius measurement are squared and can lead to large errors Not applicable in multiple jets High inter-observer variability	Zoom the image of the mitral valve and regurgitant jet Align the jet along the direction of the ultrasound beam Optimize colour-flow imaging of regurgitant jet Decrease the Nyquist limit (15–40 cm/s) Record PISA at several cardiac cycles Measure the PISA radius at mid-systole

D) 3D VC and 3D PISA (Figure 1.1.36)
- Introduction of 3DE colour mode allows acquisition of the whole regurgitant jet.
- It does not rely on assumptions about regurgitant orifice and isovelocity surface geometries and allows direct planimetry of the VC from a 3D colour data set.

E) Complementary findings in severe MR:
- E wave velocity > 120 cm/s.
- PW Doppler mitral to aortic VTI ratio > 1.4.
- systolic pulmonary vein flow reversal.

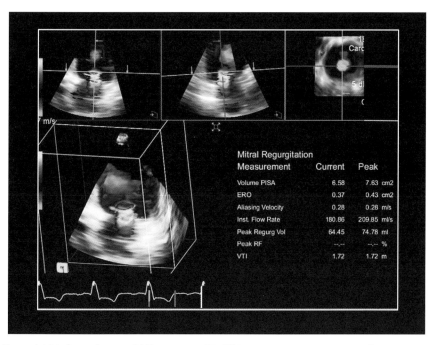

Figure 1.1.36 Quantification of MR severity by 3D PISA method. Volume rendering of the mitral regurgitant colour flow jet at mid-systole shows the complex non-circular and flat shape of the PISA.

Consequences of severe MR include:

- LA and LV dilatation (may be absent in acute MR)
- elevated PAP.

The size of left cardiac chambers, LV function, and systolic PAP must be carefully reported. Grading the severity of MR is described in Table 1.1.16.

Table 1.1.16 Grading the severity of primary MR

Parameters	Mild	Moderate	Severe
Qualitative			
MV morphology	Normal/abnormal	Normal/abnormal	Flail leaflet/ruptured PMs
Colour-flow MR jet	Small, central	Intermediate	Very large central jet or eccentric jet adhering, swirling, and reaching the posterior wall of the LA
Flow convergence zone[a]	No or small	Intermediate	Large
CW signal of MR jet	Faint/parabolic	Dense/parabolic	Dense/triangular
Semi-quantitative			
VC width (mm)	< 3	Intermediate	≥ 7 (> 8 for biplane)[b]
Pulmonary vein flow	Systolic dominance	Systolic blunting	Systolic flow reversal[c]
Mitral inflow	A wave dominant[d]	Variable	E-wave dominant (> 1.5 m/z)[e]
TVI mit/TVI Ao	< 1	Intermediate	> 1.4
Quantitative			
EROA (mm²)	< 20	20–29; 30–39[g]	≥ 40
R Vol (mL)	< 30	30–44; 45–59[g]	≥ 60
+ LV and LA size and the systolic pulmonary arterial pressure[f]			

CW, continuous wave; LA, left atrium; EROA, effective regurgitant orifice area; LV, left ventricle; MR, mitral regurgitation; R Vol, regurgitant volume; VC, vena contracta.

[a] At a Nyquist limit of 50–60 cm/s.
[b] For average between apical four- and two-chamber views.
[c] Unless other reasons of systolic blunting (atrial fibrillation, elevated LA pressure).
[d] Usually after 50 years of age.
[e] In the absence of other causes of elevated LA pressure and of mitral stenosis.
[f] Unless for other reasons, the LA and LV size and the pulmonary pressure are usually normal in patients with mild MR. In acute severe MR, the pulmonary pressures are usually elevated while the LV size is still often normal. In chronic severe MR, the LV is classically dilated. *Accepted cut-off values for non-significant left-sided chambers enlargement*: LA volume < 36 mL/m², LV end-diastolic diameter < 5 6 mm, LV end-diastolic volume < 82 mL/m², LV end-systolic diameter < 40 mm, LV end-systolic volume < 30 mL/m², LA diameter < 39 mm, LA volume < 20 mL/m².
[g] Grading of severity of organic MR classifies regurgitation as mild, moderate, or severe, and subclassifies the moderate regurgitation group into 'mild-to-moderate' (EROA for 20–29 mm² or a R Vol of 30 to 44 mL) and 'moderate-to-severe' (EROA of 30–39 mm² or a R Vol of 45–59 mL).

Lancellotti P, Tribouilloy C, Hagendorff A, et al; Scientific Document Committee of the European Association of Cardiovascular Imaging. Recommendations for the echocardiographic assessment of native valvular regurgitation: an executive summary from the European Association of Cardiovascular Imaging. *Eur Heart J Cardiovasc Imaging*. 2013 Jul;14(7):611–44. doi: 10.1093/ehjci/jet105. © European Society of Cardiology. With permission from Oxford University Press

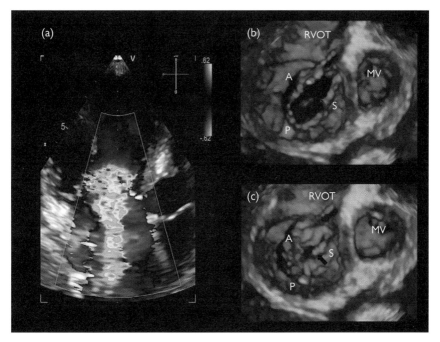

Figure 1.1.37 3DE assessment of tricuspid valve morphology in a patient with severe functional TR. (A) 2D Colour Doppler showing wide central regurgitant jet. (B) *En-face* view of the tricuspid valve from ventricular prospective at diastole demonstrating dilated tricuspid annulus, leaflets of tricuspid valve (S—septal, A—anterior, and P—posterior) and full opening of the valve. (C) *En-face* view of the tricuspid valve at mid-systole showing the coaptation defect (arrow).

Tricuspid regurgitation
Assessment of tricuspid valve morphology
- 3DE has become a valuable tool providing an *en-face* view of the valve from both atrial and ventricular prospective and dynamic assessment of valve morphology (Figure 1.1.38).

Assessment of TR severity
- Colour Doppler imaging of the regurgitant jet (Figure 1.1.37 A);
- VC (Figure 1.1.38);
- PISA method (Figure 1.1.39).

Methods of TR severity assessment are similar to those used in MR. Their accuracy is additionally affected by:

- Frequently very irregular shape of VC (Figure 1.1.40);
- High load dependency of the degree of TR;
- Significant respiratory variations of TR which may occur even under normal conditions.

Complementary findings and consequences of severe TR:

- systolic hepatic vein flow reversal (Figure 1.1.41);
- triangular shape of CW spectral Doppler tracing;
- RA and RV dilatation, dilated IVC, elevated PAP.

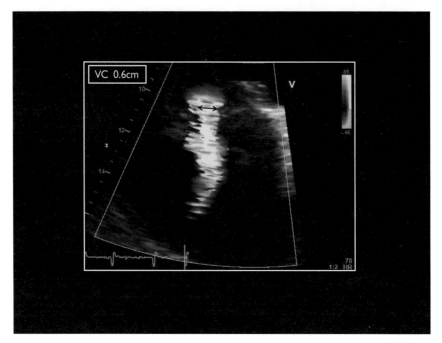

Figure 1.1.38 Measurement of VC in TR. VC are measured from zoomed image of the regurgitant jet with optimized colour scale (40–70 cm/s) immediately distal to the regurgitant orifice, perpendicular to the direction of the jet.

The assessment of systolic PAP based on peak TR jet velocity is usually inaccurate in patients with severe TR due to early equalization of pressure between RV and RA and, consequently, underestimation of the TR gradient.

Grading of TR severity is summarized in Table 1.1.17.

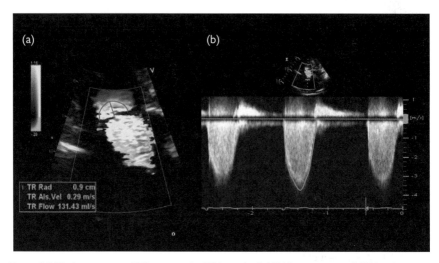

Figure 1.1.39 Assessment of TR severity by PISA method. (A) Measurement of PISA radius in zoomed image with optimized colour gain/scale. (B) Tracing of TR signal in CW Doppler.

1.1.6 Valvular morphology and function 47

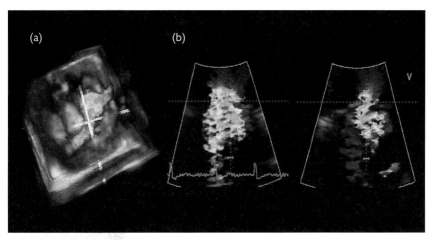

Figure 1.1.40 *En-face* view of the tricuspid regurgitant orifice by 3D colour Doppler imaging in a patient with severe functional tricuspid regurgitation, demonstrating a complex star shape of the regurgitant orifice (A) and significant difference of the jet width in two orthogonal cut planes (B) corresponding with the yellow and white lines in 3D image.

Aortic regurgitation
Assessment of AR severity

A) visual assessment of aortic valve morphology
B) Colour Doppler imaging (Figure 1.1.42A)
- AR jet width / LVOT ratio > 65% is suggestive for severe AR
C) VC
D) PISA method

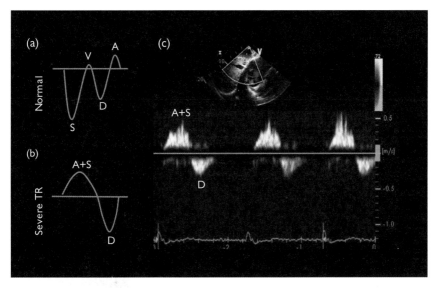

Figure 1.1.41 Assessment of hepatic vein flow by PW Doppler. Schematic illustration of normal waveform of hepatic flow (A) and biphasic waveform with systolic flow reversal in significant TR (B). (C) PW Doppler imaging of hepatic vein flow in a patient with severe TR.

Table 1.1.17 Grading the severity of TR

Parameters	Mild	Moderate	Severe
Qualitative			
Tricuspid valve morphology	Normal/abnormal	Normal/abnormal	Flail leaflet/ruptured PMs
Colour-flow TR jet[a]	Small, central	Intermediate	Very large central jet or eccentric wall-impinging jet
CW signal or TR jet	Faint/parabolic	Dense/parabolic	Dense/triangular with early peaking (peak < 2 m/s in massive TR)
Semi-quantitative			
VC width (mm)[a]	Not defined	< 7	> 7
PISA radius (mm)[b]	≤ 5	6–9	> 9
Hepatic vein flow[c]	Systolic dominance	Systolic blunting	Systolic flow reversal
Tricuspid inflow	Normal	Normal	E-wave dominant (≥ 1 m/s)[d]
Quantitative			
EROA (mm²)	Not defined	Not defined	≥ 40
R Vol (mL)	Not defined	Not defined	≥ 45
+ RA/RV/IVC dimension[e]			

CW, continuous wave; EROA, effective regurgitant orifice area; RA, right atrium; RV, right ventricle; R Vol, regurgitant volume; TR, tricuspid regurgitation; VC, vena contracta.
[a]At a Nyquist limit of 50–60 cm/s.
[b]Baseline Nyquist limit shift of 28 cm/s.
[c]Unless other reasons of systolic blunting (atrial fibrillation, elevated RA pressure).
[d]In the absence of other causes of elevated RA pressure.
[e]Unless for other reasons, the RA and RV size and IVC are usually normal in patients with mild TR. An end-systolic RV eccentricity index > 2 is in favour of severe Tr. In acute severe TR, RV size is often normal. In chronic severe TR, the RV is classically dilated. *Accepted cut-off values for non-significant right-sided chambers enlargement (measurements obtained from the optical four-chamber view)*: Mid-RV dimension ≤ 33 mm, RV end-diastolic area ≤ 28 cm², RV end-systolic area ≤ 16 cm², RV fractional area change > 32%, maximal 2D RA volume ≤ 33 mL/m².
An IVC diameter < 2.1 cm is considered normal.
Lancellotti P, Tribouilloy C, Hagendorff A, et al; Scientific Document Committee of the European Association of Cardiovascular Imaging. Recommendations for the echocardiographic assessment of native valvular regurgitation: an executive summary from the European Association of Cardiovascular Imaging. *Eur Heart J Cardiovasc Imaging*. 2013 Jul;14(7):611–44. doi: 10.1093/ehjci/jet105. © European Society of Cardiology. With permission from Oxford University Press.

E) 3DE VC/PISA assessment.
F) PHT
- This is based on the measurement of the rate of AR jet deceleration (assessed by CW Doppler) (Figure 1.1.42B).
- The rate depends not only on the severity of AR, but also on the LV end-diastolic pressure, which may be affected by LV diastolic function, blood pressure, presence of shunts, etc.
G) Diastolic flow reversal in proximal descending/abdominal aorta
   a. A complementary finding in severe AR.
   b. Brief velocity reversal in descending aorta is normal and can be seen with a stiffer aorta (i.e. in elderly patients) regardless of AR severity.
   c. Holodiastolic flow reversal with end-diastolic velocity > 20 cm/sec in proximal descending aorta is suggestive of severe AR.
   d. Diastolic flow reversal in abdominal aorta is a very specific but relatively insensitive finding in severe AR.

1.1.6 Valvular morphology and function   49

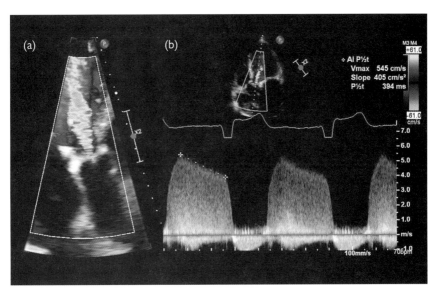

Figure 1.1.42 Assessment of AR. (A) Colour Doppler imaging of AR jet from zoomed apical 3Ch view allows to evaluate spatial orientation of the jet and jet width/LVOT ratio. (B) Measurement of PHT.

Advantages	Limitations	Tips for correct use
Easy and fast Can be used in eccentric jet Not affected by other valve regurgitation	Affected by LV compliance, blood pressure, acuity of AR, presence of shunts Complete signal difficult to obtain in eccentric jet	Measure in 5Ch or 3Ch view Align the ultrasound beam along the direction of regurgitant jet Ensure complete AR signal in spectral Doppler

Grading the severity of AR is described in Table 1.1.18.

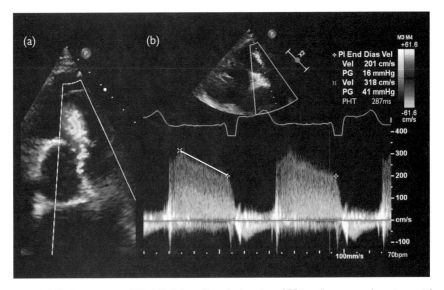

Figure 1.1.43 Assessment of PR. (A) Colour Doppler imaging of PR jet allows to evaluate its spatial orientation and jet width relative to pulmonary annulus diameter. (B) Measurement of PHT.

Table 1.1.18 Grading the severity of AR

Parameters	Mild	Moderate	Severe
Qualitative			
Aortic valve morphology	Normal/abnormal	Normal/abnormal	Abnormal/flail/large coaptation defect
Colour-flow AR jet width[a]	Small in central jets	Intermediate	Large in central jet, variable in eccentric jets
CW signal of AR jet	Incomplete/faint	Dense	Dense
Diastolic flow reversal in the descending aorta	Brief, protodiastolic flow reversal	Intermediate	Holodiastolic flow reversal (end-diastolic velocity > 20 cm/s)
Diastolic flow reversal in the abnormal aorta	Absent	Absent	Present
Semi-quantitative			
VC width (mm)	< 3	Intermediate	≥ 6
Pressure half-time (ms)[b]	> 500	Intermediate	< 200
Quantitative			
EROA (mm²)	< 10	10–19; 20–29[d]	≥ 30
R Vol (mL)	< 30	30–44; 45–59[d]	≥ 60
+ LV size[c]			

AR, aortic regurgitation; CW, continuous wave; LA, left atrium; EROA, effective regurgitant orifice area; LV, left ventricle; R Vol, regurgitant volume; VC, vena contracta.

[a] At a Nyquist limit of 50–60 cm/s.
[b] Pressure half-time is shortened with increasing LV diastolic pressure, vasodilator therapy, and in patients with a dilated compliant aorta or lengthened in chronic AR.
[c] Unless other reasons, the LV size is usually normal patients with mild AR. In acute severe AR, the LV size is often normal. *Accepted cut-off values for non-significant LV enlargement*: LV volume end-diastolic diameter < 56 mm, LV end-diastolic diameter < 82 mL/m², LV end-systolic diameter < 40 mm, LV end-systolic volume < 30 mL/m².
[d] Grading of the severity of AR classifies regurgitation as mild, moderate, or severe, and subclassifies the moderate regurgitation group into 'mild-to-moderate' (EROA for 10–19 mm or a R Vol of 20–44 mL) and 'moderate-to-severe' (EROA of 20–29 mm² or a R Vol of 45–59 mL).
Lancellotti P, Tribouilloy C, Hagendorff A, et al; Scientific Document Committee of the European Association of Cardiovascular Imaging. Recommendations for the echocardiographic assessment of native valvular regurgitation: an executive summary from the European Association of Cardiovascular Imaging. *Eur Heart J Cardiovasc Imaging.* 2013 Jul;14(7):611–44. doi: 10.1093/ehjci/jet105. © European Society of Cardiology. With permission from Oxford University Press.

Pulmonary regurgitation
Assessment of PR severity
A) Visual assessment of pulmonary valve morphology.
B) Colour-flow imaging allows the evaluation of the spatial orientation of regurgitant jet in parasternal short-axis view (Figure 1.1.43 A). Jet width > 50–65% of pulmonary annulus is a sensitive (albeit low specific) sign of severe PR.
C) Diastolic flow reversal in main PA and its branches (more specific) are sensitive signs of severe PR.
D) Dense CW Doppler PR signal with steep deceleration and early termination of diastolic flow is suggestive for severe PR.
E) PHT < 100 ms is suggestive of severe PR (Figure 1.1.43 B).

F) PR index = 100 × PR duration/diastole duration ratio. PR index < 77% is highly suggestive for significant PR (it is 100% sensitive for severe PR when combined with the presence of diastolic flow reversal in PA branch).

1.1.7 Prosthetic valves

Type (Table 1.1.19), model, size, and date of implant of the prosthetic valve to be examined are essential data which should be retrieved before the exam and included in final report.

Main echocardiographic parameters to be assessed for prosthetic valve:

- Prosthetic valve morphology, presence of thrombus/pannus
- Mobility of the cusps/discs, thickness/calcification of leaflet in bioprostheses
- Peak velocity
- Mean gradient
- VTI
- Doppler velocity index
- Effective orifice area by the continuity equation
- Presence, location, and severity of regurgitation
- LV size and function, LV hypertrophy (for prosthetic aortic and mitral valve), RV size and function, RA size, IVC size (for prosthetic tricuspid and pulmonary valve), PAP;
- Other: appearance, grade of stenosis, and regurgitation.

Table 1.1.20 summarizes the main parameters used to identify aortic valve prosthesis malfunction.

1.1.8 Endocarditis

Infective endocarditis (IE) is an inflammation of the endocardium, caused by microorganisms, and generally localized on cardiac valves.

- TTE has 60% sensitivity in diagnosis of vegetations (90% for TOE).
- *Vegetations* (oscillating masses attached on a valve, with a motion independent to that of the valve) are the main morphological findings by echocardiography in IE.
    - They are typically attached on the low pressure side of the valve, but may be located anywhere on valvular and subvalvular apparatus.
    - Large and mobile vegetations are prone to embolism as well as to valve or prosthetic obstruction.

Table 1.1.19 Types of prosthetic valves.

Biological				Mechanical
Stented	Stentless	Sutureless	Transcatheter	
Porcine bioprosthesis Pericardial bioprosthesis	Porcine bioprosthesis Pericardial bioprosthesis Aortic homograft Pulmonary autograft (Ross procedure)			Bileaflet Single tilting disk Caged ball

Table 1.1.20 Echocardiographic parameters used to identify aortic valve prosthesis malfunction

Parameters	Normal parameter	Obstruction likely	Significant obstruction
Qualitative			
Valve structure and function	Normal	Often normal	Abnormal
Morphology of spectral Doppler flow	Triangular, early peak	Triangular to intermediate	Rounded, symmetric
Semi-quantitative			
Acceleration time (ms)	< 80	80–100	> 100
Acceleration time/LV ejection time	< 0.32	0.32–0.37	> 0.37
Quantitative			
Flow dependent			
Peak velocity (m/s)	< 3	3–3.9	≥ 4
Mean gradient (mmHg)	< 20	20–34	≥ 35
Mean gradient increase during exercise	< 10	10–19	≥ 20
Mean gradient increase during follow-up	< 10	10-19	≥ 20
Flow independent			
Effective orifice area (cm^2)	> 1.1	0.8–1.1	< 0.8
Measured EOA vs Reference value	Reference value ±1DS	< Reference value – 1DS	< Reference value – 2 DS
Difference between reference and measured EOA (cm^2)	< 0.25	0.25–0.35	> 0.35
Doppler velocity index	≥ 0.35	0.25–0.34	< 0.25

Other morphological findings in IE

- Abscess: Thickened, non-homogeneous perivalvular area with echodense or echolucent appearance
- Pseudoaneurysm: pulsatile perivalvular echo-free space with flow inside by colour Doppler
- Perforation: interruption of endocardial tissue continuity traversed by colour Doppler flow
- Fistula: colour Doppler communication between two neighbouring cavities through a perforation
- Valve aneurysm: saccular bulging of valvular tissue
- Dehiscence of a prosthetic valve: paravalvular regurgitation with or without rocking motion of the prosthesis.

In addition to valve morphology, presence and degree of valve dysfunction should be accurately assessed and reported.

1.1.9 Pericardial disease

Pericardial effusion

A small amount of pericardial fluid can be present in normal conditions and can be detected as a tiny translucent space in the posterior atrioventricular junction. Usually the separation of pericardial layers is seen only during systole.

Pericardial effusions can be graded as:

- Small: pericardial layer separation ≤ 0.5 cm (< 100 ml);
- Moderate: 0.5 < pericardial layer separation ≤ 1 cm (100–500 ml);
- Large: pericardial layer separation > 1 cm (> 500 ml) (Figure 1.1.44).

Importantly, for the haemodynamic impact of pericardial effusion the rate of fluid accumulation is more important than its amount. Even relatively small pericardial effusion accumulating rapidly may cause cardiac tamponade.

Cardiac tamponade

- A life-threatening condition due to increased intrapericardial pressure above normal filling pressure of the heart.
- Main echocardiographic parameters:
  1. RA collapse during ventricular systole (time of RA collapse/time of cardiac cycle ratio > 0.34)
  2. RV free-wall collapse during ventricular diastole
  3. IVS motion toward LV during inspiration and toward RV during expiration due to reciprocal changes in ventricular volumes (increased ventricular interdependence)
  5. Respiratory variation of mitral and tricuspid velocities more than 30% and 60%, respectively
  6. IVC dilatation and blunted respiratory changes of its size
  7. Swinging heart motion
  8. In very high pericardial pressure - compression of the LA/LV

Constrictive pericarditis

- Constrictive pericarditis is characterized by impaired cardiac diastolic function due to a thickened, inflamed, adherent or calcified pericardium
- Causes include post-radiotherapy, post-surgery, as an evolution of effusive pericarditis.

Main echocardiographic parameters:

1. Pericardial thickening
2. Ventricular septal bounce and abnormal motion toward LV during inspiration and toward RV during expiration (Figure 1.1.45 A)

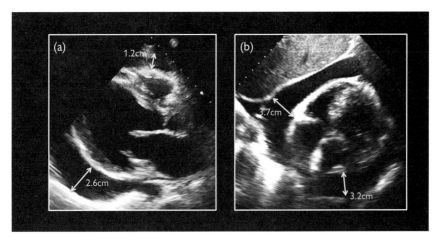

Figure 1.1.44 Large pericardial effusion. Echo-free space is seen around the heart from parasternal long axis (A) and subcostal 4Ch views (B).

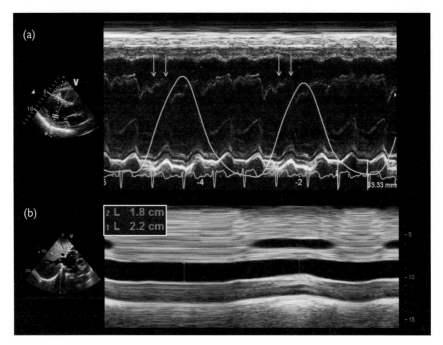

Figure 1.1.45 Echocardiographic signs of constrictive pericarditis. (A) Bright thickened pericardium close to inferolateral LV wall; abnormal motion of IVS toward LV during inspiration (arrows) and toward RV during expiration. (B) Dilated IVC dilatation with minimal changes during inspiration.

3. Decrease in mitral inflow velocities > 25% and increase in tricuspid inflow velocities > 30% during inspiration
4. LV inflow pattern with a prominent E-wave and rapid early diastolic deceleration time (< 160 ms)
5. Septal E' velocity > 7 cm/s; lateral E' velocity lower than septal E' velocity (annulus reversus); E' higher in expiration
6. Increased reversal flow during expiration in hepatic veins;
7. IVC dilatation with blunted respiratory changes of its size (Figure 1.1.45 B).

Pericardial cyst
- A benign lesion consisting of delineated insulated pericardial portion.
- Can be seen as thin-walled echo-free structure located near the heart.

Congenital absence of pericardium (total or partial)
- A rare condition. Can be seen suspected when there is an extreme levorotation of the heart with exaggerated cardiac motion.

1.1.10 Cardiac masses

Cardiac masses include tumours, thrombi, vegetations, and foreign bodies (Table 1.1.21) and require careful assessment as they may significantly affect cardiac function and be a source of cardiac embolism.

Table 1.1.21 Cardiac masses

Benign tumors	Myxoma (most common in adult population), lipoma, fibroelastoma, fibroma, etc.
Malignant tumors	Angiosarcoma (most common in adult population), rabdomiosarcoma, vena caval extension of hypernephroma, pulmonary venous extension, bronchogenic and mediastinal tumors
Thrombi	Ventricular—typically located in aneurismal sack; Atrial—frequent in atrial fibrillation/flutter
Vegetations	In IE
Iatrogenic masses	Pacemaker wires, indwelling catheter, embolized vena caval umbrella, occluders, etc.
Normal variants	RA: Eustachian valve, crista terminalis, Chiari network LA: pectinate muscles RV: moderator band, trabeculation RV: papillary muscles, false/aberrant chords, trabeculation
Others	Artefacts, reverberations from mechanical valve prosthesis

Echocardiographic characteristics of cardiac mass include:

- its site and attachment
- size and shape
- echodensity and homogenicity
- mobility
- evidence of invasiveness
- vascularization (assessed by contrast echocardiography).

In case of right cardiac mass, presence of communications between right and left cardiac chambers (i.e. patent foramen ovale, etc.) should be checked and reported as it may enable paradoxical embolization.

1.1.11 Congenital heart disease

Atrial septal defect (ASD)

- ASD is the most common adult congenital defect (20% of all congenital defects are ASDs).
- Haemodynamic changes include RV and RA dilatation, RV volume overload, reduced compliance of the LV, pulmonary hypertension (however, severe pulmonary hypertension is rare in the setting of isolated ASD).
- It is also a potential for paradoxical cardiac embolism.

ASD types:
Ostium secundum

- The most common type of ASD. It is located in central portion of the interatrial septum (Figure 1.1.46), can be single or multiple (fenestrated septum), variable in shape.
- Best echocardiographic views to detect the defect by colour Doppler are subcostal, modified apical 4Ch or parasternal short-axis view.

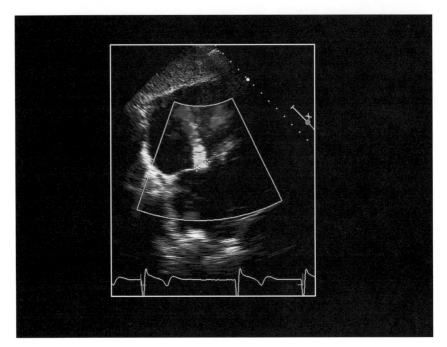

Figure 1.1.46 Ostium secundum ASD with left-to-right shunt on colour Doppler.

- TOE (particularly 3D TOE) is a valuable tool providing not only diagnostic information in patients with ASD, but also assessing parameters essential for further management, such as defect and rims sizing and exclusion of other congenital abnormalities (i.e. anomalous pulmonary venous return).

Ostium primum

- Located in the most anterior and inferior part of the interatrial septum and is a form of atrioventricular septal defect.
- Typically associated with a cleft in the anterior leaflet of the mitral valve.
- It may be associated to an additional ostium secundum defect.

Coronary sinus defect (or unroofed coronary sinus)

- A defect in the wall separating the coronary sinus from the LA.
- This is the rarest type of ASD and can be suspected in patients with enlarged coronary sinus and loss of a clear border between the coronary sinus and the LA.
- Modified (posteriorly orientated) apical 4Ch view should be used.

Sinus venosus defect

- Located on the rightward septal surface adjacent to superior or IVC drainage.
- Inferior sinus venosus defect can extend towards fossa ovalis and be mistaken for a secundum ASD.
- Defect is commonly associated with anomalous drainage of the right sided pulmonary veins (usually right upper). This type of ASD can be easily missed in TTE, which makes TOE essential for diagnosis.

Ventricular septal defect (VSD)

- The best echocardiographic views for the detection of perimembranous VSD are short-axis view at the level of great vessels and parasternal long-axis view; for muscular VSD atypical views may be useful.
VSD size:

- small < 5 mm,
- moderate 5–10 mm,
- large > 10 mm.

Small or moderate VSD are usually restrictive (with high-velocity jet across IVS > 4.5 m/sec), while large defects are non-restrictive (low velocity < 4.5 m/sec).

3DE allows an *en-face* view of the defect with accurate assessment of its morphology and measurement of its size.

Patent Ductus Arteriosus (PDA)

- PDA is a persisting communication between the descending aorta and the bifurcation of main pulmonary artery.
- PDA is present in 2% of the adult population and often associated with coarctation of the aorta and VSD.
- Echocardiography allows the assessment of PDA location, flow pattern, and haemodynamic consequences, to identify coexistent congenital abnormalities, to plan further patient management, and to provide follow-up after PDA closure.

The best echocardiographic views to identify the shunt between aorta and pulmonary artery are:

- high modified left parasternal or left infraclavicular view with slight clockwise rotation of the probe to outline both aorta and pulmonary artery;
- for confirmation: parasternal short-axis view at the level of great vessels, suprasternal and subcostal views.

PDA should be suspected in the setting of:

- dilated and hyperdynamic LV in the absence of other reasons for LV volume overload (such as AR, MR, VSD);
- diastolic reversal flow in aorta without other cause (i.e. severe AR);
- dilated pulmonary artery and its branches and pulmonary hypertension.

Aortic coarctation

- Aortic coarctation is a narrowing of the aorta typically at the junction of the aortic arch and the descending aorta just below the left subclavian artery (isthmus).
- Echocardiographic diagnosis is based on the detection of turbulent colour Doppler flow pattern at the site of coarctation and characteristic Doppler trace: high-velocity systolic flow wave profile with continuous diastolic flow (diastolic tail).
- Best echocardiographic views are high parasternal, supraclavicular, and suprasternal.

Other potential associated abnormalities:

- Bicuspid aortic valve,
- VSD,
- MV abnormalities,
- Intracranial aneurysms.

1.1.12 Pulmonary hypertension

- The evaluation of the pulmonary artery pressure (PAP) is important in the echocardiographic assessment of patients with pulmonary hypertension.
- There are several methods of echocardiographic assessment of pulmonary pressure (Table 1.1.22) including the estimation of systolic PAP by peak velocity of TR jet (Figure 1.1.47).
- More recent ESC guidance has recommended the use of tricuspid valve velocity (TRV) in addition with other markers of potential pulmonary hypertension to estimate the probability of pulmonary hypertension being present:
    - The probability of PH is classified as low / intermediate / high
    - TRV > 3.4 m/s: high probability
    - TRV ≤ 3.4 m/s: use other echocardiographic markers to assign the probability of PH
    - Two markers from different categories from Table 1.1.22 are needed to help assign the probability of PH when the TRV ≤ 3.4 m/s (Figure 1.1.48)
- Severe TR often precludes an accurate assessment of systolic PAP due to an early equalization of RV and RA pressures resulting in significant underestimation the RV-RA gradient using simplified Bernoulli equation.

Echocardiographic evaluation of patients with pulmonary hypertension includes assessment of:

- RV shape (Figure 1.1.49),
- position and motion of the IVS (Figure 1.1.49),
- estimation of the RV size
- RV systolic and diastolic function and mechanics
- RV wall motion abnormalities (i.e. McConell sign in acute pulmonary embolism).

Some echocardiographic parameters of pulmonary haemodynamics are summarised in Table 1.1.23.

1.1.13 Non-invasive haemodynamics

Echocardiography enables assessment of parameters such as stroke volume (SV), cardiac output (CO), LV filling pressures (see Figure 1.1.17 B), PAP and RA pressure

Table 1.1.22 Echocardiographic signs used to help grade the probability of PH being present

A: The Ventricles	B: Pulmonary Artery	C: Inferior vena cava and Right Atrium
Right ventricle/left ventricle basal diameter ratio > 1.0	Right ventricular outflow Doppler acceleration time < 105 ms and/or mid-systolic notching	Inferior vena cava diameter > 21 mm with decreased inspiratory collapse (< 50% with a sniff or < 20% with quiet respiration)
Flattening of the interventricular septum (left ventricular eccentricity index > 1.1 in systole or both systole and diastole)	Early diastolic pulmonary regurgitation (PR) velocity > 2.2 m/s PA diameter > 25 mm	Right atrial area (end-systole) > 18 cm²

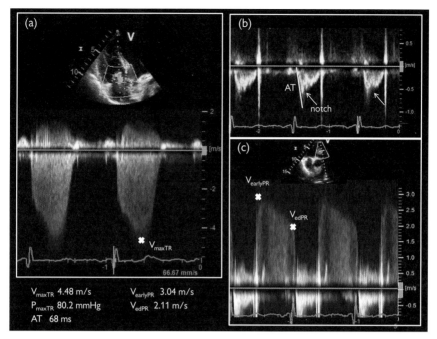

Figure 1.1.47 Echocardiographic assessment of PAP in a patient with severe pulmonary hypertension. (A) Estimation of systolic PAP by peak systolic velocity of TR jet. (B) Typical shape of RVOT flow in pulmonary hypertension by pulse wave Doppler with short acceleration time and a notching (arrow) of the curve. (C) Measurements of early proto-diastolic and end-diastolic velocity of PR necessary for calculation of mean and diastolic PAP. Abbreviations: AT—pulmonary artery flow acceleration time; dPAP—diastolic pulmonary artery pressure; mPAP—mean pulmonary artery pressure; RA—right atrium; RV—right ventricle; RVOT—RV outflow tract; sPAP—systolic pulmonary artery pressure; $V_{earlyPR}$—the early velocity of the PR jet; V_{edPR}—end-diastolic PR velocity V_{maxTR}—peak velocity of the tricuspid regurgitant jet.

SV and CO are calculated using the following formulas:

$$SV = LVOT\ area \times VTI_{LVOT} = \pi(LVOT\ diameter/2)^2 \times VTI_{LVOT}$$
$$CO = Heart\ Rate \times SV$$

The LVOT diameter is measured in a zoomed parasternal long-axis view in mid-systole at the moment of complete opening of aortic valve from the inner edge to inner edge (Figure 1.1.50 A). The LVOT VTI is measured by PW Doppler in either the apical 5Ch or 3Ch view (Figure 1.1.50 B).

Limitations which may affect the accuracy of the results are:

- LVOT has elliptical (not circular) shape in many patients (3DE planimetry may be helpful in obtaining LVOT area);
- LVOT VTI may not be accurate in irregular heart rhythm (average the VTIs of several beats);
- small errors in LVOT diameter measurements can lead to significant error in results since the radius is squared.

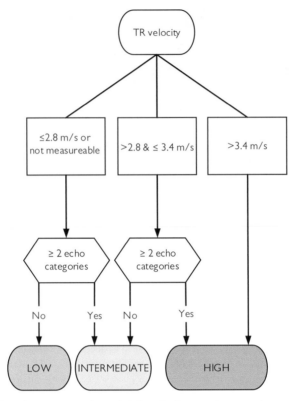

Figure 1.1.48 Flow chart to assess the probability of pulmonary hypertension.
Reproduced from Augustine DX, Coates-Bradshaw LD, Willis J, et al. Echocardiographic assessment of pulmonary hypertension: a guideline protocol from the British Society of Echocardiography. *Echo Res Pract.* 2018 Sep;5(3):G11–G24. doi: 10.1530/ERP-17-0071 with permission from Springer Nature https://creativecommons.org/licenses/by/4.0/

1.1.14 Liver congestion and venous flow, respiratory changes of the vena cava

- PW Doppler assessment of the hepatic vein flow is helpful
- Normally, hepatic venous flow include four phases (Figure 1.1.41 A): S, V, D, and A
- S and D waves indicate flow in the anterograde direction toward the heart and reflect systolic and diastolic phases
- A wave has opposite direction and corresponds with atrial contraction
- V wave may peak below, at, or above the baseline and reflects movement of tricuspid annulus back to its normal position at early diastole.
- In congestive heart failure and/or severe TR, these normal waves are absent, and due to systolic flow reversal a biphasic waveform can be detected (Figure 1.1.41 B and C).

Evaluation of IVC size and respiratory changes is another important part of TTE helping in assessment of cardiac pathology and volume status.

- IVC diameter decreases > 50% during inspiration when the negative intrathoracic pressure leads to increase in RV filling from the systemic veins.

1.1.14 Liver congestion and venous flow, respiratory changes of the vena cava 61

Table 1.1.23 Main echocardiographic parameters of pulmonary haemodynamic

Parameter	Main principles	Normal range	Pitfalls and limitations
Systolic PAP	sPAP = $4(V_{maxTR})^2$ + RA pressure	≤ 35 mmHg (or V_{TR} ≤ 2.8 m/s)	• Requires high quality spectral Doppler signal of TR. • Not applicable in patients with RVOT obstruction, pulmonary valve stenosis, prosthetic pulmonary valve, severe TR.
Mean PAP	1. mPAP = $4(V_{earlyPR})^2$ + RA pressure; 2. mPAP = 79 − (0.45 × AT); 3. mPAP = 90 − (0.62 × AT), for patients with AT < 120 ms	< 25 mmHg	• Requires high quality spectral Doppler signal of PR. • AT is dependent on heart rate, cardiac output, and position of Doppler sample volume.
Diastolic PAP	dPAP = $4(V_{edPR})^2$ + RA pressure	–	• Requires high-quality spectral Doppler signal of PR. • Less correlates with invasively measured pressure. • Less established diagnostic and prognostic value.
Mean RA pressure	1. RA pressure 3 mmHg (range, 0–5 mmHg) if IVC diameter < 2.1 cm and respiratory collapse > 50%; 2. RA pressure 15 mmHg (range, 10–20 mmHg) if IVC diameter > 2.1 cm and respiratory collapse < 50%; 3. RA pressure 8 mmHg (range, 5–10 mmHg): other combinations of IVC diameter and collapsibility index.	< 5 mmHg	• IVC may be dilated independently of PAP in specific groups (i.e. young individuals, athletes, mechanically ventilated patients; patients with narrowing of IVC-RA junction). • Requires patients' collaboration. • The estimation of RA pressure by IVC size and dynamics is encouraged for the estimation of sPAP on the basis of the TR jet velocity, rather than assuming a constant RA pressure for all patients.
Pulmonary vascular resistance	PVR = (V_{TR} / VTI_{RVOT}) × 10 + 0.16	< 1.5 WU	• Requires high-quality PW Doppler signal of RVOT flow and CW Doppler signal of TR. • Not reliable in patients with very high PVR (> 8 WU, as determined by invasive haemodynamic measurements).

Additional abbreviations: AT—pulmonary artery flow acceleration time; dPAP—diastolic pulmonary artery pressure; mPAP—mean pulmonary artery pressure; PR—pulmonary regurgitation; PVR—pulmonary vascular resistance; sPAP—systolic pulmonary artery pressure; $V_{earlyPR}$—the early velocity of the PR jet; V_{edPR}—end-diastolic PR velocity V_{maxTR}—peak velocity of the tricuspid regurgitant jet; VTI_{RVOT}—time velocity integral of RVOT flow.

- The evaluation of the inspiratory response often requires a brief sniff, as normal inspiration may not lead to significant changes.
- The diameter of the IVC and the percentage decrease in the diameter during inspiration correlate with RA pressure (see Table 1.1.23).

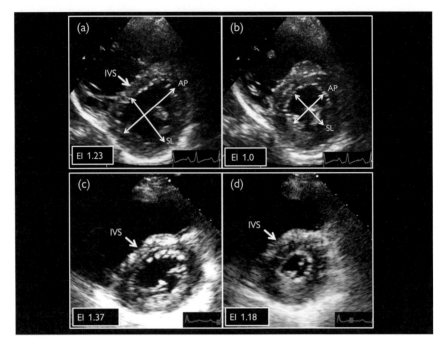

Figure 1.1.49 Assessment of the RV shape and IVS motion in parasternal short-axis view at the level of papillary muscles. (A, B) 2DE images from a patient with RV volume overload due to severe TR show the leftward septal shift and flattening during diastole with LV taking the shape of the letter 'D' (A), whereas a circular profile of LV cavity is maintained during systole (B). In a patient with pressure overload (C, D) septal flattening and deformation of the LV are maintained also during systole. Eccentricity index (EI) (LV antero-posterior diameter (AP) divided by septo-lateral (SL) diameter) value greater than 1 at end-diastole is a strong indicator of RV volume overload (A). At end-systole or during the whole cardiac cycle it suggests the RV pressure overload.

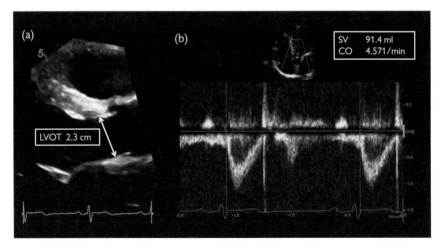

Figure 1.1.50 Echocardiographic assessment of LV SV and CO. (A) Measurement of LVOT diameter in a zoomed parasternal long-axis view. (B) LVOT VTI tracing.

Table 1.1.24 Main pathology to anticipate and to screen for in emergency echocardiography

Clinical presentation	Most common pathology	Echocardiographic assessment
Acute chest pain	Acute coronary syndrome Aortic dissection Pulmonary embolism Myopericarditis Pneumothorax	LV/RV size and global function LV/RV regional wall motion abnormalities Aortic dimensions and presence of AR PA size and pressure Pericardial effusion Signs of pericardial constriction
Acute dyspnoea	Acute decompensated heart failure Pulmonary embolism Cardiac tamponade Acute valve regurgitation/ prosthetic valve dysfunction Pneumothorax Acute coronary syndrome	LV/RV size, global and regional function Valve morphology and function Pericardial/pleural effusions Echocardiographic signs of cardiac tamponade PA size and pressure B-lines for lung congestion Detection of suspected complication of myocardial ischaemia/infarction, such as acute MR, VSD, free-wall rupture/tamponade, RV involvement, heart failure.
Haemodynamic instability/shock	Cardiogenic shock Hypovolemic shock Obstructive shock	LV/RV size and global function IVC size and respiratory variations Intravascular volume status Pericardial/pleural effusions
Chest trauma	Cardiac tamponade Aortic dissection Pneumothorax Acute valve regurgitation	Aortic dimensions and presence of AR Signs of tamponade Pericardial/pleural effusions Valve morphology and function
Cardiac arrest	Acute coronary syndrome Pulmonary embolism Cardiac tamponade	Cardiac activity (identify true asystole, electromechanical dissociation) LV/RV function Pericardial effusion/tamponade

Table 1.1.25 Normal values of aortic dimensions

Diameter	Value (mm)	Indexed to BSA (mm/m²)
Aortic annulus	< 31	< 16
Sinuses of Valsalva*	< 40	< 21
Proximal ascending aorta	< 36	< 19

* for precise assessment the aortic root diameter at the sinuses of Valsalva should be compared with special age- and BSA-related nomograms, as its size may vary significantly according to age and BSA.

Pathology to anticipate and to screen for in emergency echocardiography

Common acute presentations together with associated pathologies and echocardiographic assessment is shown in Table 1.1.24.

1.1.15 Aortic root assessment

- TTE is the first choice imaging modality for serial measurement of maximal aortic root diameters.
- Requires standardization of measurements including similar determination of edges, timing of measurements so standard procedure should be established and strictly followed.
    - Aortic annulus should be measured at peak systole from inner edge to inner edge
    - Other dimensions (aortic root and ascending aorta diameter) are measured at end-diastole from leading edge to leading edge. Normative values are listed in Table 1.1.25.
    - TOE has superior image quality, of nearly all of the ascending and descending thoracic aorta

1.2

Cardiac Magnetic Resonance Imaging

Theo Karamitsos and Chrysovalantou Nikolaidou

TABLE OF CONTENTS

- 1.2.1 Basic CMR physics 65
- 1.2.2 Types of CMR artefacts 66
- 1.2.3 CMR safety and contraindications 68
- 1.2.4 Contrast agents 69
- 1.2.5 Overview of CMR examination 69
- 1.2.6 CMR methodology 69
  - Cardiac anatomy 69
  - Cardiac function 69
  - Tissue characterization 70
  - CMR stress imaging 70
  - Blood flow assessment 71
  - MR angiography 72
- 1.2.7 CMR in specific heart diseases 73
  - Ischaemic heart disease 73
  - Heart failure 75
  - Cardiomyopathies 75
  - Hypertrophic cardiomyopathy 75
  - Dilated cardiomyopathy 76
  - Arrhythmogenic right ventricular cardiomyopathy 77
  - Restrictive cardiomyopathies 78
  - Amyloidosis 78
  - Sarcoidosis 78
  - Anderson–Fabry disease 78
  - Iron overload cardiomyopathy 78
  - Eosinophilic myocarditis 79
  - Takotsubo cardiomyopathy 79
  - Left ventricular non-compaction 79
- 1.2.8 Chemotherapy-related cardiotoxicity 79
- 1.2.9 Transplant cardiomyopathy 80
- 1.2.10 Myocarditis 80
- 1.2.11 Valvular heart disease 80
- 1.2.12 Pericardial disease 82
- 1.2.13 Cardiac and pericardial masses and tumours 82
- 1.2.14 Congenital heart disease 85
- 1.2.15 Vascular disease 87
- 1.2.16 Incidental findings 89

1.2.1 Basic CMR physics

- Magnetic Resonance Imaging (MRI) uses the magnetic properties of mostly hydrogen nuclei, radio waves, and powerful superconducting magnets to generate still and cine images of the cardiovascular system.
- CMR is generally performed at a magnetic field strength of 1.5 Tesla in clinical settings, which is about 30,000 times stronger than the earth's magnetic field.
- Hydrogen atoms in the human body are used to generate the magnetic resonance (MR) images.
- Atomic nuclei contain protons and neutrons which spin around their axis, yielding magnetic moments and causing the particles to behave like tiny bar magnets.
- Hydrogen nuclei contain a positively charged solitary proton (hydrogen-1, ^{1}H).
- When hydrogen protons are placed in a strong magnetic field, they align either toward or against the direction of the applied field.

- Opposing spins cancel each other's magnetic moments, leaving only a small number of unpaired spins that are added together to create a net magnetization vector aligned along the direction of the magnetic field.
- The spins rotate (precess) around their axis and around the magnetic field, with a frequency that is proportional to the strength of the magnetic field.
- Hydrogen nuclei are being excited intermittently by radiofrequency (RF) pulses, which must have the same frequency as the frequency with which the protons precess around their axis. This is the 'resonance' condition of MRI.
- The RF pulses deliver energy to the protons so that the net magnetization vector moves away from the direction of the applied magnetic field at an angle called the flip angle.
- When the RF pulse is removed the protons return to their original state of equilibrium. This is known as relaxation. During this process the net magnetization vector is gradually being reduced, resulting in an oscillating magnetic field that gradually decays (Free Induction Decay or FID).
- FID is detected by the receiver coils, amplified amplification, and processed to generate the MR signal. Spatial localization of the MR signal is performed by employing linear changes to the main magnetic field with the addition of so-called gradient fields.
- The signal from a given tissue (e.g. heart muscle, fat, blood) is determined by its density of hydrogen atoms (proton density), and by two distinct MR relaxation parameters:
    - Longitudinal relaxation time (T1)
    - Transverse relaxation time (T2 and T2*)
- Proton density, T1, and T2 relaxation times can vary considerably between different tissues, and these differences are used to generate contrast in MR images.
- By varying MR sequence parameters, the amount of proton density, T1 or T2 weighting in an image can be adjusted. For example:
    - In T1-weighted images, myocardial tissue is dark, whereas fat is bright. Water has low signal and appears dark.
    - In T2-weighted images fat has low signal, tissues with high water content have high signal and appear bright. T2-weighted imaging is used to detect oedema.
    - Tissues with iron overload (liver, heart) exhibit rapid fall in signal intensity and usually appear dark on T2*-weighted images.
- CMR sequences consist of a series of RF pulses, magnetic gradient field switches, and timed data acquisitions, applied in a specific order to generate the CMR image.
- Types of MR sequences are spin-echo, gradient-echo, inversion recovery, saturation recovery, fat saturation, dark blood, and navigator sequences.

1.2.2 Types of CMR artefacts

(See Figure 1.2.1)

- Motion artefacts.
    - Due to the motion of the beating heart or respiratory motion (cardiac or respiratory ghost artefacts).
    - Cardiac motion can be controlled by detecting the QRS complex of the ECG and triggering the acquisition to a specific part of the cardiac cycle (ECG gating).
    - Cardiac arrhythmias can cause mis-triggering and significant impairment in image quality.
    - Respiratory motion can be eliminated with breath-holding. Respiratory gating to the expiratory pause is commonly used in 3D imaging of the heart and vessels.

1.2.2 Types of CMR artefacts 67

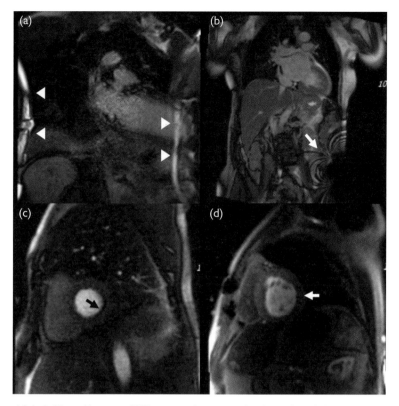

Figure 1.2.1 **A:** Vertical long-axis SSFP image with wrap artefact (arrowheads) due to inappropriately small field of view and also degraded image quality due to breathing artefact. **B:** Large artefact on a coronal localizer image due to a small metal object (safety pin). **C:** Dark rim artefact (black arrow), in contrast to a real perfusion defect (white arrow) on stress CMR perfusion imaging (D). Image courtesy of Oxford Centre for Clinical Magnetic Resonance Research (OCMR).

- Flow artefacts.
    - Due to the motion of blood. They usually appear as intraluminal loss of signal.
- Chemical shift artefacts.
    - They appear as bright and dark lines at the interfaces between fat and water.
- Aliasing or wrap-around artefacts.
    - Occur when the field of view is small, so the peripheral parts of the body wrap into the image.
    - Aliasing artefacts are also present in flow images when the actual velocity is higher than the one encoded.
- Susceptibility artefact.
    - Occur in the presence of metallic objects inside the body, where signal destruction or loss occurs, depending on the sequence.
- Inhomogeneity ('off-resonance') artefact.
    - Occur when the magnetic field is not sufficiently uniform.
- Dark rim artefact (Gibbs ringing).
    - Noted at the interface between bright (blood pool) and darker (myocardium) signal. It is usually seen during CMR perfusion imaging.

1.2.3 CMR safety and contraindications

- MRI is generally considered a safe non-invasive technique that does not expose patients nor staff to ionizing radiation.
- There is no clear relationship between MRI and subsequent health risks.
- Pregnant women can undergo a CMR scan after carefully evaluating the risk to benefit ratio.
- Potential risks associated with CMR generally arise from 3 distinct mechanisms related to MR imaging:
    - the static main magnetic field
    - gradient magnetic fields
    - pulsed RF fields
- The main risks of MRI relate to the interaction of the strong magnetic field with ferromagnetic and metal objects inside the patient's body or inside the scanner room.
- Medical material and devices are classified in three categories: MR safe, MR conditional, MR unsafe (Table 1.2.1).
- Gradient magnetic fields can induce electrical currents in electrically conductive devices and potentially cause arrhythmias. They may also induce peripheral nerve stimulation, experienced as light vibration or poking of the skin.
- Gradient magnetic fields are the main source of acoustic noise associated with an MR procedure, therefore hearing protection is always necessary.
- Pulsed RF fields may cause some heating of tissue, central venous catheters, or metallic devices such as pacemaker leads. This can result in tissue damage or an increase in pacing threshold, capture loss, or arrhythmia induction.

Table 1.2.1 Food and Drug Administration (FDA) MR safety terminology and labelling for medical devices and implants.

FDA labelling	Definition	Examples
MR safe	No known hazards in all MRI environments	Coronary artery stents, prosthetic heart valves and annuloplasty rings, most orthopaedic implants
MR conditional	Demonstrated to pose no known hazards in a specified MR environment with specified conditions of use	Some new generation cardiac pacing systems, some orthopaedic implants, most insertable cardiac monitors and loop recorders
MR unsafe	Known to pose hazard in all MRI environments	Metallic foreign objects inside the body, aneurysm clips, cochlear implants, certain types of vascular stents, most cardiac pacemakers and implantable cardioverter defibrillators (ICDs)

1.2.4 Contrast agents

- MRI contrast agents are chelates of molecules or ions with paramagnetic properties, such as gadolinium (Gd) which is mainly used in CMR imaging.
- Gadolinium-based compounds act predominantly by shortening the T1 relaxation time.
- In general, gadolinium-based contrast agents are safe, with a low incidence of adverse effects, such as nausea and vomiting, headache, or urticaria; anaphylaxis is very rare.
- Nephrogenic systemic fibrosis (NSF) is a debilitating and potentially life-threatening serious late adverse reaction which has been reported in patients at end-stage renal failure or on dialysis. MRI can be performed in patients with an estimated glomerular filtration rate (eGFR) less than 30 ml/min only when the benefits significantly outweigh the risk, and only after patient informed consent.

1.2.5 Overview of CMR examination

Careful preparation of the patient is necessary in order to obtain the best quality CMR images. This involves:

- Explaining the procedure, the breath holds, and potential symptoms or side effects from the magnetic fields or contrast agents.
- Reassuring and calming down anxious or claustrophobic patients.
- Screening the patient to exclude any contraindications to the MR environment or to contrast agent administration.
- Changing into a gown to avoid clothing with metallic components or microfibres.
- Making sure that the patient is feeling comfortable inside the scanner.
- Good ECG positioning and attachment.
- Headphones for protection from the noise and for communication.

1.2.6 CMR methodology

Cardiac anatomy

- The standard orthogonal planes (transverse/axial, coronal, sagittal) are acquired with dark and bright blood CMR techniques such as HASTE (Half-Fourier Acquisition Single-shot Turbo spin Echo) and FLASH (Fast low angle shot), or SSFP (Steady-state free precession), respectively.
- The images acquired are useful for a good overview of the size, shape, and position of the cardiac chambers, great vessels, and other anatomical structures of the chest.
- The three orthogonal planes can then be used to image the heart in the horizontal (HLA), vertical (VLA) long axes, and the short axis (SA) of the heart, as well as to plan any imaging plane specific to a particular pathology.

Cardiac function

- CMR is considered as the gold standard for the assessment of left ventricular (LV) and particularly right ventricular (RV) function in terms of accuracy and reproducibility.
- Ventricular function can be evaluated on the HLA and VLA SSFP cine images and dedicated views of the RV, and accurately assessed using the short axis cine stack of the ventricles.
- Right ventricular function can also be assessed using the transaxial RV cine stack.
- After contouring endocardial borders in end-diastole and end-systole, and epicardial borders in end-diastole or systole, cardiac function is measured using volumetric analysis software processing (Figure 1.2.2).

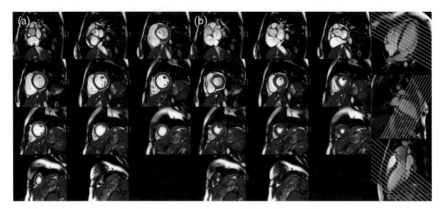

Figure 1.2.2 End-diastolic (A) and end-systolic (B) still SSFP images from multiple contiguous short-axis cine images of the left and right ventricle from base to apex used for volumetric analysis. The position of the short-axis slices is marked on the still frames of the three long-axis cine images. Image courtesy of Oxford Centre for Clinical Magnetic Resonance Research (OCMR).

Information acquired from the analysis includes:

- end-diastolic and end-systolic volumes
- stroke volume and cardiac output
- ejection fraction
- LV mass
- Myocardial deformation and strain can also be evaluated with CMR:
    - CMR tagging is the most validated technique but it is time consuming. It measures the deformation using magnetic labels/tags (black lines) that are superimposed on the myocardium at the beginning of a cine sequence.
    - Feature-tracking CMR is a new technique that allows post-processing of routinely acquired SSFP cine CMR images.

Tissue characterization

- Late gadolinium enhancement is a useful technique for differentiating between normal and diseased tissue, as well as predicting adverse outcome.
- It involves image acquisition 10–20 minutes after contrast (Gd) administration, when gadolinium has washed out of the normal myocardium and interstitial space, but persists in case of ruptured myocyte membranes and/or expansion of interstitial space.
- Normal tissue appears black, while diseased tissue appears bright (hyperenhanced).
- Novel techniques such as T1 and T2 mapping offer quantitative measures of tissue characteristics by providing pixel-wise estimates of T1 or T2 relaxation times, respectively. Each voxel can then be assigned a specific intensity value on a coloured scaled map according to its T1 or T2 value (Figure 1.2.3). T1 mapping can be performed pre-contrast (native T1) or after contrast administration (post contrast T1).

CMR stress imaging

- CMR can detect myocardial ischaemia and assess myocardial perfusion at rest and during pharmacological stress to detect CAD.
- Stress perfusion CMR detects inducible perfusion defects during vasodilator stress following the first-pass perfusion of a gadolinium-based contrast agent through the myocardium.
- In the standard protocol, 3 short axis slices are acquired during stress and are compared to images at rest at identical slice positions.

1.2.6 CMR methodology

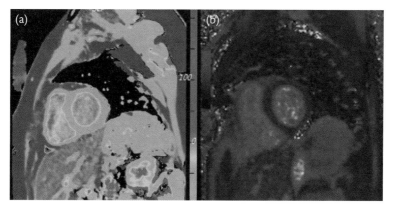

Figure 1.2.3 Mid-ventricular short axis image of normal myocardium using ShMOLLI (Shortened Modified Look-Locker Inversion Recovery) non-contrast T1 mapping. B: Normal myocardium on T2 mapping. Image courtesy of Oxford Centre for Clinical Magnetic Resonance Research (OCMR).

- Perfusion defects appear darker than the normal myocardium.
- Dark-rim artefact can mimic perfusion defects but can be usually identified by experienced readers.
- Commonly used vasodilator agents are adenosine, regadenoson or dipyridamole. Contraindications to stress perfusion are:
  - High degree (2nd or 3rd) atrioventricular block
  - Sinus bradycardia
  - Asthma or bronchoconstrictive disease
  - Severe hypotension (systolic blood pressure < 90 mmHg).
- Common side effects include dyspnea, nausea, headache, abdominal or chest pain, transient tachycardia or heart block, transient hypotension.
- Aminophylline administration may rarely be necessary to reverse persistent side effects from adenosine or regadenoson.
- Patients should avoid any products that contain caffeine (coffee, tea, chocolate, caffeine-containing beverages) and drugs that interfere with adenosine (theophylline, xanthines) for 24 hours prior to the scan.
- Dobutamine stress CMR uses the positive inotropic effects of dobutamine to detect myocardial viability (low-dose protocol) and/or inducible wall motion abnormalities (high-dose protocol) due to flow limiting coronary artery stenosis, following the same protocol as stress echocardiography. Atropine is added when the target heart rate is not reached. Contraindications to dobutamine stress are:
  - Severe systemic hypertension (≥ 220/120 mmHg)
  - Unstable angina
  - Severe aortic valve stenosis
  - Uncontrolled congestive heart failure
  - Hypertrophic obstructive cardiomyopathy
  - Complex cardiac arrhythmias including uncontrolled atrial fibrillation
  - Myocarditis, endocarditis, pericarditis.

Blood flow assessment
- Phase-contrast velocity encoded CMR allows assessment of blood flow parameters, such as visualization of the direction of flow and detection of flow acceleration or flow jets within a slice, along the slice direction ('in-plane' flow measurement).

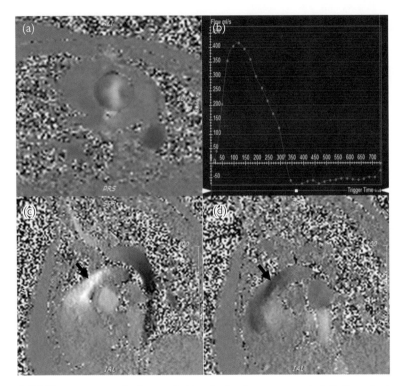

Figure 1.2.4 Phase-contrast velocity encoded imaging for flow assessment. A, B: through-plane flow at the tips of the aortic valve (red circle in A) showing the forward flow and the regurgitant flow, above and below the x-axis respectively (B), C, D: in-plane flow for assessment of the pulmonary valve. There is unobstructed forward flow through the valve (white jet, black arrow in C) and a free-flowing wide jet of pulmonary regurgitation (black jet, black arrow in D). Image courtesy of Oxford Centre for Clinical Magnetic Resonance Research (OCMR).

- It is also used for flow quantification, accurate regurgitant flow measurement and peak flow velocity measurement through the slice of interest ('through-plane' flow measurement) (Figure 1.2.4).
- The technique has a lower temporal resolution than echocardiography (25–45 msec), so it might slightly underestimate peak velocity through stenotic valves. Four-dimensional (4D) flow CMR is an emerging technique.

MR angiography

- MR angiography (MRA) for 2D or 3D image acquisitions can be performed with contrast administration (contrast-enhanced MRA) or without contrast agent (non-contrast-enhanced MRA).
- In contrast-enhanced MRA a bolus of gadolinium-based contrast agent is administered intravenously, and the images are acquired during the first passage of the contrast through the vessels of interest.
- Non-contrast-enhanced MRA relies on changes in the MR signal that are caused by the flow of blood through or within the image plane.
- Common applications of MRA include 3D angiogram of the aorta, pulmonary vein angiography, anatomy in congenital heart disease, imaging of the coronary arteries.

1.2.7 CMR in specific heart diseases

Ischaemic heart disease

CMR offers a comprehensive assessment in the setting of ischaemic heart disease by providing:

- accurate assessment of ventricular size and function
- detection of even subtle wall motion abnormalities
- evaluation of infarct size and myocardial viability.
  - On LGE sequences the signal from normal myocardium is nulled and appears black.
  - In infarcted areas, where there is expansion of the interstitial space due to myocardial death, cell membrane disruption, oedema, and/or fibrosis, gadolinium takes longer to wash out. These areas appear bright on LGE images.
  - The extent of the infarcted myocardium, starting from the endocardium (subendocardial infarction) and extending to the epicardium (transmural infarction) has been shown to be a strong predictor of viability and chance of functional recovery after revascularization.
  - When the extent of hyperenhanced regions is less than 25% the likelihood of functional recovery is more than 60%, when the infarct involves 26–50% of wall thickness there is a reasonable chance of improvement in wall contractility (around 40%), while when the infarction is near-transmural (51–75% and > 75% transmurality) there is a very low chance of improvement after revascularization (~ 10% and < 1% respectively) (Figure 1.2.5).
- detection of LV thrombus. Thrombus appears black and avascular with no contrast uptake on early or late gadolinium imaging (Figure 1.2.6).
- detection of complications of myocardial infarction
  - mechanical: myocardial rupture, ventricular septal defect, aneurysm or pseudo-aneurysm formation, papillary muscle rupture, and mitral regurgitation
  - Inflammatory: pericardial effusion, pericarditis
- detection of inducible ischaemia with stress perfusion imaging
- detection of congenital anomalies of the origin or the course of coronary arteries, or coronary artery aneurysms

In the setting of acute ischaemia / myocardial infarction CMR can evaluate:

- the presence of oedema/myocardium at risk.
  - defined as the myocardial tissue within the vascular bed distally to the culprit lesion of the infarct-related coronary artery.
  - In the acute setting the extent of ischaemic myocardium at risk can be assessed by detecting myocardial oedema using T2-weighted sequences, native T1 mapping or T2 mapping.
- microvascular obstruction and haemorrhage. CMR can reliably localize and quantify MVO as:
  - areas of hypoperfusion on first-pass rest CMR perfusion
  - areas with no gadolinium uptake which appear black inside an hyperenhanced infarcted area on early and late gadolinium imaging.
  - T1 mapping techniques can also differentiate MVO in infarcted myocardium.
  - native T1 values of areas with MVO are higher compared to those of remote myocardium but lower compared to those of infarcted myocardium.
- Intramyocardial haemorrhage (IMH) is a result of mechanical reperfusion of an infarct-related artery and of the antithrombotic therapy given to maintain the patency of lumen. Haemoglobin degradation products contain iron which has paramagnetic properties and shortens $T2^*$ relaxation time, resulting in lower signal intensities on T2 and $T2^*$ weighted imaging. T2 and $T2^*$ mapping and native T1 imaging can detect IMH, which also exhibits a T1 shortening effect

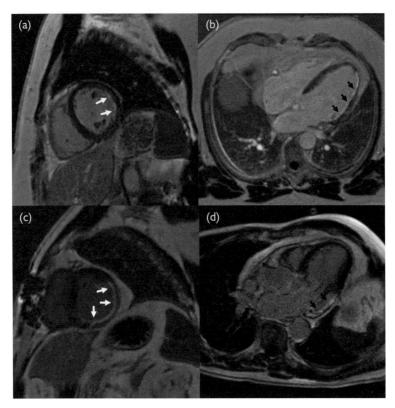

Figure 1.2.5 Late gadolinium images showing different types of myocardial infarction. A: 25% subendocardial infarction in the mid inferolateral wall, B: subendocardial infarction of the entire anterolateral wall with 50% transmurality, C: lateral wall subendocardial infarct with 75% transmurality, D: transmural infarction of the basal inferolateral wall. Image courtesy of Oxford Centre for Clinical Magnetic Resonance Research (OCMR).

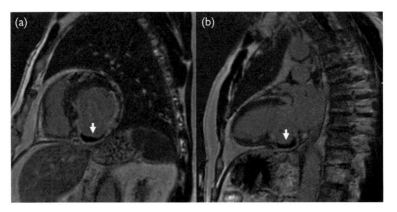

Figure 1.2.6 Layered thrombus adhered to a transmural infarction and aneurysm of the basal inferior wall seen on short axis (A) and vertical long axis (B) late gadolinium images. Image courtesy of Oxford Centre for Clinical Magnetic Resonance Research (OCMR).

Heart failure

CMR can provide unique diagnostic, prognostic, and therapeutic information in these patients. It allows for:

- accurate measurement of ventricular volumes and systolic function.
- identification of the underlying etiology of HF (ischaemic, non-ischaemic cardiomyopathy, acute myocarditis, Takotsubo cardiomyopathy, etc.)
- identification of likely reversible factors, such as myocardial viability and extent of reversible ischaemia in patients with ischaemic heart failure, valvular heart disease, cardiac sarcoidosis, Anderson–Fabry disease, iron overload cardiomyopathy, amyloidosis, pericardial constriction, etc.
- detection of myocardial scarring to guide ICD and CRT lead positioning in patients with non-ischaemic cardiomyopathy.

Cardiomyopathies

Hypertrophic cardiomyopathy

CMR provides a comprehensive assessment of the heterogeneous phenotypic appearances of hypertrophic cardiomyopathy (HCM) better than any other imaging modality. CMR helps in the diagnosis and assessment of prognosis of HCM by:

- Identifying the heterogenous HCM phenotypes, such as asymmetric septal hypertrophy, apical hypertrophy, mixed phenotypes, end-stage 'burned-out' HCM.
- Accurately measuring areas of hypertrophy and maximum wall thickness, especially when not clearly visualized on echocardiography.
- Detecting apical aneurysms and possible apical thrombus, which have significant implications for outcome and effective treatment interventions.
- Assessing mitral valve apparatus and papillary muscle/chordae tendineae abnormalities, systolic anterior motion of the mitral valve and left ventricular outflow tract (LVOT) obstruction.
- Information about the extent and location of hypertrophy and the anatomy of the mitral valve apparatus is important before septal myectomy or septal alcohol ablation. Differentiating HCM from other causes of left ventricular hypertrophy, such as hypertensive heart disease, athletic heart, as well as from non-sarcomeric diagnoses like cardiac amyloid and Anderson–Fabry disease.
- Providing an early diagnosis in genotype-positive individuals and family members of patients with HCM, especially when this will have significant clinical implications.
- **LGE in HCM:**
    - The usual LGE pattern in HCM is patchy, typically midwall, and commonly involves the hypertrophied myocardium and the LV-RV junctions, but it can also involve regions with normal wall thickness (Figure 1.2.7).
    - In cases of 'burned-out' HCM where the LV wall is typically thinned, LGE may be full thickness, mimicking myocardial infarction.
    - Extensive LGE has been shown to be predictive of arrhythmias, sudden cardiac death and end-stage systolic dysfunction.
    - LGE of ≥ 15% of LV mass is associated with a twofold increase in SCD event risk event in patients considered to be at low risk.
    - LGE in RV insertion points is not related to replacement fibrosis as in other areas of LV myocardium. More specifically, it is mainly due to expanded extracellular space containing predominantly interstitial fibrosis, adipose tissue, and disorganized myocytes (myocardial disarray), and it is not a reliable predictor of adverse outcomes.

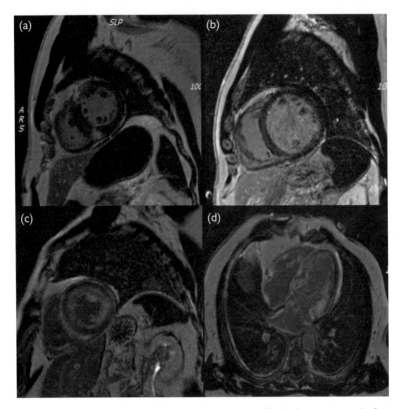

Figure 1.2.7 Typical pattern of late gadolinium enhancement of both the anterior and inferior LV-RV junctions with some patchy and hazy midwall enhancement of the hypertrophied septum in a patient with hypertrophic cardiomyopathy. B: Mid-wall fibrosis in the septum in a patient with dilated cardiomyopathy. C, D: classical LGE findings of cardiac amyloid: dark blood pool, diffuse subendocardial left and right ventricular enhancement ("zebra" sign) and diffuse atrial enhancement. LV: left ventricle, RV: right ventricle. Image courtesy of Oxford Centre for Clinical Magnetic Resonance Research (OCMR).

- **T1 mapping in HCM:**
    - Can also detect fibrosis in HCM, even when the fibrotic process is diffuse and thus may go undetected on LGE imaging.
    - In HCM pre-contrast T1 values are increased, while post-contrast T1 measurements are reduced compared to areas with normal myocardium.
    - Contrast-enhanced T1 mapping in combination with native T1 mapping enable the calculation of extracellular volume (ECV) fraction, which is increased in regions with fibrosis.

Dilated cardiomyopathy

CMR is of diagnostic and prognostic importance in patients with DCM and can help guide treatment by providing:

- Accurate measurements of LV volumes and LV ejection fraction.
- Differential diagnosis between ischaemic and non-ischaemic aetiology.
    - One third of patients with non-ischaemic DCM display a mid-wall band of enhancement mainly seen in the septum.

- Patients with ischaemic heart disease usually have extensive areas of infarction on LGE imaging.
  - Absence of LV scarring in patients with DCM cannot exclude 3-vessel ischemic heart disease with severe LV hibernation and no previous myocardial infarction.
- CMR can also recognize various forms of non-ischaemic DCM, such as infiltrative myocardial disease, myocarditis, and Takotsubo cardiomyopathy.
- Prognostic stratification:
  - LGE on CMR predicts all-cause mortality, heart failure hospitalization, and arrhythmic mortality.
  - Highest risk observed in patients with > 5–10% LGE burden.
  - A large increase in risk of death and sudden cardiac death was observed in patients with LGE in the septum compared to other locations.
  - Sudden cardiac death risk was greatest with concomitant septal and free-wall fibrosis.
  - DCM patients with no LGE have a better chance of reverse LV remodelling with treatment.
  - The presence of LGE can have implications for the choice of device therapy in DCM patients:
- ICD treatment has shown was proven benefit only in patients with LV scar
- CRT-defibrillator treatment was found superior to CRT-Pacing treatment only in patients with mid-wall fibrosis.
- Detection of intracardiac thrombus.

Arrhythmogenic right ventricular cardiomyopathy

- Arrhythmogenic right ventricular cardiomyopathy (ARVC) is a rare form of inheritable muscle disease
- It is characterized histologically by cardiomyocyte loss and progressive replacement of ventricular myocardium with adipose and fibrous tissue.
- It usually involves the right ventricle (RV), but the same pathologic abnormalities can also occur in the left ventricle and there are forms with predominant LV involvement. Therefore, the disease is increasingly being referred to as arrhythmogenic cardiomyopathy.
- The diagnosis of ARVC is challenging and is based on a combination of structural alterations, histologic, electrocardiographic, arrhythmic, and genetic features.
- The role of CMR in the diagnosis of ARVC through identifying global and/or regional dysfunction and structural alterations has been recognized in the 2010 Task Force criteria:
  - Major CMR criterion is regional RV akinesia or dyskinesia or dyssynchronous RV contraction and 1 of the following: i) Ratio of RV end-diastolic volume to BSA ≥ 110 mL/m^2 for males or ≥ 100 mL/m^2 for females, ii) RV ejection fraction ≤ 40%.
  - Minor CMR criterion is regional RV akinesia or dyskinesia or dyssynchronous RV contraction and 1 of the following: i) Ratio of RV end-diastolic volume to BSA ≥ 100 to < 110 mL/m^2 for males or ≥ 90 to < 100 mL/m^2 for females, ii) RV ejection fraction > 40% to ≤ 45%.
- CMR is considered the best imaging modality for the assessment of the RV, which can be visualized in any imaging plane.
- LGE imaging usually shows sub-epicardial/mid-wall enhancement of the LV myocardium in cases with LV involvement.
- The presence of RV enhancement on LGE correlates well with fibroadipose replacement of the myocardium and inducible ventricular arrhythmias on electrophysiologic studies.
- Tissue characterization with CMR is not considered a formal diagnostic criterion yet.

Restrictive cardiomyopathies
- Restrictive cardiomyopathies (RCM) are defined as restrictive ventricular physiology in the presence of normal or reduced diastolic volumes (of one or both ventricles), normal or reduced systolic volumes, and normal ventricular wall thickness.
- RCM may be idiopathic, familial, or result from various systemic disorders.

Amyloidosis
- CMR can identify the typical features of cardiac amyloidosis, such as concentric LV hypertrophy, thickened atrial walls, biatrial dilation, and pericardial and pleural effusions.
- Amyloid deposition alters gadolinium kinetics in the myocardium, resulting in a difficulty nulling the myocardium and a dark blood pool in LGE images.
- There is characteristic circumferential LV enhancement on LGE imaging, predominantly subendocardial but may also be transmural (Figure 1.2.7).
- Atrial involvement or in some cases RV enhancement can also be detected.
- Myocardial T1 values on native T1 mapping are significantly elevated in cardiac amyloidosis patients

Sarcoidosis
- CMR can demonstrate features of cardiac involvement, such as LV hypertrophy, septal thinning, systolic dysfunction, ventricular dilatation, as well as regions with acute inflammation using T2-weighted imaging, T1 and T2 mapping.
- LGE imaging can identify areas of myocardial damage. The typical LGE patterns include sub-epicardial and mid-wall enhancement along the basal septum and/or inferolateral wall, although subendocardial or transmural LGE has also been observed.
- Myocardial areas with LGE can help guide endomyocardial biopsy and treatment decisions regarding device therapy, as the presence of LGE on CMR imaging has been shown to correlate with increased odds of both all-cause mortality and arrhythmogenic events.

Anderson–Fabry disease
- The most common cardiac manifestation is concentric LV hypertrophy, with characteristic mid-wall basal inferolateral wall enhancement on LGE images.
- Asymmetric septal thickening and apical hypertrophy with mid-ventricular and apical scar on LGE images have also been described.
- Native T1 values on T1 mapping are very sensitive in detecting AFD because fat (glycosphingolipid) deposition significantly lowers T1 time, except for the regions with scar on LGE images which show increased T1 values.

Iron overload cardiomyopathy
- CMR is the only imaging modality that can non-invasively quantify cardiac iron overload with T2* imaging.
- For the image analysis, a full-thickness area in the mid-septum is chosen, taking care to avoid blood pool and coronary arteries in the interventricular groove.
- Normal values for T2* in 1.5 Tesla scanners are > 20 msec for the heart and > 6.3 msec for the liver.
- Myocardial T1 values on T1 mapping are lower in patients with cardiac iron loading compared to healthy controls and can help detect mild iron loading even before T2* values fall.

Eosinophilic myocarditis

- Endomyocardial inflammation due to eosinophilia can cause fibrosis and restrictive cardiomyopathy.
- It usually occurs in patients with endomyocardial fibrosis which is the most frequent form of RCM.
- It also occurs in patients with Loeffler's endocarditis or eosinophilic granulomatosis with polyangiitis (Churg–Strauss syndrome).
- CMR manifestations include:
    - Apical obliteration due to apical thrombus seen on early and late gadolinium imaging
    - Endomyocardial oedema due to inflammation detected mainly on T2-weighted imaging,
    - Circumferential subendocardial late enhancement involving mainly the apical LV segments.
    - Right ventricular involvement can also be detected.

Takotsubo cardiomyopathy

Takotsubo syndrome (TTS) is characterized by a transient wall motion dysfunction, presenting as apical ballooning or midventricular, basal, or focal wall motion abnormalities and shares common features with acute coronary syndromes, such as chest pain, ECG abnormalities, and elevated cardiac biomarkers. The right ventricle can also be involved. The condition is usually triggered by a wide range of emotional or physical triggers, affecting mainly postmenopausal women. Typical CMR findings are:

- the specific wall motion abnormalities of the syndrome
- myocardial oedema in the affected areas
- absence of significant myocardial scarring on LGE imaging.

Left ventricular non-compaction

- Left ventricular non-compaction (LVNC) is characterized by prominent LV trabeculations, deep intertrabecular recesses, and thin compacted myocardial layer.
- A non-compacted to compacted myocardium ratio > 2.3 in diastole measured in the three long axis planes (horizontal long axis, vertical long axis, LV outflow tract view) is considered the cutoff for LVNC diagnosis on CMR.
- The presence of LGE is predictive of arrhythmic events.

1.2.8 Chemotherapy-related cardiotoxicity

According to the ESC position paper on cancer treatments, cardiotoxicity is defined as a > 10 percentage points decrease in LV ejection fraction to a value below the lower limit of normal.

- CMR is used when other techniques are non-diagnostic.
- CMR can identify early myocardial oedema after cancer treatment which has been shown to have prognostic implications concerning LV function and mortality.
- Myocardial T1 and T2 mapping may have the ability to detect early myocardial tissue damage and predict LV functional deterioration.
- CMR can reliably assess valvular function and pericardial disease.

1.2.9 Transplant cardiomyopathy

The diagnostic gold standard technique for detection of graft failure is endomyocardial biopsy, which has important risks and limitations.

CMR allows for:

- A non-invasive assessment of early transplant rejection, mainly through detection of high T2 or native T1 values.
- Patients with graft failure have high ECV values.
- Identification of myocardial infarctions/scars due to allograft vasculopathy even in patients with normal or non-obstructive lesions on coronary angiogram.
- Evaluation of transplant microvasculopathy with myocardial perfusion reserve and CMR strain sequences.

1.2.10 Myocarditis

Endomyocardial biopsy (EMB) is considered the gold standard for the diagnosis of myocarditis, while CMR can support the diagnosis in clinically stable patients.

- CMR findings are consistent with the diagnosis when at least two of the proposed CMR Lake Louise Consensus Criteria for myocarditis are present:
  - Regional or global myocardial signal intensity increase (myocardium to skeletal muscle ratio ≥ 2) in T2-weighted oedema images.
  - Increased global myocardial early gadolinium enhancement ratio between myocardium and skeletal muscle in gadolinium-enhanced T1-weighted images. A global signal intensity enhancement ratio of myocardium over skeletal muscle of ≥ 4.0 or an absolute myocardial enhancement of ≥ 45% is consistent with myocarditis.
  - At least one focal lesion with non-ischaemic regional distribution in LGE imaging, in keeping with myocardial injury and/or scar. Late enhancement is typically seen as sub-epicardial and/or mid-myocardial involvement mainly of the lateral wall and less frequently of the anteroseptum, but it may be multifocal or diffuse in distribution. The sub-endocardial layer is typically spared, clearly distinguishing myocarditis from ischaemic myocardial injury (Figure 1.2.8).

Native T1, T2, and ECV mapping techniques provide comparable or even better diagnostic performance to the Lake Louise Criteria for the diagnosis of acute myocarditis and constitute promising additional diagnostic tools.

1.2.11 Valvular heart disease

Although echocardiography is the primary imaging modality for the assessment of valvular heart disease (VHD), CMR can provide significant additional diagnostic and prognostic information without the limitation of poor acoustic windows or body habitus. CMR has become the first-line investigation technique for the assessment of the pulmonary valve and of the consequences of valvular disease on right ventricular volumes and function. CMR can:

- Determine the aetiology and mechanism of valve disease.
- Quantify the severity of the valve lesion. The maximum velocity and gradient through a stenotic valve (aortic, pulmonary) are measured by phase-contrast velocity-encoded CMR.
- Provide direct planimetry of valve area at the valve tips (Figure 1.2.9).

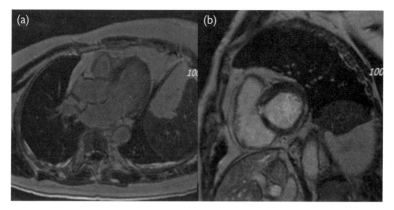

Figure 1.2.8 Typical subepicardial and midwall late gadolinium enhancement in the basal inferolateral wall in a patient with previous myocarditis. Image courtesy of Oxford Centre for Clinical Magnetic Resonance Research (OCMR).

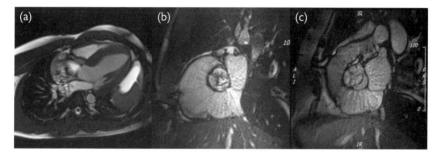

Figure 1.2.9 Left ventricular outflow tract SSFP image showing thickened aortic valve leaflets with restricted opening. B: Aortic valve view showing a bicuspid aortic valve (right and left coronary cusp fusion) with moderate aortic stenosis (valve area at the tips 1.2 cm^2). C: Aortic valve view showing a tricuspid aortic valve with mildly restricted opening (valve area by planimetry 1.6 cm^2 at the valve tips). Image courtesy of Oxford Centre for Clinical Magnetic Resonance Research (OCMR).

- Assess severity of aortic and pulmonary valvular regurgitation by through-plane flow quantification, which accurately provides the regurgitant volume and regurgitant fraction (Figure 1.2.4).
- Examine the consequences on the relevant ventricle, by providing accurate quantification of ventricular volumes and mass.
- Assess the surrounding anatomy and great vessels.
- Providing tissue characterization, which was shown to be useful for risk stratification of patients with left-sided VHD.
    - LV fibrosis is a consequence of chronic pressure and/or volume overload and cardiac remodelling caused by VHD.
    - The presence of fibrosis on LGE imaging is associated with increased mortality in patients with moderate or severe aortic stenosis and in those undergoing surgical aortic valve replacement, and with less improvement in LV systolic function.
    - Native T1 values on T1 mapping are higher in patients with symptomatic severe aortic stenosis compared with moderate and asymptomatic severe AS.
    - The presence of LGE in chronic severe mitral regurgitation is also associated with worse clinical outcomes.

1.2.12 Pericardial disease

CMR provides an excellent non-invasive imaging modality in the morphologic and functional assessment of the pericardium.

- Dark blood T1- and T2-weighted imaging with and without fat suppression is used to visualize the pericardium and surrounding structures and for measurement of pericardial thickness.
- Normal pericardium is seen as a thin (thickness less than 4 mm), curvilinear structure with low signal intensity (dark), surrounded by high-intensity (bright) pericardial and mediastinal fat on T1-weighted images.
- In cases of pericarditis or pericardial constriction the pericardial layers are usually thickened.
- Pericardial fluid and thus transudative pericardial effusion has high signal intensity on T2-weighted imaging such as SSFP, and low signal intensity on T1-weighted imaging.
- Exudates have higher signal intensity on T1-weighted imaging and low signal intensity on T2-weighted imaging.
- Haemorrhagic pericardial effusions have variable signal intensity dependent on the duration of the disease.
- T2-weighted imaging is used to detect pericardial fluid and/or pericardial oedema in cases of pericarditis, as well as associated myocardial involvement (peri-myocarditis). The inflamed pericardium appears hyperintense on T2-weighted images.
- LGE imaging can evaluate pericardial inflammation.
- Real-time cine imaging can be used to assess the haemodynamic consequences of a pericardial effusion and detect cardiac tamponade or pericardial constriction.
- CMR can assess ventricular coupling/interdependence by evaluating the changes in ventricular septal shape and motion over the respiratory cycle.

1.2.13 Cardiac and pericardial masses and tumours

Cardiac and pericardial masses are rare entities which require timely assessment, diagnosis, and appropriate treatment. CMR enables:

- Differentiation between benign and malignant tumours and diagnosis of 'pseudotumours'.
    - Intracardiac or pericardial thrombi, RV epicardial fat, lipomatous interatrial septum, pericardial cysts, or even normal anatomic variants such as the Coumadin ridge, Chiari network, or a prominent Eustachian valve can be mistaken for a mass on echocardiography.
    - Approximately 75% of primary cardiac tumours are benign, and the most common are myxomas, lipomas, papillary elastomas, rhabdomyomas, fibromas, and haemangiomas.
    - The most common pericardial benign tumours are lipoma, haemangioma, fibroma, teratoma, and paraganglioma.
    - The most prevalent malignant primary cardiac and pericardial tumours are sarcomas, mesotheliomas, and lymphomas.
- Assessment of the mass in unlimited image planes.
    - CMR can reliably assess tumour margins and invasion across tissue planes.
    - Malignant and metastatic tumours have irregular shape, heterogenous composition, and signal intensities, most commonly invade across tissue planes and are often associated with pericardial effusion.

1.2.13 Cardiac and pericardial masses and tumours 83

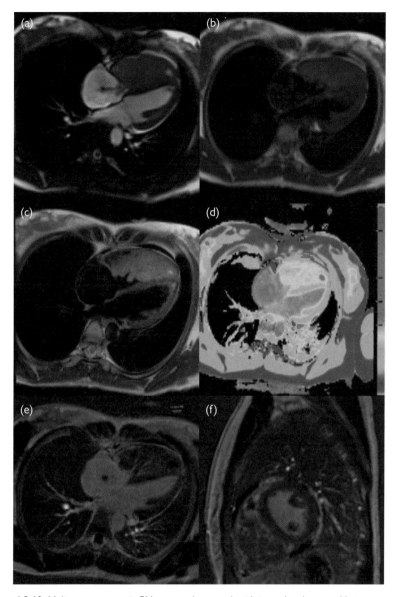

Figure 1.2.10 Malignant metastatic RV tumour (sarcoma) with irregular shape and heterogenous composition. The tumour invades the RV free wall, with prolapse of some mobile elements through the tricuspid valve into the right atrium on SSFP horizontal long axis image (A). The tumour has low signal intensity on T1-weighted imaging (B), and high signal on T2-weighted imaging (C). Heterogenous signal with increased T1 values on native T1 mapping (ShMOLLI sequence) (D), and heterogenous enhancement of the metastatic mass on late gadolinium imaging (E, F) due to variable perfusion and fibrosis. RV: right ventricle. Image courtesy of Oxford Centre for Clinical Magnetic Resonance Research (OCMR).

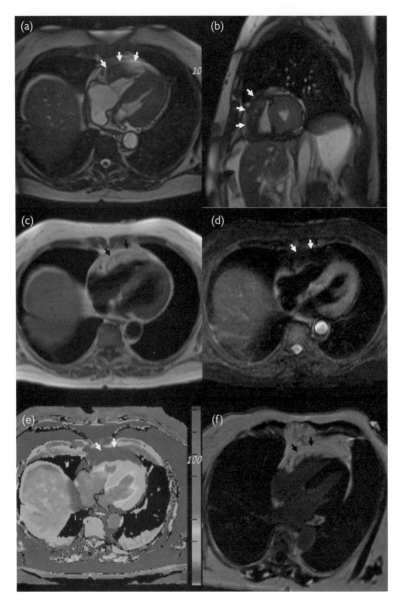

Figure 1.2.11 Benign epicardial mass (arrows) of mainly fatty composition, around the RV free wall (A) with RV compression during systole (B). The mass is bright on T1-weighted images (C), dark on T2-weighted images (D), has similar T1 values to fatty tissue on native T1 mapping (E), and high contrast uptake on LGE imaging (E). RV: right ventricle, LGE: late gadolinium enhancement. Image courtesy of Oxford Centre for Clinical Magnetic Resonance Research (OCMR).

- Tissue characterization and discrimination of different tissue characteristics. T1- and T2-weighted imaging with and without fat suppression, T1 and T2 mapping, early and late gadolinium imaging are used to differentiate tissue characteristics and predict the likely malignant nature of a cardiac mass (Figures 1.2.10 and 1.2.11):
  - Myxomas are isointense to the myocardium on T1-weighted imaging (T1-wi), hyperintense on T2-wi with heterogenous contrast uptake on LGE imaging.
  - Highly vascular tumours like haemangiomas or paragangliomas are strongly hyperintense on T2-wi with contrast uptake on LGE.
  - Lymphomas are isointense to the myocardium on T1- and T2-wi and show no or minimal contrast uptake on LGE.
  - Tumours with high fibrotic composition such as fibromas display intense hyperenhancement on LGE images.
  - Malignant tumours are usually isointense to the myocardium on T1-wi imaging, have high signal on T2-wi and most commonly heterogenous enhancement on LGE imaging.
  - Metastatic tumours, except for metastatic melanoma, have low signal intensity on T1-wi, high signal on T2-wi, and heterogenous pattern of enhancement on LGE.
  - Thrombi have low signal both on T1- and T2-wi and no contrast uptake on LGE.
  - Cysts display low signal on T1-wi, high signal on T2-wi, and no contrast uptake on LGE.
- Evaluation mass vascularity and perfusion, which is important for surgical planning.
- Monitoring mass size after chemotherapy, surgical or conservative treatment without ionizing radiation.

1.2.14 Congenital heart disease

CMR can provide:

- additional imaging in any anatomical plane and accurate serial measurements
- detailed anatomy and communications, assessment of pulmonary vein, and systemic venous drainage
- assessment of valvular flow and function in patients with congenital valvular, sub-valvular, or supra-valvular stenosis, valvular regurgitation, Ebstein anomaly, or valvular dysfunction after previous repair
- localization and quantification of shunts through atrial or ventricular septal defects (Figure 1.2.12), patent ductus arteriosus, anomalous pulmonary vein or systemic venous connections, or other types of anomalous communications
- accurate quantification of ventricular volumes and function regardless of chamber geometry
- accurate visualization and differentiation of valve phenotype in patients with bicuspid aortic valve (Figure 1.2.12)
- evaluation of the entire aorta for aortopathy, coarctation, aneurysms, dissection
- evaluation of main pulmonary trunk and branches for pulmonary stenosis or dilatation and aneurysms
- imaging of surgical conduits and baffles to evaluate their patency and function, especially in patients with Fontan circulation and atrial switch operation for transposition of the great arteries (Figure 1.2.13)

1.2 Cardiac Magnetic Resonance Imaging

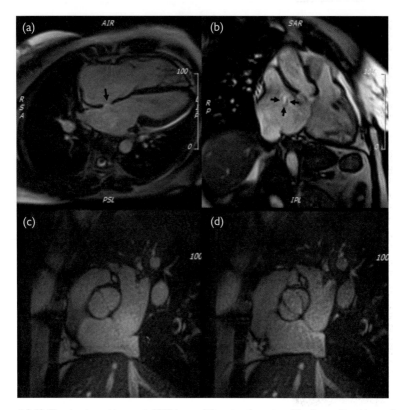

Figure 1.2.12 Top: horizontal long axis SSFP image (A) and en face view (B) of a small atrial septal defect (arrows). Bottom: "true" bicuspid aortic valve with two leaflets of equal size in diastole (C) and systole (D). Image courtesy of Oxford Centre for Clinical Magnetic Resonance Research (OCMR).

- detection of coronary artery anomalies and myocardial perfusion defects
- safe imaging in pregnant women with CHD
- tissue characterization.

A comprehensive CMR should study:

- cardiac position in the thorax (situs solitus or inversus)
- atrial arrangement (atrial situs solitus, inversus, or isomerism)
- number of functioning ventricles (univentricular or biventricular anatomy)
- atrioventricular arrangement (concordance, discordance, ambiguous connections)
- arrangement of the great vessels (transposition of the great arteries, truncus arteriosus, hemi truncus arteriosus)
- general assessment of chamber size, ventricular volumes and function, valvular function and then dedicated views and flow measurements according to each patient's anatomy and surgical repair or palliation when already performed.

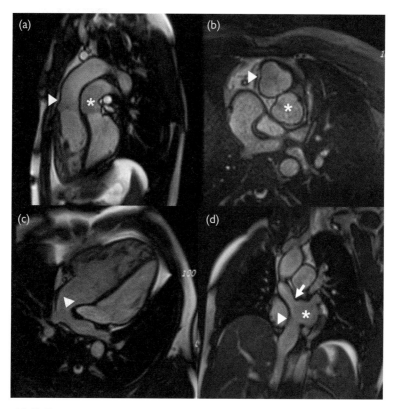

Figure 1.2.13 Typical anatomy in a patient with transposition of the great arteries post- atrial switch (Senning) operation. A, B: parallel course of the aorta (arrowhead) arising from the right ventricle and the pulmonary valve (asterisk) arising from the left ventricle. C: Modified horizontal long axis view showing the pulmonary venous baffle draining into the right atrium. D: Modified oblique sagittal view showing the superior vena cava (arrow) and inferior vena cava (arrowhead) pathways draining into the left atrium (asterisk). Image courtesy of Oxford Centre for Clinical Magnetic Resonance Research (OCMR).

1.2.15 Vascular disease

CMR with the use of static and cine anatomical imaging, MR angiography, and phase-contrast velocity-encoded imaging offers many advantages to imaging the morphology and pathology of the aorta and its branches, the pulmonary and systemic veins. Furthermore, CMR can evaluate the vascular wall for the presence of thrombus, atheroma, or inflammation (Figure 1.2.14).

- CMR can be used for the diagnosis and follow up of aortic aneurysms, dissection, and aortic coarctation before and after repair, the serial assessment in patients type B aortic dissection, and the evaluation for other associated aortic or cardiac abnormalities (Figure 1.2.15).

1.2 Cardiac Magnetic Resonance Imaging

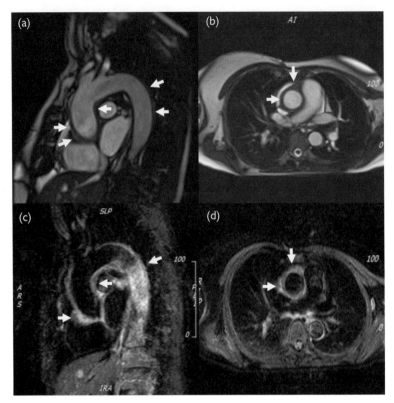

Figure 1.2.14 Aortitis: thickened aortic walls on sagittal (A) and axial (B) SSFP images (arrows), with signs of inflammation on T2-weighted imaging (C, D) in a patient with ANCA (anti-neutrophil cytoplasmic antibody) positive vasculitis. Image courtesy of Oxford Centre for Clinical Magnetic Resonance Research (OCMR).

- CMR can reveal congenital aortic variants, such as high course of the aortic arch (cervical arch), right-sided aortic arch, bovine aortic arch (common origin of the brachiocephalic and left common carotid artery—the most common aortic branching anatomical variant), and aberrant aortic branch origin and course.
- CMR can accurately visualize the number and location of the pulmonary veins, their connections to the left atrium, the shape and size of their ostium. The best method for imaging the pulmonary veins is 3D contrast-enhanced MR angiography which provides high-quality images but requires accurate timing of image acquisition to coincide the contrast bolus into the left atrium.
- CMR can detect anomalous systemic vein connections, interrupted course, and evaluate systemic vein stenosis or obstruction.

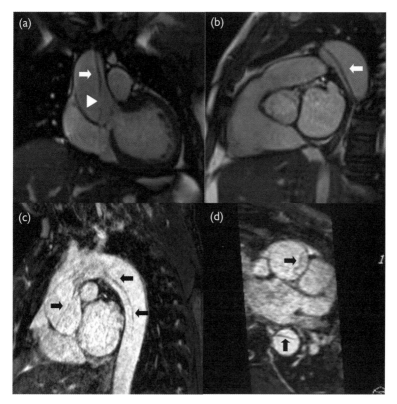

Figure 1.2.15 A, B: SSFP images showing a dissection flap (white arrows) in the ascending and descending thoracic aorta and the entry tear in the ascending aorta (arrowhead). C, D: Multiplanar reconstruction (MPR) images showing the dissection starting from the ascending aorta and extending to the descending aorta (black arrows) on sagittal (C) and axial (D) views. Image courtesy of Oxford Centre for Clinical Magnetic Resonance Research (OCMR).

1.2.16 Incidental findings

- CMR benefits from a large field of view, so many additional thoracic, neck, and upper abdominal structures are included in the images acquired.
- Extracardiac findings are common, although the majority are not clinically significant.
- The most common incidental findings are hepatic and renal cysts.

Further reading

Myerson SG, Francis J, Neubauer S. *Cardiovascular Magnetic Resonance*, 1st edn. New York: Oxford University Press, 2010.

1.3

Cardiac Computed Tomography

Jonathan Rodrigues, Benjamin Hudson, Oliver Gosling, and Kate Liang

TABLE OF CONTENTS

- 1.3.1 Overview 91
- 1.3.2 Acquisition 91
  - Intravenous contrast timing 92
  - Temporal resolution 92
  - Spatial resolution 92
  - ECG synchronization 93
  - Acquisition mode and image interrogation 95
  - Patient selection and preparation 97
- 1.3.3 Coronary artery disease 98
  - CT fractional flow reserve (CTFFR) 99
  - Calcium scoring and stenosis assessment 99
  - Bypass graft disease 100
  - Coronary stents 100
- 1.3.4 Coronary anomalies 100
- 1.3.5 Myocardial complications of CAD 101
- 1.3.6 Interventional guidance 101
  - Transcatheter valve implantation (TAVI) 101
  - Mitral valve intervention 102
- Coarctation of the aorta 102
- Pulmonary vein isolation (PVI) 102
- 1.3.7 Ventricular function 103
  - Chronic total occlusions (CTO) 103
- 1.3.8 Valvular disease and endocarditis 103
  - Valvular heart disease 103
  - Assessment of aortic valve replacement dysfunction 103
  - Prosthetic valves 104
  - Endocarditis of native and prosthetic valves 104
- 1.3.9 Cardiac masses 104
- 1.3.10 Cardiac trauma 104
- 1.3.11 Congenital heart disease 105
- 1.3.12 Pericardial disease 105
- 1.3.13 Diseases of great vessels 105
- 1.3.14 Diseases of cervical arteries and of the peripheral arteries 105

1.3.1 Overview

- Electrocardiogram-gated computed tomography (CT) offers the ability to acquire cardiac motion-free images of the cardiovascular system.
- Multi-detector computed tomography (MDCT) has high spatial and temporal resolution with the latest technology able to image the entire heart in a single heart-beat.
- It is predominantly used to assess for atherosclerotic coronary artery disease without the need for arterial puncture and is referred to as CT coronary angiography (CTCA).
- ECG-gated CT of the thoracic aorta is used in cases of suspected acute aortic syndrome and ECG-gated CT assessment of the aortic root.

1.3.2 Acquisition

Non-invasive imaging of the coronary arteries is challenging for two main reasons:

1. The heart is continually beating
2. The coronary arteries are relatively small in size
   - The coronary arteries are most stationary around end-diastole and end-systole but moving with the heart at all other times.

- This requires a high temporal resolution imaging system to rapidly capture the vessels when they are stationary.
- Given the small size, a high spatial resolution system is required to reduce partial volume-averaging and provide sufficient luminal and mural detail.

Intravenous contrast timing

To optimize contrast resolution between the coronary artery lumen and vessel wall, iodinated intravenous (IV) contrast is used.

- This is injected via a peripheral venous cannula using a power injector.
- The IV contrast bolus needs to be within the coronary arterial tree at the precise time at which they are to be imaged with CT.
- In order to achieve this, the contrast bolus timing needs to be optimized to reflect each patient's haemodynamic status.
- A common method to achieve adequate coronary opacification when performing CTCA is the test bolus technique.
- An axial image through the chest at the level of the proximal to mid ascending aorta is obtained. A small volume of IV contrast is injected with a power injector, often followed by a bolus of normal saline. After a delay, the axial image is acquired at set intervals to document an increase, peak and ultimate decrease in contrast opacification of the ascending aorta.
- Using specific post-processing software in real-time on the CT scanner console, a region of interest is then placed in the ascending aorta to determine the time to peak systemic arterial opacification for that individual patient.
- The subsequent CTCA can then be timed so that the acquisition occurs when the ascending aorta, and thus the coronary arteries, are maximally opacified.

MDCT scanners require:

- High temporal resolution (which can be thought of as similar to the shutter speed on a camera)
- High spatial resolution (which is the ability to distinguish between two objects)

Temporal resolution

- Determined primarily by rotational speed of the CT gantry and how fast the patient moves through the CT scanner.
- To increase temporal resolution either the gantry rotation speed must be increased, or the data must be acquired in less than one rotation of the gantry.
- Most modern cardiac CT scanner have a gantry rotation time of < 300 milliseconds
- Half-scan reconstruction—acquire data over c. 180° arc (c. half a rotation) and reconstruct the slices from these data, thus improving temporal resolution by 40–50%
- Fusing of data to create a meaningful image requires a regular R–R interval (Figure 1.3.1)
- Dual-source CT—images reconstructed from a quarter of a rotation by using two X-ray tubes and detectors perpendicular to each other.
- Wide-detector array CT—some vendors have large detectors 16cm or more that are sufficient to capture the entire heart without moving the patient through the scanner.

Spatial resolution

Determined by:

- Size of the detectors (0.0625–0.5 mm)
- Beam width
- Geometry and collimation (restricting X-ray beam area) amongst other factors

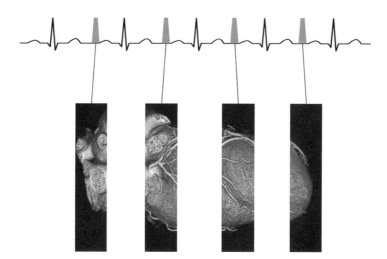

Figure 1.3.1 Data is collected from successive cardiac cycles. A regular R–R interval is needed to avoid movement artefact.

ECG synchronization
Retrospective ECG gating
- This was the traditional imaging protocol and infrequently, if at all, used on modern CT systems
- The CT beam is on during the entire duration of the scan and throughout the entire cardiac cycle (Figure 1.3.2).
- All the data are acquired and then retrospectively reconstructed, hence the name.
- This provides flexibility for CT images to be reconstructed from multiple phases of ECG R to R interval, which can help deal with coronary artery motion artefacts.
- This technique is most often used with dose modulation, where the ionizing radiation exposure is limited out of the diastolic period of the R–R interval (Figure 1.3.3).
- When the heart rate is well controlled (e.g. < 65 bpm), the heart is motion-free during ventricular diastole for the longest period of time. This represents the optimal temporal window to acquire images of the coronary arteries.
- This form of ECG gating has the additional benefit of enabling an element of dynamic valvular and ventricular functional assessment as there will be both diastolic and systolic phase data, although the latter may have increased image noise if tube current modulation has been employed outside of the diastolic window.

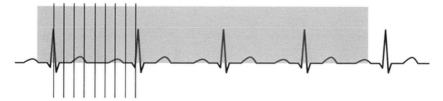

Figure 1.3.2 The R–R interval is divided into phases (%); images are usually reconstructed during diastole (70% of the R–R interval) and relative cardiac stasis.

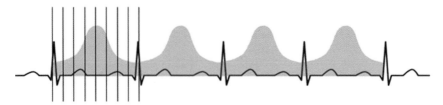

Figure 1.3.3 The X-ray tube current and therefore radiation dose is reduced during systole and increased in diastole.

Prospective gating

- This is the favoured method of triggering on modern CT scanners.
- The CT beam is only switched on for a predetermined part of the R–R interval, rather than throughout the cardiac cycle, as is the case with retrospectively gated studies (Figure 1.3.4).
- The timing of CT acquisition occurs prospectively from the R wave at either a set percentage of the R–R interval or absolute millisecond time.
- For well-controlled and stable heart rates, end-diastole at around 70% of the R–R interval is targeted.
- Some 'padding' can be added to the scan to acquire part of the R–R interval either side of 70% R–R interval to provide additional data to reconstruct in the case of motion artefact.
- Single heart-beat systems may either have an adequate MDCT detector width to cover the entire heart in one rotation, or the CT gantry pitch is sufficiently high that the region of interest passes through the CT beam in a single heart-beat.
- On scanners where single beat acquisition is not possible, or the heart rate or variability does not permit, multiple blocks or slabs are acquired (step and shoot or axial imaging) in sequence on successive or alternate cardiac cycles, until the entire volume of the heart is covered. Typically 3 to 5 blocks depending on the cranio-caudal length of the heart.
- The image blocks are then 'stitched' together. A fast and/or variable heart rate and/or respiratory motion artefact can lead to misalignment between blocks, known as 'step' artefact.
- As only data at a specific point of the cardiac cycle are acquired using this method, dynamic valvular and functional assessment cannot be performed.
- The coronary arteries are also relatively motion-free at end-systole. As heart rate increases, the total diastolic time reduces. The timing of end-systole is more consistent with elevated and irregular heart rates and performing prospective ECG triggered studies around end-systole (ranges from 180–380 ms of the R–R interval) provides the best chance to interrogate the coronary arteries in these situations.

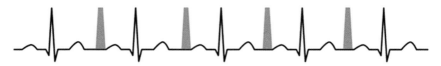

Figure 1.3.4 During prospective ECG gated acquisitions the X-ray tube current (gray line) is on for a fraction of a second during diastole.

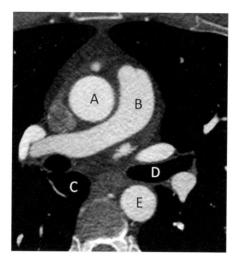

Figure 1.3.5 Axial images at the level of the pulmonary valve. A, ascending aorta; B, main pulmonary artery; C, right main bronchus; D, left main bronchus; E, descending aorta.

Acquisition mode and image interrogation
Step and shoot/axial acquisition
- Images are taken in one block equating to the size of the CT detector array width (Figures 1.3.5–1.3.9).
- The table moves to the next level of imaging, with a delay of 1 or 2 heart beats before acquiring the next block depending on heart rate.

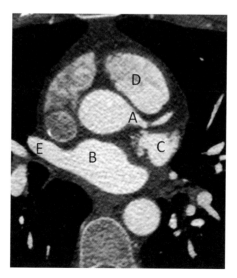

Figure 1.3.6 Axial images at the level of the left main stem. A, left main stem, B, left atrium; C, left atrial appendage; D, right ventricle; E, pulmonary vein.

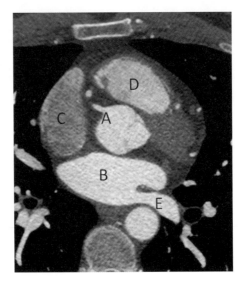

Figure 1.3.7 Axial images at the level of the aortic valve. A, ostium of RCA; B, left atrium; C, right atrium; D, right ventricle; E, pulmonary vein.

Spiral

- The table of the scanner moves continually with images acquired while the gantry rotates

Multiplanar Reconstruction (MPR)

- The sub-millimetre raw axial slice thickness can be reconstructed in coronal, sagittal and oblique imaging planes to allow multiplanar interrogation of the images (Figure 1.3.10).
- Dedicated CT coronary angiography software will segment the opacified coronary artery tree and generate curved and straightened multiplanar reformatted images.

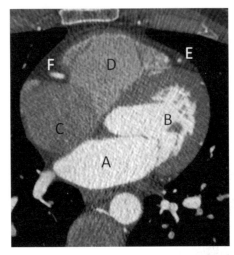

Figure 1.3.8 Axial images at the level of the mitral valve. A, left atrium; B, left ventricle; C, right atrium; D, right ventricle; E, left anterior descending artery; F, right coronary artery.

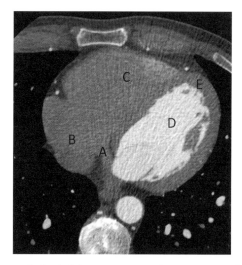

Figure 1.3.9 Axial images at the level of the coronary sinus. A, coronary sinus; B, right atrium; C, right ventricle; D, left ventricle; E, left anterior descending artery.

- Additional short axis images of the lumen, perpendicular to the longitudinal course of the epicardial coronary arteries can be created.
- Newer software, often based on artificial intelligence, is increasingly able to segment and define plaque within coronary arteries as well.

3D volume rendering/cinematic rendering

- This is a post-processing technique to generate 'real-life' 3D images of the structures acquired (Figure 1.3.11).
- These may be helpful to demonstrate anatomy and patient education, rarely used for diagnostic purposes.

Patient selection and preparation

- Good quality CT coronary angiography requires meticulous patient preparation.
- The patient should avoid caffeine and stimulants that may elevate the heart rate on the day of the study.

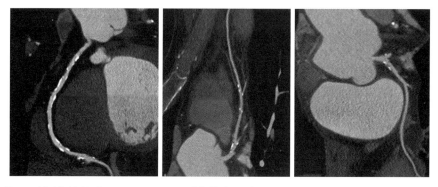

Figure 1.3.10 Multi plane reconstruction of (left) the right coronary artery, (middle) left anterior descending artery, and (right) circumflex artery.

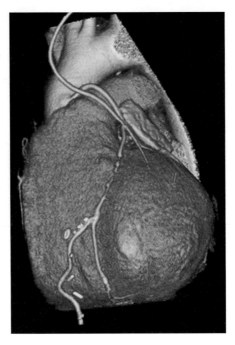

Figure 1.3.11 Multi plane reconstruction of (left) the right coronary artery, (middle) left anterior descending artery, and (right) circumflex artery.

- As the optimal heart rate for CTCA is < 60 bpm, a rate-limiting agent is often used. Most frequently, beta blockers are employed, either in the oral form taken in advance of the study and/or intravenous administration at the time of the CTCA.
- When beta blockers are contraindicated (e.g. severe asthma or severe peripheral vascular disease), ivabradine can be considered.
- Sublingual GTN should be administered (unless contraindications) to ensure optimal coronary dilation at the time of CTCA.
- It is imperative that the patient holds their breath for the duration of the scan:
  - Breath-holding instructions should be rehearsed with the patient several times prior to the scan.
  - This should be a relaxed breath hold at inspiration to minimize the chance of Valsalva manoeuvre and transient interruption of the intravenous contrast bolus.
- CT may not be the best choice of imaging in those who have a refractory tachycardia or struggle with breath holds—alternative imaging should be considered prior to referral.
- Patient body habitus can also limit diagnostic quality. Obesity increases image noise, which has a negative impact on spatial and contrast resolution. Obese patients tend to require higher tube potential (kV; the 'power' of the photons from the CT scanner) and/or tube current (mA; the 'number' of the photons from the CT scanner) to acquire diagnostic images in CT with higher effective radiation doses.

1.3.3 Coronary artery disease

- CTCA can assess for the presence or absence of coronary artery disease (CAD).
- CAD may be non-calcified, mixed morphology, or calcific.

- Current best practice includes the use of standardized reporting nomenclature (where LMS CAD is demonstrated it is typically described as <50 or >50% stenosis):
  0%—No plaque or stenosis
  1–24%—Minimal stenosis or plaque with no stenosis
  25–49%—Mild stenosis
  50–69%—Moderate stenosis
  70–99%—Severe stenosis
  100%—Total coronary occlusion
- Cardiac CT can assess for plaque morphology characteristics on cardiac CT that are associated with future acute coronary syndrome events, independent of the severity of stenosis of a particular coronary plaque—so-called vulnerable or high-risk plaque. These include:
  - Positive vessel remodelling (remodelling index >1.1)
  - Low attenuation lipid core (mean attenuation <30HU)
  - Spotty calcification (foci of spotty micro calcification)
  - The napkin ring sign (ring-like peripheral higher attenuation area with central low attenuation).
- Owing to its high negative predictive valve, CTCA originally was used in the context of low to intermediate (15–50%) pre-test probability of coronary artery disease (CAD) in stable chest pain of new onset to exclude CAD.
- The utility of CTCA in stratifying patients with CAD has also been demonstrated in the SCOT-HEART trial, which randomized patients from the rapid-access chest pain clinic to standard care or CTCA + standard care. The 5-year follow-up data show that CTCA was associated with a significantly lower rate of death from coronary heart disease or nonfatal MI at 5 years than standard care alone.
- The diagnostic performance of CTCA, and its relative cheap cost, have led to the National Institute for Health and Clinical Excellence (NICE) in 2016 in the United Kingdom to recommend CTCA as the first line test for most patients with stable chest pain of recent onset including typical and atypical chest pain and non-anginal chest pain with Q or ST-T wave changes.
- 2019 ESC guidelines for chronic coronary syndromes recommend CTCA or non-invasive functional imaging for myocardial ischaemia as the initial test for diagnosing CAD in symptomatic patients in whom obstructive CAD cannot be excluded by clinical assessment. 2021 Joint American Cardiology society guidelines recommend CTCA as a choice alongside stress testing in patients with stable chest pain and no known CAD.

CT fractional flow reserve (CTFFR)

- CT-FFR uses data from a standard cardiac CT coronary angiography scan to model blood flow and pressure in the epicardial coronary arteries.
- It uses computational fluid dynamics to generate an assessment of pressure drop across a stenosis, similar to data obtained with invasive pressure wire assessment.
- Good correlation has been demonstrated between invasive FFR and CT-derived FFR measurements, and offers the potential to reduce the demand for layered functional imaging tests after CTCA.
- As with anatomical CT coronary angiography, this relies heavily on high-quality diagnostic images to provide accurate analyses.

Calcium scoring and stenosis assessment

- Utilizes the correlation of calcification with atherosclerotic plaque disease associated with significant CAD.

- The coronary artery calcium (CAC) score, or Agatston score, quantifies calcium using a non-contrasted gated acquisition. The volume and density of the calcification are incorporated into the Agatston score.
- CAC has shown to be a robust prognostic marker in large prospective studies in asymptomatic patients. However, non-calcific CAD can occur in the context of a calcium score of zero.
- In symptomatic patients, the test is dependent on sex and age but with still high NPV (96–100%) in those with a CAC score of 0. However, using CAC as a gatekeeper to CTCA is contentious and many CTCA practitioners will proceed to CTCA regardless of CAC score, or exclusively perform CTCA in this cohort of patients.

Bypass graft disease

- In those with prior coronary artery bypass, CTCA with a wider field of view from the level of the subclavian arteries to the inferior aspect of the heart, can be used to assess graft patency and stenosis.
- The BYPASS-CTCA trial showed CTCA before ICA leads to reductions in procedure time and contrast-induced nephropathy, with improved patient satisfaction.
- CT imaging is also potentially important to define the anatomical relationship to the posterior aspect of the sternum, which would be relevant if re-do sternotomy is ever required.

Coronary stents

- CT can be used to assess stent patency, but this is not the favoured choice of investigation over invasive coronary angiography or other functional imaging.
- Images can be limited by blooming artefact resulting from stent material, which limits assessment of the lumen.
- Subtraction post-processing techniques enable the high density stent to be removed from the CTCA leaving behind the stent luminal appearances.
- The very latest photon-counting CT scanners have an extremely high spatial resolution and are capable of accurate stent assessment but this technology is not widely available at present.

Pericoronary fat attenuation index

- Inflammation drives atherosclerosis, and coronary artery inflammation inhibits adipogenesis in adjacent perivascular fat. A novel CT biomarker, the perivascular fat attenuation index (FAI), can capture coronary inflammation by mapping spatial changes of perivascular fat attenuation on CTCA.
- Perivascular FAI provides cardiac risk prediction and restratification superior to current state-of-the-art assessment in CTCA (CRISP CT study, Lancet 2018). High perivascular FAI indicates increased cardiac mortality and may guide early, targeted primary prevention and intensive secondary prevention in patients, though has not yet been recognised in international guidelines.

1.3.4 Coronary anomalies

- CTCA is excellent at demonstrating proximal coronary anatomy.
- The right coronary artery normally arises from the right-facing coronary cusp.
- The left main stem coronary artery normally arises from the left-facing coronary cusp.
- 'High riding' variant:
    - Origin from the sinotubular junction above the usual respective coronary cusp
- An inter-arterial course:

- When a coronary artery passes in between the ascending aorta and main pulmonary artery
  - May be compressed between these two vessels, conferring a potential risk of ischaemia. This is often referred to as a 'malignant' course.
  - This anatomical variant can also be associated with an intramural course, where the ostio-proximal coronary artery passes within the wall of the proximal ascending aorta.
- A sub-pulmonic/trans-septal course of the LMS or LAD:
  - From the right-facing coronary cusp
  - The vessel passes inferiorly from the origin, below the level of the pulmonary valve
  - Essentially represents a long and deep trans-septal course.
- Retro-aortic: passing posterior to the ascending aorta
- Pre-pulmonic: passing anterior to the main pulmonary artery
- Management of inter-arterial proximal coronary anatomy is challenging. Coronary re-implantation is not without significant risk. Conservative management with exercise restriction can be an option but such cases should be managed in specialist centres.
- Myocardial bridging:
  - The epicardial coronary artery passes through the myocardium over a varying length and depth.
  - Common. As coronary perfusion occurs predominantly in diastole it is not usually considered clinically relevant.
  - Altered haemodynamics superior to the segment of bridging can be a substrate for CAD. Furthermore, recently myocardial bridges have been demonstrated to lead to impaired coronary perfusion efficiency during exercise, which was due to diminished accelerating wave energy in early systole compared with controls. Additionally, there was a high prevalence of endothelial and microvascular dysfunction.

1.3.5 Myocardial complications of CAD

- Established myocardial infarction may be evident by myocardial thinning.
- Lipomatous metaplasia of a prior infarct can be often be appreciated due to the different attenuation of fat and myocardium.
- Viability assessment of prior infarction territories is currently assessed with low-dose dobutamine stress echocardiography or using cardiac MRI to assess the transmural extent of late gadolinium ischaemic pattern scar.
- A large infarct may undergo aneurysmal dilatation—which can be appreciated on gated CT. Aneurysms may demonstrate calcification, and can develop intra-aneurysmal thrombus, which is seen as a cavity filling defect that persists on delayed phase imaging.

1.3.6 Interventional guidance

Transcatheter valve implantation (TAVI)

- For detailed recommendations of TAVI planning protocols and reporting standard, the Society of Cardiovascular CT consensus paper is recommended (*J Cardiovasc Comput Tomogr*. 2019;13(1):1–20).
- ECG gated CT provides accurate measurement of the dimensions and area of aortic annulus. Some centres will acquire systolic images of the root and others will acquire both diastolic and systolic acquisitions.

- In addition to measuring the annulus, it is important to confirm the morphology of the aortic valve and describe extent and location of commissural calcification.
- CT can identify calcification extending below the annulus into the left ventricular outflow tract. Extensive calcification extending below the annulus confers increased risk of annular rupture during implantation and can represent a risk for paravalvular leak in the post-operative period.
- The height of the coronary ostia from the annulus should be documented. As the prosthesis essentially crushes the native valve leaflets against the aortic root wall, there is a risk of coronary ostial occlusion if the ostia arise in close proximity to the annulus.
- Documentation of the dimensions of the sinus of Valsalva, sinotubular junction, mid ascending aorta, and remainder of the thoracic aorta is routinely performed.
- A TAVI planning protocol will also be combined with arterial phase imaging from superior to the subclavian arteries to below the common femoral arteries. This will assess the potential routes of peripheral arterial access and should assess the presence of stenotic atherosclerotic disease in the subclavian arteries and the ilio-femoral arterial systems bilaterally, as well as the remainder of the aorta.
- It is important to assess the size and position of the TAVI and vascular access to perform the procedure.

Mitral valve intervention
- There is an increasingly recognised role of CT for pre-operative planning for mitral valve intervention to assess mitral annular anatomy and the extent of mitral annulus calcification.

Coarctation of the aorta
- CT can be used to assess the degree and location of coarctation and visualization of collateralization.
- CT can be used to help plan the interventional procedure.
- CT is also an important modality in the post-treatment surveillance of these patients, particularly in the context of stenting. CT can be performed to assess for stent patency, restenosis, and pseudo-aneurysm formation in the vicinity.

Pulmonary Vein Isolation (PVI)
- CT can be used to identify the number, size, and location of pulmonary veins prior to electrophysiology interventions via 3D volume rendered images of the left atrium.
- It can also identify adjacent structures potentially at risk of iatrogenic injury during the procedure such as the oesophagus.
- CT can also exclude left atrial appendage thrombus prior to cardioversion or ablation. Incomplete contrast mixing can occur in the appendage, particularly in patients in AF. Unopacified blood is less dense than opacified blood, which assumes a dependent position. This can mimic LAA thrombus. Delayed phase imaging and imaging the patient prone (so the denser contrast opacified blood fills the appendage) are useful techniques to exclude LAA thrombus.
- In patients undergoing left atrial appendage occlusion percutaneously, ECG gated CT can accurately characterize the appendage morphology and help determine the optimal prosthesis size.
- In patients with congenital heart disease that require devices or complex pacing, ECG gated CT to document cardiac venous anatomy (e.g. location and anatomy of the coronary sinus in congenitally corrected transposition of the great arteries) can be helpful.

1.3.7 Ventricular function

- Echocardiography and cardiac MRI are the imaging modalities of choice.
- Retrospective ECG gating can be performed to acquire ventricular morphological data throughout the cardiac cycle and provide information on LV size and ejection fraction using dedicated post-processing software, but is usually reserved for patients where information will make a treatment difference and there is an MRI contraindication.
- Accuracy is limited by the temporal resolution of images, often leading to underestimation of function and a limited ability to assess for regional wall motion abnormalities.

Chronic total occlusions (CTO)

- CT can provide information on lesion length, degree of stenosis, stump morphology, tortuosity of the proximal and distal segments, and level of calcification. There is increasing interest in using CTCA data to plan all types of coronary intervention in the chronic coronary syndrome setting.

1.3.8 Valvular disease and endocarditis

Valvular heart disease

- Echocardiography is the imaging modality of choice.
- CT can be used for anatomy, calcification, and complications of prostheses such as endocarditis, pannus, and thrombus.
- CT may identify poor opposition of the prosthetic valve and aneurysms, which may be pseudo or mycotic in nature.

Aortic valve

Stenosis

- Calcium scoring of the aortic valve has an important role in the assessment of some patients with potentially severe aortic stenosis.
- The current ESC/EACST 2021 guidelines recommend calcium score of the valve can be used to help assess severity in low flow states (see page Valvular heart disease chapter: aortic stenosis).
- There are sex-specific cut-offs for the Agatston aortic valve score and likelihood of severe stenosis:
    - Aortic Valve Calcium score thresholds:
    - Severe aortic stenosis very likely: men ≥ 3,000; women ≥ 1,600
    - Severe aortic stenosis likely: men ≥2,000; women ≥ 1,200
    - Severe aortic stenosis unlikely: men < 1,600; women < 800
- CT can also visualize consequences of stenosis (LVH in calcific stenosis and aortopathies associated with bicuspid morphology).

Assessment of aortic valve replacement dysfunction
Pannus

- Excessive endothelialization of valvular leaflets causing restricted movement resulting in stenosis and/or regurgitation

- Features on CT that favour pannus are CT attenuation of > 145 HU; usually 12 months after surgery; circular mass extending from the sewing ring, located beneath the prosthesis, can enhance and can contain calcification.

Thrombus
- Thrombus tends to have an attenuation of < 145 HU; can occur above or below the prosthesis; tends to attach to the leaflet or hinge-point and does not tend to enhance.

Regurgitation
- CT can demonstrate a valve coaptation defect.

Mitral Valve
Stenosis
- CT allows morphological information on aetiology—e.g. rheumatic changes as evidenced by leaflet thickening, commissural fusion, and chordae shortening.

Regurgitation
- CT may show a mitral valve coaptation defect but is otherwise limited in direct assessment of mitral regurgitation.

Prosthetic valves
- In those with prosthetic valves, imaging can be limited by artefact, especially in metallic valves.
- Reconstruction of the image in the midplane of the valve perpendicular to the leaflets will produce data on opening and closing angles.

Endocarditis of native and prosthetic valves
- Trans-oesophageal echocardiography remains the gold-standard investigation in the work-up of suspected endocarditis.
- There is an increasingly recognized role for PET-CT in cases of endocarditis.
- Non-cardiac sequelae of endocarditis, such as mycotic aneurysm or septic emboli, can also be seen on CT.
- Aortic abscess can be visualized as marked thickening adjacent to the aortic root.

1.3.9 Cardiac masses

- Cardiac masses can be identified on cardiac CT, but cardiac MRI offers the most advanced non-invasive tissue characterization.
- Cardiac CT can be helpful to confirm or refute the presence of thrombus as the cause of a 'cardiac mass'. Persistent filling defects on arterial phase and delayed phase imaging, and lack of enhancement, would support a diagnosis of thrombus.

1.3.10 Cardiac trauma

- CT is frequently used in the assessment of patients presenting with thoracic trauma. The modality allows rapid and accurate assessment of the great vessels, heart, and pericardium.

- Haemopericardium is depicted as a relatively high attenuation fluid collection in the pericardial space.
- CT can also demonstrate the presence of cardiac chamber laceration, pseudoaneurysm and rupture, as well as cardiac herniation through traumatic pericardial defects.
- Gated coronary CT can be used to assess for traumatic coronary artery dissections and lacerations.
- Aortic intramural haematoma, dissection and rupture are also elegantly demonstrated in the context of trauma on CT.

1.3.11 Congenital heart disease

- Anatomy is often complex in congenital heart disease with echocardiography and CMR the primary choice for imaging over CT.
- CT can be useful in imaging neonates due to the rapid acquisition time and radiation doses can be minimized.
- CT can accurately assess gross anatomy in those with congenital heart disease pre-operatively, and with monitoring of conditions such as coarctation of the aorta.
- Long-term repeated imaging with this modality is limited by cumulative radiation dose. In these cases MRI and echocardiography is preferred.
- CT is however a suitable and accurate alternative in those who cannot undertake MRI to assess quantification of ventricular volumes and function, in particular the right ventricle.
- In cases of metallic stenting (e.g. for aortic coarctation, pulmonary stenosis or baffles in atrial switch), CT may provide a greater insight than MRI, which may be degraded by significant metallic artefact.

1.3.12 Pericardial disease

- Assessment of presence, location, and size of pericardial effusions.
- Adjacent fat stranding that may suggest inflammation can also be a useful size in cases of possible acute pericarditis.
- CT is useful in pericardial calcification such as in constrictive pericarditis: > 4 mm thickness is considered abnormal.

1.3.13 Diseases of great vessels

- ECG gated CT is the first-choice investigation in suspected acute aortic syndrome.
- It is important to perform an unenhanced CT of the thoracic aorta as this helps to demonstrate acute intramural haematoma as a hyperdense crescent of the aortic wall.
- It can clearly identify pathologies such as aortic aneurysms, dissection, intra-mural haematoma, and penetrating aortic ulcers.
- CT offers structural information on congenital anomalies of the aortic arch and is particularly useful in coarctation of the aorta to assess degree of stenosis and complications of treatment (aneurysm post stent implantation/stent fracture).

1.3.14 Diseases of cervical arteries and of the peripheral arteries

- It is usually first choice in imaging of peripheral vascular disease.

- CT has a role in imaging of renal, carotid and the limb arteries prior to potential surgical and radiologically guided interventions and can provide anatomical data, including tortuosity, and visualization of pathology amenable to endovascular intervention.
- CT angiography of the neck arteries and Circle of Willis is now routinely performed in cases of suspected acute ischaemic stroke if within the time window of mechanical thrombus retrieval.

Further reading

Achenbach S, Delgado V, Hausleiter J, Schoenhagen P, Min JK, Leipsic JA. SCCT expert consensus document on computed tomography imaging before transcatheter aortic valve implantation (TAVI)/transcatheter aortic valve replacement (TAVR). J Cardiovasc Comput Tomogr. 2012 Nov-Dec;6(6):366–380. doi: 10.1016/j.jcct.2012.11.002. Epub 2012 Nov 14. PMID: 23217460.

Cury RC, Leipsic J, Abbara S, Achenbach S, Berman D, Bittencourt M, Budoff M, Chinnaiyan K, Choi AD, Ghoshhajra B, Jacobs J, Koweek L, Lesser J, Maroules C, Rubin GD, Rybicki FJ, Shaw LJ, Williams MC, Williamson E, White CS, Villines TC, Blankstein R. CAD-RADS™ 2.0 - 2022 Coronary Artery Disease - Reporting and Data System An Expert Consensus Document of the Society of Cardiovascular Computed Tomography (SCCT), the American College of Cardiology (ACC), the American College of Radiology (ACR) and the North America Society of Cardiovascular Imaging (NASCI). Radiol Cardiothorac Imaging. 2022 Sep 22;4(5):e220183. doi: 10.1148/ryct.220183. PMID: 36339062; PMCID: PMC9627235.

Curzen N, Nicholas Z, Stuart B, Wilding S, Hill K, Shambrook J, Eminton Z, Ball D, Barrett C, Johnson L, Nuttall J, Fox K, Connolly D, O'Kane P, Hobson A, Chauhan A, Uren N, Mccann G, Berry C, Carter J, Roobottom C, Mamas M, Rajani R, Ford I, Douglas P, Hlatky M. Fractional flow reserve derived from computed tomography coronary angiography in the assessment and management of stable chest pain: the FORECAST randomized trial. Eur Heart J. 2021 Oct 1;42(37):3844–3852. doi: 10.1093/eurheartj/ehab444. PMID: 34269376; PMCID: PMC8648068.

Gulati M, Levy PD, Mukherjee D, Amsterdam E, Bhatt DL, Birtcher KK, Blankstein R, Boyd J, Bullock-Palmer RP, Conejo T, Diercks DB, Gentile F, Greenwood JP, Hess EP, Hollenberg SM, Jaber WA, Jneid H, Joglar JA, Morrow DA, O'Connor RE, Ross MA, Shaw LJ. 2021 AHA/ACC/ASE/CHEST/SAEM/SCCT/SCMR Guideline for the Evaluation and Diagnosis of Chest Pain: A Report of the American College of Cardiology/American Heart Association Joint Committee on Clinical Practice Guidelines. Circulation. 2021 Nov 30;144(22):e368–e454. doi: 10.1161/CIR.0000000000001029. Epub 2021 Oct 28. Erratum in: Circulation. 2021 Nov 30;144(22):e455. Erratum in: Circulation. 2023 Dec 12;148(24):e281. PMID: 34709879.

Knuuti J, Wijns W, Saraste A, Capodanno D, Barbato E, Funck-Brentano C, Prescott E, Storey RF, Deaton C, Cuisset T, Agewall S, Dickstein K, Edvardsen T, Escaned J, Gersh BJ, Svitil P, Gilard M, Hasdai D, Hatala R, Mahfoud F, Masip J, Muneretto C, Valgimigli M, Achenbach S, Bax JJ; ESC Scientific Document Group. 2019 ESC Guidelines for the diagnosis and management of chronic coronary syndromes. Eur Heart J. 2020 Jan 14;41(3):407–477. doi: 10.1093/eurheartj/ehz425. Erratum in: Eur Heart J. 2020 Nov 21;41(44):4242. PMID: 31504439.

NIfHaC, E. Recent-onset chest pain of suspected cardiac origin: assessment and diagnosis. London: National Institute for Health and Care Excellence (NICE); 2016 Nov 30. PMID: 32065740.

SCOT-HEART Investigators; Newby DE, Adamson PD, Berry C, Boon NA, Dweck MR, Flather M, Forbes J, Hunter A, Lewis S, MacLean S, Mills NL, Norrie J, Roditi G, Shah ASV, Timmis AD, van Beek EJR, Williams MC. Coronary CT Angiography and 5-Year Risk of Myocardial Infarction. N Engl J Med. 2018 Sep 6;379(10):924–933. doi: 10.1056/NEJMoa1805971. Epub 2018 Aug 25. PMID: 30145934.

Stirup J, Williams M, Bull R. Nicol E. *Oxford Specialist Handbooks in Cardiology: Cardiovascular Computed Tomography*. Oxford: Oxford University Press, 2019.

1.4

Nuclear Techniques

Nik Sabharwal and Katharine Thomas

TABLE OF CONTENTS

1.4.1　Overview　107
1.4.2　Radiation protection　108
1.4.3　Myocardial perfusion scintigraphy　108
　　　　Cameras and isotopes　109
　　　　Principles of stress　110
　　　　Stress protocols　110
　　　　Image acquisition, reconstruction, and display　111
　　　　Image interpretation　113
　　　　Clinical value　113
　　　　Limitations of myocardial perfusion scintigraphy　116
　　　　Reporting of myocardial perfusion scintigraphy　116
1.4.4　Equilibrium radionuclide ventriculography　116
1.4.5　Positron emission tomography　117
1.4.6　Hybrid imaging　117
1.4.7　Other nuclear cardiology investigations　118
　　　　DPD scintigraphy　118
　　　　Imaging of sympathetic innervation　118
　　　　Radiolabelled leucocyte scintigraphy　118
　　　　Macro aggregated albumin (MAA) for quantification of pulmonary perfusion and right-to-left shunting　118
　　　　Imaging of pulmonary embolism　119
1.4.8　The future　119

1.4.1 Overview

The term 'nuclear cardiology' encompasses several main types of scan:

1) Myocardial perfusion scintigraphy (MPS)
2) Radionuclide ventriculography (RNV)
3) Positron emission tomography (PET)
4) Other nuclear cardiology investigations
    - As a basic principle all these techniques use a camera designed to detect radioactive particles emitted from medical isotopes
    - MPS provides a functional and ischaemic assessment of the left ventricle. It is sometimes known as 'thallium scan', 'MIBI scan', or 'Myoview™ scan' depending on the isotope in question
    - RNV produces data on the left and sometimes right ventricular function through assessment of ventricular volumes. This is sometimes known as a multi-gated acquisition (MUGA) scan
    - PET determines myocardial viability through the assessment of glucose metabolism
    - RNV has been available since the 1970s
    - Planar (fixed head) MPS started soon after, with single photon emission computed tomography (SPECT) beginning in the 1980s and ECG gated SPECT in the 1990s
    - Much of the impressive evidence base is from old studies with early technology

- Recent developments have allowed nuclear cardiology techniques to regain some of the ground that has passed over to alternative, and complementary, imaging techniques
- The practice of nuclear medicine investigations is closely governed by ionizing radiation regulations
- All UK practitioners of nuclear medicine must hold valid certification under the Ionising Radiation (Medical Exposure) Regulations 2017 (IRMER)
- Consultants with responsibility for overseeing a UK nuclear cardiology service should hold an Administration of Radioactive Substances Advisory Committee (ARSAC) certificate.

1.4.2 Radiation protection

- Lifetime risk of cancer is approximately 1:3 (30%)
- Annual UK background radiation exposure is 2.6 mSv
- A typical MPS study exposes the patient to between 6–14 mSv of ionizing radiation depending on the isotope used
- The long term carcinogenic effects of radiation are difficult to accurately determine; however, the following examples are helpful:
    - For a stress-redistribution thallium-201 study the injected dose would be approximately 80 MBq, with an effective dose equivalent of 14 mSv. The lifetime risk of cancer would increase by 1:1429 (0.0007%) on a background lifetime cancer risk of 30%
    - For a 1-day Tc-99m tetrofosmin study the injected dose would be approximately 1000 MBq with an effective dose equivalent of 8 mSv. The lifetime risk of cancer would increase by 1:2667 (0.0004%) on a background lifetime cancer risk of 30%
- Doctors and technologists performing the tests do not need to wear any protective clothing apart from everyday clinical gloves when handling the isotopes
- Badge monitoring is mandatory but rarely reveals excessive exposure during routine practice
- The isotopes are held under lead shielding
- Employees in the UK have a dose limit of 20 mSv/year.
- Dose reference limits (DRLs) are the maximum recommended injected radiation doses
- Doses are usually adjusted according to body weight
- These limits are often not achieved due to adherence to as low as reasonably achievable (ALARA) principles.

1.4.3 Myocardial perfusion scintigraphy

- Myocardial perfusion scintigraphy (MPS) is a robust and well-validated technique for the diagnosis and assessment of CAD
- The technique uses rest and peak stress images to determine resting myocardial perfusion, inducible defects, and functional information which help to determine prognosis and guide therapeutic options
- Myocardial uptake of tracer will be homogenous in absence of myocardial infarction or ischaemia
- Levels of uptake will vary in the presence of significant coronary artery disease with reduced or absent uptake in affected areas
- Matched defects in rest and stress images indicate non-viable myocardium

- Normal tissue at rest with defects at stress indicate areas of ischaemic but viable myocardium
- A paradoxical worsening of defect in the rest study may indicate that the area is supplied by an unobstructed coronary artery that has been previously obstructed
- The use of MPS as an initial diagnostic tool for intermediate-risk patients has been cemented with its appearance in NICE 2010 guidance for the investigation of suspected coronary disease
- The use of MPS was retained in NICE 2016 guidance update
- The NICE guidelines do not differentiate between MPS, DSE, or CMR
- Local expertise is crucial for a successful service
- Typical evidence-based indications include:
    - Assessment of atypical chest pain
    - Identification of ischaemic territory and burden pre-revascularization
    - Assessment of symptoms post-revascularization
    - Assessment of the residual ischaemic burden post MI
    - Risk assessment before non-cardiac surgery, e.g. vascular and transplant surgery
    - Evidence of hibernating myocardium in LV systolic dysfunction
    - Identification of ACS in those presenting with acute chest pain.
- MPS has also been validated in 'special' sub groups:
    - Women
    - Diabetics
    - The elderly
- In all of these groups, MPS provides superior diagnostic and prognostic value over conventional risk factor variables and exercise test results.

Cameras and isotopes

- Technetium-99m (^{99m}Tc) and thallium-201 (^{201}Tl) continue to be the only used tracers for MPS
- Research into newer tracers is ongoing but progress has been slow
- Thallium is an older radioisotope the use of which has been in decline until recently
- Thallium redistributes freely between the blood pool and the myocardial cells via the Na$^+$/K$^+$ ATPase mechanism
- Technetium-99m has been a popular addition to nuclear cardiology
- The technetium is bound to either sestamibi or tetrofosmin before it is injected and it is then retained in intact cardiac myocytes
- Unlike thallium, these agents do not allow redistribution with the blood pool
- Thallium-201 has a half-life of 73 h
- The technetium-99m agents have a half-life of 6 h, which allows for up to two injections in one day
- Photons are emitted at characteristic energies, which are detected as scintillations on the NaI crystal within the heads of the gamma camera
- Thallium is cheaper but must be delivered ready to use to the hospital from the cyclotron
- Technetium isotopes can be reconstituted by hospital pharmacists from an onsite generator (delivered on a weekly basis)
- New scanners are reducing the time to image and the radiation dose
- Cadmium-zinc-telluride (CZT) gamma cameras are revolutionizing MPS with acquisition times as short as 2–3 minutes and with improved image quality
- CZT cameras can provide stress only doses of 1 mSv
- This hardware solution coupled with innovative software (resolution recovery) has shifted MPS back into the spotlight

- Technetium-based isotopes have suffered from erratic supply lines in the last few years and these new developments are extremely important
- This technology also allows new tracers to be developed and older discarded tracers to be resurrected.

Principles of stress
- MPS acquires images at rest and at peak stress. The stressor may be:
    - Physiological: treadmill, bicycle
    - Pharmacological: regadenoson, adenosine, dipyridamole, dobutamine
    - Other: pacing, mental (rarely used in clinical practice)
- Treadmill stress testing tends to follow the Bruce or modified Bruce protocols
- Bicycle stress involves starting at 25 W and increasing every 3 min by 25 W
- Both these physiological stressors also provide invaluable symptom, HR/BP, and ECG data, which cannot be so easily assessed with pharmacological stress
- Ideally physiological stress should be the default stressor for all patients attending a nuclear cardiology department
- The vasodilator stress agents are regadenoson, adenosine or dipyridamole
- Adenosine acts on A1 receptors causing coronary vasodilatation
- It has a very short half-life and is therefore given as a 6-minute infusion, with the isotope injected during the infusion
- Dipyridamole reduces the uptake and inhibits breakdown of endogenous adenosine
- Peak hyperaemia is seen 2–3 min after a 4-min infusion of dipyridamole, at which point the isotope is injected
- With relatively reduced flow down a stenosed vessel and hyperaemia through normal arteries, areas of hypoperfusion are revealed
- Both agents can cause bronchospasm and are not used if significant bradycardia or second- and third-degree heart block are present
- They are also antagonized by caffeine and theophyllines, which must be avoided for at least 12 hours prior to administration
- Regadenoson is a newer cardiac specific A2a receptor angonists which is given as a non-weight adjusted bolus
- There are much lower rates of bronchospasm and bradycardia and this agent is not contraindicated in mild or moderate airways disease
- An alternative agent is dobutamine, which acts as a beta agonist, increasing both heart rate and coronary flow. Atropine may be required to augment the tachycardia and reduce vagally mediated side effects (as per stress echocardiography)
- Isotope is injected at peak heart rate
- Dobutamine should be used with caution in unstable coronary disease or after recent MI and is unlikely to give good results in those patients receiving beta blockers

Stress protocols
- See Figure 1.4.1
- Protocols differ depending on whether thallium or technetium is used
- Thallium is injected at peak stress with imaging completed within 10–15 min following cessation of stress
- The redistribution acquisition is performed 4 h later, which allows the isotope to equilibrate with the blood pool, to provide a 'rest' scan
- If this redistribution scan identifies areas of hypoperfusion then a further image acquisition can be performed 24 h later to ensure that severe prolonged ischaemia is excluded

1.4.3 Myocardial perfusion scintigraphy

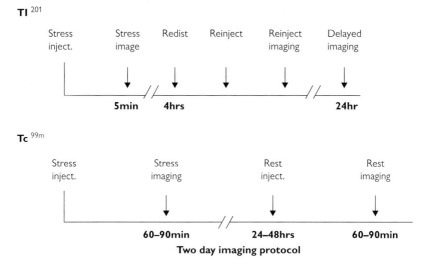

Figure 1.4.1 Typical scanning protocols.

- Occasionally there is need for a re-injection of thallium to identify hibernating myocardium
- This occurs at 4 h post stress and is followed by immediate image acquisition
- Technetium protocols are simpler as there is no redistribution (or washout) of tracer with the blood pool
- Isotope is injected at peak stress and at rest
- Protocols using peak-stress injections first are usually preferred, as a normal stress study precludes the need for the rest scan
- The best configuration is a 2-day protocol, which allows the activity from the first injection to have completely disappeared
- This protocol is not suitable for those patients travelling long distances, and therefore the one-day stress–rest protocol is also available
- With a one-day protocol the activity of the first injection is usually 3 times lower than the second injection, thus any residual activity from the first injection is 'drowned out' by the second one.
- Sublingual GTN is administered before the rest injections to augment resting flow and reduce any latent ischaemia

Image acquisition, reconstruction, and display

- The patient is positioned under the gamma camera (see Figure 1.4.2), which usually has two heads
- The heads can image in a 'planar' (fixed) position or can rotate around the patient through 180° (SPECT)
- Planar acquisition has effectively been superseded by SPECT, which is now routinely ECG gated to provide regional and global LV functional assessment
- 3D reconstruction is also possible using gated SPECT
- Reconstructed SPECT images are displayed by convention in three orthogonal planes: short axis from apex to base, vertical long axis from septum to lateral wall, and horizontal long axis from inferior to anterior wall
- The stress images are placed in a row above the corresponding rest images. The count activity is shown with a continuous colour scale (see Figure 1.4.3).

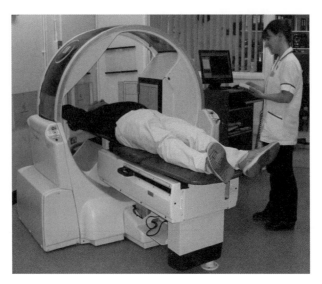

Figure 1.4.2 Typical dedicated cardiac gamma camera. It has a small footprint with no claustrophobia. Patient is able to lie flat and rest whilst image acquisition in process. Members of staff routinely sit in room to keep patient company and do not require lead shielding.

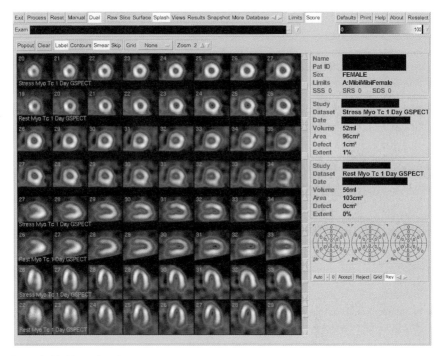

Figure 1.4.3 Normal study.

Image interpretation

See Figures 1.4.3, 1.4.4, and 1.4.5 for a normal study, diaphragmatic attenuation, and infarct/ischaemia.

- ECG gated SPECT allows detection of regional wall motion abnormalities and quantification of LV volumes
- Regional wall motion or thickening defects can be described in the same manner as for echocardiography (see Figures 1.4.4 and 1.4.5)
- Rest and stress scans are compared to identify areas of abnormal uptake, which is further quantified by extent, severity, and distribution, to assess the total ischaemic burden
- Dilatation of LV during rest and stress indicate LV dysfunction whereas dilatation of LV during stress only (transient ischaemic dilatation) suggests a large ischaemic burden
- Semi-quantitative scoring systems and measures are available, which have been validated. The most commonly used is the summed stress score
- The overall burden of ischaemia can be quantified by the proprietary software within most systems, presented as a percentage and risk stratified accordingly (see Table 1.4.1)
- Attenuation correction can be considered but may in turn create its own artefacts

Clinical value

- A normal myocardial perfusion scan result confers an annual cardiovascular adverse event rate of less than 1% per annum for medium-to-high risk pre-test probabilities (see Figure 1.4.6)
- In the low-to-medium risk patients this prognostic benefit is conferred for at least 5 years
- A small defect is low risk, representing a MACE rate < 3% per year

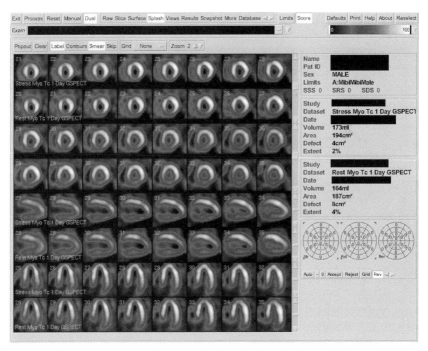

Figure 1.4.4 Diaphragmatic attenuation. Note uniform reduced counts along inferior wall, present both at rest and in stress. The gated study confirms normal wall thickening, which excludes a fixed inferior wall infarct.

1.4 Nuclear Techniques

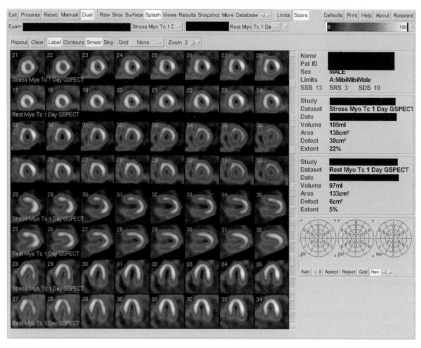

Figure 1.4.5 Abnormal study. There is evidence of a moderate-sized inferior infarct with additional small volume of stress induced ischaemia in the anterior wall.

Table 1.4.1 Quantified burden of ischaemia.

Extent of ischaemia	Percentage of myocardium at risk	Myocardial segments at risk (out of 17)
Small	5–10	1–2
Medium	10–20	2–3
Large	> 20	≥ 4

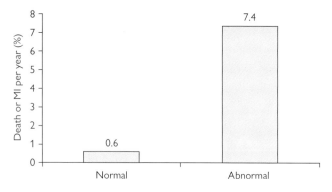

Figure 1.4.6 Cardiac event rates in 12,000 patients with normal or abnormal stress sestamibi scans.
Reproduced from Iskander S, Iskandrian AE. Risk assessment using single-photon emission computed tomographic technetium-99m sestamibi imaging. *J Am Coll Cardiol.* 1998 Jul;32(1):57–62. doi: 10.1016/s0735-1097(98)00177-6 with permission from Elsevier.

1.4.3 Myocardial perfusion scintigraphy 115

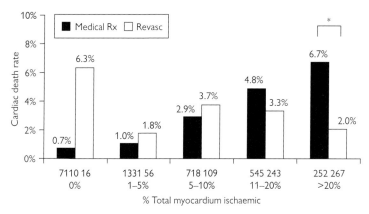

Figure 1.4.7 Annual cardiac death rate according to the percentage of myocardium with inducible hypoperfusion, stratified by management (10,627 patients followed for mean 2 years).
Adapted from Hachamovitch et al. *Circ.* 2003
Reproduced from Hachamovitch R, Hayes SW, Friedman JD, et al. Comparison of the short-term survival benefit associated with revascularization compared with medical therapy in patients with no prior coronary artery disease undergoing stress myocardial perfusion single photon emission computed tomography. *Circulation.* 2003 Jun 17;107(23):2900–7. doi: 10.1161/01.CIR.0000072790.23090.41 with permission from Wolters Kluwer.

- Patients with a low risk MPS and an exercise capacity of more than ten metabolic equivalents (METS) have a cardiac death rate of < 0.1% per year
- Ischaemic defects greater than 10% of the myocardium are associated with a 4.8% cardiac death rate; > 20% ischaemia is associated with a 6.7% cardiac death rate if treated medically (see Figure 1.4.7)
- LV dilatation or drop in LVEF post stress is an adverse sign and provides incremental prognostic value over quantitative SPECT
- An LV ejection fraction of < 45% confers a worse prognosis in the context of inducible defects, especially if the end systolic volume is > 70 ml (cardiac death rate 7.9%/year) (see Figure 1.4.8)
- A blunted heart rate in response to vasodilator stress is an independent risk factor of cardiac mortality
- Increased lung uptake of thallium is a further indirect indicator of severe ischaemic burden
- An analysis of published data using all tracers demonstrated a sensitivity of 73–94% and a specificity of around 90% for the detection of angiographically significant stenoses

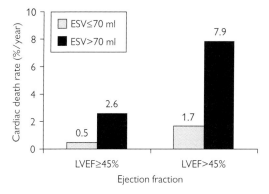

Figure 1.4.8 The prognostic value of combined LVEF and ESV after gated SPECT.
Reproduced from Sharir T, Germano G, Kavanagh PB, et al. Incremental prognostic value of post-stress left ventricular ejection fraction and volume by gated myocardial perfusion single photon emission computed tomography. *Circulation.* 1999 Sep 7;100(10):1035–42. doi: 10.1161/01.cir.100.10.1035 with permission from Wolters Kluwer.

- A meta-analysis of pharmacological stress echocardiography reported a sensitivity of 85–86% with a specificity of 86–89%.

Limitations of myocardial perfusion scintigraphy
- Ionizing radiation is required (although doses are acceptable in most populations). Modern solid state cameras require lower injected doses.
- MPS can struggle with ECG gating patients with uncontrolled AF; in these patients the LVEF may be inaccurate
- LBBB is a challenge with regards to interpretation
- Renal or hepatic dysfunction, obesity, claustrophobia, or metal implants are *not* a contraindication to the test.

Reporting of myocardial perfusion scintigraphy
Look at referral indication, PMH, and type/quality of stress.

- Assess quality of images (extra-cardiac activity, attenuation from diaphragm/breast)
- Defects at rest represent infarct; assess viability
- Assess peak-stress images; matched defects = infarct, mismatch = ischaemia
- Look at global and regional LV function.

Formulate report, giving diagnosis, estimate of prognosis, and answer to clinical question.

1.4.4 Equilibrium radionuclide ventriculography

- Equilibrium radionuclide ventriculography (ERNV) uses planar (fixed head) imaging to reproducibly measure the LVEF
- Unlike all other techniques, RNV does not rely on endocardial border edge detection (c.f. MPS, TTE, CMR, and CT)
- This technique relies on accurately quantifying radiolabelled RBCs in their passage through the LV (and RV) cavity.
- The blood pool is pre-treated with stannous pyrophosphate, which diffuses into red blood cells (RBCs)
- The blood pool is then labelled using technetium-99m, which binds to the stannous ions intra-cellularly
- Multiple gated cardiac cycles are acquired (up to 32 slices per cardiac cycle) and merged (hence alternative term 'multi-gated acquisition'), giving an accurate and reproducible assessment of overall LV function
- This procedure is therefore less suitable for patients with poorly controlled atrial fibrillation or very frequent extrasystoles
- Clearly modern echocardiography is the first-line test for the assessment of LV function; however, the main strength of RNV is its reproducibility
- Advances in gamma camera technology have led to dose reduction
- A modern refinement of RNV allows for ECG gated SPECT analysis rather than planar imaging
- This allows for assessment of both LVEF and RVEF with again a high degree of accuracy and reproducibility
- Radionuclide ventriculography is useful in serial assessment of LVEF in patients before and during cardiotoxic chemotherapy

- Phase mapping can be undertaken to assess regionality. This has limited use in patients with aneurysms and LBBB. Dyssynchrony can be clearly identified by this method which can be utilized pre and post CRT device implant.

1.4.5 Positron emission tomography

- Positron emission tomography (PET) uses ^{18}F-fluorodeoxyglucose (FDG) to detect changes in glucose metabolism.
- These changes are an indicator of myocardial viability.
- This test is usually combined with an assessment of myocardial perfusion.
- Perfusion-metabolic mismatches (greater than 7%) indicate hibernating viable myocardium that could benefit from revascularization.
- Myocardial perfusion assessments can be performed using the tracers ^{13}Nitrogen ammonia or ^{15}Oxygen water.
- These tracers require an on site cyclotron which limits availability.
- The recent introduction of ^{82}Rubidium, which does not require a cyclotron, is likely to expand the use of PET myocardial perfusion throughout the world.
- There is growing interest in another new tracer, ^{18}F-flupiridaz, which can be produced at a cyclotron off site.
- ^{18}F-flurpiridaz appears to increase sensitivity, have fewer artefacts, and thus allow a lower radiation dose.
- However there are cost implications with these new tracers.
- FDG–PET is considered the gold standard for the assessment of myocardial viability but use of specialist isotopes and expensive co-incidence detection cameras limit its use to specialist centres.
- The use of FDG-PET has expanded to include assessment of inflammation and infection (endocarditis and device related) though there also remains a role for radiolabelled leucocyte scintigraphy with SPECT (Section 1.4.7).
- Inflammation and infection causes increased metabolism of glucose leading to increased uptake of ^{18}F-fluorodeoxyglucose.
- FDG-PET is used to identify cardiac sarcoidosis through intra- and extra cardiac inflammation.
- It can also be used to monitor disease progression in cardiac sarcoidosis and response to immunosuppression.
- FDG-PET provides excellent sensitivity in detection of prosthetic valve endocarditis.
- Molecular imaging with cardiac PET (including micro-calcification with ^{18}F-NaF) is at the forefront of understanding processes at the cellular level.

1.4.6 Hybrid imaging

- SPECT and PET offer information regarding function and perfusion of the heart.
- MRI and CT provide detailed information of the anatomy of the heart, and CT exquisitely delineates the coronary arteries.
- Hybrid imaging combines these data sets to allow the addition of cardiac anatomy to functional imaging to improve diagnostic yield.
- This provides essentially a complete one-stop assessment for patients with suspected coronary artery disease (CAD).
- Modalities include SPECT-CT, PET-CT, and PET-MRI.

- Combining myocardial perfusion scans and CTCA has shown prognostic benefit in those with known or suspected CAD.
- Images can be acquired on one machine or on individual machines and then fused off line.
- Attenuation correction must be performed to ensure data sets are combined without error.
- Hybrid imaging is associated with higher doses of radiation exposure to the patient and principles of ALARA must always be followed.

1.4.7 Other nuclear cardiology investigations

DPD scintigraphy
- The use of ^{99m}Tc-3,3-diphosphono-12,2-propranodicarboxylic acid (DPD) bone scans has emerged recently as a promising tool for identification of TTR amyloidosis.
- Cardiac uptake of DPD occurs in the presence of transthyretin (TTR) amyloidosis
- Severity is graded using the Perugini grading system: 0 (negative) to 3 (strongly positive).
- DPD scintigraphy is a highly sensitive non-invasive tool for the detection of TTR amyloidosis.
- It is important to check for the absence of monoclonal protein in the serum and urine.

Imaging of sympathetic innervation
- Sympathetic nerve terminals are more sensitive to ischaemia than myocardium.
- ^{123}Iodine-metaiodobenyzlguanidine (mIBG) is an isotope that acts as a false neurotransmitter to the sympathetic nervous system.
- It identifies areas of myocardium that have been denervated through myocardial injury or ischaemia.
- These areas remain denervated even after revascularization.
- The lack of cardiac uptake is a marker of adverse prognosis for sudden cardiac death and progression of heart failure in patients with LV systolic dysfunction
- mIBG has been available for many years for non-cardiac imaging but is likely to become an integral tool in the risk assessment of patients with both ischaemic and non-ischaemic heart failure.

Radiolabelled leucocyte scintigraphy
- Radiolabelled leucocyte scintigraphy involves the labelling of leucocytes with ^{99m}Technetium.
- Scintigraphy acquisitions are performed following injection of radiolabelled leucocytes.
- The area of infection or inflammation will show uptake of leucocytes which is greater than background uptake and which increases over time.
- This form of imaging is very specific for detection of PVE (a difficult diagnosis to confirm) and is recommended alongside FDG-PET for detection of prosthetic valve endocarditis (which is highly sensitive).
- Leucocyte scintigraphy can also be used for detection of myocardial abscesses.

Macro aggregated albumin (MAA) for quantification of pulmonary perfusion and right-to-left shunting
- As a historical note: prior to widespread availability and popularity of agitated saline microbubble echocardiography, right-to-left and left-to-right shunting could be demonstrated through scintigraphy.
- This was performed using ^{99m}Technetium-macro aggregated albumin (MAA).
- With left-to-right shunt there is prolonged pulmonary washout.

- With right-to-left shunt there is extra-pulmonary uptake and may be detected in organs such as the brain and the kidneys.
- This method of imaging can also be used to quantify pulmonary perfusion by comparison of radioactivity in each lung.

Imaging of pulmonary embolism

- Planar V/Q scans and CTPA are first line for investigation of pulmonary embolism.
- V/Q scans are performed in two phases.
- Ventilation (V scan) is demonstrated through inhalation of radionuclides in gaseous form such as Xenon or Technetium.
- Perfusion (Q scan) is demonstrated through intravenous administration of ^{99m}Technetium-macro aggregated albumin (MAA).
- A ventilation-perfusion mismatch indicates pulmonary embolism.
- V/Q SPECT is superior to planar V/Q imaging and of similar efficacy to CTPA.
- Planar V/Q and V/Q SPECT should be considered first line when radiation dose is of concern to the patient, e.g. in pregnant or lactating women.
- There is an emerging role for the hybrid imaging method of V/Q SPECT-CT to investigate pulmonary embolism.
- Early data suggest V/Q SPECT-CT may be most accurate with a sensitivity of 97% and specificity of 100% compared to V/Q SPECT which has a sensitivity of 97% and a specificity of 88%.

1.4.8 The future

- MPS likely to increase its 'workhorse' role for routine ischaemia detection.
- An increasing role for hybrid imaging.
- Increasing role for PET and labelled leucocyte imaging for detecting sites of infection, especially with prosthetic valves and implanted cardiac devices.

Further reading

Sabharwal N. State of the art in nuclear cardiology. *Heart*. 2017;10:790–9. doi:10.1136/heartjnl-2015-308670

Sabharwal N, Arumugam P, Kelion A. *Nuclear Cardiology*. 2e Oxford: Oxford University Press, 2017.

Underwood SR et al. Myocardial perfusion scintigraphy: the evidence. *Eur J Nucl Med Mol Imaging*. 2004 Feb;31(2):261–91. doi: 10.1007/s00259-003-1344-5. PMID: 15129710; PMCID: PMC2562441.

CHAPTER 2

CORONARY ARTERY DISEASE

2.1

Acute Coronary Syndrome

Mark Mariathas, and Florence Mouy

TABLE OF CONTENTS

- 2.1.1 Pathophysiology of acute coronary syndrome (ACS) 123
  - Atherosclerotic plaque rupture 123
  - Vulnerable plaque characteristics 124
  - Effect of shear stress 124
  - Patient characteristics 124
  - Atherosclerotic plaque erosion 124
- 2.1.2 Non-atherosclerotic causes of ACS 124
  - Variant angina 124
  - Spontaneous Coronary Artery Dissection 125
  - Takotsubo cardiomyopathy 126
  - Coronary artery embolism 126
- 2.1.3 Diagnostic criteria of ACS 126
- 2.1.4 ACS risk scores 127
- 2.1.5 Diagnostic techniques in the management of a patients with ACS 127
  - Electrocardiogram 127
  - High-sensitivity cardiac troponin (hs-cTN) and other biomarkers 127
  - Echocardiography 128
  - Non-invasive imaging 128
- 2.1.6 Universal definition of myocardial injury and myocardial infarction 129
- 2.1.7 Pharmacotherapy in ACS 130
  - Antiplatelet agents 130
  - Pre-treatment and duration of antiplatelet therapy 132
  - Antiplatelet therapy and non-cardiac surgery 135
  - Antiplatelet therapy and CABG 135
  - Anticoagulants 135
  - Fibrinolytic therapy 137
  - Other medication 137
- 2.1.8 Diagnostic coronary angiography and revascularization 139
  - Timing of an invasive approach 139
  - Selective invasive strategy 139
  - Multivessel disease 139
  - Coronary artery bypass grafting (CABG) 140
  - Specific situations 140
- 2.1.9 Early and late complications of ACS and their management 140
  - LV dysfunction 140
  - LV aneurysm 140
  - LV thrombus 140
  - Secondary mitral valve regurgitation 141
  - Papillary muscle rupture 141
  - Free wall rupture 141
  - Ventricular septal rupture 141
  - Pericarditis 142
  - Arrhythmias 142
- 2.1.10 Impact of co-morbidities in ACS 142
  - Heart failure and cardiogenic shock 142
  - Diabetes mellitus 143
  - Chronic kidney disease 143
  - Cancer 143
  - Anaemia 143
  - Thrombocytopenia 144
  - The older person 144
  - Frailty 144

2.1.1 Pathophysiology of acute coronary syndrome (ACS)

Atherosclerotic plaque rupture

- Plaque rupture is the commonest atherosclerotic event that leads to clinically relevant arterial ischaemia.
- It is an area of plaque with fibrous cap disruption whereby the overlying thrombus is in continuity with the necrotic core.

- Fracture of the fibrous cap allows platelets, circulating clotting factors, and inflammatory cells to come into contact with the thrombogenic necrotic core and promote thrombus formation.

Vulnerable plaque characteristics
- Thin-capped plaques (defined by Virmani and colleagues as < 65 μm thick). These lesions are most prone to cap disruption, thrombus formation, and subsequent clinical events
- Large necrotic lipid-rich core
- High macrophage numbers
- Paucity of smooth muscle cells
- Intraplaque haemorrhage

Effect of shear stress
- The most important dynamic that defines likelihood of rupture is the balance between tangential stresses exerted on the fibrous cap by luminal blood flow and the innate mechanical strength of the cap itself; a change in either one of these factors can shift the balance towards cap rupture.

Patient characteristics
- Thrombophilic propensities of individual patients are important in determining the extent of thrombosis and may be affected by lifestyle factors such as cigarette smoking.
- Platelet function: platelet interaction with the endothelium, circulating coagulant factors, and inflammatory cells is of key importance in the promotion of thrombus in association with plaque rupture.

Atherosclerotic plaque erosion
- Plaque erosion is far less well understood than rupture.
- It contributes to about a third of all sudden thrombotic coronary deaths identified on post-mortem studies.
- Loosely defined as luminal thrombus in an arterial segment without evidence of plaque rupture.
- Typical plaque characteristics underlying erosions are stenotic fibrous lesions with little or no atheromatous core; the endothelium is usually absent at the site of erosion.
- Erosions are more common in young men and women < 50 years old and are associated with smoking, especially in premenopausal women.

2.1.2 Non-atherosclerotic causes of ACS

Variant angina
First described by Prinzmetal in 1959, variant angina (or Prinzmetal's angina) can be differentiated from typical angina by the following:

- The angina is not brought on by exertion and exercise, with stress tests often negative.
- During an episode of pain, patients typically present with ST elevation, which is usually transient.
- The pain occurs at the same time of the day, often waking the patient up from sleep.

It has subsequently been shown that the mechanism behind variant angina is spasm of epicardial coronary arteries. Often the symptoms are quickly alleviated by nitrates. During episodes patients can suffer from arrhythmias, which can be fatal, it is therefore imperative to consider variant angina as a differential in patients suffering with rest pain and syncope. Apart from cigarette smoking, traditional risk factors for atherosclerosis do not apply to variant angina. As opposed to typical angina, exertion is not a precipitant of variant angina. Precipitants include hyperventilation and exposure to the cold.

Historically the diagnosis of variant angina has been based on the following clinical features;

- Rest angina
- Transient ST elevation
- Resolution with administration of nitrates

More recently provocative spasm testing has been used by clinicians to help establish a diagnosis of variant angina. This is undertaken with the aid of coronary angiography. Provocation tests have been reported to have sensitivity of 90% with a specificity of 99%.

Treatment of variant angina includes:

- Avoidance of known precipitants such as smoking
- Short-acting nitrates for an acute episode and long acting nitrates for prevention
- Calcium channel blockers are also known effective treatment for variant angina

Spontaneous Coronary Artery Dissection

Spontaneous coronary artery dissection (SCAD) is estimated to cause 0.1–0.4% of cases of ACS. In SCAD there is disruption to the arterial wall causing a separation of the intima from the outer vascular wall. As a result of this intramural haematoma develops, which eventually forms a false lumen. Often in patients with SCAD, non-affected coronary artery segments will be smooth and appear disease free on angiography.

Patients with SCAD tend to be younger (mean age of 43) and the vast majority are female. Predisposing factors include postpartum, connective tissue disease, fibromuscular dysplasia, and hormonal therapy.

SCAD based on angiography can be divided into three types;

- Type 1: Longitudinal filling defect, which represents the luminal flap. There is the appearance of a double lumen on angiography. 29% of all SCAD are type 1.
- Type 2: Due to intramural haematoma there are long smooth tubular lesion, there is no visible dissection plane. The hallmark is disease free segments followed by an abrupt reduction in vessel lumen for a long segment, typically more than 30 mm. This is the most common type (67%).
- Type 3: Multiple focal tubular lesions that can be mistaken for atherosclerotic lesions. The diagnosis can only be made with the assistance of intracoronary imaging. Only 4% of SCAD are type 3.

The coronary arterial walls of patients with SCAD are fragile and prone to catheter-induced dissections, therefore the coronary ostia of these patients should be intubated carefully to minimize the risk of catheter-induced dissections.

Non-invasive management of patients with SCAD is recommended. Of patients with SCAD treated conservatively, 10% require invasive treatment by day 4 of their presentation, highlighting the importance of careful and relatively long in-hospital observation. The latest ESC guidelines recommend PCI in SCAD only when there are ongoing symptoms and signs of myocardial ischaemia, a large area of the myocardium is in jeopardy or there is reduced anterograde flow. Although the long-term prognosis for patients with SCAD is good, up to 27% of patients will have further events.

Takotsubo cardiomyopathy

Takotsubo cardiomyopathy (TCM) is an episode of acute heart failure that can often present as an ACS. The clinical course of patients with TCM is heterogeneous which can range from benign to life-threatening. Classical TCM presents with an LAD-syndrome ECG pattern accompanied with apical ballooning of the LV.

The following novel diagnostic criteria has been put forward by the International Takotsubo Registry:

- Transient acute LV dysfunction that presents not only with apical ballooning but also involving mid and basal walls in a focal motion abnormality.
- An emotional or physical trigger can precede a TCM.
- New ECG abnormalities, not only anterior ST elevation.
- Moderate elevation of cardiac biomarkers.
- Neurological disorders such as stroke, subarachnoid haemorrhage, or seizures can trigger a TCM.
- More common in post-menopausal women.

The basis of treatment of patients with TCM once ACS has been ruled out is based on supportive treatment. The lack of evidence on treatment of TCM and the reversibility of the LV dysfunction currently supports this approach. Acute complications of TCM included cardiogenic shock and LV outflow tract obstruction. In the long term it is unclear whether patients with TCM should receive treatment for LV dysfunction. However, all patients with TCM should be followed up to ensure LV recovery, treatment of any complications, and detection of recurrences.

Coronary artery embolism

Coronary artery embolism (CE) is a known cause of acute myocardial infarction with unobstructed coronary arteries on angiography. The prevalence of CE in patients with ST elevation myocardial infarctions has been reported to be from 4–13%. It is associated with prosthetic aortic and mitral valves, atrial fibrillation, dilated cardiomyopathy, neoplasia, and atrial septal defects. In some cases, patients appear to be in a prothrombotic state. The long-term outcome in patients with CE is worse than expected when their traditional risk factors are taken into consideration.

2.1.3 Diagnostic criteria of ACS

The spectrum of ACS represents the clinical expression of atherosclerotic plaque pathology.
At one end of the spectrum is occlusive thrombus associated with plaque rupture or erosion causing epicardial coronary obstruction and transmural infarction.
At the other end is slow, progressive coronary luminal obstruction caused by increasing plaque bulk. Typically this produces increasing symptoms of ischaemia at decreasing workload or rest.
The European Society of Cardiology has categorized ACS patients into two major groups:

- Patients with typical acute chest pain and persistent (> 20 min) ST segment elevation on the ECG. This is termed ST elevation Myocardial Infarction (STEMI) and generally reflects an epicardial coronary occlusion.
- Patients with acute chest pain but without persistent ST segment elevation. They have transient or persistent ST segment depression or T wave inversion, flat T waves, pseudo-normalization of T waves, or no ECG changes at presentation. If this is associated with a rise in cardiac biomarkers, then this is termed a non-ST elevation ACS (NSTE-ACS).
- If the patient has ischaemic chest pain without a rise in cardiac biomarkers, they may be labelled as having unstable angina.

- Since the introduction of the high-sensitivity cardiac troponin assay (hs-cTn) into clinical practice there has been an increase in the detection of MI with a comparable reduction in the detection of unstable angina.

2.1.4 ACS risk scores

The GRACE (Global Registry of Acute Coronary Events) Score is a prospectively studied scoring system to risk stratify patients with diagnosed ACS to estimate their in-hospital and 6-month to 3-year mortality. The score can be calculated using web and app calculators: www.outcomes-umassmed.org/risk_models_grace_orig.aspx
ESC guidelines (ACS) 2023 recommend utilizing the GRACE risk score models and measuring BNP or NT-proBNP plasma concentrations to gain prognostic information. Serial measurement of high-sensitivity cardiac troponin is also recommended for the estimation of prognosis.

2.1.5 Diagnostic techniques in the management of a patients with ACS

Electrocardiogram
- First-line investigation in the work up of a patient with suspected ACS is a 12-lead electrocardiogram (ECG).
- It should be performed within 10 minutes of arrival in hospital or if pre-hospital it should be undertaken at the first point of contact with medical staff.
- In 30% of cases the 12-lead ECG will be normal.
- If the ECG is normal but ongoing ischaemia is suspected, additional leads such as V7–V9 should be recorded.
- ST elevation on an ECG corresponding to a myocardial territory should result in the activation of pathway to mandate immediate reperfusion.
- Where possible comparison with previous ECGs (if available) should be undertaken.
- Patients with LBBB and a high level of suspicion of ischaemia should be treated as a STEMI.
- The Sgarbossa criteria can be used when assessing the need for immediate cardiac catheterization in patients with LBBB.
- In haemodynamically stable patients with LBBB, the hs-cTn result on admission should be used to risk stratify patients and help decide who requires immediate cardiac catheterization.
- More than 50% of patients with LBBB or RBBB presenting with acute chest pain will be found to have diagnosis other than MI.

High-sensitivity cardiac troponin (hs-cTN) and other biomarkers
- All patients with suspected NTE-ACS should have a biomarker of cardiomyocyte damage measured.
- The biomarker of choice should ideally by hs-cTn.
- This is the most sensitive and specific biomarker of cardiomyocyte injury available to clinicians.
- A hs-cTn level above the 99th percentile with a dynamic change is compatible with a diagnosis of MI.
- Rises in troponin can now be detected within 1 hour of the onset of symptoms when using the high sensitivity assays.

- Troponin levels remain elevated for several days.
- The development of the high sensitivity assays has allowed for the rapid 'rule in' and 'rule out' of MI in patients presenting with acute chest pain.
- This leads to better efficiency within the emergency department for the admission and discharge of patients with chest pain.
- The ESC currently recommends the use of 0/1 hr and 0/2 hr.
- This is based on two notions:
    - Rising hs-cTn levels increase the probability that the cause is an MI.
    - Early changes over 1 and 2 hours can be used as proxies for changes which will occur over 3 and 6 hours.
- Each assay has specific hs-cTn values which are used in these algorithms.
- Using these algorithms ensures a negative predictive value of at least 99% and a positive predictive value of at least 70%.
- Patients who fall in the 'rule in' arm of the algorithm are in the general suitable for cardiac catheterization and admission to the coronary care unit.
- Some patients who do not fall in the 'rule in' or 'rule out' arms are observed with a repeat hs-cTn measured at 3 hours and echocardiography the next recommended steps.
- When using hs-cTn levels to diagnose, it is important remember other factors which can influence hs-cTn levels such as age, gender, and renal function.
- It is also important to remember that 10–15% of patients who have their 1 hr blood sample taken will either have had a very low 0 hr level (ie MI ruled out without 1 hr level) or have presented more than 3 hours from the onset of symptoms (therefore do not require a further hs-cTn level).
- Other biomarkers that can be used in conjunction with troponin levels included CK-MB, myosin-binding protein C, and copeptin.
- Currently cardiac troponin is the gold standard biomarker for the diagnosis of MI.

Echocardiography

- Transthoracic echocardiography is very useful when assessing a patient with acute chest pain.
- Regional wall motion abnormalities can be very useful in helping to diagnose ongoing ischaemia, and risk assess patients as to whether coronary angiography is indicated.
- Furthermore, transthoracic echocardiography can help diagnose alternative causes for the patient's presentation such as pulmonary embolism, acute aortic dissection, and pericardial effusion.
- Echocardiography can also provide an estimation of LV function which is extremely important in the management and prognosis of patients admitted with ACS. Ideally this should be done before discharge.
- If echocardiography is suboptimal/inconclusive, cardiac MRI can be considered.

Non-invasive imaging

- In patients with suspected ACS but with non-elevated (or uncertain) hs-cTn, no ECG changes and no recurrence of pain, incorporating CTCA or a non-invasive stress imaging test as part of the initial work-up should be considered.
- Patients with a significant burden of ischaemia (> 10% ischaemic myocardium) are at lower risk of death and MI with revascularization as opposed to medical therapy.
- In patients with poor LV function, myocardial viability assessment (typically with a cardiac MRI) may help to guide appropriateness of revascularization.

Computed tomography coronary angiography (CTCA)
- CTCA is excellent in excluding significant CAD due to high negative predictive values (NPV).
- It produces moderate positive predictive values (PPVs), i.e. only approximately 50% of stenoses classified as significant on CTCA are associated with ischaemia on interrogation during coronary angiography.
- CT derived fractional flow reserve measurements (CTFFR) is relatively new technology, which has demonstrated good correlation with invasive FFR. This offers the potential to reduce the demand for layered functional imaging tests after CTCA.

Stress echocardiography
- Stress echocardiography involves exercise on a treadmill or bicycle ergometer. If unable to physically exercise, then a pharmacological stressor such as dobutamine may be used.
- Intravenous contrast agents help to identify the true endocardial border, making inducible regional wall motion abnormalities easier to detect.
- The technique has a pooled sensitivity of 80–85% and specificity of 84–86%.

Myocardial perfusion scintigraphy (MPS)
- MPS has a sensitivity of 85–90% and specificity of 70–75%.
- ECG gating may improve these parameters in women, diabetics, and elderly patients.

Cardiac MRI (CMR)
- Perfusion imaging identifies myocardium subtended by significantly stenosed coronary arteries.
- Following administration of a vasodilator (typically adenosine), the dynamic passage of a contrast agent (typically gadolinium) is imaged through the cardiac chambers and myocardium. The hypoperfused myocardium is exposed relative to a normal segment.
- Recent meta-analysis has shown a 91% sensitivity and 81% specificity of this technique.
- Myocardial viability can be assessed by late gadolinium enhancement (LGE). This is based on the principle that an irreversibly damaged myocardium holds up gadolinium for longer than a normally functioning myocardium, appearing brighter on T1-weighted images.

Positron emission tomography
- Positron emission tomography is expensive and limited to a few UK centres.
- The technique has a sensitivity of 92% and specificity of 85% in the detection of CAD.

2.1.6 Universal definition of myocardial injury and myocardial infarction

The fourth universal definition of myocardial infarction (2018) states that the term myocardial injury should be used when there is evidence of elevated cardiac troponin values (cTn) with at least one value above the 99th percentile upper reference limit (URL). The myocardial injury is considered acute if there is a rise and/or fall of cTn values.

The term acute myocardial infarction should be used when there is acute myocardial injury with clinical evidence of acute myocardial ischaemia and with detection of a rise and/or fall of (cTn) values with at least one value above the 99th percentile URL and at least one of the following:

- Symptoms of myocardial ischaemia
- New ischaemic ECG changes
- Development of pathological Q waves

- Imaging evidence of new loss of viable myocardium or new regional wall motion abnormality in a pattern consistent with an ischaemic aetiology
- Identification of an intracoronary thrombus by angiography or autopsy

Classification

Myocardial infarction can be further classified into the following:

- Type 1: Spontaneous myocardial infarction related to atherosclerotic plaque disruption (rupture, ulceration, erosion, or dissection).
- Type 2: Myocardial infarction as a result of an imbalance between myocardial oxygen supply and demand (unrelated to acute coronary atherothrombosis). Examples include coronary artery spasm, tachyarrhythmias, and anaemia.
- Type 3: Cardiac death with symptoms suggestive of myocardial ischaemia accompanied by presumed new ischaemic ECG changes or ventricular fibrillation. Includes MI detected by autopsy.
- Type 4a: PCI related MI ($\leq$ 48 h after the index procedure): Elevation of cTn values $> 5 \times$ 99th percentile URL in patients with normal baseline values or a rise of cTn values $> 20\%$ if the baseline values are elevated and are stable or falling in addition to objective markers of MI such as regional wall motion abnormalities or angiographical evidence of a complication.
- Type 4b: Stent thrombosis (either seen on angiography or postmortem) with a cardiac biomarker above the 99th percentile URL.
- Type 5: CABG related MI ($\leq$ 48 h after the index procedure): Elevation of cardiac biomarker values $> 10 \times$ 99th percentile URL in patients with normal baseline cTn values.

2.1.7 Pharmacotherapy in ACS

Antiplatelet agents

- The mainstay of early pharmacological treatment consists of antiplatelet and antithrombotic agents.
- Pharmacological inhibition of platelet function has been shown to have both symptomatic and prognostic benefit in patients with ACS.

Acetylsalicylic acid (aspirin)

- Irreversible inhibition of cyclooxygenase (mainly COX-1) reduces thromboxane A2 production thereby reducing platelet aggregation. Large doses can lead to inhibition of COX-2, which may offer some anti-inflammatory effect.
- Aspirin is recommended for all patients without contraindications at an initial oral loading dose of 150–300 mg, followed by a daily maintenance dose of 75–100 mg long term.
- Inhibition of COX1 can reduce the production of protective prostaglandins in the stomach, making gastrointestinal (GI) ulceration more likely. GI intolerance, including bleeding, is the major reason for discontinuation.

$P2Y_{12}$ inhibitors

- Clopidogrel, prasugrel, and ticagrelor inhibit the $P2Y_{12}$ subtype of the ADP platelet receptor.

Clopidogrel

- Clopidogrel is a pro-drug that is converted to its active metabolite by hepatic cytochrome enzyme (CYP3A4) pathway.
- This may explain why some patients do not achieve expected levels of platelet inhibition and may be prone to further thrombotic events including catastrophic stent thrombosis.

2.1.7 Pharmacotherapy in ACS

- The CURE trial showed additive benefit to conventional therapy in treatment of NSTE-ACS, reducing major adverse cardiovascular events (MACE) rates from 11.4% to 9.3% (p < 0.0001)
- The trade-off was an increase in major bleeding from 2.7% to 3.7% (p = 0.001).
- The CLARITY trial showed additive benefit to aspirin alone in STEMI patients receiving fibrinolytic therapy.
- The ARMYDA-2 trial showed a reduction in cardiovascular events in patients undergoing PCI who received a 600-mg loading dose as opposed to 300 mg up to 8 h pre-procedure

Prasugrel

- Prasugrel is also a pro-drug but its pharmacodynamics differ to clopidogrel.
- It is converted to its active form faster and more consistently; it gives more reliable platelet inhibition.
- TRITON-TIMI 38 showed that, in a large cohort of ACS patients undergoing PCI, patients receiving prasugrel had lower rates of the combined endpoints of MACE (9.9% vs 12.1%; p < 0.0001) than those receiving clopidogrel at 15 months.
- Within this there was a significant reduction in non-fatal MI but no difference in rates of death or stroke.
- As expected, this was offset by an increase in significant bleeding complications in the prasugrel group.
- The loading dose of prasugrel is 60 mg followed by a daily maintenance dose of 10 mg (reduce to 5 mg if body weight < 60 kg or aged ≥ 75 years).
- Prior stroke is a contraindication.
- Prasugrel should be considered in preference to ticagrelor for NSTE-ACS patients who proceed to PCI.

Ticagrelor

- Ticagrelor is an oral, reversible direct acting inhibitor of the $P2Y_{12}$ ADP receptor.
- Since it is active in its native form it has a more rapid onset and achieves more pronounced platelet inhibition than clopidogrel.
- The PLATO trial showed that in a large cohort of ACS patients, treatment with ticagrelor reduced the incidence of MACE at 12 months as compared to patients treated with clopidogrel (9.8% vs 11.7%; p < 0.001).
- Importantly there was significantly lower mortality in the ticagrelor group.
- Interestingly there was no difference in the rate of overall major bleeding between the two groups but there was an increase in the rate of non-CABG-related bleeding in the ticagrelor group (4.5% vs 3.8%; p = 0.03).
- The loading dose of ticagrelor is 180 mg followed by a maintenance dose of 90 mg twice daily.
- Ticagrelor is contraindicated in patients with a history of intracranial bleeding.
- Non-exertional dyspnoea (typically described as sudden and unexpected air hunger or unsatisfied inspiration) has been reported in 10–20% of patients on ticagrelor. This often resolved with continued treatment. Discontinuation of ticagrelor due to dyspnoea was 0.9% in the PLATO trial.

Cangrelor

- Intravenous adenosine triphosphate (ATP) analogue that binds reversibly with high affinity to the $P2Y_{12}$ receptor.
- Immediate effect (2 minutes) with short plasma half-life (offset 30–60 minutes).
- Typically utilized in $P2Y_{12}$ receptor naive ventilated patients undergoing PCI (e.g. out-of-hospital cardiac arrests survivors).

Glycoprotein IIb/IIIa inhibitors (abciximab/eptifibatide/tirofiban)
- Glycoprotein IIb/IIIa inhibitors bind to fibrinogen and von Willebrand factor thus blocking the final common pathway of platelet activation.
- Upstream initiation in high-risk ACS patients in whom coronary anatomy is not known is no longer recommended. Patients with recurrent ischaemia should undergo urgent coronary angiography.
- GP IIb/IIIa antagonists should be considered for bail-out during PCI if there is evidence of no-reflow or a thrombotic complication.

Pre-treatment and duration of antiplatelet therapy
- Typically following a diagnosis of ACS, patients are commenced immediately on dual antiplatelet therapy (DAPT)—see Figure 2.1.1 for a summary of default antithrombotic therapy regimens in ACS in patients without an indication for OAC.

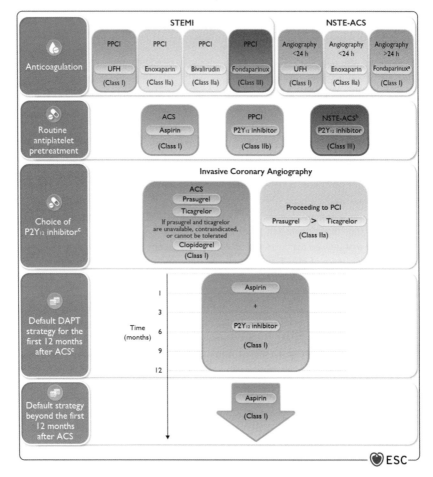

Figure 2.1.1 Recommended default antithrombotic therapy regimens in acute coronary syndrome patients without an indication for oral anticoagulation.

Reproduced from Byrne RA, Rossello X, Coughlan JJ, et al; ESC Scientific Document Group. 2023 ESC Guidelines for the management of acute coronary syndromes. *Eur Heart J*. 2023 Oct 12;44(38):3720–3826. doi: 10.1093/eurheartj/ehad191. © European Society of Cardiology. With permission from Oxford University Press.

Table 2.1.1 Major and minor criteria for high bleeding risk according to the Academic Research Consortium for High Bleeding Risk at the time of percutaneous coronary intervention.

Major criteria	Minor criteria
	Age > 75 years
Anticipated use of long-term oral anticoagulation[a]	
Severe or end-stage CKD (eGFR < 30 ml/min)	Moderate CKD (eGFR 30–59 ml/min)
Haemoglobin < 11 g/dL	Haemoglobin 11–12.9 g/dL for men and 11–11.9 g/dL for women
Spontaneous bleeding requiring hospitalization or transfusion in the past 6 months or at any time, if recurrent	Spontaneous bleeding requiring hospitalization or transfusion within the past 12 months not meeting the major criterion
Moderate or severe baseline thrombocytopenia[b] (platelet count < 100 × 10^9/L)	
Chronic bleeding diathesis	
Liver cirrhosis with portal hypertension	Long-term use of oral non-steroidal anti-inflammatory drugs or steroids
Active malignancy[c] (excluding non-melanoma skin cancer) within the past 12 months	
Previous spontaneous ICH (at any time) Previous traumatic ICH within the past 12 months Presence of a brain arteriovenous malformation Moderate or severe ischaemic stroke[d] within the past 6 months	Any ischaemic stroke at any time not meeting the major criterion
Non-deferrable major surgery on dual antiplatelet therapy	
Recent major surgery or major trauma within 30 days before percutaneous coronary intervention	

Reproduced from Byrne RA, Rossello X, Coughlan JJ, et al; ESC Scientific Document Group. 2023 ESC Guidelines for the management of acute coronary syndromes. *Eur Heart J.* 2023 Oct 12;44(38):3720–3826. doi: 10.1093/eurheartj/ehad191. © European Society of Cardiology. With permission from Oxford University Press.

- Ticagrelor or prasugrel (in addition to aspirin) is usually preferred to clopidogrel. Clopidogrel is recommended in patients requiring concomitant anticoagulation and may be considered in older patients (particularly if they have a high bleeding risk—see Table 2.1.1 for bleeding risk criteria).
- DAPT is recommended for 1 year unless there are contraindications such as excessive bleeding risk.
- P2Y$_{12}$ inhibitor monotherapy can be considered as an alternative to aspirin monotherapy for long-term treatment.
- Pre-treatment with a P2Y$_{12}$ receptor inhibitor in patients with a working diagnosis of STEMI can be considered. In those with a working diagnosis of NSTE-ACS, who are likely to undergo early invasive strategy (< 24 h from admission), pre-treatment with a P2Y$_{12}$ receptor inhibitor is not recommended. In those with a working diagnosis of NSTE-ACS who are likely to undergo later invasive strategy (> 24 h), pre-treatment with a P2Y$_{12}$ receptor inhibitor can be considered depending on bleeding risk.

Shortened and extended antiplatelet therapy

- In patients who are event-free after 3–6 months of DAPT and who are not high ischaemic risk, single antiplatelet therapy (SAPT, preferably with a $P2Y_{12}$ receptor inhibitor) should be considered.
- In patients with a high bleeding risk (PRECISE-DAPT score of ≥ 25), aspirin or $P2Y_{12}$ receptor inhibitor monotherapy after 1 month of DAPT can be considered.
- In patients requiring oral anticoagulation, withdrawing antiplatelet therapy at 6 months while continuing anticoagulation can be considered.
- De-escalation of antiplatelet therapy (eg prasugrel/ticagrelor to clopidogrel to reduce bleeding risk) in the first 30 days after an ACS event is not recommended.
- Adding a second antithrombotic agent to aspirin for extended long-term secondary prevention should be considered in patients with a high risk of ischaemic events (see Table 2.1.2) and without increased risk of major bleeding. Options are rivaroxaban 2.5 mg bd (for patients with CAD or symptomatic PAD at high risk of ischaemic events), Ticagrelor 60 mg/90 mg bd, clopidogrel or prasugrel (post MI in patients who have tolerated DAPT for 1 year)

Table 2.1.2 Risk criteria for extended treatment with a second antithrombotic agent.

High thrombotic risk (Class IIa)	Moderate thrombotic risk (Class IIb)
Complex CAD and at least 1 criterion	**Non-complex CAD and at least 1 criterion**
Risk enhancers	
Diabetes mellitus requiring medication	Diabetes mellitus requiring medication
History of recurrent MI	History of recurrent MI
Any multivessel CAD	Polyvascular disease (CAD plus PAD)
Polyvascular disease (CAD plus PAD)	CKD with eGFR 15–59 ml/min/1.73 m^2
Premature (< 45 years) or accelerated (new lesion within a 2-year time frame) CAD	
Concomitant systemic inflammatory disease (e.g. human immunodeficiency virus, systemic lupus erythematosus, chronic arthritis)	
CKD with eGFR 15–59 ml/min/1.73 m^2	
Technical aspects	
At least 3 stents implanted	
At least 3 lesions treated	
Total stent length > 60 mm	
History of complex revascularization (left main, bifurcation stenting with ≥ 2 stents implanted, chronic total occlusion, stenting of last patent vessel)	
History of stent thrombosis on antiplatelet treatment	

Reproduced from Collet JP, Thiele H, Barbato E, et al; ESC Scientific Document Group. 2020 ESC Guidelines for the management of acute coronary syndromes in patients presenting without persistent ST-segment elevation. *Eur Heart J.* 2021 Apr 7;42(14):1289–1367. doi: 10.1093/eurheartj/ehaa575. © European Society of Cardiology. With permission from Oxford University Press.

Antiplatelet therapy and non-cardiac surgery
Should DAPT be required to be stopped for non-cardiac surgery that cannot be postponed:

- Aspirin should continue uninterrupted.
- Peri-operative cessation of the $P2Y_{12}$ inhibitor may be reasonable 1 month after PCI if the risk and consequences of a recurrent ischaemic event (e.g. stent thrombosis) was felt to be less severe than the risk of bleeding on DAPT. Various factors including stent type, extent of stenting etc need to be considered (most current generation drug eluting/coated stents facilitate 1 month of DAPT).
- Surgery should be performed in centres where there is 24-hour cardiac catheterization lab availability.

Antiplatelet therapy and CABG
- In unstable NSTE-ACS (ongoing ischaemia or haemodynamic instability) patients requiring CABG, surgery should be performed urgently irrespective of antiplatelet therapy.
- In stable patients who have critical anatomy or high-risk features urgent surgery should be performed within 24 hours irrespective of antiplatelet therapy.
- In stable patients without critical anatomy or high-risk features, postponing surgery for at least 3 days after discontinuation of ticagrelor, at least 5 days after clopidogrel, and at least 7 days after prasugrel should be considered.
- Some surgeons will operate on clopidogrel. Aspirin should be continued through surgery.
- Bridging therapy with a glycoprotein IIb/IIIa inhibitor or cangrelor can be used in patients who have recently had drug-eluting stent implantation where cessation of dual antiplatelet therapy is necessitated.
- If DAPT has been stopped to undergo CABG, DAPT should be resumed after surgery for at least 12 months.

Anticoagulants
Unfractionated heparin
- Antithrombotic effects achieved through a number of different pathways most importantly by accelerating the effect of antithrombin on factor Xa.
- Due to poor subcutaneous absorption, intravenous administration is the route of choice.
- A narrow therapeutic window means regular APTT monitoring is mandatory.
- Anticoagulant of choice during PCI.

Low molecular weight heparin
- The antithrombotic effect of low molecular weight heparin (LMWH) is achieved through inhibition of factors IIa and Xa.
- Its major advantages over UFH are in ease of administration, as there is almost complete subcutaneous absorption, and a predictable weight-adjusted dose–effect relationship.
- There is a lower incidence of heparin-induced thrombocytopenia with LMWH as opposed to UFH.
- Due to partial renal excretion, dose adjustment or alternative anticoagulants should be used in patients with significant impairment of renal function.
- FRISC trial demonstrated significant reduction in death and re-infarction in ACS patients treated with LMWH versus placebo (2.5% vs 6%; $p < 0.05$).
- A large meta-analysis of trials comparing LMWH to UFH (21,946 patients) showed that whilst there was no significant difference in death at 30 days between the two, there was a significant reduction in the combined endpoint of death or MI for patients treated with LMWH (10.1% vs 11%; $p < 0.05$). There was no significant difference in major bleeding between the two groups.

Factor Xa inhibitors (fondaparinux)
- Fondaparinux is a synthetic pentasaccharide inhibitor of factor Xa.
- It has 100% bioavailability after subcutaneous injection and a standard dosing of 2.5 mg is recommended for all patients with ACS.
- As with LMWH, excretion is mainly renal and therefore care is advised in patients with significant renal impairment.
- OASIS-5 trial of 20,078 patients showed that fondaparinux was non-inferior to LMWH at preventing future MACE following NSTE-ACS, with the added advantage of halving major bleeds (2.2% vs 4.1% p < 0.001).

Antiplatelet therapy in patients on long-term oral anticoagulants
- Duration of triple therapy should be limited and dependent on the indication for anticoagulation, ischaemic, and bleeding risk.
- The current default strategy recommended by the ESC is as follows (see Figure 2.1.2):
    - Triple antithrombotic therapy (TAT) consisting of an oral anticoagulant (OAC) and DAPT for 1 week, then dual antithrombotic therapy (DAT) for 12 months (which can be

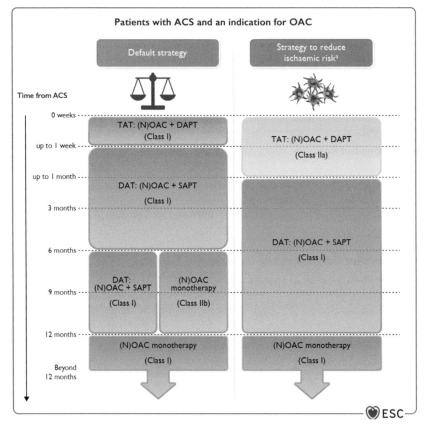

Figure 2.1.2 Antithrombotic regimens in patients with acute coronary syndrome and an indication for oral anticoagulation.

Reproduced from Byrne RA, Rossello X, Coughlan JJ, et al; ESC Scientific Document Group. 2023 ESC Guidelines for the management of acute coronary syndromes. *Eur Heart J.* 2023 Oct 12;44(38):3720–3826. doi: 10.1093/eurheartj/ehad191. © European Society of Cardiology. With permission from Oxford University Press.

shortened to 6 months in those with high bleeding risk) with OAC and single antiplatelet therapy (SAPT), followed by OAC monotherapy lifelong.
- In patients with high ischemic risk, TAT should be prolonged for up to 1 month, followed by DAT for up to 12 months.
- The recommended antiplatelet in SAT is clopidogrel.
- Non-vitamin K antagonist oral anticoagulants (NOACs) are preferred over vitamin K antagonists (VKA). In cases where VKA are mandated (e.g. mechanical prosthetic valves), the same default strategy is recommended with TAT for 1 week, then DAT for up to 12 months.
- In ACS patients undergoing CABG, TAT should be avoided, and DAT should be resumed after CABG as soon as possible.
- Routine use of a proton pump inhibitor is recommended.

Fibrinolytic therapy

- The benefit of fibrinolytic therapy is well established as compared to routine medical therapy, with 30 deaths prevented per 1000 patients treated.
- Early fibrinolysis (< 2 h) is supported by meta-analysis of 22 relevant trials.
- The original fibrinolytic agents were derived from bacterial Streptococcus species; the most common being streptokinase.
- Another group of drugs uses recombinant biotechnology to manufacture tissue plasminogen activator (TPA) using cell culture. These groups are known as recombinant TPA (or rTPA; commonly alteplase, tenecteplase, and urokinase). These drugs break down the cross-links between fibrin molecules, dissolving the fibrin strands which make up blood clots.
- Because of the potential for non-specific fibrin breakdown and a systemic lytic state, there is a significant risk of uncontrolled bleeding.
- Fibrinolytic therapy is commonly contraindicated absolutely in patients with a history of intracranial haemorrhage or recent ischaemic stroke, transient ischaemic attack, head injury or brain surgery, recent internal bleeding or bleeding disorders.
- Relative contraindications are numerous and necessitate a weighing-up of risks vs benefits
- Intracranial haemorrhage occurs in approximately 1% of the treated population, with age, female gender, low BMI, and previous CVA increasing that risk. Significant non-cerebral bleeds occur in 5–15% of patients.

Other medication

Beta blockers

- Beta blockers have been consistently shown to have a beneficial effect in patients with ACS.
- ISIS-1 and MIAMI trials demonstrated a significant mortality benefit in patients with STE-ACS, although these trials were performed before the advent of modern reperfusion therapy.
- Data suggest that beta blockers have beneficial effects for some years post MI, with a mortality benefit seen up to 3 years.
- Although contemporary data are somewhat lacking, meta-analysis has suggested a 13% relative risk reduction in NSTE-ACS patients progressing to STE-ACS when treated with beta blockers.

Statins

- In all subgroups of patients with CAD, statins improve outcomes.
- As well as their beneficial effect on altering the lipid profile, it is increasingly clear that statins have other powerful anti-inflammatory or pleiotropic effects.
- The benefits of statins can be demonstrated very early after ACS, suggesting that these non-cholesterol lowering properties are dominant in this context.

- Studies such as MIRACL, PROVE-IT, and IDEAL have demonstrated clinical benefit for early aggressive statin therapy in ACS.
- The effect of statins is largely mediated by favourably altering the lipid profile of patients in favour of HDL and reducing LDL.
- PROVE-IT trial showed a significant reduction in both measured LDL levels and clinical endpoints in patients taking 80 mg atorvastatin versus those taking 40 mg pravastatin (22.4% vs 26.3%; p = 0.005).
- In patients already on lipid-lowering therapy before admission, this should be intensified either by increasing the dose of the statin and/or by adding in another lipid-lowering agent (e.g. ezetimibe).
- The aim is to achieve an LDL-C level of < 1.4 mmol/L and to reduce LDL-C by ≥ 50% from baseline (ESC guidelines). If this is not achieved on maximally tolerated statin therapy and ezetimibe, additional lipid-lowering therapy is recommended. ESC guidelines recommend the addition of a PCSK9 inhibitor. UK guidelines recommend the addition of bempedoic acid, inclisiran, or a PCSK9 inhibitor.

ACE inhibitors

- ACE inhibitors prevent conversion of angiotensin I to angiotensin II.
- They are potent vasoconstrictors and prevent aldosterone release.
- Benefit to patients with CAD both with or without LV systolic dysfunction has been shown:
    - HOPE trial showed that in patients with preserved LV function and CVD, patients taking 10 mg ramipril had a significant reduction in death, MI, and stroke at 5 years as compared to placebo (14% vs 17.8%; p < 0.001).
    - The benefit of ACE inhibition was seen at 2 years and continued to increase over time, suggesting that long-term therapy is the gold standard for patients with CVD.
    - SMILE trial showed that in patients with LV dysfunction after an anterior MI, those randomized to receive an ACE inhibitor had a significant reduction in death and CCF at 6 weeks as compared to placebo (7.1% vs 10.6%; p = 0.018).

Angiotensin receptor blockers

- Angiotensin receptor blockers (ARBs) block the angiotensin II AT1 receptor producing benefits similar to ACE inhibitors.
- Unlike ACE inhibitors they do not inhibit the breakdown of bradykinin, which causes cough and discontinuation of treatment in up to a quarter of patients:
    - The ONTARGET trial demonstrated non-inferiority of telmisartan as compared to ramipril in the reduction of cardiovascular endpoints in patients with established CVD.
    - With equivalent benefit this leaves ARBs mainly for patients who are ACE inhibitor intolerant.

Colchicine

- The anti-inflammatory agent colchicine has been shown to improve outcomes in patients with acute and chronic coronary syndromes.
- In the Colchicine Cardiovascular Outcomes Trial (COLCOT), which enrolled 4745 patients with a recent ACS event, low-dose colchicine (0.5 mg daily) was associated with a significant reduction of the primary composite endpoint (CV death, resuscitated cardiac arrest, MI, stroke, or urgent revascularization) in comparison to placebo.
- The ESC suggests using low-dose colchicine (0.5 mg once daily) in ACS, particularly if other risk factors are insufficiently controlled or if recurrent cardiovascular disease events occur under optimal therapy.

2.1.8 Diagnostic coronary angiography and revascularization

Timing of an invasive approach
Immediate approach

- An immediate approach is indicated in patients presenting with ACS and the following features
    - Persistent ST segment elevation
    - ST segment depression in leads V1–V3 (especially when the terminal T wave is positive) and/or ST-segment elevation in V7–V9 (highly suggestive of posterior coronary artery occlusion)
    - ST segment depression ≥ 1mm in ≥ 6 surface leads (inferolateral ST depression) with ST elevation in AVR and/or V1 (suggestive of multivessel ischaemia or left main coronary artery occlusion)
    - Recurrent dynamic ST segment or T wave changes, particularly with intermittent ST segment elevation
    - Haemodynamic instability
    - Cardiogenic shock
    - Recurrent/refractory chest pain despite optimal medical management
    - Life-threatening arrhythmias
    - Mechanical complications of MI
    - Acute heart failure related to ACS

Early invasive approach

- ICA is indicated within 24 hours for the following patients (high risk criteria):
    - Confirmed diagnosis of NSTE-ACS based on current recommended ESC hs-cTn algorithms
    - Dynamic ST-segment or T wave changes
    - Transient ST-segment elevation
    - GRACE score > 140
- Data from RCTs have shown that an early invasive approach:
    - Is not associated with a reduction in death, non-fatal MI, or stroke in unselected NSTE-ACS patients.
    - Is associated with a reduction in recurrent/refractory ischaemia and hospital stay.
- An early approach is advocated in patients with at least one of the high risk criteria.

Selective invasive strategy

Patients who do not meet the immediate or early invasive approach criteria (generally patients with clinical suspicion for NSTE-ACS and non-elevated troponins or patients with elevated troponins not meeting the criteria for MI), the strategy can be tailored based on the degree of clinical suspicion.

For patients with a high index of suspicion for unstable angina, an inpatient invasive strategy is recommended. Conversely, for patients with a low index of suspicion, a selective invasive approach is recommended. Non-invasive tests, e.g. CTCA or functional/stress tests should be considered.

Multivessel disease

- In stable STE-ACS patients undergoing PPCI, complete revascularization (culprit lesion and non-infarct related arteries) is recommended either during the index PCI procedure or within 45 days.

- In patients with NSTE-ACS, data from British Cardiovascular Society have shown that single stage complete revascularization is associated with lower cumulative mortality rates when compared to culprit only PCI (n = 21857, 22.5% vs 25.9%, p = 0.0005) with a median follow up at 4.1 years (Rathod et al.).
- Furthermore, the SMILE trial has shown a single stage complete revascularization approach is associated with a lower rate of cardiovascular and cerebrovascular events when compared to multi-stage complete revascularization.
- It is important to remember the benefits of a single complete revascularization procedure must be weighed against the complexity of the CAD when risk assessing these patients.

Coronary artery bypass grafting (CABG)

- 5–10% of NSTE-ACS patients require CABG.
- CABG is typically undertaken during the same inpatient stay. The timing of surgery is based on individual and institutional factors.
- The risk of ischaemia due to suboptimal antiplatelet therapy whilst waiting CABG is 0.1%, whereas the perioperative bleeding complications associated with antiplatelet agents is 10%.
- DAPT should stop prior to CABG and resumed after surgery for at least 12 months.

Specific situations

- Patients with ongoing ischaemia are recommended to have ICA with a view to revascularization within 2 hours of admission to hospital.
- Routine immediate angiography after resuscitated cardiac arrest is not recommended in haemodynamically stable patients without persistent ST-segment elevation (or equivalents).
- Transport of patients with out of hospital cardiac arrests to a cardiac arrest centre according to local protocols should be considered.
- Echocardiography can help in comatose patients with diagnosing alternative diagnoses such as PE or acute aortic dissection.
- Evaluation of neurological prognosis (no earlier than 72 h after admission) is recommended in all comatose survivors after cardiac arrest.

2.1.9 Early and late complications of ACS and their management

LV dysfunction

- Most frequent complication of ACS.
- Patients may be asymptomatic or have significant heart failure.
- Diagnosis is usually made on transthoracic echocardiography.

LV aneurysm

- Can occur in up to 5% of patients presenting with ACS.
- Results from large transmural infarctions with subsequent adverse remodelling leading to the formation of LV aneurysms.
- No mortality benefit from surgical intervention has been shown but can be considered in patients with large aneurysms and uncontrolled heart failure.

LV thrombus

- Known complication of an anterior MI.
- Consider CMR or contrast echo to detect.

- Oral anticoagulation (warfarin or NOAC) is recommended for 3–6 months, with consideration of echo features, bleeding risk, and concomitant use of antiplatelet drugs.

Secondary mitral valve regurgitation
- In the context of ACS, secondary (functional) mitral valve regurgitation is due to LV remodelling leading to displacement of the papillary muscles, leaflet tethering and annular dilatation.
- Traditionally this is a late complication in individuals who have extensive postero-lateral infarction.
- Can be improved through revascularization and medical therapy.
- In non-responders surgery is indicated. Although this improves both survival and LV function when compared to medical therapy, the outlook is still relatively poor.

Papillary muscle rupture
- Typically occurs 2–7 days post infarction and leads to acute mitral regurgitation
- It usually presents as hemodynamic collapse with associated dyspnoea, pulmonary oedema, and cardiogenic shock.
- Diuretic and vasodilator/inotropic support with intra-aortic balloon pump insertion can serve as a bridge towards surgical intervention.
- Mortality is high at 25%.

Free wall rupture
- Occurs in less than 1% of ACS cases.
- Typically occurs in the first week post infarction with sudden pain and/or cardiovascular collapse. Hemopericardium and tamponade invariably occur and is often fatal.
- Risk factors for the development of free wall rupture include increasing age, lack of revascularization and delayed fibrinolysis.
- Partial sealing of the rupture can occur through thrombus formation. This may allow enough time for the passage of a pericardial drain with a view to definitive surgery in the form of ventricular repair with a pericardial patch.
- Mortality is in the order of 25–75%.

Ventricular septal rupture
- Can present acutely with heart failure and cardiogenic shock.
- A loud pansystolic murmur is the hallmark clinical sign in the subacute phase.
- Can occur from 24 hours to several days post infarction.
- Diagnosis is usually made on transthoracic echocardiography.
- When there is a significant right to left shunt, patients usually present with acute onset right heart failure.
- Intra-aortic balloon pumps can serve as a bridge towards definitive surgical treatment.
- The use of diuretics and vasodilators should be undertaken with caution.
- There is no clear consensus on the timing of surgical intervention.
- The survival rates in those who are intervened on early is poor, and this should be weighed against the delay in intervention. Although the survival rates are better in those who have a delayed surgical intervention, there is the increased risk of rupture extension and death when taking this approach.

Pericarditis

- Early pericarditis post infarction can occur and usually transient.
- Late pericarditis (Dressler's syndrome) typically presents 1–2 weeks post infarction, this immune-mediated response is thought to occur as a result of myocardial necrosis leading to pericardial tissue damage.
- In the primary PCI era the event of early and late pericarditis is rare.
- A combination of anti-inflammatory medication (ESC recommends high-dose aspirin or NSAIDs) for 2–4 weeks with colchicine for 3 months.

Arrhythmias

- Atrial fibrillation (AF) is the most common supraventricular arrhythmia in patients with ACS. Prompt treatment is required for AF causing acute haemodynamic instability, with electrical cardioversion being the preferred approach. Adequate rate control can be achieved by administration of beta blockers depending on the presence of HF and low ejection fraction. For patients with low LVEF, amiodarone or digoxin could be used (preferably amiodarone). In cases of hypotension, digoxin is preferred over amiodarone or beta blockers.
- 6-8% of patients with STEMI develop haemodynamically significant VT or VF. The typical arrhythmia presentation is unstable, frequently polymorphic, and relatively fast VT, often degenerating into VF. Urgent reperfusion is most important as ischaemia is often the trigger for these arrhythmias. Early administration of intravenous or oral beta blockers reduces the incidence of malignant arrhythmias. Sustained VT/VF late after reperfusion (> 48 h) requires an evaluation for ICD implantation for secondary prevention of sudden cardiac death.
- In cases of bradyarrhythmias with haemodynamic compromise, intravenous positive chronotropic medication (adrenaline, vasopressin, and/or atropine) is recommended. If this fails, temporary pacing is recommended. Implantation of a permanent pacemaker is recommended when high-degree AV block does not resolve within a waiting period of at least 5 days after MI.

2.1.10 Impact of co-morbidities in ACS

Heart failure and cardiogenic shock

- There is up to fourfold increase in mortality in ACS patients with acute heart failure compared to ACS patients without acute heart failure.
- The diagnosis of ACS in patients with acute heart failure can be difficult, particularly due to incidence of myocardial injury in patients with acute heart failure, which can occur in patients with non-obstructive coronary artery disease and also obstructive coronary artery disease.
- Coronary revascularization should be based on the relevance of coronary artery stenoses to the patient's LV function.
- Ideally decisions on revascularization in these patients should be made by the Heart Team once all the relevant investigations have been undertaken.
- Cardiogenic shock (CS) occurs in around 4% of ACS cases.
- Major causes include acute severe mitral regurgitation, mechanical complications, and acute heart failure related to ischaemia.
- 80% of patients with CS have multivessel disease.
- The CULPRIT-SHOCK trial, which looked at culprit only versus complete revascularization in ACS patients with CS, found the risk of all cause death to be lower in the culprit only group (RR 0.84, 95% CI 0.72–0.98, P = 0.03).

- The use if intra-aortic balloon pumps (IABP) should be considered in ACS related mechanical complications. Routine use is not recommended in CS without mechanical complications.
- In selected patients with ACS and CS, short-term mechanical circulatory support (e.g. Impella device, ECMO) may be considered depending on patient age, comorbidities, neurological function, and the prospects for long-term survival and predicted quality of life.

Diabetes mellitus
- Patients with diabetes more frequently have multifocal coronary artery disease and present with atypical symptoms.
- It has been shown that ACS patients with diabetes have worse clinical outcomes.
- Both ticagrelor and prasugrel have been shown to have higher absolute risk reductions compared to clopidogrel in the diabetic ACS population.
- All ACS patients should have blood glucose monitoring during their hospital stays. It is however important to take into account the glycaemic effect an acute event can cause when diagnosing diabetes in ACS patients.
- Glucose-lowering therapy should be considered in patients with ACS with persistent hyperglycaemia, while episodes of hypoglycaemia should be avoided.

Chronic kidney disease
- Patients with chronic kidney disease (CKD) have a worse prognosis than their ACS counterparts with normal renal function, and in addition less commonly receive evidence-based treatments in the form of medical and invasive treatments.
- In patients with CKD, a rise in cardiac biomarkers could also be due to chronic myocardial injury.
- Patients with CKD are less likely to receive invasive treatment despite a reduced 1-year mortality in patients treated with invasive approach.
- As renal function declines the benefits of an invasive approach decline, with no benefit seen in patient with an eGFR less than 15 ml/min/1.73^2 or receiving dialysis.
- In patients with an eGFR of less than 15 ml/min/1.73^2, there are insufficient data to support the safety and efficacy of $P2Y_{12}$ receptor inhibitors.

Cancer
- Patients with a history of cancer should be treated like all other ACS patients, but the management of ACS patients with active cancer has some specific issues that need to be taken into consideration.
- Given that they are considered to be high bleeding risk, the preferred $P2Y_{12}$ inhibitor for ACS patients with active cancer is clopidogrel.
- Invasive management of ACS is recommended in patients with cancer, as long as the prognosis is > 6 months or, irrespective of the prognosis, if the patient is unstable.
- A temporary interruption of cancer therapy is recommended in patients in whom the cancer therapy is suspected to be a contributing cause of ACS.

Anaemia
- Anaemia is a common problem for many ACS patients.
- Patients with anaemia, in the ACS setting, have an increased risk of mortality, major bleeding, and further MI.
- Choice of medical therapy should be tailored towards bleeding safety.
- Should invasive revascularization be required in these patients, the newer generation of drug-eluting stents (DES) should be used, as there is data for shorter DAPT use with the modern DES.

Thrombocytopenia

- Thrombocytopenia is defined as a platelet count of ≤ 100,000/ml or a relative drop of 50% or more.
- It is also an independent predictor of poorer outcomes including death, major bleeding events, and thrombotic events.
- Thrombocytopenia is more encountered when glycoprotein (GP) IIb/IIIa inhibitors such as abciximab and tirofiban
- Patients given GP IIb/IIIa inhibitors should have their platelet count checked within 8–12 hours of the medication being administered, at the onset of bleeding complications and at 24 hours after administration.
- The infusion of GP IIb/IIIa should be stopped if the platelet count falls below 100,000/ml or there is relative drop of 50% or more.
- Platelet infusions are recommended in the setting of thrombocytopenia with active bleeding.
- Further supportive treatment can be given in the form of fresh frozen plasma, cryoprecipitate, corticosteroids, and immunoglobulins.
- Heparin-induced thrombocytopenia (HIT) occurs in 0.5–3% of patients treated with unfractionated heparin (UFH).
- Typically occurs 5–10 days after heparin use or within hours for patients who have previously been treated with heparin.
- This is a prothrombotic disorder that can potentially be fatal.
- Treatment with non-heparin-based anticoagulants, such as argatroban danaparoid, are recommended.
- All heparin should be discontinued.

The older person

- Advancing age is associated with more atypical presentations of ACS.
- Furthermore, Hs-cTn elevations not due to ACS are more common in the aging population. This can make diagnosing ACS in the older population challenging.
- It is also well established that age is a risk factor for both in-hospital and 6 month mortality.
- Decision-making on whether an invasive approach to treating the older ACS population should be made with a review of a number of factors including the ischaemic and bleeding risks, co-morbidities, life expectancy, quality of life, and cognitive impairment.

Frailty

- Frail patients have been shown to have more complex CAD, have longer lengths of stay in hospital, and have higher risk of death.
- Despite this, frail patients are less likely to receive ACS dedicated pharmacology and invasive treatments.
- No data are available to guide how these patients should be managed. The ESC recommends using a holistic approach to individualize interventional and pharmacological treatments after careful evaluation of the risks and benefits.
- Currently frail patients are treated on a case-by-case scenario with an evaluation of the risks and benefits of any treatment strategy considered.

Further reading

Byrne RA, Rossello X, Coughlan JJ, Barbato E, Berry C, Chieffo A, Claeys MJ, Dan GA, Dweck MR, Galbraith M, Gilard M, Hinterbuchner L, Jankowska EA, Jüni P, Kimura T, Kunadian V, Leosdottir M, Lorusso R, Pedretti RFE, Rigopoulos AG, Rubini Gimenez M, Thiele H, Vranckx P,

Wassmann S, Wenger NK, Ibanez B; ESC Scientific Document Group. 2023 ESC Guidelines for the management of acute coronary syndromes. *Eur Heart J*. 2023 Oct 12;44(38):3720–826. doi: 10.1093/eurheartj/ehad191

Collet JP, Thiele H, Barbato E, Barthélémy O, Bauersachs J, Bhatt DL, Dendale P, Dorobantu M, Edvardsen T, Folliguet T, Gale CP, Gilard M, Jobs A, Jüni P, Lambrinou E, Lewis BS, Mehilli J, Meliga E, Merkely B, Mueller C, Roffi M, Rutten FH, Sibbing D, Siontis GCM; ESC Scientific Document Group. 2020 ESC Guidelines for the management of acute coronary syndromes in patients presenting without persistent ST-segment elevation. *Eur Heart J*. 2021 Apr 7;42(14):1289–367. doi: 10.1093/eurheartj/ehaa575

Ibanez B, James S, Agewall S, Antunes MJ, Bucciarelli-Ducci C, Bueno H, Caforio ALP, Crea F, Goudevenos JA, Halvorsen S, Hindricks G, Kastrati A, Lenzen MJ, Prescott E, Roffi M, Valgimigli M, Varenhorst C, Vranckx P, Widimský P; ESC Scientific Document Group. 2017 ESC Guidelines for the management of acute myocardial infarction in patients presenting with ST-segment elevation: The Task Force for the management of acute myocardial infarction in patients presenting with ST-segment elevation of the European Society of Cardiology (ESC). *Eur Heart J*. 2018 Jan 7;39(2):119–77. doi: 10.1093/eurheartj/ehx393

Lemkes JS, Janssens GN, van der Hoeven NW, Jewbali LSD, Dubois EA, Meuwissen M, Rijpstra TA, Bosker HA, Blans MJ, Bleeker GB, Baak R, Vlachojannis GJ, Eikemans BJW, van der Harst P, van der Horst ICC, Voskuil M, van der Heijden JJ, Beishuizen A, Stoel M, Camaro C, van der Hoeven H, Henriques JP, Vlaar APJ, Vink MA, van den Bogaard B, Heestermans TACM, de Ruijter W, Delnoij TSR, Crijns HJGM, Jessurun GAJ, Oemrawsingh PV, Gosselink MTM, Plomp K, Magro M, Elbers PWG, van de Ven PM, Oudemans-van Straaten HM, van Royen N. Coronary Angiography after Cardiac Arrest without ST-Segment Elevation. *N Engl J Med*. 2019 Apr 11;380(15):1397–407. doi: 10.1056/NEJMoa1816897

Neumann FJ, Sousa-Uva M, Ahlsson A, Alfonso F, Banning AP, Benedetto U, Byrne RA, Collet JP, Falk V, Head SJ, Jüni P, Kastrati A, Koller A, Kristensen SD, Niebauer J, Richter DJ, Seferovic PM, Sibbing D, Stefanini GG, Windecker S, Yadav R, Zembala MO; ESC Scientific Document Group. 2018 ESC/EACTS Guidelines on myocardial revascularization. *Eur Heart J*. 2019 Jan 7;40(2):87–165. doi: 10.1093/eurheartj/ehy394. Erratum in: Eur Heart J. 2019 Oct 1;40(37):3096

Rathod KS, Koganti S, Jain AK, Astroulakis Z, Lim P, Rakhit R, Kalra SS, Dalby MC, O'Mahony C, Malik IS, Knight CJ, Mathur A, Redwood S, Sirker A, MacCarthy PA, Smith EJ, Wragg A, Jones DA. Complete Versus Culprit-Only Lesion Intervention in Patients With Acute Coronary Syndromes. *J Am Coll Cardiol*. 2018 Oct 23;72(17):1989–99. doi: 10.1016/j.jacc.2018.07.089

Redwood S, Curzen N, Thomas M (eds). *Oxford Textbook of Interventional Cardiology*. Oxford: Oxford University Press, 2010.

Sardella G, Lucisano L, Garbo R, Pennacchi M, Cavallo E, Stio RE, Calcagno S, Ugo F, Boccuzzi G, Fedele F, Mancone M. Single-Staged Compared With Multi-Staged PCI in Multivessel NSTEMI Patients: The SMILE Trial. *J Am Coll Cardiol*. 2016 Jan 26;67(3):264–72. doi: 10.1016/j.jacc.2015.10.082

Thiele H, Akin I, Sandri M, Fuernau G, de Waha S, Meyer-Saraei R, Nordbeck P, Geisler T, Landmesser U, Skurk C, Fach A, Lapp H, Piek JJ, Noc M, Goslar T, Felix SB, Maier LS, Stepinska J, Oldroyd K, Serpytis P, Montalescot G, Barthelemy O, Huber K, Windecker S, Savonitto S, Torremante P, Vrints C, Schneider S, Desch S, Zeymer U; CULPRIT-SHOCK Investigators. PCI Strategies in Patients with Acute Myocardial Infarction and Cardiogenic Shock. *N Engl J Med*. 2017 Dec 21;377(25):2419–32. doi: 10.1056/NEJMoa1710261

Thygesen K, Alpert JS, Jaffe AS, Chaitman BR, Bax JJ, Morrow DA, White HD; Executive Group on behalf of the Joint European Society of Cardiology (ESC)/American College of Cardiology (ACC)/American Heart Association (AHA)/World Heart Federation (WHF) Task Force for the Universal Definition of Myocardial Infarction. Fourth Universal Definition of Myocardial Infarction (2018). *J Am Coll Cardiol*. 2018 Oct 30;72(18):2231–64. doi: 10.1016/j.jacc.2018.08.1038

2.2

Chronic Coronary Syndrome

Phillip Freeman and Majd Protty

TABLE OF CONTENTS

- 2.2.1 Pathogenesis of atherosclerosis 147
- 2.2.2 Risk factors for atherosclerosis 149
- 2.2.3 Coronary physiology 151
- 2.2.4 Myocardial ischaemia, stunning, hibernation, and viability 151
- 2.2.5 Prognosis of chronic coronary syndromes and risk stratification 152
- 2.2.6 Clinical assessment of known or suspected chronic coronary syndrome 153
  - Angina pectoris 153
  - Differential diagnosis of chest pain 154
  - Non-cardiac causes of chest pain 154
- 2.2.7 Investigation of suspected chronic coronary syndrome 156
  - Assessment of pre-test probability and clinical likelihood of coronary artery disease 156
  - Selecting appropriate testing (ESC Guidelines 2019) 156
  - Selecting appropriate testing (UK NICE Guidelines 2016) 158
- 2.2.8 Management of chronic coronary syndromes 159
  - Lifestyle recommendations 159
  - Pharmacological management 159
- 2.2.9 Coronary revascularization 161
  - PCI vs CABG 161
- 2.2.10 Angina without obstructive disease in the epicardial coronary arteries 162
  - Microvascular angina 162
  - Vasospastic angina 163
- 2.2.11 Alternative interventions for chronic refractory angina 163

2.2.1 Pathogenesis of atherosclerosis

A graphical representation of the development of atherosclerosis is shown in Figure 2.2.1.

- Atherosclerosis is a chronic and multifocal immuno-inflammatory, fibroproliferative disease of medium- and large-sized arteries, mainly driven by lipid accumulation and macrophage deposition/uptake of oxidized Low-Density Lipoproteins (oxLDL) leading to formation of 'foam cells'
- Develops over many decades, first evident in the second decade of life
- Basic knowledge of the normal arterial structure is required in order to understand the process of underlying atherogenesis (see Figure 2.2.2)
- Progression of atherosclerosis is unpredictable and is impacted by well-characterized risk factors
- Coronary plaque progression is complex and heterogeneous
- Initial lipid deposition is triggered by activation of endothelial cells and recruitment of inflammatory leucocytes such as monocytes and T lymphocytes, via chemo-attractant and adhesion molecules
- Monocytes within the plaque transform into macrophages and scavenge modified lipoproteins, becoming lipid-laden foam cells
- Foam cells play an important role in the dynamics of the plaque through release of cytokines including tissue factor, tumour necrosis factor α (TNF α), interleukins, and metalloproteinases
- Further recruitment of leucocytes is driven by release of inflammatory cytokines and growth factors, with additional effects on smooth muscle cell migration and proliferation

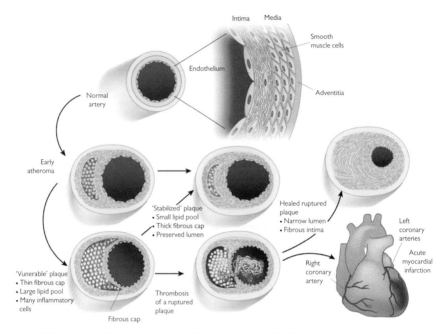

Figure 2.2.1 Graphical representation of the development of atherosclerosis from infancy to adulthood.
Reproduced from Libby, P. Inflammation in atherosclerosis. *Nature* 420, 868–874 (2002). https://doi.org/10.1038/nature01323 with permission from Springer.

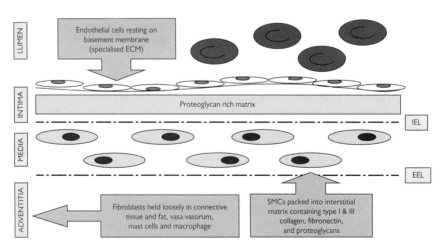

Figure 2.2.2 An illustration of the normal composition of the arterial wall. ECM, extracellular matrix; IEL, internal elastic lamina—a further layer of ECM composed primarily of elastin fibres which acts as a barrier to the transport of high molecular weight molecules between intima and media; SMC, smooth muscle cells—packed between the internal and external elastic laminae, predominantly orientated in a circumferential pattern; EEL, external elastic lamina

- Ultimately plaques consist of fibrous, calcific, lipidic, and necrotic components—vulnerability is discussed in Chapter 2.1 (ACS)
- Arterial remodelling is bidirectional—initially the vessel compensates for the accumulation of plaque through outward expansion (positive remodelling) and ultimately plaque accumulation overtakes vessel expansion and luminal narrowing develops.

2.2.2 Risk factors for atherosclerosis

Risk factors for atherosclerosis are shown in Table 2.2.1.

Male gender
- In the UK, 1 in 5 men die from coronary disease under the age of 75 (one in seven women).
- After the menopause, female risk increases greatly, with a 55-year-old woman having an identical risk of cardiovascular death to a 45-year-old man.

Genetic predisposition
- Increased risk associated with a family history of early ischaemic heart disease (IHD) (male < 55 years and female < 65 years) ranges between 1.5 and 1.7 times the normal population and is independent of other risk factors.
- There appear to be vulnerable genotypes, which are intrinsically related to the pathophysiology of IHD, i.e. those affecting dyslipidaemia, endothelial dysfunction, diabetes, and hypertension.
- Candidate genes have been investigated, but in isolation have little effect on overall risk stratification above that of traditional risk factors.

Smoking
- Smoking accelerates atherosclerosis through:
    - Increase in blood pressure and sympathetic tone
    - Reduction in myocardial oxygen supply
    - Oxidation of LDL
    - Impairment of endothelial function through disruption of nitric oxide synthesis
    - Spontaneous platelet aggregation
- Smoking cessation offers the greatest impact in preventative cardiology, with a reduction in cardiac mortality of 30–40%.

Hypertension
- Prevalence of hypertension increasing
- Systolic and diastolic pressure are important determinants of risk.

Table 2.2.1 Risk factors for atherosclerosis.

Conventional	Novel
Male gender	hs-CRP
Genetic predisposition	Homocysteine
Smoking	Fibrinogen/fibrin
Hypertension	Lipoprotein (a)
Hyperlipidaemia	
Diabetes	

- Reduction in SBP of 10 mmHg or in DBP of 5 mmHg reduces all major CV events by ~20%, all-cause mortality by 10–15%, stroke by ~35%, coronary events by ~20%, and heart failure by ~40% (ESC Guidelines 2018).
- ESC Guidelines 2018 recommend commencing lifestyle modifications as first-line therapy in all patients with hypertension.
- If executed well, low salt diet (DASH diet) and exercise are often highly effective
- Pharmacological therapy to be commenced immediately in patients with Grade 2–3 hypertension, and in Grade 1 patients with high risk of CVD (additional risk factors, or 10-year SCORE risk calculation of > 5%), renal disease or hypertension-mediated organ damage.

Hyperlipidaemia

- Raised total cholesterol and LDL-C levels are positively associated with ischaemic heart disease (IHD) mortality
    - For each 1 mmol/L reduction in LDL-C levels, a 10% reduction in all-cause mortality and 23% reduction in coronary events is observed.
- Inverse relationship between high density lipoprotein (HDL) level and vascular risk—attributed to 'reverse cholesterol transport'
- Elevated triglyceride levels are associated with increased CVD risk
- Low HDL and high triglycerides level are components of the metabolic syndrome
- ESC Guidelines on dyslipidaemia 2016 describe treatment targets based on cardiovascular risk as calculated by the SCORE system.
    - Very high risk: < 1.8 mmol/L LDL-C
    - High risk: < 2.6 mmol/L LDL-C
    - Low to moderate risk: < 3.0 mmol/L

Diabetes and metabolic syndrome

- Diabetes is a potent risk factor for CAD and is associated with a high burden of atherosclerosis
- Hyperglycaemia is associated with microvascular dysfunction and insulin resistance appears to promote atherosclerosis
- Presence of the metabolic syndrome elevates risk of CAD
- A number of definitions exist for metabolic syndrome, but all include glucose intolerance, raised triglycerides, low HDL levels, hypertension, microalbuminuria, small dense LDL particles, and central obesity
- ESC Guidelines on Diabetes (2013) recommend a tight glycaemic control with an HbA1c less than 7% (or 53 mmol/mol).

Novel risk factors

- Large numbers of novel risk factors for CVD have been considered
- Widespread adoption of these risk factors is often limited by a combination of paucity of data and the lack of a standardized commercial assay for measurement/detection
- High sensitivity C-reactive protein (hs-CRP), lipoprotein (a), and homocysteine have the greatest amount of data supporting their value in risk assessment
- Hs-CRP:
    - Is a marker of inflammation but may also directly influence plaque vulnerability
    - Its role in risk assessment that is most likely limited to individuals with moderate or high risk, defined by conventional risk factors

- Homocysteine:
  - Homocysteine is a sulfhydryl-containing amino acid derived from demethylation of dietary methionine
  - A genetic defect in methionine metabolism can result in severe hyperhomocysteinaemia and associates with premature CAD
  - In the general population, elevated homocysteine levels tend to associate with poor dietary intake of folic acid
  - Elevated homocysteine levels are linked with an increased incidence of premature CAD and rate of venous thromboembolism
- Lipoprotein(a)—Lp(a):
  - Lipoprotein (a) is composed of an LDL particle with its apolipoprotein B-100 component linked to apolipoprotein (a)
  - Lipoprotein (a) is a complex molecule and has over 25 heritable forms
  - Lipoprotein shares many of the structural characteristics with plasminogen, strengthening the link with atherothrombosis.

2.2.3 Coronary physiology

- Coronary blood flow at rest forms approximately 5% of cardiac output
  - In 50% of people, flow in the RCA > LCA
  - In 20%, flow in LCA > RCA
  - In 30% flow in LCA = RCA
- The majority of coronary blood flow occurs during diastole, where the myocardial pressure drops below the diastolic pressure within the coronary arterioles allowing flow.
  - This hydrostatic pressure drops as the arteriole traverses from epicardium to endocardium
  - This is why the endocardium is most at risk of ischaemia
  - Factors that shorten diastole (e.g. tachyarrhythmia) impact on coronary flow and therefore may lead to ischaemia.
- Mechanisms that affect coronary luminal area directly impact on blood flow, and therefore oxygen delivery, these include:
  - Arteriolar autoregulation in response to pressure within vessels
  - Local metabolites such as adenosine and nitric oxide (both dilators)
  - Nervous regulation through sympathetic and parasympathetic stimulation
    - alpha adrenoreceptors: vasoconstriction →↓flow downstream
    - beta adrenoreceptors: ↑contractility →↑stroke volume →↑cardiac output →↑coronary blood flow
    - acetylcholine (vagus n.) →minimal vasodilation
  - Pathological factors impacting on luminal area such as atherosclerosis and thrombosis impair blood flow and lead to myocardial ischaemia

2.2.4 Myocardial ischaemia, stunning, hibernation, and viability

Myocardial ischaemia

- Myocardial ischaemia is commonly driven by:
  - Coronary atherosclerosis
  - Coronary vasoconstriction
  - Coronary artery thrombosis
- Ischaemia is the result of a mismatch between oxygen demand and supply and a cascade of events that ensues (see Figure 2.2.3)

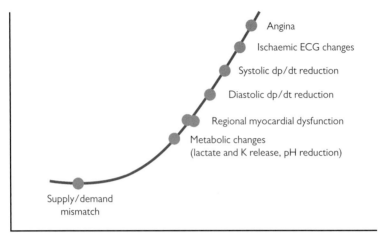

Figure 2.2.3 'The ischaemic cascade'. Sequence of events following mismatch between oxygen supply and demand.

- Initially ischaemia impacts at a cellular level with cell swelling, glycogen depletion, and apoptosis; ongoing tissue hypoxia results in ATP depletion, increased lactate levels, and acidosis
- Myocardial contractility diminishes and the loss of intracellular potassium and a reduction in the transmembrane potassium gradient drives ECG change
- Ischaemic chest pain is a late feature; an afferent pathway of non-medullated small sympathetic nerve fibres runs parallel to coronary arteries and enters the spinal cord from C8–T4
- Impulses are transmitted to corresponding spinal ganglia and then through the spinal cord to the thalamus and cerebral cortex
- Angina pectoris, like other pain of visceral origin, is often poorly localized and is commonly referred to the corresponding segmental dermatomes.

Myocardial stunning, hibernation, and viability

- *Stunning:* A term proposed over three decades ago to refer to areas of the myocardium with depressed contractility as a consequence of ischaemic insults with a short duration.
    - Such areas are expected to recover spontaneously within a few days.
- *Hibernation/Viability:* Often the two terms are (confusingly) used interchangeably in the literature to refer to areas of the myocardium which are dysfunctional at rest, but not scarred, and therefore have the potential for functional recovery upon revascularization. Such dysfunction is a consequence of severe and sustained reduction in coronary blood flow.
    - The consensus is to use the term *hibernation* 'retrospectively', i.e. dysfunctional myocardium which *has* improved following revascularization
    - Whereas *viability* is to be used 'prospectively', i.e. dysfunctional myocardium which *may* improve if revascularized

2.2.5 Prognosis of chronic coronary syndromes and risk stratification

- Prognostic information is derived from clinical assessment and subsequent investigations. The main factors that influence prognosis are left ventricular function and severity of coronary disease.

- Clinical evaluation: adverse prognosis implied by presence of heart failure symptoms, peripheral vascular disease, obesity, and metabolic syndrome.
  - Limited correlation between symptoms and severity
  - Risk scores (e.g. Framingham) were not designed for a population with symptoms, and therefore have limited value
- Assessment of LV function (e.g. echo/CMR): Mortality increases as LVEF declines.
  - 12-year survival rate of patients with LVEF > 50%, 35–49%, and < 35% were 73%, 54%, and 21%, respectively
- Non-invasive stress tests:
  - Exercise ECG: High risk indicated by ST segment depression ≥ 1 mm at Bruce stage 1, slow ST depression recovery (> 5 min) after exercise, less than 4 METs achieved, abnormal blood pressure response, or Duke treadmill score ≤ –11
  - Stress myocardial scintigraphy: High risk features are multiple and/or large and/or severe reversible perfusion defects, stress-induced left ventricular dilation, stress-induced lung thallium-201 uptake
  - Stress echocardiography: Multiple and/or large and/or severe regional wall motion abnormalities, stress-induced left ventricular dilatation
- Coronary angiography: Extent of atherosclerosis found to be a better predictor of poor outcome than severity. Consequently, higher risk with multi-vessel disease (e.g. 3-vessel disease carries 50% risk of mortality at 12 years in CASS registry) particularly if proximal LAD affected (5-year survival 54% in 3-vessel disease with > 95% LAD stenosis, compared to 79% in 3-vessel disease without LAD stenosis).
  - Limited value in using scores that quantify extent of disease (e.g. SYNTAX)

2.2.6 Clinical assessment of known or suspected chronic coronary syndrome

Angina pectoris

- Anginal chest pain:
  - Is constricting discomfort in the front of the chest, or in the neck, shoulders, jaw, or arms
  - Is precipitated by physical exertion
  - Is relieved by rest or GTN within about 5 minutes

The presence of all 3 features above is described as 'typical anginal pain'. The presence of 2 out of 3 is described as 'atypical angina' and 0–1 out of 3 is 'non-anginal pain'

- Characteristically involves build-up of pain—crescendo in nature
- 'Shooting' or 'stabbing' pain that reaches maximum intensity fast is more likely musculoskeletal or neural in origin
- Location:
  - Classically retrosternal or just left of midline with heavy radiation bilaterally (left arm + right arm) and into neck and lower jaw
  - In the arms the discomfort or heaviness can be bilateral. Note Levine's sign, which is one or two clenched fists held over the sternum
- Exacerbators of anginal chest pain include:
  - Exercise
  - Emotional stress
  - Anxiety
  - Anger

> **BOX 2.2.1 CANADIAN CARDIOVASCULAR SOCIETY (CCS) FUNCTIONAL CLASSIFICATION OF ANGINA PECTORIS**
>
> **I** Ordinary physical activity, such as walking and climbing stairs, does not cause angina. Angina results from strenuous or rapid or prolonged exertion at work or recreation.
>
> **II** Slight limitation of ordinary activity. Walking or climbing stairs rapidly, walking uphill, walking or climbing after meals, in cold, in wind, or when under emotional stress, or only during the few hours after awakening. Walking more than two blocks on the level and climbing more than one flight of ordinary stairs at a normal pace and under normal conditions.
>
> **III** Marked limitations of ordinary physical activity. Walking one to two blocks on the level and climbing more than one flight under normal conditions.
>
> **IV** Inability to carry on any physical activity without discomfort—anginal syndrome may be present at rest.
>
> Reproduced from 'Letter: Grading of angina pectoris', L. Campeau, *Circulation* 54, 522–3, copyright 1976, with permission of Wolters Kluwer Health.

- Lying down—angina decubitus
- After meals—post-prandial angina
- Extreme heat/cold
- Anaemia
- Thyrotoxicosis
- Hypoxia

• Response to GTN cannot always be used as a marker of cardiac chest pain as it induces widespread smooth muscle relaxation. GTN may relieve pain secondary to oesophageal spasm or biliary colic.

• The severity of anginal symptoms has been classified as outlined in Box 2.2.1.

Differential diagnosis of chest pain

• Differential diagnostic list for chest pain is extensive (Table 2.2.2)
• Suspecting a diagnosis of cardiac chest pain should not immediately exclude other (at times critical) differential diagnoses
• Appropriate diagnosis requires effective history taking, examination, and investigation
• Investigation should augment not replace physician–patient communication.

Non-cardiac causes of chest pain

Respiratory

• Commonly sharp and localized, with exacerbation through inspiration or coughing (often described as pleuritic)
• Pain in the shoulder tip suggests irritation of the diaphragmatic pleura
• History, including assessment of risk factors for venous thrombo-embolism, associated symptoms (cough, sputum), and signs on examination required for assessment of aetiology.

Gastrointestinal

• 'Heartburn' secondary to gastrointestinal irritation sometimes difficult to distinguish from cardiac chest pain
• Patients often suffer with oesophageal spasm which can respond well to sublingual nitrates (smooth muscle)

Table 2.2.2 Differential diagnosis of chest pain.

System	Diagnosis
Cardiac	
Ischaemic origin	Angina pectoris
	Aortic stenosis
	Hypertrophic cardiomyopathy
	Aortic regurgitation
	Severe systemic hypertension
	Severe pulmonary hypertension
Non-ischaemic origin	Aortic dissection
	Pericarditis/myopericarditis
	Mitral valve prolapse
Respiratory	Pneumonia
	Pneumothorax
	Pulmonary embolism
	Pleurisy
Gastrointestinal	Oesophageal reflux
	Oesophageal rupture
	Oesophageal spasm
	Peptic ulcer disease
	Gallbladder disease
	Pancreatitis
Neuromusculoskeletal	Degenerative joint disease of cervical/thoracic spine
	Costochondritis (Tietze's syndrome)
	Thoracic outlet syndrome
	Trauma/musculoskeletal injury
Psychogenic	Anxiety (Da Costa's syndrome)
	Depression
Infectious	Herpes zoster

- Classically symptoms may associate with meals or a recumbent position
- Burning quality with associated belching is common, and symptoms often can be relieved with use of antacids.

Neuro-musculoskeletal

- Often difficult to distinguish from cardiac chest pain
- Reliant upon thorough history taking, with particular emphasis on precipitating factors, the duration of symptoms, and localization
- Thorough patient examination will aid differentiation of neurological causes for pain

- Antecedent history of trauma/injury, prolonged duration of pain, exacerbation of symptoms with movement or respiration, reproduction of pain on palpation, and pinpoint localization of discomfort all increase the likelihood of a musculoskeletal aetiology
- Chest pain relating to nerve impingement is likely to be confined to specific dermatomes and may involve associated paraesthesia.

Psychogenic/Functional
- Many terms exist to describe psychogenic chest pain, including: Da Costa's syndrome, soldier's heart, effort syndrome, and cardiac neurosis
- All listed as 'somatoform autonomic dysfunction' by the World Health Organization in the ICD-10 classification
- Physical manifestation of anxiety disorder—classically symptoms include:
  - Sharp or stabbing left submammary chest pain
  - Palpitations
  - Breathlessness/hyperventilation.
  - Symptoms often occurs at rest and there is usually no relationship to exertion
  - Symptoms may occur for long periods of time over 30 minutes and sometimes days

2.2.7 Investigation of suspected chronic coronary syndrome

The approach for the initial diagnostic management of patients with angina and suspected coronary disease is illustrated in Figure 2.2.4.

Assessment of pre-test probability and clinical likelihood of coronary artery disease

The likelihood of obstructive CAD is influenced by the prevalence of the disease in the population studied, as well as by clinical features of an individual patient.
Table 2.2.3 shows pre-test probabilities (PTP) of obstructive coronary disease in 15,815 symptomatic patients according to age, sex, and the nature of their symptoms in a pooled analysis of contemporary data.

Selecting appropriate testing (ESC Guidelines 2019)
- Selection of the appropriate diagnostic test is based on the clinical likelihood of CAD and other patient characteristics that influence test performance, local expertise, and the availability of tests.
- Coronary CTA is the preferred test in patients with a lower range of clinical likelihood of CAD, no previous diagnosis of CAD and characteristics associated with a high likelihood of good image quality (e.g. sinus rhythm, low heart rate).
- Non-invasive functional tests for ischaemia typically have better rule in power and are associated with fewer downstream referrals for invasive coronary angiography (ICA) compared with anatomical imaging. Functional imaging is recommended if CTA shows CAD of uncertain significance or is non-diagnostic.
- Coronary CTA complemented by CT-based FFR combines anatomical and functional assessment and has been shown in patients with extensive CAD to be non-inferior to ICA and FFR for decision-making and the identification of targets for revascularization.
- Proceeding directly to ICA should be considered in a patient with a high clinical likelihood of CAD, symptoms unresponsive to medical therapy or typical angina at a low level of exercise, and an initial clinical or non-invasive evaluation that indicates a high event risk.
- The definitions of high event risk for different test modalities is illustrated in Table 2.2.4.

2.2.7 Investigation of suspected chronic coronary syndrome

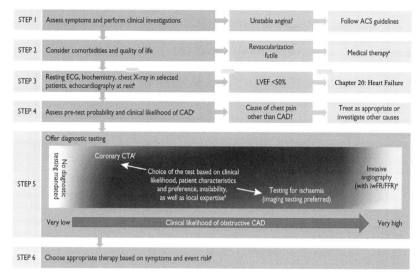

Figure 2.2.4. Approach for the initial diagnostic management of patients with angina and suspected coronary artery disease. [a]If the diagnosis of CAD is uncertain, establishing a diagnosis using non-invasive functional imaging for myocardial ischaemia before treatment may be reasonable. [b]May be omitted in very young and healthy patients with a high suspicion of an extracardiac cause of chest pain, and in multimorbid patients in whom the echocardiography result has no consequence for further patient management. [c]Consider exercise ECG to assess symptoms, arrhythmias, exercise tolerance, BP response, and event risk in selected patients. [d]Ability to exercise, individual test-related risks, and likelihood of obtaining diagnostic test result. [e]High clinical likelihood and symptoms inadequately responding to medical treatment, high event risk based on clinical evaluation (such as ST-segment depression, combined with symptoms at a low workload or systolic dysfunction indicating CAD), or uncertain diagnosis on non-invasive testing. [f]Functional imaging for myocardial ischaemia if coronary CTA has shown CAD of uncertain grade or is non-diagnostic. [g]Consider also angina without obstructive disease in the epicardial coronary arteries.

Reproduced from Knuuti J, Wijns W, Saraste A, et al; ESC Scientific Document Group. 2019 ESC Guidelines for the diagnosis and management of chronic coronary syndromes. Eur Heart J. 2020 Jan 14;41(3):407–477. doi: 10.1093/eurheartj/ehz425. © European Society of Cardiology. With permission from Oxford University Press.

Table 2.2.3 Pre-test probability of finding obstructive coronary artery disease based on a patient's symptoms, age and sex.

Age	Typical		Atypical		Non-anginal		Dyspnoea[a]	
	Men	Women	Men	Women	Men	Women	Men	Women
30–39	3%	5%	4%	3%	1%	1%	0%	3%
40–49	22%	10%	10%	6%	3%	2%	12%	3%
50–59	32%	13%	17%	6%	11%	3%	20%	9%
60–69	44%	16%	26%	11%	22%	6%	27%	14%
70+	52%	27%	34%	19%	24%	10%	32%	12%

[a]In addition to the classic Diamond and Forrester classes, patients with dyspnoea only or dyspnoea as the primary symptom are included. The regions shaded dark green denote the groups in which non-invasive testing is most beneficial (PTP > 15%). The regions shaded light green denote the groups with PTPs of CAD between 5% and 15%, in which, testing for diagnosis may be considered after assessing the overall clinical likelihood based on the modifiers of PTPs presented in Figure 2.2.5.
Adapted from ESC Guidelines 2019 for the diagnosis and management of chronic coronary syndromes.

Table 2.2.3 shows pre-test probabilities (PTP) of obstructive coronary disease in 15,815 symptomatic patients according to age, sex, and the nature of their symptoms in a pooled analysis of contemporary data.

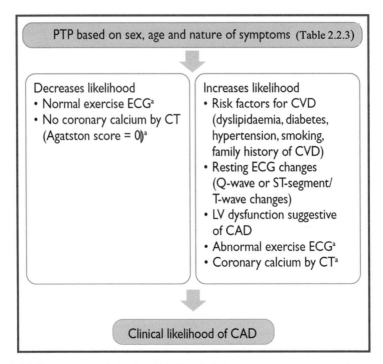

Figure 2.2.5 Determinants of the clinical likelihood of obstructive coronary artery disease.
[a]When available.
Adapted from ESC Guidelines 2019 for the diagnosis and management of chronic coronary syndromes.
Reproduced from Knuuti J, Wijns W, Saraste A, et al; ESC Scientific Document Group. 2019 ESC Guidelines for the diagnosis and management of chronic coronary syndromes. *Eur Heart J*. 2020 Jan 14;41(3):407–477. doi: 10.1093/eurheartj/ehz425. © European Society of Cardiology. With permission from Oxford University Press.

Selecting appropriate testing (UK NICE Guidelines 2016)

The UK NICE guidelines (updated 2016) for recent-onset chest pain of suspected cardiac origin: assessment and diagnosis recommend for people presenting with stable chest pain:

Table 2.2.4 Definitions of high event risk for different test modalities in patients with established chronic coronary syndromes.

Exercise ECG	Cardiovascular mortality > 3% per year according to Duke Treadmill Score
SPECT or PET perfusion imaging	Area of ischaemia ≥ 10% of the left ventricle myocardium
Stress echocardiography	≥ 3 of 16 segments with stress-induced hypokinesia or akinesia
CMR	≥ 2 of 16 segments with stress perfusion defects or ≥3 dobutamine-induced dysfunctional segments
Coronary CTA or ICA	Three-vessel disease with proximal stenoses, LM disease, or proximal anterior descending disease
Invasive functional testing	FFR ≤ 0.8, iwFR ≤ 0.89

CTA—computed tomography angiography; CMR—cardiac magnetic resonance; ECG—electrocardiogram; FFR—fractional flow reserve; ICA—invasive coronary angiography; iwFR—instantaneous wave-free ration (instant flow reserve); LM—left main; PET—positron emission tomography; SPECT—single-photon emission computed tomography.
Reproduced from Knuuti J, Wijns W, Saraste A, et al; ESC Scientific Document Group. 2019 ESC Guidelines for the diagnosis and management of chronic coronary syndromes. *Eur Heart J*. 2020 Jan 14;41(3):407–477. doi: 10.1093/eurheartj/ehz425. © European Society of Cardiology. With permission from Oxford University Press.

- First-line: Offer CT coronary angiography (CTCA) in patients with typical or atypical angina or in those patients with non-anginal symptoms but 12-lead resting ECG indicates ST-T changes or Q waves
- For people with confirmed CAD (previous MI, revascularization, previous angiography), offer non-invasive functional testing when there is uncertainty about whether chest pain is caused by myocardial ischaemia.
- Third-line: Offer invasive coronary angiography when the results of non-invasive functional imaging are inconclusive.

2.2.8 Management of chronic coronary syndromes

Lifestyle recommendations
- Smoking cessation
- Healthy diet high in vegetables, fruit, and wholegrains. Limit saturated fat to < 10% of total intake and alcohol to < 100 g/week or 15 g/day
- Moderate physical activity 30–60 min most days
- Obtain and maintain a healthy weight < 25 kg/m²
- Exercise-based cardiac rehabilitation, cognitive behavioural interventions, and involvement of multidisciplinary healthcare professionals are recommended to help individuals achieve a healthy lifestyle
- Psychological interventions recommended to improve symptoms of depression
- Annual influenza vaccination recommended, especially in the elderly

Pharmacological management
Anti-ischaemic drugs
General principles:
- Short-acting nitrates are recommended in all.
- First line treatment is indicated with beta blockers (BB) or calcium channel blockers (CCB). BBs preferred if recent MI or heart failure with reduced EF.
- Combination of BB and CCB (dihydropyridine) recommended if symptoms not controlled.
- Second-line treatment options (in combination with BB and/or CCB) are long-acting nitrates, ranolazine, ivabradine, nicorandil, or trimetazidine.

Short-acting nitrates
- Spray acts more rapidly than sublingual nitroglycerin.
- Advise patient to rest in a sitting position when taking to avoid collapse from hypotension, take 0.3–0.6 mg tablet sublingually not swallowed or 0.4 mg spray to the tongue every 5 mins until pain disappears or a maximum of 1.2 mg taken within 15 minutes. If angina persists, immediate medical attention required.
- Can be administered for prophylaxis before physical activity.

Long-acting nitrates
- Nitrates are exogenous source of vasodilator nitric oxide.
- Dilate large coronary arteries and arterioles > 100 μm, enhancing collateral supply and relieving dynamic stenoses/coronary spasm. Also reduce afterload and preload of the heart, reducing myocardial oxygen demand.
- Can be administered orally or transdermally through slow-release patches.

- Chronic use produces tolerance with loss of efficacy—requires prescription of nitrate free/low interval (10–14 hours)—modified release preparations overcome this problem.
- Common side effects are headache, hypotension, and flushing.
- Contraindications include severe aortic stenosis, hypertrophic obstructive cardiomyopathy, and co-administration of phosphodiesterase inhibitors (e.g. sildenafil) or riociguat.

Beta-receptor antagonists (beta blockers)
- Beta blockade results in reduced oxygen demand through a reduction in heart rate and blood pressure, and myocardial contractility. Also lengthens diastolic filling time through slowing myocyte relaxation, enhancing myocardial perfusion.
- Multiple indications for use. Good evidence of prognostic benefit in patients with recent MI and heart failure with reduced EF. Also beneficial for treatment of arrhythmias and hypertension. (Drug choice in patients with angina pectoris is often determined by the presence of concomitant conditions.)
- Protective benefits in patients without prior or recent MI (> 1 year) or heart failure less well established (no proven mortality benefit).
- Chronic therapy leads to an increased beta-receptor density and consequently abrupt withdrawal can result in exacerbation of angina and MI.
- Adjust dose to limit heart rate to 55–60 bpm.
- Common side effects are bradycardia, heart block, fatigue, depression, bronchospasm, peripheral vasoconstriction, impotence, masking of hypoglycaemic symptoms, nightmares.

Calcium channel antagonists
- Calcium channel blockade primarily induces peripheral vasodilation and a reduction in peripheral vascular resistance.
- Two groups within the family—dihydropyridines and non-dihydropyridines (NDHPs)—the NDHPs (e.g. verapamil) have an additional effect on nodal tissue with a resultant reduction in heart rate and myocardial contractility.
- Anti-anginal properties include the reduction of afterload, and negative chronotropic and inotropic effect.
- Combination of NDHPs (particularly verapamil) with beta blockers not advised due to the risk of bradycardia and heart block. NDHPs also not advised in heart failure.
- Side effects of dihydropyridines are related to vasodilatory effects: e.g. headache and ankle oedema.

Ranolazine
- Ranolazine acts through modulating the trans-cellular late sodium current. It indirectly prevents the calcium overload via an effect on sodium-dependent calcium channels.
- Unique to other antianginals as does not affect blood pressure or heart rate.
- Side effects include dizziness, nausea, and constipation. Also causes prolongation of the QT interval.

Ivabradine
- Ivabradine selectively inhibits the pacemaker I_f current in a dose-dependent manner. Blocking this channel reduces cardiac pacemaker activity, slowing the heart rate and allowing more time for blood to flow to the myocardium.
- Similarity between the I_f channels and I_h ion channels found in the retina can lead to visual field disturbance. Other side effects include bradycardia and headache.

Nicorandil

- Nicorandil is a potassium channel activator (opens mitochondrial ATP-sensitive potassium channels) with a nitrate component and has both arterial and venous vasodilating properties.
- Side effects include headache, flushing, nausea, vomiting, and potentially severe skin, oral, intestinal, and mucosal ulceration.
- Avoid in patients with heart failure or those with diverticular disease.

Trimetazidine

- Has haemodynamically neutral side-effect profile.
- Contraindicated in Parkinson's disease and other motion disorders (e.g. tremor, restless legs).

Event prevention drugs

- Low-dose aspirin recommended in patients with a previous MI or revascularization (clopidogrel if aspirin intolerant).
- Statins are recommended in all patients with chronic coronary syndrome. Combination with other lipid lowering therapies recommended if targets not achieved.
- ACE-inhibitors recommended if a patient has other conditions (heart failure, hypertension, diabetes) and should be considered in chronic coronary syndrome patients at very high risk of cardiovascular events.

2.2.9 Coronary revascularization

The aim of revascularization (by PCI or CABG) is to either improve survival or diminish/eradicate symptoms.
Indications for revascularization in patients with stable angina or silent ischaemia (from 2018 ESC/EACTS Guidelines on Myocardial Revascularisation)
For prognosis:

- LMS or proximal LAD stenosis > 50%*.
- Two or three vessel disease with stenosis > 50%* with impaired LV function (LVEF ≤ 35%).
- Proven large area of ischaemia (> 10% LV) or abnormal invasive FFR (< 0.75).
- Single remaining patent coronary artery with stenosis > 50%*.
* With documented ischaemia or a haemodynamically relevant lesion defined by FFR ≤ 0.80 or iwFR ≤ 0.89, or > 90% stenosis in a major coronary vessel.

For symptoms:
- Haemodynamically significant stenosis* with limiting angina despite optimal medical therapy (including lifestyle and dietary changes).

PCI vs CABG

- Recent evidence (ISCHAEMIA trial 2020) suggests that PCI in patients with stable symptoms and moderate–severe ischaemia does not alter survival compared to medical therapy but is effective in reducing symptoms and spontaneous MI (increased periprocedural MI of uncertain significance, patients with left main disease and LVEF ≤ 35% were excluded).
- CABG trials have demonstrated improved 5-year survival rates in the following groups:
    - Significant (>70%) left main stenosis
    - Significant (>70%) proximal stenoses of the three major vessels
    - Significant (>70%) stenosis of two major vessels including the proximal LAD
    - The presence of LV dysfunction increases the absolute prognostic advantage of CABG

SYNTAX score

- Independent predictor of MACE in PCI but not CABG.
- Based on the angiographic complexity, the SYNTAX score can be used to categorize patients SYNTAX score tertiles: a low risk category (SYNTAX score < 22), an intermediate risk category (SYNTAX score 23–32) and an increased risk category (SYNTAX score ≥ 33)
- In the SYNTAX trial, patients were randomized to PCI with TAXUS drug-eluting stents or CABG—no significant difference in outcome out to 3 years for patients with low scores, higher MACE rates in PCI cohort for higher scores driven mainly by need for repeat revascularization

SYNTAX score II

- Combines clinical variables (age, creatinine clearance, LVEF, left main stem disease, gender, COPD, PVD) with the anatomical SYNTAX score, providing expected 4-year mortality for both CABG and PCI
- This tool can be utilized to recommend PCI only, CABG only, or equipoise in treatment based on long-term mortality

The EuroSCORE

- Initially validated to predict surgical mortality.
- 17 simple questions regarding patient, cardiac, and operative factors.
- Independent predictor of MACE in studies for both PCI and CABG.

The Society of Thoracic Surgeons (STS) score

- Validated in surgical patients only.
- It is extensive and includes operative, demographic, patient, and haemodynamic factors.

The Heart Team

- Team based approach to optimize the management of complex patients, particularly in light of new devices/approaches/evidence.
- Composition varies across institutions, but with respect to decisions on revascularization the heart team is expected to include the Cardiac Surgeon, Interventional Cardiologist, and the Primary Cardiologist who is familiar with the complexities of the case beyond the coronary anatomy.
- Patient factors such as the patient's status, co-morbidities, and wishes should be used in combination with the SYNTAX scores to help guide decision
- With evolving PCI technologies, the evidence of PCI vs CABG will continue to grow, but current evidence suggests that in patients with complex coronary disease (e.g. left main stem disease or high SYNTAX score), long-term outcome from CABG is superior to PCI, primarily driven by reduced rates of revascularization and infarction.

2.2.10 Angina without obstructive disease in the epicardial coronary arteries

Microvascular angina

- Characterized by:
    - Typical symptoms of angina
    - 'Ischaemic-like' changes on ECG during angina or stress testing

- Normal coronary arteries on angiography
  - No evidence of artery spasm or systemic disease known to cause microvascular dysfunction
- Also known as cardiac syndrome X
- No clear data on prevalence or incidence, but may be found in 10–30% undergoing coronary angiography for anginal chest pain.
- Mechanisms not clearly defined but relate to endothelial dysfunction, impaired vasodilator function, and increased vasoconstrictor activity.
- Appear to be associated with abnormal adrenergic activity, insulin resistance, inflammation, and oestrogen deficiency (in women)
- Leads to reduced coronary flow reserve (CFR)
- Increased risk of major adverse cardiovascular events and quality of life is often considerably restricted
- Treat in similar way to angina. Small studies suggest benefit with ACE inhibitors, statins, xanthine derivatives, and oestrogens (in women).

Vasospastic angina

- Also known as Prinzmetal angina and caused by vascular spasm
- Occurs at rest, and can be associated with ST segment elevation
- Epidemiology is unclear, estimated at 1–2% of patients with transient angina attacks.
- Diagnosed by recording transient ECG changes during angina attack. If not possible, ambulatory ECG monitoring may be used.
- Some patients may require intracoronary acetylcholine provocation testing
- Prognosis: Higher risk of sudden cardiac death in multi-vessel spasm and in patients with spasm-related arrhythmias.
- Treatment: Calcium channel blockers and nitrates. Avoid beta blockers (can lead to spasm by shifting adrenergic stimulation to alpha receptors).

2.2.11 Alternative interventions for chronic refractory angina

- Refractory angina is defined as ongoing symptoms significantly limiting activity (CCS 3–4) not sufficiently controlled by maximal medical therapy and with no revascularization options.
- Possible treatment options include (all Class IIb):
  - Coronary sinus constriction with a reducer device
  - Spinal cord stimulation (SCS): Some evidence in reducing symptoms and re-hospitalizations. No life-threatening complications reported.
  - Enhanced external counterpulsation: Contraindicated in severe LV dysfunction, uncontrolled hypertension, aortic stenosis, significant aortic regurgitation, peripheral vascular disease, and anticoagulation.

Further reading

Camm AJ, Lüscher TF, and Serruys PW (eds). *The European Society of Cardiology Textbook of Cardiovascular Medicine*. Oxford: Oxford University Press, 2009.

Collet C, Onuma Y, Andreini D, Sonck J, Pompilio G, Mushtaq S, La Meir M, Miyazaki Y, de Mey J, Gaemperli O, Ouda A, Maureira JP, Mandry D, Camenzind E, Macron L, Doenst T, Teichgraber U, Sigusch H, Asano T, Katagiri Y, Morel MA, Lindeboom W, Pontone G, Luscher TF, Bartorelli

AL, Serruys PW. Coronary computed tomography angiography for heart team decision-making in multivessel coronary artery disease. *Eur Heart J* 2018;39:3689–98.

Juarez-Orozco LE, Saraste A, Capodanno D, Prescott E, Ballo H, Bax JJ, Wijns W, Knuuti J. Impact of a decreasing pre-test probability on the performance of diagnostic tests for coronary artery disease. *Eur Heart J Cardiovasc Imaging* 2019; doi: 10.1093/ehjci/jez054

Knuuti J, Wijns W, Saraste A, Capodanno D, Barbato E, Funck-Brentano C, Prescott E, Storey RF, Deaton C, Cuisset T, Agewall S, Dickstein K, Edvardsen T, Escaned J, Gersh BJ, Svitil P, Gilard M, Hasdai D, Hatala R, Mahfoud F, Masip J, Muneretto C, Valgimigli M, Achenbach S, Bax JJ; ESC Scientific Document Group. 2019 ESC Guidelines for the diagnosis and management of chronic coronary syndromes. *Eur Heart J*. 2020 Jan 14;41(3):407–77. doi: 10.1093/eurheartj/ehz425

Maron DJ, Hochman JS, Reynolds HR, Bangalore S, O'Brien SM, Boden WE, Chaitman BR, Senior R, López-Sendón J, Alexander KP, Lopes RD, Shaw LJ, Berger JS, Newman JD, Sidhu MS, Goodman SG, Ruzyllo W, Gosselin G, Maggioni AP, White HD, Bhargava B, Min JK, Mancini GBJ, Berman DS, Picard MH, Kwong RY, Ali ZA, Mark DB, Spertus JA, Krishnan MN, Elghamaz A, Moorthy N, Hueb WA, Demkow M, Mavromatis K, Bockeria O, Peteiro J, Miller TD, Szwed H, Doerr R, Keltai M, Selvanayagam JB, Steg PG, Held C, Kohsaka S, Mavromichalis S, Kirby R, Jeffries NO, Harrell FE Jr, Rockhold FW, Broderick S, Ferguson TB Jr, Williams DO, Harrington RA, Stone GW, Rosenberg Y; ISCHEMIA Research Group. Initial Invasive or Conservative Strategy for Stable Coronary Disease. *N Engl J Med*. 2020 Apr 9;382(15):1395–407. doi: 10.1056/NEJMoa1915922. Epub 2020 Mar 30. PMID: 32227755; PMCID: PMC7263833.

Neumann FJ, Sousa-Uva M, Ahlsson A, Alfonso F, Banning AP, Benedetto U, Byrne RA, Collet JP, Falk V, Head SJ, Jüni P, Kastrati A, Koller A, Kristensen SD, Niebauer J, Richter DJ, Seferovic PM, Sibbing D, Stefanini GG, Windecker S, Yadav R, Zembala MO; ESC Scientific Document Group. 2018 ESC/EACTS Guidelines on myocardial revascularization. *Eur Heart J*. 2019 Jan 7;40(2):87–165. doi: 10.1093/eurheartj/ehy394. Erratum in: *Eur Heart J*. 2019 Oct 1;40(37):3096. PMID: 30165437.

Recent-onset chest pain of suspected cardiac origin: assessment and diagnosis. London: National Institute for Health and Care Excellence (UK); 2010. Updated 2016 CIH

2.3

Cardiac Catheterization

Daniel McKenzie and Paul Brady

TABLE OF CONTENTS

2.3.1 Principles of radiation physics and safety regulations 165
2.3.2 Catheterization laboratory equipment 166
2.3.3 Vascular access 166
　　Radial 166
　　Femoral 168
2.3.4 Coronary anatomy 169
　　Normal aortic root anatomy 169
　　Normal coronary course and nomenclature 170
　　Common native vessel variations 170
　　Vein grafts 170
　　Coronary anomalies 170
2.3.5 Coronary angiography: catheter selection and views 174
　　Left coronary artery 174
　　Right coronary artery 174
　　Internal mammary artery 174
　　Vein grafts 174
　　Coronary angiography: Views 176
2.3.6 Indications for coronary angiography and PCI 179
2.3.7 Invasive functional assessment and intracoronary imaging 179
　　Pressure wire assessment 179
　　Intravascular ultrasound 181
　　Optical coherence tomography 182
2.3.8 Complications of coronary angiography and PCI 182
　　Consent 182
　　Vascular complications 182
　　Contrast-related complications 183
　　Coronary complications 184
2.3.9 Right heart catheterization and cardiac haemodynamics 185
　　Measurements 185
　　Cardiac output 188
　　Stroke volume 189
　　Systemic and pulmonary vascular resistance 189
　　Shunts 189
　　Valve assessments 189
　　Other conditions 192

2.3.1 Principles of radiation physics and safety regulations

- Coronary angiography uses X-rays that pass from a posteriorly positioned radiation source though the patient to an anteriorly positioned image intensifier, both of which are mounted on a 'C-arm' to facilitate imaging in different planes.• An X-ray is a form of ionizing radiation at the short-wavelength end of the electromagnetic spectrum.
- In the UK, all medical staff performing fluoroscopy must undergo mandatory 'Ionising Radiation (Medical Exposure) Regulations' (IR(ME)R) training.
- All staff working in the catheter lab are required by law to wear a dosimeter so that the total radiation doses can be audited with the aim to keep the radiation dose 'as low as reasonably achievable/practicable'.
- Radiation-related adverse effects are categorized as deterministic effects, i.e. there is a predictable linear relationship between an adverse event and the radiation dose, or stochastic

effects, i.e. more random events that may occur even after a single exposure and/or after many years.
- It is very important that operators are aware of the inverse-square law of radiation ($1/x^2$) which means that doubling the distance from the radiation source reduces the radiation dose by a factor of 4. Tubing should therefore be routinely used to enable operators to stand as far away from the radiation source as possible.
- Strategies to reduce radiation exposure dose include:
  - Wearing appropriate lead aprons, thyroid shields, shin guards and glasses.
  - Using appropriate lab-based protection including transparent lead glass shield and lead drapes around the procedure table.
  - Avoiding prolonged periods using steep views known to increase radiation scatter, e.g. steep left caudal views.
  - Avoid excessive cineangiography acquisitions when possible.
  - Use lower frame rate when possible, e.g. frame rates of 7.5 frames/s.
  - Reducing image field by collimation when possible.

2.3.2 Catheterization laboratory equipment

- Patient safety during invasive coronary angiography is a key priority and there should be continuous monitoring of the electrocardiogram, systemic arterial pressure, and pulse oxygen saturation throughout the procedure.
- A blood gas analyser is also required as analysis of arterial and venous blood gases is often very important, particularly in the context of right heart catheterization.
- Immediate access to cardiorespiratory resuscitation equipment, oxygen, and advanced life support medication must be available in case of cardiac arrest or critical haemodynamic instability.
- Although less commonly used due to advancements in non-invasive imaging, the use of an automated injector system to perform ventriculography and/or aortography may be required in certain situations, e.g. when considering Takotsubo cardiomyopathy as the diagnosis.
- Ventriculography is normally performed in the right anterior oblique projection with a pigtail catheter positioned in left ventricle using a 30–40 mL bolus of contrast via a mechanical pump at 10–15 mL/s. This enables rapid evaluation of left ventricular function and assessment of mitral valve regurgitation.
- An aortogram is normally performed in the left anterior oblique projection with a pigtail catheter positioned in the aortic root using a 30–40 mL bolus of contrast via a mechanical pump at 15–20 mL/s.

2.3.3 Vascular access

Radial

- Has become the preferred route in the UK (BCIS audit figures).
- Once the learning curve is climbed the obvious advantages outweigh the disadvantages (see Table 2.3.1).
- The RIVAL trial has shown significantly fewer vascular complications for the radial route and better outcomes in the STEMI patient subgroup among those procedures performed by radial experts.

Table 2.3.1 Advantages and disadvantages of the radial approach.

Advantages	Disadvantages
Earlier ambulation	Operator learning curve
Fewer vascular complications	Vessel spasm
Safer in anticoagulated patients	Vasovagal reactions
	Too small for > 7F sheaths or IABP use
	Potential difficulties accessing arterial grafts
	Anatomical abnormality, e.g. radial loop/subclavian tortuosity

- In addition, the MATRIX trial demonstrated that in patients with ACS, there was a significant reduction in major bleeding and all-cause mortality with transradial access compared to transfemoral access.
- ESC guidelines on myocardial revascularization (2018) recommend using transradial access first line (class 1 level A recommendation).
- The hand usually benefits from a dual blood supply from the radial and ulnar arteries (Figure 2.3.1).
- The clinical benefit of performing the modified Allen's or Barbeau's test to assess ulnar flow into the palmar arch is unclear.

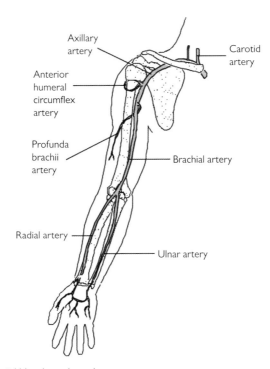

Figure 2.3.1 Arterial blood supply to the arm.
© EMIS, from http://www.patient.co.uk/diagram/Arteries-Of-The-Arm.htm

- In the Allen's test, both arteries are compressed and the patient clenches and releases their hand into a fist. The hand will blanch. In a positive Allen's test the colour returns to normal after release of the ulnar artery, thus confirming dual supply. This may also be performed using pulse oximetry plethysmography.
- Strategies to minimize radial spasm include:
  - Adequate local anaesthetic
  - Use of smaller 5F sheaths and catheters
  - Administration of a 'radial cocktail', often of nitrate and verapamil.
  - Routine administration of heparin is advised to minimize radial artery thrombosis and occlusion in the ensuing weeks (3000–5000 units).

Femoral

The femoral route may be used for a variety of reasons:

- Failed radial approach
- Absent radial pulse
- Possible IABP requirement
- Procedure mandating 8F sheath (e.g. 2-stent bifurcation, rotablation)
- Complex graft anatomy
- The artery is palpated and punctured two fingers-breadths below the inguinal ligament (see Figure 2.3.2).
- Fluoroscopic screening of a radio-opaque instrument (needle or forceps) over the intended puncture site can help identify optimal puncture height (mid-femoral head)
- Ultrasound guidance is recommended where available.
- Punctures above the ligament risk subsequent inability to adequately apply compression post removal and increase the risk of a retroperitoneal bleed. The greater calibre of the femoral artery means that use of vasodilators and heparin is not routinely mandated.

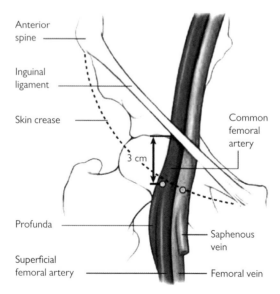

Figure 2.3.2 Relevant anatomy to femoral artery and vein puncture.
Reproduced from Zipes, D., Libby, P., Bonow, R., Braunwald, E, Braunwald's Heart Disease, © 2005 with permission from Elsevier.

2.3.4 Coronary anatomy

- Invasive coronary angiography remains the gold standard test for imaging the coronary arteries, if done properly.
- Acquisition is of a 2D image. Multiple views are necessary to image every section of each artery in orthogonal planes.
- Each angiogram will require the operator to adapt the next manoeuvre or view throughout the procedure to gain all the information required.
- Expertise in this process will come with experience but the foundations of good coronary angiography are a sound knowledge and understanding of anatomy (normal and abnormal).

Normal aortic root anatomy

- Normally the coronary ostia arise from the sinus above the respective aortic cusps.
- The ostia are best profiled and engaged in the LAO view (see Figure 2.3.3).

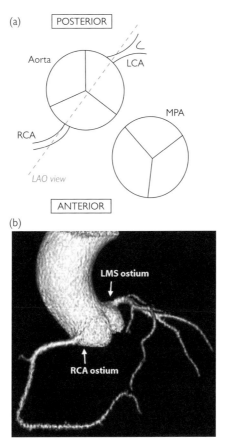

Figure 2.3.3 Coronary ostia anatomy. (a) Diagrammatic cross-sectional view of LAO projection and (b) 3D computed tomography reconstruction representing this view for optimal ostial profiling and engagement. LAO, left anterior oblique; MPA, main pulmonary artery; RCA, right coronary artery, LCA, left coronary artery.

Reproduced from Manghat NE, Morgan-Hughes GJ, Marshall AJ, Roobottom CA. Multidetector row computed tomography: imaging congenital coronary artery anomalies in adults. *Heart.* 2005 Dec;91(12):1515–22. doi: 10.1136/hrt.2005.065979 with permission from BMJ.

Normal coronary course and nomenclature

The right coronary artery (see Figure 2.3.4)

- The right coronary artery (RCA) arises anteriorly from the right aortic sinus and descends in the right atrioventricular groove.
- The proximal portion (1) gives rise to the conus and sinus node branches.
- The middle third (2) extends to the acute margin (the sharp angle between the sternocostal and diaphragmatic surfaces of the heart) at which point the distal third (3) continues on the inferior surface.
- In 70% of cases it bifurcates at the interventricular groove and gives rise to the posterior descending artery (PDA; 4), thus conferring dominance (supplying the inferior septum and notably the posteromedial papillary muscle) and a posterior left ventricular branch (pLV; 16).

The left coronary system (see Figure 2.3.5).

- The left coronary system arises posteriorly as the left main stem (LMS; 5) from the left aortic sinus and branches behind the main pulmonary artery (MPA) into the left anterior descending (LAD; 6–8) and circumflex arteries (Cx; 11–15).
- Occasionally there is also an intermediate branch (17) that originates between the LAD and Cx.
- The proximal LAD (6) runs up to the origin of the first septal branch.
- Branching diagonals (9,10) serve the lateral LV wall.
- The Cx descends in the left atrioventricular groove (11,13) and gives off posterior obtuse marginal (OM) branches (12,14) and, in 10% of cases, the PDA, and is thus dominant.
- In approximately 20% of cases there is co-dominance with the RCA.

Common native vessel variations

- The LMS may be absent, with either a 'shotgun' origin to the LAD and LCx arteries, or these arteries may be separate entirely; the former may be obvious from dye reflux but the latter should be actively sought, with a sinus injection if suspected.
- In approximately 10% cases the RCA may have a high and/or anterior origin, which can be difficult to intubate.

Vein grafts

See Figure 2.3.6.

- This 3D cardiac CT AP reconstruction demonstrates the usual origins and courses of saphenous vein coronary bypass grafts (SVG).
- The graft to the RCA usually arises from the lateral aortic wall (above the native RCA) with a vertical course and is hence best engaged in the LAO or AP views
- Grafts to the LAD and Cx arteries usually arise anteriorly and traverse the MPA as shown. Their engagement is often aided by an RAO view

Coronary anomalies

Coronary artery arising from wrong sinus

- RCA arising from LC sinus, aberrant course.
- LCA arising from RC sinus, aberrant course.

2.3.4 Coronary anatomy 171

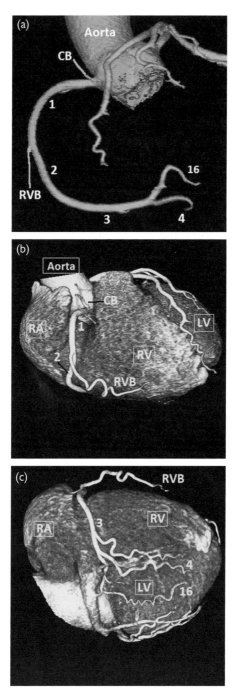

Figure 2.3.4 3D rendered CT image of the coronary tree demonstrating the right coronary artery (a) and 3D reconstruction in AP view (b) and inferior view (c), showing AHA-defined segments and arterial course. See text. CB, conus branch; RVB, right ventricular branch.

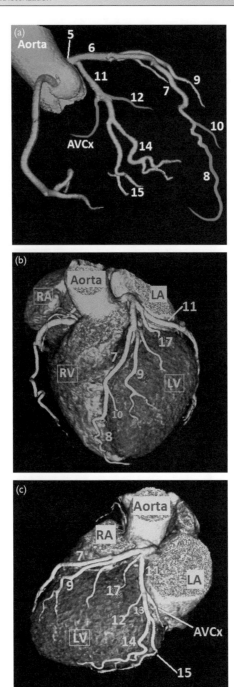

Figure 2.3.5 3D rendered CT image of the coronary tree showing the left coronary system (a) and a 3D CT image in LAO cranial view (b) and posterior view (c), showing AHA-defined segments and arterial course. See text. AVCx, atrioventricular circumflex branch.

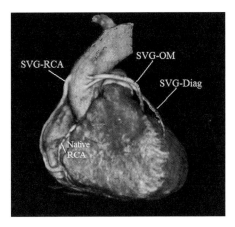

Figure 2.3.6 3D computed tomography reconstruction in AP view showing common anatomy of bypass grafts. SVG, saphenous vein graft.

Branch of coronary arising from wrong sinus

- LCx arising from RC sinus, aberrant course.
- LAD arising from RC sinus, aberrant course.

Single coronary artery

- Arising from LC sinus, aberrant RCA.
- Arising from RC sinus, aberrant LCA.

The course of the proximal aberrant artery is critical: is it interarterial, i.e. between aorta and main pulmonary artery (see Figure 2.3.7) and subject to compression with possible ischaemia and dysrhythmias (with the associated risk of sudden death)? In the presence of symptoms, ischaemia testing is sought and treatment may be surgical re-implantation.

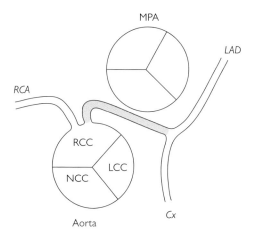

Figure 2.3.7 Diagrammatic representation of anomalous LCA (shaded) arising from right coronary cusp (RCC) with inter-arterial course. MPA, main pulmonary artery.

Anomalous coronary artery arising from pulmonary artery
- Whilst very rare as a group, anomalous origin of the left coronary artery arising from the pulmonary artery (ALCAPA) is by far the most common form (90%)
- Most present with infarction, sudden death, or heart failure and untreated 1-year mortality is 90%.
- Management is surgical reimplantation into the aorta.

2.3.5 Coronary angiography: catheter selection and views

Left coronary artery
- See Figure 2.3.8a.
- A Judkins left catheter (e.g. JL4) is usually employed to engage the left coronary ostium.
- The primary (distal) curve engages and the secondary curve stabilizes on the opposite aortic wall.
- The number refers to the distance in centimetres between the two curves. Hence a JL5/JL6 catheter may be required if the aorta is dilated.
- If access is via the right radial artery, the steeper angle of approach usually mandates using a shorter JL3.5 catheter.

Right coronary artery
- See Figure 2.3.8b.
- A Judkins right catheter (JR4) is usually employed for both femoral and radial approaches.
- It requires steady clockwise rotation.
- Femorally, a William's catheter is a commonly used alternative (or an Amplatz right (AR) catheter radially).
- Larger roots may require a JR5/6 or an AR catheter.

Internal mammary artery
- See Figure 2.3.8c.
- Pass the internal mammary artery (IMA) catheter over wire into ascending aorta.
- Withdraw J-wire into catheter.
- Rotate catheter anticlockwise until pointing up.
- Pull back until it engages the left subclavian artery ('3rd click').
- Pass J-wire beyond left IMA ostium, then catheter.
- Dragging back usually engages the left IMA with some rotational adjustment.
- A similar technique will engage the right IMA, after manoeuvring the catheter via the innominate artery ('1st click') to the right subclavian artery.

Vein grafts
Right-sided vein grafts are best engaged in LAO or AP view (see Figure 2.3.9a).
- JR4 will often click into ostium upon dragging up from RCA engagement.
- Beware, if downward ostium; a JR4 catheter may point into roof and graft will only appear as stump.
- A Multipurpose A (MPA) catheter is usually better (or right coronary bypass (RCB) catheter).
- If reach needed use an Amplatz left (AL) catheter.

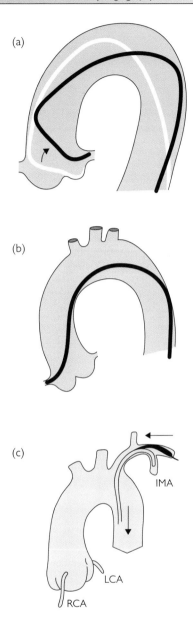

Figure 2.3.8 Catheter engagement. (a) left coronary artery engagement, (b) right coronary artery engagement, (c) internal mammary artery engagement.
Reproduced from Zipes, D., Libby, P., Bonow, R., Braunwald, E, Braunwald's Heart Disease, © 2005 with permission from Elsevier.

The RAO view is often helpful to locate left-sided vein grafts (Figure 2.3.9b).

- Rotate JR4 to point towards sternal wires (anteriorly).
- Slide slowly up and down aorta until catches (may need rotational adjustment).
- If reach is needed use AR2/AL1/LCB catheters.

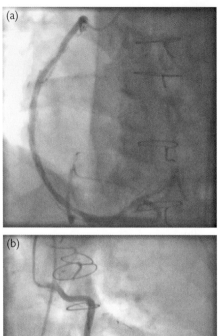

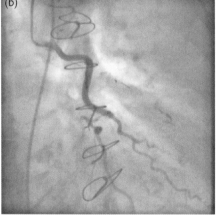

Figure 2.3.9 Vein graft engagement. (a) Right-sided vein graft engagement, (b) Left-sided vein graft engagement.

General points for graft cases:

- If vein grafts are difficult to find or there is no operation note, an aortogram may prove useful.
- Right femoral artery approach is often the default for angiography of graft patients.
- With practice, the left radial is an excellent approach for left IMA and vein graft cases.
- Indeed, intubation of the former is usually made easier.

Coronary angiography: Views

- There are several standard views of left and right coronary systems.
- Good angiography is not simply a matter of acquiring each of them in every patient.
- One 2D acquisition is useless without the other complementary views.
- Each angiogram is a dynamic process of image selection.
- Some will not need all views, and some will need further modified views.
- The diagrams can therefore only be a guide.

2.3.5 Coronary angiography: catheter selection and views

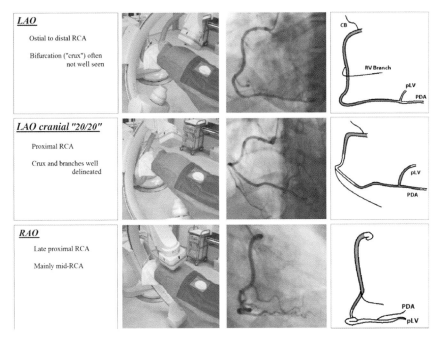

Figure 2.3.10 Standard RCA angiographic views and angiograms. Left-hand boxes show coronary anatomy best highlighted in each view, represented diagrammatically by shaded area in right-hand boxes. CB, conus branch; RV, right ventricular branch; pLV, posterior left ventricular branch; PDA, posterior descending artery.

- They show the position of the C-arm during acquisition, juxtaposed with the corresponding angiographic image and a diagrammatic representation showing the specific anatomy best shown in that view (shaded).

Right coronary artery—see Figure 2.3.10
Left coronary artery—see Figure 2.3.11

Left ventriculography
- A pigtail catheter is advanced down onto the aortic valve (with the introducer wire pulled back into the catheter) so that is curls up slightly.
- It may pass straight through. If not, with some rotation upon slow withdrawal, it will often prolapse through.
- Advancing the wire within the catheter may encourage prolapse, or the valve can be crossed with the wire J-tip prior to advancing the catheter.
- Further strategies include using a soft-tipped straight wire via either a pigtail or AL1 catheter (particularly in aortic stenosis) to direct a course through the valve
- After measuring LV end-diastolic pressure, a pump is used to give about 35 ml of contrast into the LV over 3 seconds, to assess function and regional wall motion as Figure 2.3.12 illustrates.
- The pigtail should then be withdrawn whilst recording, to measure the pullback gradient across the aortic valve.
- It should be noted this is a peak-to-peak gradient (approximates to the mean echo gradient); similar readings may be made invasively using a pressure wire if the valve is difficult to cross.
- These data may be useful to corroborate echocardiographic findings if the latter are not clear-cut.

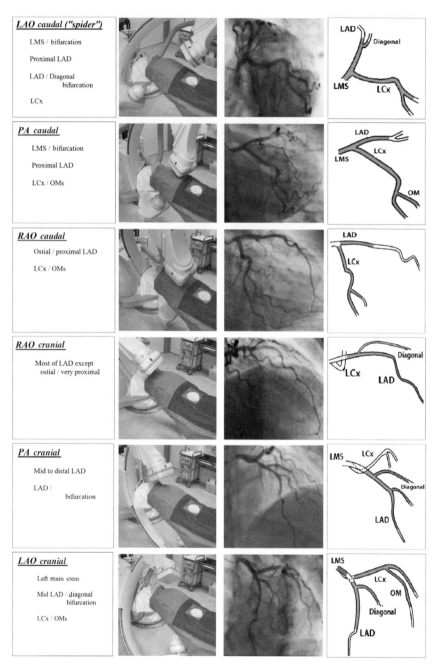

Figure 2.3.11 Standard LCA angiographic views and angiograms. Left-hand boxes show coronary anatomy best highlighted in each view, represented diagrammatically by shaded area in right boxes.

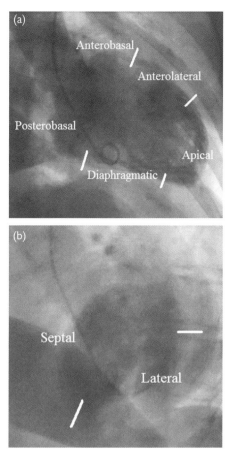

Figure 2.3.12 Left ventricular angiography in the RAO (a) and LAO (b) views showing profiled LV territories.

2.3.6 Indications for coronary angiography and PCI

See Chapters 2.1 and 2.2.

2.3.7 Invasive functional assessment and intracoronary imaging

Pressure wire assessment

- Coronary pressure-derived Fractional Flow Reserve (FFR) and Instantaneous wave Free Ratio (iFR) are currently the standard of care for the functional assessment of lesion severity in patients with intermediate-grade (30–70% angiographic) stenosis.
- ESC guidelines on myocardial revascularization (2018) recommend FFR or iFR first line in the assessment of the haemodynamic significance of intermediate-grade stenosis (class 1 level A recommendation)
- These guidelines also recommend that FFR-guided PCI should be considered in patients with multivessel disease under-going PCI (class IIa level B recommendation).

- Over 21,000 pressure wire assessment cases were performed in the UK in 2017–18 BCIS Audit year, compared to 5000 in 2007-8.

Definition:
- FFR is the maximal blood flow in the presence of a stenosis divided by the theoretical maximal flow in the absence of the stenosis. It assumes resistance from vascular bed to be minimal and constant during maximal hyperaemia (see Figure 2.3.13)

In the lab:
- Administer heparin and intracoronary nitrate.
- The pressure wire transducer (located at the proximal end of a 3 cm radio-opaque tip) is equalized (synchronized) with simultaneous aortic pressure just out of the guide catheter in the coronary ostium.
- Wire passed across the lesion.
- Adenosine, ideally via intravenous infusion (at 140 mg/kg/min) or as an intracoronary bolus is administered.
- Hyperaemia achieved: fall in blood pressure/heart block/symptoms.
- iFR measurement does not require administration of adenosine
- Functional significance is defined as FFR ≤ 0.80 or iFR ≤ 0.89
- Distal lesions, microvascular disease, and collaterals may confound the results.

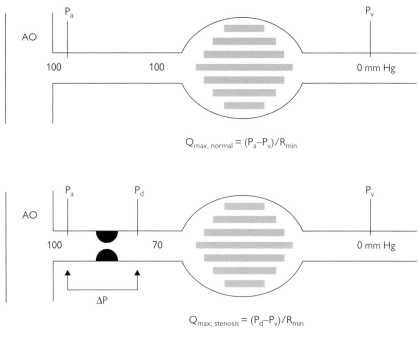

Figure 2.3.13 Diagrammatic representation of the measurement of fractional flow reserve. P_a, mean aortic pressure; P_d, mean distal coronary pressure; P_v, mean central venous pressure; AO, aorta; $Q_{max, normal}$, maximal achievable myocardial flow in normal coronary artery; Qmax, stenosis, maximal achievable myocardial flow in the presence of a stenosis; R_{min}, minimal resistance of the myocardial vascular bed.

Reprodcued from Pijls NH, De Bruyne B. Coronary pressure measurement and fractional flow reserve. *Heart*. 1998;80(6):539–542. doi:10.1136/hrt.80.6.539 with permission from BMJ.

Table 2.3.2 Post PCI FFR and subsequent events rates and FFR.

FFR	Subsequent event rate (%)
< 0.8	29.3
0.8–0.9	20.9
0.9–0.95	6.2
> 0.95	4.9

Evidence:

- The DEFER study investigated the effect of stenting non-significant lesions. Not only did it show it was safe to leave lesions with an FFR > 0.75, it also showed a higher MI and CABG rate in those patients stented with FFRs > 0.75.
- The FAME trial used FFR to guide revascularization in MVD. The primary end-point of death, MI, and TVR were significantly lower in the FFR group as compared to the angiographically guided group.
- Registry data shows that repeat FFR measurements immediately post-stenting are associated with subsequent event rates as shown in Table 2.3.2.
- Two large randomized controlled trials, DEFINE FLAIR and SWEDEHEART, have demonstrated the equivalent clinical utility of iFR to direct management strategy compared to FFR.

Intravascular ultrasound

- Intravascular ultrasound (IVUS) was initially a research tool but is now an everyday diagnostic technique giving histological information on vessel wall, luminal size, plaque morphology, and stent placement.
- There is a growing evidence base supporting the use of IVUS and meta-analysis data from randomized and observational studies suggest better clinical outcomes with IVUS-guided versus angiography-guided PCI.
- The ESC guidelines on myocardial revascularization (2018) recommend that IVUS should be considered to assess the severity of unprotected left main stem lesions (class IIa level B recommendation).
- These guidelines also recommend that IVUS or Optical Coherence Tomography (OCT) should be used for stent optimization in selected patients (class IIa level B recommendation).

In the lab:

- Administer heparin and intracoronary nitrate.
- Pass transducer along standard guidewire into the coronary beyond the lesion.
- Pullback of device produces a cross-sectional ultrasound map.

Main indications:

- Assessment of angiographically ambiguous lesions.
- Accurate vessel sizing pre-intervention.
- Ensuring optimal stent deployment.
- Left main/bifurcation intervention.
- Investigation of stent failure.
- Recognition of dissection and thrombus.

Optical coherence tomography

- Optical coherence tomography (OCT) uses infrared light to gain near-histological cross-sectional coronary imaging.
- 10 times the resolution of IVUS.
- Limited by penetration depth and the need for flush with contrast during acquisition.
- Hence OCT may be less useful in larger vessels or for ostial lesions
- The ESC guidelines on myocardial revascularization (2018) recommend IVUS or OCT for stent optimization in selected patients (class IIa level B recommendation).

2.3.8 Complications of coronary angiography and PCI

Consent

- An understanding of the procedure and its possible complications is essential in order to gain informed consent (see Table 2.3.3).
- Complication rates are approximate in the UK and centre-specific data should be provided if possible.
- Clearly these will vary according to patient-specific factors.

Vascular complications

Retroperitoneal haemorrhage

- Usually related to femoral puncture but may be spontaneous as a result of adjunctive pharmacology.
- Presentation may simply be with unexplained hypotension. A high index of suspicion is required.
- Hence any such presentation post-angiography should be aggressively investigated, usually via a CT scan.
- Management: supportive (fluid resuscitation +/− blood transfusion), may require reversal of anticoagulation. Interventional/surgical treatment rarely indicated.

Haematoma

- Associated with:
    - Femoral punctures
    - Long procedures
    - Large sheath (IABP use)
    - Anticoagulation

Table 2.3.3 Complications and approximate incidences for consent purposes.

Complication	Treatment	Diagnostic	PCI
Vascular access damage[a]	Blood transfusion/surgical repair	< 0.1%	Variable
Abnormal heart rhythm	DCCV/drugs	< 0.2%	—
Reduced kidney function	Usually observation	Rare	Rare
Contrast reaction	Usually observation	< 0.1%	< 0.1%
Coronary damage	Stent or emergency CABG	< 0.2%	1%[b]
Stroke	Specialist care	< 0.2%	< 1%
Death	—	< 0.1%	< 1%

[a]Radial, much higher if femoral access and/or complex PCI, up to 10% [b]MI approx 1%, emergency CABG <0.1%.

- Removal technique
- Patient factors (Hypertension, obesity, PVD)
- The femoral sheath can usually be removed in the lab if no heparin was given, otherwise after 4 h or once ACT < 150 s
- Manual pressure for 10 minutes by an experienced member of staff is necessary on sheath removal followed by a few hours of recumbency
- Vascular closure devices are used to facilitate ambulation but have not been proven to reduce complications post angiography/PCI
- The Angioseal™ device uses an intraluminal anchor to sandwich the arteriotomy with a collagen plug, which completely dissolves over 90 days.
- Suture-based devices such as the Perclose™ aim to attain surgical closure without impinging upon the lumen
- Haematoma management: Manual pressure. May be aided by clamping devices such as the Femostop™

Pseudoaneurysm

- This may occur after femoral (or radial) punctures and will present as a tender pulsatile swelling over the arteriotomy site with an audible bruit.
- Blood collects in a tear between the adventitia and media and is diagnosed with Doppler ultrasound.
- Some may spontaneously resolve but the risk is of expansion, local impingement, and rupture and distal embolization.
- Hence if flow persists into the pseudoaneurysm it will need treating.
- Management: Doppler-guided compression (with success rates of only 30–62% on anticoagulation), ultrasound-guided thrombin injection (success rates of 90–100% and rare complications), or (particularly for larger pseudoaneurysms), surgical repair.

Limb ischaemia

- Occurrence is rare.
- More associated with femoral route (e.g. closure device lifting plaque in diseased artery) and IABP use.
- Compartment syndrome via radial route is very rare. Surgical intervention is often necessary.

Contrast-related complications
Anaphylaxis

- May not be obvious but should always be considered with unexplained tachycardia and hypotension and a rash should be sought.
- Management: depending upon severity is with intravenous steroids, chlorpheniramine, fluids, and intramuscular adrenaline.

Contrast-induced nephropathy

- There is no everyday diagnostic test available to diagnose contrast-induced nephropathy (CIN) but it is usually manifest as deteriorating renal function 48–72 hours post-exposure, although this may occur for other reasons.
- Management: there is limited clinical evidence to show improved clinical outcomes using N-acetylcysteine, sodium bicarbonate, or iso-osmolar contrast.
- Pre-hydration is essential in patients with reduced eGFR (< 60 ml/min)
- In patients with moderate or severe CKD, low or iso-osmolar contrast media is recommended. The volume of contrast should be minimized (as low as possible, preferably total contrast volume < 3.7× eGFR)

- Traditionally it has been recommended to withhold metformin for 48 hours before elective angiography or PCI due to the risk of lactic acidosis if renal function deteriorates. However, as this risk is low, checking renal function after angiography in patients on metformin and withholding the drug when renal function deteriorates is an acceptable alternative.

Coronary complications
Coronary dissection
- This may be catheter induced, related to balloon dilatation/stent deployment, or caused by instrumentation of the vessel with adjunctive tools (e.g. rotational/laser atherectomy or intracoronary imaging catheter). Coronary guidewires can also cause dissection, but this is rare with standard workhorse wires.
- Early appreciation is essential to avert acute vessel closure.
- Management: if extensive dissection, coverage with a stent may be required

No reflow
- May occur after ballooning or stent deployment.
- Occurs in the presence of a patent coronary lumen and is a reflection of microvascular obstruction, which may be appreciated by abnormal myocardial blush.
- Associated with thrombotic lesions (e.g. STEMI)
- Management: intracoronary nitrate, adenosine, verapamil, or sodium nitroprusside—injection into distal vessel via a microcathether, aspiration, or dual lumen catheter is preferred. GIIb/IIIa drugs should also be considered.

Coronary perforation/rupture
- Coronary perforation can be caused by disruption of the vessel wall secondary to instrumentation, for example, balloon angioplasty, stenting or atherectomy, or can occur distally secondary to coronary guidewire exit.
- The clinical consequences of a coronary perforation are clearly dependent on the location and extent of the disruption.
- Large vessel perforation is usually obvious upon image acquisition in the lab, but a guide wire exit perforation may not become apparent until the patient returns to the ward where the accumulating pericardial blood becomes clinically evident.
- Management: depends on type and extent of perforation. The first step is always balloon tamponade of the vessel to stop further extravasation of blood. Haemodynamic support, emergency pericardial drainage and a blood transfusion may be required.
- Review of antithrombotic and anticoagulant therapy is also important—GPIIbIIIa inhibitor infusions should stop and consideration given to *partial* reversal of heparin in some situations (very high ACT or distal guidewire exit perforation).
- If there is persistent extravasation of blood from a large vessel perforation, implantation of a covered stent is required.
- Distal embolization of fat, coil, thrombin, or autologous clotted blood is required if there is persistent leak from guidewire exit perforation

Stent embolization
- Rare, but dislodging from the delivery system may occur at the guide catheter tip or whilst traversing through struts of another stent in a bifurcation procedure.
- Management: retrieval using partially inflated balloons or snare devices.
- Embolization into the wider circulation does not tend to cause problems.

In-stent restenosis

- Patients typically present some months later with recurrent angina: 'clinical restenosis'.
- Management: depends on aetiology, which should be assessed with intracoronary imaging (IVUS or OCT).
- If under-expansion is present, balloon optimization with a larger non-compliant balloon is required. If under-expansion is resistant to balloon expansion (e.g. due to calcium), adjunctive modification tools are required (cutting balloon, laser or rotational atherectomy, intravascular lithotripsy).
- Neo-intimal proliferation can be treated with cutting balloons and/or laser therapy and then a drug-eluting balloon used to recoat the original stent struts.
- For BMS restenosis, a DES may be used to cover. There is also some evidence for the use of drug-coated balloons.
- Aggressive ISR in DES, particularly in the setting of MVD or diabetes will usually require referral for CABG.

Stent thrombosis

- Early stent thrombosis (ST) occurs within 30 days and is mostly likely related to premature cessation of DAPT or stent under-sizing/deployment.
- Late ST can occur years later and is associated with delayed endothelialization
- Patient factors associated with stent thrombosis are renal failure, smoking, and diabetes.
- Outcome: 60% suffer acute MI and mortality is > 15%.
- Large-scale registries show that with contemporary antiplatelet therapies and new generation DES (thinner struts with biocompatible polymer), the rate of stent thrombosis is 0.2–0.6% per year.
- In direct comparison to first-generation DES, contemporary evidence supports the use of new-generation DES which have been shown to be safer than first-generation DES and BMS.

2.3.9 Right heart catheterization and cardiac haemodynamics

Measurements

Right and left heart pressure measurements provide important information in the assessment and diagnosis of many cardiac conditions and circulatory shock. It is essential that it is done properly, and an appreciation is needed of the normal pressures and waveforms (Table 2.3.4 and Figure 2.3.14).

- Right heart catheterization is typically performed from the right femoral vein but can also be performed via the right internal jugular or basilic veins.

Table 2.3.4 Normal chamber haemodynamic pressures.

Chamber	Peak-systolic	End-diastolic	Mean
RA	—	—	2–8
RV	17–32	2–8	—
MPA	17–32	4–13	9–19
PCWP	—	—	2–12
LV	90–140	5–12	—
Aorta	—	—	70–105

Reproduced from *Cardiovascular Haemodynamics for the Clinician*, ed. George Stouffer, copyright 2008 with permission from John Wiley and Sons.

2.3 Cardiac Catheterization

- A calibrated, flushed Swan–Ganz (or MPA) catheter is passed into the RA and directed across the tricuspid valve into the RV. It is carefully manipulated into the main pulmonary artery then advanced further into a subsegmental branch whilst watching the pressure trace until 'wedging' occurs (see Figure 2.3.14). This pulmonary capillary wedge pressure (PCWP) is taken to equate to left atrial pressure.
- Getting an accurate 'wedge' is important. An accurate reading is represented by a typical PCWP pressure waveform (see Figure 2.3.16). Oxygen saturations levels of > 90% (or similar to arterial saturations) in blood taken from a 'wedged' catheter is supportive of a good 'wedge' position.
- A pigtail catheter in the LV allows simultaneous LVEDP/PCWP readings (to measure gradient of mitral stenosis).
- On pulling back, recording of the pulmonary artery pressure is made and a recorded pullback across the pulmonary valve will reveal any gradient.
- Simultaneous right and left ventricular pressures trace can be recorded (for changes of constriction) before withdrawing to right atrium.
- The pigtail catheter can then be withdrawn across the aortic valve to assess for a gradient.
- If cardiac output and shunt calculations are necessary, O2 saturation samples should be taken from each chamber (PA, RV, high RA, mid RA, low RA, SVC, IVC, and aorta).
- Cardiac output can also be measured directly using the thermodilution technique with a Swan–Ganz catheter.

The Wiggers diagram (Figure 2.3.15) shows the temporal relationship of the ECG and chamber pressures. When attempting to 'wedge' the right heart catheter, angiographic screening beyond entry to the bronchial artery branch is not often helpful. One should look for the change in pressure wave from that of the pulmonary artery to the classic wedge appearance of left atrial pressure

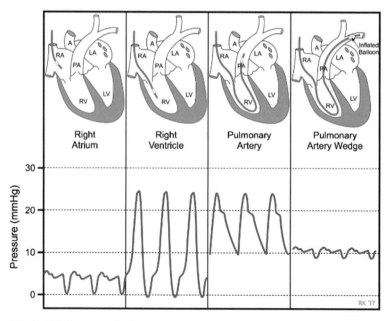

Figure 2.3.14 Right heart catetherization pressure waveforms
Taken from: https://www.cvphysiology.com/Heart%20Failure/HF008
Reproduced from Stouffer, G., ed., Cardiovascular Hemodynamics for the Clinician, © 2008 with permission from John Wiley and Sons.

2.3.9 Right heart catheterization and cardiac haemodynamics   187

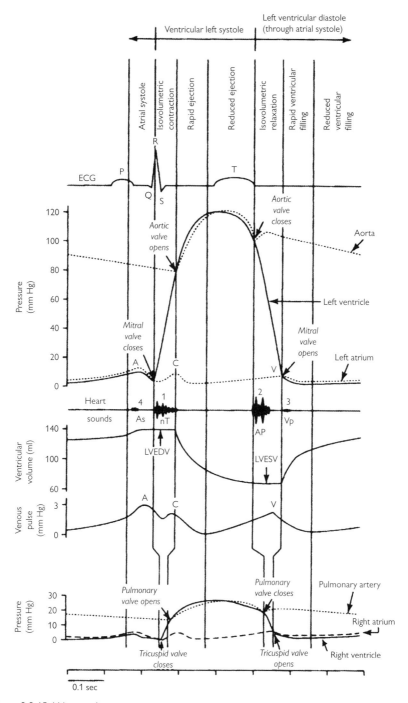

Figure 2.3.15 Wiggers diagram.
Reproduced with permission from Richard E. Klabunde, *Cardiovascular Physiology* (2023), Pulmonary Capillary Wedge Pressure, https://cvphysiology.com/heart-failure/hf008 Copyright: Richard E Klabunde [accessed on 12th December 2023].

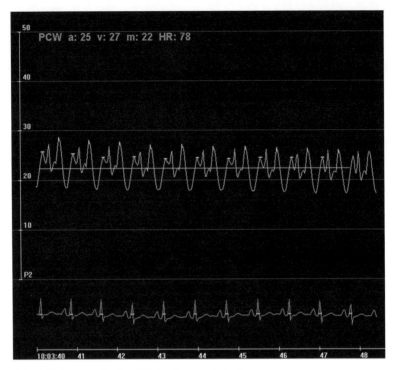

Figure 2.3.16 Pulmonary Capillary Wedge Pressure Waveform
Courtesy of Dr. Kevin Carson, Consultant Cardiologist, Royal United Hospital Bath NHS Foundation Trust, UK

characterized by the A wave (atrial contraction, absent in AF), C wave (ventricular contraction, with subsequent retrograde movement of mitral apparatus), and V wave (peak atrial filling just prior to mitral valve opening).

Cardiac output

Cardiac output (CO) can be measured in the catheter lab using the Fick principle or Thermodilution. The formula for the Fick principle is:

$$CO(l/min) = \frac{O_2 \text{ consumption}}{A - VO_2 \text{ difference}} = \frac{130 \times BSA}{1.36 \times Hb \times 10 \times (SaO_2 - SvO_2)}.$$

Standard oxygen consumption is 130 mls/min; BSA, body surface area (m²); 1.36 mm oxygen is held per gram of haemoglobin; Hb, g/dl haemoglobin (multiplied by 10 to convert to litres), and SaO_2/SvO_2 is expressed as a fraction.

Thermodilution method to calculate cardiac output:

- 10 ml of cold saline is injected through the proximal port of a Swan–Ganz catheter into the RA. Temperature is simultaneously measured in the MPA.
- The area under the thermodilution curve is inversely proportional to cardiac output, which is calculated by a computer.

Cardiac index (CI) compares CO between patients of different size and is obtained by dividing CO by the BSA. It is normally between 2.5 and 4.0 l/min. Hence from this data it is possible to derive the stroke volume and the systemic and pulmonary vascular resistance (SVR, PVR).

Stroke volume

$$CO = SV \times HR \text{ hence } SV = \frac{CO}{HR}$$

Systemic and pulmonary vascular resistance

SVR = (mean aortic pressure − mean RA pressure)/cardiac output

Normal range: 9–20 Wood units (700–1600 dynes.sec.cm^{-5})

PVR = (mean PA pressure − mean PCWP)/cardiac output

Normal range: ≤ 3 Wood units

SVR and PVR can be expressed as dynes.sec.cm^{-5} (Wood units × 80)

PVR is important in transplant assessments as it quantifies the afterload the transplanted RV will need to overcome.

Shunts

The ratio of pulmonary (Q_p) to systemic (Q_s) blood flow aims to quantify a shunt:

$$\frac{Q_p}{Q_s} = \frac{\text{Arterial sat} - \text{Mixed venous sat}}{\text{Pulm vein sat} - \text{Pulm artery sat}} = \frac{SAO_2 - MVO_2}{PVO_2 - PAO_2}.$$

- The mixed venous saturation should be taken from the chamber preceding the shunt.
- So for a VSD, the RA should be used.
- For an ASD, the IVC and SVC according to the formula: ((3 × SVC) + IVC) ÷ 4.
- Generally speaking Q_p/Q_s ratios of 1–1.5 are observed, 1.5–2.0 suggest closure should be considered, and >2.0 indicate closure unless there is a clear contraindication.
- An example calculation is given in Figure 2.3.17.

$$\frac{Q_p}{Q_s} = \frac{98-67}{98-83} = \frac{31}{15} = 2.06$$

Valve assessments

Aortic stenosis

- It should be remembered that echocardiographic-derived data will not correlate with pullback gradients in the lab.
- In Figure 2.3.18, the peak-to-peak gradient from pullback is shown by the dotted arrow, the peak instantaneous gradient from echocardiography by the solid arrow, and the shaded area is the mean pressure gradient.
- It is possible to calculate aortic valve area in the lab using:

$$\text{Gorlin Formula: } \frac{CO/(SEP \times HR)}{44.3 \times \sqrt{\text{(mean pressure gradient)}}}$$

$$\text{Hakki Formula: } \frac{CO}{\sqrt{\text{(peak-to-peak pressure gradient)}}}$$

- There are sources of error, including the presence of significant AR and LV impairment.

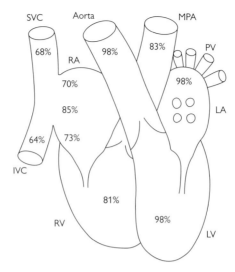

Figure 2.3.17 Diagrammatic representation of results of saturation run during left and right heart catheterisation. There is an atrial septal defect with a significant left to right shunt at the mid-RA level.

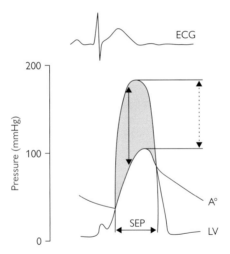

Figure 2.3.18 Comparison of invasive and echocardiograph-derived haemodynamics in a patient with AS. SEP, systolic ejection period.

Reproduced from Brown, J., Morgan-Hughes, N., Aortic stenosis and non-cardiac surgery, Continuing Education in Anaesthesia Critical Care & Pain, Volume 5, Issue 1, February 2005, Pages 1–4, https://doi.org/10.1093/bjaceaccp/mki001 with permission from Oxford University Press.

Mitral stenosis

- Characteristic findings are:
- Increased LA pressure
- Persistent diastolic LA/LV gradient

- Increased right heart pressures
- Prominent A wave on atrial tracings
- Decreased slope of y-descent on LA trace (slowed LV filling)
- The mean pressure gradient and the mitral valve area quantify severity of the lesion (see Table 2.3.5)
- The latter may be calculated in the lab using the Gorlin formula (see Figure 2.3.19):

$$\frac{CO/(DFP \times HR)}{37.7 \times \sqrt{(\text{mean pressure gradient})}}.$$

Table 2.3.5 Parameters of severity of mitral stenosis.

Severity of MS	Mean gradient	MVA
Mild	0–5 mmHg	>1.5 cm²
Moderate	5–10 mmHg	1–1.5 cm²
Severe	>10 mmHg	<1 cm²

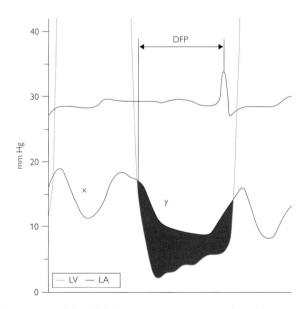

Figure 2.3.19 Simultaneous LV and PCW pressures in a patient with mitral stenosis. Shaded area is the transmitral gradient. (DFP, diastolic filling period).
Reproduced from Zipes, D., Libby, P., Bonow, R., Braunwald, E, Braunwald's Heart Disease, © 2005 with permission from Elsevier.

Table 2.3.6 Causes of pulmonary hypertension and normal left atrial pressures

Parenchymal lung disease (cor pulmonale)	Primary pulmonary hypertension
Chronic thromboembolic disease	Collagen vascular disease
Congenital heart shunts	Sarcoidosis
Obstructive sleep apnoea	Toxins/drugs
Collagen vascular disease	HIV

Reproduced from *Cardiovascular Haemodynamics for the Clinician*, ed. George Stouffer, copyright 2008 with permission from John Wiley and Sons.

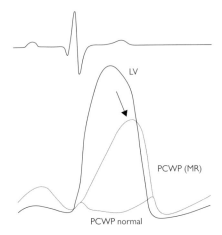

Figure 2.3.20 Simultaneous LV and PCWP tracing in acute severe MR. Note prominent V wave during systole (arrow).

Mitral regurgitation

- Characteristic findings are:
    - Increased right heart pressures
    - Prominent V waves on PCWP trace (not sensitive/specific)
    - Bifid systolic PAP peak (a reflected V wave)
    - Raised LVEDP, SV, lowered CO
- These will be most marked in acute MR in the context of a normal sized, hyperdynamic LV (see Figure 2.3.20)
- As chronic MR decompensates with dilating LV and reducing LV function, right heart pressures will elevate but V waves may not be prominent.

Other conditions
Pulmonary hypertension

- Many cardiac conditions can cause pulmonary hypertension but in the absence of a raised PCWP, other conditions must be considered, as in Table 2.3.6.

Restrictive cardiomyopathy/constrictive pericarditis

- Both conditions usually present with insidious predominant right-sided heart failure and are difficult to distinguish clinically, using echo or haemodynamic data (see Table 2.3.7 and Figure 2.3.21).
- Of note, radiation therapy can cause both conditions

Table 2.3.7 Causes of constrictive pericarditis and restrictive cardiomyopathy and distinguishing haemodynamic findings.

	Constrictive pericarditis	Restrictive cardiomyopathy
Causes	Post-pericarditis	Amyloidosis/carcinoid
	Post-cardiac surgery	Haemochromatosis/sarcoid
	Radiation therapy	Metabolic storage diseases
	Tuberculosis	Metastasis/radiation
LV systolic function	May be normal	May be reduced
PA systolic pressure	Usually < 50 mmHg	May be > 50 mmHg
RV/LV systolic pressure	Discordant	Concordant
RVEDP/LVEDP separation	< 5 mmHg[a]	> 5 mmHg
RVEDP/RV systolic pressure	> 1/3	< 1/3
Kussmaul's sign	Present[b]	Absent

[a]Hypovolaemia may cause equalization of diastolic pressures in a normal heart and false negative results if constrictive pericarditis is present, hence intravenous fluid challenge during procedure is essential, [b]i.e. RA pressure does not decrease with inspiration.
Reproduced from *Cardiovascular Haemodynamics for the Clinician*, ed. George Stouffer, copyright 2008 with permission from John Wiley and Sons.

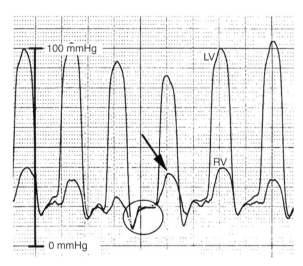

Figure 2.3.21 Ventricular pressure tracings with respiration in constrictive pericarditis showing ventricular discordance where peak RV pressure rises and peak LV pressure drops during inspiration (arrow) and equalization of RV and LV EDP, the 'square root' or 'dip and plateau' sign (circled).
Reproduced with permission from Nishimura RA. Constrictive pericarditis in the modern era: a diagnostic dilemma. *Heart*. 2001 Dec;86(6):619–23. doi: 10.1136/heart.86.6.619. with permission from BMJ Publishing Group Ltd.

Further reading

Camm AJ, Lüscher TF, Serruys P (eds). *The European Society of Cardiology Textbook of Cardiovascular Medicine*. Oxford: Oxford University Press, 2009.

Ibanez B, James S, Agewall S, Antunes MJ, Bucciarelli-Ducci C, Bueno H, Caforio ALP, Crea F, Goudevenos JA, Halvorsen S, Hindricks G, Kastrati A, Lenzen MJ, Prescott E, Roffi M, Valgimigli M, Varenhorst C, Vranckx P, Widimský P; ESC Scientific Document Group. 2017 ESC Guidelines for the management of acute myocardial infarction in patients presenting with ST-segment elevation: The Task Force for the management of acute myocardial infarction in patients presenting with ST-segment elevation of the European Society of Cardiology (ESC). *Eur Heart J*. 2018 Jan 7;39(2):119–77. doi: 10.1093/eurheartj/ehx393.

Ludman PF. BCIS Audit Report—adult interventional procedures, 2018–2019. https://www.bcis.org.uk/

Neumann FJ, Sousa-Uva M, Ahlsson A, Alfonso F, Banning AP, Benedetto U, Byrne RA, Collet JP, Falk V, Head SJ, Jüni P, Kastrati A, Koller A, Kristensen SD, Niebauer J, Richter DJ, Seferovic PM, Sibbing D, Stefanini GG, Windecker S, Yadav R, Zembala MO; ESC Scientific Document Group. 2018 ESC/EACTS Guidelines on myocardial revascularization. *Eur Heart J*. 2019 Jan 7;40(2):87–165. doi: 10.1093/eurheartj/ehy394. Erratum in: *Eur Heart J*. 2019 Oct 1;40(37):3096.

Norrell M, Perrins J, Meier B, Lincoff AM. *Essential Interventional Cardiology*. Saunders Elsevier, 2008.

Stouffer GA. *Cardiovascular Haemodynamics for the Clinician*. John Wiley & Sons, 2008.

Zipes DP, Libby P, Bonow RO, Braunwald E. *Braunwald's Heart Disease: A Textbook of Cardiovascular Medicine*. Saunders Elsevier, 2004.

CHAPTER 3

VALVULAR HEART DISEASE

3.1

Epidemiology

Sarah Hudson and Daniel X Augustine

3.1.1. Changes with time

The Western world:

- Degenerative disease is the most common cause (mainly calcific aortic valve disease and degenerative mitral valve disease).
- Rheumatic is the second most common: young immigrants or older patients exposed during childhood to rheumatic fever.

Developing countries:

- Rheumatic is the most frequent cause.

3.2

Aortic Valve Disease

Sarah Hudson and Daniel X Augustine

TABLE OF CONTENTS

3.2.1 Anatomy 199
3.2.2 Aortic regurgitation 199
   Aetiology 199
   Pathophysiology 200
   Natural history 200
   Symptoms 200
   Examination 201
   Investigations 201
   Management 202
   Follow-up 203
3.2.3 Aortic stenosis 203
   Aetiology 203
   Pathophysiology 204
   Natural history 204
   Symptoms 205
   Examination 205
   Investigations 206
   Management 207
   ESC guideline 2021 recommendation 208
   ACC/AHA 2020 guideline recommendations 208
   Special populations 210

3.2.1 Anatomy

- The aortic valve usually has three cusps, which overlap each other by 1 mm
- The lines where the valve cusps meet are known as the commissures
- The sinus of Valsalva surrounds the aortic valve cusps and acts to pool blood to allow improved coronary flow during diastole
- The cusps and associated sinus are named with the associated coronary artery that arises from it (right, left, and non).
- 1–2% of the population have two cusps (bicuspid valve). This increases risk of aortic valve disease and aortic dilation. Patients with this should have an echo every 3–5 years in the absence of stenosis and their first-degree relatives should have a screening echo.

3.2.2 Aortic regurgitation

Aetiology
Primary valve disease
- Degenerative valve disease is the most common form in the Western world, accounting for approximately two-thirds of cases
- Bicuspid valve is affected in 15–30%
- Rheumatic disease is the most common form in developing countries
- Endocarditis causes 10% of cases

- Rarer causes:
  - Trauma
  - Drugs, e.g. fenfluaramine
  - Radiation

Disease of the aorta

Most often due to:

- Systemic hypertension
- Aortic dissection
- Aortitis
- Connective tissue disease:
  - Marfan syndrome
  - Ankylosing spondylitis
  - Ehlers–Danlos syndrome
  - Pseudoxanthoma elasticum

Pathophysiology

Acute severe aortic regurgitation

- There is an abrupt increase in end diastolic volume whilst a normal left ventricular size is maintained. The ventricle is unable to dilate acutely to compensate for this increased volume and there is a reduction in forward-stroke volume, causing increased end diastolic pressure and acute pulmonary oedema.
- Commonest cause is infective endocarditis. Aortic dissection is a less frequent cause.

Chronic severe aortic regurgitation

- Slowly increasing end diastolic volume causes a gradual increase in LV size
- Increase in LV wall stress occurs together with initial compensatory myocardial hypertrophy
- The combination of hypertrophy and increased LV volumes increases stroke volume—net forward flow is maintained despite the regurgitant lesion and so patients may remain asymptomatic for some time
- Decompensation and symptoms occur due to the onset of LV dysfunction leading to an inability to maintain the stroke volume.

Natural history

- Acute severe AR: poor prognosis unless surgical correction used
- Asymptomatic severe AR with preserved LV function
  - Development of LV dysfunction: < 1.3% per year
  - Sudden death < 0.2% per year
  - Development of symptoms with LV dysfunction or death < 4.3% per year
- Predictors of outcome in these individuals include:
  - Age
  - End systolic volume
  - Ejection fraction.

Symptoms

- Symptoms of heart failure: dyspnoea, orthopnoea, and paroxysmal nocturnal dyspnoea
- Palpitations due to tachycardia or premature beats can occur
- Angina (in the absence of coronary artery disease) may be seen due to reduced myocardial perfusion pressure or as a result of subendocardial ischemia due to left ventricular hypertrophy.

Examination
Peripheral signs
- Water hammer or Corrigan pulse:
    - Initial distension of the peripheral arteries occurs due to increased stroke volume and an elevation in systolic pressure
    - The regurgitation leads to a fall in pressure and rapid collapse of the arteries and a low diastolic pressure (creating a wide pulse pressure)
- Other findings associated with a hyperdynamic pulse include:
    - Traube's sign: systolic and diastolic sounds heard over femoral arteries
    - Duroziez sign: systolic and diastolic bruit heart over femoral arteries
    - DeMusset's sign: head bobbing with heart beat
    - Quincke's pulse: capillary pulsations in finger tips.

Precordial palpation
- As a consequence of left ventricular enlargement the apical pulse is displaced laterally and is more diffuse.

Cardiac auscultation
- Heart sounds:
    - A third heart sound (gallop) is heard due to severe LV systolic impairment in decompensated disease
- Heart murmur:
    - High-pitched diastolic murmur is audible following A2; best heard in the third/fourth intercostal space at the left sternal edge
    - The duration of the murmur in diastole correlates with severity of regurgitation
    - Austin Flint murmur is a mid-to-late diastolic murmur audible at the apex due to anterior mitral valve leaflet displacement from the regurgitant flow and also turbulence due to mixing of the antegrade mitral flow with retrograde aortic flow
    - An ejection systolic murmur can often be heard, similar to that of aortic stenosis, due to the increased stroke volume across the aortic valve.

Investigations
Chest radiograph
- Cardiomegaly.

Electrocardiogram
- Changes due to increase in left ventricular size or hypertrophy (increasing amplitude of the QRS complex) with or without repolarization abnormalities may be seen.

Echocardiography
See also Chapter 1.1.6.

Cardiac catheterization
- The 2021 ESC/EACTS guidelines recommend cardiac catheterization only be used for assessment of ventricular function and valvular regurgitation in patients where non-invasive tests are inconclusive or discordant with clinical findings.
- It is usually undertaken to establish the presence of coronary artery disease prior to aortic valve surgery

Table 3.2.1 Echocardiographic parameters for assessing severity in aortic regurgitation.

	Vena contracta	Regurgitant volume	Regurgitant fraction	AR/LVOT ratio	EROA	Pressure half time
Mild	< 0.3 cm	≤ 30 ml	≤ 30%	< 25%	≤ 0.1 cm²	> 500 ms
Severe	> 0.6 cm	≥ 60 ml	≥ 50%	≥ 65%	≥ 0.3 cm²	< 200 ms

Cardiac MRI

- ESC/EACTS guidelines (2021) state that cardiac MRI should be used to assess AR in those with suboptimal echocardiography. CMR allows quantification of left ventricular function, stroke volumes, assessment of regurgitant volume, and assessment of the ascending aorta.

Exercise stress testing

- Symptoms are an indication for surgery in severe AR and exercise testing may be required to provoke these.

Management

Figure 3.2.1

Medical management

- ACE inhibitors (vasodilatation) or dihydropiridines may provide symptomatic improvement.

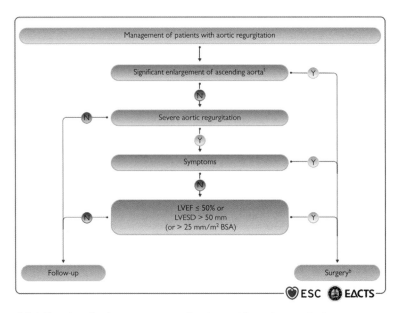

Figure 3.2.1 Flowchart for the management of patients with aortic regurgitation.
Reproduced with permission from Vahanian A, Beyersdorf F, Praz F, et al; ESC/EACTS Scientific Document Group. 2021 ESC/EACTS Guidelines for the management of valvular heart disease. *Eur Heart J*. 2022 Feb 12;43(7):561–632. doi: 10.1093/eurheartj/ehab395. © European Society of Cardiology. With permission from Oxford University Press

Surgical management

Severe aortic regurgitation: indications for surgery:

- Symptomatic
- Asymptomatic but with LV ejection fraction ≤ 50% or LV end systolic diameter > 50 mm (or > 25 mm/m² BSA in patients with small body size).
- Patients undergoing CABG or surgery of the ascending aorta or another valve
- Surgery may be considered in asymptomatic patients with severe AR with LVESD > 20 mm/m² BSA or resting LVED ≤ 55% if surgery is at low risk (IIb recommendation)
- Surgery may be considered in asymptomatic patients with LVEDD > 65 mm and with progressive enlargement in size of LV or progressive decrease in LVEF.
    - Aortic root or tubular ascending aortic aneurysm surgery:
    - When surgery is primarily indicated for the aortic valve, replacement of the aortic root or tubular ascending aorta should be considered when ≥ 45 mm (especially in the presence of a bicuspid aortic valve).
- Aortic root surgery if (irrespective of the severity of aortic regurgitation):
    - Aortic diameter ≥ 45 mm:
        - Marfan syndrome and additional risk factors (FH of aortic dissection or personal history of spontaneous vascular dissection); severe AR or MR; desire for pregnancy; uncontrolled systemic arterial hypertension; aortic size increase > 3 mm/yr)
        - TGFBR1 or TGFBR2 mutation (including Loeys–Dietz)—may consider surgery at 40 mm in TGFRB2 or women with low BSA or severe extra-aortic features
    - Aortic diameter ≥ 50 mm: In the presence of a bicuspid valve with additional risk factors or coarctation; patients with Marfan syndrome without additional risk factors
    - Aortic diameter ≥ 55 mm: All other patients

Follow-up

- Mild–moderate AR should have clinic review yearly and echocardiography every 2 years
- Asymptomatic severe AR should have 3–6-monthly follow up after initial examination, and then if all is stable 1-yearly follow up is sufficient
- In those with a dilated aortic root (> 40 mm), follow up with CT or CMR is recommended

3.2.3 Aortic stenosis

Aetiology

Supravalvular aortic stenosis

This is a form of congenital heart disease. There are two main forms:

- Constriction of a thickened ascending aorta at the superior aspect of the sinuses of Valsalva ('hour glass deformity'): 60–75%
- Diffuse narrowing along the ascending aorta: 25–40%.

Valvular aortic stenosis

Causes include:

- Calcific 'degenerative' aortic stenosis—accounts for 80% of cases in the West
- A congenitally abnormal valve (unicuspid or bicuspid) with superimposed calcification
- Rheumatic valve disease.

- Rare causes include:
  - Familial hypercholesteraemia: lipid infiltration causes thickening of the aortic cusps
  - Hyperparathyroidism: characterized by disturbed mineral metabolism and associated inflammation/calcification of the aortic cusps
  - Paget's disease: increased cardiac output causes increased turbulence across the valve, increasing the incidence of calcific aortic stenosis
  - Lupus erythematosus: characterized by thickening of valvular leaflets and distortion with fibrocalcific nodules.
  - Fabry disease
  - Ochronosis: accumulation of homogentisic acid, dark staining of valves (alkaptonuria)
  - Post radiation therapy

Subvalvular aortic stenosis

- Subvalvular aortic stenosis usually results from a variety of fixed lesions such as a thin membrane (most common) or a thick fibromuscular ridge.

Pathophysiology
Calcific degenerative disease

This is characterized by:

- Subendothelial accumulation of low density lipoprotein (LDL) and subsequent production of angiotensin II together with inflammation of T lymphocytes and macrophages
- Local production of proteins causing tissue calcification and activation of inflammatory signalling pathways (such as tumour necrosis factor alpha, C reactive protein, and the complement system)
- Microscopic accumulation of extracellular calcification in the early disease stage, progression as disease advances culminating in areas of frank bone formation in end-stage disease.

Rheumatic valve disease

- Rheumatic valve disease is characterized by fusion of the commissures between the leaflets with a small central orifice.

Natural history

Age at presentation:

- Rheumatic disease often presents early: second to fourth decades
- Bicuspid valve-associated stenosis: fifth to sixth decades
- Degenerative calcific trileaflet stenosis: seventh to eighth decades
- Overall, 4–5% of people over 65 years of age will have aortic stenosis.

Asymptomatic patients with severe aortic stenosis:

- Rate of sudden death without surgery is less than 1% per year
- Likelihood of remaining free from cardiac death and aortic valve replacement at 1, 2, and 5 years was approximately 80%, 63%, and 25% respectively
- In symptomatic patients, average survival following symptom onset is 2–3 years and there is a high risk of sudden death.

Symptoms
Heart failure
- Obstructed outflow causes increase in LV filling pressures and compensatory hypertrophy
- As diastolic dysfunction progresses there is an inability of the LV to sustain cardiac output during exercise
- Systolic heart failure occurs late and can often be an end-stage finding.

Pre-syncope/syncope
This reflects decreased cerebral perfusion and may manifest due to:

- Exercise-induced vasodilation in conjunction with a fixed obstruction resulting in hypotension
- Transient bradyarrhythmia or arrhythmia such as atrial fibrillation post exertion
- Increased left ventricular (LV) pressures causing stimulation of LV baroreceptors and then a fall in arterial pressures causing reduced venous return.

Angina
Angina occurs in up to two-thirds of patients. In those without underlying coronary artery disease, angina can occur via several mechanisms:

- Increased left ventricular mass causing increased oxygen demand
- Compression of intra myocardial coronary arteries from prolonged contraction
- Outflow obstruction causing a compensatory tachycardia to augment cardiac output but with reduced diastolic coronary perfusion time.

Examination
Carotid pulse palpation
- Slow rising, low volume pulse due to prolonged ejection through the narrowed aortic valve and decreased stroke volume.

Precordial palpation
- A sustained apex due to outflow obstruction. In later stages as LV failure occurs the cardiac impulse becomes displaced.

Cardiac auscultation
Heart sounds:

- Aortic valve closure becomes progressively delayed with progression, and S2 is soft and single (occurring simultaneously with P2)
- In severe AS S2 may disappear—specific but not sensitive
- Fourth heart sound due to vigorous left atrial contraction into a stiff non-compliant LV
- Bicuspid valve: an aortic ejection click may be heard following S1 in the early stages of aortic stenosis when the leaflets have some stiffness but are still mobile

Heart murmur:

- Classically an ejection systolic murmur is audible, loudest at the base of the heart in the second right intercostal space and radiating to the carotid arteries
- With increasing severity the maximum outflow and gradient occur late in systole; later murmurs signify worse disease.

Investigations

Chest radiograph
- Usually normal until decompensation occurs.
- With advancing disease calcification of the aortic valve leaflets and dilatation of the ascending aorta can be seen.

Electrocardiogram
- LVH, with or without repolarization changes, is seen in approximately 80% with severe aortic stenosis.

Echocardiography
Echocardiography is the main diagnostic tool used. See Chapter 1.1.6

ESC guidelines define 4 categories of aortic stenosis based on echo findings:

- High-gradient aortic stenosis:
  - Valve area ≤ 1 cm², mean gradient ≥ 40 mmHg
  - Severe aortic stenosis assumed irrespective of LVEF and flow
- Low-flow, low gradient aortic stenosis with reduced ejection fraction:
  - Valve area ≤ 1 cm², mean gradient < 40 mmHg, EF <5 0%, stroke volume index ≤ 35 ml/m²
  - Here there is a need to establish if reduced valve area is due to 'true' severe aortic stenosis or a consequence of impaired left ventricular function with reduced valve opening ('pseudo-severe').
  - Low-dose dobutamine stress echocardiography (DSE) can help differentiate:
    - True aortic stenosis: there is little change in valve area (< 0.2 cm²) but increasing aortic valve gradient
    - Pseudo-severe aortic stenosis: an increase in aortic valve area to > 1.0 cm² with flow normalization
    - During low-dose DSE an increase in stoke volume by > 20% is a sign of contractile reserve and associated with better prognosis
    - In the absence of contractile reserve then calcium score br MSCT can be helpful (score ≥ 3000 (men) or ≥ 1600 (women) make severe AS very likely)—see below also.
- Low flow, low gradient aortic stenosis with preserved ejection fraction
  - valve area ≤ 1 cm², mean gradient < 40 mmHg, EF ≥ 50%, stroke volume index ≤ 35 ml/m²
  - Typically hypertensive elderly patients with small ventricle size and LVH
  - Diagnosis is difficult and requires careful review of images and consideration for other explanations for echo findings
  - Calcium score by MSCT can be useful:
    - Severe aortic stenosis very likely: men > 3,000; women > 1,600
    - Severe aortic stenosis likely: men > 2,000; women > 1,200
    - Severe aortic stenosis unlikely: men < 1,600; women < 800
- Normal flow, low gradient aortic stenosis with preserved ejection fraction:
  - Valve area ≤ 1 cm², mean gradient < 40 mmHg, EF ≥ 50%, stroke volume index > 35 ml/m²
  - In general these patients have only moderate stenosis

On average the various echocardiographic parameters of aortic stenosis progress as follows:
- Valve area declines by 0.1 cm^2 per year
- Aortic valve gradient increases by 7 mmHg per year
- Aortic valve velocity increases by 0.25 m/s per year.

Exercise tolerance test

- Exercise tolerance test is used in the risk stratification of the asymptomatic individual by monitoring the development of symptoms and for abnormal haemodynamic changes with exercise (fall in resting blood pressure with exercise or failure to augment resting blood pressure by >10 mmHg)
- ST depression during exercise is common in asymptomatic patients and has no known prognostic significance
- The test is contraindicated in symptomatic patients.

Cardiac catheterization

- Cardiac catheterization is usually undertaken to establish the presence of coronary artery disease prior to surgery.
- LV catheterization to assess severity of aortic stenosis is only indicated in patients where non-invasive tests are inconclusive.

Cardiac computed tomography

- Multislice cardiac computed tomography (CT) is able to provide quantitative estimation of the amount of valvular calcification. It may have a role in low flow, low gradient AS with preserved ejection fraction.
- It allows assessment of the ascending aorta.

Cardiac magnetic resonance

- Cardiac magnetic resonance (CMR) is able to detect the presence of aortic stenosis, the antegrade velocity, and allows assessment of the ascending aorta.

Management
Medical management

- The development of symptoms, or progressive worsening haemodynamic parameters, are indications for surgery
- The role of medical therapy is to alleviate symptoms of advanced disease such as heart failure.

Intervention

- In symptomatic patients, valve replacement is recommended for all unless there are severe comorbidities resulting in intervention being unlikely to improve quality of life or survival.
- Interventional options are surgical aortic valve replacement (SAVR), transcatheter aortic valve implantation (TAVI), or balloon valvuloplasty
- Balloon valvuloplasty is a 'bridging' option only
- Decision between SAVR or TAVI is patient-specific and evolving:
    - Factors which favour TAVI selection include age ≥ 75 yrs, euroSCORE II > 8%, frailty, previous cardiac surgery, porcelain aorta, sequalae of chest radiation, severe chest deformation or scoliosis, or high likelihood of severe patient–prosthesis mismatch.
    - In the elderly with extreme surgical risk TAVI is superior to medical management.

- In the elderly with high or intermediate surgical risk TAVI is non-inferior to SAVR
- In those with low surgical risk the PARTNER 3 trial has shown favourable outcome for TAVI when compared with SAVR after 2 years of follow-up. Longer follow-up outcomes is desirable in this cohort.
- TAVI has a higher risk of vascular complications, paravalvular regurgitation, and need for pacemaker, whilst SAVR has a higher risk of severe bleeding, AKI, and development of AF.
- Risk of stroke is similar for TAVI or SAVR.
- SAVR can be indicated in asymptomatic patients, whilst TAVI is not.

ESC guideline 2021 recommendation

- Asymptomatic patients:
    - In all patients, intervention is recommended if:
        - Reduced LV function (EF < 50%) without another cause
        - Symptoms during ETT
        - Intervention should be considered if:
            - LVEF < 55% without another cause
            - sustained fall in BP (> 20 mmHg) during ETT
    - In low-risk asymptomatic patients, consider intervention if:
        - Markedly calcified valve with a rapid increase in velocity of ≥ 0.3 m/s per year
        - Mean gradient ≥ 60 mmHg or Vmax > 5m/s
        - Markedly elevated BNP levels (> 3× normal range without other explanation)
        - BNP levels > 3× age and sex corrected normal range without other explanation
- Symptomatic patients and likely to benefit from intervention:
    - SAVR is recommended in younger patients who are low risk for surgery (< 75 years and EuroSCORE II < 4%) or in patients who are operable and unsuitable for transfemoral TAVI
    - TAVI is recommended in older patients (≥ 75 years) or in those who are high risk (EuroSCORE II > 8%) or unsuitable for surgery and suitable for TF TAVI

ACC/AHA 2020 guideline recommendations

1. Symptomatic and asymptomatic patients with severe AS and any indication for AVR who are < 65 years of age or have a life expectancy > 20 years: SAVR
2. Symptomatic patients 65–80 years with severe AS and have no anatomic contraindication to transfemoral TAVI, either SAVR or transfemoral TAVI is recommended after shared decision-making about the balance between expected patient longevity and valve durability
3. Symptomatic patients with severe AS who are > 80 years of age or for younger patients with a life expectancy < 10 years and no anatomic contraindication to transfemoral TAVI, transfemoral TAVI is recommended in preference to SAVR
4. Asymptomatic patients with severe AS and an LVEF < 50% who are ≤ 80 years and have no anatomic contraindication to transfemoral TAVI, the decision between TAVI and SAVR should follow the same recommendations as for symptomatic patients listed in points 1–3 above
5. Asymptomatic patients with severe AS and an abnormal exercise test, very severe AS, rapid progression, or an elevated BNP, SAVR is recommended in preference to TAVI
6. For patients with an indication for AVR for whom a bioprosthetic valve is preferred but not suitable for transfemoral TAVI, SAVR is recommended

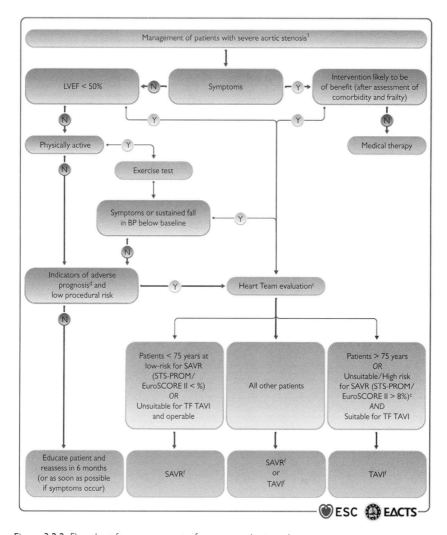

Figure 3.2.2 Flowchart for management of severe aortic stenosis.
Reproduced with permission from Vahanian A, Beyersdorf F, Praz F, et al; ESC/EACTS Scientific Document Group. 2021 ESC/EACTS Guidelines for the management of valvular heart disease. *Eur Heart J.* 2022 Feb 12;43(7):561–632. doi: 10.1093/eurheartj/ehab395. © European Society of Cardiology. With permission from Oxford University Press.

7. Symptomatic patients of any age with severe AS and a high or prohibitive surgical risk, TAVI is recommended if predicted post-TAVI survival is > 12 months with an acceptable quality of life
8. Symptomatic patients with severe AS for whom predicted post-TAVI or post-SAVR survival is < 12 months or for whom minimal improvement in quality of life is expected, palliative care is recommended after shared decision-making, including discussion of patient preferences and values.
9. In critically ill patients with severe AS, percutaneous aortic balloon dilation may be considered as a bridge to SAVR or TAVI.

Special populations

Aortic valve replacement should be considered in patients requiring coronary artery bypass grafting with at least moderate aortic stenosis

Follow-up

- Asymptomatic severe aortic stenosis: follow up every 6 months
- Moderate aortic stenosis: yearly
- Young patients with mild AS and no significant calcification: 2–3 years
- Figure 3.2.2 shows a flow chart for the most recent ESC guidelines.

3.3

Mitral valve disease

Sarah Hudson and Daniel X Augustine

TABLE OF CONTENTS

3.3.1 Anatomy 211
3.3.2 Mitral regurgitation 211
　　Aetiology 211
　　Pathophysiology 212
　　Natural history 212
　　Symptoms 212
　　Examination 212
　　Investigations 213
　　Management 213
　　TEER in patients with severe symptomatic MR 215
　　Follow-up 215
3.3.3 Mitral stenosis 215
　　Aetiology 215
　　Pathophysiology 217
　　Natural history 217
　　Symptoms 217
　　Examination 217
　　Investigations 218
　　Management 219
　　Follow-up 221

3.3.1 Anatomy

The mitral valve consists of two leaflets (anterior and posterior).

- Each leaflet has three scallops, with A1 and P1 being adjacent to the antero-lateral commissures; A3 and P3 are adjacent to the postero-medial commissures
- The valve leaflets are supported by the mitral valve annulus
- The leaflets are attached to the papillary muscles by chordae tendinae.

3.3.2 Mitral regurgitation

Aetiology

Primary mitral regurgitation

Main causes:

- Degenerative MR—most common cause
- Infective endocarditis
- Rheumatic valve disease
- Trauma causing ruptured chordae

Other causes:

- Connective tissue diseases—Marfan, Ehlers–Danlos
- Carcinoid

- Drug-induced
- RA/SLE

Secondary mitral regurgitation
Main causes:

- Ischemic heart disease
- LV systolic dysfunction: annular dilatation can occur due to left ventricular enlargement causing poor leaflet coaptation.

Pathophysiology
Acute severe mitral regurgitation
- If the left ventricle and atrium have not had a chance to adapt to the MR, its compliance is usually normal (and there has been no compensatory LVH)
- Acutely: forward stroke volume and cardiac output are reduced
- Increased LA volumes cause a marked rise in LA pressure, which is reflected back to the pulmonary circulation
- Cardiogenic shock can quickly develop. Tachycardia occurs to try to compensate for the fall in left ventricular ejection volume, and the ventricle can appear 'hyperdynamic'.

Chronic severe mitral regurgitation
- The LV adapts to the chronic increase in LV volume by enlarging to deliver a larger stroke volume (whilst systolic function is maintained)
- Eccentric LVH contributes to the increase in LV size whilst better LA compliance allows moderation of left atrial pressure, a feature not seen in acute severe mitral regurgitation
- Patients may remain asymptomatic for some time.

Natural history
Acute severe mitral regurgitation
- Without intervention acute severe mitral regurgitation carries a poor prognosis.

Chronic asymptomatic mitral regurgitation
- With medical management, end points and 5-year rates are:
    - Death from any cause: 22%
    - Death from cardiac causes: 14%
    - Cardiac events (cardiac cause death, heart failure, or new AF): 33%
- Predictors of poor outcome include ERO, left atrial dilatation, LV enlargement, and reduced LV ejection fraction.

Symptoms
- Exertional dyspnoea
- Palpitations due to AF

Examination
Precordial palpation
- Chronic MR (LV dilatation)—apex pulse laterally displaced
- Acute MR—the apex beat is hyperdynamic and not displaced
- Apical thrill indicates severe disease.

Cardiac auscultation

- Heart sounds:
    - S1 can be reduced as the mitral valve leaflets do not coapt properly
    - Wide splitting of S2 can happen as A2 occurs earlier due to the reduced LV ejection time
    - In patients with pulmonary artery hypertension, P2 will be increased and delayed, further accentuating splitting of S2
    - In severe MR with LV systolic impairment, the increased flow into a dilated left ventricle produces an S3
- Heart murmur:
    - Holosystolic murmur is most easily audible at the apex, radiating to the axilla
    - With mitral valve prolapse a systolic click occurs in mid–late systole (time of maximum prolapse) when the chordae are under peak tension
    - In acute MR (fall in LV filling pressure together with the acutely raised LA pressure): intensity of the murmur does not correlate with severity.

Investigations
Chest radiograph

- Chronic severe MR: LV and LA dilatation
- Acute severe MR: Normal cardiac silhouette with evidence of pulmonary congestion.

Electrocardiogram

- LV hypertrophy and LA dilation
- AF is common
- In ischaemic MR, ischaemic features are most commonly inferolateral.

Echocardiogram

See Chapter 1.1.6

Cardiac catheterization

- This is usually undertaken to establish the presence of coronary artery disease prior to mitral valve surgery. Haemodynamic measures should be undertaken only when non-invasive tests are inconclusive.

Cardiac MRI

- If there is a discrepancy between echocardiographic and clinical findings then CMR allows calculation of MR regurgitant volumes and ERO as well as LV/LA size and LV function.

Management
Medical management

- Acute MR:
    - Management is aimed at stabilizing haemodynamics in preparation for surgery
    - Nitrates and diuretics can reduce filling pressures
    - Sodium nitroprusside reduces afterload and regurgitant fraction
    - Inotropic agents/intra-aortic balloon pump may be needed in those with cardiogenic shock
- Chronic asymptomatic MR:
    - There are no long-term studies to indicate any prognostic benefit from the use of vasodilators in patients with chronic MR and preserved LV ejection fraction

In those with symptoms, optimal medical therapy for heart failure in line with guidelines should be given

Surgical/percutaneous management of primary mitral regurgitation (ESC guidelines 2021)

Acute severe mitral regurgitation
- In symptomatic patients urgent surgery is recommended

Chronic severe primary mitral regurgitation
- Mitral valve repair is preferred to valve replacement
- If repair not possible then replacement is undertaken (ideally with chordal preservation)

Symptomatic severe primary mitral regurgitation
- Surgery is recommended in patients who are operable and not high risk.
- Transcatheter edge-to-edge repair (TEER) may be considered in patients who fulfil the echocardiographic criteria of eligibility and who are judged inoperable or at high surgical risk by the Heart Team

Asymptomatic severe primary mitral regurgitation
ESC guidelines recommend surgery in the following circumstances (Figure 3.3.1):

- LV ejection fraction ≤ 60% and/or LV end systolic diameter ≥ 40 mm (IB)

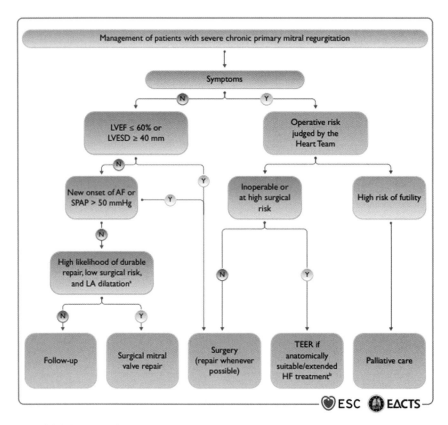

Figure 3.3.1 Flowchart for management of severe chronic primary mitral regurgitation.
Reproduced with permission from Vahanian A, Beyersdorf F, Praz F, et al; ESC/EACTS Scientific Document Group. 2021 ESC/EACTS Guidelines for the management of valvular heart disease. *Eur Heart J.* 2022 Feb 12;43(7):561–632. doi: 10.1093/eurheartj/ehab395. © European Society of Cardiology. With permission from Oxford University Press.

Surgery should be considered (IIa) if:
- atrial fibrillation secondary to MR
- systolic pulmonary artery pressure > 50 mmHg at rest
- significant LA dilation (LA volume ≥ 60 ml/m^2 or diameter ≥ 55 mm in sinus rhythm)

Transcatheter edge-to-edge repair (TEER)
- May be considered in patients with symptomatic severe primary mitral regurgitation who fulfil echocardiographic criteria and judged inoperable/high surgical risk by the Heart Team

Functional mitral regurgitation
- In patients with functional (or secondary) mitral regurgitation the papillary muscles, chordae, and valve leaflets are normal. Major causes of functional mitral regurgitation are ischaemia, any cause of a dilated ventricle and secondary to chronic atrial fibrillation which causes LA enlargement and annular dilatation. The management of patients with chronic secondary mitral regurgitation is shown in Figure 3.3.2.
- Note that lower thresholds may be applied to define severe secondary MR compared to primary
- First-line treatment is optimal medical management of heart failure.
- Valve intervention is generally not an option when LVEF is < 15%

Surgical/percutaneous management of severe secondary mitral regurgitation (ESC guidelines 2021)
- Surgery indicated in those undergoing CABG or other cardiac surgery
- Surgery is recommended if patients remain symptomatic despite optimal medical therapy, including CRT if indicated, and has to be decided by a structured collaborative Heart Team
- Patients who remain symptomatic but who are not appropriate for surgery, TEER should be considered

TEER in patients with severe symptomatic MR
- TEER in patients with severe symptomatic secondary MR has been evaluated in 2 RCTs—COAPT and MITRA-FR.
- These showed TEER to be safe and effectively reduce MR up to 3 years.
- There were conflicting results however—MITRA-FR showed no impact of MitraClip implantation on all-cause mortality or HF hospitalization compared to OMT, whilst COAPT showed substantially reduced hospitalization for HF and all-cause mortality at 2 years.
- Additional studies are needed to identify which patients would benefit most from TEER

Follow-up
- Asymptomatic patients with severe MR and LVEF > 60%: Echo and clinical follow up every 6 months
- Moderate MR: Annual clinic review and echocardiography every 1–2 years

3.3.3 Mitral stenosis

Aetiology
Rheumatic heart disease is responsible for the majority of cases. Rarer causes include:

- Degenerative mitral valve disease
- Mucopolysaccharidosis

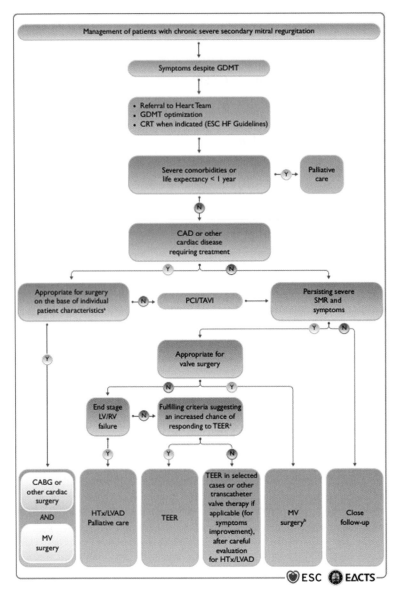

Figure 3.3.2 Flowchart for management of severe chronic secondary mitral regurgitation.
Reproduced with permission from Vahanian A, Beyersdorf F, Praz F, et al; ESC/EACTS Scientific Document Group. 2021 ESC/EACTS Guidelines for the management of valvular heart disease. *Eur Heart J*. 2022 Feb 12;43(7):561–632. doi: 10.1093/eurheartj/ehab395. © European Society of Cardiology. With permission from Oxford University Press.

- Gout
- Lupus erythematosus
- Stenosis due to obstruction from vegetations or tumour.

Pathophysiology

- Leaflets thicken with a loss of normal valve morphology due to deposition of fibrin
- As disease progresses there is fusion of the leaflet commissures and thickening/shortening of the chordae tendinae
- Ultimately calcification of the mitral valve apparatus
- Reduced LV diastolic filling and subsequently left atrial pressures increase
- A diastolic pressure gradient between the LA and LV exists
- Increase in LA pressure is transmitted through the pulmonary circulation causing an increase in pulmonary capillary and arterial pressures
- Pulmonary oedema ensues as the pulmonary capillary wedge pressure approaches 25 mmHg
- With chronic mitral stenosis, LV systolic dysfunction occurs in around 25% of cases
- Atrial fibrillation is common in advanced disease due to:
    - Chronically increased LA size
    - The fibrotic effects of rheumatic disease on the left atrium and intermodal and interatrial tracts as well as damage to the sinus node.

Natural history

- MS is a slowly progressive disease and patients remain asymptomatic for years
- Disease progression has been noted to increase following the onset of symptoms
- The mean rate of progression is estimated to be 0.1 cm^2 per year and the mean interval between rheumatic fever and the onset of symptoms is 16–20 years
- In symptomatic patients, without intervention 5-year survival rates were estimated at 44%.

Symptoms

The normal mitral valve area is 4–6 cm^2 and clinical symptoms may occur with moderate narrowing (< 2 cm^2). The most frequent symptoms encountered are:

- Dyspnoea
    - Left ventricular systolic dysfunction
    - Inability to increase left ventricular ejection with increased physiological demands
- Palpitations
    - Atrial fibrillation is commonly seen with advanced disease
- Haemoptysis—rare
    - Increased LA pressures causing rupture of thin dilated bronchial veins
    - Pulmonary oedema causing pink frothy sputum
- Dsyphonia/hoarseness
    - Compression of the recurrent laryngeal nerve by the dilated LA (Ortners syndrome)
- Oedema/ascites
- Embolic events
    - Presenting feature in 20% of cases

Examination

Precordial palpation

- In advanced disease an apical diastolic thrill may be palpable
- With pulmonary hypertension a right ventricular heave and palpable S2 occurs.

Cardiac auscultation
Opening snap
- Due to leaflet tip fusion—rapid initial opening of the valve followed by a sudden reduction in motion
- In more advanced stenosis the increasing LA pressure brings mitral valve opening earlier and reduces the interval between S2 and the opening snap

First heart sound
- In non-calcified MS the leaflets are still patent at the onset of ventricular contraction and S1 is loud
- As the leaflets become more restricted due to calcification their movement is limited and S1 is soft

Second heart sound
- P2 is loud in those with pulmonary hypertension

Heart murmur
Low-pitched diastolic rumble loudest at the apex

- The duration of the murmur correlates with disease severity
- In severe MS the increased LA to LV pressure gradient and longer duration of blood flow across the mitral valve results in longer murmur duration
- Right heart failure
- Chronically raised pulmonary pressures are reflected by signs of right-sided heart failure with changes in the JVP, peripheral oedema, and sometimes ascites present.

Investigations
Chest radiograph
- Enlarged left atrium with a double contour
- Straightening of left heart border
- Calcification of the mitral valve annulus
- Pulmonary congestion.

Electrocardiogram
Common ECG features seen include:

- Broad and bifid P wave due to left atrial enlargement and hypertrophy
- Atrial fibrillation
- Changes due to pulmonary hypertension: right ventricular hypertrophy, right axis deviation.

Echocardiogram
See Chapter 1.1.6

Exercise stress test/stress echocardiography
- In patients who have symptoms but whose parameters of severity do not correlate, stress testing may be considered to estimate heart rate, blood pressure response, transmitral gradient, and pulmonary artery pressure at rest and upon stress

Management
Medical management
- Diuretics
- Beta blocker/rate-controlling calcium antagonist/ivabradine
- Anticoagulation with warfarin for:
    - AF/pAF
    - history of systemic embolism
    - dense spontaneous contrast seen on echo
    - LA > 60 ml/m² or diameter > 50 mm

Note in patients with severe MS DCCV or ablation are not indicated as they do not durably restore sinus rhythm.

Surgical management
If possible percutaneous mitral commissurotomy (PMC) is performed. The suitability for this procedure depends on the mobility of the leaflet and degree of thickening/calcification. One such scoring system is the Wilkins score (see Table 3.3.1).

Symptomatic Rheumatic MS (valve area ≤ 1.5 cm²)
See Figure 3.3.3. PMC for those who are symptomatic without unfavourable characteristics and those where surgery is contraindicated/high risk

Table 3.3.1 Wilkins classification.

Grade	Mobility	Subvalvular thickening	Thickening	Calcification
1	Highly mobile valve with only leaflet tips restricted	Minimal thickening just below the mitral leaflets	Leaflets near normal in thickness	A single area of increased echo brightness
2	Leaflet mid and base portions have normal mobility	Thickening of chordal structures extending to one-third of the chordal length	Mid-leaflets normal, considerable thickening of margins (5–8 mm)	Scattered areas of brightness confined to leaflet margins
3	Valve continues to move forward in diastole, mainly from the base	Thickening extended to distal third of the chords	Thickening extending through the entire leaflet (5–8 mm)	Brightness extending into the mid-portions of the leaflets
4	No or minimal forward movement of the leaflets in diastole	Extensive thickening and shortening of all chordal structures extending down to the papillary muscles	Considerable thickening of all leaflet tissue (> 8–10 mm)	Extensive brightness throughout much of the leaflet tissue

Scores > 8 are not suitable for PMC. Reproduced from Padial LR, Abascal VM, Moreno PR, Weyman AE, Levine RA, Palacios IF. Echocardiography can predict the development of severe mitral regurgitation after percutaneous mitral valvuloplasty by the Inoue technique. *Am J Cardiol.* 1999 Apr 15;83(8):1210–3. doi: 10.1016/s0002-9149(99)00061-2 with permission from Elsevier..

Percutaneous mitral commissurotomy has a failure rate of 1–15%, a mortality of 0–3%. It results in severe MR in 2–10% and causes a residual intra-atrial septal defect in up to 80% of cases, most of which close spontaneously.

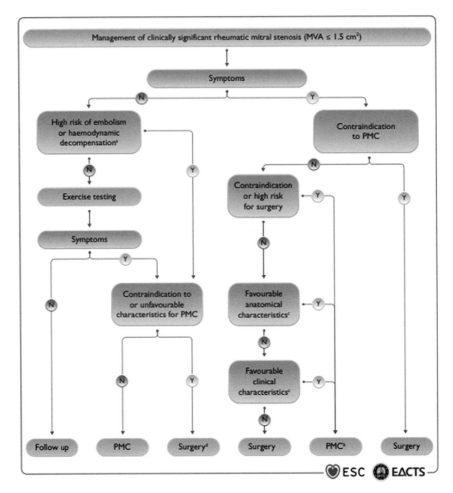

Figure 3.3.3 Flowchart for management of clinically significant rheumatic mitral stenosis.
Reproduced with permission from Vahanian A, Beyersdorf F, Praz F, et al; ESC/EACTS Scientific Document Group. 2021 ESC/EACTS Guidelines for the management of valvular heart disease. *Eur Heart J.* 2022 Feb 12;43(7):561–632. doi: 10.1093/eurheartj/ehab395. © European Society of Cardiology. With permission from Oxford University Press

- Contraindications to PMC: left atrial thrombus, > mild MR, severe or bi-commissural calcification, absence of commissural fusion, other indication for cardiac surgery
- Unfavourable anatomical or clinical characteristics, defined as the presence of several of the following:
    - Clinical characteristics
        - Old age
        - History of PMC
        - NYHA IV
        - Permanent AF
        - Severe pulmonary hypertension

- Anatomic characteristics
  - Echo score > 8
  - Cornier score 3 (calcification of any extent seen on fluoroscopy)
  - Severe tricuspid regurgitation
  - Very small valve area

Valve replacement for those with:

- Contraindications to PMC
- Unfavourable anatomical characteristics, unfavourable clinical characteristics for PMC.

Asymptomatic Rheumatic MS (valve area ≤ 1.5 cm^2)

Intervention is indicated in:

1) Patients with high risk of embolism (history of systemic embolism, dense spontaneous contrast in LA or new onset AF) or high risk of haemodynamic decompensation (systolic pulmonary artery pressure > 50 mmHg at rest, need for major non-cardiac surgery or desire for pregnancy)
2) Patients who have symptoms on exercise testing.

PMC is the preferred approach if they do not have any unfavourable clinical or anatomical characteristics.

If PMC not possible, they should be considered for surgery, if operative risk is low, and they have symptoms at a low level of exercise.

Degenerative MS with mitral annular calcification

- Echo assessment of severity is difficult as the usual parameters lack validation
- Mean transmitral gradient has been shown to have prognostic valve
- If intervention is planned CT is necessary to assess degree and location of calcification
- Degenerative MS cannot be treated by PMC as there is no commissural fusion
- Surgery/transcatheter approaches are high risk and evidence from RCT is lacking

Follow-up

In asymptomatic patients with significant MS yearly follow-up is recommended. For moderate MS, or post PMC, follow up is every 2-3 years.

3.4

Tricuspid valve disease

Sarah Hudson and Daniel X Augustine

TABLE OF CONTENTS

3.4.1 Anatomy 223
3.4.2 Tricuspid regurgitation 223
　　Aetiology 223
　　Pathophysiology 224
　　Natural history 224
　　Symptoms 224
　　Examination 224
　　Investigations 224

3.4.3 Tricuspid stenosis 225
　　Aetiology 225
　　Pathophysiology 225
　　Symptoms 225
　　Examination 226
　　Investigations 227
　　Management 227

3.4.1 Anatomy

- The valve is made up of three cusps: anterior, posterior, and septal
- Chordae tendinae attach the cusps to papillary muscles on the septum and right ventricular free wall and the valve is seated in its own annulus.

3.4.2 Tricuspid regurgitation

Aetiology
Primary tricuspid regurgitation

This is as a consequence of a disruption to the valve, papillary muscles, or chordae. Causes include:

- Infective endocarditis
- Trauma from pacemaker lead
- Rheumatic valve disease
- Carcinoid syndrome
- Ebstein's anomaly
- Drug induced

Functional tricuspid regurgitation:

This accounts for the majority of cases (> 90%) and is due to RV pressure or volume overload. Causes include:

- Pulmonary hypertension from left sided heart disease (commonest cause)
- Cor pulmonale

- Primary pulmonary hypertension
- ASD causing volume overload
- Intrinsic disease of the RV—ischaemic or cardiomyopathic

Pathophysiology
- In mild–moderate TR the RA adapts relatively well (good compliance)—patients remain asymptomatic for some time
- Onset of symptoms usually coincides with the onset of right-sided heart failure
- RA decompensates with the increasing volumes
- It is reflected by high right atrial pressure and increased right ventricular pressures/volume overload.

Natural history
- Primary TR—poor prognosis unless corrected
- Functional TR—remain asymptomatic for some time and the degree of TR may improve as RV failure improves.

Symptoms
- Symptoms of right-sided heart failure or the underlying disease process.

Examination
Jugular veins
- Elevation of right atrial pressure causes distension of the jugular veins and the JVP has characteristic features.

Palpation
- A right ventricular heave may be present due to RV dilatation and raised pulmonary pressures
- Right heart failure:
    - This manifests by the presence of peripheral oedema and ascites
    - Hepatomegaly
    - Pulsatile hepatomegaly can be present in severe TR.

Cardiac auscultation
- Heart sounds:
    - P2 component is increased with pulmonary hypertension
    - Third heart sound occurs with right heart failure and a dilated right ventricle
- Heart murmur:
    - A pan systolic murmur is heard, loudest in the left sternal border and accentuated by inspiration

Investigations
Chest radiograph
- Cardiomegaly

Electrocardiogram
- If TR is due to right ventricular infarction then ischaemic changes may be seen inferiorly/posteriorly

- If TR is due to pulmonary hypertension then features of right ventricular hypertrophy may exist (right axis deviation, tall R waves V1 and V2, right bundle branch block).

Echocardiogram
See Chapter 1.1.6

Medical
- Diuretics
- Addition of aldosterone antagonist may be considered

Surgical
- ESC guidelines (20121) recommend early repair (rather than valve replacement) prior to irreversible RV dysfunction
- Current recommendations for TV surgery due to TR:
    - Recommended in patients with:
        - Severe primary or secondary TR who are undergoing left sided valve surgery
        - Severe isolated primary TR without severe RV dysfunction
    - Should be considered in patients with:
        - Mild or moderate primary TR who are undergoing left sided valve surgery
        - Mild or moderate secondary TR with a dilated annulus (≥ 40 mm or > 21 mm/m^2) who are undergoing left sided valve surgery
        - Asymptomatic isolated severe primary TR and RV dilation who are appropriate for surgery

Severe secondary TR who are symptomatic or have RV dilation, in the absence of severe RV or LV dysfunction or severe pulmonary hypertension. Transcatheter treatment of symptomatic secondary severe TR may be considered in inoperable patients. Figure 3.4.1 is a flow diagram for the management of tricuspid regurgitation.

3.4.3 Tricuspid stenosis

Aetiology
- Rheumatic valve disease (most common)
- Congenital atresia or stenosis of valve
- Carcinoid
- Right atrial tumours
- Drug induced
- Bacterial endocarditis.

Pathophysiology
- Persistent pressure gradient between the right atrium and right ventricle—increases during inspiration and exercise (as venous return increases)
- Pressure gradient of up to 5 mmHg is sufficient to cause an increase in mean right atrial pressure.

Symptoms
- Fatigue due to obstruction of tricuspid flow limiting cardiac output.

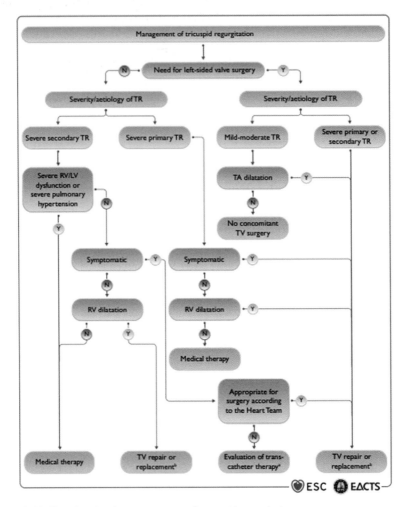

Figure 3.4.1 Flowchart for the management of tricuspid regurgitation.
Reproduced with permission from Vahanian A, Beyersdorf F, Praz F, et al; ESC/EACTS Scientific Document Group. 2021 ESC/EACTS Guidelines for the management of valvular heart disease. *Eur Heart J*. 2022 Feb 12;43(7):561–632. doi: 10.1093/eurheartj/ehab395. © European Society of Cardiology. With permission from Oxford University Press.

Examination

- Jugular venous pressure: large A wave and rate of Y descent
- Signs of pulmonary hypertension and right heart failure: hepatomegaly/hepatic pulsation, ascites, peripheral oedema, right ventricular parasternal heave.

Auscultation

- Heart sounds:
    - Opening snap localized to lower left sternal border
    - S2. Loud P2 in pulmonary hypertension

- Heart murmur:
    - Low-frequency diastolic murmur audible at the lower left sternal border, fourth intercostal space.

Investigations
Chest radiograph
- Right atrial dilatation and right ventricular enlargement may be evident.

Electrocardiogram
- Right atrial hypertrophy
- Atrial fibrillation is a common presentation.

Echocardiogram
See Chapter 1.1.6

Management
Medical management
- Diuretics when heart failure present

Surgical management
- Current ESC recommendations (2021) for surgical intervention in those with TS are:
  Severe TS (±TR) with symptoms
  Severe TS (±TR) in patient undergoing left-sided valve intervention.
- Percutaneous balloon dilatation can be attempted in cases of pure tricuspid stenosis (TS)
- Due to the higher risk of thrombosis, biological prostheses are the preferred choice

3.5

Pulmonary valve disease

Sarah Hudson and Daniel X Augustine

TABLE OF CONTENTS

3.5.1 Anatomy 229
3.5.2 Pulmonary regurgitation 229
   Aetiology 229
   Pathophysiology 229
   Symptoms 229
   Examination 230
   Investigations 230
   Management 230
3.5.3 Pulmonary stenosis 230
   Aetiology 230
   Pathophysiology 231
   Natural history 231
   Symptoms 231
   Examination 231
   Investigations 231
   Management 232
   Follow-up 232

3.5.1 Anatomy

- The pulmonary valve (PV) consists of three cusps: anterior, left, and right.

3.5.2 Pulmonary regurgitation

Aetiology
- Pulmonary hypertension
- Tetralogy of Fallot
- Infective endocarditis
- Rheumatic heart disease
- Carcinoid.

Pathophysiology
- The regurgitation occurs usually by one of the following mechanisms:
  - Dilatation of the pulmonary valve ring
  - Acquired alteration of the valve leaflet morphology
  - Congenital absence or malformation of the valve
  - Increasing regurgitation causing RV volume overload.

Symptoms
- Dyspnoea
- Fatigability

- Right-sided heart failure: oedema
- Symptoms related to the underlying disease process.

Examination
- Raised jugular venous pressure
- Precordial palpation
    - Right ventricular heave may be palpable due to pulmonary hypertension
- Cardiac auscultation
- Heart sounds:
    - Loud delayed P2 in the presence of pulmonary hypertension
    - Absent P2 if regurgitation is due to congenitally absent valve or surgical resection
- Heart murmur:
    - Classically there is a high-pitched early diastolic murmur audible in the left upper sterna area.

Investigations
Chest radiograph
- Features of pulmonary hypertension/right heart failure may be present.

Electrocardiogram
- Features reflect increasing RV volume and pressure overload: right bundle branch block (RBBB), right axis deviation, right atrial dilatation, and RVH.

Echocardiogram
See Chapter 1.1.6

Management
Medical
- Treatment of the underlying cause (e.g. with secondary pulmonary hypertension)
- Treatment of heart failure.

Surgical
- When symptoms continue despite medical therapy then surgical intervention can be considered either by surgical reconstruction or valve replacement.

3.5.3 Pulmonary stenosis

Aetiology
- Congenital pulmonic stenosis
- Congenital rubella syndrome
- Tetralogy of Fallot
- Noonan syndrome
- Supravalvular/subvalvular pulmonic stenosis.

Pathophysiology
- Fibrous thickening and fusion of the commisures. Two main morphological types exist:
    - Commissural fusion leaving an effectively bicuspid pliable valve (90%)
    - No commissural fusion but valves are dysplastic and thickened
- The obstruction leads to right ventricular hypertrophy and pulmonary hypertension
- Increasing right heart pressures in the presence of a patent foramen ovale (PFO) or septal defect will cause cyanosis
- Ultimately right ventricular failure will ensue.

Natural history
- Symptoms usually begin in those with mild pulmonary stenosis (PS)
- With moderate pulmonary stenosis both medical and surgical treatment has been shown to be effective
- Severe pulmonary stenosis, when detected early in life, will require surgical treatment to avoid right ventricular failure.

Symptoms
- Asymptomatic or may present with exertional dyspnoea progressing to symptoms of right heart failure
- Exercise induced symptoms—inability to augment pulmonary flow during physical activity. May present as syncope or chest pain
- Palpitations are common due to atrial arrhythmias.

Examination
In severe pulmonary stenosis several key clinical features are apparent.

Precordial palpation
- A left parasternal lift indicates a prominent right ventricular systolic impulse.

Cardiac auscultation
- Heart sounds:
    - Systolic ejection click is audible if leaflets are thin and pliable
    - Splitting of the second heart sound may occur due to delay in the pulmonary component
    - A right fourth heart sound due to right ventricular hypertrophy and a 'stiff' ventricle
- Heart murmur:
  Ejection systolic murmur loudest at the left upper sternal edge.

Investigations
Chest radiograph
- Dilatation of the main pulmonary artery may be evident together with reduced vascular pulmonary markings.

Electrocardiogram
- Depending on the severity of obstruction the following may be present: P pulmonale, RVH, right axis deviation.

Echocardiogram
See Chapter 1.1.6

Cardiac MRI
- Can be very useful to get accurate flow measures.

Management
- Balloon valvuloplasty is the preferred option (if leaflets are pliable) when peak gradient > 50 mmHg with symptoms, or > 60 mmHg without (AHA guidelines)
- Valve replacement is usually reserved for dysplastic/calcified leaflets or in those with significant PR.

Follow-up
- Mild PS: every 3–5 years
- Moderate: 2 years
- Severe: yearly

3.6

Mixed and multi-valvular disease

Shaun Robinson

TABLE OF CONTENTS

3.6.1 Echocardiographic assessment of mixed and multi-valve disease 235
3.6.2 Aortic or pulmonary stenosis with concomitant 235
 AR or PR 235
 MR or TR 235
 MS or TS 236
3.6.3 Aortic or pulmonary regurgitation with concomitant 236
 AS or PS 236
 MR or TR 237
 MS or TS 237
3.6.4 Mitral or tricuspid stenosis with concomitant 237
 MR or TR 237
 AS or PS 238
 AR or PR 239
3.6.5 Mitral or tricuspid regurgitation with concomitant 239
 MS or TS 239
 AS or PS 240
 AR or PR 240
 Impact of concomitant co-morbidities 241
3.6.6 Symptoms 241
3.6.7 Management and follow-up of patients with multi-valvular disease 242

- Primary heart valve disease is typically isolated to a single valve and with usually a single pathology of regurgitation or stenosis (e.g. myxomatous mitral valve degeneration or senile aortic valve calcification).
- Mixed and multiple valve disease accounts for 20% of patients with native valve disease and 17% of patients undergoing valve surgery

More common multi-valvular disease aetiologies:

- rheumatic valve disease
    - despite the association of rheumatic valve disease with mitral stenosis (MS), mitral regurgitation is the most common initial pathology with MS developing in the later stages. Multi-valve disease occurs with the development of aortic regurgitation and eventually stenosis. As rheumatic valve disease progresses, increased left atrial pressure leads to pulmonary hypertension, dilated right heart chambers, and consequently tricuspid regurgitation secondary to annular dilation.
- calcific degenerative disease
    - prior to the development of valve stenosis, thickening of the cusp/leaflet tips inhibits adequate coaptation and causes regurgitation, usually mild or moderate in severity.
- infective endocarditis
    - valve destruction secondary to endocarditis leads to regurgitation. Multi-valve involvement is present in around 20% of all endocarditis cases and portends a worse prognosis.

- chamber remodelling and annular dilation
  - annular dilation secondary to chronic atrial fibrillation is a common cause of concomitant tricuspid and mitral regurgitation.

Less common multi-valvular disease aetiologies:

- radiotherapy-based cancer treatment (typically mediastinal/thoracic)
- autoimmune inflammatory responses
- ergot-derived agonists and anorectic agents
- connective tissue disorders
- non-cardiac systemic diseases
- carcinoid heart disease
- congenital heart abnormalities

Normal valve function is defined by:

- unrestricted cusp/leaflet excursion to allow flow through the valve at low velocity and without obstruction.
- competent closure to prevent retrograde flow when the valve is shut

Progressive valvular dysfunction (whether stenosis or regurgitation) will eventually lead to abnormal loading (volume and/or pressure overload) and adverse remodelling of cardiac chambers. In cases of isolated stenosis or regurgitation (and with otherwise normal cardiac structure and function), the degree of chamber volume and/or pressure overload reflects the severity of valve disease and alters trans-valvular flow dynamics with predictability that enables the diagnosis of disease severity:

- **aortic stenosis (AS) and pulmonary stenosis (PS)**—progressive increase in afterload and therefore raised systolic pressure within the associated ventricle leads to high pressure difference between the ventricle and connecting vessel and high transvalvular velocities.
- **aortic regurgitation (AR) and pulmonary regurgitation (PR)**—when low volume, regurgitant flow through the aortic valve (AV) or pulmonary valve (PV) does not increase ventricular diastolic pressure and a high pressure difference remains between the Ao/PA and associated ventricle throughout diastole. Because flow velocity is determined by the pressure difference, regurgitant velocity is maintained throughout diastole. However, when regurgitant volume is high, ventricular diastolic pressure increases as volume increases, resulting in a rapid decrease in the pressure difference between the ventricle and associated vessel. The rapid decrease in pressure difference leads to a rapid decrease in regurgitant flow velocity.
- **mitral stenosis (MS) and tricuspid stenosis (TS)**—progressive obstruction of forward flow through either the mitral valve (MV) or tricuspid valve (TV) results in volume and consequently pressure overload of the associated atrium. The increase in atrial pressure leads to a greater pressure difference between the atria and ventricle and is reflected by increased transvalvular flow velocity when the valve opens
- **mitral regurgitation (MR) and tricuspid regurgitation (TR)**—when MR or TR volume is high, atrial volume and consequently pressure is increased, leading to high velocity antegrade flow when the valve reopens in diastole.

The abnormal loading conditions associated with mixed (concomitant stenosis and regurgitation of a single valve) and multi-valve disease (pathology of multiple valves) alters chamber pressures such that trans-valvular flow dynamics may no longer reflect the degree of disease severity.

Before performing echocardiography, it is important to bear in mind the following factors:

- Severe valve disease may reduce the SV and therefore gradient across another stenotic valve.

- Concomitant regurgitation increases anterograde flow and pressure gradient across a stenotic valve, thereby potentially leading to overestimation of stenosis severity.
- If transvalvular flow volumes are unequal, the continuity equation is inapplicable.
- Aortic or pulmonary valve disease may induce/increase mitral or tricuspid regurgitation, respectively.
- Left-sided valvular lesions may induce pulmonary hypertension, tricuspid annular dilatation, and tricuspid regurgitation.
- Methods derived from pressure half-time assessment assume a fixed rate of LV relaxation for all patients and therefore may be invalid in the presence of altered LV compliance/relaxation.

3.6.1 Echocardiographic assessment of mixed and multi-valve disease

Although the 'recommended' echo measures provide accurate estimates of valve disease parameters, alterations in loading conditions associated with mixed valve disease may result in discordance between two parameters of the same pathology, regurgitant volume and estimated regurgitant orifice area (EROA) for example. Each echocardiographic parameter should therefore be considered in the context of the associated loading conditions.

3.6.2 Aortic or pulmonary stenosis with concomitant

AR or PR

Haemodynamics

- for a given AV or PV valve area, the trans-valvular pressure difference, and therefore flow velocity, will increase as stroke volume (SV) increases and decrease as SV decreases. Therefore, because of the associated increase in ventricular SV, AR or PR will increase the transvalvular pressure gradient across a stenotic valve.

Echocardiographic assessment

- Not recommended
    - **Peak velocity and peak/mean pressure gradient**—are influenced by variations in SV and transvalvular flow. Parameters of transvalvular velocity and pressure gradient are therefore overestimated in the setting of moderate+ AR or PR. Although peak gradient may not be reflective of the true degree of AS in the setting of AR, it remains an important prognosticating factor and should be quoted.
- Recommended
    - **Effective orifice area (EOA) and dimensionless index**—estimates of EOA and dimensionless index are independent of variations in SV and flow and therefore remain accurate for the estimation of AS severity

MR or TR

Haemodynamics

- severe MR or TR decreases ventricular afterload by additional systolic off-loading of the ventricle into the atria, thereby reducing ventricular forward SV. The reduction in flow volume through the AV or PV secondary to severe MR or TR therefore causes a reduction of the pressure gradients across the valve.

Echocardiographic assessment

- Not recommended
  - **Peak velocity and peak/mean pressure gradient**—are influenced by variations in SV and transvalvular flow. Parameters of transvalvular velocity and pressure gradient may be underestimated when severe MR or TR cause reduced ventricular SV.
- Recommended
  - **EOA and dimensionless index**—estimates of EOA and dimensionless index are independent of variations in SV and flow and are therefore remain accurate for the estimation of AS severity.

MS or TS
Haemodynamics

- the reduced ventricular filling associated with severe MS or TS leads to reduced ventricular SV. The pressure gradient across the AV or PV is consequently reduced.

Echocardiographic assessment

- Not recommended
  - **Peak velocity and peak/mean pressure gradient**—are influenced by variations in SV and transvalvular flow. Parameters of transvalvular velocity and pressure gradient may be underestimated when severe MS or TS reduce ventricular SV.
- Recommended
  - **EOA and dimensionless index**—estimates of EOA and dimensionless index are independent of variations in SV and flow and therefore remain accurate for the estimation of AS severity.

3.6.3 Aortic or pulmonary regurgitation with concomitant

AS or PS
Haemodynamics

- AR and PR flow are determined by the regurgitant orifice size and pressure difference between the vessel and associated ventricle. When severe AS or PS cause pressure overload of the ventricle and consequently raised diastolic pressures, the diastolic pressure difference between the vessel and ventricle is reduced. This reduction in pressure difference will cause pressures to equalise more rapidly with a progressive reduction in regurgitant flow velocity and volume throughout diastole.

Echocardiographic assessment

- Not recommended
  - **P½t**—the reduction in vessel-ventricle diastolic pressure difference results in more rapid equalisation of pressures and shortens the P½t, therefore overestimating AR or PR severity.
- Recommended
  - **VC**—is much less flow dependent and not significantly affected by the alterations in ventricular diastolic pressure
  - **PISA**—PISA estimates of regurgitant volume and regurgitant orifice area (EROA) are much less flow dependent and are not affected by the rate of pressure equalization.

MR or TR

Haemodynamics

- severe AR or PR may lead to dilation of the ventricle with an associated increase in MV or TV annular diameter. Consequently, MR or TR secondary to annular dilation may be associated with severe AR or PR.

Echocardiographic assessment

- Not recommended
    - **P½t**—severe MR or TR may result in a more rapid rise in LV filling pressure, due to increased ventricular preload, and may therefore increase the rate of pressure equalisation between the Ao/Pa and associated ventricle. P½t may therefore overestimate AR/PR severity in the setting of severe MR or TR.
    - **Volumetric estimate of regurgitant volume**—as the volumetric method of estimating regurgitant volume assumes that the difference in SV between the LV/RV outflow tract and MV/TV represents the AR/PR regurgitant volume, any increase in MV/TV SV secondary to MR or TR will negate the difference in SV and will therefore lead to an underestimate of true regurgitant volume.
- Recommended
    - **VC** and **PISA**—are much less flow dependent and are not affected by the rate of pressure equalization.

MS or TS

Haemodynamics

- although ventricular underfilling and consequently lower filling pressures secondary to severe MS or TS, could, theoretically, lead to a very slight increase in the diastolic pressure difference between the vessel and associated ventricle and may consequently increase AR or PR volume, normal fluctuations in systemic BP or PAP and variations in heart rate (HR) have a far greater influence on AR or PR volume than the effects of MS or TS.

Echocardiographic assessment

- Not recommended
    - **P½t**—the rate of pressure equalisation may be influenced by alterations in ventricular filling volume and diastolic pressures. P½t may be inaccurate in the setting of severe MS or TS.
- Recommended
    - **VC** and **PISA**—are much less flow dependent and are not affected by the rate of pressure equalization.

3.6.4 Mitral or tricuspid stenosis with concomitant

MR or TR

Haemodynamics

- the already raised atrial pressure secondary to MS or TS is raised further by additional volume loading from MR or TR during systole. The additional pressure-load secondary to MR or TR results in an increased transvalvular pressure gradient and therefore higher transvalvular forward flow velocity when the valve opens in diastole.

Echocardiographic assessment

- Not recommended
    - **mean pressure gradient**—is influenced by variations in SV and transvalvular flow. Parameters of mean pressure gradient are therefore overestimated in the setting of moderate+ MR or TR.
    - **Mitral/Tricuspid valve area (M/TVA) by P½t**—the P½t method assumes that the rate of pressure decay is determined solely by the MV/TV orifice area. However, when atrial pressure is elevated further due to concomitant MR/TR, the altered atrial compliance alters the rate of pressure decay such that the P½t is no longer accurate for estimation of orifice area.
    - **M/TVA by continuity**—the continuity method of estimating M/TVA assumes that the SV passing through the MV/TV is equal to the SV through LV/RVOT. Since MR/TR increase the trans-mitral/tricuspid SV and therefore the measured velocity-time integral (VTI), the M/TVA is underestimated and stenosis severity overestimated by continuity method in the presence of MR/TR.
- Recommended
    - **MVA by 2D planimetry**—planimetry of the M/TVA is independent of load and flow conditions and therefore remains accurate in the setting of mixed and multi-valve disease. 2D planimetry is limited by 2D image quality and off-axis imaging however.
    - **MVA by 3D planimetry**—3D planimetry overcomes the issues of off-axis 2D imaging and is considered the gold-standard for estimations of M/TVA.

AS or PS

Haemodynamics

- MS and TS severity is typically defined by the magnitude of the consequent atria-ventricular (trans-valvular) pressure difference. However, when ventricular diastolic pressure is increased secondary to advanced AS or PS, the trans-valvular pressure difference is reduced and the degree of MS or TS is underestimated.

Echocardiographic assessment

- Not recommended
    - **mean pressure gradient**—is assumed to reflect the degree of MS/TS, where high atrial pressure and high transvalvular pressure gradient suggest severe stenosis and low atrial pressure and low transvalvular pressure difference suggest mild MS/TS. When AS or PS lead to elevated ventricular diastolic pressure, the atria-ventricular, and consequently transvalvular pressure difference, is reduced leading to underestimation of MS/TS severity.
    - **M/TVA by P½t**—when severe AS/PS raises ventricular diastolic pressure, the time taken for atrial and ventricular pressures to equalise shortens, leading to a shortened P½t with consequently overestimated M/TVA and underestimated stenosis severity.
- Recommended
    - **M/TVA by continuity**—because AS/PS does not lead to a mismatch in SV, the continuity method of estimating M/TVA remains accurate.
    - **MVA by 2D planimetry**—planimetry of the M/TVA is independent of load and flow conditions and therefore remains accurate in the setting of mixed and multi-valve disease. 2D planimetry is limited by 2D image quality and off-axis imaging however.
    - **MVA by 3D planimetry**—3D planimetry overcomes the issues of off-axis 2D imaging and is considered the gold standard for estimations of M/TVA.

AR or PR
Haemodynamics
- the increase in ventricular diastolic volume secondary to AR or PR increases ventricular diastolic pressures. This increase in ventricular diastolic pressure reduces the atria-ventricular pressure difference and therefore trans-valvular pressure gradient

Echocardiographic assessment
- Not recommended
    - **mean pressure gradient**—when AR or PR leads to raised ventricular diastolic pressure, the atria-ventricular, and consequently transvalvular pressure difference, is reduced leading to underestimation of the degree of MS/TS.
    - **Mitral valve area (MVA) by P½t**—when AR/PR raises ventricular diastolic pressure, the time taken for atrial and ventricular pressures to equalize shortens and leads to a shortened P½t with consequently overestimated M/TVA and underestimated stenosis severity.
    - **MVA by continuity**—the continuity method of estimating M/TVA assumes that the SV passing through the MV/TV is equal to the SV through LV/RVOT. Since AR/PR increase the SV through the LV/RVOT and, therefore, the measured velocity-time integral (VTI), the M/TVA is overestimated and stenosis severity underestimated by continuity method.
- Recommended
    - **MVA by 2D planimetry**—planimetry of the M/TVA is independent of load and flow conditions and therefore remains accurate in the setting of mixed and multi-valve disease. 2D planimetry is limited by 2D image quality and off-axis imaging however.
    - **MVA by 3D planimetry**—3D planimetry overcomes the issues of off-axis 2D imaging and is considered the gold standard for estimations of M/TVA.

3.6.5 Mitral or tricuspid regurgitation with concomitant MS or TS
Haemodynamics
- MR and TR volume is determined by the size of the regurgitant orifice and the pressure difference driving the regurgitant flow between the ventricle and atria. Therefore, for a given regurgitant orifice size the regurgitant volume will increase when the ventricular-atria pressure difference increases and decrease when the pressure difference decreases. Severe MS and TS increase atrial pressure, consequently decreasing the ventricle–atria pressure difference and may reduce MR or TR volume
- Not recommended
    - **Haemodynamic indicators of flow**—because MS/TS lead to further increase in atrial pressure, the trans-valvular E velocity, E/A ratio and pulmonary/hepatic vein flow profiles cannot be reliably interpreted as indicators of MR/TR severity.
- Recommended
    - **PISA**—PISA estimates are much less flow dependent and not affected by increases in atrial pressure associated with MS/TS
    - **Continuity**—although the continuity method of assessing regurgitant volume is applicable, it should be combined with estimates of M/TVA rather than measures of annular diameter

- **Vena Contracta**—VC estimates are much less flow dependent and not affected by increases in atrial pressure associated with MS/TS

AS or PS
Haemodynamics
- increases in the systolic pressure difference between the ventricle and atria will increase the MR or TR volume. Therefore, for a given MR or TR regurgitant orifice size, MR or TR volume will increase secondary to AS or PS related increases in ventricular systolic pressure

Echocardiographic assessment
- Not recommended
  - **Haemodynamic indicators of flow**—trans-valvular E velocity, E/A ratio, and pulmonary/hepatic vein flow profiles may be influenced by raised ventricular diastolic pressures secondary to advanced AS/PS.
- Recommended
  - **PISA**—PISA estimates of regurgitant volume and EROA are much less flow dependent and remain accurate in the setting of raised ventricular systolic pressure secondary to AS/PS.
  - **Continuity**—the continuity method of assessing regurgitant volume is applicable
  - **Vena Contracta**—VC estimates are much less flow dependent and not affected by increases in ventricular systolic pressure associated with AS/PS
  - **N.B.**—because MR/TR volume is determined by the regurgitant orifice size and ventricular to atria pressure difference, increasing ventricular systolic pressure secondary to AS/PS will lead to increasing regurgitant volume without significant changes in orifice area. EROA is therefore a more accurate indicator of true MR/TR severity in this scenario since regurgitant volume will decrease with reduction in ventricular systolic pressure.

AR or PR
Haemodynamics
- increases in the ventricular diastolic volume secondary to AR or PR will increase ventricular filling pressures and consequently decrease the diastolic pressure difference between the ventricle and atria. The combined increase in ventricular preload and diastolic pressure may result in ventricular dilation and a decrease in trans-mitral flow velocities in diastole.

Echocardiographic assessment
- Not recommended
  - **Haemodynamic indicators of flow**—trans-valvular E velocity, E/A ratio and pulmonary/hepatic vein flow profiles may be influenced by raised ventricular diastolic pressures secondary to advanced AR/PR.
  - **Continuity**—because AR/PR increases the SV through the LV/RVOT, the continuity method of assessing regurgitant volume is not applicable.
- Recommended
  - **PISA**—PISA estimates of regurgitant volume and EROA are much less flow dependent and remain accurate in the setting of raised ventricular diastolic pressure secondary to AR/PR.
  - **Vena Contracta**—VC estimates are much less flow dependent and not affected by increases in ventricular systolic pressure associated with AR/PR.

Impact of concomitant co-morbidities
Hypertension
- Increased systolic pressure within the Ao or PA may lead to a reduction in the pressure gradient across the AV or PV and therefore an underestimation of AS/PS severity. For a given regurgitant orifice size, AR/PR volume will also vary according to fluctuations in Ao/PA pressures, increasing as pressures increases and vice-versa.
- Raised ventricular systolic pressure (whether secondary to systemic or pulmonary HTN or AS/PS) increases the ventricular–atria systolic pressure difference and will increase MR or TR volume.

Ventricular diastolic dysfunction
Raised ventricular diastolic pressures secondary to diastolic dysfunction will:
- Decrease the pressure difference between the Ao/Pa and ventricle, in turn leading to more rapid pressure equalisation and overestimation AR/PR severity when assessed by P½t.
- Decrease the pressure difference between the atria and ventricle, in turn leading to more rapid trans-mitral/tricuspid diastolic pressure equalisation. This will lead to overestimation of orifice area and consequent underestimation of MS/TS severity when assessed by mean pressure gradient and P½t.

Anaemia
- Increased SV and cardiac output secondary to anaemia results in increased transvalvular flow velocities and may lead to overestimated transvalvular pressure gradients during the assessment of AS/PS

Obesity
- Parameters of valve area indexed to body surface area (BSA) should be considered in context of the patient size. Extremes of BSA can lead to under or over estimation of valve disease severity.

3.6.6 Symptoms

- Symptoms of co-morbidities should be excluded before symptomatic valve disease is confirmed.
- Further assessment by stress echocardiography may help differentiate symptoms of diastolic dysfunction and concomitant coronary artery disease from non-severe valve disease.
- Non-severe mixed/multi-valve disease or the addition of co-morbidities may lead to haemodynamic loading conditions and symptoms that are equivalent to severe single valve disease.
  - In the setting of mixed AV disease (AR+AS), a systolic transvalvular pressure gradient > 64 mmHg is an important prognosticating factor and identifies severe mixed valve disease.
  - Similarly, in the setting of mixed MV disease (MR+MS), a trans-mitral diastolic pressure gradient exceeding 10 mmHg indicates severe valve disease
  - Combined systemic hypertension and moderate AS may result in a ventricular afterload and symptoms equivalent to severe AS. This does not indicate severe valve disease however and medical optimisation of HTN is recommended.
- Increased LV systolic pressure secondary to severe AS will increase MR volume due to the increased LV–LA systolic pressure difference. Secondary MR typically reduces following AVR due to the reduction of LV systolic pressure. Pre-op echo assessment should consider MR severity in the context of high LV systolic pressure

3.6.7 Management and follow-up of patients with multi-valvular disease

- Symptomatic severe mixed valve disease remains an indication for intervention.
- The management and follow-up of patients with mixed valve disease should be in accordance with mixed valve disease severity.
- Patients with confirmed severe asymptomatic mixed valve disease (as outlined above) should undergo echo and clinical review at 6-month intervals to reassess symptom status and for adverse ventricular remodelling.
- Stress echocardiography is recommended to confirm symptom free status and, where feasible, should be utilised for surveillance of asymptomatic severe valve disease.
- More than mild regurgitation is a contra-indication to balloon mitral or aortic valvuloplasty.

3.7

Prosthetic valves

Sarah Hudson and Daniel X Augustine

TABLE OF CONTENTS

3.7.1 Biological prosthesis 243
3.7.2 Mechanical valve 243
3.7.3 Choice of prosthetic valve 243
3.7.4 Anticoagulation 244
3.7.5 Haemodynamics of prosthetic valves 245

3.7.1 Biological prosthesis

- Do not require long-term anticoagulation
- Homograft/autograft
- Xenograft, e.g. porcine valve
- Bioprosthesis: uses biological tissue (usually harvested from the pericardial sac of either horses or cows) that is sewn into an artificial stent.

3.7.2 Mechanical valve

- Require long-term anticoagulation
- Ball and cage (Starr–Edwards)
- Tilting disc: a singular disc suspended within a frame
- Bileaflet (e.g. Carbomedics): two leaflets hinged in the centre of the prosthesis.

3.7.3 Choice of prosthetic valve

- The choice of prosthesis type should be individualized

Favours Mechanical Prosthesis	Favours Bioprosthesis
Desire of the informed patient	
No contraindication to anticoagulation	Contraindication to anticoagulation or likely poor compliance with anticoagulation
Age < 60 needing AVR	Age > 65 needing AVR
Age < 65 needing MVR	Age > 70 needing MVR

Favours Mechanical Prosthesis	Favours Bioprosthesis
Life expectancy > 10 yrs for whom redo surgery would be high risk	Low likelihood and/or low operative risk of future redo valve surgery
Already has a mechanical prothesis in a different position	Reoperation for mechanical valve thrombosis despite good anticoagulant control
Already on long-term anticoagulation for high risk thromboembolism	Young woman contemplating pregnancy
Patients at risk of accelerated valve deterioration (Age < 40 yrs; hyperparathyroidism; haemodialysis)	Those whose life expectancy is lower than durability of the bioprosthesis

3.7.4 Anticoagulation

- The target INR for mechanical valves depends on a combination of prosthesis thrombogenicity and patient related risk factors (see Table 3.7.1).

Management of anticoagulant therapy in special circumstances

- If a patient with a mechanical valve undergoes PCI after ACS, recommended antithrombic/antiplatelet therapy is one week triple therapy (warfarin, aspirin and clopidogrel), then warfarin and a single antiplatelet (preferably clopidogrel) to 12 months, then warfarin alone (See figure 3.7.1).
- In patients undergoing surgery, it is recommended not to interrupt oral anticoagulation for most minor surgical procedures and those procedures where bleeding can be easily controlled
- In patients undergoing major surgical procedures which require an INR < 1.5, bridging with low molecular weight heparin or I.V. unfractionated heparin should occur. If UFH is used, the infusion stopping 6 hours before surgery.
- In women with mechanical valves who become pregnant, anticoagulation is particularly important as pregnancy is a prothrombotic state.

Table 3.7.1 Anticoagulation for prosthetic valves.

Prosthesis thrombogenicity[a]	Patient-related risk factors[b]	
	No risk factor	≥ 1 risk factor
Low	2.5	3.0
Medium	3.0	3.5
High	3.5	4.0

[a] Prosthesis thrombogenicity: low = Carbomedics, Medtronic Hall, Medtronic Open-Pivot, ATS, St Jude Medical, On-X, Sorin bicarbon. medium = other bileaflet valves; high = Lillehei–Kaster, Omniscience, Starr–Edwards, Bjork–Shiley, and other tilting-disc valves.

[b] Patient-related risk factors: mitral or tricuspid valve replacement; previous thrombo-embolism; atrial fibrillation; MS of any degree; LVEF < 35.

Reproduced with permission from Vahanian A, Beyersdorf F, Praz F, et al; ESC/EACTS Scientific Document Group. 2021 ESC/EACTS Guidelines for the management of valvular heart disease. *Eur Heart J*. 2022 Feb 12;43(7):561–632. doi: 10.1093/eurheartj/ehab395. © European Society of Cardiology. With permission from Oxford University Press

- In patients requiring < 5 mg/day warfarin, OAC throughout pregnancy and a change to UFH before delivery is favoured
- In patients requiring higher warfarin doses, switching to LMWH during the first trimester with anti-Xa monitoring is recommended, switching back to warfarin in the second trimester before changing to UFH prior to delivery

3.7.5 Haemodynamics of prosthetic valves

- Different types of prosthetic valves have different haemodynamics, affected by their mechanism of opening (consider the different flows resulting from tilting discs compared to tissue leaflets), whether they are stented or unstented, sutured or sutureless, and their effective orifice area. Consequently, the expected transvalvular pressure gradient and effective orifice area is different for each type and size of valve. The partition values for native valve stenosis do not apply to replacement valves.
- Transprosthetic gradients are measured using continuous-wave Doppler echocardiography and the simplified Bernoulli equation:

$$\Delta P = 4 \times V^2$$

Where v is the maximal transprosthetic velocity. Irrespective of the position (AV, MV, TV or PV), transprosthetic pressure gradient is a load dependent parameter and therefore under or overestimated in low or high flow conditions respectively.

- The dimensionless index (DI) for aortic prosthetic valves is the ratio of the VTI in the LVOT to the VTI through the prosthetic AV. The normal value of this is ≥ 0.3
- For prosthetic mitral valves, the DVI is calculated by dividing the transprosthetic flow VTI by the LVOT VTI. For a normally functioning prosthetic mitral valve this should be < 2.2.
- In bileaflet mechanical valves, the central orifice is often smaller than the 2 lateral offices so a Doppler through this may result in an overestimation of the transvalvular gradient
- When assessing valve function by echocardiography, the effective orifice area should be calculated and compared to the expected parameter for the valve *in situ*.

Complications
Prosthetic valve thrombosis
Obstructive left-sided thrombus:

- Identified on echocardiography by a decrease in estimated effective orifice area on serial studies, commonly associated with a simultaneous increase in transvalvular pressure gradient. Any degree of regurgitation through a bioprosthetic valve is abnormal and identifies valve dysfunction. Although 'closure jets' are a normal finding with mechanical valve replacements, an increase in regurgitation (without significant increase in ventricular or aortic pressure) may be an indication of leaflet thrombus preventing complete valve closure.
- If haemodynamically unwell—consider surgery if available; if no immediate surgery available, proceed with fibrinolysis
- If haemodynamically well and recent inadequate anticoagulation, give heparin ± aspirin (regular follow-up if this is successful). If unsuccessful (according to repeat echocardiography) then ideally proceed to surgery; if patient too high risk for surgery, proceed with fibrinolysis
- If haemodynamically well and recent adequate anticoagulation, proceed to surgery. If too high risk for surgery, proceed with fibrinolysis.
- A flow diagram for the management of mechanical prosthetic thrombosis is shown in Figure 3.7.2.

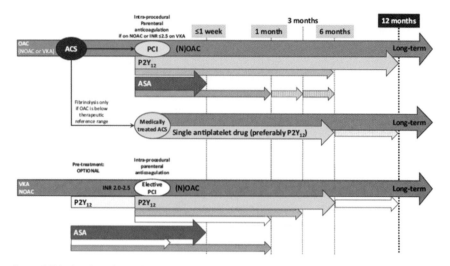

Figure 3.7.1 Antithrombotic therapy in patients with indication to OAC and ACS/PCI.
Reproduced with permission from Vahanian A, Beyersdorf F, Praz F, et al; ESC/EACTS Scientific Document Group. 2021 ESC/EACTS Guidelines for the management of valvular heart disease. *Eur Heart J.* 2022 Feb 12;43(7):561–632. doi: 10.1093/eurheartj/ehab395. © European Society of Cardiology. With permission from Oxford University Press.

Non-obstructive left-sided thrombus:

- Optimize anticoagulation, repeat echocardiography, and follow up for evidence of thromboembolism (either clinically or cerebral imaging) (see Figure 3.7.1).
- If evidence of thromboembolism and
    - ≥ 10 mm thrombus: proceed to surgery (or fibrinolysis if surgery risk high)
    - < 10 mm thrombus: optimize anticoagulation and proceed to surgery (or fibrinolysis if high risk) if thrombus persists and there is evidence of recurrent thromboembolism
- If no evidence of thromboembolism and large thrombus (≥ 10 mm): optimize anticoagulation and proceed to surgery (if not high risk) if thrombus persists or there is evidence of recurrent thromboembolism (if high risk for surgery then fibrinolysis).

Haemolysis and paravalvular leak

- Current ESC recommendations are to recommend reoperation if there is haemolysis requiring repeated blood transfusions or if the leak is related to endocarditis.
- Medical therapy, including iron supplementation, beta blockers, and erythropoietin, is indicated in patients with severe haemolytic anaemia when contraindications to surgery are present. Transcatheter closure of a paravalvular leak is feasible.

Prosthesis–patient mismatch

- Prosthesis–patient mismatch occurs when the effective orifice area of the replacement valve is insufficient for the patient's cardiac output requirements and occurs when the implanted valve is too small for the patient habitus.
    This results in higher transvalvular gradients, worse functional class, increased risk of hospitalization, and higher short- and long-term mortality rates

3.7.5 Haemodynamics of prosthetic valves

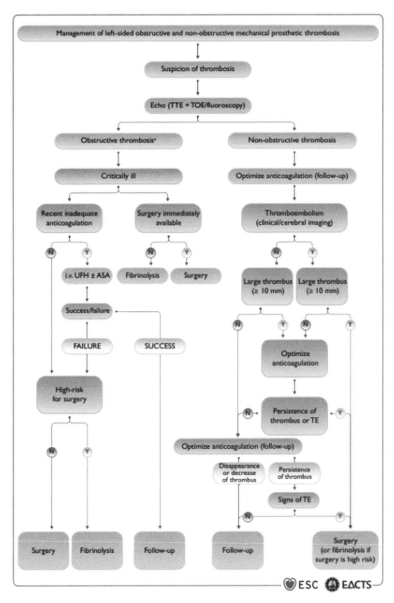

Figure 3.7.2 Flowchart for management of obstructive and non-obstructive left sided mechanical prosthetic thrombosis.

Reproduced with permission from Vahanian A, Beyersdorf F, Praz F, et al; ESC/EACTS Scientific Document Group. 2021 ESC/EACTS Guidelines for the management of valvular heart disease. *Eur Heart J*. 2022 Feb 12;43(7):561–632. doi: 10.1093/eurheartj/ehab395. © European Society of Cardiology. With permission from Oxford University Press.

- To resolve, further surgery with a larger valve would be needed; this requires careful risk/benefit analysis.

Structural valve degeneration

- This is an acquired bioprosthetic abnormality defined as deterioration of the leaflets or support structures resulting in thickening, calcification, or tearing with eventual associated valve haemodynamic dysfunction.
- Meta-analyses have shown SVD commonly begins 8 years after implantation, with increased rate after 10 years.
- SVD may result in either stenosis or regurgitation. The early echocardiographic indications of bioprosthetic valve degeneration are increased echogenicity of the leaflet/cusp tips but with unrestricted excursion and is often associated with trace/mild regurgitation.
- Percutaneous balloon interventions should be avoided in the treatment of stenotic left-sided bioprostheses.

Follow-up of prosthetic valves
Echo surveillance:

- Bioprosthesis and homografts: yearly
- TAVI: yearly from implant
- Endocarditis: as per guidelines—see Chapter 3.8
- When prosthetic valve dysfunction is identified, repeat echo in 6 months is recommended to assess for rapid progression.

Further reading

2021 ESC/EACTS Guidelines for the management of valvular heart disease. *Eur Heart J*. 2021 Aug 28:ehab395.

Baumgartner H, Falk V, Bax JJ, De Bonis M, Hamm C, Holm PJ, Iung B, Lancellotti P, Lansac E, Muñoz DR, Rosenhek R, Sjögren J, Mas PT, Vahanian A, Walther T, Wendler O, Windecker S, Zamorano JL. 2017 ESC/EACTS Guidelines for the Management of Valvular Heart Disease. *Rev Esp Cardiol (Engl Ed)*. 2018 Feb;71(2):110. English, Spanish. doi: 10.1016/j.rec.2017.12.013. PMID: 29425605.

Camm J, Lüscher TF, Serruys PW (eds). *The European Society of Cardiology Textbook of Cardiovascular Medicine*, 2nd edn. Oxford: Oxford University Press, 2009.

ChambersJ, Gardbi M, Nieman K, Myerson S, Pierard LA, Habib G, Zamorano JL, Edvardsen T, Lancellotti P. Appropriateness criteria for the use of cardiovascular imaging in heart valve disease in adults: a European Association of Cardiovascular Imaging report of literature review and current practice. *Eur Heart J*. 2017;18:489–98.

Lancellotti P, Tribouilloy C, Hagendorff A, Moura L, Popescu BA, Agricola E, Monin J-L, Pierard LA, Badano L, Zamorano JL; European Association of Echocardiography. European Association of Echocardiography recommendations for the assessment of valvular regurgitation. Part 1: aortic and pulmonary regurgitation (native valve disease). *Eur J Echocard*. 2010; 11: 223–44.

Leeson P, Monteior C, Augustine D, Becher H. *Echocardiography*, 3rd edn. Oxford: Oxford University Press, 2020.

3.8

Infective endocarditis

Bernard Prendergast, James Harrison, and James Tomlinson

TABLE OF CONTENTS

- 3.8.1 Definition 249
- 3.8.2 Epidemiology 249
- 3.8.3 Classification and terminology 250
- 3.8.4 Microbiology 251
- 3.8.5 Pathophysiology 251
- 3.8.6 Diagnosis 252
- 3.8.7 Prognosis 259
- 3.8.8 Antibiotic treatment 260
- 3.8.9 Outpatient parenteral antibiotic therapy (OPAT) 262
- 3.8.10 Surgical treatment 263
- 3.8.11 Infective endocarditis affecting cardiac implantable electronic devices (CDRIE) 264
- 3.8.12 Non-bacterial thrombotic endocarditis (NBTE) 265
- 3.8.13 Multidisciplinary management 265
- 3.8.14 Antibiotic prophylaxis 267
- 3.8.15 What's new in the European Society of Cardiology guidelines (2023) 268

3.8.1 Definition

Infective endocarditis (IE) is an infection of the endocardium of the heart. It may involve:

- One or more valves (native or prosthetic)
- Pacemaker/defibrillator leads
- Septal defects
- Mural endocardium (rare)

3.8.2 Epidemiology

- Despite significant advances in diagnosis and treatment, IE remains a dangerous disease
- People at highest risk:
    - Previous surgical valve replacement (or repair using prosthetic material)
    - Previous transcatheter valve implantation
    - Congenital heart disease (CHD): untreated cyanotic CHD or any type of CHD repaired with prosthetic material (shunts, conduits or other prosthesis)
    - Previous IE
    - Ventricular assist devices
- Annual incidence of 15–60 per million (significant geographic variation):
    - Male:female 2:1
    - Significant increase with age

- Epidemiological profile has changed in recent decades (particularly in developed nations) due to evolving risk factors:
    - Rheumatic heart disease now rare
    - Increasing elderly population with native valve disease
    - More patients with prosthetic valves and cardiac devices
    - Increasing intravenous drug abuse
    - More nosocomial infection (related to invasive procedures, haemodialysis)
    - *Staphylococcus aureus* has overtaken oral streptococci as the most common pathogen in high income countries

3.8.3 Classification and terminology

IE may be classified in several ways:
According to location of infection and presence/absence of intracardiac material:

- Left-sided native valve IE (NVE)
- Left-sided prosthetic valve IE (PVE)
- Early PVE < 1 year after surgery
- Late PVE > 1 year after surgery
- Right-sided IE
- Cardiac device-related IE (CDRIE) (pacemaker, defibrillator)

According to mode of acquisition:

- Healthcare associated IE
    - Nosocomial: signs/symptoms of IE developing > 48 h after hospitalisation
    - Non-nosocomial: signs/symptoms of IE developing < 48 h after hospitalisation in a patient with healthcare contact
    - Home-based nursing or i.v. therapy, haemodialysis, or i.v. chemotherapy < 30 days before onset of IE
    - Hospitalisation in acute care facility < 90 days before onset of IE
    - Resident in nursing home or long-term care facility
- Community-acquired IE: signs/symptoms of IE developing < 48 h after admission in a patient not fulfilling the criteria for healthcare associated IE
- Intravenous drug abuse (IVDU)-related IE

Active IE:

- Persistent fever and positive blood cultures
- Active inflammatory morphology found at surgery
- Patient still receiving antibiotic therapy
- Histopathological evidence of active IE

Recurrence:

- Relapse: repeat IE caused by the same microorganism < 6 months after the initial episode—should prompt search for a persistent source of infection and consideration of surgical therapy
- Reinfection: infection with a different microorganism or repeat IE caused by the same microorganism > 6 months after the initial episode

3.8.4 Microbiology

Infective endocarditis with positive blood cultures (85% of cases)

- Mainly staphylococci, streptococci, and enterococci
    - Staphylococci: *S. aureus* (more commonly NVE), coagulase-negative staphylococci (more commonly PVE)
    - Streptococci:
        - Oral (formerly viridians) streptococci: *S. sanguis*, *S. mitis*, *S. salivarius*, *S. mutans*, *Gemella morbillorum*—almost always respond to penicillin G
        - *S. milleri* or *S. anginosus* group: *S. anginosus*, *S. intermedius*, *S. constellatus*—tendency to abscess formation and haematogenous dissemination, requiring longer duration of antibiotic therapy
        - Former nutritionally variant streptococci: *Abiotrophia* and *Granulicatella*—often penicillin-resistant
        - Group D streptococci: *S. gallolyticus* (formerly *S. bovis*), *S. equinus*—commensals of the human gastrointestinal tract (investigation should include colonoscopy to exclude colonic malignancy); usually sensitive to penicillin G
    - Enterococci: *E. faecalis*, *E. faecium*, *E. durans*

Infective endocarditis with negative blood cultures as a result of prior antibiotic treatment

- Antibiotics for unexplained fever before blood cultures performed
- Blood cultures may remain negative for many days
- Causative organisms most commonly antibiotic sensitive oral streptococci or coagulase-negative staphylococci (CoNS)

Infective endocarditis with negative blood cultures due to fastidious organisms

- *Abiotrophia* and *Granulicatella* (formerly nutritionally variant streptococci)
- Gram-negative HACEK organisms (*Haemophilus*, *Actinobacillus*, *Cardiobacterium*, *Eikenella*, *Kingella*)
- Brucella
- Fungi

Infective endocarditis with negative blood cultures due to intracellular organisms (5% of cases)

- *Coxiella burnetii*
- *Bartonella*
- *Chlamydia*
- *Tropheryma whipplei*
- Diagnosis relies on serological testing, cell culture or gene amplification.

3.8.5 Pathophysiology

Endothelial damage:

- Normal valve endothelium is resistant to colonization and infection
- Mechanical disruption of endothelium results in:
    - Exposure of underlying extracellular matrix proteins

- Production of tissue factor
- Deposition of fibrin and platelets
- Bacterial adherence and vegetation formation
- Endothelial damage may result from:
    - Turbulent blood flow
    - Cardiac instrumentation (catheters, pacing/defibrillator leads)
    - Inflammation (rheumatic carditis)
    - Degenerative changes (particularly in the elderly)

Transient bacteraemia:
- Magnitude and ability of pathogen to adhere to damaged endothelium are both important
- Occurs after invasive procedures (particularly dental procedures)
- However, also occurs following chewing or tooth brushing (short duration and low magnitude) resulting in annual cumulative exposure thousands to millions times greater than that caused by tooth extraction. This may explain why most cases of IE are unrelated to invasive procedures.

3.8.6 Diagnosis

- IE remains a diagnostic challenge (see Figures 3.8.1, 3.8.2, 3.8.3)
- Clinical history is very variable, depending on causative microorganism, presence/absence of pre-existing cardiac disease, and mode of presentation
- May present as acute, rapidly progressive infection or sub-acute/chronic disease with non-specific symptoms and low-grade fever
- As a result, patients may present to a variety of specialists
- Early involvement of a cardiologist and infectious diseases specialist is recommended. A high index of suspicion is more important than strict adherence to diagnostic criteria, although the ESC has developed modified diagnostic criteria that are superior to conventional diagnostic criteria (e.g. Duke's modified criteria) (Box 3.8.1). Repeat echocardiography, blood cultures and multi-modality imaging are recommended if a high clinical suspicion of IE persists in 'possible' or 'rejected' cases.

> **BOX 3.8.1 DEFINITIONS OF THE 2023 EUROPEAN SOCIETY OF CARDIOLOGY MODIFIED DIAGNOSTIC CRITERIA OF INFECTIVE ENDOCARDITIS**
>
> **Clinical criteria**
> - **Major criteria:**
>   (i) *Blood culture positive for IE*
>   a) Typical microorganism for infective endocarditis from two separate blood cultures
>   - Oral streptococci, *Streptococcus gallolyticus* (formerly *S. bovis*), HACEK group, *S. aureus, E. faecalis*
>   b) Microorganism consistent with infective endocarditis from continuously positive blood cultures:
>   - At least 2 blood cultures drawn more than 12 h apart or
>   - All of 3 or a majority of 4 or more separate blood cultures, with first and last drawn at least 1 h apart
>   c) Single positive blood culture for *C. burnetii* or phase I IgG antibody titre > 1:800

(ii) *Imaging positive for IE*
- Valvular, perivalvular/periprosthetic and foreign material anatomic and metabolic lesions characteristic of IE detected by any of the following imaging techniques:
- Echocardiography (TTE and TOE)
- Cardiac CT
- [18F]-FDG-PET/CT(A)
- WBC SPECT/CT

- **Minor criteria:**
  (i) *Predisposition: predisposing heart condition or intravenous drug use*
  (ii) *Fever: ≥ 38.0°C (100.4°F)*
  (iii) *Embolic vascular dissemination (including 'silent' dissemination, i.e. those detected by imaging only):*
  - Major systemic and pulmonary emboli/infarcts and abscess
  - Mycotic aneurysms
  - Intracranial ischaemic/haemorrhagic lesions
  - Conjunctival haemorrhages
  - Janeway's lesions

  (iv) *Immunologic phenomena:*
  - Glomerulonephritis
  - Oslers nodes and Roth spots
  - Rheumatoid factor

  (v) *Microbiologic evidence:*
  - Positive blood culture not meeting major criterion or
  - Serologic evidence of active infection with organism consistent with infective endocarditis

IE Classification (at admission and during follow-up):

Definite
- 2 major criteria, or
- 1 major and 3 minor criteria, or
- 5 minor criteria.

Possible
- 1 major criteria and 1 or 2 minor criteria, or
- 3–4 minor criteria

Rejected
- Does not meet criteria for 'definite' or 'possible' infective endocarditis at admission with or without a firm diagnosis

- IE should be suspected in the following clinical situations:
  - New regurgitant heart murmur
  - Embolic events of unknown origin
  - Sepsis of unknown origin (particularly if caused by a typical IE organism)
  - Fever (seen in up to 90% of IE cases) associated with:
    - Intracardiac prosthetic material (prosthetic valve, pacemaker/defibrillator, congenital heart disease repair)

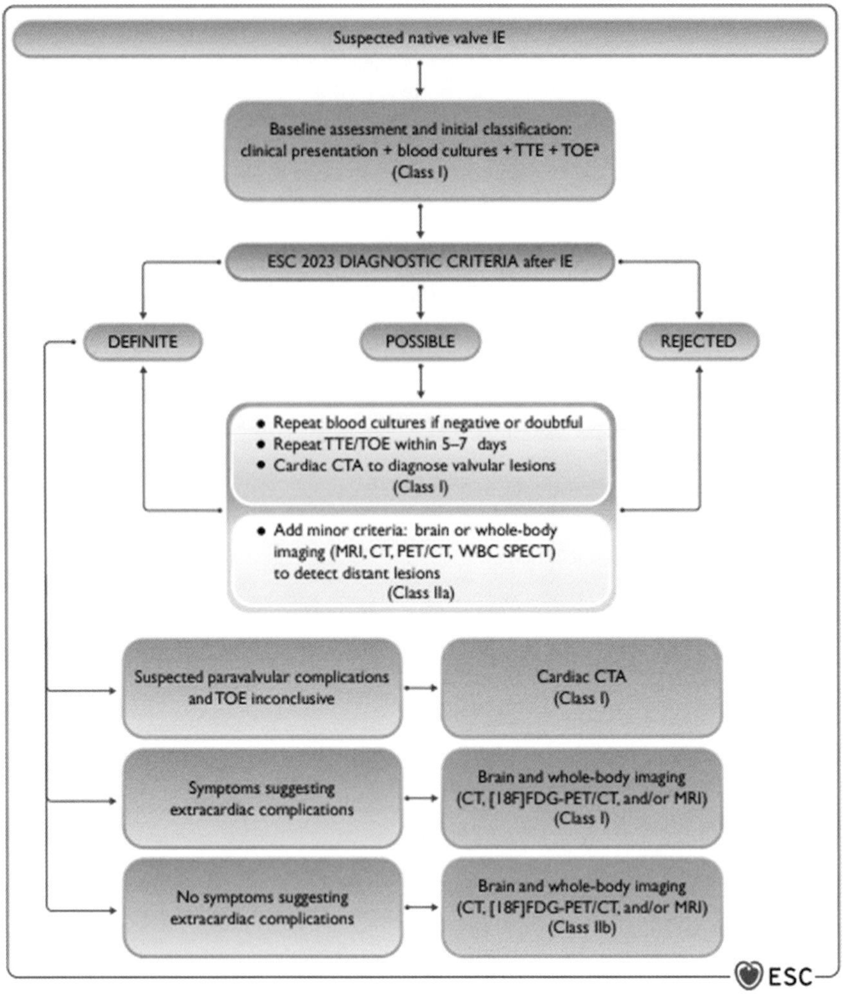

3.8 Infective endocarditis

Figure 3.8.1 European Society of Cardiology 2023 algorithm for diagnosis of NVE.

[a] TOE for diagnosis and to detect perivalvular complications in all cases (unless right-sided NVE when TTE quality is good quality and conclusive).

Delgado V, Ajmone Marsan N, de Waha S, et al; ESC Scientific Document Group. 2023 ESC Guidelines for the management of endocarditis. *Eur Heart J*. 2023 Oct 14;44(39):3948–4042. doi: 10.1093/eurheartj/ehad193. © European Society of Cardiology. With permission from Oxford University Press.

- Previous IE
- Known valve or congenital heart disease
- Immunocompromise
- Intravenous drug abuse
- Recent invasive procedure
- Congestive heart failure
- New conduction disturbance
- Positive blood cultures with typical I organism
- Positive serology for chronic Q fever (*Coxiella burnetii*)
- Embolic event
- Roth spots, splinter haemorrhages, Janeway lesions, Osler's nodes

- Focal or non-specific neurological signs/symptoms
- Pulmonary embolism or infiltration (right-sided IE)
- Peripheral abscesses of unknown cause
- Poor appetite, weight loss
- Elevated C-reactive protein or erythrocyte sedimentation rate, leukocytosis, anaemia, and microscopic haematuria (these lack specificity and are not included in current diagnostic criteria)
* Fever may be absent in the elderly and immunocompromised, after antibiotic therapy, and in IE caused by less virulent or atypical organisms.

ESC diagnostic algorithm

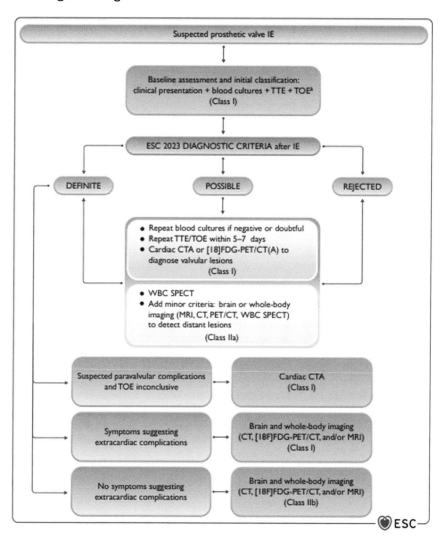

Figure 3.8.2 European Society of Cardiology 2023 algorithm for diagnosis of prosthetic valve infective endocarditis.
[a] TOE for diagnosis and to detect perivalvular complications in all cases (unless right-sided NVE when TTE quality is good quality and conclusive).
Delgado V, Ajmone Marsan N, de Waha S, et al; ESC Scientific Document Group. 2023 ESC Guidelines for the management of endocarditis. *Eur Heart J.* 2023 Oct 14;44(39):3948–4042. doi: 10.1093/eurheartj/ehad193. © European Society of Cardiology. With permission from Oxford University Press.

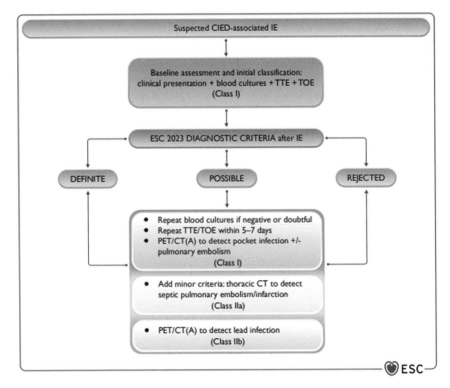

Figure 3.8.3 European Society of Cardiology 2023 algorithm for diagnosis of cardiac device-related infective endocarditis.

Delgado V, Ajmone Marsan N, de Waha S, et al; ESC Scientific Document Group. 2023 ESC Guidelines for the management of endocarditis. *Eur Heart J*. 2023 Oct 14;44(39):3948–4042. doi: 10.1093/eurheartj/ehad193. © European Society of Cardiology. With permission from Oxford University Press.

Echocarditis (See Chapter 1.1.8)

- Should not be used indiscriminately—the exception is *Staphylococcus aureus* bacteraemia (which has potential devastating consequences), where routine echocardiography should be considered, irrespective of the presence/absence of other features of IE
- A negative TTE with good image quality is sufficient if clinical suspicion of IE is low
- In all other circumstances, TTE is the initial imaging modality of choice when there is a suspicion of IE, but should be followed promptly by TOE if IE is confirmed or still suspected
- TOE is recommended in patients with a prosthetic heart valve or intracardiac device is present when there is a clinical suspicion of IE
- If initial TOE negative, this should be repeated after 5–7 days if clinical suspicion of IE remains (earlier if *Staphylococcus aureus* bacteraemia)
- TOE should be considered in all patients with suspected IE (even in those with positive TTE), except isolated right-sided native valve IE with good TTE images and unequivocal echocardiographic findings
- If TOE positive, follow-up echocardiography is mandatory to monitor the response to treatment and detect complications

- Repeat TTE and/or TOE should be considered during the follow up of uncomplicated IE and is recommended as soon as a new complication of IE is suspected (new murmur, embolism, persisting fever and bacteraemia, heart failure, abscess, AV block)
- TOE is advised in stable patients prior to switching from intravenous to oral antibiotic therapy
- Intra-operative echocardiography is recommended in all cases of IE requiring surgery
- TTE and/or TOE is recommended at completion of therapy

Computed Tomography (CT)

Can be used:

- As an alternative to invasive angiography when planning surgery in haemodynamically stable patients with aortic vegetations
- To detect valve lesions and confirm diagnosis of native and prosthetic IE (if TOE is inconclusive or not feasible)
- To detect abscesses, pseudoaneurysms and fistulae
- To diagnose paravalvular or peri-prosthetic complications in PVE (if echocardiography inconclusive)
- To define aortic valve and aortic root anatomy
- To look for suspected cerebral lesions (if MRI not feasible)
- To detect distant lesions and extra-cardiac sources of bacteraemia—whole-body CT can detect alternative foci of infection though [18F]FDG positron emission tomography/computed tomography (PET/CT) is preferred

Magnetic resonance imaging (MRI)

- Increases the likelihood of detecting cerebral complications of IE (higher sensitivity than CT)
- Diagnosis of spinal lesions—spondylodiscitis, vertebral osteomyelitis
- Cardiac MRI has low spatial resolution and is limited in its ability to diagnose IE and cardiac complications (compared with cardiac CT)

Nuclear imaging (PET/SPECT)

- [18F]FDG-positron emission tomography (PET)/CT (angiography) and white blood cell (WBC) single photon emission tomography (SPECT)/CT are supplementary imaging techniques in IE
- Increase diagnostic yield and sensitivity, and reduce the rate of misdiagnosis
- Detection of PVE and CDRIE (if echocardiography inconclusive)
- Detection of embolic and metastatic infection

Microbiological diagnosis

- Blood cultures:
    - Remain the cornerstone of diagnosis
    - Three sets (aerobic and anaerobic) taken at 30-minute intervals are usually sufficient
    - Should be taken before starting antibiotic therapy
    - Sampling from central venous lines should be avoided due to high risk of contamination
    - No rationale for delaying sampling to coincide with peaks of fever (bacteraemia is usually constant)
    - A single positive blood culture may be a contaminant and should be viewed with caution
    - Blood cultures should be repeated after 48–72 h to check effectiveness of treatment
    - In culture-negative IE, antibiotics should be withdrawn and blood cultures repeated

- Histological/immunological examination:
    - Pathological examination of surgically resected tissue
    - Serological testing—*Coxiella burnetii*, *Bartonella* species, *Legionella pneumophila*, *Brucella* species, *Mycoplasma* species, *Aspergillus* species
    - Blood PCR—*Staphylococcus aureus*, *Tropheryma whipplei*, fungi, *Escherichia coli*, *Streptococcus galloyticus*, *Streptococcus mitis*, *Enterococci*
- Blood culture negative endocarditis (BCNIE)
    - Accounts for up to 30% of all cases
    - *Brucella* spp/*Bartonella* spp/legionella
        - Blood cultures, serology, culture, immunohistology, and PCR of surgical material
    - Coxiella burnetti
        - Serology (IgG phase 1 > 1:800), tissue culture, immunohistology, and PCR of surgical material
    - Trophyerma whipplei
        - Histology and PCR of surgical material
    - Legionella spp.
- Blood cultures, serology, culture, immunohistology, and PCR of surgical material
    - Fungi
        - Blood cultures, serology, culture, and PCR of surgical material
    - Mycoplasma
        - Blood cultures, serology, PCR of surgical material

Complications

- Frequent and often severe
- Cardiac complications:
    - Heart failure (in 50–60% of cases)
    - Acute valvular regurgitation (stenosis much less common)
        - Abscess
        - Pseudoaneurysm
        - Fistula
        - Peri-prosthetic dehiscence
        - Ventricular septal defect
        - Conduction abnormalities
            - Mainly first-/second- and third-degree AV block
            - Bundle branch block (rarely)
        - Acute coronary syndrome
        - Myocarditis
        - Pericarditis
- Non-cardiac complications:
    - Embolic events (20–50% of cases; silent in 20%)
        - Mainly spleen (infarcts / abscess) and brain (infectious aneurysm; meningitis; TIA/CVA; haemorrhage)
        - Lungs (in right-sided and device-related IE)
        - More likely with larger and more mobile vegetations
            - Major bleeding—interruption of antiplatelet and/or anticoagulant therapy is recommended (including intracranial haemorrhage).

- Acute renal failure—multifactorial causes:
  - Immune complex and vasculitic glomerulonephritis
  - Renal infarction
  - Heart failure
  - Antibiotic toxicity or related to imaging contrast
- Musculoskeletal
  - Arthralgia, myalgia, back pain
  - Peripheral arthritis
  - Pyogenic vertebral osteomyelitis
  - Spondylodiscitis

Management of neurological complication

- If indicated, surgery is recommended without delay after a silent embolism or transient ischaemic attack
- Neurosurgery or endovascular therapy is recommended for large, enlarging or ruptured intracranial infectious aneurysms
- Postpone surgery for at least 1 month following intracranial haemorrhage
- Following stroke without coma or cerebral haemorrhage, proceed with surgery if ongoing heart failure, uncontrolled infection, abscess or persistent high embolic risk
- Investigate for intracranial infectious aneurysms in those with neurological symptoms
- Thrombolysis is not recommended in IE-related embolic stroke, but mechanical thrombectomy may be considered if expertise and time permit.

Management of musculoskeletal complications

- Musculoskeletal complications of IE include spondylodiscitis and vertebral osteomyelitis
- MRI or PET/CT should be used to identify musculoskeletal manifestations of IE
- TTE/TOE is recommended to exclude IE in patients with spondylodiscitis and/or septic arthritis with positive blood cultures for typical IE microorganisms
- > 6 weeks of antibiotic therapy should be considered in patients with osteoarticular IE-related lesions caused by difficult to treat microorganisms (e.g. *S. aureus* or *Candida* spp.) and/or complicated by severe vertebral destruction or abscesses.

3.8.7 Prognosis

- In-hospital mortality 10–26%
- Predictors of poor outcome:
  - Patient characteristics:
    - Older age
    - PVE
    - Insulin-dependent DM
    - Significant comorbidity (e.g. frailty, immunosuppression, renal or pulmonary disease)
  - Presence of complications:
    - Heart failure
    - Renal failure
    - Stroke

- Septic shock
- Cerebral haemorrhage
  - Causative organism:
    - *S. aureus*
    - Fungi
    - Non-HACEK gram-negative bacilli
  - Echocardiographic findings:
    - Peri-annular complications
    - Severe left-sided valve regurgitation
    - Low left ventricular ejection fraction
    - Pulmonary hypertension
    - Large vegetations
    - Severe prosthetic dysfunction
    - Premature mitral valve closure (and other signs of elevated left ventricular end-diastolic pressure)

3.8.8 Antibiotic treatment

- Early involvement of an infectious diseases expert is mandatory
- Key principles of antibiotic therapy in IE are:
  - Bactericidal agents
  - Synergistic antibiotic combinations
  - High doses
  - Prolonged duration
- Local guidelines should be used at all times, but suggested regimens are as follows:

Oral streptococci and *Streptococcus gallolyticus* (formerly S. bovis) group
Fully susceptible to penicillin (mean inhibitory concentration (MIC) < 0.125 mg/l)

- Standard treatment (4 weeks):
  - Penicillin G 12–18 million U/day i.v. in 4–6 doses *or*
  - Amoxicillin 100–200 mg/kg/day i.v. in 4–6 doses *or*
  - Ceftriaxone 2 g/day i.v./i.m. in 1 dose
- 2-week treatment:
  - Penicillin G 12–18 million U/day i.v. in 4–6 doses *or*
  - Amoxicillin 100–200 mg/kg/day i.v. in 4–6 doses *or*
  - Ceftriaxone 2 g/day i.v./i.m. in 1 dose *with*
  - Gentamicin 3 mg/kg/day i.v./i.m. in 1 dose *or*
  - Netilmicin 4–5 mg/kg/day i.v. in 1 dose

Penicillin allergy

- Vancomycin 30 mg/kg/day i.v. in 2 doses (for 4 weeks)

Relatively resistant to penicillin (MIC 0.125–2 mg/l)

- Standard treatment (4 weeks):
  - Penicillin G 24 million U/day i.v. in 4–6 doses *or*
  - Amoxicillin 12g day i.v. in 6 doses *or*

- Ceftriaxone 2 g/day i.v./i.m. in 1 dose *with*
- Gentamicin 3 mg/kg/day i.v./i.m. in 1 dose (for 2 weeks)

Penicillin allergy
- Vancomycin 30 mg/kg/day i.v. in 2 doses (for 4 weeks) *with*
- Gentamicin 3 mg/kg/day i.v./i.m. in 1 dose (for 2 weeks).

Staphylococcus species
- *Native valves:*
  - Methicillin-susceptible staphylococci:
    - Flucloxacillin 12 g/day i.v. in 4–6 doses *or*
    - Cefazolin 6 g/day i.v. in 3 doses (for 4–6 weeks)
  - Penicillin allergy/methicillin-susceptible staphylococci:
    - Cefazolin 6 g/day i.v. in 3 doses (for 4–6 weeks)
    - Methicillin-resistant staphylococci:
    - Vancomycin 30–60 mg/kg/day i.v. in 2–3 doses
- *Prosthetic valves:*
  - Methicillin-susceptible staphylococci:
    - Flucloxacillin 12 g/day i.v. in 4–6 doses or Cefazolin 6 g/day i.v. in 3 doses (for ≥ 6 weeks) *with*
    - Rifampicin 900 mg/day i.v. or p.o. in 3 doses (for ≥ 6 weeks) *and*
    - Gentamicin 3 mg/kg/day i.v./i.m. in 1–2 doses (for 2 weeks)
  - Penicillin allergy/methicillin-susceptible:
  - Cefazolin 6 g/day i.v. in 3 doses (for ≥ 6 weeks) *with*
  - Rifampicin 900 mg/day i.v. or p.o. in 3 doses (for ≥ 6 weeks) *and*
  - Gentamicin 3 mg/kg/day i.v./i.m. in 1–2 doses (for 2 weeks)
    - Methicillin-resistant staphylococci:
      - Vancomycin 30–60 mg/kg/day i.v. in 2–3 doses (for ≥ 6 weeks) *with*
      - Rifampicin 900–1200 mg/day i.v. or orally in 2–3 doses (for ≥ 6 weeks) *and*
      - Gentamicin 3mg/kg/day i.v./i.m. in 1–2 doses (for 2 weeks)

Enterococcus species
- Beta-lactam and gentamicin susceptible:
  - Amoxicillin 200 mg/kg/day i.v. in 4–6 doses *or*
    - Ampicillin 12 g/day i.v. in 4–6 doses *with*
    - Ceftriaxone 4 g/day i.v. in 2 doses (for 6 weeks) *or*
    - Gentamycin 3 mg/kg/day i.v. or i.m. in 1 dose (for 2 weeks).
  - If penicillin allergic:
    - Vancomycin 30/mg/day i.v. in 2 doses (for 6 weeks) *with*
    - Gentamicin 3 mg/kg/day i.v. or i.m. in 1 dose (for 2 weeks).

Blood culture-negative IE
- *Brucella:* doxycycline 200 mg/day + cotrimoxazole 960 mg/12 h + rifampicin 300–600 mg/day for ≥ 3–6 months (all oral)
- *Coxiella burnetii:* doxycycline 200 mg/day + hydroxychloroquine 200–600 mg/day for > 18 months (all oral)
- *Bartonella:* doxycycline 100 mg/12 h orally for 4 weeks + gentamicin 3 mg/kg/day i.v. for 2 weeks

- *Legionella*: levofloxacin 500 mg/12 h i.v. or orally for ≥ 6 weeks or clarithromycin 500 mg/12 h i.v. for 2 weeks then orally for 4 weeks + rifampicin 300–1200 mg/day
- *Mycoplasma*: levofloxacin 500 mg/12 h i.v. or orally for ≥ 6 months
- *Tropheryma whipplei*: doxycycline 200 mg/day plus hydroxychloroquine 200–600 mg/day orally for ≥ 18 months

Gram-negative bacteria
- HACEK related
    - Standard treatment: ceftriaxone 2 g/day (NVE 4 weeks; PVE 6 weeks)
- Non-HACEK related
    - Early surgery plus:
    - At least 6 weeks of bactericidal combinations of beta lactams and aminoglycosides (sometimes with additional quinolones or cotrimoxazole)

Empirical treatment (before or without pathogen identification)
- Community acquired native valves and prosthetic valves ≥ 12 months following surgery:
    - Penicillin tolerant:
        - Ampicillin 12 g/day i.v. in 4–6 doses *with*
            - Ceftriaxone 4 g/day i.v. or i.m. in 2 doses *or*
            - Flucloxacillin 12 g/day i.v. in 4–6 doses *and*
        - Gentamicin 3 mg/kg/day i.v. or i.m. in 1 dose
    - Penicillin allergic:
        - Cefazolin 6 g/day i.v. in 3 doses *or*
            - Vancomycin 30 mg/kg/day i.v. in 2 doses *with*
        - Gentamicin 3 mg/kg/day i.v. or i.m. in 1 dose
- Early prosthetic valve or nosocomial or non-nosocomial healthcare-associated IE
    - Vancomycin 30 mg/kg/day i.v. in 2 doses *or*
    - Daptomycin 10 mg/kg/day i.v. in 1 dose *with*
    - Gentamicin 3 mg/kg/day i.v. or i.m. in 1 dose *and*
    - Rifampicin 900–1200 mg/day i.v. or orally in 2–3 doses

3.8.9 Outpatient parenteral antibiotic therapy (OPAT)

- Outpatient parenteral or oral antibiotic treatment should be considered:
    - In patients with left-sided IE caused by *Streptococcus* spp., *E. faecalis*, *S. aureus*, or CoNS who have received appropriate i.v. antibiotic treatment for at least 10 days (or at least 7 days after cardiac surgery).
    - In patients who are clinically stable with no signs of abscess formation or valve abnormalities requiring surgery.
- But should not be used in patients with IE caused by difficult-to-treat microorganisms and/or additional high-risk features:
    - Abscess formation (intra- or extra-cardiac)
    - Severe valve regurgitation
    - Valve abnormalities or other severe conditions requiring surgery
    - Liver cirrhosis (Child–Pugh B or C)
    - Severe CNS emboli

- Severe post-surgical complications
- IVDU

3.8.10 Surgical treatment

- Almost 50% of patients with IE will undergo surgery
- Early surgery recommended in those with:
    - Heart failure
    - Abscess
    - Perivalvular complications
    - Embolism

Indications for early surgery
'Emergency' surgery (within 24 h)
- Heart failure
- Aortic/mitral IE or PVE with severe acute regurgitation, obstruction, or fistula causing refractory pulmonary oedema or shock

'Urgent' surgery (within 3–5 days)
Heart failure
- Aortic/mitral or PVE with severe regurgitation or obstruction causing symptoms of HF or echocardiographic signs of poor haemodynamic tolerance
- Severe valvular regurgitation, obstruction or fistula causing refractory pulmonary oedema or cardiogenic shock

Uncontrolled infection
- Locally uncontrolled infection and abscess, false aneurysm, fistula, enlarging vegetation, prosthetic dehiscence or new conduction disturbance (AV block)
- Fungi or multi-resistant organisms
- Persistent fever and positive blood cultures at 7–10 days despite appropriate antibiotic therapy and adequate control of septic metastatic foci (extra-cardiac infection excluded)
- Prosthetic valve endocarditis caused by staphylococci or non-HACEK gram-negative bacteria

Prevention of embolism
- Aortic/mitral or prosthetic vegetation > 10 mm in size and the following:
    - one or more embolic events (which may be silent and detected radiologically) despite appropriate antibiotic therapy
    - associated with severe stenosis or regurgitation and low operative risk
    - other indications for surgery
- Aortic/mitral or prosthetic vegetation > 30 mm (associated with high risk of neurological complications)

'Early' surgery (after 1–2 weeks of antibiotic therapy)
- PVE caused by staphylococci or non-HACEK gram-negative bacteria
- Early PVE (within 6 months of index surgery) with new valve replacement and complete debridement

Surgical treatment of right-sided infective endocarditis

When possible, tricuspid valve repair should be performed instead of valve replacement. Surgery is recommended in:

- Persistent vegetation with respiratory insufficiency requiring ventilatory support after recurrent pulmonary emboli
- Persistent tricuspid vegetations > 20 mm after recurrent pulmonary emboli
- Right heart failure due to severe TR with poor response to diuretics
- Patients with simultaneous involvement of left-heart structures

Consider surgical treatment if:

- Microorganisms difficult to eradicate or bacteraemia for > 7 days

Perioperative management of conduction disease

- Immediate pacemaker implantation should be considered in IE patients with complete heart block who are undergoing valve surgery in the presence of factors predicting persistent high degree AVB:
    - Pre-operative conduction abnormality
    - *S. aureus* infection
    - Aortic root abscess
    - Tricuspid valve involvement
    - Previous valve surgery

Coronary angiography prior to surgery

- Pre-operative invasive coronary angiography is recommended in men > 40 years, post-menopausal women, and patients with a high risk of CAD (history of CAD or at least 1 cardiovascular risk factor)
- CT coronary angiography may be used as an alternative in haemodynamically stable patients with (A) large aortic vegetation which could be dislodged during cardiac catheterization, or (B) need for emergency surgery
- Valve surgery without pre-operative coronary anatomy assessment should be considered in emergency situations, regardless of CAD risk

3.8.11 Infective endocarditis affecting cardiac implantable electronic devices (CDRIE)

- *Investigations*
    - Three or more blood cultures
    - Lead-tip culture
    - TOE (independent of TTE) regardless of blood culture findings
    - Consider intra-cardiac echo and/or [18F]F-FDG PET/CT
- *Treatment*
    - Initiate empirical antibiotic therapy for CDRIE once 3 sets of blood cultures have been obtained (ensuring coverage of methicillin-resistant staphylococci and Gram-negative bacteria)
    - Complete hardware extraction (device and leads) without delay in definite CDRIE (with initial empirical antibiotic therapy)

- Extended antibiotic treatment following extraction (4–6 weeks in the presence of septic emboli or prosthetic valves)
- Consider complete hardware removal if occult infection without another source
- Consider complete hardware extraction in those with NVE or PVE (with no evidence of device infection)
- Consider complete hardware extraction in cases of valvular IE, even without definite lead involvement
- *Device removal*
  - Percutaneous extraction preferred
  - Surgical extraction if percutaneous extraction incomplete or impossible, or vegetation > 20 mm
- *Reimplantation*
  - Defer if possible to allow a few days/weeks of antibiotics until signs and symptoms of infection have abated and blood cultures are negative (for at least 72 hours if vegetations are absent or at least 2 weeks if vegetations are present)
  - Reimplantation is recommended at a site remote from the previous generator
  - Temporary ipsi-lateral active fixation strategy may be considered in pacemaker-dependent patients who need antibiotics prior to implantation
  - Temporary pacing is not recommended
  - Routine antibiotic prophylaxis is recommended prior to device implantation

3.8.12 Non-bacterial thrombotic endocarditis (NBTE)

- NBTE (marantic endocarditis; Libman–Sacks endocarditis or verrucous endocarditis) is characterized by sterile vegetations (made of fibrin and platelet aggregates on cardiac valves)
- Bacteraemia or valve destruction unusual
- Associated with several diseases: e.g.,
  - Systemic lupus erythematosus with antiphospholipid antibodies (Libman–Sacks endocarditis)
  - Autoimmune disorders
  - Hypercoagulable states
  - Tuberculosis
- Features of NBTE include:
  - Vegetations unresponsive to antibiotics
  - Multiple systemic emboli
- Management:
  - Treat underlying cause
  - Anticoagulation (although poor supporting evidence)
  - Indications for valve surgery as for IE (including recurrent thromboembolism)

3.8.13 Multidisciplinary management

- IE requires a collaborative approach involving an 'Endocarditis Team' (Figure 3.8.4)
- Endocarditis Team should include cardiologists, cardiac surgeons and infectious disease specialists (or microbiologists)

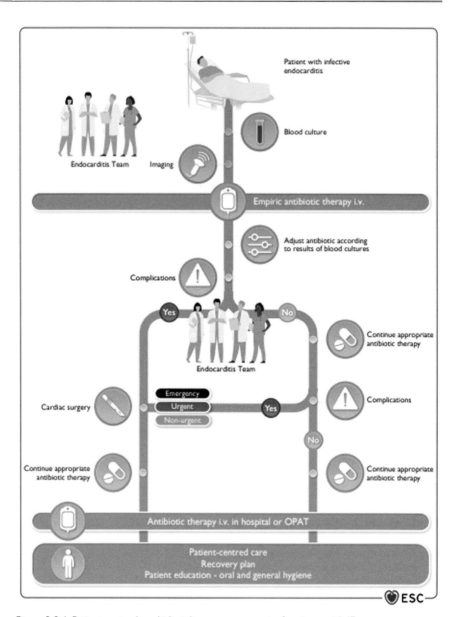

Figure 3.8.4 Patient-centred, multidisciplinary management of patients with IE.
Delgado V, Ajmone Marsan N, de Waha S, et al; ESC Scientific Document Group. 2023 ESC Guidelines for the management of endocarditis. *Eur Heart J.* 2023 Oct 14;44(39):3948–4042. doi: 10.1093/eurheartj/ehad193. © European Society of Cardiology. With permission from Oxford University Press.

- Expertise in multi-modality imaging (echocardiography, CT, MRI and PET) is essential
- Electrophysiologists, congenital heart disease specialists, neurologists and neurosurgeons may be involved for discussion of individual cases
- Regular meetings to discuss management
- Complicated IE (heart failure, abscess, embolic or neurological complications, congenital heart disease) should be discussed at an early stage and managed in a centre with facilities for immediate surgery

3.8.14 Antibiotic prophylaxis

- The evidence in favour is limited—no randomised trial
- Many cases of IE arise in those without known pre-existing valvular heart disease—and with no clear preceding invasive medical or dental procedure
- *Staphylococcus aureus* is the most common organism (with fewer cases due to oral streptococci)
- International organizations have updated their guidelines in the past decade and a careful approach is required to explain these changes to patients (many of whom are aware of the dangers of IE and have taken antibiotic prophylaxis for years
- Peri-procedural antibiotic prophylaxis is recommended for surgical or transcatheter implantation of a prosthetic valve, cardiac device or other intravascular prosthesis

Antibiotic regimens

- Single dose 30–60 min before procedure (Table 3.8.1).
- Dental procedures requiring manipulation of the gingival or periapical region of the teeth or perforation of the oral mucosa are defined as high-risk procedures.

Table 3.8.1 Guidelines from the European Society of Cardiology for antibiotic prophylaxis before dental procedures.

	Antibiotics (Single-dose 30–60 min before procedure)
Penicillin tolerant	Amoxicillin 2 g orally or i.v. Ampicillin 2 g i.m. or i.v. Cefazolin or ceftriaxone 1 g i.m. or i.v.
Penicillin allergic	Clarithromycin 500 mg orally Doxycycline 100 mg orally Cefazolin or ceftriaxone 1 g i.m. or i.v. (if no history of anaphylaxis, angioedema, or urticaria with penicillin-based antibiotics)

3.8.15 What's new in the European Society of Cardiology guidelines (2023)

- The ESC IE guidelines have been recently updated (see Further Reading)
- Antibiotic prophylaxis is recommended:

Before cardiac device implantation (covering S. *aureus*)

- In high-risk patients (including those patients with ventricular assist devices) undergoing high-risk procedures (dental extraction, oral surgical procedures and those involving manipulation of the gingival or periapical region of the teeth)

Antibiotic prophylaxis is no longer indicated for native valve disease

- Antibiotic prophylaxis may be considered in heart transplant recipients and high-risk patients undergoing invasive diagnostic or therapeutic procedures involving the respiratory, gastrointestinal, genitourinary tract, skin or musculoskeletal systems (Table 3.8.2).
- Specific diagnostic algorithms emphasise the use of multi-modality imaging for the detection and diagnosis of NVE, PVE and CDRIE (Figures 3.8.1, 3.8.2, 3.8.3)
    - Echocardiography is the primary imaging modality for the diagnosis of IE, although use of other techniques is encouraged for the assessment of cardiac involvement (cardiac CT, [18F]FDG-PET/CT, or WBC SPECT/CT) or detection of remote lesions (cerebral MRI, whole-body CT and/or PET/CT)
    - Echocardiography may have limited utility in patients with PVE and CDRIE and multi-modality imaging is strongly recommended to confirm a diagnosis of IE
    - Brain and whole body multi-modality imaging (whole-body CT, [18F]FDG-PET and/or MRI) is recommended in symptomatic patients with NVE and PVE to detect peripheral lesions and demonstrate minor diagnostic criteria
    - Brain CT or MRA is recommended in patients with IE and suspected infective cerebral aneuryms
- Multi-modality imaging may be considered as a screening tool in asymptomatic patients.

Non-antibiotic prevention of infective endocarditis

The risk of IE can be mitigated by simple general measures in high- and intermediate risk patients (Figure 3.8.5):

- Wound disinfection
- Eradication (or reduction) of chronic bacterial carriage
- Curative antibiotics for bacterial infection
- Strict infection control for at-risk procedures

Table 3.8.2 Classification of individuals at high risk of IE.

High-risk patients	<ul><li>Previous IE</li><li>Prosthetic valve or prosthetic material used for valve repair (including transcatheter valve)</li><li>Untreated cyanotic congenital heart disease</li><li>Congenital heart disease repaired with prosthetic material (for 6 months in the absence of residual defects or valve prostheses, indefinite if residual defect)</li><li>Ventricular assist device</li></ul>

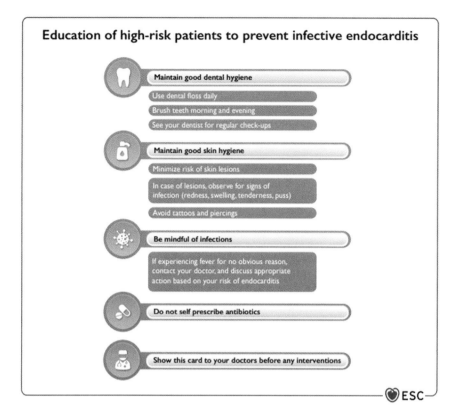

Figure 3.8.5 Education of high-risk patients to prevent IE.
Delgado V, Ajmone Marsan N, de Waha S, et al; ESC Scientific Document Group. 2023 ESC Guidelines for the management of endocarditis. *Eur Heart J.* 2023 Oct 14;44(39):3948–4042. doi: 10.1093/eurheartj/ehad193. © European Society of Cardiology. With permission from Oxford University Press.

- Avoid unnecessary invasive procedures (including intravenous cannulae and urinary catheters)
- Patient education on preventative measures (with particular emphasis on dental health) and the risk of recurrence
- Addiction treatment for patients with IVDU-related IE

Further reading

Delgado V, Marsan N.A, de Waha S, Bonaros N, Brida M, Burri H, Caselli S, Doenst T, Ederhy S, Erba P.A, Foldager D, Fosbøl E.L, Kovac J, Mestres C.A, Miller I.O, Miró J.M, Pazdernik M, Pizzi M.N, Quintana E, Rasmussen T.B, Ristić A.D, Rodés-Cabau J, Sionis A, Zühlke L.J and Borger M.A. 2023 ESC Guidelines for the management of endocarditis: Developed by the task force on the management of endocarditis of the European Society of Cardiology (ESC) Endorsed by the European Association for Cardio-Thoracic Surgery (EACTS) and the European Association of Nuclear Medicine (EANM). *Eur Heart J.* 2023;44(39):3948–4042, https://doi.org/10.1093/eurheartj/ehad193

CHAPTER 4

RHYTHM DISORDERS

4.1

The electrocardiogram

S M Afzal Sohaib and Mark Elliott

TABLE OF CONTENTS

4.1.1 The mechanisms and anatomy of electrical activity in the heart 273
4.1.2 The ECG and electrical vectors throughout the cardiac cycle 275
4.1.3 Common artefacts and lead reversal ECGs 278
4.1.4 The ECG in patients with cardiac pathology 278
  Chamber hypertrophy 278
  Ischaemia and infarction 283
  Pre-excitation 292
  Cardiac ion channel dysfunction 292
  Other repolarization disturbances 294
  Pericarditis, pericardial effusion, myocarditis 297
  Arrhythmogenic cardiomyopathy 298
  Pacemaker, ICD and CRT devices 299
4.1.5 Arrhythmia definitions 299
4.1.6 Investigate a patient with palpitations 300
  Long-term ambulatory ECG 300
  Exercise ECG testing 301

4.1.1 The mechanisms and anatomy of electrical activity in the heart

Cellular and molecular mechanisms

- The membrane potential of a cardiac myocyte is dependent on flow through ion channels, chiefly sodium channels, L-type and T-type Ca^{2+} channels, and various K^+ channels
- The resting potential of a myocyte is polarized (i.e. the inside of the cell is negative compared to the extracellular space)
- Depolarization occurs when there is an influx of cations, resulting in the intracellular space becoming positive in comparison to the extracellular space
- This causes a rise in intracellular Ca^{2+} levels which triggers myocyte contraction
- After several hundred milliseconds, the inward depolarizing currents are outweighed by outward repolarizing currents (mainly through K^+ channels), and the membrane potential repolarizes to its polarized resting state
- The depolarization current spreads from one myocyte to the next via gap junctions resulting in a wave of depolarization spreading across the cardiac muscle
- The action cardiac action potential is divided into 4 phases (figure 4.1.1):

Phase 0, depolarization
Upon reaching the threshold membrane potential rapid Na^+ channels open and positive Na^+ ions enter the cell

Phases 1–3, repolarization

Phase 1: starts with rapid outward K⁺ current; resulting in a fast early repolarization
Phase 2 (plateau phase): due to opening of Ca^{2+} channels, inward Na^+ and Ca^{2+} currents balance the outward K^+ currents. The cell is refractory to any stimulus in this phase
Phase 3: due to opening of 'delayed rectifier' outward K^+ channels, outward currents exceed inward currents

Phase 4, resting phase

No net movement of ions; the cell is fully excitable

Anatomy and physiology of the conducting system

- The conduction system of the heart ensures the wave of depolarization spreads in a specific way to allow efficient sequential contraction of the atria and ventricles
- The conduction properties of different cardiac tissue in this system depends on the presence of different ion channels in the membrane:
    - Rapidly conducting tissue (atrial and ventricular myocytes and the His–Purkinje system) relies on voltage-gated Na^+ channels, which allow rapid influx of cations and depolarization of the cell
    - Slow conduction tissue (the sino-atrial (SA) and atrio-ventricular (AV) nodes) lack the Na^+ channels responsible for rapid Na^+ influx, relying on the slower Ca^{2+} influx for depolarization

Sinus node

- A collection of specialized cells located in the right atrial sulcus terminalis, between the superior vena cava and right atrium (RA)
- Pacemaker (P) cells have the ability to depolarize spontaneously due to the possession of HCN (hyperpolarization-activated cyclic nucleotide-gated) channels that are open at resting membrane potentials, allowing slow influx of Na^+ and K^+ ions (the *'funny current'* (I_f))

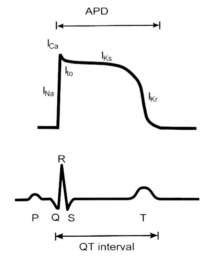

Figure 4.1.1 Diagram showing schematic human ventricular action potential (above) and corresponding surface ECG trace (below). The main currents (I) involved during each stage is shown on the upper image. Action potential duration (APD) is analogous to the QT interval seen on surface ECG recording
Reproduced from Amanfu RK, Saucerman JJ. Cardiac models in drug discovery and development: a review. *Crit Rev Biomed Eng.* 2011;39(5):379–95. doi: 10.1615/critrevbiomedeng.v39.i5.30.

- These P cells have regular spontaneous depolarization (automaticity) to initiate the depolarization, activation, and subsequent contraction of the surrounding atrial myocardial cells
- Blood supply usually from a branch that arises from proximal right coronary artery

Atrial conduction

- Electrical impulses propagate through the atrial tissue and pathways of preferential conduction from the right atrium to the AV node as well as to the left atrium
- Normal atrial conduction occurs in the sequence of high right atrium, mid right atrium, low right atrium, atrioventricular junction, and coronary sinus
- Intra-atrial conduction delay leads to a broad P wave—this may be largely due to enlarged atrial size and is often associated with congenital heart disease, e.g. endocardial cushion defects and Ebstein's anomaly

Atrioventricular node

- Located in the low atrial septum, anterior to the ostium of coronary sinus and above the insertion of the septal leaflet of the tricuspid valve, in the anatomically defined Triangle of Koch
- It accounts for the major component of time in normal AV conduction
- Delays in the AV node account for the major source of prolonged AV conduction
- AV conduction varies greatly with autonomic influence
- Blood supply from AV nodal artery, a branch of the posterior descending artery, which arises from the right coronary artery (80%) or from the circumflex artery (20%)
- HCN channels are also found in the AV node and His–Purkinje system, allowing these cells to takeover pacemaker activity, at slower rates, if the SA node is diseased or suppressed

Bundle of His

- Passes through the annulus fibrosus and penetrates the membranous interventricular septum before division of the left and right bundle branches
- Blood supply predominantly from the AV nodal artery, and sometimes from the septal perforators from the left anterior descending coronary artery

Infra-His conduction

- Right bundle branch crosses the anterior part of the interventricular septum and reaches the apex of the right ventricle and the base of the anterior papillary muscle
- Left bundle branch is less anatomically discrete and 'fans' into an anterior (superior) and a posterior (inferior) fascicle
- The bundle branches ramify and give rise to the endocardially located terminal Purkinje fibres, ensuring the activation of both ventricles

4.1.2 The ECG and electrical vectors throughout the cardiac cycle

- The electrical activity of the heart can be detected at skin level by electrodes, which allow the formation of the ECG
- Each skin electrode produces a signal comprising the amplitude of the electrical activity and its direction, called a vector
- The 12-lead ECG is created from 10 electrodes:
    - 6 chest electrodes correspond to leads V1–V6, which represent the electrical activity of the heart in the horizontal plane

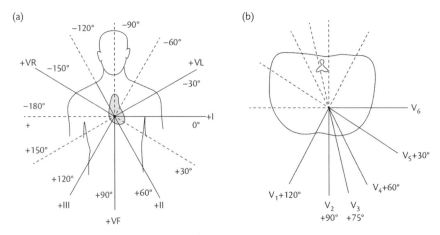

Figure 4.1.2 (a) Bailey's hexaxial system of the six leads of frontal plane. (b) Position of the positive and negative pole in the six precordial leads
Reproduced from the *ESC Textbook of Cardiovascular Medicine 3rd edition*, ed. John Camm, Thomas Lüscher, Gerald Maurer and Patrick Serruys, copyright 2018 with permission of Oxford University Press

- Information from 4 limb electrodes (RA, LA, LL, RL) are combined to produce 3 limb leads (I, II, and III) and three augmented limb leads (VR, VL, and VF), which represent the electrical activity of the heart in the coronal, or frontal, plane (see Figure 4.1.2)
- The normal ECG comprises a P-wave, QRS complex, and T-wave, as well as the intervals between them
- These represent different parts of the cardiac cycle (as outlined in Table 4.1.1)

Table 4.1.1 Stages of the cardiac cycle by surface ECG.

P-wave	Atrial depolarization; best evaluated in lead II and V1
PR interval	Time taken for electrical wave to travel from SA node, across the atria and through the AV node; normal is 120 ms to 200 ms
Q-wave	Small negative deflection after the P-wave and represents depolarization of the interventricular septum; best appreciated in the lateral leads
R-wave	The first positive deflection after the P-wave; represents ventricular depolarization
S-wave	Negative deflection after the R wave representing depolarization of the Purkinje fibres
J point	The point at which the QRS complex meets the ST-segment; a distinct upward deflection at this point is called a J-wave or Osborn wave
ST segment	The period that the ventricles are depolarized
T wave	Ventricular repolarization
QT interval	Total duration of ventricular depolarization and repolarization; most commonly measured in lead II; normal QT interval is > 350 ms in all, and < 440 ms in men, < 460 ms in women
U wave	Small upward deflection after the T-wave; hypothesized to represent repolarization of the interventricular septum; prominent U wave usually pathological

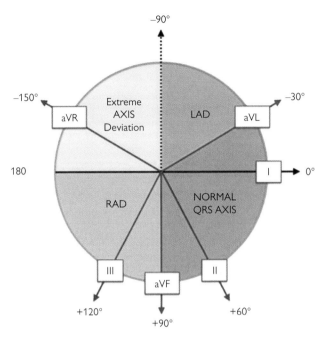

Figure 4.1.3 Calculation of cardiac axis using the limb leads (LAD = left axis deviation, RAD = right axis deviation)
Source data from https://litfl.com/ecg-axis-interpretation/

- The overall direction of the main depolarization wave across the myocardium (QRS complex) is referred to as the cardiac axis and can be calculated using the limb leads (see Figure 4.1.3)
- Cardiac axis can be estimated using direction of the QRS complex in leads I, II, and III or aVF (see Table 4.1.2)
- Changes in the QRS axis can represent changes in the physical shape of the heart (e.g. ventricular hypertrophy), abnormal conduction system or areas of previous infarction (outlined in Table 4.1.3)

Table 4.1.2 Estimation of the cardiac axis using leads I, II, and III or aVF.

	Normal Axis (0 to +30°)	Left Axis Deviation (0 to –30°)	Right Axis Deviation (+90° to +180°)	Extreme Axis Deviation (–90° to –180°)
Lead I	Positive	Positive	Negative	Negative
Lead II	Positive	Negative	Positive	Negative
Lead III or aVF	Positive	Negative	Positive	Negative

Table 4.1.3 Main causes of left and right axis deviation.

Left Axis Deviation	Right Axis Deviation
Normal variant	Normal variant
Left anterior fascicular block	Left posterior fascicular block
Left bundle branch block	Right ventricular hypertrophy
Left ventricular hypertrophy	Acute lung disease (e.g. pulmonary embolus)
Inferior myocardial infarction	Chronic lung disease
Ectopic ventricular rhythms	Lateral myocardial infarction
Pre-excitation syndromes	Ectopic ventricular rhythms
	Pre-excitation syndromes

4.1.3 Common artefacts and lead reversal ECGs

- Artefacts are signals on the ECG that are not derived from intrinsic myocyte electrical activity and there are various causes for this (see Box 4.1.1)
- Incorrect electrode placement can result in an abnormal appearance of the surface ECG that does not represent underlying pathology; REVERSE is a useful mnemonic to detect common limb lead reversals (see Table 4.1.4)

4.1.4 The ECG in patients with cardiac pathology

Chamber hypertrophy

- *Left atrial (LA) enlargement:*
  - Caused by LA pressure overload (e.g. mitral stenosis, LV systolic or diastolic dysfunction) or volume overload (e.g. mitral regurgitation, ventricular septal defect)
  - The main ECG criteria are a P-wave duration of > 110 ms +/− a notched or bifid P-wave (called 'P-mitrale', see Figure 4.1.4)

> **BOX 4.1.1 COMMON CAUSES OF SIGNAL ARTEFACT ON AN ECG**
>
> Patient movement
> Tremor or muscle activity
> Pacing spikes
> ICD or external defibrillator firing
> Neuro-stimulator
> Diathermy
> Poor skin to electrode contact (e.g. hair)
> Electrode or lead malfunction

Table 4.1.4 REVERSE—a mnemonic for ECG evidence of lead malposition.

	Abnormal ECG Finding	Potential Lead Mal-position
R	R wave is positive in lead aVR	Reversal of left arm and right arm electrodes
E	Extreme axis deviation: QRS axis between 180° and –0° (negative R wave in lead I, positive R wave in aVF)	Reversal of left arm and right arm electrodes
V	Very low (< 0.1 mV) amplitude in isolated limb lead (isolated 'flat' lead)	Reversal of right leg and left arm or right arm electrodes
E	Exchanged amplitude of the P waves (P wave in lead I greater than in lead II)	Reversal of left arm and left leg electrodes
R	R wave abnormal progression in the precordial leads	Reversal of chest leads (V1–V6)
S	Suspect dextrocardia (negative P wave, QRS and T wave in lead I; right axis deviation; positive R wave in aVR; absent R wave progression in precordial leads)	Reversal of left arm and right arm electrodes
E	Eliminate noise and interference (artefact mimicking tachycardia or ST changes)	

Source data from Baranchuk A, Shaw C, Alanazi H, Campbell D, Bally K, Redfearn DP, Simpson CS, Abdollah H. Electrocardiography pitfalls and artifacts: the 10 commandments. *Crit Care Nurse*. 2009 Feb;29(1):67–73. doi: 10.4037/ ccn2009607.

- The Morris index for defining LA enlargement by ECG criteria:
  - The amplitude of a negative P-wave multiplied by its duration = > 0.03
  - Is associated with increased risk of developing atrial fibrillation
- *Right atrial (RA) enlargement:*
  - Causes include pulmonary hypertension, right ventricular failure, tricuspid regurgitation, and some congenital heart diseases (e.g. atrial septal defect (ASD), tetralogy of Fallot, pulmonary stenosis, or Epstein's anomaly)

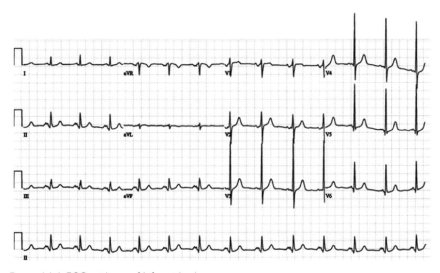

Figure 4.1.4 ECG evidence of left atrial enlargement
Reproduced from Tan LL, Teo SG, Poh KK. ECG P wave abnormalities. *Singapore Med J*. 2013 Jan;54(1):4–7; quiz p.7. doi: 10.11622/smedj.2013002 with permission from Wolters Kluwer.

Table 4.1.5 The different ECG voltage criteria for detecting left ventricular hypertrophy.

Name	Criteria
Gubner	R-wave lead I + S-wave lead III ≥ 2.5 mV
Sokolow–Lyon	S-wave V1 + R-wave lead V5/6 ≥ 3.5 mV
Cornell	R-wave aVL + S-wave lead V3 > 2.8 mV (men)
	R-wave aVL + S-wave lead V3 > 2.0 mV (women)

Adapted from the *ESC Textbook of Cardiovascular Medicine*, 3rd edn, ed. John Camm, Thomas Lüscher, Gerald Maurer, and Patrick Serruys, copyright 2018 with permission of Oxford University Press.

- In acquired heart disease is characterized by a peaked P-wave (> 2.5 mm in height) with right P wave axis deviation (also called 'P-pulmonale'), (see Figure 4.1.5)
- In congenital heart disease is often characterized by peaked P-wave (> 2.5 mm in height) with left P wave axis deviation (also called 'P-congenitale')
- Often associated with the QRS morphology of RV hypertrophy (see below)
- *Left ventricular hypertrophy (LVH):*
    - Can be caused by primary muscle disease (e.g. hypertrophic cardiomyopathies) or any condition that increases left ventricular afterload (e.g. systemic hypertension or aortic stenosis)
    - The LV accounts for the majority of the total cardiac mass. As a result the main representation of LVH on the ECG is an increase in QRS voltage (see Figure 4.1.6)
    - Multiple voltage criteria have been proposed and are summarized in Table 4.1.5
    - These criteria have poor sensitivity and specificity for LVH: many patients with proven moderate LVH have normal ECGs, whilst some patients meeting ECG voltage criteria for LVH in fact have normal LV size and wall thickness on imaging
    - ECG voltage criteria for LVH has, however, been shown to be an independent predictor of poor cardiovascular outcome even if the LV mass on imaging is normal. This may be related to muscle fibrosis, ischaemia, or inflammation

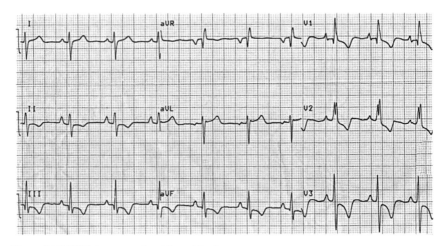

Figure 4.1.5 ECG demonstrating right atrial enlargement
https://www.ecgquest.net/diagnosis/right-atrial-enlargement/?order=asc

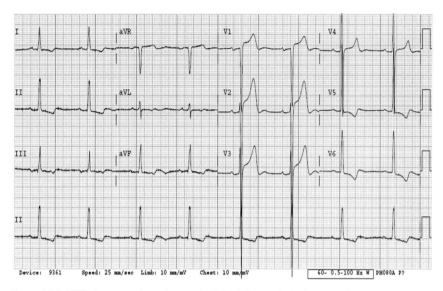

Figure 4.1.6 ECG demonstrating voltage criteria for left ventricular hypertrophy
https://litfl.com/left-ventricular-hypertrophy-lvh-ecg-library/

Table 4.1.6 Romhilt–Estes Score for left ventricular hypertrophy; ≥ 5 points = definite LVH; ≥ 4 points = probable LVH.

	Assessment	Score
Amplitude	R or S wave in limb leads ≥ 2.0 mV *or* S-wave V1/2 ≥ 3.0 mV *or* R-wave in V5/V6 ≥ 3.0 mV	3 points
ST-T segment pattern	ST segment depression in opposite direction to QRS complex	Without digitalis = 3 points With digitalis = 1 point
Left atrial involvement	Terminal negativity of P-wave in V1 ≥ 0.10 mV *and* ≥ 0.04 ms	3 points
Left axis deviation	≥ −30°	2 points
QRS duration	≥ 90 ms	1 point
Intrinsicoid deflection	≥ 50 ms in V5–V6	1 point

N.B. *Intrinsicoid deflection* represents the early phase of ventricular depolarization and is defined as the time from the beginning of the QRS complex to the peak of the R-wave. Adapted from the *ESC Textbook of Cardiovascular Medicine*, 3rd edn, ed. John Camm, Thomas Lüscher, Gerald Maurer, and Patrick Serruys, copyright 2018 with permission of Oxford University Press.

- Other ECG features of LVH include:
  - leftward QRS axis deviation
  - mild QRS duration prolongation
  - left atrial enlargement
  - repolarization abnormalities, e.g. J-point depression, down-sloping ST depression, and asymmetric T-wave inversion in left chest leads; commonly referred to as 'left ventricular strain'

Table 4.1.7 The different ECG voltage criteria for detecting right ventricular hypertrophy.

Name	Criteria
Lewis	(R-wave lead I + S-wave lead III) − (S-wave lead I + R-wave lead III) is < 15 mm
Sokolow-Lyon	R-wave lead V1 + S-wave in lead V5/V6 is > 10.5 mm
Butler-Leggett	(Max R or R' in lead V1/V2) + (Max S in lead I or V6) − (S-wave in V1) is > 6 mm

Adapted from the *ESC Textbook of Cardiovascular Medicine*, 3rd edn, ed. John Camm, Thomas Lüscher, Gerald Maurer, and Patrick Serruys, copyright 2018 with permission of Oxford University Press.

- These features have been combined to produce the Romhilt–Estes score (see Table 4.1.6)
• Right ventricular hypertrophy (RVH):
  - Can be caused by pulmonary hypertension, pulmonary valve disease, and some congenital heart diseases (e.g. ASD, tetralogy of Fallot)
  - As the right ventricle is smaller than the left, RVH generally has to be severe before significant changes in the QRS complex appear on the ECG (see Figure 4.1.7)
  - Various QRS voltage criteria for RVH are summarized in Table 4.1.7
  - Other ECG features of RVH include:
    • right QRS axis deviation
    • mild QRS duration prolongation
    • right atrial enlargement
    • repolarization abnormalities, e.g. ST-depression and T-wave inversion in right-sided

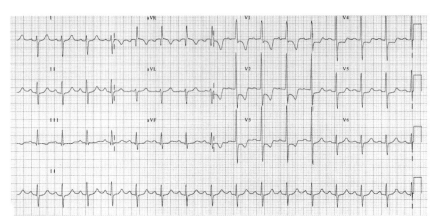

Figure 4.1.7 ECG demonstrating right ventricular hypertrophy
https://litfl.com/wp-content/uploads/2018/08/ECGH-RVH-Right-ventricular-hypertropy-RV-Strain.jpg

chest leads (V1–V3), commonly referred to as 'right ventricular strain'

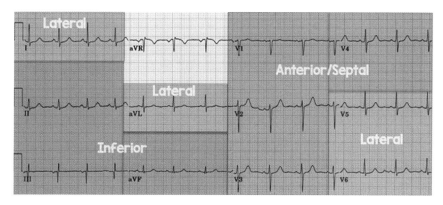

Figure 4.1.8 Myocardial regional wall territories by 12 lead ECG
https://www.grepmed.com/images/2848/localization-cardiology-diagnosis-coronary-artery-ekg-map

Ischaemia and infarction

- In the context of myocardial ischaemia due to epicardial coronary artery occlusion or narrowing, ECG leads correspond to myocardial regional walls, and thus coronary artery territories (see Figure 4.1.8)
- This can enable assessment of the potential culprit artery effected if regional ECG changes are seen, though there are well-recognized variations in coronary anatomy that will affect the accuracy of this ECG assessment (see Figure 4.1.8)
- ECG changes in an ST-elevation myocardial infarction (MI):
    - ECG changes evolve as ischaemia persists resulting in infarction and necrosis (see Figure 4.1.9)
    - ST segment deviation occurs because ischaemia lowers the membrane potential of cardiac myocytes, shortens the duration of the action potential, and changes the shape of the plateau phase of the action potential (see Figure 4.1.10)
    - This results in a voltage gradient between ischaemic and normal cardiac tissue, causing abnormal current flow

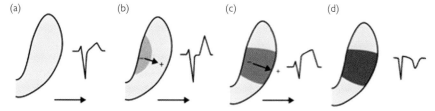

Figure 4.1.9 The ECG morphology explains the different degrees of ischaemia that appear sequentially following total coronary occlusion. (a) ECG with no previous ischaemia; (b) Predominating ischaemia in the sub-endocardial area (T wave is symmetrical and often higher than normal with a longer QT interval); (c) If ischaemia is severe and become transmural, ST elevation appears; (d) If ischaemia persists, transmural necrosis appears and is expressed as the Q wave of necrosis and a negative T wave left intra-ventricular patterns (window effect of Wilson)
(Reproduced from the *ESC Textbook of Cardiovascular Medicine 3rd edition*, ed. John Camm, Thomas Lüscher, Gerald Maurer and Patrick Serruys, copyright 2018 with permission of Oxford University Press)

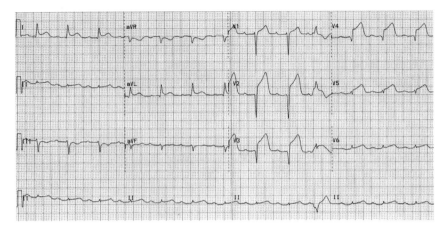

Figure 4.1.10 ECG demonstrating an anterior ST elevation myocardial infarction
https://litfl.com/anterior-myocardial-infarction-ecg-library/

- In severe, transmural ischaemia, net current flow runs away from ischaemic tissue, causing depression of the isoelectric line during the resting polarized state and the appearance of ST segment elevation in overlying electrodes during ventricular depolarization
- If ischaemia persists, tissue becomes necrotic (infarction) resulting in loss of the R-wave and development of pathological Q-waves as the dead tissue acts as a 'window' through which the skin electrodes detect the R-wave from the contralateral wall

ST-elevation MI (STEMI) equivalents:
1. Posterior STEMI:
    - No standard 12-lead ECG electrodes directly overlie the posterior wall of the left ventricle
    - During a posterior MI, dominant R-waves and ST-depression are seen in leads V1–V3
    - This is the equivalent of Q-waves and ST-elevation being seen in the opposite direction by the anterior leads
    - The diagnosis is best confirmed with a posterior ECG, applying leads V7–V9 sequentially around the chest wall after lead V6 (see Figure 4.1.11)
    - Usually seen in association with an inferior STEMI (in right dominant circulations) or lateral STEMI (in left dominant circulations)
2. Right ventricular infarction:
    - Complicates 40% of inferior STEMIs and important to detect as can cause preload sensitive hypotension
    - ST elevation often present in lead V1, in addition to inferior leads
    - Confirmed with a right-sided ECG with mirror placement of precordial leads (V1R–V6R) which will show ST elevation in leads V4R–V6R (see Figure 4.1.12)
3. Left bundle branch block (LBBB):
    - New onset LBBB in the context of MI is usually secondary to a large anterior or anteroseptal infarct resulting in damage to the extensive conduction system of the left ventricle
    - Pre-existing LBBB makes interpretation of the ECG in a patient with suspected MI difficult, including when due to right ventricular pacing (see Figure 4.1.13)
    - Sgarbossa's criteria (see Table 4.1.8) help determine the likelihood of STEMI in the context of LBBB with a score ≥ 3 having 90% specificity but low (36%) sensitivity for diagnosis of MI

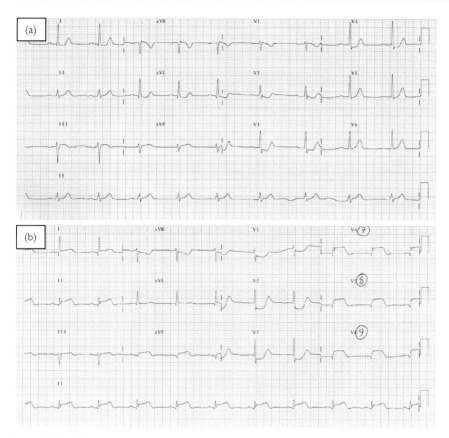

Figure 4.1.11 ECGs demonstrating a posterior ST elevation myocardial infarction, with A. demonstrating ST depression V2-V4 and reciprocal ST elevation in leads II, III and aVF, and B. demonstrating the use of sequential V7–V9 lead placement to identify the ST elevation evident in the posterior wall
https://litfl.com/posterior-myocardial-infarction-ecg-library/

ECG changes in non ST-elevation MI (NSTEMI), a sub-total vessel occlusion:
- Ischaemia is usually limited to the sub-endocardium, resulting in current flow from the sub-endocardial to sub-epicardial tissue
- This causes upward deviation of the isoelectric line at rest, resulting in apparent ST segment depression in overlying electrodes during left ventricular depolarization
- T-wave inversion also occurs due to changes in ventricular repolarization

Table 4.1.8 Sgarbossa's criteria for assisting with diagnosis of myocardial infarction in pre-existing left bundle branch block (score of ≥ 3 more likely to represent myocardial infarction).

Criteria	Points
ST elevation ≥ 1 mm in a lead with a positive QRS complex (concordance)	5
Concordant ST depression ≥ 1 mm in lead V1, V2, or V3	3
ST elevation ≥ 5 mm in a lead with a negative (discordant) QRS complex	2

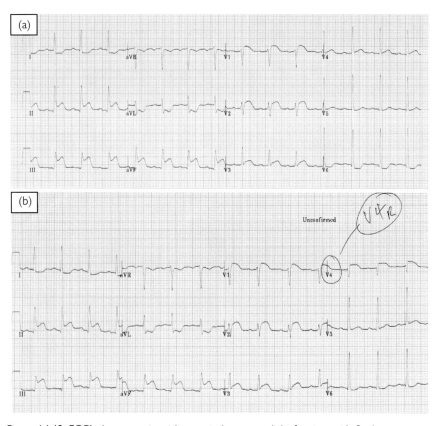

Figure 4.1.12 ECG's demonstrating right ventricular myocardial infarction, with **A.** demonstrating ST elevation in leads II, III, aVF, and extending to leads V1-3, and **B.** utilising right sided ECG leads with ST elevation seen also in V4R-V5R.
https://litfl.com/right-ventricular-infarction-ecg-library/

- In healthy tissue, the epicardial myocytes have a shorter action potential than endocardial myocytes and so the negative repolarization current travels away from overlying electrodes, producing a positive deflection (T-wave)
- In sub-endocardial ischaemia, the action potential of diseased myocytes is shortened, causing the depolarization current to change direction and producing a negative T-wave in overlying electrodes
- Patients with NSTEMI may have apparently normal ECGs

Stable coronary disease (i.e. chronic coronary syndrome):
- Patients classically only develop ischaemia when myocardial demand increases (i.e. during exercise) and so the resting ECG is often normal (in the absence of previous significant infarction)
- ECG changes may only develop during stress, which is the basis of the traditional exercise ECG test
- Resting ECG may provide evidence of ischaemia (ST segment depression and T-wave inversion) or previous transmural infarction (Q-waves and loss of R-wave)

Conduction disturbances

Left bundle branch block (LBBB) and right bundle branch block (RBBB):

BOX 4.1.2 THE CLASSICAL ECG APPEARANCE AND CAUSES OF LEFT BUNDLE BRANCH BLOCK (LBBB) AND RIGHT BUNDLE BRANCH BLOCK (RBBB); *STEMI = ST ELEVATION MYOCARDIAL INFARCTION*

LBBB	RBBB
ECG changes: • QRS duration ≥ 120 ms • Broad notched or slurred R wave in leads I, aVL, V5, and V6 • Absent q waves in leads I, V5, and V6 • ST and T waves usually opposite in direction to QRS (discordance) • Positive T wave in leads with upright QRS may be normal (positive concordance)	**ECG changes:** • QRS duration ≥ 120 ms • rsr', rsR', or rSR' in leads V1 or V2. The R' or r' deflection is usually wider than the initial R wave • S wave duration > R wave duration or > 40 ms in leads I and V6
Causes: Ischaemic heart disease Acute anterior STEMI Aortic stenosis Dilated cardiomyopathy Degenerative conduction system disease Hypertension	**Causes:** Normal variant Right ventricular hypertrophy or dilatation (e.g. chronic lung disease; pulmonary embolism) Ischaemic heart disease or acute MI (supplied by first and second septal branches of left anterior descending coronary artery) Cardiomyopathies Degenerative conduction system disease

- Both represent a conduction block at ventricular level of either the left or right bundle branches
- If a bundle branch is blocked, depolarization of the corresponding ventricle is achieved through the interventricular septum via the contralateral ventricle, which distorts the normal appearance of the QRS complex, and causes prolongation of this to > 120 ms
- Septal repolarization dominates over the delayed ventricular depolarization resulting in ST segment and T-wave changes
- The classical ECG appearances and causes of RBBB and LBBB are shown in Box 4.1.2, with ECG examples in Figure 4.1.14 and 4.1.15
- In partial RBBB or LBBB, the altered QRS morphology is seen without significant prolongation of the QRS duration (typically 110–120 ms duration)
- Intermittent RBBB or LBBB are often rate related (i.e. seen during periods of tachycardia or bradycardia)

Hemi-fascicular block:

- The left bundle is divided further into the anterior and posterior fascicles, and conduction disease can affect either or both of these
- ECG features of left anterior hemi-block:
  - Left axis deviation (frontal plane QRS axis between −45° and −90°)
  - qR pattern in lead aVL

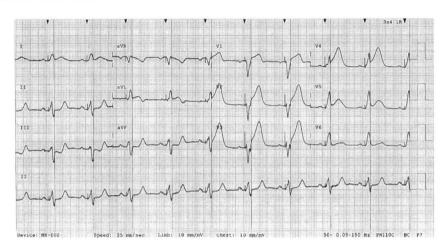

Figure 4.1.13 ECG example of right ventricular pacing with associated left bundle branch block and super-added anterior ST elevation meeting Sgarbossa's criteria for diagnosis of MI
https://litfl.com/sgarbossa-criteria-ecg-library/

- R-peak time in lead aVL of ≥ 45 ms
- QRS duration < 120 ms
- ECG features of left posterior hemi-block:
    - Right axis deviation (frontal plane QRS axis between 90° and 180°)
    - rS pattern in leads I and aVL
    - qR pattern in leads III and aVF
    - QRS duration < 120 ms

Other types of intraventricular conduction delay:

- Non-specific intraventricular conduction delay:
    - QRS duration > 110 ms but ECG criteria for RBBB or LBBB not met
- Bilateral RBBB and LBBB:
    - Alternating RBBB and LBBB seen on ECG or rhythm strip; implies impending complete heart block

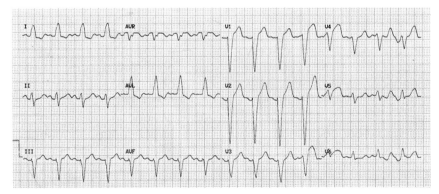

Figure 4.1.14 ECG demonstrating typical left bundle branch block
https://litfl.com/left-bundle-branch-block-lbbb-ecg-library/

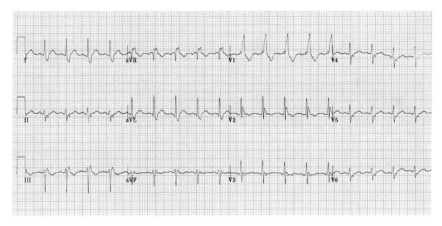

Figure 4.1.15 ECG example of right bundle branch block (RBBB) and left anterior hemi-block (also termed bi-fascicular block). Sinus rhythm with left axis deviation with a qR pattern in aVL, and typical RBBB
https://litfl.com/bifascicular-block-ecg-library/

- Bi-fascicular block:
    - RBBB with either left anterior hemi-block (Figure 4.1.15) or right anterior hemi-block
- Tri-fascicular block:
    - RBBB with alternating left anterior hemi-block and right anterior hemi-block (i.e. disease of all three fascicles)
    - Bi-fascicular block with prolonged PR interval is often erroneously referred to as tri-fascicular block and can be explained by bi-fascicular block with delayed conduction in either the bundle of His or in the remaining fascicle (see Figure 4.1.16)

Atrioventricular (AV) block:

- First-degree AV block:

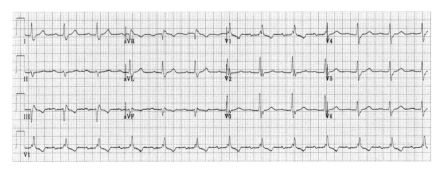

Figure 4.1.16 ECG demonstrating right bundle branch block, left posterior hemi-block, and first degree heart block (prolonged PR interval); often erroneously referred to as "tri-fascicular block"
https://litfl.com/trifascicular-block-ecg-library/

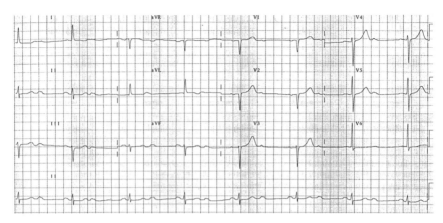

Figure 4.1.17 ECG demonstrating 2:1 atrioventricular block, with alternating conducted and non-conducted P waves
https://litfl.com/av-block-2nd-degree-fixed-ratio-blocks/

- Prolonged PR interval (> 200 ms) due to delayed conduction through the AV node or His–Purkinje system; QRS morphology is usually normal
- Second-degree AV block:
  - Mobitz type 1 (Wenckebach):
    - progressively prolonging PR interval before a non-conducted P-wave
    - may be physiological (e.g. high vagal tone) or due to disease at the AV node
    - low risk of progression to complete heart block
  - Mobitz type 2:
    - fixed PR interval with intermittent non-conducted P-wave and usually due to disease of the His–Purkinje system
  - 2:1 AV block:
    - alternating conducted and non-conducted P-waves (see Figure 4.1.17)
    - can be Mobitz 1 (at the AV node) or Mobitz 2 (below the AV node)
  - High-grade AV block:

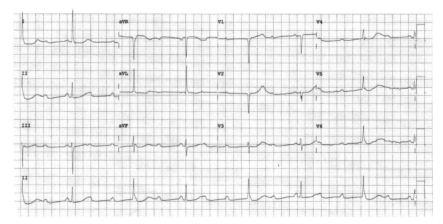

Figure 4.1.18 ECG demonstrating third degree (complete) atrioventricular block

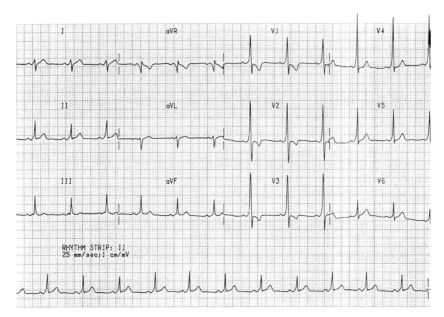

Figure 4.1.19 ECG demonstrating an accessory pathway: short PR interval and classic up-slurring R wave, termed a delta wave
https://litfl.com/pre-excitation-syndromes-ecg-library/

- P:QRS ratio of 3:1 or higher, which results in marked bradycardia
• Third-degree (complete) AV block:
  - Complete dissociation between P waves and QRS complexes with the atrial rate exceeding the ventricular rate (see Figure 4.1.18)

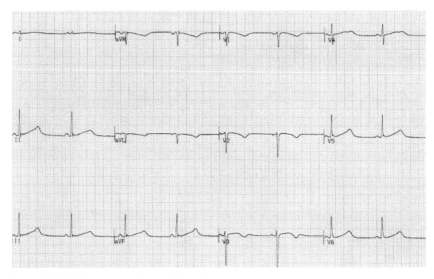

Figure 4.1.20 ECG example of long QT syndrome
https://litfl.com/qt-interval-ecg-library/

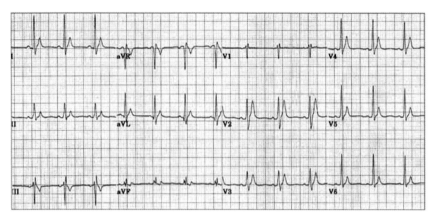

Figure 4.1.21 ECG example of short QT syndrome
https://www.ecgquest.net/diagnosis/short-qt-syndrome/

- The escape rhythm varies in rate and stability according to the location of the block: a narrow QRS and ventricular rate of 40–60 suggests a more stable junctional escape rhythm, a broad QRS and ventricular rate of 20–40 suggests a more unstable escape rhythm coming from the ventricular myocardium
- Failure of the escape rhythm results in Stokes–Adams attacks or sudden cardiac death

Pre-excitation

- Refers to premature activation of the ventricles due to conduction via an alternative route than the AV node, termed an accessory pathway
- Accessory pathways are discussed in more detail in section 4.4.2, but the most common form is Wolf–Parkinson–White, in which the resting ECG will typically have a short PR interval (< 120 ms) and broad QRS duration due to the presence of a delta wave (see Figure 4.1.19). ECG changes can be intermittent and vary according to the relative sympathetic and vagal tone, which affects the speed of AV nodal conduction

Cardiac ion channel dysfunction

Long QT syndrome (LQTS):

- An inherited arrhythmia disorder characterized by prolonged repolarization and increased risk of ventricular arrhythmias—(see Figure 4.1.20) discussed in detail in section 4.8.2

Short QT syndrome (SQTS):

- An inherited channelopathy characterized by shortened repolarization phase and increased risk of AF, syncope, and sudden cardiac death—discussed in detail in section 4.8.5
- ECG shows short (< 330 ms) QTc (see Figure 4.1.21)

Brugada ECG pattern:

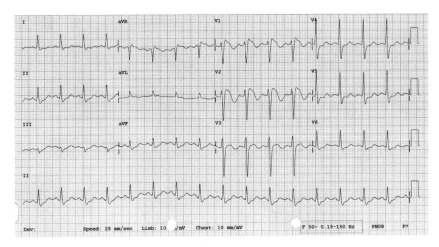

Figure 4.1.22 ECG example of type 1 Brugada pattern
https://litfl.com/what-is-brugada-syndrome/

- An inherited channelopathy causing increased risk of ventricular arrhythmias that classically occur during sleep or with fever—discussed in detail in section 4.8.3
- Three main ECG patterns recognized, found in more than one of leads V1–V3 (see Figures 4.1.22 and 4.1.23):
  1. Type 1: ≥ 2 mm J point elevation with coved ST-segment elevation and negative T-wave
  2. Type 2: ≥ 2 mm J point elevation with saddle-shaped ST-segment elevation and positive or biphasic T-wave
  3. Type 3: either coved or saddle-shaped ST-segment elevation < 1 mm

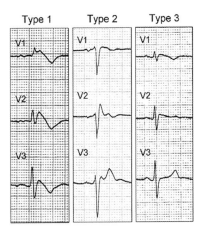

Figure 4.1.23 Demonstration of the varying QRS and T wave morphologies of Brugada types 1 to 3

Reproduced from Napolitano, C., Priori, S.G. Brugada syndrome. *Orphanet J Rare Dis* 1, 35 (2006). https://doi.org/10.1186/1750-1172-1-35 with permission from Springer Nature https://creativecommons.org/licenses/by/4.0/.

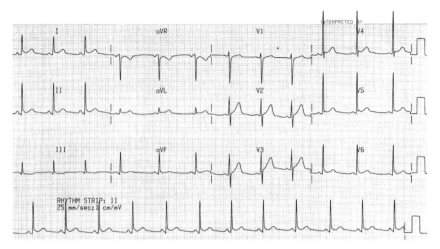

Figure 4.1.24 ECG example of global early repolarisation
https://litfl.com/benign-early-repolarisation-ecg-library/

Early repolarization (ER):

- ER pattern is a relatively common variant on the ECG (see Figure 4.1.24), but in rare cases can be associated with ventricular fibrillation and sudden cardiac death
- Discussed in more detail in section 4.8.6 but is defined on ECG as J-point elevation ≥ 1 mm in two adjacent leads with either a slurred or notched morphology (also known as a J-wave)

Other repolarization disturbances

Electrolytes abnormalities:

- Hyperkalaemia:
  - Causes the resting membrane potential of cardiac myocytes to become less negative (i.e. partial depolarization); this inactivates some of the voltage-gated sodium channels resulting in slowed conduction through the myocardium
  - This initially causes repolarization abnormalities, which is followed by bradycardia and conduction abnormalities
  - ECG changes progress as extracellular potassium concentration increases:
    - Peaked T-waves
    - PR prolongation with flattened or absent P-waves
    - AV node block or other conduction blocks
    - QRS widens resulting in a sine wave, before ventricular standstill or ventricular fibrillation
- Hypokalaemia:
  - Causes hyperpolarization of the myocyte resting membrane potential; this has several effects including deactivation of the repolarizing outward potassium current, resulting in increased myocyte excitability
  - ECG changes progress as extracellular potassium concentration decreases (see Figure 4.1.25):
    - Increased P-wave amplitude and duration
    - Prominent U wave (best seen in leads V4–V6); merging of T-wave and U-wave can cause apparent QTc prolongation
    - ST segment depression with flattened or inverted T-waves

> **BOX 4.1.3 DRUGS CAUSING QT PROLONGATION**
>
> **Anti-microbials:**
> - Macrolides (erythromycin, clarithromycin)
> - Moxifloxacin
> - Fluconazole / ketoconazole
>
> **Antiarrhythmics:**
> - Class I agents (flecainide, quinidine)
> - Class III agents (amiodarone, dronedarone, sotalol)
>
> **Anti-psychotics:**
> - Typical (haloperidol, chlorpromazine)
> - Atypical (risperidone, quetiapine, clozapine)
>
> **Anti-depressants:**
> - Tricyclics (amitriptyline, dosulepin, doxepin, clomipramine, imipramine, lofepramine)
> - SSRIs (citalopram, escitalopram)
>
> **Anti-emetics:**
> - Ondansetron
> - Droperidol
> - Domperidone
>
> **Others:**
> - Some anti-retrovirals
> - Some anti-malarials
> - Protein kinase inhibitors

- Increased atrial and ventricular ectopics with risk of supraventricular or ventricular re-entrant tachycardia
- Hypercalcaemia:
  - Causes decrease in the duration of phase 2 of the myocyte action potential (due to more rapid Ca^{2+} influx)
  - Results in short QTc interval on ECG
  - Other ECG changes that can be seen include:
    - PR prolongation
    - ST-elevation in V1–V2 (Brugada-like pattern)
    - T-wave changes
- Hypocalcaemia:
  - Causes prolongation of phase 2 of the myocyte action potential due to delayed calcium influx
  - Results in QTc prolongation on the ECG and typically normal T-wave morphology
  - Arrhythmia is uncommon, but Torsades de Pointes can occur
- Hypomagnesaemia:
  - Causes a variety of non-specific ECG changes, similar to those found in both hypokalaemia and hypocalcaemia

Anti-arrhythmic and other drugs:

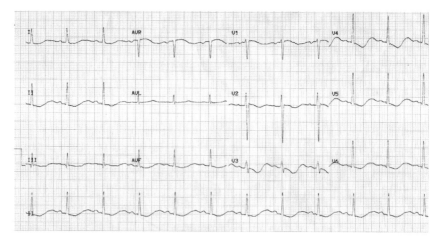

Figure 4.1.25 ECG example of hypokalaemia, with ST depression, T wave inversion, prominent U waves and long QU interval
https://litfl.com/hypokalaemia-ecg-library/

- Digoxin:
    - Has multiple effects on cardiac myocytes including:
        - Increasing intracellular calcium, causing increased automaticity/excitability
        - Increased vagal tone, causing delayed conduction through the AV node
    - At therapeutic levels, digoxin causes changes in the ECG:
        - PR prolongation
        - QTc shortening
        - Concave ST depression ('reverse-tick') best seen in lateral leads
    - At toxic levels, digoxin can result in various arrhythmias:
        - Increased automaticity causes frequent PVCs, atrial arrhythmias, ventricular tachycardias (including bi-directional ventricular tachycardia), and ventricular fibrillation
        - Increased vagal tone causes: sinus bradycardia, sinus arrest or sinoatrial exit block, and any form of AV node block
- Drugs that prolong QTc interval (main drugs listed in Box 4.1.3):
    - Many antiarrhythmic and non-cardiac drugs can block the I_{KR} current, resulting in delayed repolarization, prolonged QTc on ECG, and risk of ventricular arrhythmias (classically Torsades de Pointes)
    - Risk of arrhythmia is increased by:
        - Concomitant use of more than one drug
        - Underlying cardiac disease causing QTc prolongation (including congenital LQTS)
        - Electrolyte abnormalities (particularly hypokalaemia)

Hypothermia:

- Causes slowed conduction through all cardiac tissue
- Results in bradycardia and prolongation of all intervals on the ECG (PR, QRS, QT)
    - A classical ECG feature is J-point elevation (known as J-wave or Osborne wave) whose height is proportional to the severity of hypothermia

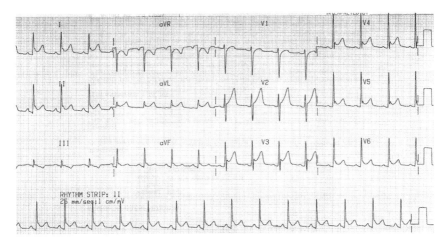

Figure 4.1.26 ECG example of global saddle shaped ST elevation and PR depression, in keeping with acute pericarditis
https://litfl.com/pericarditis-ecg-library/

Pericarditis, pericardial effusion, myocarditis

Acute pericarditis:

- ECG changes occur due to inflammation of the epicardium
- Typically there are 4 stages of ECG changes (though only seen in 50% of cases, see Figure 4.1.26)
    - Stage 1 (first hours to days): diffuse concave ST-elevation and PR depression (except in leads aVR and V1 where the opposite can occur)
    - Stage 2 (first few weeks): normalization of ST and PR segments
    - Stage 3 (duration not well documented): diffuse T-wave inversion

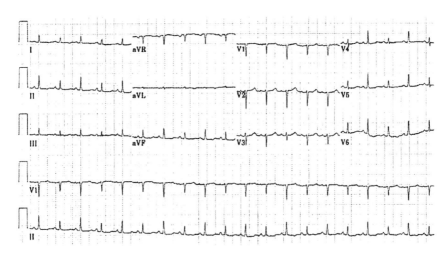

Figure 4.1.27 ECG demonstrating classical triad of sinus tachycardia, low voltage QRS complexes and "electrical alternans" seen in massive pericardial effusion / cardiac tamponade
https://litfl.com/ecg-findings-in-massive-pericardial-effusion/

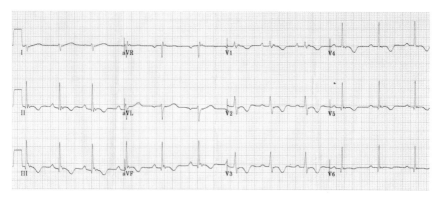

Figure 4.1.28 ECG demonstrating the associated T wave inversion, prolonged S wave in the absence of right bundle branch block, and epsilon wave seen in arrhythmogenic right ventricular cardiomyopathy
https://litfl.com/arrhythmogenic-right-ventricular-cardiomyopathy-arvc/

- Stage 4: normalization of the ECG
- ST elevation in pericarditis differs from STEMI in several ways:
    - Concave/saddle-shaped and < 5 mm
    - Associated with PR depression (88% sensitivity if present)
    - Usually diffuse (not related to coronary territories)
    - Not associated with reciprocal ST depression (except in aVR and V1)
    - Associated T-wave inversion takes longer to develop

Pericardial effusion:

- Classical triad of ECG findings in a massive pericardial effusion (usually associated with cardiac tamponade, see Figure 4.1.27):
    1. Sinus tachycardia
    2. Low voltage ECG (defined as QRS amplitude in all limb leads < 5 mm *or* QRS amplitude in all chest leads < 10 mm) due to attenuation of ECG signal by pericardial fluid
    3. 'Electrical alternans' (cyclic beat-to-beat shift in the QRS axis or amplitude) due to mechanical swinging of the heart in a large pericardial effusion

Myocarditis:

- Can cause a variety of non-specific ECG findings
- May have features of acute pericarditis in diffuse myo-pericarditis
- May have features of acute myocardial infarction due to inflammatory myocardial damage
- Associated with risk of complex ventricular and, less commonly, atrial arrhythmias

Arrhythmogenic cardiomyopathy

- An inherited condition where ventricular myocytes are gradually replaced by fibro-fatty tissue—discussed in detail in section 5.2
- ECG features that contribute towards formal diagnosis (> 85% of patients have at least one feature) include (see Figure 4.1.28):
    - T-wave inversion in leads V1–V3 in the absence of complete RBBB (Note, T-wave inversion in leads V5–V6 suggest LV involvement)

- Prolonged S-wave up-stroke (interval from nadir of S-wave to end of QRS ≥ 50 ms in absence of complete RBBB)
- Epsilon wave (a positive deflection at the end of the QRS complex) in leads V1–V3
- Ventricular tachycardias in ARVC are classically of LBBB pattern with superior axis (i.e. negative in leads II, III, and aVF)

Pacemaker, ICD, and CRT devices

- Normal device function:
  - Paced rhythms are important to identity on the ECG and can make interpretation of other pathology difficult
  - Pacing spikes may be seen prior to the P-wave or QRS complex, however these can be small, particularly in bipolar leads, or due to the filter settings of the ECG machine
  - Most pacemakers are programmed in demand mode (only pacing when required, i.e. certain parameters met), and therefore the ECG may show intermittent pacing or intrinsic rhythm depending on intrinsic rate and pacemaker settings
- Right ventricular pacing is characterized on ECG by:
  - LBBB pattern (due to delayed activation of the LV through the septum)
  - Superior QRS axis (i.e. negative in leads II, III, and AVL) when right ventricular (RV) lead is in the apex
  - Inferior QRS axis (i.e. positive in leads II, III, and AVL) when RV lead is in the septum
- Biventricular pacing causes a more variable ECG appearance as vectors from the RV lead and LV lead impulses are combined:
  - There are multiple possible positions for the LV lead in the coronary venous system leading to many possible ECG appearances
  - In general, a functioning LV lead will result in a dominant R wave in V1
- The Sgarbossa criteria (see Table 4.1.8 and Figure 4.1.13) can be used to help with the diagnosis of STEMI in patients with a paced rhythm

4.1.5 Arrhythmia definitions

Bradycardia: heart rate < 60 bpm

Sinus node disease: failure of the SA node to maintain a sufficient heart rate. Manifests as chronic sinus bradycardia, junctional escape rhythm, sinus pauses or chronotropic incompetence

'Heart block'/Atrioventricular (AV) block: disease at or below the AV node causing typical ECG changes +/− bradycardia. Divided into first, second, and third degree

Tachycardia: heart rate > 100 bpm

Narrow complex tachycardia: heart rate > 100 bpm, QRS complexes < 120 ms

Broad complex tachycardia: heart rate > 100 bpm, QRS complexes > 120 ms

Supraventricular tachycardia (SVT): tachycardia that requires structures above the bundle of His in order to be maintained. Includes:
  - *Sinus tachycardia*: sinus rhythm > 100 bpm
  - *Inappropriate sinus tachycardia*: resting sinus tachycardia, or intermittent rapid acceleration in heart rate to sinus tachycardia, without an identifiable cause
  - *Atrioventricular nodal re-entrant tachycardia (AVNRT)*: SVT caused by re-entry circuit within the AV node

- *Atrioventricular re-entrant tachycardia (AVRT)*: SVT caused by re-entry circuit involving accessory pathways (APs) and (usually) the AV node
  - Persistent junctional reciprocating tachycardia (PJRT) is a rare variant of AVRT usually found in childhood; often refractory to pharmacological therapy
- *Atrial tachycardia*: regular atrial arrhythmia > 100 bpm originating outside the SA node. May be focal or re-entrant and includes atrial flutter
- *Atrial fibrillation*: irregularly irregular atrial arrhythmia, usually arises from the pulmonary veins

Ventricular tachycardia (VT): tachycardia arising from below the bundle of His, in the ventricular muscle or the conduction system, independent of atrial/AV nodal conduction

- *Non-sustained VT*: lasting for > 3 beats and < 30 seconds
- *Sustained VT*: lasting for > 30 seconds
- *Monomorphic VT*: QRS complex morphology is the same from beat to beat, implying the tachycardia arises from a single focus or a single circuit
- *Polymorphic VT*: QRS complexes vary in morphology from beat to beat, implying the arrhythmia arises from multiple different foci
- *Ventricular fibrillation (VF)*: rapid and irregular ventricular activation with variation in QRS amplitude and cycle length (usually > 350 bpm)

4.1.6 Investigate a patient with palpitations

- *Palpitations* = a patient reported sensation of feeling a fast, fluttering, or pounding heartbeat
- Many causes for these, including non-arrhythmic (e.g. stress, anxiety, exercise) or arrhythmic (e.g. brady or tachy-arrhythmia)
- All patients presenting should be assessed with a clinical history (including relevant family history and potential offending medications), examination, and 12-lead ECG
- Further assessment should include assessment of non-cardiac causes of arrhythmia (e.g. full blood count to check for anaemia, thyroid function, electrolytes, etc.)
- Further cardiac assessment should include an echocardiogram to assess for structural heart disease +/− rhythm monitoring (discussed below)
- Abnormal resting 12-lead ECG, family history, or syncope, increase the likelihood of a cardiac arrhythmic cause and highlight the potential for a more malignant process and should prompt strong consideration of further assessment, even in presence of normal echocardiogram (e.g. with cardiac MRI, prolonged rhythm monitoring or an invasive electrophysiological study)
- Where exercise-induced arrhythmia is reported, a supervised exercise ECG may be considered

Long-term ambulatory ECG

- Multiple ambulatory ECG recording devices are available for the detection of intermittent arrhythmias
- Options vary according to duration of recording, patient acceptability and number of leads recorded:
  - Holter monitors (24–48 hrs); can be 3-lead or 12-lead ECGs
  - Adhesive 'patch ECG monitors' (up to 14 days); 1- or 2-lead ECG
  - External loop recorder (up to 4 weeks); records events when triggered by patient (only suitable for symptomatic arrhythmias); 1-lead ECG

- Smartphone based ECG recording; patient records 1-lead ECG during symptomatic period
    - Mobile cardiac telemetry (continuous monitoring); usually 3-lead ECG
    - Implantable loop recorder (up to 3 years); continuous 1-lead recording
- Indications for ambulatory monitoring include:
    - Unexplained syncope
    - Unexplained palpitations
    - Detection of atrial fibrillation after cryptogenic stroke
    - Evaluation of accessory pathway conduction properties and detection of paroxysmal atrial fibrillation in WPW syndrome
    - Assessment of non-ischaemic cardiomyopathy if tachyarrhythmia suspected
    - Risk stratification (non-sustained ventricular tachycardia and ventricular ectopy) in cardiomyopathies
    - Diagnosis of intermittent ECG changes in pre-excitation syndromes or channelopathies
    - Assessment of response to treatment (e.g. post-AF ablation)
- Limitations of ambulatory monitoring:
    - Short recording duration limits detection of infrequent arrhythmias
    - Single lead (or 3-lead) ECGs lack ability to locate and specify arrhythmias
    - Prolonged monitoring often not well tolerated by patient
    - Electrodes can detach or cause skin irritation

Exercise ECG testing

- Historically used as a first-line diagnostic test for patients with low-intermediate risk of stable coronary disease, but due to relatively low sensitivity has been replaced by CT coronary angiography and functional imaging
- Can be used to determine prognosis in patients with known coronary disease; e.g. the Duke treadmill score, which incorporates:
    1. Maximal ST segment deviation (mm)
    2. Degree of angina
    3. Duration of exercise
- Other indications include:
    - Evaluation of inducible arrhythmias (e.g. VT)
    - Evaluation of functional capacity (e.g. in heart failure)
    - Evaluation of haemodynamic response to exercise (e.g. in valvular heart disease)
    - Evaluation of treatment response (e.g. post coronary intervention)
- Contraindications:
    - Patient factors (e.g. arthritis, poor mobility, peripheral vascular disease)
    - Resting ECG changes that limit interpretation (e.g. LBBB, paced rhythm, LVH with ST changes)
    - Unstable coronary disease or recent MI
    - Symptomatic severe aortic stenosis
    - Uncontrolled symptomatic heart failure
    - Acute myocarditis
    - Severe hypertension (systolic blood pressure > 200 mmHg, diastolic > 110 mmHg)
    - Severe pulmonary hypertension
- Criteria for stopping the test:
    - Protocol-based (i.e. patient has reached target heart rate)
    - Patient factors (onset of limiting symptoms/fatigue)

- Development of significant ECG changes (e.g. ST-segment changes, new BBB, or arrhythmias)
• Complications:
  - Although rare, there is small risk of myocardial infarction, sustained arrhythmias, and death (approximately 1 in 10,000)
  - Risks can be minimized by:
    • Careful history and examination prior to test
    • Careful interrogation of resting ECG
    • Continuous ECG monitoring during test and recovery period
    • Access to resuscitation equipment and emergency drugs
    • Attention to exercise protocol end-points
    • Supervision by appropriate trained personnel
    • Attention to patient symptoms

Further reading

Baranchuk A, Shaw C, Alanazi H, Campbell D, Bally K, Redfearn DP, Simpson CS, Abdollah H. Electrocardiography pitfalls and artifacts: the 10 commandments. *Crit Care Nurse*. 2009 Feb;29(1):67–73. doi: 10.4037/ccn2009607. PMID: 19182282

Camm AJ, Lüscher TF, Maurer M, Serruys PW (eds). *The European Society of Cardiology Textbook of Cardiovascular Medicine. ESC Textbook of Cardiovascular Medicine*, 3rd edn. Oxford: Oxford University Press, 2018

Mark DB, Shaw L, Harrell FE Jr, Hlatky MA, Lee KL, Bengtson JR, McCants CB, Califf RM, Pryor DB. Prognostic value of a treadmill exercise score in outpatients with suspected coronary artery disease. *N Engl J Med*. 1991 Sep 19;325(12):849–53. doi: 10.1056/NEJM199109193251204. PMID: 1875969

Steinberg JS, Varma N, Cygankiewicz I, Aziz P, Balsam P, Baranchuk A, Cantillon DJ, Dilaveris P, Dubner SJ, El-Sherif N, Krol J, Kurpesa M, La Rovere MT, Lobodzinski SS, Locati ET, Mittal S, Olshansky B, Piotrowicz E, Saxon L, Stone PH, Tereshchenko L, Turitto G, Wimmer NJ, Verrier RL, Zareba W, Piotrowicz R. 2017 ISHNE-HRS expert consensus statement on ambulatory ECG and external cardiac monitoring/telemetry. *Heart Rhythm*. 2017 Jul;14(7):e55–e96. doi: 10.1016/j.hrthm.2017.03.038

Surawicz B, Childers R, Deal BJ, Gettes LS, Bailey JJ, Gorgels A, Hancock EW, Josephson M, Kligfield P, Kors JA, Macfarlane P, Mason JW, Mirvis DM, Okin P, Pahlm O, Rautaharju PM, van Herpen G, Wagner GS, Wellens H; American Heart Association Electrocardiography and Arrhythmias Committee, Council on Clinical Cardiology; American College of Cardiology Foundation; Heart Rhythm Society. AHA/ACCF/HRS recommendations for the standardization and interpretation of the electrocardiogram: part III: intraventricular conduction disturbances: a scientific statement from the American Heart Association Electrocardiography and Arrhythmias Committee, Council on Clinical Cardiology; the American College of Cardiology Foundation; and the Heart Rhythm Society. Endorsed by the International Society for Computerized Electrocardiology. *J Am Coll Cardiol*. 2009 Mar 17;53(11):976–81. doi: 10.1016/j.jacc.2008.12.013. PMID: 19281930

4.2

Transient loss consciousness

Boon Lim and Katharine Thomas

TABLE OF CONTENTS

4.2.1 Overview and glossary of terms 303
4.2.2 Prevalence 303
4.2.3 Classification and pathophysiology 305
  Cardiac syncope 305
  Reflex syncope (neurally mediated) 305
  Orthostatic hypotension 306
  Psychogenic pseudo-syncope 307
4.2.4 Evaluation of patients 307
  Purpose 307
4.2.5 Investigations 309
  Carotid sinus massage (CSM) 309
  Orthostatic challenge: active standing 310
  Orthostatic challenge: tilt testing 310
  Echocardiography 311
  Electrocardiographic monitoring 311
  Exercise stress test 311
  Smartphone applications 312
  Electrophysiology study 312
4.2.6 Treatment options 312
  Reflex and orthostatic hypotension 312
  Cardiac syncope 313
4.2.7 Driving regulations 314

4.2.1 Overview and glossary of terms

- The terminology in patients with transient loss of consciousness (TLOC) and related symptoms is very muddled, and the use of the same terms by different doctors/in different settings can lead to a different diagnosis
- Getting the terminology right is a major part of getting the assessment and the treatment right (see Box 4.2.1)
- 'Syncope' is often used synonymously with TLOC, and this is quite wrong, as TLOC has many possible aetiologies, only one of which is syncope
- **Syncope** = a *transient loss of consciousness (TLOC) due to global cerebral hypoperfusion characterized by rapid onset, short duration, and spontaneous complete recovery*
- **Pre-syncope** = a *state that resembles the prodrome of syncope but which is not followed by loss of consciousness*

4.2.2 Prevalence

- Frequent: 30% experience at least one episode of TLOC with a peak between the ages of 10 and 30 years
- First episode commonly occurs in patients presenting between 10 and 30 years, but frequency increases with age, with a much more rapid increase after 70 years
- The 10-year cumulative incidence of syncope is 11% for both men and women at age 70–79, and 17% and 19% respectively for men and women at age ≥ 80
- Approximately one-third of patients have recurrences of syncope at three years of follow-up

BOX 4.2.1 GLOSSARY

TLOC	A **transient** loss of consciousness.
Blackout	A **transient** loss of consciousness, and a term used commonly by patients, relatives, and neurologists.
Syncope	A **transient** loss of consciousness (TLOC) due to **global cerebral hypoperfusion** characterized by **rapid onset, short duration,** and **spontaneous complete recovery.**
Presyncope	A state that resembles the prodrome of syncope but which is not followed by loss of consciousness.
Convulsive syncope	An episode of syncope that results in seizure activity, typically due to significant cardio-inhibition or profound fall in blood pressure. Reflex Anoxic Seizures (RAS) are a form of convulsive syncope which occurs typically in younger children. Pacing is not necessarily recommended for convulsive syncope.
Psychogenic pseudosyncope	If occurs with convulsive features, this is termed psychogenic non-epileptic seizures (PNES). This term implies that syncope has occurred in the absence of any BP or heart rate changes and without electrical brain discharges associated with epilepsy.
Collapse	An abrupt loss of postural control, with or without TLOC.
Fall	An episode of collapse where there is no TLOC, and contributory factors include musculoskeletal infirmity, inability to adjust against gravity when over-balancing, failure of postural aids, e.g. a walking stick.
Apparent fall	Up to 30% of falls are actually TLOC with collapse interpreted by the patient or the doctor as a fall. Patients may forget the blackout or choose to minimize it. A proportion of these patients need pacing.
Epilepsy attack	This is defined by the International League Against Epilepsy as 'transient occurrence of signs and/or symptoms due to abnormal excessive or synchronous neuronal activity in the brain'.
Epilepsy	A chronic neurological condition characterized by recurrent epileptic seizures.
Seizure	An episode of TLOC accompanied by convulsive features. Syncope may be convulsive, and be accompanied by abrupt collapse, abnormal limb movements, tongue-biting, and incontinence due to cerebral anoxic irritation. Generalized epilepsy may also be accompanied by these features. 'Seizure' should not be used to imply that the mechanism of TLOC is epilepsy.

4.2.3 Classification and pathophysiology

- TLOC can be classified as traumatic (caused by concussion) and non-traumatic (caused by syncope, epileptic seizures, psychogenic blackouts, and other rare miscellaneous causes, e.g. cataplexy)
- Syncope is the most common subset of TLOC
- Syncope is caused by cerebral hypoperfusion, which largely results from a fall in systemic blood pressure (BP), but can also be associated with a fall in heart rate
- Experience from tilt testing shows that a decrease in systolic BP to below 60 mmHg is associated with syncope
- Systemic BP is the product of cardiac output and total peripheral vascular resistance, and a fall in either component can contribute to syncope, though there is usually an element of both components
- Interruption in cerebral blood flow for only 6–8 seconds is sufficient to cause total LOC
- A number of mechanisms are involved in regulating systolic BP and in maintaining cerebral perfusion:
    - Arterial baroreceptor-induced adjustment of heart rate, cardiac contractility, systemic vascular resistance
    - Renin-angiotensin and vasopressin induced vasoconstriction
    - Renal–body–fluid pressure control system
    - Cerebrovascular *autoregulation*
- The prodromal symptoms which occur prior to syncope may include: palpitations, shortness of breath, feeling hot and sweaty, dizziness, nausea, fatigue, chest pain; some of these symptoms may be explained by sympathetic activation prior to the occurrence of syncope
- Reflex syncope is by far the most common cause of TLOC, and can mimic an epileptic seizure if there are convulsive features
- Cardiac syncope should always be considered and ruled out during the initial assessment, as this can be associated with significant morbidity and death

Cardiac syncope

- Arrhythmia:
    - Bradycardia: sick sinus syndrome, atrioventricular (AV) block, drug-induced, electrolyte abnormalities
    - Tachycardia: supraventricular, ventricular
    - Drug-induced or electrolyte disturbance: bradycardia/tachycardia
- Structural disease:
    - Valvular disease, acute myocardial ischemia, hypertrophic cardiomyopathy, cardiac masses, pericardial disease/tamponade, anomalous coronary arteries
    - Others: pulmonary embolus, acute aortic dissection, pulmonary hypertension

Reflex syncope (neurally mediated)

- Reflex syncope is a heterogeneous group of disorders caused by withdrawal of sympathetic innervation and/or vagal hyperactivity, causing either vasodilatation, bradycardia/asystole, or a mixture of both
- Usually proceeded by prodromal symptoms, and often has an identifiable trigger

- Prodromal symptoms are usually caused by an appropriate rise in sympathetic tone immediately preceding the reflex syncope episode, and may include: dizziness, shortness of breath, palpitations, feeling hot and sweaty, chest pain, nausea, anxiety
- Can be classified according to cardiovascular response to reflex, or trigger
- Response
    - Vasodepressor type: vasodilatation predominates
    - Cardioinhibitory type: bradycardia or asystole predominates (this does not necessarily mandate pacing)
    - Mixed type: both mechanisms are involved
- Trigger:
    - Vasovagal
        - Mediated by emotional distress, fear, pain
        - Mediated by orthostatic stress
    - Situational
        - Cough, sneeze, gastrointestinal stimulation (e.g. swallow, defecation, visceral pain), post-prandial, micturition, post-exercise, others (e.g. laughter, bass instrument playing, weightlifting)
    - Carotid sinus syncope
    - Atypical forms (without apparent triggers and/or atypical presentation)

Orthostatic hypotension

- Classical orthostatic hypotension is defined by BP decrease ≥ 20 mmHg and/or 10 mmHg in diastolic pressure, or a decrease in systolic to < 90 mmHg, within 3 min of standing, *associated with symptoms*
- Common in elderly, those with autonomic dysfunction (i.e. diabetes) or on polypharmacy for hypertension

Sub-types

- Initial orthostatic hypotension
    - BP decrease immediately upon standing up, ≤ 30 s
    - Can be diagnosed with active stand test in clinic
- Delayed (progressive) orthostatic hypotension
    - Common in the elderly
    - BP decrease slowly upon standing, 3–30 min
    - Reflex bradycardia 'vagal' may be present or absent
    - Diagnosis usually made by tilt table test
    - Syncope common, particularly if impaired cerebral auto-regulation (leading to minimal prodrome)
- Reflex syncope triggered by standing
    - Common in the young and healthy, women > men
    - Syncope often preceded by prodromal symptoms (symptoms related to sympathetic activation prior to syncope)
- Postural orthostatic tachycardia syndrome (POTS)
    - The precise mechanism is uncertain though may be due to inadequate venous return or excessive blood venous pooling
    - There is an orthostatic increase in heart rate by > 30 bpm or to > 120 bpm within 10 minutes of active standing, in the absence of orthostatic hypotension and *associated with typical clinical symptoms*

- Associated with dizziness, palpitation, fatigue, 'brain fog', and pre-syncope, but can coexist with reflex syncope
- Common in young females
- Can be associated with benign hypermobility syndrome (Ehlers–Danlos Syndrome Type III)

Aetiology

- Primary autonomic failure
    - Pure autonomic failure, multiple system atrophy, Parkinson's disease with autonomic failure, Lewy body dementia
- Secondary autonomic failure
    - Diabetes, amyloidosis, uraemia, spinal cord injuries
- Drug induced orthostatic hypotension
    - Alcohol, vasodilators, diuretics, beta blockers, phenothiazine, antidepressants
- Volume depletion
    - Haemorrhage, diarrhoea, vomiting, etc.

Psychogenic pseudo-syncope

- A difficult-to-diagnose condition, often missed for many years
- Due to an episode of TLOC in the absence of haemodynamic compromise or epileptic waveform activity in brain
- Clues in the history are: frequent attacks (i.e. several times a day), eyes always closed during attacks, previous psychosocial history including abuse, neglect, depression
- Can coexist with true vasovagal syncope or pre-syncope, with sympathetic activation in the pre-syncopal phase often a trigger for psychogenic pseudo-syncope
- Can be diagnosed on tilt table testing: The patient is often seen to slump against the tilt bed straps abruptly, head leaning forwards or to the side, without a drop in BP or HR (often associated with a rise in HR)
- Similar aetiology to Psychogenic Non-Epileptic Seizures (PNES), but without any convulsive movements

4.2.4 Evaluation of patients

- Careful and thorough history taking in patients admitted with syncope is essential
- Initial evaluation alone (*history, examination, and 12-lead ECG*) is often sufficient to establish a diagnosis in > 75% of cases
- Despite the wide ranges of causes of syncope, definite diagnosis can often be established during the first clinical encounter

Purpose

- Consider all causes of collapse (abrupt loss of postural control)
- Confirm that TLOC did occur, though be aware that a proportion of patients will be unaware they lost consciousness
- Establish by careful history-taking that syncope/pre-syncope occurred
- Establish aetiology
- Undertake risk stratification

Diagnose syncope
- History:
  - LOC complete? Transient with rapid onset and short duration? Spontaneous complete recovery? Loss of postural tone? Prodromal symptoms?
  - Past history of syncope: childhood faints in school, pain, strong emotions
  - Triggers: prolonged standing, dehydration, heat, strong emotions, pain, coughing, micturition

Establish aetiology
- History:
  - Circumstances: posture position, activity, predisposing factors
  - Symptoms at onset: autonomic symptoms including sweatiness, pallor, shortness of breath, palpitations, anxious, nausea
  - Symptoms at offset and how rapid recovery is
  - History from eyewitness can be important—asking eyewitness to 'demonstrate' event can be more helpful than 'describe'
  - Past history: cardiac disease, neurological disease, medication, family history
- Examination
  - Physical examination
  - Orthostatic blood pressure measurements (lying and standing BP for 3 minutes)
  - Cardiac examination: exclusion of aortic stenosis or any other significant cardiac finding (heart failure, bradycardia)
- Investigation
  - *In all patients:* **12-lead ECG**
  - *In selected cases*:
    - Carotid sinus message (patients > 40 years old)
    - Echocardiography
    - Tilt table test
    - Ambulatory ECG monitor: in-hospital telemetry, Holter, implantable loop recorder
    - Exercise test
    - CT pulmonary angiogram
- Further evaluation in cases of doubt about the mechanism of TLOC:
  - Neurological evaluation
  - Psychiatric/psychological evaluation
  - Some tests will only be needed when there is clearly an electrical or structural cardiac abnormality, and it is deemed very likely to be the cause of TLOC
  - Cardiac catheterization
  - Electrophysiological study

Risk stratification
- Patients should be risk stratified on presentation, with three main questions:
  - Is there a serious underlying cause?
  - Is there a risk of a life-threatening outcome?
  - Does the patient require admission to hospital?

- High risk features:

    Cardiovascular:
    - New onset chest discomfort, breathlessness, abdominal pain, cardiac history of heart failure/myocardial infarction or headache
    - Syncope occurring during effort or supine (predictors of arrhythmia as a cause)
    - Abrupt onset palpitations prior to syncope
    - Syncope resulting in injury
    - Undiagnosed systolic murmur on examination
    - Abnormal 12-lead ECG
        - Major: acute ischemia, Mobitz II second- and third-degree AV block, slow atrial fibrillation or sinus bradycardia (< 40 bpm) or pauses > 3 seconds associated with symptoms in the absence of physical training, bundle branch block/intraventricular conduction delay/ventricular hypertrophy/Q waves consistent with ischemic heart disease or cardiomyopathy, ventricular tachycardia (sustained or non-sustained), dysfunction of PPM/ICD, long QT interval, Brugada pattern ECG (type 1)
        - Minor (high risk if history suggestive of arrhythmic syncope): Mobitz I second-degree AV block, first-degree heart block, inappropriate slow atrial fibrillation or sinus bradycardia (40–50 bpm) without symptoms, paroxysmal SVT or AF, pre-excited QRS complex, short QT interval, ARVC or atypical Brugada pattern ECG (type II)
    - History of cardiovascular disease especially structural disease, ventricular arrhythmia, and heart failure
    - Syncope that occurs without warning, in the sitting position, or in those with a family history of sudden cardiac disease under 40 years in age are minor features that are considered high risk if associated with structural heart disease or an abnormal ECG

    Neurological
    - Features that strongly suggest epilepsy: tonic-clonic movements at the onset, facial cyanosis, head-turning, lateral tongue-biting, incontinence (faecal), prolonged recovery
    - A history of brain injury (birth/infection/infarction/tumour/traumatic etc.)
    - New or evolving neurological deficit

    Other
    - Unexplained systolic BP < 90 mmHg
    - Suggestion of gastrointestinal bleed on rectal examination
    - Hypoxia

N.B. Patients with high-risk features should not be discharged from hospital

4.2.5 Investigations

Table 4.2.1 outlines the clinical features suggestive of diagnosis on initial evaluation

Carotid sinus massage (CSM)

- Indicated in patients > 40 years with unexplained aetiology after initial evaluation
- There is a risk of TIA or stroke with this procedure (0.24% in pooling of four large studies)
- Diagnostic if syncope is reproducible in the presence of asystole > 3 s *and/or* a fall in systolic BP > 50 mmHg *and* reproduces symptoms
- If cardio-inhibition is observed and correlated to symptoms, this is termed carotid sinus syndrome (CSS): refer for pacemaker therapy

Table 4.2.1 Clinical features suggestive of diagnosis on initial evaluation.

Type of syncope	Clinical features
Reflex syncope (neurally mediated)	Absence of heart disease Long history of recurrent episodes Triggers, e.g. stress, sound, smell, or pain Provoked by dehydration, prolonged standing, or crowded, hot places Prodromal symptoms prior to syncope During a meal or post-prandial After exertion
Orthostatic hypotension	Preceded by standing up Temporal relation to taking medication Prolonged standing or crowded, hot places Presence of autonomic neuropathy, diabetes, or Parkinsonism Standing after exertion
Cardiovascular syncope	Structural cardiac disease Family history of unexplained sudden death or channelopathy During exertion or supine Abnormal ECG: • Bifascicular block, QRS duration ≥ 120 ms, Mobitz I/II second-degree AV block, complete heart block • Inappropriate bradycardia or sinus pause ≥ 3 s • Non-sustained VT • Pre-excited QRS complexes • Long or short QTc intervals • Early repolarization • Brugada ECG pattern • ARVC ECG pattern • Ischemic changes

Orthostatic challenge: active standing

- Can be easily done in clinic and should form part of standard syncope assessment with history, examination, and ECG
- Recommended methodology
    - Manual intermittent BP measurement with lying and active standing for 3 min
    - Continuous beat-to-beat non-invasive BP measurement may be helpful if in doubt or to capture short-lived BP variations such as in initial orthostatic hypotension
- Diagnostic, when symptoms reproduced with
    - Progressive and sustained fall of a systolic BP of ≥ 20 mmHg or diastolic BP ≥ 10 mmHg, or:
    - Drop of a systolic BP to < 90 mmHg

Orthostatic challenge: tilt testing

- Should be done in conjunction with history taking and clear assessment of patient symptoms prior to tilt, to understand and report whether or not the patient's clinical symptoms are reproduced on tilt
- Used traditionally in patients with unexplained single syncopal episode in high-risk settings after cardiac syncope has been excluded
- Patients likely to have reflex syncope have the highest yield. Tilt testing may be considered in patients with orthostatic hypotension or POTS, and it is a useful test for discriminating between delayed orthostatic hypotension and reflex syncope

- It can be useful where it is thought a patient may gain confidence from having their symptoms reproduced. Often the clear communication of a diagnosis and education about mechanisms during pre-syncope and syncope allows the patient to fully engage in the conservative strategies to improve symptoms
- It is useful in suspected psychogenic blackouts when suggestibility to a psychogenic blackout can be used to reproduce symptoms during tilt (while monitoring ECG, BP, and ideally EEG), or to differentiate syncope with jerking movements from epilepsy

Diagnostic criteria

- Induction of reflex hypotension/bradycardia with reproduction of symptom is diagnostic
- Induction of reflex hypotension/bradycardia without reproduction of symptom may be diagnostic

Recommended methodology

- Patient usually fasted
- Supine pre-tilt phase of > 5 min
- BP should ideally be measured using non-invasive continuous HR and BP monitoring
- CSM can be performed in the supine and head-up position
- Tilt angle between 60° and 70°
- Passive phase of ≥ 20 min
- For nitroglycerine challenge, a fixed dose of 300–400 μg sublingually administered in the upright position after 20 minutes of passive phase tilt, followed by a further 15 minutes of active tilt
- Patients should correlate symptoms during tilt testing to the spontaneous clinical symptoms

Echocardiography

- Not routinely indicated if the history, examination, and 12-lead ECG indicate a clear diagnosis of reflex syncope
- May play an important role in risk stratification if there is suspicion of cardiac syncope
- Useful in patients with severe aortic stenosis, obstructive cardiac tumours or thrombi, pericardial tamponade or aortic dissection as the cause of syncope
- Exercise stress echocardiography can be useful in detection of left ventricular outflow tract obstruction in patients with HCM

Electrocardiographic monitoring

- **In-patient telemetry** for high-risk patients where cardiac syncope and arrhythmia are suspected
- **Holter monitor** for patients with frequent symptoms, continued for 1 week as appropriate
- **Implantable loop recorders (ILRs)** for long term implantable monitoring, indicated
    - Where the diagnosis remains unclear and symptoms are infrequent
    - In patients with high-risk symptoms, but in whom a comprehensive evaluation did not demonstrate a cause of syncope or lead to specific treatment

Exercise stress test

- Indicated in patients who have experienced episodes of syncope during and shortly after exertion
- If Mobitz type II second-degree or third-degree AV block develops during exercise the test is diagnostic even without syncope

- To rule out tachycardia during exercises (SVT, VT)
- In those patients who develop syncope after exertion, consider modifying exercise test with abrupt cessation in exercise, followed by standing for 3 minutes to observe for reflex syncope (post-exercise reflex syncope)

Smartphone applications

- There are little data to support use of smart phone in detecting ECG changes during syncope
- Photoplethysmography (PPG) sensors (green-light technology) record data related to blood flow, which arises following cardiac contraction, and may introduce a lag in heart rate sensing
- Impedance based sensors (e.g. Alivecor Kardia) may be useful to detect real-time single lead ECG but the challenge is getting patients to record a trace during syncope
- Home video recordings of syncope is extremely useful. Patient's relatives/friends should be advised to record the whole body for the duration of syncope, once the patient has been positioned in a safe environment

Electrophysiology study

- Positive results occurred predominantly in patients with structural heart disease (previous myocardial infarction or other scar-related conditions)
- Less important as diagnostic test with development of prolonged ECG monitoring
- May have a role in specific clinical situations suspected to cause syncope
  - Asymptomatic sinus bradycardia
  - Bi-fascicular bundle branch block
  - Suspected tachycardia

4.2.6 Treatment options

Reflex and orthostatic hypotension
Lifestyle measures

- Important to appreciate that syncope can be a transient symptom and not necessarily a disease
- However must also realize the potential impact of syncope on the patient's lifestyle
- Education and reassurance regarding benign nature of condition is essential
- Trigger avoidance
- Avoidance of volume depletion
- Sufficient salt and water intake is useful in orthostatic hypotension (2–3 litres of oral fluid intake per day and 6 g of NaCl)
- Ensure all hypotensive therapy has been discontinued (i.e. anti-hypertensives, nitrates, diuretics, neuroleptic antidepressants, dopaminergic drugs)
- Specific treatment aside from education and reassurance is often unnecessary

Physical counter-pressure manoeuvres

- Isometric muscle contractions increase arterial blood pressure and cardiac output
- Useful in reflex syncope/vasovagal syncope
- Leg crossing, hand grip, arm tensing
- Tilt training, i.e. progressively prolonged periods of enforced upright posture
- Compression stockings

Pharmacological therapy

- This is adjunctive therapy to salt and water intake
- Midodrine (alpha agonist): this drug is by far the most useful in reflex syncope. Start with 2.5 mg tds, to be taken first thing in morning, and every 4 hours after, with no doses after 6 p.m. (to avoid nocturnal supine hypertension)
- Midodrine may also be effective in conditions with autonomic failure
- Fludrocortisone may be effective in reducing syncopal recurrences in young patients with low normal BP
- Beta blockers are considered inappropriate in reducing syncope occurrences (N.B. clinicians may wish to consider discontinuing beta blocker therapy if present and clinically appropriate)
- Other drugs have been tried, but without conclusive evidence of efficacy: paroxetine, ivabradine, octreotide, theophylline

Cardiac pacing

- Only recommended where brady-arrhythmia or asystole is the predominant cause of syncope
- Can consider in patients with recurrent syncope reproducible by carotid sinus massage, associated with ventricular asystole of > 3 s
- Early trials used tilt-testing response for pre-implant selection and showed sub-optimal benefit from pacing
- More recent trials (ISSUE 2 and 3) using ILR guided pacemaker implantation produced a greater degree of benefit
- Asystole during tilt-testing does not necessarily signify adverse prognosis
- There is a suggestion from an ISSUE 3 sub study that tilt test positive patients (with *hypotensive susceptibility*) are less likely to benefit from pacemaker implantation, even in the context of documented asystole during a clinical event
- **In reflex syncope, pacing should only be considered** in patients with recurrent severe vasovagal syncope who show prolonged asystole during ECG recording and after failure of other therapeutic options
- The risk vs. benefit must be carefully considered, particularly in younger patients who are likely to need several pacemaker box changes during their lifetimes

Cardiac syncope
Cardiac pacing

- In the presence of confirmed brady-arrhythmia, cardiac pacing is the first-line treatment
- Indications and choice of pacing mode (as per guidelines) are outlined in chapter 4.3

Address underlying pathology

- Treatment should also focus on any underlying cardiac pathology driving arrhythmias, e.g.
    - Valve intervention in severe aortic stenosis
    - Consideration of electrophysiology study (EPS) and ablation in tachy-arrhythmia

Implantable cardioverter defibrillator

- As per guidelines for ICD implant (see section 4.9)
- Patients with previous MI, poor LVEF, and syncope may have syncopal VT. These patients have a 1-year mortality of 44%

- ICDs are indicated in patients with syncope due to VT and EF < 35% and in patients with syncope and previous MI where VT is induced during an EPS

4.2.7 Driving regulations

- TLOC is an important cause of incapacitation whilst driving
- Driving regulations differ between countries; knowledge of local protocols is imperative
- ESC recommendations are shown in Table 4.2.2
- The doctor's duty is to advise his/her patient when they should cease to drive and the consequences of not following this advice
- In the UK, it is sensible to check DVLA guidance contemporaneously during the patient's clinical visit. A recent change in the guideline made a distinction between syncope during sitting (DVLA notification needed) compared to standing (DVLA does not need to be notified) for typical vasovagal syncope. See section 4.10.3 for further details on UK DVLA guidance.
- A diagnosis of cough syncope results in a driving ban until attacks have been successfully controlled

Table 4.2.2 Recommendations concerning driving regulations (ESC).

Diagnosis	Group 1 (private drivers)	Group 2 (professional drivers)
Cardiac arrhythmias		
Medical treatment	After successful treatment established	After successful treatment established
Pacemaker implant	After 1 week	After appropriate function is established
Successful catheter ablation	After successful treatment established	After long-term success is confirmed
ICD implant	Primary prevention: driving must cease for 2 weeks. Secondary prevention: driving must cease for 3 months	Permanent restriction for both primary and secondary prevention
Reflex syncope		
Single/mild	No restrictions	No restriction unless it occurred during high-risk activity*
Recurrent and severe*	After symptoms are controlled	Permanent restriction unless effective treatment has been established
Unexplained syncope	No restrictions unless absence of prodrome, occurrence during driving, or presence of severe structural heart disease	After diagnosis and appropriate therapy is establishes

*Neurally mediated syncope is defined as severe if it is very frequent, or occurring during the prosecution of a 'high-risk' activity, or recurrent or unpredictable in 'high-risk' patients

Further reading

Brignole M, Auricchio A, Baron-Esquivias G, Bordachar P, Boriani G, Breithardt OA, Cleland J, Deharo JC, Delgado V, Elliott PM, Gorenek B, Israel CW, Leclercq C, Linde C, Mont L, Padeletti L, Sutton R, Vardas PE; ESC Committee for Practice Guidelines (CPG), Zamorano JL, Achenbach S, Baumgartner H, Bax JJ, Bueno H, Dean V, Deaton C, Erol C, Fagard R, Ferrari R, Hasdai D, Hoes AW, Kirchhof P, Knuuti J, Kolh P, Lancellotti P, Linhart A, Nihoyannopoulos P, Piepoli MF, Ponikowski P, Sirnes PA, Tamargo JL, Tendera M, Torbicki A, Wijns W, Windecker S; Document Reviewers, Kirchhof P, Blomstrom-Lundqvist C, Badano LP, Aliyev F, Bänsch D, Baumgartner H, Bsata W, Buser P, Charron P, Daubert JC, Dobreanu D, Faerestrand S, Hasdai D, Hoes AW, Le Heuzey JY, Mavrakis H, McDonagh T, Merino JL, Nawar MM, Nielsen JC, Pieske B, Poposka L, Ruschitzka F, Tendera M, Van Gelder IC, Wilson CM. 2013 ESC Guidelines on cardiac pacing and cardiac resynchronization therapy: the Task Force on cardiac pacing and resynchronization therapy of the European Society of Cardiology (ESC). Developed in collaboration with the European Heart Rhythm Association (EHRA). *Eur Heart J.* 2013 Aug;34(29):2281–329. doi: 10.1093/eurheartj/eht150. Epub 2013 Jun 24. PMID: 23801822

Brignole M, Moya A, de Lange FJ, Deharo JC, Elliott PM, Fanciulli A, Fedorowski A, Furlan R, Kenny RA, Martín A, Probst V, Reed MJ, Rice CP, Sutton R, Ungar A, van Dijk JG; ESC Scientific Document Group. 2018 ESC Guidelines for the diagnosis and management of syncope. *Eur Heart J.* 2018 Jun 1;39(21):1883–948. doi: 10.1093/eurheartj/ehy037. PMID: 29562304

Camm J, Lüscher TF, Maurer G, Serruys PW (eds). *The European Society of Cardiology Textbook of Cardiovascular Medicine*, 3rd edn. Oxford: Oxford University Press, 2018.

Josephson ME. *Clinical Cardiac Electrophysiology: Techniques and Interpretation*, 5th edn. Philadelphia, USA: Lippincott, Williams & Wilkins, 2015.

4.3

Bradycardia and pacemakers

Richard Bond and Howell Williams

TABLE OF CONTENTS

4.3.1 Bradycardia classification and indications for pacing 317
- Bradycardia 317
- Sinoatrial (SA) node disease 318
- Atrioventricular (AV) conduction disease 319
- Bundle branch block (BBB) 320

4.3.2 Approach to bradycardia 320
- Aims 320
- History and evaluation 323
- Investigation 323
- Acute Treatment 323
- Clinical implication of electrophysiology study (EPS) in patients with suspected conduction disturbances 324

4.3.3 Permanent pacemakers 324
- Pacemaker nomenclature 324
- Basic pacing concepts 325
- Complications of pacemaker implantation 327
- Optimal pacing mode 327
- Magnet mode 328
- Pacemaker syndrome 328

4.3.4 Pacemaker troubleshooting 329
- Pacemaker mediated tachycardia (PMT) 329
- Failure to pace 329
- Failure to capture 330
- Oversensing 330
- Undersensing 331
- Practical considerations 331
- Pacemaker follow-up 333

4.3.1 Bradycardia classification and indications for pacing

Bradycardia

- Defined as inappropriately low heart rate in relation to age, gender, activity level, and physical training status
- Can be caused by intrinsic conduction system disease or extrinsic factors
- Intrinsic disease is caused by:
  - Age-related idiopathic fibrosis (most common)
  - Ischaemia
    - Acute MI—often transient if reperfusion achieved
    - Chronic ischaemia—accelerated fibrosis (similar pathology to idiopathic fibrosis)
  - Cardiomyopathy
  - Infiltrative disease (e.g. cardiac amyloid, sarcoidosis, haemochromatosis)
  - Collagen vascular disease (e.g. systemic lupus erythematosus, rheumatoid arthritis)
  - Myotonic muscular dystrophy
  - Congenital disease
  - Surgical damage (AV conduction may be damaged during surgical aortic valve replacement or catheter ablation for arrhythmias; SA node disease is common in the donor heart following orthotopic transplant)

- Ablation therapy
- Infectious disease (e.g. endocarditis, typhoid, diphtheria, Chagas disease)
- Extrinsic factors include:
  - Drugs (primarily antiarrhythmics)
  - Increased vagal tone (e.g. carotid sinus hypersensitivity, vasovagal syncope)
  - Non-cardiac illness (e.g. hypothermia)
  - Physical training
  - Vagal hyper-reactivity (e.g. reflex syncope)
  - Electrolyte imbalance (e.g. hypokalaemia or hyperkalaemia)
  - Metabolic disturbances (e.g., hypothyroidism, anorexia nervosa)
  - Neurological disorders (e.g. raised intracranial pressure)
  - Obstructive sleep apnoea

Sinoatrial (SA) node disease

- Classically defined as sinus node rate < 60 bpm with normal P waves before each QRS complex
- Usually a benign finding and often asymptomatic, or may present with:
  - symptoms related to sinus pauses (e.g. pre-syncope, syncope)
  - symptoms related to chronic sinus bradycardia and chronotropic incompetence (e.g. fatigue, reduced exercise tolerance)
- SA node disease may present with *sinoatrial (SA) exit block and sinus arrest*
  - Sinus pause of > 150% of cardiac cycle length
  - May be due to failure of sinus node impulse or failure of the impulse to exit the sinus node and reach the atrium (SA exit block)
  - SA block will appear as multiples of baseline P–P interval on ECG
- SA node disease may also present with *junctional rhythm*
  - Absence of sinus node activity and hence no P waves visible prior to QRS complexes
  - Narrow QRS complexes that typically originate in the AV node
  - Ventricular rate typically slower than in sinus rhythm
  - Often paroxysmal, with sinus bradycardia at other times
  - May be asymptomatic or may present with dizziness or exertional fatigue
- SA node disease may also present with *tachycardia-bradycardia syndrome:*
  - patients with intact AV conduction who develop a paroxysmal atrial arrhythmia (incidence of new onset AF in SA node disease is ~5% per year) are tachycardic during the arrhythmia and bradycardic when in sinus rhythm
  - typically observed as a sinus pause or sinus bradycardia following the cessation of the paroxysmal supraventricular tachycardia
  - due to overdrive suppression of the sinus automaticity during the tachycardia phase
  - treatment may involve pacing to manage bradycardia followed by rate controlling medications to treat the tachycardia. An alternative option to this is ablation to reduce the tachycardia burden and therefore reduce the requirement for rate control medications, which may offer an alternative to avoid pacemaker implantation. The latest ESC Pacing and CRT guidelines (2021) give a IIa recommendation to AF ablation to avoid pacing in this clinical scenario, but this will of course take account of patient factors such as patient preference, age, frailty, and AF duration
- SA node disease may also present with *chronotropic incompetence*. This is an inability of the SA node to appropriately increase heart rate in response to exertion. This causes exertional symptoms, including fatigue, shortness of breath, and occasionally syncope

- The incidence of coexistent advanced AV conduction disease among patients with SA node disease is ~5–10% and the natural history of SA node disease is generally more benign than AV conduction disease, with slow progression expected over several decades
- There is no evidence that pacing prolongs survival in patients with SA node disease; overall survival and the risk of sudden cardiac death are similar in patients with SA node disease to the general population

Atrioventricular (AV) conduction disease

- AV conduction disturbances can be classified by criteria combining implications about anatomic site, mechanism, and prognosis
    - Traditionally they are classified as first-, second-, or third-degree block
    - Depending on the anatomical point of the conduction defect can be described as supra-Hisian, intra-Hisian, or infra-Hisian
    - ECG examples given in chapter 4.1
- May be asymptomatic, or present with:
    - symptoms related to pauses (e.g. pre-syncope, syncope)
    - symptoms related to chronic bradycardia (e.g. fatigue, reduced exercise tolerance)
    - worsening of co-morbid conditions (e.g. worsening angina, heart failure symptoms)

First-degree block (prolonged conduction):

- PR interval > 200 ms on the surface ECG
- Excellent prognosis, requires pacing only under exceptional circumstances (PR interval 350–400 ms, with loss of AV synchrony causing symptoms)

Second-degree block (intermittent conduction):

- Failure to conduct one or more atrial stimuli to the ventricles
- *Mobitz type 1*: progressive prolongation of the PR interval until a P wave is not conducted to the ventricles; often asymptomatic
- *Mobitz type 2*: constant PR interval with either constant block (e.g. 2:1, 3:1 block) or intermittent non-conducted P waves
    - Although this is traditionally an indication for pacing irrespective of symptoms, caution must be applied when paroxysmal episodes are seen in young patients with high vagal tone who are very unlikely to require pacing

Third-degree block (no conduction):

- Complete dissociation of P waves and QRS complexes

Important note: distinction between paroxysmal AV block caused by intrinsic disease vs often benign and reversible AV block caused by increased vagal tone is important:

- Paroxysmal AV block caused by increased vagal tone rarely requires pacing—it may be associated with specific activities (e.g. micturition, phlebotomy) and is typically seen on the surface ECG as gradual slowing of sinus rate and AV conduction, followed by transient sinus arrest or complete AV block
- Paroxysmal AV block caused by intrinsic disease is usually sudden onset and should be managed in the same way as persistent AV block
    - Although no randomized controlled trials comparing pacing to conservative management in high-degree AV block have been performed, observational studies suggest pacing improves survival in this cohort

- There is considerable overlap in the location of the disturbances and pattern of block. Surface ECG also may not be able to identify the site of block:
  - First-degree heart block: commonly occurs at the level of the atrium, AV node, intra-His or infra-His regions
  - Second-degree heart block: virtually never occurs in the atrium
    - Type 1 second degree commonly occurs at the level of the AVN and uncommonly at the intra- or infra-His levels
    - Type 2 second degree commonly occurs below the level of AVN, in the intra-His or infra-His levels
  - Third-degree heart block: commonly occurs at the levels of AVN, intra-His or infra-His

Bundle branch block (BBB)

- Conduction delays can occur at any level between the His and Purkinje system
- The vast majority of patients with BBB do not require pacing for bradycardic indications; however, there are certain patients who may benefit:
  - *Tri-fascicular block:*
    - Represents evidence of advanced AV conduction system disease affecting all three fascicles (right bundle branch, left anterior and left posterior fascicles)
    - Technically only true 'complete tri-fascicular block' if evidence of complete (third-degree) AV block
    - The following manifestations on the surface ECG are often taken as tri-fascicular block (they do represent significant conduction system disease, but technically represent 'incomplete tri-fascicular block' unless an EPS proves AV node involvement in infra-His):
      - RBBB, left axis deviation, and first-degree heart block
      - LBBB and first-degree heart block
      - RBBB with alternating left anterior hemi-block and right anterior hemi-block (i.e. disease of all three fascicles)
    - Pacing can be considered in appropriate patients (usually older patients) with tri-fascicular block who present with symptoms suggestive of bradycardia, even without documented evidence of a direct causal relationship (see Box 4.3.1)
  - *Bi-fascicular block:*
    - Disease in the AV conduction system that manifests on the surface ECG as complete RBBB with either left anterior (more common) or left posterior fascicular block (see Figure 4.3.1)
    - Pacing is usually not required and should be approached in the same way as pacing for BBB (see Box 4.3.1)
  - *Right or left bundle branch block:*
    - With the exception of alternating left and right BBB, pacing is rarely required (see indications below)

4.3.2 Approach to bradycardia

Aims

- Identify inappropriate bradycardia
- Assess impact of bradycardia upon quality of life

BOX 4.3.1 BRADYCARDIA INDICATIONS FOR PERMANENT PACING (BASED ON ESC GUIDELINES FOR PACING AND CRT (2021) AND SYNCOPE (2018))

Sinus node disease
- Pacing is indicated when symptoms documented to be caused by bradycardia, sinus arrest or sinoatrial block (class I[B])
- Pacing is indicated in patients with tachycardia-bradycardia syndrome in order to correct the bradyarrhythmia and enable pharmacological treatment, unless ablation of the tachyarrhythmia is preferred (class I[B])
- In patients who present with chronotropic incompetence and have clear symptoms during exercise, DDD pacing (pacing nomenclature described in section 4.3.3) with rate-responsive pacing should be considered (class IIa[B])
- AF ablation should be considered as a strategy to avoid pacemaker implantation in patients with AF-related bradycardia or symptomatic sinus pauses after AF conversion, taking account of the clinical situation (class IIa[C])
- Pacing may be considered when symptoms are likely to be caused by bradycardia, but the evidence is not conclusive (class IIb[C])
- In patients with syncope, pacing may be considered when asymptomatic pauses > 6 s due to sinus arrest is documented (class IIb[C])
- *N.B. in practice even longer sinus pauses are sometimes tolerated without pacing, especially in younger patients with high vagal tone*

Atrioventricular block
- Pacing is indicated in paroxysmal or persistent third-degree and Mobitz II second-degree block irrespective of symptoms (class I[C])
- Pacing is indicated in patients with atrial arrhythmia and permanent or paroxysmal third- or high-degree AV block, irrespective of symptoms (class I[C])
- Pacing should be considered in patients with Mobitz I second-degree block in whom symptoms have been documented to be caused by bradycardia, or who have undergone an EPS showing that the level of block is intra- or infra-Hisian (class IIa[C]). In practice it is rare for patients with Mobitz I block to require pacing or undergo EPS
- In patients with AV block, dual chamber DDD pacing should be considered over single chamber ventricular pacing to avoid pacemaker syndrome and improve quality of life (class IIa[A])
- Pacing should be considered in patients with persistent symptoms similar to those of pacemaker syndrome and clearly attributable to first-degree AVB (PR > 0.3 s) (class IIa[C])
- Neuromuscular diseases (e.g. myotonic muscular dystrophy, Kearns–Syre syndrome, etc.) with second- or third-degree AV block
- Second- or third-degree AV block:
  - Post catheter ablation of the AV junction
  - Post valvular surgery when the block is not expected to resolve (especially if the block is still present 5 days post-operatively)

Bundle branch block
- Pacing is indicated in alternating left and right BBB irrespective of symptoms (class I[C])
- Pacing is indicated in patients with unexplained syncope, bifasicular block and a positive EP study (defined as HV interval ≥ 70 ms, or second-/third-degree intra- or infra-Hisian

block demonstrated with incremental atrial pacing or with drug challenge (class 1[B]). In practice it is rare to for patients with BBB alone to require pacing or undergo EPS
- Pacing may be considered in selected patients with unexplained syncope and bifascicular block without a prior EPS (usually elderly, frail, high-risk, and/or recurrent syncope) (class IIb [B])
- Pacing is not recommended for asymptomatic BBB or bifascicular block (class III[B])

Reflex syncope
- Pacing is indicated in to reduce recurrent syncope in patients aged > 40 years with severe, recurrent, unpredictable reflex syncope who have: spontaneous documented symptomatic pauses > 3 s or asymptomatic pauses > 6 s, or cardioinhibitory carotid sinus hypersensitivity, or asystolic syncope during tilt testing (class I[A])
- Pacing may be considered to reduce syncope recurrence in patients with the clinical features of adenosine-sensitive syncope (class IIb[B])
- Pacing is not indicated in the absence of a documented cardioinhibitory reflex (class III[B])

Reversible causes
- Permanent pacing is not required in patients with sinoatrial node disease or atrioventricular block that is due to reversible causes (class III)

Others
- After transcatheter aortic valve implantation (TAVI), permanent pacing is recommended if:
  - Complete or high-grade AV block 24–48 hours post procedure (class I[B])
  - New onset alternating BBB (class I[C])
  - Patient with pre-existing RBBB develops further conduction disturbance (class IIa[B])
- Neuromuscular diseases (e.g. myotonic muscular dystrophy) with first-degree AV block (PR > 240 ms) or QRS >120 ms (class IIb[C]) or with any second- or third-degree AV block (class I[C])
- In Kearns–Sayre Syndrome, pacing should be considered in patients who have any evidence of AV block (first-, second-, third-degree block, BBB, fascicular block) (class IIa[C])
- Congenital third-degree AV block with:
  - Symptoms
  - Mean daytime ventricular rate < 50 bpm
  - Ventricular dysfunction
  - Wide QRS escape rhythm
  - Complex ventricular ectopy
  - Abrupt ventricular pauses more than three times of the basic cycle length of the escape rhythm
  - Prolonged QTc interval
- N.B. In patients with *LMNA* gene mutations who fulfil conventional pacing criteria or have prolonged PR with LBBB, ICD implantation with pacing capabilities should be considered if prognosis ≥ 1 year.

Glikson M, Nielsen JC, Kronborg MB, et al; ESC Scientific Document Group. 2021 ESC Guidelines on cardiac pacing and cardiac resynchronization therapy. *Eur Heart J.* 2021 Sep 14;42(35):3427–3520. doi: 10.1093/eurheartj/ehab364. © European Society of Cardiology. With permission from Oxford University Press
Brignole M, Moya A, de Lange FJ, et al; ESC Scientific Document Group. 2018 ESC Guidelines for the diagnosis and management of syncope. *Eur Heart J.* 2018 Jun 1;39(21):1883–1948. doi: 10.1093/eurheartj/ehy037. © European Society of Cardiology. With permission from Oxford University Press

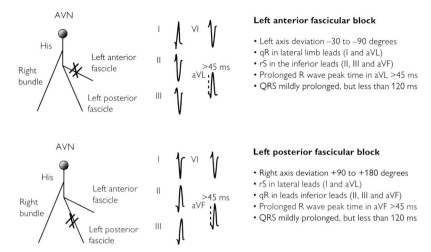

Figure 4.3.1 Left anterior and left posterior fascicular blocks

- Assess risk of serious complication such as syncope, heart failure, arrhythmia with embolic risk, or sudden death

History and evaluation

- Identify symptoms of inappropriate bradycardia, which is failure to respond to physiological demand. This leads to chronotropic incompetence which presents with breathlessness, fatigue, syncope
- Identify and correct potentially reversible causes of bradycardia such as drugs, ischemia, metabolic or electrolyte disturbances
- In the absence of reversible causes, drug therapy or cardiac pacing may be required

Investigation

- 12-lead ECG, bloods, carotid sinus message
- Ambulatory ECG (Holter, event recorder, implantable loop recorder)
- Electrophysiological testing has a potential role in:
    - Assessing sinus node function
    - Assessing the level of the block along the conduction system
    - Risk stratification in asymptomatic patients with bifascicular block or trifascicular block

Acute treatment

- Acute treatment is only required for patients with evidence of haemodynamic compromise
- Medical therapy includes boluses of atropine and an infusion of isoprenaline (can be given peripherally; note this drug may not be effective in third-degree AV block)
- Non-pharmacological therapy includes transcutaneous pacing, temporary transvenous pacing systems, permanent transvenous pacing and epicardial pacing (e.g. post-cardiothoracic surgery)
- Temporary transvenous pacing can be performed via internal jugular, axillary/subclavian or femoral access. A relatively high rate of complications has been observed in case series, including infection, haematoma, arterial puncture, pneumothorax, haemothorax, and pericardial effusion/tamponade secondary to cardiac perforation

- Externalized pacing (permanent pacing equipment (generator and ventricular lead) with the generator placed externally; used on a temporary basis) may offer a safer alternative to temporary pacing wires
  - N.B. A disadvantage vs temporary wire is that the rate, sensitivity, and output can only be changed by staff with pacemaker interrogation equipment and training

Clinical implication of electrophysiology study (EPS) in patients with suspected conduction disturbances

Sinus node dysfunction

- Normal corrected sinus node recovery time (cSNRT) < 550 ms
- Marked prolongation of cSNRT and an absence or blunted response to atropine and exercise suggest impaired sinus node function

Atrioventricular conduction

- Identification of concealed His extrasystoles, which may render part of the conduction system refractory resulting in first- or second-degree AV block
- More accurate determination of the site or sites of conduction block, AV node, intra-His and infra-His, especially in the presence of coexistent bundle branch block
- Atrial pacing or introduction of premature stimuli may reveal latent prolongation or failure of conduction (which may be physiological or pathological)

Intraventricular conduction

- In patients with bi- or trifascicular block, His-ventricular (H–V) conduction time >100 ms (normal H–V is 35–55 ms), or the demonstration of intra- or infra-His block during incremental atrial pacing at a rate of < 150 bpm, is predictive for the development of high-grade AV block
- Electrophysiology study allows the determination of VA conduction, accessory pathway, and risk of ventricular arrhythmia, which may uncover a different cause for the symptoms than bradyarrhythmia

4.3.3 Permanent pacemakers

- Europe implants approximately 1000 new pacing systems per million population per annum
  - In the UK, 'syncope' or 'pre-syncope' is the indication for pacing in 70% of cases
- Indications for a permanent pacemaker are outlined in Box 4.3.1
- Where indicated, patients should receive a permanent pacemaker as soon as possible after presentation (ideally without temporary pacing)

Pacemaker nomenclature

- Pacemaker function is described using a series of letters that refer to their functionality, with each letter in turn referring to the following:
  - Chamber-paced: O (none), A (atrium), V (ventricle), D (dual), S (single)
  - Chamber-sensed: O (none), A (atrium), V (ventricle), D (dual), S (single)
  - Response to sensing: O (none), T (triggered), I (inhibited), D (dual)
  - Rate modulation: O (none), R (rate modulation)
  - Multisite pacing: O (none), A (atrium), V (ventricle), D (dual)

(The S is only used by device companies)

Basic pacing concepts
Unipolar versus bipolar pacing
- Figures 4.3.2 and 4.3.3 outline the differences between these two pacing circuits
- Unipolar pacemakers have larger signals and so more visible pacing spikes on the surface ECG, vs bipolar pacemakers, which have smaller signals and the pacing spike can be difficult to identify on the surface ECG
- Unipolar devices are more susceptible to electrical interference, i.e. myopotentials, than bipolar pacemakers
- Pacemakers programmed as unipolar will stop pacing during generator change once the generator has been taken out of the pocket due to the circuit's reliance on contact with the tissue
    - If a patient is pacing dependent, programme as bipolar or if not possible consider temporary pacing during the procedure

Stimulation threshold
- This is the minimum amount of energy and duration required to reliably capture and depolarize the myocardium
- There is an exponential relationship between the stimulus amplitude and pulse-duration–strength-duration curve (see Figure 4.3.4)
- At short pulse durations a small change is associated with a large change in threshold whereas at longer pulse durations there is only a small change in threshold
- Threshold can be affected by:
    - Type of lead
    - Distance between electrode and tissue
    - Health of tissue in contact with the electrode
    - Antiarrhythmic drugs (AADs)

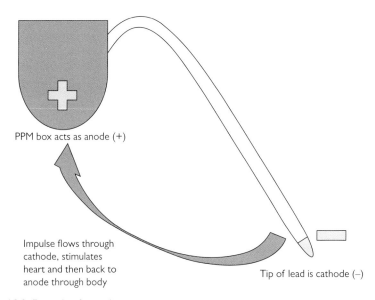

Figure 4.3.2 Example of unipolar pacing

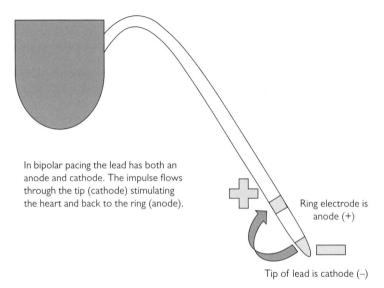

Figure 4.3.3 Example of bipolar pacing

- The relationship between threshold, pulse duration, lead impedance, and energy required to pace (higher energy means reduced battery longevity) is given by:

$$E = \frac{V^2}{R} \times PD$$

where E=energy, V=threshold, R=lead impedance, PD=pulse duration

- If V and PD are increased then energy required to pace increases and the battery will run out faster
- A higher lead impedance will reduce the energy required to pace and is beneficial for battery longevity
- Ventricular lead should have a threshold < 1 V at implant (unless active fixation, where higher thresholds are initially accepted and usually reduce over 24 h)
- The atrial lead threshold should be < 1.5 V at implantation

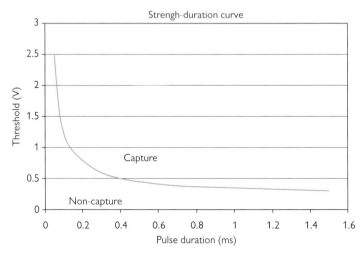

Figure 4.3.4 Strength–duration curve. Relationship between pulse duration and threshold. Measurements above the curve result in capture whereas below the line there is non-capture

- The safety margin for threshold programmed to the device is usually 2–3 times higher than implant threshold
- Some devices have internal algorithms that can recheck the threshold on a day-to-day basis and change the output each day, therefore adding extra safety, increasing battery longevity, and highlighting a problem sooner

Lead impedance

- Impedance varies between manufacturers and is usually < 1000 Ω, but high impedance leads are now available to increase battery life
- Impedance can be thought of in simple terms as equal to resistance (R) and can be estimated by Ohm's law:

    $V = IR$
    where V = potential difference between poles (Volts), I = current, R = resistance

- However, in reality total pacing impedance is determined by a number of factors:
    - A very low impedance is usually due to failure of the insulation (reduced resistance due to current escape)
    - A high impedance occurs with lead fracture (increasing resistance)

Sensing and sensitivity (terms can confuse)

Sensing:

- A pacemaker must be able to *sense* intrinsic cardiac activity and discriminate these from other forms of electrical interference, e.g. myopotentials, far-field cardiac events
- It senses the potential difference between the two electrodes, e.g. the two electrodes (distal tip and proximal ring) at the tip of the lead in a bipolar system
- The ventricular lead should have minimum R wave sensing of > 5 mV and the atrial lead should have minimum P wave sensing of > 2 mV

Sensitivity:

- The minimum amplitude of signal that the device is programmed to register as a *sensed event* (signals smaller in amplitude are ignored), e.g. a programmed sensitivity of 2 mV is more sensitive (higher sensitivity) than 5 mV (lower sensitivity)
- Smaller amplitude signals require a lower programmed value of sensitivity for detection (higher sensitivity)
- To increase sensitivity and treat 'undersensing', the value is lowered to sense smaller amplitude signals
- To treat 'oversensing', the sensitivity is decreased (i.e. the value sensed is increased) to avoid sensing inappropriately

Complications of pacemaker implantation

- Complications include infection (1%), haematoma, lead displacement (2–4%), pneumothorax with subclavian / axillary vein approach (1–2%), haemothorax, cardiac perforation (< 0.5%)

Optimal pacing mode

- Current evidence supports dual-chamber pacing with minimization of RV pacing, and where needed supporting chronotropic response to exercise
- In normal atrial activity, atrial-based pacing has been shown to be haemodynamically superior to ventricular-based pacing and is associated with a lower incidence of AF and heart failure
- A key priority of dual-chamber pacing is to minimize RV pacing. RV apical pacing produces dyssynchrony (LBBB) and produces electrical remodelling of the LV. This may lead to LV dysfunction

- The DAVID trial showed an increase in death and hospitalization for heart failure in patients who had an ICD and DDD pacing at 70 bpm compared to those who had backup pacing at 40 bpm. Patients in the study who experienced > 40% right ventricular pacing had a higher incidence of heart failure and death
- Chronotropic incompetence is failure to increase heart rate to 70–85% predicted and can be diagnosed by an exercise test. It can also be suspected by reviewing the pacemaker histograms (i.e. assess for heart rate variability across time)
- Rate response (R) can be programmed in situations of sinus node disease with chronotropic incompetence
    - Rate-adaptive sensors detect increased patient movement and respiratory rate
    - Some measure the QT interval, which decreases with exercise and increased sympathetic tone
    - The closed loop system also measures changes in cardiac contractility at the lead tip and requires a bipolar lead
    - Each of these parameters enables an increase in ventricular rate in response
- Recommended modes depending on indication:

    Isolated sinus node disease and no AV conduction disturbance: AAIR—as annual incidence of second- or third-degree AV block < 1%. In modern practice most operators implant a dual chamber system and use a device algorithm that minimizes V pacing, such as mode switching from AAI to DDD

    Sinus node and AV conduction disturbance: DDDR

    Paroxysmal AF/AT: DDI/DDD with mode switching
    - Mode switching is the ability of the pacemaker to switch from one mode to another in response to initiation and termination of a paroxysmal atrial tachycardia (AT); e.g. in sinus rhythm the pacemaker will operate in DDD mode but when an AT is sensed it will switch to VVI or DDI where there is no atrial tracking

    AV block or bi/tri-fascicular block: DDDR

    Long-standing persistent AF: VVIR

Magnet mode
- Placing a magnet over the generator converts the pacemaker to asynchronous mode (i.e. DOO, VOO) and the pacemaker will pace at a programmed rate without sensing or inhibition
- The magnet rate varies according to company and battery life
- This can be useful to assess permanent pacemaker function at the bedside, assess battery status if manufacturer parameters are known, and can also be used to treat oversensing if a programmer is not immediately available
- Placing a magnet over an ICD generator will inhibit shock therapy but not pacing function; as a result it is a useful acute treatment for inappropriate shocks

Pacemaker syndrome
- Usually occurs in patients with intact sinus node and ventricular pacing alone (i.e. VVI, but can occur with DDI pacing)
- Most symptoms relate to the loss of AV synchrony, with the loss of contribution from atrium to cardiac output and also VA conduction. Effectively, this can result in contraction of the atria when the mitral valve is closed
- Symptoms include SOB, chest pain, nausea, dizziness, fatigue, and chest fullness
- Hypotension can occur with ventricular pacing
- Management usually requires restoration of AV synchrony and consideration should be given to upgrading the system to DDD with the addition of an atrial lead

4.3.4 Pacemaker troubleshooting

- Pacemaker malfunctions include the following:
  - Pacemaker mediated tachycardia
  - Failure to pace
  - Failure to capture
  - Oversensing
  - Undersensing

Pacemaker-mediated tachycardia (PMT)

- PMT is a re-entry arrhythmia in which the dual-chamber pacemaker acts as the anterograde limb of the tachycardia and the His–Purkinje–AV system as the retrograde pathway (see Figure 4.3.5)
- PMT is distinct from a pacemaker-facilitated tachycardia due to high rate ventricular pacing (dual chamber) whilst tracking an atrial arrhythmia
- Usually caused by a premature ventricular extrasystole leading to VA conduction. The sensed atrial beat leads to pacing in the ventricle and a re-entrant mechanism is set up. The maximum rate is limited by the pacemaker's programmed upper rate limit
- PVARP (post-ventricular atrial refractory period) can be extended to prevent PMT, and many pacemakers automatically extend the PVARP temporarily at the onset of a PMT
- A magnet can also be used to diagnose and treat PMT, as sensing is inhibited and asynchronous pacing takes place

Failure to pace

- Pacing does not occur despite an indication to pace

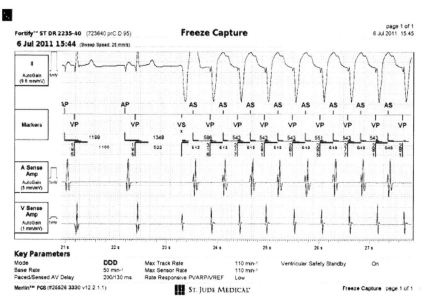

Figure 4.3.5 Example of pacemaker mediated tachycardia. A ventricular ectopic beat conducts retrogradely through the AV node producing a retrograde P-wave, which is sensed. This is then followed by a paced beat and so on. The retrograde P-wave can be seen in the T-wave on the surface ECG
Reproduced by kind permission of Richard Chambers of St Jude Medical Inc.

- Can be due to a battery at end of life, a lead or lead insulation fracture, oversensing, or cross-talk (which is where the atrial output is sensed by a ventricular lead in a dual-chamber pacer, which inhibits ventricular pacing)
- If the patient is symptomatic or there is no underlying rhythm then acute treatment including temporary pacing may be required
- CXR is required to assess lead position, position of pin in header, and for lead fracture, which occurs most commonly at the clavicle or first rib
- Pacing check will assess battery life, lead impedances, and sensing parameters
- A very low impedance is usually due to failure of the insulation, whilst a high impedance occurs with lead fracture
- Will require lead reposition or a new lead if fracture or insulation failure
- Cross-talk can be temporarily managed by magnet application and subsequently extension of the ventricular blanking period

Failure to capture

- Loss of pacemaker capture occurs when there is appropriate output but no atrial or ventricular depolarization; may be seen as a pacing spike on ECG with no associated paced complex
- This may be intermittent or persistent
- Most problems occur at the pacemaker lead/tissue interface, e.g. lead dislodgment
- Increase in the pacing threshold occurs with:
  - Lead maturation within a few weeks following lead placement
  - Fibrosis
  - Drug therapy (e.g. flecainide)
  - Electrolyte abnormalities
  - Myocardial infarction or ischaemia at the lead tip
- Mechanical problems that can cause failure to capture include
  - Fracture of the lead
  - Insulation breaks
  - Poor lead connection in header of the generator
- Requires a pacemaker check (to assess pacing threshold and lead impedance) and CXR
- If the threshold is high then pacing outputs can be increased temporarily, and it is worth trying unipolar pacing
- Usually requires lead revision or replacement

Oversensing

- Occurs when either non-cardiac or cardiac electrical activity is sensed inappropriately and pacing is inappropriately inhibited
- Sensing of this electrical activity can inhibit the ventricular output if sensed on the ventricular channel or can trigger a ventricular output if sensed on the atrial channel
- Unipolar systems are more susceptible
- Can be caused by muscular activity, electromagnetic interference (MRIs), fractured lead insulation, or oversensing of intrinsic P or T waves (see Figure 4.3.6)
- Diagnosis requires analysis of ECG and pacemaker interrogation
- Treatment requires reducing the sensitivity to a level that avoids oversensing whilst still sensing intrinsic cardiac depolarizations
- T wave oversensing can also be managed by increasing the ventricular refractory period
- Programming to an asynchronous mode or magnet application can be a temporary solution

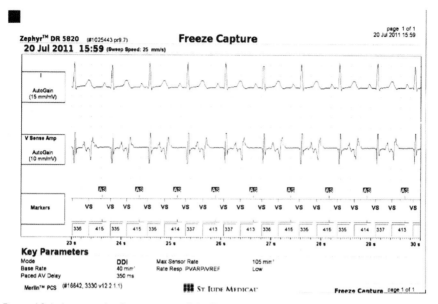

Figure 4.3.6 An example of oversensing of the T-wave.
Reproduced by kind permission of Richard Chambers of St Jude Medical Inc.

Undersensing

- This represents a lack of sensing of intrinsic cardiac electrical activity (see Figure 4.3.7)
- An inadequate intra-cardiac signal can lead to undersensing, usually more of a problem in the atrium
- At implant aim for P wave of > 1.5 ms and R wave of > 5 ms
- Undersensing can be a result of lead dislodgement, lead insulation breaks, cardiac arrhythmias, electrolyte abnormalities, and infarction/ischaemia at lead/tissue interface
- Treated by programming an enhanced sensitivity (decreasing the sensing level)
- *Functional undersensing* can occur and is normal pacemaker function. For example, a premature ventricular complex (PVC) occurring in the programmed refractory period (blanking period) will not be sensed and pacing output will not be inhibited. This can be managed by shortening the refractory period

Practical considerations

Driving

- See section 4.10.3

Mobile phones

- Can rarely affect pacemaker functioning if held in close proximity
- Patients are advised to hold the phone on the opposite side to the PPM and not to carry it in a pocket overlying the PPM

Diathermy

- During surgery, diathermy use and power output should be kept to a minimum, using short bursts and keeping away from the device. However, diathermy is routinely used during pacemaker extractions as lead damage is less likely than with scalpels

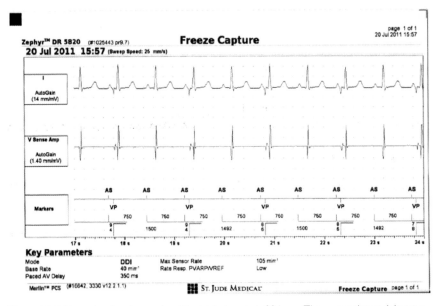

Figure 4.3.7 Example of undersensing. The intrinsic rate is 80 bpm. The pacemaker is delivering pacing spikes at the base rate of 40 bpm resulting in fusion as it is not sensing the normal underlying ventricular rhythm. The markers show VP (V pace) at 40 bpm with no VS (V sense).
Reproduced by kind permission of Richard Chambers of St Jude Medical Inc.

- Bipolar diathermy is generally safe if it is not applied to the region of the PPM, though PPM should be checked after the procedure
- A programmer or magnet should be kept close by to allow asynchronous pacing in case of PPM inhibition
- With unipolar diathermy the other electrode should be placed well away from the device so that it does not lie between electrodes, e.g. on the leg

Defibrillation

- Defibrillation pads should be placed as far away from the device as possible to avoid damage or re-setting of the device. The PPM should be checked afterwards to ensure normal function

MRI

- All manufacturers now produce MRI conditional pacemakers but the strength of magnet (measured in Teslas) needs to be checked before the patient has an MRI and the device may require specific programming (to fixed-output mode) prior to the scan
- There is now also a large body of evidence demonstrating that patients with non-MRI conditional ('legacy') devices can also be scanned safely, as long as specific imaging protocols are followed
    - Patients with non-MRI conditional devices should therefore now have the same access to MRI as all other patients

Airport metal detectors

- Patients should always carry their PPM identity card
- The possibility of adverse events is low
- Patients are advised to walk quickly through gates or request a pat-down by security staff

Pacemaker follow-up

- All patients with a pacemaker are typically followed up on an annual basis, enabling detection of impending device related issues, timing of generator change, optimizing device function and assessment of other arrhythmias
- A typical follow-up will assess:
    - device longevity
    - monitoring lead thresholds and impedance (if changing over time, i.e. rising or falling, this will lead to further assessment of cause and planning of potential new lead); when tracking this the frequency of follow-up appointments is typically increased
    - device detected arrhythmias
    - heart rate charts to look at variability
    - percentage of ventricular pacing, and assess for any optimization (e.g. lengthening AV delay) to be done to reduce RV pacing
    - monitor wound

Further reading

Brignole M, Moya A, de Lange FJ, Deharo JC, Elliott PM, Fanciulli A, Fedorowski A, Furlan R, Kenny RA, Martín A, Probst V, Reed MJ, Rice CP, Sutton R, Ungar A, van Dijk JG; ESC Scientific Document Group. 2018 ESC Guidelines for the diagnosis and management of syncope. *Eur Heart J*. 2018 Jun 1;39(21):1883–948. doi: 10.1093/eurheartj/ehy037. PMID: 29562304

Glikson M, Nielsen JC, Kronborg MB, Michowitz Y, Auricchio A, Barbash IM, Barrabés JA, Boriani G, Braunschweig F, Brignole M, Burri H, Coats AJS, Deharo JC, Delgado V, Diller GP, Israel CW, Keren A, Knops RE, Kotecha D, Leclercq C, Merkely B, Starck C, Thylén I, Tolosana JM; ESC Scientific Document Group. 2021 ESC Guidelines on cardiac pacing and cardiac resynchronization therapy. *Eur Heart J*. 2021 Sep 14;42(35):3427–520. doi: 10.1093/eurheartj/ehab364. PMID: 34455430

Issa ZF, Miller JM, Zipes DP. *Clinical Arrhythmology and Electrophysiology*, 2nd edn. Elsevier, 2012.

4.4

Supraventricular tachycardia

Richard Bond, Howell Williams, Christopher N. Floyd, and Alexander Carpenter

TABLE OF CONTENTS

4.4.1 Tachyarrhythmia mechanisms and pharmacology of antiarrhythmic drugs 335
    Tachyarrhythmia mechanisms 335
    Pharmacology of antiarrhythmic drugs 336
4.4.2 Supraventricular tachycardia classification and management 340
    ECG diagnosis of narrow complex tachycardia 340
    Pathophysiology of a re-entrant tachycardia 340
    AVNRT 342
    AVRT and accessory pathways 344
    Special notes 350
4.4.3 Electrophysiology study principles and invasive SVT management 350
    EPS features of AVNRT 351
    3D electro-anatomic mapping 353

4.4.1 Tachyarrhythmia mechanisms and pharmacology of antiarrhythmic drugs

Cardiac action potential
- Understanding the cardiac action potential (discussed in chapter 4.1) is important to understand the three main mechanisms for tachyarrhythmias (outlined below), as well as the mechanism of antiarrhythmic drug therapy

Tachyarrhythmia mechanisms
Re-entry
- Most common mechanism for arrhythmias (AVNRT, AVRT, atrial flutter, VT)
- Requires two pathways with different electrophysiological properties (conduction and refractoriness); one pathway conducts quicker and has a longer refractory period and the other conducts slower but has a shorter refractory period
- Each involved pathway of the circuit must be capable of conducting an impulse in an anterograde and retrograde direction
- Initiated by a premature impulse

Automaticity
- Not common (automatic ATs, automatic junctional tachycardia, automatic VT)
- Automaticity is the ability of cardiomycetes to spontaneously depolarise
- Abnormal acceleration of phase 4 of the action potential produces an early depolarization
- Often have metabolic causes, e.g. ischaemia, hypoxia, hypokalaemia, hypomagnesaemia, high sympathetic tone

Triggered activity

- Produced by abnormal fluxes of positive ions into cardiac cells producing an afterdepolarization during late phase 3 or early phase 4
- If the afterdepolarizations are large enough they can cause another action potential to be generated
- Can cause digitalis toxic arrhythmias, Torsade de Pointes, and some VTs that respond to calcium channel blockers (CCBs)

Pharmacology of antiarrhythmic drugs

- Antiarrhythmic medications are used to control or suppress pathological arrhythmia, usually tachyarrhythmia
- This is achieved by altering the electrical properties on a cellular or tissue level to disrupt specific arrhythmia mechanisms
- It is worth noting, however, that this can indirectly promote other forms of arrhythmia (e.g. amiodarone-induced QT prolongation)
- The Vaughan–Williams classification (Table 4.4.1) describes antiarrhythmic medication in terms of their differential effects on ion channels and the cardiac action potential

Class I antiarrhythmics (Na⁺ channel blockers)

- Class I antiarrhythmics display Na^+ channel blocking behaviour
- As the fast sodium current is responsible for the rapid upstroke of the cardiac action potential (AP), its blockade can lead to potentially arrhythmogenic AP prolongation, which manifests as QRS or QT prolongation on the surface ECG
- Therefore, class I drugs should be avoided in the presence of pre-existing QT prolongation or conduction system disease

Class IA

- Block K^+ channels as well as fast Na^+ channels, prolonging action potential and slowing refractoriness

Table 4.4.1 The Vaughan–Williams classification of antiarrhythmic drugs.

Vaughan–Williams class	Mechanism	Antiarrhythmic drugs
Ia	Intermediate-action Na^+ channel blockade	Ajmaline, disopyramide, procainamide, quinidine
Ib	Rapid-action Na^+ channel blockade	Lignocaine, mexiletine, phenytoin
Ic	Slow-action Na^+ channel blockade	Encainide, flecainide, propafenone
II	Beta-adrenergic blockade	Atenolol, bisoprolol, carvedilol, metoprolol, nadolol, nebivolol, propranolol
III	K^+ channel blockade	Amiodarone*, dofetilide, dronedarone, ibutilide, sotalol**, vernakalant***
IV	Ca^{2+} channel blockade	Diltiazem, verapamil

*: amiodarone also demonstrates class I, II, and IV activity; **sotalol also demonstrates class II activity; ***: vernakalant also demonstrates class I activity

- Act in both atria and ventricles and therefore can be used to treat both atrial and ventricular arrhythmias
- Relevant side effects:
  - All class IA drugs are proarrhythmic
  - Quinidine can cause significant GI upset
  - Procainamide can cause agranulocytosis
  - Disopyramide has significant anticholinergic side effects

Class IB

- Decrease duration of action potential and therefore reduce refractory periods
- Have little effect in the atria and are therefore only useful for ventricular arrhythmias
- Lidocaine can only be given IV because of first-pass metabolism
- Relevant side effects:
  - Low potential for a proarrhythmia action
  - Class IB agents mainly cause neurological and GI side effects
  - Lignocaine is negatively inotropic
  - Gingival hyperplasia is common with phenytoin

Class IC

- Significantly reduce conduction velocity, and do not significantly affect action potential duration
- Effective for both atrial and ventricular arrhythmias
- Torsades de Pointes is very rarely seen with Class IC agents, with proarrhythmic effect due to re-entrant VT
- Class IC agents should not be given to patients with IHD or LV systolic impairment
  - The Cardiac Arrhythmia Suppression Trial (CAST) showed increased mortality in patients receiving flecainide or encainide following MI
- Flecainide demonstrates '*use dependence*', becoming progressively more active as the heart rate increases, which is a desirable property for a drug used to treat tachyarrhythmia
- It is sometimes used as part of a rhythm-control or 'pill in the pocket' strategy in AF
  - However, as noted above, there is a potential for AP prolongation, with this lengthening of the action potential promoting slowing of a re-entrant tachy-arrhythmia circuit
  - If a patient with paroxysmal AF experiencing palpitations is, in fact, experiencing an episode of atrial flutter (typically a macro-re-entrant circuit around the cavotricuspid isthmus), then flecainide has the potential to slow this re-entrant rhythm significantly
  - In such patients there is a risk that the cycle length of such a re-entrant arrhythmia could slow to the point at which their AV node (particularly in young patients with 'slick' AV nodes) is able to conduct this fast arrhythmia into the ventricle, leading to potentially dangerous rapid ventricular activity
  - For this reason, flecainide is usually co-prescribed with a beta blocker to reduce the likelihood of rapid AV conduction

N.B. Class I antiarrhythmic drugs, particularly ajmaline, are used as part of 'provocation testing' to demonstrate a Type 1 ECG pattern diagnostic of Brugada syndrome:

- In the most common genetic variants of Brugada syndrome, dysfunction of sodium channels responsible for the rapid upstroke of the action potential can lead to dangerous ventricular arrhythmia
- Therefore, outside a provocation-testing setting (and arguably even within), these drugs can be dangerous for patients with this condition

Class II antiarrhythmics (beta blockers)

- The beta-adrenergic receptor is present throughout the body in multiple organs and throughout the autonomic nervous system, and stimulation of the receptor leads to positive cardiac inotropic and chronotropic effects
- Beta blockers (BBs) work by blunting the arryhthmogenic action of catecholamines, and sympathetic innervation is greatest in the SA and AV nodes, where they have the greatest effect
- Phase 4 depolarization is blunted, automaticity is decreased, and HR is slowed
- In the AV node, BBs produce a marked slowing in conduction and a prolongation in refractory periods
- Those in the heart and lungs are predominantly β2 receptors: BBs antagonize the action of β-adrenergic receptors, and those which are predominantly selective for β2 receptors are referred to as 'cardio-selective'
- BBs have multiple uses in cardiovascular medicine: antiarrhythmic or rate-controlling medication, anti-hypertensive agents, cardiac remodelling in HFrEF, and IHD (both ACS and CCS)
- In arrhythmia, BBs are commonly used to slow cardiac conduction, to suppress or to manage arrhythmia—they are used in both atrial and ventricular arrhythmia
- Suppression of β2-adrenergic receptors reduces cardiac automaticity (i.e. the propensity of individual cardiac myocytes to spontaneously depolarize) and this can reduce associated arrhythmic mechanisms such as triggered activity or ectopy
- The effects of BBs on slowing conduction velocity and prolonging the action potential also have the effect of slowing and suppressing re-entrant arrhythmia
- BBs are useful in preventing arrhythmias in congenital LQTS
- Finally, slowing of conduction at the AVN makes BB therapy the first-line choice when pursuing a ventricular rate-control strategy in atrial arrhythmia (e.g. AF)
- BBs are generally safe and well tolerated:
    - Their use in COPD was previously contraindicated. New evidence, however, suggests significant overall benefit in these patients (who typically have high cardiovascular risk) unless they are acutely wheezy. Similar caution should be used in other patients with acute airways dysfunction
    - Typically, non-cardiac side effects such as wheeze, flushing, tiredness, or peripheral vasoconstriction may be more common with less-cardioselective beta blockers such as atenolol or propranolol

N.B. BBs also have a role in management of hypertension, although their use is not first line, IV BB can be used for management of hypertensive emergencies, with labetalol favoured due to its additional alpha adrenoreceptor blockade (i.e. for the management of hypertensive crises in pregnancy)

Class III antiarrhythmics

- Increase the duration of the action potential, usually by blocking K$^+$ channels, and increase refractory periods
- Used for atrial and ventricular arrhythmias

Amiodarone

- A potent antiarrhythmic which, although used widely, demonstrates questionable efficacy across a range of indications
- It produces effects across Vaughan-Williams classes I–IV, including:
    - Prolonging the repolarization phase of the action potential
    - Prolonging atrial and ventricular refractory periods
    - Slowing conduction of the sinoatrial and atrioventricular nodes and across cardiac tissue
    - β-adrenergic inhibition
- Generally considered effective for reducing episodes of VT and VF, and is moderately effective in maintaining SR in AF/flutter, however:

- Rhythm-control therapy with amiodarone provided no additional benefit over rate-control in patients with AF in the AFFIRM study, and there was a significant excess of adverse drug events in the rhythm-control group
  - Given the significant burden of potential side effects and questionable efficacy, its use in management of narrow-complex tachycardia should be avoided in the majority of cases
  - While demonstrating poor efficacy in acute pharmacological termination of VT, its role likely lies as an adjunct to improving the success of DCCV
  - Long-term use in selected patients at ongoing risk of VT with or without an ICD *in-situ*, although the evidence for this is conflicting and ablation therapy will be a preferable option for many in this at-risk group
- The effect of amiodarone on prolonging the action potential via various mechanisms can cause significant and potentially dangerous QT prolongation, particularly in those with pre-existing QT prolongation, whether inherited or acquired
  - Exercise caution in the presence of existing conduction disease or QT prolongation
- Multiple well documented non-cardiac side effects include: hyper- or hypo-thyroidism, pulmonary fibrosis, corneal micro-deposits, deranged liver function or fibrosis, photosensitivity (~20% of patients) or blue-grey discolouration of the skin, taste disturbances and peripheral neuropathy
- Other, less common side effects: haematological, movement and vasculitis disorders
- Metabolized and excreted hepatically, the average half-life is ~60 days, and is an inhibitor of the cytochrome P450 family of iso-enzymes and therefore subject to numerous drug interactions
- IV amiodarone can cause transient hypotension. Importantly, the infusion should only be administered via a sufficiently large-bore peripheral cannula or ideally, a central cannula to minimize the risk of tissue extravasation, which can lead to profound tissue necrosis

Sotalol

- Produces prolongation of the action potential in both the atria and ventricles, and has a class II action as well
- While acting chiefly as a K^+ channel blocker, it also demonstrates non-selective BB activity
- Has been used widely for management of tachyarrhythmias such as AF and to reduce incidence of VT in at-risk patients
- Its use is somewhat limited by potential for profound dose-dependent QT prolongation and significant bradycardia, with the risk of life-threatening Torsades de Pointes increasingly significantly with higher doses

Class IV antiarrhythmics

- The non-dihydropyridine CCBs inhibit the calcium channel responsible for depolarization in the SA and AV node, where they reduce automaticity, slow conduction, and increase the refractory period
- CCBs can suppress early or delayed afterdepolarizations
- CCBs can be used for atrial tachyarrhythmias, and verapamil is very good at terminating narrow complex tachycardias, and are particularly helpful if BBs are contra-indicated
- Verapamil can be effective as pharmacological therapy for AV node re-entrant tachycardia (AVNRT) and occasionally in structurally normal heart VT, e.g. RVOT VT and fascicular VT, although they are not good for terminating typical re-entrant VT and have been associated with serious adverse effects
- Side effects:
  - Verapamil and diltiazem are negative inotropes and can produce bradycardia and hypotension, considered dangerous in those with impaired LV function (in particular if LVEF is <40%)
  - Verapamil can also cause constipation

Other antiarrhythmic medication
- Digoxin is a cardiac glycoside which is negatively dromotropic, i.e. it slows conduction across the AV node
- This effect is useful in attempts to slow the ventricular rate during atrial arrhythmia
- Due to its effect on shortening the effective refractory period, it is likely to promote occurrence of AF, and thus should be avoided in a rhythm-control approach
- Digoxin should be used with caution if there are concurrent electrolyte abnormalities:
  - Hypokalaemia can predispose to digoxin toxicity, as digoxin and K^+ bind to the same site at the Na^+/K^+ ATPase ion channel
  - Therefore reduced plasma K^+ leads to increased digoxin binding and enhanced therapeutic and toxic effects
- Digoxin is renally excreted and therefore requires caution in those with renal impairment, whether acute or chronic, as there is heightened risk of accumulation and toxicity

4.4.2 Supraventricular tachycardia classification and management

Remember the definition of SVT: a tachycardia that requires structures above the bundle of His in order to be maintained

- Common SVTs include:
  - Atrioventricular nodal re-entry tachycardia (AVNRT)
  - Atrioventricular re-entrant tachycardia (AVRT)
  - Atrial tachycardia (AT)
  - Atrial fibrillation (AF)
  - Atrial flutter
- This section will focus on AVNRT and AVRT, chapters 4.5 and 4.6 cover atrial fibrillation and atrial flutter

ECG diagnosis of narrow complex tachycardia
- The 12-lead ECG helps in differentiating SVT diagnoses (see Figure 4.4.1)
- These can be divided according to RP duration, with 'long RP' defined as RP (onset of the R wave to the onset of next P wave), longer then the interval from that same P wave to the next R wave, and vice versa for 'short RP'
- *Long RP tachycardias*
  - Sinus tachycardia/inappropriate sinus tachycardia
  - Atrial tachycardia
  - Atypical AVNRT
  - AVRT (less commonly long RP)
- *Short RP tachycardias*
  - Typical AVNRT
  - AVRT (more commonly short RP)

Pathophysiology of a re-entrant tachycardia
- Both AVNRT and AVRT are *re-entrant tachycardias*
- Re-entry describes a continuous and repetitive propagation of electrical activation in a circular path
- Figure 4.4.2 below demonstrates the three criteria for re-entry:
  1. Unidirectional block of a potential circular path is required for initiation

4.4.2 Supraventricular tachycardia classification and management

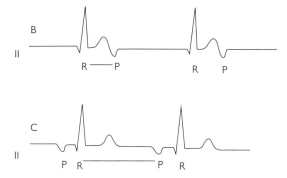

Figure 4.4.1 Descriptive terminology of SVT. A, normal SR; B, short RP tachycardia with RP < PR interval; C, long RP tachycardia with RP ≥ PR.

Reproduced from Lee KW, Badhwar N, Scheinman MM. Supraventricular tachycardia—part I. *Curr Probl Cardiol*. 2008 Sep;33(9):467–546. doi: 10.1016/j.cpcardiol.2008.06.002 with permission Elsevier.

2. A wave of electrical activation travels repeatedly in a single direction around the pathway
3. The resultant tachycardia should be terminated by blockade of one limb of the pathway
- To favour re-entry:
    - Two pathways must be linked (e.g. the AV node and an accessory AV pathway)
    - These two pathways must have different conduction velocities and different refractory characteristics
    - 'Timing' is critical ('*excitable gap*')
- Slower pathways have shorter RPs and fast pathways have longer RPs (useful analogy: a fast sprint requires greater recovery time than a gentle stroll)
- A premature complex that finds the faster pathway refractory will instead travel via the slower pathway (see Figure 4.4.2), and if it then reaches the faster pathway during the 'critical time' when it has recovered from refractoriness, it can travel back retrogradely
- By the time it comes round to the slower pathway, which has now recovered from refractoriness, re-entry will continue

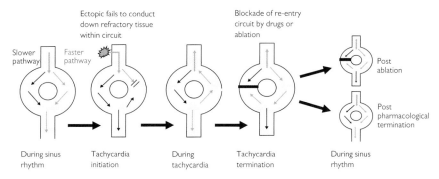

Figure 4.4.2 Schematic demonstrating re-entry. The faster conduction pathway (grey) has a longer refractory period than the slower pathway (black). Following a critically timed premature electrical impulse, the fast pathway tissue is **refractory**, whilst the slower pathway is **not refractory** and is able to conduct. By the time the impulse has travelled around to the fast pathway, it has recovered and is able to conduct retrogradely, thus instigating re-entry. Blockade of either limb of the pathway will terminate the tachycardia

> **TIP**
>
> The pathophysiological nature of AV re-entry gives rise to the characteristic description in the history of 'sudden onset and sudden offset' palpitations, reflecting the critically timed beats of initiation and termination, often from atrial or ventricular extras. This history is often distinct from the more gradually onset and offset of non-re-entrant or focal tachycardia, as described

AVNRT

Background

- Most common SVT
- Commonly manifests in second and third decades of life although there is a second peak in incidence between 60–80 due to changes in conduction properties of slow and fast pathways
- Twice as common in females as males
- Typically presents with fast regular palpitations that are sudden onset and sudden offset
- Re-entry tachycardia caused by a circuit within the AV node
- Requires *dual AV node physiology* as the underlying arrhythmia substrate, something which is found in up to 20% of the general population:
  - Two (or more) pathways through the AV node with differing electrophysiological properties
  - One pathway conducts faster than the other—hence the description of fast and slow pathways (see Figure 4.4.3)

Pathophysiology

- In SR, impulses travel down both the fast and slow pathways, meeting in the slow pathway
- In typical AVNRT, an ectopic beat generates an impulse that travels down the slow pathway:
  - The slow pathway conducts more slowly, but repolarizes more quickly, than the fast pathway
  - When the ectopic impulse arrives, the slow pathway has repolarized (i.e. ceased to be refractory) before the fast pathway

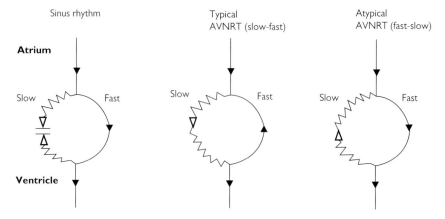

Figure 4.4.3 Schematic illustration of AV nodal re-entry

Reproduced from Lee KW, Badhwar N, Scheinman MM. Supraventricular tachycardia—part I. *Curr Probl Cardiol.* 2008 Sep;33(9):467–546. doi: 10.1016/j.cpcardiol.2008.06.002 with permission Elsevier.

- The impulse therefore travels down the slow pathway and back up the fast pathway (which has now had time to repolarize)—see 'tachycardia initiation' in Figure 4.4.2
- ECG appearance is short RP as retrograde conduction to the atrium is fast, via the fast pathway
- Typical AVNRT accounts for ~90% of AVNRTs
• In atypical AVNRT (remaining 10%), the impulse either travels down the fast pathway and back up the slow pathway, or forms a re-entry circuit within two separate slow pathways (not shown above)
    - ECG appearance is long RP as retrograde conduction to the atrium is slow, via the slow pathway

> **TIP**
>
> *Symptomatic neck pulsation in tachycardia is suggestive of typical AVNRT—simultaneous activation of atria and ventricles, seen in about 50% of AVNRT patients*

ECG features

- Narrow complex tachycardia
- Rate can vary from 120 to 250 bpm
- Typical AVNRT—short RP interval, or P wave buried in the QRS complex and not visible (example seen in Figure 4.4.4)
    - May be seen as a pseudo r' in V1 or pseudo s in the inferior leads (both features suggestive of AVNRT)
- Atypical AVNRT—long RP interval
- If seen, the P waves are almost always negative in the inferior leads (retrograde activation of the atria from bottom to top, away from the inferior leads)

Management

- Acute management involves blockade of the AV node, which blocks part of the re-entry circuit and terminates the tachycardia:
    - Vagal manoeuvres (e.g. blow into a 10 ml syringe)

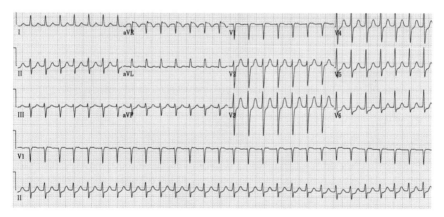

Figure 4.4.4 Usual ECG pattern of typical AVNRT. 12-lead ECG shows a regular narrow complex tachycardia (sweep speed 25 mm/sec). Note the pseudo r' in V1 (arrow) and accentuated S waves in II, III, aVF (arrow) suggestive of AVNRT

- Adenosine in escalating dose as required to achieve AV node blockade
  - Transplant recipients and pregnant women may be more sensitive, start with a lower dose
  - Contraindicated in severe asthma, long QT syndrome, second- and third-degree AV block
- AV node blockade may also be achieved with CCBs (verapamil first choice) or BBs
- DC cardioversion if drug therapy fails
• Longer term management may be invasive, pharmacological, or conservative. An invasive approach is considered **low risk and likely to be curative**, and is therefore first line in the majority of cases
• Management strategies:
  - *Invasive*: electrophysiological study +/− catheter ablation (see section 4.4.3)
    - High cure rate (~95–99%) and ESC recommended first line if recurrent episodes (*Class I[B]*)
    - Radiofrequency or cryoablation aiming to ablate the slow pathway
    - Main risk is iatrogenic complete AV block requiring a pacemaker (important as majority of patients are young and therefore much higher risk of a pacing complication during their lifetime)
  - *Pharmacological*: verapamil used either regularly or as 'pill in the pocket' is most common choice; beta blockers or class 1 antiarrhythmics may also be used. May be helpful in highly symptomatic patients awaiting ablation
  - *Conservative*: 'watch and wait' approach if very infrequent/short-lived episodes, guided by patient choice

AVRT and accessory pathways
Definitions
- *Accessory pathway* (AP): an additional connection between the atria and ventricles that is able to conduct electrical impulses
- *Pre-excitation*: a surface ECG manifestation of an AP that allows AV conduction to occur faster than it can through the AV node. This leads to activation of some of the ventricular myocardium via the AP rather than via the AV node with typical ECG changes (short PR interval, delta wave). This also known as Wolff–Parkinson–White pattern
- *Wolff–Parkinson–White syndrome*: pre-excitation on the surface ECG *with symptoms* suggestive of tachyarrhythmia, or documented tachyarrhythmia, and caused by conduction down the accessory pathway
- *AVRT*: atrioventricular re-entrant tachycardia—a macro re-entrant SVT with a re-entry circuit that involves an AP
- *Pre-excited AT/AF*: AT or AF that conducts from atria to ventricles wholly or partially through an AP. APs that are capable of rapid AV conduction can allow very rapid ventricular rates in this setting, which can be life-threatening

Background
- AVRT is a re-entry tachycardia caused by a circuit involving the AV node and an AP (there are rare cases of multiple pathways that allow pathway–pathway re-entrant circuits that are not discussed in detail here). APs can conduct electrical impulses:
  - Antegradely only: atrium to ventricle only (< 5%)
  - Retrogradely only: ventricle to atrium only (~30%)
  - Bidirectionally: atrium to ventricle and ventricle to atrium (~60%)

- Pathways may be further divided into:
  - Manifest: APs that are capable of antegrade conduction, and so evident as pre-excitation on the surface ECG in sinus rhythm
  - Concealed: APs that are capable of only retrograde conduction and are therefore not seen on the surface ECG in sinus rhythm
- APs are twice as common in men as in women and usually become manifest in the first year of life
- The prevalence of manifest APs with pre-excitation on the surface ECG in the general population is 0.15% to 0.25%; the prevalence of concealed APs is not known
- Most patients with APs are asymptomatic but may present with symptoms due to arrhythmia. The two commonest arrhythmias in patients with APs are AVRT and AF (increased incidence of AF vs general population)
  - AVRT presents with paroxysmal sudden onset/offset palpitations
  - AF may present with palpitations, or with symptoms consistent with haemodynamic compromise (syncope or aborted sudden cardiac death)
- Incidence of sudden cardiac death in patients with pre-excitation on their surface ECG is low, ranging from 0% to 0.39% per year in case series
- APs vary in location—in descending order of frequency (see Figure 4.4.8):
  (i) Left free wall
  (ii) Left posterior wall
  (iii) Left or right postero-septal wall
  (iv) Right free wall
  (v) Antero-septal region
- The anatomical position influences the likelihood of successfully ablating the pathway

Pathophysiology of tachycardia

- Myocytes in the accessory pathway rapidly conduct due to the presence of voltage-gated Na^+ channels, and therefore some ventricular myocytes are activated early, prior to the conduction through the AV node and the His–Purkinje system
- AVRT can be divided as follows (see Figure 4.4.5):
  - Orthodromic (~95% of AVRTs):
    - Antegrade (A to V) conduction occurs through the AV node and retrograde (V to A) conduction occurs through an AP
    - Usually a narrow complex tachycardia as A to V conduction occurs via the specialized conduction system, but may be broad if pre-existing or rate-related BBB is present
    - May be caused by an AP that conducts bi-directionally in which case pre-excitation is likely to be present on the resting ECG in sinus rhythm, or an AP that only conducts retrogradely (a concealed AP) in which case pre-excitation will not be present on the ECG in sinus rhythm

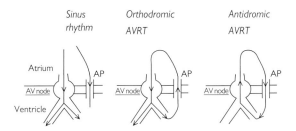

Figure 4.4.5 Orthodromic vs antidromic AVRT
Reproduced from Lee KW, Badhwar N, Scheinman MM. Supraventricular tachycardia—part I. *Curr Probl Cardiol.* 2008 Sep;33(9):467–546. doi: 10.1016/j.cpcardiol.2008.06.002 with permission Elsevier.

4.4 Supraventricular tachycardia

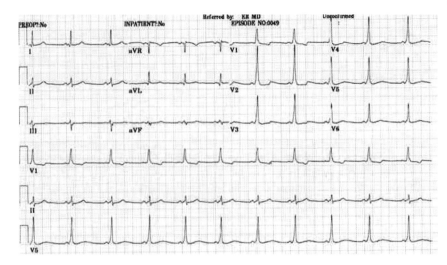

Figure 4.4.6 12-lead ECG demonstrating clear ventricular pre-excitation, with a strongly positive delta wave and R wave in lead V1 (wave-front moving from left to right across the chest leads suggests left sided) and a small negative delta wave in the lateral limb leads I and aVL (i.e. wave-front passes away from lateral LV wall) suggesting this is a left lateral AP

- Antidromic (~5% of AVRTs):
  - Antegrade (A to V) conduction occurs through an AP and retrograde (V to A) conduction occurs through the AV node
  - Usually a broad complex tachycardia as A to V conduction does not occur via the specialized conduction system
  - May be caused by an AP that conducts bi-directionally or antegradely only—in both cases, pre-excitation is likely to be present on the surface ECG during sinus rhythm

ECG features
- ECG features of manifest APs in sinus rhythm (see Figure 4.4.6):
  - Short PR interval
  - Broad QRS with delta waves
  - Often more obvious with right-sided pathways (AP closer to the SA node so the ventricle pre-excites earlier relative to left sided AP)
  - Localization of the AP can be estimated from the surface ECG, e.g. positive delta and R wave in V1 likely left sided as the ventricular depolarization wave-front moves from left to right across the chest leads (see Figure 4.4.6)
  - Relative conduction velocity of the AV node can influence the degree of pre-excitation, which can thus be intermittent (slicker AVN conduction means less pre-excitation)
- Orthdromic AVRT
  - Regular narrow complex tachycardia
  - Rate 150–250 bpm
  - Usually short RP interval
- Antidromic AVRT
  - Regular broad complex tachycardia
  - Rate may be rapid, up to 250 bpm
  - Usually long RP interval (retrograde V to A conduction is slow via the AV node)

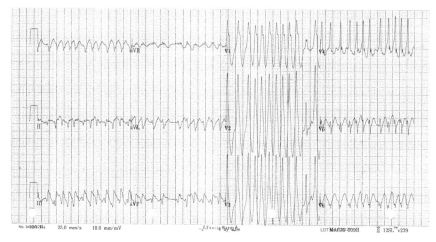

Figure 4.4.7 ECG showing pre-excited AF; note the short RR interval (shortest approx. 160 ms). V1 positive thus likely left sided AP (wave-front from left to right), and probably left lateral (negative in limb lead I)

- Pre-excited AF (see Figure 4.4.7)
    - Irregularly irregular broad complex tachycardia
    - Only occurs in patients with APs that are capable of antegrade conduction (manifest pathways)
    - Ventricular rate is dependent on the antegrade conduction properties of the AP—if the AP is capable of very rapid antegrade conduction (typically < 250 ms at EP study—see below) this can lead to VF and sudden cardiac death

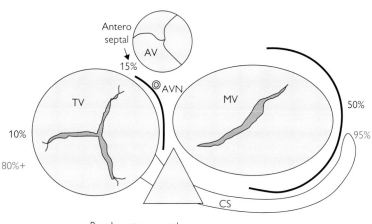

Figure 4.4.8 Schematic demonstrating the relative frequency of AP on the AV ring (black) along with the likelihood of successful ablation (dark grey). Note most pathways are left-sided and lateral. Antero-septal pathways are close to the normal conduction system and thus provide a challenge to treat with catheter ablation without causing harm

Modified with kind permission from Dr CB Pepper

Management
Acute management of AVRT
- Blockade of either the AV node or the AP to block part of the re-entry circuit, which should terminate the tachycardia
  - Vagal manoeuvres (e.g. blow into a 10 ml syringe)
  - Adenosine in escalating dose as required to achieve AV node blockade
    - Small risk of inducing AF with adenosine, with subsequent pre-excited AF and rapid ventricular rates—wise to keep a defibrillator nearby
  - Verapamil, diltiazem, and beta blockers may also be used to block the AV node but with caution in patients with manifest APs due to risk of pre-excited AF (see below)
  - Class 1 agents such as flecainide may also be used—preferentially block the AP rather than the AV node
- DC cardioversion if drug therapy fails

Long term management of AVRT
- Ablation of the AP is first line therapy in symptomatic patients with documented AVRT or palpitations that have not been captured and pre-excitation on their ECG (curative in ~90–95%); *class I[B]*
  - The location of the AP affects success rates at ablation (see Figure 4.4.8)
  - Main risk associated with APs that are close to the AV node is damage to the AV node causing AV block requiring a pacemaker (again an important consideration for younger patients)
- Pharmacological therapy for patients who cannot or choose not to undergo ablation:
  - Patients with pre-excitation on their resting ECG: oral flecainide or propafenone (if no ischaemic or structural heart disease); *class IIb [B]*
  - Patients without pre-excitation on their resting ECG: beta blockers, calcium channel blockers, or flecainide can safely be used; *class IIa [B]*

Acute management of pre-excited AF
- Usual ABC approach with prompt DCCV if evidence of haemodynamic compromise
- Flecainide may chemically cardiovert AF to SR and is safe to use in pre-excited AF as it will usually preferentially slow conduction via the AP and therefore slow the ventricular rate during AF. Flecainide has a class IIb indication in the ESC guidelines, while ibutilide and procainamide have a class IIa recommendation (in the UK, flecainide is the most commonly used agent)
- If flecainide fails—DCCV under conscious sedation
- AV node blocking drugs are *contraindicated*—may reduce conduction via the AV node and increase conduction via the AP, which can increase the ventricular rate and cause haemodynamic instability

Long term management of pre-excited AF
- Anticoagulation based on CHA_2DS_2-VASc score
- Ablation of the AP is the first-line management and is usually done as an inpatient following acute admission with pre-excited AF
- Pharmacological therapy for patients who cannot or choose not to undergo ablation involves either procainamide (*IIa[B]*) or flecainide (*IIb[B]*). Amiodarone is not recommended (*III[B]*)

Risk stratification
- Challenging but important as patients with APs that are capable of rapid antegrade conduction are at risk of sudden cardiac death (SCD) due to pre-excited AF with rapid ventricular rates that degenerate into VF
- Overall risk of SCD among all-comers with pre-excitation on ECG is low (0–0.39% per year in case series)
- There is no risk of SCD from concealed APs that can only conduct retrogradely
- There is a higher risk of SCD among patients with antegradely conducting APs and the following:
    - Proof of rapid antegrade conduction at EPS (shortest pre-excited RR interval < 250 ms)
    - Shortest RR interval < 200 ms during AF (i.e. HR > 300 bpm)
    - Inducible AVRT at EPS
    - Multiple APs
    - Documented AF and AVRT
    - Ebstein's anomaly
- Non-invasive tests such as exercise treadmill testing or drug challenges with flecainide/ajmaline are considered unreliable in the risk stratification of APs, but may be considered

Treatment strategy in asymptomatic pre-excited ECG
- Treatment strategy in asymptomatic pre-excited ECG (i.e. not WPW syndrome) is considered controversial:
    - EP study has not been routinely recommended unless patients are deemed to be in high-risk categories, though it is increasingly becoming routine in some centres due to the uncertainty in non-invasive risk stratification and the relatively low-risk nature of invasive EPS (< 1%)
    - 2019 ESC guidelines rate level of evidence for EPS (+/− catheter ablation if high risk features seen) for asymptomatic patients as *I[B]* for those with a high risk occupation or athletes, and *IIa[B]* for all others
- Initial evaluation of patients with echo to look for structural abnormalities such as Ebstein's anomaly, a period of monitoring to look at rate profile and asymptomatic AF, as well as a treadmill test to look for sudden disappearance of delta waves; these may give some information about risk stratification, but are poorly predictive (*IIb[B]*)
- Presence of multiple pathways, rapidly conducting AP, and inducibility of AVRT or AF during EPS are felt to be most predictive of future events, though none is perfect
- Current guidelines could be summarized as:
    - It is reasonable to offer an EP study for risk stratification to all (*ACC/AHA/ESC class IIa, level of evidence B*)
    - Ablation favoured if:
        - Documented arrhythmia (AF or AVRT)
        - High-risk features at EPS
        - Occupation threatened by diagnosis, e.g. pilots
        - LV impairment due to dyssynchrony induced by AP
    - Avoid ablation if:
        - Asymptomatic and none of above
        - Patient declines
        - High-risk of complications, e.g. anteroseptal pathways and minimal symptoms
    - Note that the risk of AV block is low with cryo-ablation

Special notes
Mahaim physiology
- A misnomer, but sometimes used to describe an AV bypass tract (accessory pathway) on the right side with decremental conduction properties acting as an accessory His–Purkinje system
- Presents with a broad QRS AVRT (usually LBBB, as inserts into the right ventricle)

Lown-Ganong-Levine syndrome
- Short PR interval and normal QRS (caused by a peri-nodal accessory pathway or enhanced AV nodal conduction)

Persistent junctional reciprocating tachycardia (PJRT)
- An incessant form of long RP tachycardia due to an atypical AV junction bypass tract (atypical as the AP has decremental retrograde conduction properties)
- ECG features are thus similar to AT and its relentless nature (due to a large excitatory gap) can result in tachycardiomyopathy if left untreated
- Most common in childhood, may be refractory to pharmacological therapy

N.B. Decremental conduction = the gradual decrease in the stimuli and response along a pathway of conduction

4.4.3 Electrophysiology study principles and invasive SVT management

- An EPS enables the identification and electrical mapping of both normal and abnormal circuits and pathways within the heart
- The typical EP study consists of insertion of two to four electrodes (within catheters), usually via the femoral veins
- Standard positions are the high right atrium, coronary sinus, His bundle, and the right ventricle, providing electrical insight into the:
  - Right atrium
  - Left atrium (and ventricle)
  - AV junction
  - Both ventricles (see Figure 4.4.9)
- Timing intervals between these sites are measured, with cycle lengths and timings expressed in milliseconds rather than beats per minute (600 ms is 100 bpm, 300 ms is 200 bpm, and so on)
- Different protocols and mapping are employed depending on the indication for the EPS and detailed discussion of these is beyond the scope of this chapter
- Common protocols involve either programmed stimulation with burst pacing; a drive train of 8–10 beats at a fixed cycle length of ~< 100 ms of the intrinsic cycle length, or an extra-stimulus technique; a drive train of 6–10 fixed cycle length stimuli with an added on extra-stimulus at the end (S1–S2 protocol)
- The extra-stimulus at the end (the S2) can be brought forward by 10–20 ms until the refractory period (P) is reached (known as decremental coupling intervals); additional extra-stimuli (S3 or S4) can also be added, for example in VT stimulation studies
- The ECG and intracardiac electrogram recordings used during an EPS are viewed at a slower rate than conventional surface ECGs, and so QRS complexes appear broader

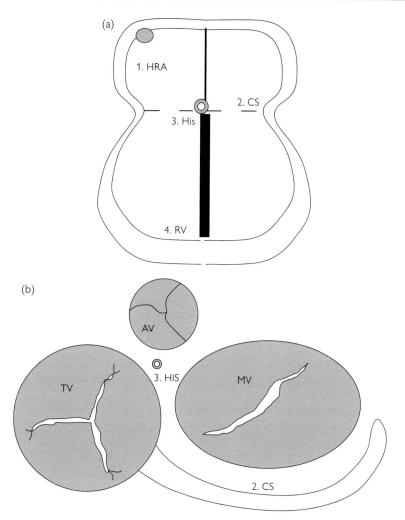

Figure 4.4.9 Schematic of four-chamber heart and AV ring, demonstrating typical positions of diagnostic EP catheters. (HRA = high right atrium, CS = coronary sinus, RV = right ventricle, AV = aortic valve, TV = tricuspid valve, MV = mitral valve)

EPS features of AVNRT

- Figure 4.4.10 demonstrates the dual AV node physiology (fast pathway and slow pathway) that is required for AVNRT
- Pacing is delivered in the RA or the LA (via coronary sinus catheter) with a progressively shorter cycle length (i.e. progressively faster bpm, or atrial pacing with 10 ms decremental coupling intervals of the extra-stimulus)
- This leads to atrial activation with AV conduction via both the fast and slow pathways, with a short AH (atrium to His) interval due to rapid conduction via the fast pathway (the His signal in Figure 4.4.10 is best appreciated on the His 1–2 channel)
- Remember, the fast pathway depolarizes more quickly but **repolarizes more slowly** than the slow pathway

4.4 Supraventricular tachycardia

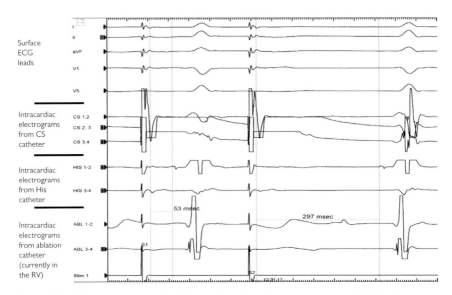

Figure 4.4.10 EP study demonstrating AH jump (jump from fast to slow pathway). A1H1=53ms, A2H2=297ms. Note echo beat representing retrograde fast pathway activation on last recorded electrogram. CS=coronary sinus catheter, His=His catheter, ABL=ablation catheter (in right ventricle)

- Eventually, an RA pacing spike is delivered that reaches the AV node while the fast pathway is still refractory, but the slow pathway is not. The fast pathway therefore cannot conduct, but the slow pathway can
- This leads to an 'AH jump'—a sudden lengthening of the AH interval (normally needs to be > 50 ms)—as conduction from A to H is now dependent on the slow pathway. In Figure 4.4.10, the AH interval increases from 53 msec to 297 msec

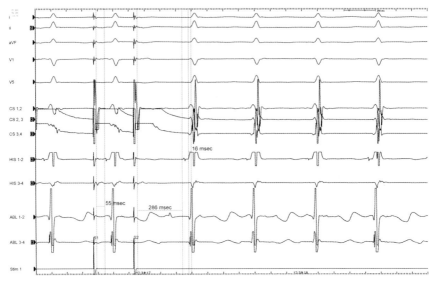

Figure 4.4.11 Initiation of AVNRT with AH jump. A1H1=55ms, A2H2=286ms, VA time=16ms. CS=coronary sinus catheter, His=His catheter, ABL=ablation catheter in right ventricle

- This finding means dual AVN physiology is present but does not necessarily mean the clinical tachycardia is AVNRT (the AH interval is the time it takes the atrial impulse to travel to and through the AVN)
- A diagnostic feature of AVNRT is initiation of tachycardia following a critical interval with an 'AH jump'
- Figure 4.4.11 demonstrates initiation of an AVNRT during EPS, following another AH jump

3D electro-anatomic mapping

- One of the most significant advances in cardiac EP was the evolution of 3D electro-anatomic mapping (EAM) techniques, which allows recording of the intra-cardiac electrical activation and propagation in relation to anatomical structures
- These rapidly evolving systems have been proven to reduce radiation dose (fluoroscopy time) and procedure time as well as increasing the success rates of more complex procedures
- Commonly used mapping systems include:

CARTO® (Biosense Webster – example in Figure 4.4.12)

Function: magnetic sensor in catheter tip allows localization within external magnetic field

Strengths: accurate reconstruction and activation mapping; user-friendly propagation maps; simultaneous anatomic, activation, and voltage acquisition; scar and tagging functions

Weaknesses: Only compatible with own brand diagnostic and ablation catheters, limited utility for non-sustained arrhythmia

EnSite NavX® (St Jude Medical)

Function: catheter located through voltage impedance changes relative to skin patches

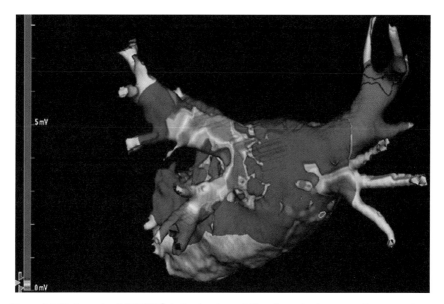

Figure 4.4.12 Example of CARTO® derived endocardially collected voltage map demonstrating regions of left atrial scar

(Taken from http://what-when-how.com/cardiac-arrhythmias-new-considerations/novel-technologies-for-mapping-and-ablation-of-complex-arrhythmias-electrophysiology-study-of-the-heart-mapping-procedure-cardiac-arrhythmias-part-2/)

Strengths: accurate anatomical reconstruction; ability to locate and display multiple catheters at once; compatibility with any catheter; simultaneous multi-electrode collection of activation, voltage, and anatomical mapping

Weaknesses: limited utility with non-sustained arrhythmia, prone to reference shift

EnSite Array; non-contact mapping (St Jude Medical)

Function: a balloon covered in 64 electrodes producing high-density virtual unipolar array to rapidly map electrical signals off a single beat; 'non-contact mapping'

Strengths: useful in non-sustained or poorly tolerated arrhythmia

Weaknesses: accuracy depends on activation being within a certain distance from the balloon; prone to reference shifts; balloon can be obtrusive to ablation if small chamber

Further reading

Brignole M, Moya A, de Lange FJ, Deharo JC, Elliott PM, Fanciulli A, Fedorowski A, Furlan R, Kenny RA, Martín A, Probst V, Reed MJ, Rice CP, Sutton R, Ungar A, van Dijk JG; ESC Scientific Document Group. 2018 ESC Guidelines for the diagnosis and management of syncope. *Eur Heart J*. 2018 Jun 1;39(21):1883–948. doi: 10.1093/eurheartj/ehy037. PMID: 29562304

Brugada J, Katritsis DG, Arbelo E, Arribas F, Bax JJ, Blomström-Lundqvist C, Calkins H, Corrado D, Deftereos SG, Diller GP, Gomez-Doblas JJ, Gorenek B, Grace A, Ho SY, Kaski JC, Kuck KH, Lambiase PD, Sacher F, Sarquella-Brugada G, Suwalski P, Zaza A; ESC Scientific Document Group. 2019 ESC Guidelines for the management of patients with supraventricular tachycardia. The Task Force for the management of patients with supraventricular tachycardia of the European Society of Cardiology (ESC). *Eur Heart J*. 2020 Feb 1;41(5):655–720. doi: 10.1093/eurheartj/ehz467. PMID: 31504425

Echt DS, Liebson PR, Mitchell LB, Peters RW, Obias-Manno D, Barker AH, Arensberg D, Baker A, Friedman L, Greene HL, et al. Mortality and morbidity in patients receiving encainide, flecainide, or placebo. The Cardiac Arrhythmia Suppression Trial. *N Engl J Med*. 1991 Mar 21;324(12):781–8. doi: 10.1056/NEJM199103213241201. PMID: 1900101

Issa ZF, Miller JM, Zipes DP. *Clinical Arrhythmology and Electrophysiology*, 2nd edn. Elsevier, 2012.

Nielsen AO, Pedersen L, Sode BF, Dahl M. β-blocker therapy and risk of chronic obstructive pulmonary disease—A Danish nationwide study of 1·3 million individuals. *EClinicalMedicine*. 2019 Jan 29;7:21–6. doi: 10.1016/j.eclinm.2019.01.004. PMID: 31193622; PMCID: PMC6537528

4.5

Atrial fibrillation

Kim Rajappan and Dan Raine

TABLE OF CONTENTS
4.5.1 Definition 355
4.5.2 Classification 355
4.5.3 Epidemiology 356
4.5.4 Associated morbidity and mortality 356
4.5.5 Natural history and pathophysiology 357
4.5.6 Pre-disposing conditions 357
4.5.7 Diagnostic assessment 358
4.5.8 Management 359
   Anticoagulation 359
   Risk factor modification 361
   Rate control 361
   Rhythm control 362
   Catheter ablation 364
   Surgical/hybrid ablation 365
4.5.9 Special situations 366
   Wolff–Parkinson–White syndrome 366
   Pregnancy 366
   Post-operative AF 367
   Familial atrial fibrillation 367
4.5.10 Atrial fibrillation summary 367

4.5.1 Definition

- A supraventricular tachyarrhythmia with uncoordinated atrial electrical activation and consequently ineffective atrial contraction
- On the surface ECG, AF is characterized by irregularly irregular R–R intervals, absence of distinct repeating P waves, and/or irregular atrial activation (Figure 4.5.1). ECG documentation is required to establish a *clinical* diagnosis, which can include a single-lead ECG tracing
- Patients can be asymptomatic or can experience symptoms including chest pain, palpitations, dyspnoea, fatigue, and dizziness
- Atrial high rate episodes (AHRE) or subclinical AF refer to episodes detected through cardiac implanted electronic devices, or wearable technologies suggesting AF, but not yet confirmed on ECG

4.5.2 Classification

- AF can be classified into five categories based on the clinical presentation and arrhythmia duration:
   1. *First diagnosed AF*: Irrespective of arrhythmia duration and symptomatic burden
   2. *Paroxysmal AF*: Self-terminating episodes (last > 30 s and usually cardioverts within 48 hours but can last up to 7 days)
   3. *Persistent AF*: Episodes last longer than 7 days including those that are terminated by pharmacological or electrical cardioversion (after ≥ 7 days)

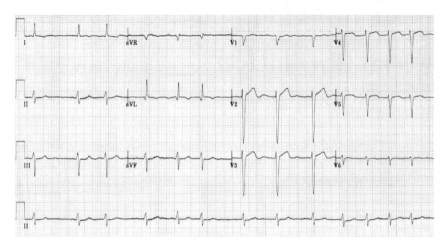

Figure 4.5.1 12 lead ECG demonstrating atrial fibrillation
Image taken from LITFL: https://litfl.com/atrial-fibrillation-ecg-library/

4. *Long-standing Persistent AF:* Continuous AF lasting ≥ 12 months when it has been decided to pursue a rhythm control strategy
5. *Permanent AF:* AF accepted by patient and physician—'rate control strategy'

4.5.3 Epidemiology

- AF is the most common sustained cardiac arrhythmia encountered in clinical practice and affects 1–2% of the general population
- Among people of European descent, the lifetime risk of developing AF after age 40 is 26% for men and 23% for women
- Modifiable risk factors include hypertension, diabetes mellitus, obesity, endurance exercise, obstructive sleep apnoea, thyroid disease, and alcohol consumption
- Non-modifiable risk factors include age, sex, family history, race, chronic kidney disease, and other types of heart and valvular disease

4.5.4 Associated morbidity and mortality

- AF is associated with increased mortality (predominantly cardiovascular) due to sudden death, heart failure, or stroke. It is also associated with increased hospitalization
- The overall rate of ischaemic stroke in patients with non-valvular AF is approximately 5% per year, which is two to seven times greater than in patients in sinus rhythm
- 20–30% of strokes are attributed to AF and stroke may be the initial presentation of AF
- Quality of life is impaired in AF independent of other cardiovascular conditions
- Impaired left ventricular systolic function is found in 20–30% of patients with AF
- AF may be the cause of LVSD, especially in the setting of an uncontrolled ventricular rate, or may be a manifestation of an underlying cardiomyopathy
- Cognitive decline and vascular dementia can develop in patients with AF even in the presence of anticoagulation. The proposed mechanism is recurrent thromboembolism which is reflected as white matter lesions on cerebral imaging

4.5.5 Natural history and pathophysiology

- The pathophysiology of AF is complex and involves multiple factors including:
    - *Triggers*, which are responsible for initiating AF
    - A *substrate*, which is necessary for AF maintenance
    - And *perpetuators*, which underline the progression of the arrhythmia from paroxysmal to persistent forms
- The trigger mechanisms include focal enhanced automaticity and triggered activity secondary to intracellular calcium dysregulation
- The muscular sleeves of the pulmonary veins are the commonest location for focal triggers that initiate and/or sustain AF
- Activation of the parasympathetic and sympathetic nervous system also plays a role in maintaining AF
- The concept of 'AF begets AF' remains a cornerstone in our understanding of the natural history of AF progression; whereby an increasing AF burden is associated with progressive atrial remodelling which can contribute to the persistence of AF
- Persistent AF leads to electrical, structural, and contractile remodelling of the atria via oxidative stress, inflammation, myofibroblast activation, and atrial dilatation
- Electrical remodelling correlates with shortening and increased dispersion of atrial refractory periods which contributes to the persistence of AF
- Remodelling can be electrical (e.g. changes in action potential duration) but later in the process can be structural (e.g. fibrosis), involving shortening of the atrial action potential duration and refractoriness. This may prevent calcium overload-induced cell death but the reduction in wave length contributes to AF recurrence
- Reduced atrial contractile function persists for several weeks after restoration of sinus rhythm ('atrial stunning') and is a reason to maintain anticoagulation in the first weeks after cardioversion
- AF also induces atrial fibrosis resulting in slowed conduction and electrical isolation of atrial cardiomyocytes, further maintaining AF or provoking recurrence
- Chronic dilatation of the atria secondary to chronic pressure or volume overload may induce the structural changes that predispose to AF, e.g. secondary to valvular disease or heart failure
- High-level endurance sports may predispose to AF via chronic atrial dilatation
- Protein mutations seen in inherited cardiomyopathies such as the long and short QT syndromes may cause AF

4.5.6 Pre-disposing conditions

- **Hypertension**—occurs in approximately two-thirds of patients. ACE inhibitors and ARBs most effective in preventing incident AF in hypertensive patients
- **Heart failure**—30% of AF patients NYHA class II–IV. AF is found in 30–40% of heart failure patients (50% of NYHA IV patients). May be cause or consequence of AF, and ACEi and BBs may prevent new-onset AF
- **Tachycardia-cardiomyopathy**—LV dysfunction caused by AF with fast ventricular response; LV function may be restored with adequate rate control or return to sinus rhythm
- **Valvular heart disease**—especially mitral stenosis and mitral regurgitation. Some degree of valvular disease in 30% of AF patients

- **Cardiomyopathies**—high risk of AF. Includes hypertrophic cardiomyopathy, dilated cardiomyopathy, arrhythmogenic right ventricular cardiomyopathy as well as 'channelopathies' such as long and short QT syndromes and Brugada syndrome
- **Atrial septal defects (ASDs)**—associated with AF in 10–15% of patients. AF may be due to pressure and volume overload due to septal defect itself or common abnormality, e.g. genetic cause
- **Other congenital defects**—patients with single ventricles, atrial repair, transposition of the great arteries, or Fontan procedure are at especially high risk of AF
- **Coronary artery disease**—present in 20% of AF patients. Unclear if CAD itself predisposes to AF—association may be secondary to other shared risk factors, e.g. heart failure, hypertension. AF indicates poor prognosis after MI
- **Obesity**—25% of AF patients
- **Chronic kidney disease**—present in 10–15% of patients
- **Diabetes mellitus**—20% of AF patients
- **COPD**—10–15% of AF patients
- **Sleep apnoea**—associated with increased atrial pressure and dilatation
- **Thyroid dysfunction**—hyperthyroidism and hypothyroidism may cause AF

4.5.7 Diagnostic assessment

- Comprehensive medical history and examination, assessing for:
    - Concomitant conditions associated with AF (outlined above), e.g. thyroid disease, hypertension, valvular heart disease, and diabetes mellitus
    - AF pattern and symptoms; AF can have a significant impact on quality of life scores, and use of the modified EHRA symptom scale (see Table 4.5.1) is recommended in clinical practice and research studies to quantify AF-related symptoms (*Class I [C]*)
    - Assessment of stroke risk
    - AF related complications, e.g. LV dysfunction, thromboembolism
- 12-lead ECG:
    - Look for evidence of structural or pre-existing conduction disease such as ischaemic changes suggestive of previous MI, LVH, bundle branch block, ventricular pre-excitation, cardiomyopathy, and other arrhythmias that may provoke AF

Table 4.5.1 Modified European Heart Rhythm Association AF symptom scale.

Modified EHRA Score	Symptoms	Description
1	None	Asymptomatic
2A	Mild	Normal daily activity not affected
2B	Moderate	Normal daily activity not affected but patient troubled by symptoms
3	Severe	Normal daily activity affected
4	Disabling	Normal daily activity discontinued

Wynn GJ, Todd DM, Webber M, Bonnett L, McShane J, Kirchhof P, Gupta D. The European Heart Rhythm Association symptom classification for atrial fibrillation: validation and improvement through a simple modification. *Europace*. 2014 Jul;16(7):965–72. doi: 10.1093/europace/eut395. © European Society of Cardiology. With permission from Oxford University Press

- Opportunistic screening for silent AF is important and cost-effective, particularly in older populations (age > 65 years)
- Transthoracic echo to guide management:
  - Atrial dimensions, LV function, valvular heart disease
  - Structural heart disease both increases risk of AF developing, and reduces the likelihood of a successful rhythm-control strategy
- Holter monitoring—diagnosis of paroxysmal AF, or for assessment of ventricular rate control in persistent AF
  - By accepted convention, an episode lasting at least 30 seconds is diagnostic
- Blood tests—full blood count, renal and thyroid function, BNP, coagulation profile
- Exercise testing—to determine ventricular rate control during exercise in symptomatic patients with normal resting heart rate

4.5.8 Management

- AF management combines treatments with prognostic benefit (anticoagulation and treatment of co-existing cardiovascular conditions) and symptomatic benefit (rate and rhythm control)
- It is recommended that this is a multidisciplinary, integrated approach which includes shared decision making with the patient and incorporate the relative risks and benefits of various interventions depending on individual patient comorbidities and symptom burden
  - As highlighted, the presence of coexistent structural heart disease both increases the risk of AF, and reduces the likelihood of a successful rhythm-control strategy
- This has been recently summarized as ABC—**A**nticoagulation/**A**void stroke, **B**etter symptom management, and **C**ardiovascular and **C**omorbidity optimization

Anticoagulation

- Oral anticoagulation can prevent the majority of ischaemic strokes in patients with AF and has been shown to increase life expectancy
- It is superior to no treatment or aspirin and the clinical benefit is almost universal with the exception of patients at very low stroke risk
- The introduction of the CHA_2DS_2-VASc score has simplified the decision-making process for starting anticoagulation in patients with AF (see Table 4.5.2)
- In general, patients without clinical risk factors for stroke do not need anticoagulation, whilst patients with stroke risk factors (i.e. CHA_2DS_2-VASc score of ≥ 1 for men and ≥ 2 for women) are likely to benefit from anticoagulation (see Table 4.5.3)
- The potential benefits of anticoagulation should be balanced against the patients' bleeding risk (which can be assessed using risk scores such as HAS-BLED)
- Stroke and bleeding risk scores overlap and a high bleeding risk score should not generally necessitate withholding anticoagulation. Rather, modifiable bleeding risk factors, e.g. uncontrolled hypertension, labile INR, concurrent medication predisposing to bleeding (e.g. antiplatelet drugs and non-steroidal anti-inflammatories), and excess alcohol intake should be addressed
- Non-vitamin K antagonist oral anticoagulants (NOACs) including the direct thrombin inhibitor dabigatran and the factor Xa inhibitors (apixaban, rivaroxaban, and edoxaban) are suitable alternatives to vitamin K antagonists (e.g. warfarin) for stroke prevention in AF. These act at different points in the coagulation cascade
- A meta-analysis of the pivotal studies of warfarin vs higher-dose NOACs showed that NOACs reduced the risk of stroke or systemic embolism by 19% compared to warfarin,

Table 4.5.2 CHA$_2$DS$_2$-VASc Score comprising clinical risk factors for stroke, transient ischaemic attack, and systemic thromboembolism.

Risk Factor	Points
Congestive Heart Failure	1
Hypertension	1
Age ≥ 75 years	2
Diabetes Mellitus	1
Previous **S**troke, Transient Ischaemic Attack, or Thromboembolism	2
Vascular disease (previous myocardial infarction, peripheral artery disease or aortic plaque	1
Age 65–74 years	1
Sex (female)	1

Hindricks G, Potpara T, Dagres N, et al; ESC Scientific Document Group. 2020 ESC Guidelines for the diagnosis and management of atrial fibrillation developed in collaboration with the European Association for Cardio-Thoracic Surgery (EACTS): The Task Force for the diagnosis and management of atrial fibrillation of the European Society of Cardiology (ESC) Developed with the special contribution of the European Heart Rhythm Association (EHRA) of the ESC. *Eur Heart J.* 2021 Feb 1;42(5):373–498. doi: 10.1093/eurheartj/ehaa612. © European Society of Cardiology. With permission from Oxford University Press

which was driven by a significant reduction in haemorrhagic stroke. Mortality was 10% lower in patients on NOACs and intracranial haemorrhage was halved, whilst gastrointestinal bleeding was more frequent (RR 1.25)
- NOACs are therefore recommended in preference to warfarin in patients with non-valvular AF who are eligible for a NOAC. However, warfarin is recommended for stroke prevention in patients with moderate-to-severe mitral stenosis or mechanical heart valves in light of the elevated risk of thromboembolism observed with NOACs in this patient cohort
- Percutaneous **left atrial appendage occlusion** is non-inferior to warfarin for stroke prevention in AF patients with moderate stroke risk and is associated with a lower bleeding

Table 4.5.3 Adjusted stroke rate according to CHA$_2$DS$_2$-VASc score.

CHA$_2$DS$_2$-VASc Score	Patients (n = 7329)	Adjusted stroke rate (%/year)
0	1	0
1	422	1.3
2	1230	2.2
3	1730	3.2
4	1718	4
5	1159	6.7
6	679	9.8
7	294	9.6
8	82	6.7
9	14	15.2

Hindricks G, Potpara T, Dagres N, et al; ESC Scientific Document Group. 2020 ESC Guidelines for the diagnosis and management of atrial fibrillation developed in collaboration with the European Association for Cardio-Thoracic Surgery (EACTS): The Task Force for the diagnosis and management of atrial fibrillation of the European Society of Cardiology (ESC) Developed with the special contribution of the European Heart Rhythm Association (EHRA) of the ESC. *Eur Heart J.* 2021 Feb 1;42(5):373–498. doi: 10.1093/eurheartj/ehaa612. © European Society of Cardiology. With permission from Oxford University Press

risk. It is currently reserved for patients with a high bleeding risk and/or contraindication to oral anticoagulant therapy
- Antiplatelet monotherapy is not recommended for stroke prevention in AF patients, regardless of stroke risk

Warfarin
- Warfarin inhibits the synthesis of vitamin K-dependent clotting factors as well as coagulation regulators protein C, protein S, and protein Z
- It is important to note that during initial commencement of warfarin therapy, there is a paradoxical prothrombotic effect due to a reduction in the levels of endogenous antithrombotic factors protein C and protein S. This can be mitigated by use of low doses or brief cover with other anticoagulation therapy; commonly low molecular weight heparin (LMWH)
- Warfarin is also commonly used for anticoagulation following implantation of metallic prosthetic valves. No other anticoagulant types are licensed for this indication, although intravenous unfractionated heparin (UFH) is commonly used. Limited evidence suggests weight-adjusted (usually twice-daily) dosing of LMWH is likely to be as safe as UFH
- Warfarin metabolism varies significantly between individuals and is affected by genetic factors, other medications, foods, and the level of serum-albumin binding
- Warfarin is dependent on hepatic CYP metabolism and therefore subject to interactions with CYP inhibitors or inducers

Risk factor modification
- Modifiable risk factors associated with AF are:

• Obesity	• Diabetes Mellitus
• Obstructive Sleep Apnoea	• Alcohol
• Hypertension	• Endurance Training

- These modifiable risk factors share a common pathophysiology in that they all cause electrical and structural remodelling in the atria which increases the likelihood of AF initiation and persistence
- The ARREST-AF cohort study evaluated the impact of weight loss and risk factor management in patients undergoing catheter ablation for AF. In this observational study, aggressive management of risk factors associated with AF resulted in an improvement in AF symptoms and a fivefold greater likelihood of maintaining sinus rhythm following catheter ablation over a 42-month follow-up period
- Interrogation for clinical signs of obstructive sleep apnoea should be considered in all AF patients

Rate control
- Ventricular rate control is an integral part of AF management and is often associated with a significant improvement in AF-related symptoms
- Lenient rate control (i.e. resting heart rate < 110 bpm) is recommended initially based on the results of the RACE II trial, which reported no difference in clinical events between patients with persistent AF who were randomized to strict (< 80 bpm at rest and < 110 bpm during moderate exercise) vs lenient rate control
- Beta blockers (BBs) or rate limiting calcium-channel antagonists (e.g. diltiazem/verapamil) are recommended first line due to their rapid onset of action and effectiveness at high sympathetic tone (Figure 4.5.2)

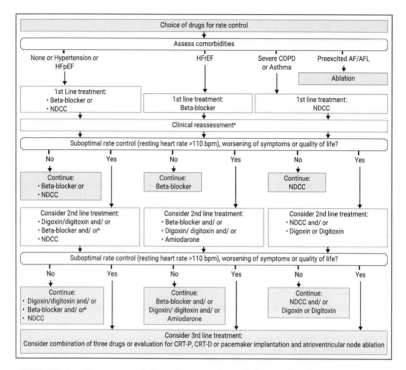

Figure 4.5.2 Choice of rate control drugs (HFrEF = heart failure with reduced ejection fraction, HFpEF = heart failure with preserved ejection fraction, AFL = atrial flutter, COPD = chronic obstructive pulmonary disease, NDCC = non dihydropyridine calcium channel blockers, CRT-P/D = cardiac resynchronisation therapy pacemaker / defibrillator)

Hindricks G, Potpara T, Dagres N, et al; ESC Scientific Document Group. 2020 ESC Guidelines for the diagnosis and management of atrial fibrillation developed in collaboration with the European Association for Cardio-Thoracic Surgery (EACTS): The Task Force for the diagnosis and management of atrial fibrillation of the European Society of Cardiology (ESC) Developed with the special contribution of the European Heart Rhythm Association (EHRA) of the ESC. *Eur Heart J.* 2021 Feb 1;42(5):373–498. doi: 10.1093/eurheartj/ehaa612. © European Society of Cardiology. With permission from Oxford University Press

- BBs are probably better for thyrotoxic or post-MI patients
- Diltiazem and verapamil should be avoided in patients with impaired left ventricular systolic function due to their negative inotropic effects (EF < 40%)
- Digoxin can be added to BBs or rate limiting CCBs if satisfactory rate control has not been achieved in the presence of normal or impaired LV function, but is mostly effective on resting heart rate only. It has no role in AF if SR is restored
- Avoid AV nodal-blocking drugs in those with pre-excitation as they will have no effect on the accessory pathway (use i.v. sodium channel blockers, such as flecainide, instead)
- Amiodarone can be used for both rhythm and rate control in patients who are critically ill or have acute decompensated heart failure

Rhythm control

- A rhythm control strategy is indicated for patients with AF predominantly to reduce AF-related symptoms and improve quality of life
- To date, all trials comparing rhythm versus rate control with appropriate anticoagulation in patients with AF have yielded neutral outcomes, predominantly using cardioversion or antiarrhythmic medication for rhythm control

- The EAST-AFNET 4 and CABANA trials investigated whether early comprehensive rhythm control therapy in the form of catheter ablation and antiarrhythmic drugs leads to a reduction in major cardiovascular events. Results from CABANA showed no overall mortality/morbidity benefit at 5 years from ablation, however sub-analyses of the data suggest there may be some benefit, and this was a single-blinded study with a reasonable amount of cross-over between groups which will have impacted the results
- Ablation in some patients with heart failure with reduced ejection fraction may have significant mortality benefits and reduce hospitalization (CASTLE-AF study)
- In the short term (if AF onset < 24 h) two-thirds will spontaneously revert to sinus rhythm
- Pharmacological cardioversion restores sinus rhythm in approximately 50% of patients with recent onset AF:
  - **Flecainide** and **propafenone** are effective but their use is restricted to patients *without structural heart disease*. These should be prescribed in combination with an AV-blocking drug to prevent fast ventricular rates if atrial flutter occurs. 'Pill in the pocket' strategy, using flecainide or propafenone loading doses within 5 min of PAF onset, has been shown to reduce hospitalizations
  - **Amiodarone** can be used in patients with ischaemic heart disease and/or heart failure
  - **Ibutilide** (class III antiarrhythmic) has been shown to cardiovert around 50% of recent onset AF patients within 90 min but is more effective at converting atrial flutter
  - **Sotalol** not effective for acute cardioversion. It may facilitate conversion to sinus rhythm but can cause Torsades de Pointes
- Electrical cardioversion restores sinus rhythm faster and more effectively than antiarrhythmic drugs and is associated with shorter hospitalization
  - It is the method of choice in patients with new-onset AF associated with haemodynamic compromise
  - The higher the impedance, the less current delivered, and transthoracic impedance is determined by body habitus, skin/electrode interface, and position of electrode paddles
  - Antero-posterior paddle position may be more successful at electrically cardioverting patients than the sterno-apical position
  - If cardioversion is unsuccessful with maximum energy in both positions, reconsider appropriateness of rhythm control strategy. If appropriate to pursue, consider using antiarrhythmic therapy before a further attempt as this is evidenced to increase success rates (e.g. if an elective patient, consider loading with flecainide or oral amiodarone and returning in 4 to 6 weeks for further attempt)
  - Unless < 48 hours from definite AF episode onset patients should have ≥ 3 weeks of anticoagulation pre-DCCV, or a TOE to assess for LA clot
  - All patients should have 4 weeks of anticoagulation post-DCCV regardless of stroke risk (due to 'atrial stunning' discussed previously)
  - AF recurrence risks are higher in the first months post cardioversion and antiarrhythmics should therefore be continued in patients at high risk of recurrence
  - Factors increasing recurrence risk are age, increased duration of AF prior to cardioversion, previous recurrences, structural heart disease (in particular increased LA size or reduced LV function), and underlying cardiac disease
- In the longer-term, maintenance of SR in patients who have demonstrated preponderance to AF is challenging and success rates can be low—after cardioversion around 25–50% patients will have a recurrence of AF within 1–2 months and thereafter the recurrence rate is approximately 10% per year
- Antiarrhythmic drug therapy approximately doubles the likelihood of maintaining sinus rhythm compared with no therapy. However, there is no appreciable effect on mortality or the incidence of cardiovascular events, and therefore the decision to initiate long-term

4.5 Atrial fibrillation

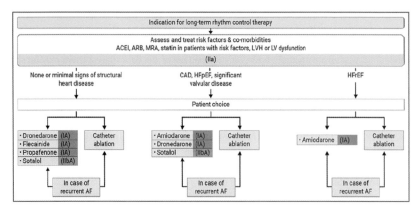

Figure 4.5.3 Long-term rhythm control therapy (ACEi = Angiotensin-converting-enzyme inhibitor, ARB = angiotensin receptor blocker, MRA = mineralocorticoid receptor antagonist, CAD = coronary artery disease)

Reproduced from Hindricks G, Potpara T, Dagres N, et al; ESC Scientific Document Group. 2020 ESC Guidelines for the diagnosis and management of atrial fibrillation developed in collaboration with the European Association for Cardio-Thoracic Surgery (EACTS): The Task Force for the diagnosis and management of atrial fibrillation of the European Society of Cardiology (ESC) Developed with the special contribution of the European Heart Rhythm Association (EHRA) of the ESC. *Eur Heart J.* 2021 Feb 1;42(5):373–498. doi: 10.1093/eurheartj/ehaa612. © European Society of Cardiology. With permission from Oxford University Press

antiarrhythmic drug therapy should take into account the symptomatic burden of AF as well as patient preferences and possible drug side effects
- The choice of antiarrhythmic drug is dependent on the relative safety of the drug, cardiovascular comorbidity, and patient choice (Figure 4.5.3)
- ECG recording during the initiation of antiarrhythmic drug therapy should be considered to monitor heart rate, detect QRS and QT interval prolongation, and the occurrence of AV block
- In practice, BBs are often used as first-line therapy because of their safety, their AV node effect during AF with fast ventricular response, and, in those with CCF, BBs may reduce the incidence of new onset AF. They may be slightly better than placebo at preventing AF recurrence post cardioversion, and there is no evidence that any one BB is better than another for prevention of AF

Catheter ablation

- Since the seminal paper by Haissaguerre et al. describing the role of triggered activity from the muscular sleeves of the pulmonary veins in initiating paroxysmal AF, catheter ablation has developed from an experimental procedure into a common treatment for symptomatic AF
- Catheter ablation is effective in restoring and maintaining sinus rhythm in patients with symptomatic paroxysmal and persistent AF and is generally used as a second-line treatment after failure of or intolerance to antiarrhythmic drug therapy. In such patients, catheter ablation is more effective than antiarrhythmic drug therapy
- In experienced high-volume centres, complication rates are similar with catheter ablation and antiarrhythmic drugs and therefore catheter ablation can be offered as a first-line treatment for symptomatic paroxysmal AF, especially in the setting of a structurally normal heart
- Pulmonary vein isolation (PVI) is the cornerstone of catheter ablation for AF and can be achieved by wide area circumferential ablation using radiofrequency energy, cryoballoon, or more recently pulsed-field ablation with similar reported outcomes. Given access to the left atrium is required, procedures involve a trans-septal puncture from right to left atrium
- PVI was initially shown to be beneficial in patients with PAF. Success rates vary between 70–90% according to department experience, with 30% of patients requiring a second procedure.

More recently, PVI alone has also been shown to be non-inferior to more extensive ablation strategies in patients with persistent AF. Success rates are lower in patients with persistent AF (50–80% depending on arrhythmia duration and burden of left atrial fibrosis) with 50% of patients requiring a second procedure
- Insufficient data is currently available to recommend the routine use of left atrial substrate ablation strategies (i.e. linear ablation, complex fractionated atrial electrograms (CFAEs), ganglionic plexi, dominant frequency mapping and rotors) in addition to PVI as a first procedure for patients with persistent AF. However, these adjunctive strategies can be considered in patients with recurrent AF after the initial ablation procedure and in those with extensive left atrial fibrosis identified at the first ablation procedure
- In a systematic review of 83,236 patients who had undergone catheter ablation for AF, Gupta et al. reported a 2.9% incidence of peri-procedural complications. The most important severe complications are stroke (< 1%), cardiac tamponade (1–2%), atrio-oesophageal fistula (< 0.5%) and death (< 0.2%). Less severe complications include vascular injury (1–2%), pulmonary vein stenosis (< 1%), and persistent phrenic nerve palsy (1–2%) which is more commonly observed with cryoballoon therapy

Pacemaker and AV node ablation

- A 'Pace and Ablate' strategy (which combines pacemaker implantation and ablation of the AV node) can also be used, although this should be reserved for patients who have ongoing AF-related symptoms despite pharmacological attempts at rhythm and/or rate control as it is irreversible and renders the patient pacing dependent.
- The choice of pacing therapy (right ventricular vs biventricular) depends on the patient's individual characteristics and left ventricular function (see sections 4.3 and 4.10 for further details)

Drugs post left atrial ablation

- AF or atrial tachycardia incidence is 45% in first 3 months after LA ablation despite antiarrhythmic medication
- Early recurrence may be transient and related to inflammation secondary to radiofrequency injury and may subside after 3 months when the inflammation has resolved and autonomic regulation has been restored
- Thus antiarrhythmic therapy is often used for the first 1–3 months post ablation and is associated with a 30% increase chance of remaining in sinus rhythm
- Should continue anticoagulation post ablation for a minimum of 2 months and then maintain if CHA_2DS_2-VASc score ≥ 2

Surgical/hybrid ablation

- The Cox Maze III 'cut and sew' procedure involves creating surgical incisions to divide the atria into smaller compartments to abort or block potential anatomical re-entrant circuits so that AF cannot be initiated or maintained (Figure 4.5.4)
- Prasad et al. reported that 76% of patients maintained sinus rhythm off antiarrhythmic drugs at 5-year follow-up following the Cox Maze III procedure; however there is a higher incidence of permanent pacemaker implantation (OR 1.26, 95% CI 1.07–1.49)
- AF surgery was originally reserved for patients undergoing concomitant cardiac surgery although advances in radiofrequency and cryoablation technology have made it possible to perform safely and effectively via a mini-thoracotomy approach
- To facilitate the creation of durable transmural ablation lesions, hybrid strategies have emerged which combine surgical epicardial and catheter based endocardial ablation. Preliminary experience has shown promise although the procedural time and rates of bleeding complication are higher
- Hybrid AF procedures combine a minimally invasive epicardial non-sternotomy ablation (not requiring cardiopulmonary bypass) with a percutaneous endocardial approach. They can be

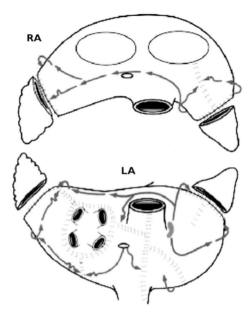

Figure 4.5.4 Original cut-and-sew Cox Maze procedure III. RA (right atrium): Excision of right atrial appendage, free wall incision, linear incision from superior vena cava to inferior vena cava (IVC) and from IVC to tricuspid valve annulus. LA (left atrium): Excision of left atrial appendage, pulmonary vein encirclement with extension to mitral valve annulus, and atrial septal incision

Reproduced from Weimar T, Schena S, Bailey MS, Maniar HS, Schuessler RB, Cox JL, Damiano RJ Jr. The cox-maze procedure for lone atrial fibrillation: a single-center experience over 2 decades. *Circ Arrhythm Electrophysiol.* 2012 Feb;5(1):8–14. doi: 10.1161/CIRCEP.111.963819 with permission from Wolters Kluwer.

performed as a single intervention or sequentially, when the endocardial catheter mapping and, if needed additional ablations are done within 6 months after the epicardial procedure. This is generally reserved for selected, symptomatic patients with long-standing persistent AF

4.5.9 Special situations

Wolff–Parkinson–White syndrome
- As discussed in section 4.4, most accessory pathways (AP) do not have decremental properties and thus patients with pre-excitation are at risk of rapid conduction across the AP, which may degenerate into VF and sudden cardiac death
- As a result of this significant associated risk with pre-excited AF, ablation is the recommended first line treatment

N.B. *See chapter 4.4 for a more detailed discussion on accessory pathways*

Pregnancy
- AF in pregnancy rare
- Avoid all antiarrhythmic medication if possible
- DC cardiovert if haemodynamic compromise (safe in all stages of pregnancy)
- BBs may be harmful in first trimester
- Amiodarone has harmful foetal effects

- Warfarin teratogenic so avoid in first trimester and for 1 month before due date (typically use LMWH or UFH instead)
- Currently NOACs should be avoided in pregnancy and in women planning a pregnancy

Post-operative AF
- Peak incidence 2–4 days post cardiac surgery
- Atrial flutter and ATs also common
- BBs effective at preventing AF especially if given peri-operatively
- Amiodarone and sotalol also effective at preventing post-op AF
- Most post-op AF spontaneously converts to sinus within 24 h
- Amiodarone or DCCV can be used to cardiovert patients who develop AF post-surgery
- Long-term anticoagulation should be considered in patients with AF after cardiac surgery at risk for stroke, considering individual stroke and bleeding risk

Familial atrial fibrillation
- AF presence in multiple family members or occurrence at an early age should raise the possibility of a genetic cause, e.g. as the primary feature in a family with a *LMNA* variant or BrS
- The underlying genetic factors identified to date are similar to those for other rhythm disorders, i.e. affecting cardiac potassium and sodium channels

4.5.10 Atrial fibrillation summary

AF is characterized by uncoordinated atrial electrical activation and consequently ineffective atrial contraction, with diagnosis confirmed with an ECG
- AF is the most common sustained cardiac arrhythmia encountered in clinical practice and affects 1–2% of the general population. It is associated with increased mortality (predominantly cardiovascular) due to sudden death, heart failure, and stroke
- Management of AF combines treatments with prognostic benefit (anticoagulation and treatment of coexisting cardiovascular conditions) and symptomatic benefit (rate and rhythm control)
- Oral anticoagulation (warfarin or NOACs) can prevent the majority of ischaemic strokes in patients with AF and has been shown to increase life expectancy
- NOACs are recommended in preference to warfarin in eligible patients due to the lower risk of haemorrhagic stroke and systemic embolism and the 10% reduction in mortality compared to warfarin.
- NOACs should not be used in patients with moderate-to-severe mitral stenosis or mechanical heart valves in light of the elevated risk of thromboembolism
- Risk factor modification in the form of weight loss and aggressive management of hypertension, diabetes mellitus, obstructive sleep apnoea, and excessive alcohol consumption is associated with a fivefold greater likelihood of maintaining sinus rhythm following catheter ablation
- Ventricular rate control is an integral part of AF management and is often associated with a significant improvement in symptoms. A resting heart rate < 110 bpm is recommended initially
- Rhythm control is indicated for patients with AF predominantly to reduce AF-related symptoms and improve quality of life. To date, all trials comparing rhythm versus rate control with appropriate anticoagulation have yielded neutral outcomes in terms of mortality
- Catheter ablation is effective in restoring and maintaining sinus rhythm in patients with paroxysmal and persistent AF and is generally used as a second-line treatment after failure of

or intolerance to antiarrhythmic drug therapy. In such patients, it has been shown to be more effective than antiarrhythmic drug therapy
- In experienced high-volume centres, catheter ablation can be offered as a first-line treatment for paroxysmal AF especially in selected patients in the setting of a structurally normal heart
- Surgical ablation was originally reserved for patients undergoing concomitant cardiac surgery but can now be considered independently via a minimally invasive approach. A hybrid strategy combining surgical epicardial and catheter based endocardial ablation is also in use in selected patients

Further reading

Allessie M, Ausma J, Schotten U. Electrical, contractile and structural remodeling during atrial fibrillation. *Cardiovasc Res.* 2002 May;54(2):230–46. doi: 10.1016/s0008-6363(02)00258-4. PMID: 12062329

Calkins H, Hindricks G, Cappato R, Kim YH, Saad EB, Aguinaga L, Akar JG, Badhwar V, Brugada J, Camm J, Chen PS, Chen SA, Chung MK, Cosedis Nielsen J, Curtis AB, Davies DW, Day JD, d'Avila A, Natasja de Groot NMS, Di Biase L, Duytschaever M, Edgerton JR, Ellenbogen KA, Ellinor PT, Ernst S, Fenelon G, Gerstenfeld EP, Haines DE, Haissaguerre M, Helm RH, Hylek E, Jackman WM, Jalife J, Kalman JM, Kautzner J, Kottkamp H, Kuck KH, Kumagai K, Lee R, Lewalter T, Lindsay BD, Macle L, Mansour M, Marchlinski FE, Michaud GF, Nakagawa H, Natale A, Nattel S, Okumura K, Packer D, Pokushalov E, Reynolds MR, Sanders P, Scanavacca M, Schilling R, Tondo C, Tsao HM, Verma A, Wilber DJ, Yamane T; Document Reviewers:. 2017 HRS/EHRA/ECAS/APHRS/SOLAECE expert consensus statement on catheter and surgical ablation of atrial fibrillation. *Europace.* 2018 Jan 1;20(1):e1–e160. doi: 10.1093/europace/eux274. PMID: 29016840; PMCID: PMC5834122

Hindricks G, Potpara T, Dagres N, Arbelo E, Bax JJ, Blomström-Lundqvist C, Boriani G, Castella M, Dan GA, Dilaveris PE, Fauchier L, Filippatos G, Kalman JM, La Meir M, Lane DA, Lebeau JP, Lettino M, Lip GYH, Pinto FJ, Thomas GN, Valgimigli M, Van Gelder IC, Van Putte BP, Watkins CL; ESC Scientific Document Group. 2020 ESC Guidelines for the diagnosis and management of atrial fibrillation developed in collaboration with the European Association for Cardio-Thoracic Surgery (EACTS). *Eur Heart J.* 2021 Feb 1;42(5):373–498. doi: 10.1093/eurheartj/ehaa612. PMID: 32860505

Packer DL, Mark DB, Robb RA, Monahan KH, Bahnson TD, Poole JE, Noseworthy PA, Rosenberg YD, Jeffries N, Mitchell LB, Flaker GC, Pokushalov E, Romanov A, Bunch TJ, Noelker G, Ardashev A, Revishvili A, Wilber DJ, Cappato R, Kuck KH, Hindricks G, Davies DW, Kowey PR, Naccarelli GV, Reiffel JA, Piccini JP, Silverstein AP, Al-Khalidi HR, Lee KL; CABANA Investigators. Effect of catheter ablation vs antiarrhythmic drug therapy on mortality, stroke, bleeding, and cardiac arrest among patients with atrial fibrillation: The CABANA Randomized Clinical Trial. *JAMA.* 2019 Apr 2;321(13):1261–74. doi: 10.1001/jama.2019.0693. PMID: 30874766; PMCID: PMC6450284

Ruff CT, Giugliano RP, Braunwald E, Hoffman EB, Deenadayalu N, Ezekowitz MD, Camm AJ, Weitz JI, Lewis BS, Parkhomenko A, Yamashita T, Antman EM. Comparison of the efficacy and safety of new oral anticoagulants with warfarin in patients with atrial fibrillation: a meta-analysis of randomised trials. *Lancet.* 2014 Mar 15;383(9921):955–62. doi: 10.1016/S0140-6736(13)62343-0. Epub 2013 Dec 4. PMID: 24315724

Van Gelder IC, Groenveld HF, Crijns HJ, Tuininga YS, Tijssen JG, Alings AM, Hillege HL, Bergsma-Kadijk JA, Cornel JH, Kamp O, Tukkie R, Bosker HA, Van Veldhuisen DJ, Van den Berg MP; RACE II Investigators. Lenient versus strict rate control in patients with atrial fibrillation. *N Engl J Med.* 2010 Apr 15;362(15):1363–73. doi: 10.1056/NEJMoa1001337. Epub 2010 Mar 15. PMID: 20231232

4.6

Atrial flutter

Kim Rajappan and Dan Raine

TABLE OF CONTENTS

4.6.1 Introduction 369
4.6.2 ECG characteristics 370
4.6.3 Correlation with other atrial arrhythmias 370
4.6.4 Treatment 371
4.6.5 Atypical atrial flutter 371
4.6.6 Atrial tachycardia 372
     ECG features 373
     Features at electrophysiology study 373
4.6.7 Atrial flutter summary 373

4.6.1 Introduction

- Atrial flutter is a macro re-entrant atrial arrhythmia that can occur in either atrium and can be 'typical' or 'atypical'
- Right atrial flutter is the most common and is characterized by a regular atrial rate and constant P wave morphology
- '*Typical*' counter-clockwise right atrial flutter is a macro re-entrant circuit that travels through the cavotricuspid isthmus (CTI) in a counter-clockwise direction (Figure 4.6.1)

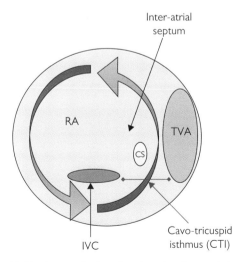

Figure 4.6.1 Right atrial (RA) schematic looking from lateral wall towards interatrial septum. The diagram shows typical counter-clockwise RA flutter, which is CTI dependent. CTI ablation eliminates the critical isthmus of conduction thereby terminating and preventing further episodes of typical RA flutter (TVA = tricuspid valve annulus, CS = coronary sinus, IVC = inferior vena cava)

4.6.2 ECG characteristics

- These can vary widely, though classically there is no isoelectric point due to continuous atrial activity
- *Typical* counter-clockwise RA flutter has a negative saw tooth pattern in the inferior leads as atrial depolarization travels from the CTI up the inter-atrial septum
- Positive flutter waves are typically seen in lead V1 as the depolarization wavefront travels from the septum to the anterior RA (Figure 4.6.2)
- Note that not all CTI-dependent atrial flutters have a counter-clockwise pattern of atrial activation. A CTI-dependent RA flutter going the other way (i.e. clockwise) is still 'typical' (CTI-dependent), but clockwise; the P-wave axis is now positive in the inferior leads, as atrial depolarization progresses down the inter-atrial septum towards the CTI in a clockwise fashion. This is sometimes called 'reverse typical', or 'typical clockwise RA flutter'
- This arrhythmia has the opposite ECG characteristics to counter-clockwise RA flutter with positive flutter waves in the inferior leads and negative flutter waves in lead V1
- The intra-cardiac cycle length for typical RA flutter is usually 200 ms (300 bpm) although this can be altered by right atrial dilatation, fibrosis, and antiarrhythmic drugs

4.6.3 Correlation with other atrial arrhythmias

- Atrial flutter can occur in similar clinical scenarios to atrial fibrillation (AF) and can be triggered by atrial tachycardia or AF
- It is also common for AF and atrial flutter to coexist in the same patient. After CTI ablation, 22–50% of patients have been reported to develop AF over a mean follow up of 14–30 months
- Risk factors for developing AF after CTI ablation (discussed below) include prior AF, impaired left ventricular function, structural or ischaemic heart disease and left atrial dilatation
- AF may be 'organized' to atrial flutter by antiarrhythmic drugs including flecainide and amiodarone

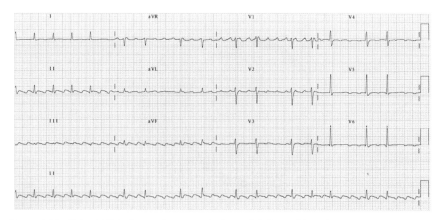

Figure 4.6.2 12-lead ECG of typical counter-clockwise RA flutter. Note the negative saw-tooth pattern in the inferior leads as atrial depolarization moves up the main muscle bulk of the inter-atrial septum from the low CTI (see figure 4.31), and positive flutter waves in V1, as the depolarisation wavefront moves from the septal side (back) to the front of the RA

From LITFL: https://litfl.com/atrial-flutter-ecg-library/

4.6.4 Treatment

- As with AF, a discussion with patients regarding the relative merits of rate vs rhythm strategies is recommended, though rate control can prove more challenging and rhythm control strategies are generally more effective
- Intravenous or oral beta blockers, diltiazem, or verapamil can be used to control the ventricular rate in patients who are haemodynamically stable (again, diltiazem and verapamil should be avoided in presence of significant LVSD)
- Electrical cardioversion is recommended for patients who are haemodynamically unstable or do not respond to pharmacological therapy, and can be considered as part of a rhythm control strategy in other patients
- Class 1C drugs (such as flecainide) can retard the atrial conduction velocity (i.e. flutter rate can reduce) but do not necessarily prolong the AV nodal RP:
  - This can lead to an increased likelihood of 1:1 AV conduction, and a sudden increase in ventricular rate
  - Patients don't like this and it could even be life threatening
- CTI ablation is recommended in patients with atrial flutter who are symptomatic, and/or refractory to pharmacological rate/rhythm control, and can be considered in patients who develop atrial flutter on antiarrhythmic drugs used for the treatment of AF. The success rates for CTI ablation in typical RA flutter are 90–95%
  - It involves delivering high-dose radiofrequency energy into a thick structure
  - The trabeculation and anatomical variations in the CTI mean success rates can never be 100%
  - Non-CTI-dependent atrial flutter is difficult to ablate and success rates vary from 50% to 88% (see below)
  - Patients do not necessarily need to be in atrial flutter at the time of ablation
- Patients with atrial flutter are thought to have the same risk of thromboembolism as patients with AF; therefore, recommendations for anticoagulation mirror those used for AF
- Similarly, with respect to electrical cardioversion, this can be performed without formal anticoagulation within the 48-hour period after onset of atrial flutter. However, if there is uncertainty regarding the time of onset, or it has been sustained for more than 48 hours, patients should be anticoagulated for a minimum of three weeks prior to electrical cardioversion

4.6.5 Atypical atrial flutter

- A macro re-entrant atrial tachyarrhythmia that is not dependent on conduction through the cavotricuspid isthmus (CTI)
- A number of circuits have been described including:
  - Peri-mitral flutter—around the mitral valve annulus
  - Roof dependent flutter—re-entry involving the left atrial roof
  - Around regions of scarring in the right or left atrium
- Atypical atrial flutter typically occurs in patients with atrial scarring from previous cardiac surgery or catheter ablation but can also occur with other forms of heart disease or be idiopathic
- Atypical atrial flutter can coexist with typical RA flutter in the same patient and can involve the presence of multiple re-entrant circuits. The re-entrant circuits can be macro re-entrant (> 2 cm in diameter) or micro re-entrant (≤ 2 cm in diameter), the latter of which may be indistinguishable from a focal atrial tachycardia

- In patients with previous cardiac surgery or catheter ablation, the flutter wave morphology on the 12-lead ECG is not a reliable predictor of whether the flutter circuit involves the CTI, and a definitive diagnosis requires intra-cardiac mapping
- Micro- or macro re-entrant left atrial tachycardias occur in approximately 5% of patients after catheter ablation for AF, however, they are observed less frequently if ablation is limited to PVI alone
- On the other hand, these arrhythmias are more common in patients with longstanding persistent AF, dilated left atria or when linear lesions have been used
- In addition, focal ablation at sites of complex fractionated atrial electrograms (CFAEs) without anchoring the lesions to a non-conducting neighbouring area can create an arrhythmogenic substrate responsible for future micro re-entrant atrial tachycardias
- Detailed activation and entrainment mapping with guidance from electroanatomical mapping systems is required for successful ablation of these left atrial tachycardias with success rates in the region of 90%
- Many of the organized atrial tachyarrhythmias observed within the three-month period after AF ablation will not recur later on, and are simply a reflection of the healing phase following ablation. Further catheter ablation should be deferred until after up to a 3-month period has elapsed unless the arrhythmias are refractory to antiarrhythmic drug therapy and electrical cardioversion

TIP

A macro re-entrant tachycardia circuit = sites > 2 cm apart are entrained in 'the circuit' vs focal tachycardia where it originates at a point source with centrifugal spread which may be due to re-entry (micro re-entry)

4.6.6 Atrial tachycardia

- Atrial tachycardia (AT) can be focal (micro) or macro-re-entrant, and can be multifocal
- AT can be 'incision related', i.e. scar related, following surgery or catheter ablation—it is increasingly seen as an unfortunate and difficult-to-treat complication of extensive LA ablation for AF
- Multifocal ATs are common in patients with COPD (defined as 3 distinct P-wave morphologies present—see Figure 4.6.3)
- Focal ATs are often (approximately 50%) adenosine sensitive

TIP

Termination of SVT with adenosine therefore does not exclude AT (but AT is less likely to terminate than AVNRT or AVRT)

- Antiarrhythmic drugs are generally considered first line, as AT can be more of challenge in the EP lab
- Useful agents include:
  - Beta blockade to reduce ventricular rate as well as automatic and triggered features
  - Stabilizing agents such as flecainide or amiodarone, although consideration will have to be given to side-effect profile on an individual basis

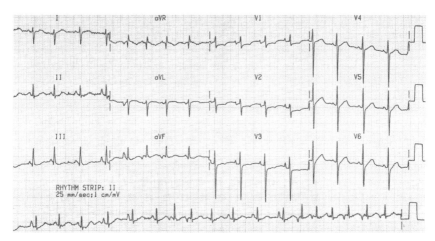

Figure 4.6.3 Rapid, irregular rhythm with multiple P-wave morphologies (best seen in the rhythm strip), as well as features in keeping with chronic pulmonary disease, including right axis deviation, dominant R wave in V1 and deep S wave in V6 suggest right ventricular hypertrophy due to cor pulmonale

Taken from https://litfl.com/multifocal-atrial-tachycardia-mat-ecg-library/

- Catheter ablation can be challenging (discussed below), though has a role for those unable to or unwilling to take/tolerate AADs, or in whom AADs have failed

ECG features
- Usually long RP tachycardia; often will be > 1:1 A:V
- Variation in cycle length
- Variation in VA (RP) time
- Morphology of P wave can be useful to localize the AT (e.g. negative P wave in inferior leads suggests origin from low down in the atria; negative in V1 suggests RA)

Features at invasive electrophysiology study (EPS)
- Usually started with extra stimulus pacing or burst overdrive pacing in the atrium, but often need isporenaline to initiate
- Can be unpredictable and difficult to initiate and sustain during EPS, thereby making mapping challenging
- Mapping AT has improved through use of 3D electro-anatomical mapping systems, particularly if multiple ATs
- These considerations make catheter ablation less likely to be successful and generally a second-line choice after drug therapy has failed

4.6.7 Atrial flutter summary

- Right atrial flutter is the commonest form of macro re-entrant atrial arrhythmia
- 'Typical' right atrial flutter involves conduction through the cavotricuspid isthmus

- Catheter ablation of the cavotricuspid isthmus is recommended in patient with atrial flutter who are either symptomatic or refractory to pharmacological rate control with success rates of 90–95%
- Atypical atrial flutter does not involve conduction through the cavotricuspid isthmus and typically occurs in the presence of atrial scarring from previous cardiac surgery or catheter ablation
- Atrial flutter is considered to have the same thromboembolic risk as AF and therefore, the recommendations for anticoagulation are the same for both arrhythmias

Further reading

Roberts-Thomson KC, Kistler PM, Kalman JM. Focal atrial tachycardia I: clinical features, diagnosis, mechanisms, and anatomic location. *Pacing Clin Electrophysiol*. 2006 Jun;29(6):643–52. doi: 10.1111/j.1540-8159.2006.00413.x. PMID: 16784432

4.7

Ventricular arrhythmia

Richard Bond and Howell Williams

TABLE OF CONTENTS

4.7.1 Diagnosis of ventricular tachycardia 375
    Patient characteristics 376
    ECG characteristics 376
4.7.2 Management of ventricular tachycardia 378
    Acute management of VT 378
    Polymorphic VT 380
    'Normal heart' VT 381
    Long-term management of VT 381
4.7.3 Specific conditions that predispose to VT 382

4.7.1 Diagnosis of ventricular tachycardia

- The differential diagnosis and prevalence among all-comers with broad complex tachycardia (BCT) (Figure 4.7.1) is:
    - VT (~80%)
    - SVT with aberrancy (aberrance = pre-existing or rate-related BBB ~15–20%)
        - AF/AT/AVNRT/orthodromic AVRT
    - Pre-excited tachycardia (~1–6%)
        - Antidromic AVRT (i.e. AVRT where antegrade conduction is via the pathway and retrograde conduction via the AV node; the more typical orthodromic AVRT has antegrade conduction over the AV node and is narrow)
        - Pre-excited AF/AT

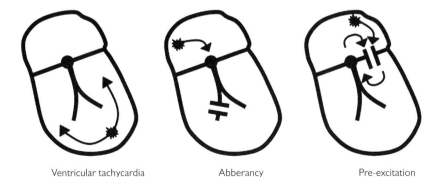

    Ventricular tachycardia   Abberancy   Pre-excitation

Figure 4.7.1 Diagram demonstrating the initial site of activation in the three causes of a regular broad complex tachycardia. In aberrancy and pre-excitation the rhythm us supra-ventricular whereas in VT it is from within the ventricle

- Differentiating between these involves assessment of patient characteristics and ECG characteristics

Patient characteristics

- Age
  - BCT in patients > 35 years old is more likely to be VT, < 35 years old is more likely to be SVT
- Structural heart disease, especially coronary disease
  - BCT in these patients is much more likely to be VT
- The presence or absence of symptoms may not be helpful—VT does not always cause 'worse' symptoms or haemodynamic compromise

ECG characteristics

- See Figure 4.7.2.
- AV dissociation—diagnostic of VT (i.e. pathognomonic)
  - P waves seen that are unrelated to and slower than the ventricular rate
  - Fusion beats: the independent P waves are timed so that they are able to penetrate the AV node and begin depolarizing down the His–Purkinje system, but the VT continues and the two complexes fuse together
  - Capture beats: the independent beats timed perfectly to activate the His–Purkinje system and depolarize the entire ventricular myocardium before the next beat of VT
- QRS duration—broader QRS favours VT
  - > 160 ms in LBBB pattern
  - > 140 ms in RBBB pattern

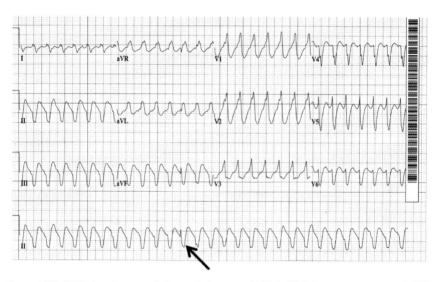

Figure 4.7.2. ECG showing several diagnostic features of VT: 1. QRS duration approximately 200 ms. 2. The arrow points to a fusion beat which demonstrates independent p wave activity. 3. The morphology is 'RBBB like' (positive in V1, negative in V6) but the appearance is highly atypical, with a deep S wave in V6, suggesting the left ventricle is origin for the VT. 4. The inferior leads are negative further localizing the origin of the VT to the inferior portion of the left ventricle. 5. aVR is positive and the frontal ECG axis is 210 degrees

- However:
  - If the BCT QRS is narrower than the SR QRS, that is suggestive of VT. This is because an SVT with aberrancy QRS would be at least as broad as the QRS in SR as both use the same conduction pathway and a conduction defect on a resting ECG will not rectify itself during tachycardia
  - There is also a specific form of VT called fascicular VT that has a relatively narrow QRS (see below)
- QRS morphology
  - If the BCT is SVT with aberrancy, it should appear as a *typical* LBBB or RBBB
    - In RBBB this means an RsR′ pattern with the R′ larger than the R wave and a relatively small S wave in V6
    - In LBBB this means a sharp initial downwards deflection in V1 and a positive deflection in V6
  - If the BCT QRS morphology is exactly the same as the QRS morphology in sinus rhythm, this favours SVT with pre-existing aberrancy
  - The morphology of the VT can be used to give clues as to where the VT originates. If the VT has a 'LBBB-like' morphology then it implies the right ventricle was activated first, and vice versa for 'RBBB-like' morphology
- QRS axis
  - Marked axis deviation favours VT
    - aVR predominantly positive (this indicates that activation is unlikely to be coming antegradely through the AV node and therefore the tachycardia is more likely to be VT)
    - 'Northwest axis'—negative in lead I and aVF
  - A significant axis change from the sinus to BCT ECG points to VT (as it represents a new focus of initiation vs when in SR)
  - The axis can also be used to give clues to the origin of the VT. If the inferior leads are positive the VT must originate superiorly and propagate downwards and vice versa (i.e. if the inferior leads are negative the VT originated inferiorly and propagates superiorly)
- Chest lead concordance
  - If all the chest leads show a negative deflection, there is negative concordance, which demonstrates that the impulse is initiated in the apex and therefore the rhythm must be VT (see Figure 4.7.3)
  - If all the chest leads show a positive deflection (positive concordance) it implies that the rhythm may be VT originating from the left basal area, but it is also possible that the rhythm is an SVT with conduction across a left-sided pathway
  - Note that concordance means that the predominant QRS deflection is in the same direction in all the chest leads, i.e. in positive concordance all the chest leads are positive
- Ventricular ectopics (VEs) on ECG in SR
  - Multiple VEs on the resting ECG in SR that are identical in morphology to the BCT QRS complexes favours VT
- The morphology of the ECG
  - Compare the BCT with the ECG in sinus rhythm. If the morphology of the BCT is identical to that in SR it is likely the diagnosis is SVT with pre-existing branch block, i.e. aberrancy (see Figure 4.7.4)

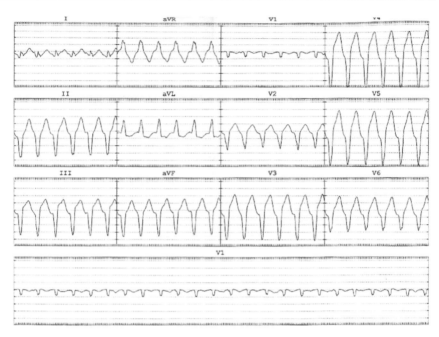

Figure 4.7.3 ECG demonstrating negative concordance across the chest leads, i.e. V1–V6 all have a predominantly negative deflection. This rhythm was mapped to the apex of the left ventricle on EP study

4.7.2 Management of ventricular tachycardia

Acute management of VT
- There is a clear differentiation between patients with haemodynamic compromise and those who are haemodynamically stable
- Haemodynamic compromise (typically defined as SBP < 90 mmHg):
    - During cardiac arrest, follow ALS guidelines (see section 6.2)
    - During VT with shock (i.e. hypotension, impaired organ perfusion) urgent DCCV is advised. If there is time, involve anaesthetic support for conscious sedation
    - Appropriate medical therapy should then be initiated and reversible factors addressed as below to prevent recurrence
- Haemodynamically stable:
    - Both pharmacological and DC cardioversion are options
    - Pharmacological cardioversion may be achieved with:
        - Fascicular VT (see below) = verapamil (Class I)
        - Outflow tract VT: IV beta blockers, usually IV metoprolol in practice (Class I)
        - Other VT:
            - 1st-line = IV procainamide (Class IIa)
            - 2nd-line = IV amiodarone ((Class IIb) can be irritant to peripheral veins and extravasation can cause tissue damage - give centrally if central access is available but do not delay therapy just to insert a CVC, which also has risks in the emergency setting

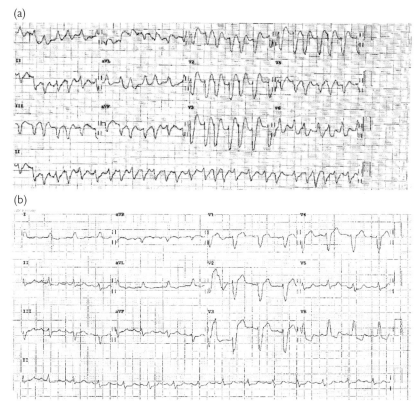

Figure 4.7.4 ECG of patient with AF, before and after returning to sinus rhythm. A. ECG showing an irregular broad complex tachycardia demonstrating that it is AF. The LBBB morphology is also typical with a sharp downstroke in V1 and positivity in V6. aVR is negative and the axis is − 60°, which is consistent with LBBB. B. This ECG is in the same patient after they have returned to sinus rhythm. It can be seen that the QRS morphology is the same confirming that the original rhythm was AF with pre-existing LBBB

- IV lignocaine is useful in VT associated with acute ischemia and when amiodarone has failed. Also useful if acute VT ablation is planned—short half-life and therefore less likely to render VT 'non-inducible' at EP study than amiodarone, which can prevent successful ablation
- If pharmacological cardioversion fails, proceed to DC cardioversion as above
- Reversible factors should also be sought and addressed:
  - Electrolyte derangement (aim for K^+ > 4.5, Mg^{2+} level ~1.0)
  - Ischaemia—VT in the context of acute ischemia is an indication for urgent coronary angiogram +/− proceed
  - Cessation of culprit medications—sympathomimetics, e.g. dobutamine (can it be reduced or discontinued), QT-prolonging drugs if polymorphic VT
- If an ICD is *in-situ*, access the anti-tachycardia pacing (ATP) and shock functions (see also chapter 4.9)

- Confirm appropriately diagnosed VT and not AF/SVT or lead oversensing, which should each be addressed if present
- If pharmacological therapy fails, successful ATP may prevent the need for DC cardioversion
- Consider a temporary increase in pacing rate to suppress ectopy and reduce VT recurrence
- Recurrent VT in patients with an ICD *in-situ* leading to multiple therapies ('VT storm') is highly distressing for them
- Initial application of a magnet to the ICD (to disable therapies and temporarily stop shocks) is often helpful—the VT may be haemodynamically stable giving time for medical therapy to work without further shocks
  - Recurrent VT despite pharmacological therapy and DC cardioversion may be terminated with general anaesthesia and intubation
  - Rarely, temporary pacing wires have been inserted to allow overdrive pacing (equivalent of delivering ATP in patients with ICDs), then pacing at a faster rate than intrinsic rhythm to suppress ectopy
  - Lastly, urgent VT ablation may be considered in refractory cases, and such patients should be escalated to the local referral centre
- Once stabilized, transfer to CCU for monitoring and further care
- Subsequent work-up depends on the cause of VT. The majority of patients will require:
  - Transthoracic echo
  - Coronary angiogram
  - Cardiac MRI (especially useful if no ischemic cause is found)
  - +/− EP investigation for rarer causes, e.g. Brugada Syndrome, CPVT (see below)

Polymorphic VT

- VT with QRS complexes that vary in morphology from beat to beat, implying the tachycardia arises from multiple different foci
- Polymorphic VT without QT prolongation:
  - Most common cause is acute ischaemia (chronic ischaemia with scar usually causes monomorphic VT due to stable re-entry around the scar)
  - Management as for other forms of VT but strong consideration should be given to urgent revascularization
- Polymorphic VT with QT prolongation:
  - Associated with inherited or acquired (usually medication) causes of QT prolongation
  - Usually caused by a ventricular ectopic falling on the T wave of the preceding ventricular activation ('R on T' phenomenon)
  - May also result from severe bradycardia, e.g. in context of high-grade AV block, which prolongs the QT interval
  - Management:
    - Urgent correction of electrolyte abnormalities (K^+ and Mg^{2+}—reasonable to give empirical Mg^{2+} as it is so important)
    - Beta blockers if no bradycardia present
    - Urgent pacing (often temporary) or isoprenaline infusion if significant bradycardia is present

TIP
The term 'Torsades de Pointes' should be reserved for the specific combination of QT prolongation with a distinct form of polymorphic VT in which the axis of ventricular complexes moves progressively from beat to beat in such a way that there is a transition from positive to negative complexes within a single ECG lead. Torsades de Pointes VT is often initiated by a 'short–long–short' sequence: a ventricular ectopic beat leads to a compensatory pause before the next sinus beat; this pause means that the QT interval of the next sinus beat is further prolonged; a further ectopic beat therefore has a greater chance of falling within the end of the T wave and leading to the 'R on T' phenomenon and resulting in polymorphic VT

'Normal heart' VT
- VT can occur in patients with structurally normal hearts who do not have any of the arrhythmia syndromes described above
- The rhythm is generally much more stable and requirement for an ICD (discussed later) is very rare
- Right ventricular outflow tract (RVOT) VT:
    - Originates from RV outflow tract (rarely the LVOT)
    - ECG in VT shows BCT with LBBB-like pattern, positive in the inferior leads
    - May terminate with adenosine or verapamil, also safe to use beta blockers or amiodarone acutely
    - Differentiated from VT associated with ARVC by normal ECG and imaging (TTE/CMR). Multiple VT morphologies are also more likely to represent arrhythmogenic cardiomyopathy rather than 'normal heart' VT
    - VT ablation usually successful in patients in whom medical therapy does not work or is poorly tolerated
    - ICDs are not normally required
- Fascicular VT
    - Arises from the fascicles of the LV and has a relatively narrow QRS (120–140 ms)
    - Left posterior fascicle most common
        - ECG shows RBBB and left axis deviation
    - Left anterior fascicle less common
        - ECG shows RBBB and right axis deviation
    - May terminate with verapamil, often not sensitive to adenosine
    - Long-term management either with beta blockers or calcium channel blockers, with catheter ablation for patients in whom medical therapy does not work or is poorly tolerated

Long-term management of VT
- This will differ depending on the cause of VT
- Four broad categories
    i) Correct reversible factors, e.g. revascularization in the acute setting, optimal medical therapy for heart failure
    ii) Pharmacological therapy
        - Anti-arrhythmic therapy
        - Oral beta blockers appropriate in most cases

- Oral amiodarone (caution re: side effects with long-term use)
- Oral class 1 agents, e.g. mexiletine

Medical heart failure therapy
- All four key medical heart failure drug classes (B blocker, ARNI/ ACE-I / ARB, MRA and SGLT2i) reduce the occurrence of ventricular arrhythmias in patients with heart failure with reduced ejection fraction. These medications also improve quality of life, reduce hospitalisation and reduce mortality in this population.

iii) Secondary prevention ICD (see section 4.9)
- These have revolutionized long-term VT management and have been proven to be more effective than medical therapy alone in multiple RCTs

iv) VT ablation
- This is a helpful adjunct for patients with recurrent VT despite initial measures. It can also help to avoid the use of long term amiodarone therapy in selected patients

4.7.3 Specific conditions that predispose to VT

Cardiomyopathies
- Any form of cardiomyopathy places an individual at increased risk of ventricular arrhythmia
- In particular, these include:
    - Ischaemic cardiomyopathy
    - Dilated (non-ischaemic) cardiomyopathy
    - Hypertrophic cardiomyopathy
    - Arrhythmogenic (right) ventricular cardiomyopathy
- A more detailed summary of these conditions can be found in chapter 5.2, and of sudden cardiac death (SCD) risk assessment and management in chapter 6.3

Cardiac ion channel dysfunction
- Recognized causes of ventricular arrhythmia include:
    - Long QT syndrome
    - Brugada syndrome
    - Catecholaminergic polymorphic VT
    - Short QT syndrome
    - Early repolarization syndrome

Further reading

Issa ZF, Miller JM, Zipes DP. *Clinical Arrhythmology and Electrophysiology*, 2nd edn. Elsevier, 2012.

Zeppenfeld K, Tfelt-Hansen J, de Riva M, Winkel BG, Behr ER, Blom NA, Charron P, Corrado D, Dagres N, de Chillou C, Eckardt L, Friede T, Haugaa KH, Hocini M, Lambiase PD, Marijon E, Merino JL, Peichl P, Priori SG, Reichlin T, Schulz-Menger J, Sticherling C, Tzeis S, Verstrael A, Volterrani M; ESC Scientific Document Group. 2022 ESC Guidelines for the management of patients with ventricular arrhythmias and the prevention of sudden cardiac death. Eur Heart J. 2022 Oct 21;43(40):3997–4126. doi: 10.1093/eurheartj/ehac262. PMID: 36017572.

4.8

Cardiac ion channel dysfunction

Richard Bond, Howell Williams, Victoria McKay, and Stewart Brown

TABLE OF CONTENTS

4.8.1 Cardiac ion channel dysfunction 383
4.8.2 Long QT syndrome (LQTS) 383
   LQTS Sub-types 384
   Management 385
   Additional genetics 385
4.8.3 Brugada syndrome 386
   Management 387
   Additional genetics 387
4.8.4 Catecholaminergic polymorphic VT 388
   Management 388
   Additional genetics 388
4.8.5 Short QT syndrome 389
   Management 389
   Genetics 389
4.8.6 Early repolarisation syndrome 389

4.8.1 Cardiac ion channel dysfunction

- Genetic mutations affect the function of ion channel subunits or proteins that regulate ion channel function. This results in an increased risk of arrhythmias with a variety of environmental triggers.
- Genetic counselling is recommended for anyone undergoing genetic testing
- Preimplantation genetic testing should be discussed with women of child-bearing age

4.8.2 Long QT syndrome (LQTS)

- Inherited cardiac channelopathy caused by genetic variants in Na^+ and K^+ channels
- It is the most common inherited arrhythmia syndrome affecting 1 in 2000 individuals
- LQTS is suspected with a corrected QT (QTc) > 480 ms or in the context of unexplained syncope with a QT interval of > 460 ms (in the absence of secondary causes of QT prolongation), preferably measured at 60–70 bpm to minimise error from correction algorithms
- LQTS is diagnosed by any one of:
   - QTc > 480 ms on repeated 12 lead ECGs
   - LQTS risk score > 3 (also known as the Schwartz score, described in Table 4.8.1)
   - Confirmed pathogenic LQTS genetic mutation, irrespective of QTc duration
   - Importantly, normal QTc does not exclude LQTS as 20–40% of patients have a normal QTc at rest
- Risk of cardiac events increases by 5–15% for every 10 ms increase in QTc. Patients with QTc > 500 ms have a significantly higher risk of cardiac events
- Exercise testing should be performed to assess for QT prolongation >480ms in minute four of recovery

Table 4.8.1 The modified LQTS score (also known as the Schwartz score) for the diagnosis of Long QT Syndrome. A score of more than 3 is considered diagnostic of LQTS.

Criterion	Points
ECG findings	
QTc, ms > 480	3
QTc, ms 460–469	2
QTc, ms 450–459 in male patient	1
Torsade de Pointes	2
T-wave alternans	1
Notched T wave in 3 leads	1
Low heart rate for age	0.5
Clinical history	
Syncope with stress	2
Syncope without stress	1
Congenital deafness	0.5
Family history	
A. Family members with definite LQTS	1
B. Unexplained sudden cardiac death < 30 y in an immediate family member	0.5

LQTS Sub-types

- LQTS 1-3 (Figure 4.8.1) account for majority (80–90%) of cases. LQT1 and LQT2 each make up 40–45% of cases, though 15 different genetic mutations have been described (LQT1–LQT15).
- LQT1
  - Autosomal dominant, loss of function variants in the *KCNQ1* gene causing reduction in I_{KS} current
  - 45% of all gene-positive LQTS cases
  - Characterised by polymorphic VT triggered by exercise, swimming, or emotion
  - Associated with wide, broad-based T-waves
- LQT2
  - Autosomal dominant, K+ channel mutation with loss of function variants in the *KCNH2* gene causing reduction in I_{KR} current

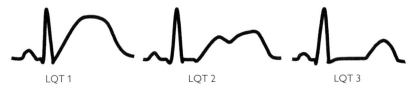

Figure 4.8.1 Examples of QT morphology in LQT 1–3

- 45% of gene-positive LQTS cases
- Cardiac events (syncope, cardiac arrest, SCD) occur during rest or exercise, particularly during the post-partum period, and are characteristically triggered by abrupt sounds such as alarm clocks
- Associated with low amplitude and notched T waves
* LQT3
  - Autosomal dominant, Na⁺ channel mutation with gain of function variants in the *SCN5A* gene (loss of function variants in *SCN5A* cause Brugada syndrome) causing an increase in late I_{Na} current
  - 5% of gene-positive LQTS cases, with higher risk of SCD compared to other genotypes
  - Cardiac events (syncope, cardiac arrest, SCD) occur at rest or during sleep
  - Associated with a long ST segment and peaked T-wave

Management

* Management involves pharmacological therapy and risk stratification for SCD
  - Lifestyle: avoid genotype/LQTS sub-type specific triggers
  - Pharmacological:
    * Non-selective beta blockers reduce cardiac events (syncope, cardiac arrest, SCD) and should be considered in all genotype positive patients, irrespective of QT interval
    * Avoid hypokalaemia and all QT-prolonging drugs (list at www.crediblemeds.org, useful to inform patients about this website)
    * Mexiletine reduces cardiac events in LQT3
  - Risk stratification for SCD:
    * Primary prevention ICD may be considered in asymptomatic high risk patients, using the 1-2-3 LQT risk calculator (*IIb B*) which combines the QT interval length and genotype
    * Secondary prevention: ICD should be offered to patients who experience aborted SCD (*IB*), or who are symptomatic despite medication (*IC*)
    * Left cardiac sympathetic denervation may be considered in patients who experience ICD therapies despite beta blockers, or who cannot take beta blockers (IC)

Additional genetics

* LQTS is clinically highly variable and has incomplete penetrance
* Romano–Ward Syndrome was the historical name given to the autosomal dominant form of LQTS but is now rarely used in clinical practice
* Jervell–Lange–Nielsen syndrome is an autosomal recessive condition characterised by LQTS and congenital sensorineural deafness, caused by heterozygous variants in *KCNQ1*
* Andersen-Tawil syndrome (LQT7) is caused by *KCNJ2* loss of function variants and affects 1 per million. It is characterised by ventricular arrhythmias (bidirectional), dysmorphologies, and periodic paralysis. There is a prominent U wave which can help distinguish it from other channelopathies. Beta blockers and flecainide reduce ventricular arrhythmias. ICDs are indicated after aborted cardiac arrest of poorly tolerated VT.
* Testing identifies variants in about 70% of families
* Genetic testing is important in facilitating cascade testing in families and guiding treatment. Beta blockers should be offered in genotype positive patients, regardless of QT interval. Beta blockers are effective in LQT1 and 2, but not 3. Mexiletine is effective in LQT3
* Misinterpretation of ECGs and genetic test results can result in undue anxiety, unnecessary lifestyle changes, insurance or occupation-related issues, and inappropriate ICD implantation

4.8.3 Brugada syndrome

- Inherited cardiac channelopathy caused by mutation affecting the Na^+ channel.
- Genetic testing for *SCN5A* variants is recommended.
- Prevalence of the Brugada ECG pattern is ~0.6% in Europeans
- Characterised by typical ECG changes and an increased risk of ventricular arrhythmias and SCD
- Patients may present with syncope, nocturnal laboured respiration with agitation, 'seizures' (e.g. 'febrile seizures' in children), and/or aborted SCD—all related to episodes of ventricular arrhythmia (commonly VF or polymorphic VT)
- There may be a family history of SCD before age 45
- Ventricular arrhythmias occur during sleep but may also be triggered by fever, medical drugs (e.g. class 1 agents), or recreational drugs (alcohol excess, cocaine use)
- Brugada syndrome is diagnosed using the Shanghai criteria (Table 4.8.2)
- There are three Brugada ECG patterns (Figure 4.8.2)
- Type 1 ECG is diagnostic:
    - ST segment elevation with type 1 morphology ≥ 2 mm in one or more leads among the right precordial leads (V1 and or V2) positioned in either the 2nd, 3rd, or 4th intercostal space

Table 4.8.2 Proposed Shanghai Score System for Diagnosis of Brugada Syndrome.

	Points
I. ECG* (12-lead/ambulatory)	
A. Spontaneous type 1 Brugada ECG pattern at nominal or high leads	3.5
B. Fever-induced type 1 Brugada ECG pattern at nominal or high leads	3
C. Type 2 or 3 Brugada ECG pattern that converts with provocative drug challenge	2
II. Clinical history†	
A. Unexplained cardiac arrest or documented VF/polymorphic VT	3
B. Nocturnal agonal respirations	2
C. Suspected arrhythmic syncope	2
D. Syncope of unclear mechanism/unclear etiology	1
E. Atrial flutter/fibrillation in patients <30 yrs without alternative etiology	0.5
III. Family history	
A. First- or second-degree relative with definite BrS	2
B. Suspicious SCD (fever, nocturnal, Brugada aggravating drugs) in a first- or second-degree relative	1
C. Unexplained SCD <45 yrs in first- or second-degree relative with negative autopsy	0.5
IV. Genetic test result	
A. Probable pathogenic mutation in BrS susceptibility gene	0.5

SCD = sudden cardiac death; VF = ventricular fibrillation; VT = ventricular tachycardia.
* One item from this category must apply.
† Only award points once for highest score within this category. Score (requires at least 1 electrocardiographic (ECG) finding): >3.5 points: probable and/or definite Brugada syndrome (BrS); 2 to 3 points: possible BrS; <2 points: nondiagnostic.

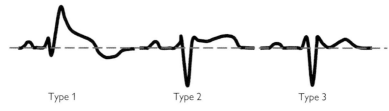

Figure 4.8.2 Example of Brugada ECGs in the right precordial chest leads

- This may occur either spontaneously or with provocation with class 1c Na⁺ channel blockers (e.g. ajmaline or flecainide—ajmaline is preferred in the UK due to short half-life)
- Type 2 and type 3 Brugada patterns may convert to a type 1 pattern on sodium channel provocation. High lead placement may increase in the sensitivity in detecting the Brugada ECG pattern
- Some Brugada patients also develop AF or AV block
- Malignant ventricular arrhythmias occur in 13.5% of patients per year in those with a previous cardiac arrest, 3.2% in patients with previous syncope, and 1% in asymptomatic patients. Those who have a Brugada pattern only with sodium channel blockade have a low risk of ventricular arrhythmias

Management

- Avoid precipitating factors including certain drugs (see list at www.brugadadrugs.org, useful to inform patients about this website), promptly treating fever, and avoiding large carbohydrate meals late at night
- The risk of SCD is related to the following risk factors:
  - Previous aborted cardiac arrest or ventricular arrhythmia
  - Family history SCD
  - Spontaneous type 1 ECG pattern
  - Syncope
  - Male sex
  - Presence of AF or sinus node disease
- ICD treatment is recommended for symptomatic Brugada syndrome
  - Primary prevention: ICD is not indicated in the absence of arrhythmias or symptoms
  - Secondary prevention: all patients with sustained VT or aborted SCD should be offered an ICD (Class I C)
    - ICD implant should be considered in patients with spontaneous type 1 Brugada pattern and history of syncope
  - Quinidine should be considered in patients with Brugada syndrome who qualify for an ICD but have a contraindication, decline, or have recurrent ICD shocks (Class IIa C)
- Pharmacological treatment of VT storm is different in Brugada syndrome
  - Isoprenaline infusion or quinidine are recommended by the ESC (IIa C)
  - VT ablation may help to prevent recurrence
- Implantable loop recorders may be implanted when syncope is unexplained, ICDs should be considered when syncope is thought to be arrhythmic.

Additional genetics

- Brugada Syndrome demonstrates incomplete penetrance and variable expressivity
- The combination of a low yield of positive genetic tests and a highly variable clinical picture suggests that Brugada syndrome is not purely a monogenic disease

- It's likely that in some families an accumulation of several single nucleotide variants (SNV) results in the Brugada phenotype. These SNVs may modulate the sodium channel function which may either increase or decrease the severity of phenotype
- Genetic testing reveals a pathogenic variant in 20–30% of cases, most of which are due to *SCN5A* loss of function variants. Other causative variants seem to modulate or affect the same sodium channel as the *SCN5A* gene
- The risk of ventricular arrhythmias is higher in patients with *SCN5A* loss of function variants than *SCN5A* non-loss of function variants

4.8.4 Catecholaminergic polymorphic VT

- Rare but malignant inherited condition (usually autosomal dominant but may also be recessive) that predisposes to polymorphic or bidirectional VT, often during physical or emotional stress
- Onset is usually in childhood with syncope or cardiac arrest but can present in adult life, as late as the fourth decade
- Prevalence is estimated to be 1:10,000
- Most common subtype is CPVT1, caused by mutation in ryanodine receptor (*RYR2* variant) that leads to excess intracellular Ca^{2+} release and arrhythmias
- Examination and cardiac imaging are both normal, though sinus bradycardia and prominent U-waves are occasionally seen on the ECG
- VT may be provoked on supervised exercise testing or Holter monitoring
- CPVT diagnostic criteria are either one of:
    - Exercise or emotion induced bidirectional or polymorphic VT in the presence of a structurally normal heart and normal ECG
    - Confirmed pathogenic genetic variant

Management

- Lifestyle:
    - Avoid competitive sports, strenuous exercise, and stressful environments
- Pharmacological:
    - Non-selective beta blockers are recommended for all patients with CPVT. They may be offered to gene positive asymptomatic family members
    - Flecainide should be considered as a second-line agent for patients who experience syncope, documented VT or ICD therapies despite beta blockers
- Risk stratification for SCD:
    - Primary prevention: ICD is not routinely recommended for primary prevention
    - Secondary prevention: ICD should be offered to all patients who experience cardiac arrest, or have sustained VT or syncope despite medication.
- Left cardiac sympathetic denervation may be considered for patients who experience recurrent VT despite optimal pharmacological therapy

Additional genetics

- 60% of patients have a *RYR2* variant which is autosomal dominant
- *RYR2* variants affect the cardiac ryanodine receptor function and cause a reduction in calcium release from the sarcoplasmic reticulum during diastole
- Variants in the *CASQ2* gene (which regulates the RyR2 receptor) are autosomal recessive but cause a more severe phenotype and make up about 5% of positive tests

- Homozygotes (or compound heterozygotes, with different variants on each of the two alleles of *CASQ2*) are severely affected whereas heterozygotes may be mildly affected or asymptomatic
- 80% of patients have a positive genetic test result

4.8.5 Short QT syndrome

- Very rare inherited arrhythmia syndrome characterised by consistently short QTc (< 360 ms), often with tall peaked T waves
    - Diagnosed if QTc ≤360 ms and ≥1 of (i) a pathogenic mutation, (ii) family history of SQTS, (iii) survival from a VT/VF episode in the absence of heart disease
- Propensity to AF
- High risk of SCD
- It is very rare with only ~150 families affected worldwide
- One third of patients present with SCD, the others present with presyncope, syncope, and AF, with a slight predominance of lethal events in male patients
- Although SQTS can be a genetic condition, a shortened corrected QT interval can be caused by electrolyte imbalance and drug therapy

Management

- The low incidence limits the strength of recommendations
    - ESC guidelines recommend ICD in all patients with documented sustained VT or survivors of aborted cardiac arrest, and to consider ICD for other patients on a case-by-case basis
- Quinidine may be trialled as medical therapy in asymptomatic patients with a family history of SCD, and those who refuse an ICD
- Isoprenaline may be considered in SQTS patients with an electrical storm

Genetics

- Genetically, SQTS demonstrates an autosomal dominant inheritance pattern with high penetrance
- It is caused by variants in the same genes as LQTS but with opposing consequences, i.e. variants that cause a gain of function of potassium channels or loss of function of sodium or calcium channels
- Pathogenic variants can be divided into two main groups:
    - Increased potassium current (SQT1–3): short QTc with peaked T-waves and short or absent ST segment
    - Reduced L-type calcium current (SQT4–5): short QTc with ST elevation (may be a combined short QT/Brugada syndrome)
- The yield from genetic testing is 20–30%

4.8.6 Early repolarisation syndrome

- Early repolarization (ER) has traditionally been considered benign but recent case control studies have associated early repolarization in the inferior and/or lateral leads with an increased risk of SCD

- ER is defined on ECG as J-point elevation ≥ 1 mm in two adjacent inferior/lateral leads with either a slurred or notched morphology
- *ER syndrome* is diagnosed in a patient resuscitated from polymorphic VT or VF without any heart disease, with an ER pattern in the inferior and/or lateral leads
- ER pattern affects 6% of adults and is more common in young males
- Yield and utility of genetic testing is low
- The location of ER on the ECG has been shown to predict risk of SCD:
  Type 1: ER in the lateral precordial leads; common among healthy, male athletes and most likely benign
  Type 2: ER in the inferior or inferolateral leads; moderately increased risk of SCD
  Type 3: ER globally in the inferior, lateral and right precordial leads; associated with the highest relative risk of SCD
  Type 4: J point elevation in leads V1–V2 (seen in Brugada syndrome)
- Survivors of cardiac arrest with ER syndrome should be offered an ICD. The risk of recurrence is 27%
- Qunidine and milrinone may reduce the recurrence of VF. Isoprenaline is used to treat VT storm. Ablation of ventricular ectopics arising from the Purkinje system can also reduce further ventricular arrhythmias
- There are currently no indications for primary prevention ICDs or pharmacotherapy, however ICD implantation or quinidine may be considered in individuals with ER, arrhythmic syncope and additional risk features (J waves >2 mm, dynamic changes in J point and ST morphology) or a family history of premature SCD

Further reading

Issa ZF, Miller JM, Zipes DP. *Clinical Arrhythmology and Electrophysiology*. 2nd edn. Elsevier, 2012.

Hosseini SM, Kim R, Udupa S, Costain G, Jobling R, Liston E, Jamal SM, Szybowska M, Morel CF, Bowdin S, Garcia J, Care M, Sturm AC, Novelli V, Ackerman MJ, Ware JS, Hershberger RE, Wilde AAM, Gollob MH; National Institutes of Health Clinical Genome Resource Consortium. Reappraisal of Reported Genes for Sudden Arrhythmic Death: Evidence-Based Evaluation of Gene Validity for Brugada Syndrome. *Circulation*. 2018 Sep 18;138(12):1195–205. doi: 10.1161/CIRCULATIONAHA.118.035070. PMID: 29959160; PMCID: PMC6147087

Priori SG, Wilde AA, Horie M, Cho Y, Behr ER, Berul C, Blom N, Brugada J, Chiang CE, Huikuri H, Kannankeril P, Krahn A, Leenhardt A, Moss A, Schwartz PJ, Shimizu W, Tomaselli G, Tracy C. HRS/EHRA/APHRS expert consensus statement on the diagnosis and management of patients with inherited primary arrhythmia syndromes: document endorsed by HRS, EHRA, and APHRS in May 2013 and by ACCF, AHA, PACES, and AEPC in June 2013. *Heart Rhythm*. 2013 Dec;10(12):1932–63. doi: 10.1016/j.hrthm.2013.05.014. Epub 2013 Aug 30. PMID: 24011539

Wellens HJ. Electrophysiology: Ventricular tachycardia: diagnosis of broad QRS complex tachycardia. *Heart*. 2001 Nov;86(5):579–85. doi: 10.1136/heart.86.5.579. PMID: 11602560; PMCID: PMC1729977

Zeppenfeld K, Tfelt-Hansen J, de Riva M, Winkel BG, Behr ER, Blom NA, Charron P, Corrado D, Dagres N, de Chillou C, Eckardt L, Friede T, Haugaa KH, Hocini M, Lambiase PD, Marijon E, Merino JL, Peichl P, Priori SG, Reichlin T, Schulz-Menger J, Sticherling C, Tzeis S, Verstrael A, Volterrani M; ESC Scientific Document Group. 2022 ESC Guidelines for the management of patients with ventricular arrhythmias and the prevention of sudden cardiac death. Eur Heart J. 2022 Oct 21;43(40):3997–4126. doi: 10.1093/eurheartj/ehac262. PMID: 36017572.

4.9

Implantable cardioverter defibrillator

Richard Bond and Howell Williams

TABLE OF CONTENTS

- 4.9.1 Introduction and main trials 391
- 4.9.2 Indications 392
- 4.9.3 Arrhythmia detection and programming 393
  - Defibrillation threshold 393
  - Shock vectors 394
  - Arrhythmia detection 396
  - Programming 396
  - SVT discrimination 398
- 4.9.4 Device therapy 398
  - Pacing 398
  - Antitachycardia pacing (ATP) 399
  - Shock therapy 399
- 4.9.5 Alternative device positioning 399

Subcutaneous ICDs 399
Wearable ICDs 402
- 4.9.6 Device interrogation and follow-up 402
  - Box plots 402
  - Intracardiac electrograms 403
- 4.9.7 Complications and deactivation 403
- 4.9.8 ICD troubleshooting 404
  - Multiple *appropriate* shocks 404
  - Shock therapy fails to cardiovert arrhythmia 405
  - *Inappropriate* shocks 407
  - Ventricular arrhythmias without therapy being delivered 407

4.9.1 Introduction and main trials

- The frequency of ICD implants is increasing; the majority of ICD implants in the UK are for secondary prevention of SCD, though UK implant rate is lower than many similar European countries and is likely to increase in the future
- Several landmark trials have established a role for ICDs in primary prevention
- Careful counselling is recommended prior to implantation as the incidence of complications from ICDs is up to 20% (including long-term lead dysfunction and inappropriate shock therapy, although the rate of this is decreasing with improved lead longevity and the use of less aggressive ICD settings) and there are important lifestyle implications, e.g. driving (see section 4.10.3)
- In their simplest form they may have a single lead to the right ventricle or they may be dual-chamber or biventricular
- The two essential features of all ICDs are:
  - To detect ventricular arrhythmias
  - Then deliver appropriate therapy

Secondary prevention trials

AVID study: ICD versus antiarrhythmic drugs (AADs, amiodarone or sotalol):

- Trial featured survivors of cardiac arrest or poorly tolerated VT
- Significant decrease in mortality in the ICD group: RRR of 39±20%, 27±21%, and 31±21% at 1, 2, and 3 years respectively

- The benefit of an ICD was more marked in patients with an LVEF ≤ 35%

CASH study: patients with prior cardiac arrest:

- Randomized to metoprolol, amiodarone, propafenone, or ICD implant
- 23% non-significant trend towards decreased mortality in the ICD group compared to AADs. The propafenone arm was stopped early due to an increase in mortality.

Primary prevention trials

MADIT study: patients with coronary artery disease, LV systolic dysfunction with EF < 35%, non-sustained ventricular tachycardia (NSVT) and inducible VT at EPS:

- Randomized to ICD versus conventional medical treatment (most commonly amiodarone)
- ICD use decreased mortality by 54% in patients with ischaemic cardiomyopathy

MADIT II study: patients with previous MI and EF < 30%—NSVT or EP testing was not required:

- Randomized to ICD versus conventional medical therapy
- 31% reduced mortality in the ICD cohort after an average follow-up period of 20 months

SCD HeFT study: patients with NYHA II/III heart failure and LVSD (EF < 35%) irrespective of aetiology (ischaemic and non-ischaemic):

- Randomised to conventional medical therapy plus placebo versus amiodarone versus ICD
- Amiodarone equal to placebo in reducing mortality
- ICD implantation reduced mortality by 23%

DEFINITE trial: patients with non-ischaemic cardiomyopathy and frequent ventricular ectopics or NSVT:

- Randomised to conventional medical therapy versus medical therapy plus ICD
- Significant reduction in SCD and a trend toward reduction of overall mortality rates

4.9.2 Indications

- ESC guideline recommendations:
    - Primary prevention ICD recommended in all patients with symptomatic ischaemic heart failure and should be considered for those with non-ischaemic pathology, NYHA II–III and LVEF ≤ 35% despite ≥ 3 months of optimal medical therapy (OMT), i.e. beta blockers, ARNI / ACE-I / ARB, MRA and SGLT2i who are expected to survive at least 1 year with good functional status
        - *Class I A* for ischaemic aetiology
        - *Class IIa A* for non-ischaemic aetiology
    - Primary prevention ICD should be considered in patients with CAD, NYHA class I, and LVEF ≤30% despite ≥3 months of OMT (*Class IIa B*)
    - Primary prevention ICD should be considered in patients with CAD, LVEF ≤40% despite ≥3 months of OMT, and NSVT if they have inducible sustained monomorphic VT at EP study (Class IIa B)
    - Secondary prevention ICD in patients with a reasonable expectation of survival (> 1 year) with a good functional status and:
        - Aborted arrhythmic SCD
        - Documented VF or haemodynamically compromised VT without a reversible cause, or < 48 hours after MI in a patient on chronic optimal medical therapy (*Class I A*)

- Recurrent sustained VT (not < 48 hours after MI) who are receiving chronic optimal medical therapy and have a normal LVEF (*Class IIa C*)
- Should be considered if haemodynamically tolerated sustained monomorphic VT and an LVEF ≥40% if VT ablation fails, is not available, or is not desired (*Class IIs C*)
  - Primary and secondary prevention ICDs may be considered in patients with arrhythmias and primary arrhythmia syndromes—*these are discussed in detail in chapters 4.8 and 6.3 on predisposing conditions to sudden cardiac death*
- Of note, the evidence demonstrating benefit of primary prevention ICDs in heart failure with reduced ejection fraction (HFrEF) is more powerful among patients with an ischaemic cause of LV impairment than non-ischaemic causes of LV impairment
- *DANISH trial* from 2016 was a large RCT that investigated the role of ICDs in non-ischaemic HFrEF:
  - Non-ischaemic HFrEF with LVEF < 35% randomized to OMT +/− CRT vs OMT +/− CRT plus ICD (note CRT rate same (58%) in both groups)
  - Primary outcome death from any cause was the same in both groups
  - Subgroup analysis showed significant mortality benefit from ICDs among patients < 68 years old, with no significant mortality benefit among patients > 68 years old
  - Difference presumably caused by older patients dying of non-cardiac causes before gaining benefit from ICD
- Many operators therefore take age into account when discussing the benefits of primary prevention ICDs with patients who have non-ischaemic causes of HFrEF

NICE guidelines (UK) for ICD implant

- NICE incorporate discrimination based on QRS duration in primary prevention device therapy (see Box 4.9.1)
- Commonest indication for primary prevention ICD is HFrEF:
  - LVEF ≤ 35%, despite OMT as the EF will often improve with OMT, especially in non-ischaemic DCM
    - No specific duration of OMT recommended by NICE, ESC recommend at least 3 months
  - LVEF ≤ 35% due to ischaemic heart disease at least 6 weeks after acute MI (due to the potential for improvement in LV systolic function over this time period)

4.9.3 Arrhythmia detection and programming

Defibrillation threshold

- Defibrillation threshold (DFT) is the minimum amount of energy required to reliably defibrillate the heart. If this is tested, most centres ensure there is a safety margin of 10 J below the maximum output of the device: the defibrillation safety margin (DSM). Although most centres do not perform this now, it can be useful for right sided devices (see shock vectors and Figure 4.9.1) or when previous shocks have failed and if the device has been revised
- DSM testing may be omitted at implant and tested at a later date if needed (e.g. non-anticoagulated AF)
- Normokalaemia is important
- VF can be induced by the device via (i) direct current shock, (ii) shock on the T wave (overdrive pacing for 12 beats followed by a shock on the T wave), (iii) burst pacing or stimulating the heart at 50 Hz

> **BOX 4.9.1 NICE GUIDANCE ON ICDS (2014)**
>
> **Secondary prevention**
>
> ICDs are recommended for people who:
> - Have survived a cardiac arrest due to either VT or VF
> - Have spontaneous sustained VT causing syncope or significant haemodynamic compromise
> - Have sustained VT without syncope or cardiac arrest, and also have an associated reduction in LV systolic function to LVEF ≤ 35%, with symptoms that are no worse than NYHA III
>
> **Primary prevention**
>
> ICDs (with or without CRT) are recommended for people who:
> - Have heart failure with reduced ejection fraction to LVEF ≤ 35% and associated BBB with QRS duration ≥ 120 ms
> - Have heart failure with reduced ejection fraction to LVEF ≤ 35% and QRS duration < 120 ms if there is a high risk of sudden cardiac death (factors suggesting a higher risk of SCD include ischaemic aetiology of heart failure, NSVT, certain causes of non-ischaemic LV impairment, e.g. lamin cardiomyopathy)
>   - In patients with NYHA class IV symptoms, ICD generally not indicated
> - Have arrhythmia syndromes that pre-dispose to VT and SCD (including HCM, LQTS, Brugada syndrome, arrhythmogenic cardiomyopathy)
> - Have congenital heart disease and have had corrective surgery, who have a high risk of SCD
>
> Reproduced from NICE guidelines—Technology appraisal guideline [TA314], June 2014

- The device is tested whilst the ventricular lead sensitivity is set to its highest setting; it can only detect ventricular fibrillation signals with a voltage greater than 1 mV. The test is performed in the 'worst-case scenario' for the device, as the normal detection is set to > 0.3 mV once the test is finished
- Once VF is induced most ICDs will rely on the programmed settings to detect the arrhythmia, diagnose it, and deliver therapy. It is possible that defibrillation will not occur; it is important that the patient is connected to an external defibrillator so that rescue shocks can be delivered in this situation
- The device should be programmed to deliver backup right ventricular pacing after shock therapy as some patients may become bradycardic after shock therapy
- If a patient requires subsequent DSM testing, 5 min should be left to allow for full haemodynamic recovery
- Lack of appropriate defibrillation safety margin = any DFT within 10 J of the device's maximum delivered energy output. Dual coil (SVC and RV shocking coils) rather than single coil leads (RV coil only) may help. Options include changing the shocking vector (dual coil) or polarity and, ultimately, moving the lead position. Some AADs, including amiodarone, can increase the DFT dramatically. Sotalol can lower the DFT

Shock vectors

- Dual coil leads were common and many patients with ICDs have dual coil leads.
- However, they are now rarely implanted due to the increased risk from device extraction
    - Fibrous adherence of the SVC coil to the SVC wall increases the risk of SVC damage during extraction
    - This can cause significant haemorrhage and is life threatening

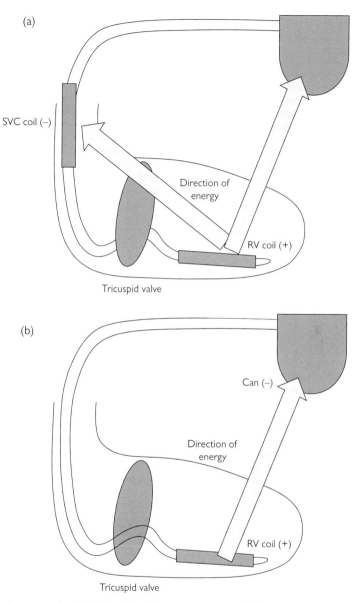

Figure 4.9.1 When a shock is delivered to the heart, energy travels from the positive pole to the negative pole. In defibrillation leads with two coils, the SVC coil can be turned on or off. The RV coil is positive and the SVC coil or can is negative. Changing the direction of energy across the heart can make defibrillation more effective. Polarity can be reversed so that the SVC coil or can becomes positive and the RV coil is negative. In a single coil ICD the circuit is between the RV coil and can. Note that most ICDs are implanted with atrial pacing leads that have not been included above

Arrhythmia detection

- ICDs diagnose arrhythmias by counting intervals on the intra-cardiac electrogram (EGM) and using the morphology of the ventricular EGM
- The rhythms recognized are supraventricular rhythms (including sinus rhythm, SVT, AF/flutter), VT and VF. The device recognizes them from the cycle length or intervals (R–R interval) measured in milliseconds (as well as other criteria or 'discriminators'—discussed below)
- Cycle length = 60,000 ÷ rate (bpm), e.g. SR = 60–100 bpm = 1000–600 ms
- The ICD averages a number of cycle lengths to make a diagnosis. The number of cycle lengths required to make a diagnosis can be programmed by the operator but is usually around 12
- After a therapy has been delivered (i.e. anti-tachycardia pacing (ATP) or shock) the device then can 'redetect' to check the therapy was successful. The number of cycle lengths analysed now is less. If unsuccessful the device can deliver further therapy
- Therapy an ICD can offer: bradycardia pacing, ATP, low and high output shocks
- The physician will program the device to have different *detection zones* (see Figure 4.9.2)

Programming

- The aim is to detect dangerous sustained ventricular arrhythmias whilst avoiding inappropriate therapy or therapy for a non-sustained arrhythmia
- Avoid shocking atrial arrhythmias or sinus tachycardia (young and active patients): SVT versus VT discrimination programming algorithms should be switched on
- Atrial lead will aid discrimination of atrial arrhythmias (AV synchrony) but simultaneous paroxysmal atrial and ventricular arrhythmia are possible; very fast ventricular rates (> 200–220 bpm) irrespective of origins are interpreted as ventricular arrhythmia for safety
- Devices are typically set up with 'VF zone' and 'VT zones', which can be graded according to how the device will respond (see below)
- For the VF zone, the device simply monitors the ventricular R–R intervals. If it measures enough beats with a short enough cycle length (i.e. a fast enough rate) such as 300 ms (200 bpm) the device diagnoses VF and begins instigating therapy **without looking at other criteria**
- If the rate is slower and there are sufficient R–R intervals within the VT zone the device will then examine the rhythm according to several different algorithms to determine whether it is an SVT or a VT (see below for further discriminators)
- A single trial of ATP whilst or before charging to a shock, even in the VF zone (likely fast VT), can be effective and prevent shocks
- ATP delivered via both left and right ventricular leads (in CRT devices) is more effective than right ventricular ATP alone. ATP is delivered at a high voltage, typically 7.5 V to try to penetrate the VT circuit
- Long QT is prone to Torsade de Pointes and may not result in lack of consciousness. Torsade de pointes is often self-terminating and may be remarkably well tolerated. The detection interval is prolonged, with the aim that the patient does not receive unnecessary shock therapy. Atrial pacing at 80–90 bpm shortens the QT interval and prevents the occurrence of long–short intervals
- Secondary prevention: ICD therapy can be tailored to the clinical VT.
- Primary prevention: several trials have demonstrated the importance of multiple pulses of ATP, longer arrhythmia detection times and therapy only at higher ventricular rates in reducing the number of shocks that patients receive. These include the PAIN-FREE trials and MADIT-RIT. Typically therapy is only programmed at a ventricular rate >185bpm. An example of ICD therapy programming zones is:

4.9.3 Arrhythmia detection and programming

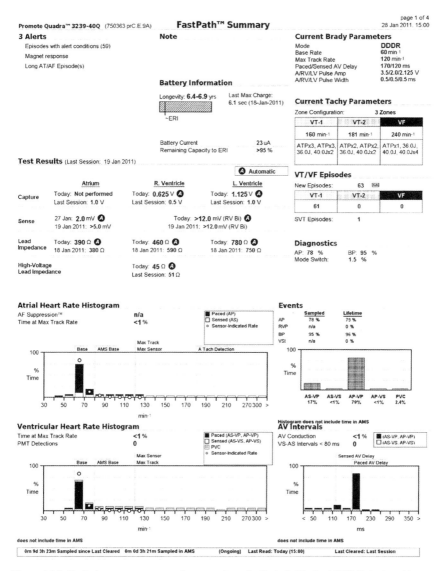

Figure 4.9.2 Typical summary page on interrogation of a St. Jude Medical CRT-D device; this particular patient has two VT zones and a VF zone

Reproduced by kind permission of Richard Chambers of St Jude Medical Inc.

- VF zone: >240bpm, ATP while charging then shocks
- VT zone: 188 – 240bpm, eight pulses of ATP followed by shocks (ESC recommends the slowest tachycardia therapy zone programmed should be at ≥188bpm (*Class I A*))
- Monitor zone: at user discretion, will record arrhythmias at this rate but will not deliver therapy. An example rate zone is 160-188bpm.
• In patients with structural heart disease (primary and secondary prevention), ESC recommends the programming of at least one ATP therapy in all tachyarrhythmia zones (*Class I A*)

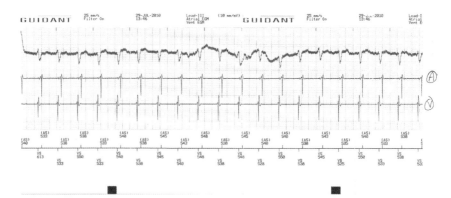

Figure 4.9.3 Supraventricular tachycardia. This patient was seen in the ICD clinic with this arrhythmia at a rate of approximately 110 bpm. There is VA conduction (A sense follows V sense). The rhythm was monitored, as it was below the programmed detection parameters for the VT-1 zone. This was terminated with IV adenosine

SVT discrimination

- SVT discriminators are algorithms programmed into the VT zones. They cannot be programmed for the VF zone
- Different companies will have different algorithms based around the same themes
- *Rate branch* (only possible in dual chamber ICDs): compares atrial to ventricular rate. If V < A or V = A the device assumes an atrial arrhythmia or sinus tachycardia respectively and inhibits therapy. If V > A the device assumes VT and delivers therapy
- *Interval stability*: this discriminator compares R–R interval stability. If R–R intervals are stable, the ICD diagnoses VT. If the R–R intervals are unstable (irregular) the device assumes AF and inhibits therapy (Figure 4.9.4)
- *Sudden onset*: sinus tachycardia builds up gradually vs VT starting suddenly
- *Chamber of onset*: (only possible in dual chamber ICDs): onset in the V is suggestive of ventricular arrhythmia and in the A suggests supraventricular arrhythmia
- *Morphology discrimination*: compares the patient's own sinus QRS complex to the QRS complexes during a tachycardia. If approximately 60% of the QRS complexes match then an SVT is diagnosed. If the device cannot match the current QRS complexes then VT is diagnosed
- These algorithms can be used alone or combined

4.9.4 Device therapy

Pacing

- All transvenous ICDs have pacing capabilities (important to consider likelihood of pacing need in decision-making of transvenous vs subcutaneous system)
- Backup bradycardia support; if no conduction issues i.e. anticipated left at a low base rate, e.g. 40 bpm with avoidance of atrial arrhythmia tracking, (i.e. DDI)
- Ventricular pacing prevents long pauses that occur after a shock; in some patients it is the post-shock pause rather than the primary arrhythmia that causes syncope

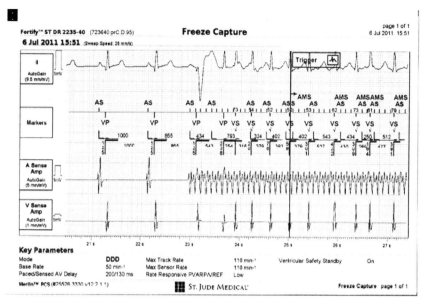

Figure 4.9.4 Onset of atrial fibrillation recorded by ICD
Reproduced by kind permission of Richard Chambers of St Jude Medical Inc.

Antitachycardia pacing (ATP)

- See Figure 4.9.5. ATP only works on monomorphic VT involving a re-entry circuit
- Pacing occurs at a rate faster than the VT (shorter cycle length), with the aim being to deliver an appropriately timed stimulus to enter into the VT re-entry circuit in such a way that it disrupts the circuit and terminates the tachycardia
- *Burst pacing*: sequence of paced beats at the same cycle length (around 88% of the tachycardia cycle length)
- *Ramp pacing*: burst of pacing with increasing pacing rate (decreasing cycle length, normally each paced beat 10 ms faster than last)
- *Scanning*: changing the cycle length from one burst to the next, allowing a burst to be delivered and, if the VT persists, the next burst to be delivered at a faster rate

Shock therapy

- See Figure 4.9.6. In a dual coil system the SVC coil can be programmed on or off; the electrical circuit is formed from the RV coil to both the SVC coil and the ICD can, or the ICD can alone
- The amount of energy an ICD is capable of delivering varies by make and model, and the energy to be delivered in shock therapy is pre-programmed and can be adjusted (often around 35J)

4.9.5 Alternative device positioning

Subcutaneous ICDs (S-ICDs)

- Traditional transvenous access to the right heart in some patients is difficult/not possible. In addition, there is a relatively high failure rate of transvenous ICD leads (up to 10%).

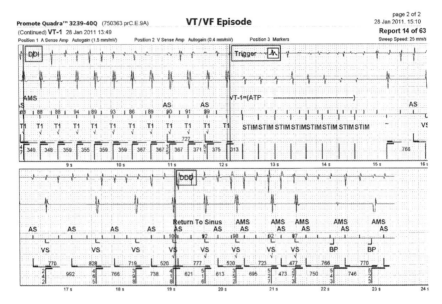

Figure 4.9.5 Anti-tachycardia pacing. A rhythm is detected in the VT-1 zone. All 12 intervals fall into this zone and so the device labels this 'VT' and initiates therapy. ATP is delivered and the device believes sinus rhythm is restored. Underlying rhythm is actually AF

Reproduced by kind permission of Richard Chambers of St Jude Medical Inc.

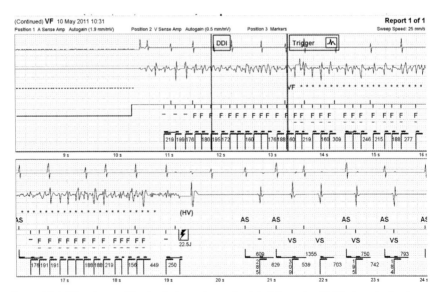

Figure 4.9.6 VF is detected by the device and so a shock is delivered at 22.5 J; sinus rhythm is restored

Reproduced by kind permission of Richard Chambers of St Jude Medical Inc.

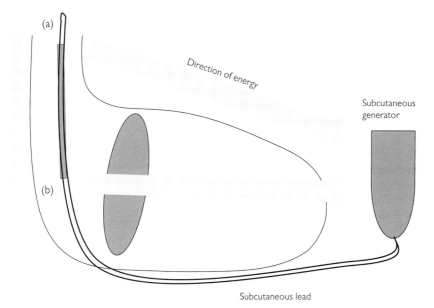

Figure 4.9.7 Schematic of S-ICD. The generator is paced subcutaneously in the 5th axillary space in between the left anterior and mid-axillary line. There are three electrodes - the generator, one on the distal tip of the lead (A in diagram) and one on the proximal part of the lead (B in diagram). There are three different options for shock vectors, indicated by the arrows

Furthermore, if devices become infected then extraction is required. Extracting a transvenous device has important risks that are not present when extracting subcutaneous ICDs
- Alternative options to infraclavicular transvenous systems include:
  - Femoral transvenous ICDs (abdominal generator placement, high risk of infection, very rarely used)
  - Epicardial ICDs (significantly more invasive than transvenous systems, high failure rate, very rarely used)
  - Subcutaneous ICDs (S-ICDs)
- S-ICDs are placed on the left anterior chest wall, entirely subcutaneously, outside of the thoracic cavity (see Figure 4.9.7)
- They have the additional benefit of avoiding transvenous lead complications (no risk of pneumothorax, RV perforation/tamponade at implant, greatly reduced risk associated with lead extraction). This is particularly relevant for young patients who are more like to suffer lead complications over the lifetime of their device(s)
- They are not suitable among the following groups:
  - Patients who require bradycardia pacing as well as ICD therapy—they do not have pacing capability, although transcutaneous pacing can be delivered for up to 30 s after a shock to prevent prolonged post-cardioversion pauses
  - Patients who are likely to require ATP—S-ICDs cannot deliver ATP
  - Patients who require CRT as well as ICD therapy
- Long term data, as well comparative RCT data vs transvenous ICDs, is lacking. However, several prospective trials have shown that S-ICDs are effective in preventing sudden death
- The largest of these is the *EFFORTLESS S-ICD* registry, which reported 3.1 +/− 1.5 yr follow-up data in ~1000 patients, demonstrating:

- Procedural complications 4.1% at 30 days and 8.4% at 360 days
- Inappropriate shocks in 11.7% after 3 years
- Appropriate shocks in 13.5% after 5 years
  - Cardioversion success for discrete spontaneous VT/VF 97.4%
- ESC guidelines recommend S-ICD should be considered:
  - In patients with an indication for ICD when bradycardia pacing, ATP and CRT are not required (*class IIa, level of evidence C*)
  - Or may be considered if venous access is challenging, after the removal of a transvenous ICD for infection, or in young patients (*class IIb, level of evidence C*)

Wearable ICDs

- These are wearable devices that can be removed—an external defibrillator with leads and electrodes attached to a vest
- No RCT data but case series and registries have demonstrated successful treatment of VT/VF
- Can be considered in patients with a transient indication for an ICD:
  - Severe LV systolic impairment that is expected to recover (peri-partum cardiomyopathy, myocarditis, early post-MI phase (*Class IIb B*))
  - Bridge to cardiac transplant
  - Bridge to permanent ICD (*Class IIa C*)

4.9.6 Device interrogation and follow-up

- Routine follow up every 6 months, either in an ICD clinic or via remote download of data over phone lines/internet, e.g. the 'care-link' system
  - ESC recommends remote monitoring where possible to reduce the incidence of inappropriate shocks (*class I B*)
- Interrogation and appropriate follow up as soon as possible within normal working hours for a single shock in an otherwise well patient
- If there have been multiple shocks or the patient is otherwise unwell they should be admitted via the A&E department and assessed urgently
- Interrogation of the device should enable the physician to determine if the shock was appropriate or inappropriate
- ICD setup can be changed to avoid inappropriate shocks
- The findings of interrogation can guide drug management to avoid both appropriate and inappropriate shocks
- There are two essential components to look at when examining an event: the box plot and the electrograms recorded by the device

Box plots

- Box plots show the R–R and A–A intervals for each of the leads (note that in a single chamber device there will only be R–R intervals)
- Look at the onset (see Figure 4.9.8): it is sudden, suggesting VT vs gradual, suggesting sinus tachycardia or AF with poor rate control
- Look at regularity of the rhythm: regular rhythm suggests VT, versus irregular for AF
- Look at the discordance between the V rate and A rate:
  - If there are more Vs than As this shows the rhythm is ventricular
  - It should be noted that an equal number of Vs and As could be an AVRT, AVNRT, atrial tachycardia, sinus tachycardia, or VT with 1:1 retrograde conduction

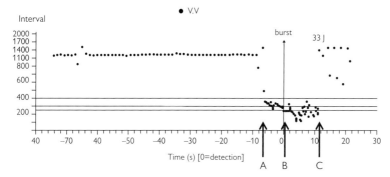

Figure 4.9.8 Box plot from a single chamber ICD (no data from the atrium). **A.** Sudden onset of a regular tachycardia with an R–R interval of 310 ms (i.e. a rate around 194 bpm). This falls within the VT zone (programmed to an R–R interval of 300–400 ms). **B.** The time at detection is set at 0 s. At this point burst ATP is delivered marked 'burst'. This results in eight regular beats that have a shorter R-R interval (and are therefore faster) than the VT—these are the burst pacing beats. **C.** After the burst pacing has finished the rhythm becomes irregular and the cycle length shortens with R–R intervals of around 200 ms (i.e. 300 bpm); this indicates that the burst pacing has degenerated the rhythm to VF. This is correctly detected and the device delivers a shock which restores sinus rhythm (this is annotated with '33J' indicating the energy of the shock). At this point the R–R interval returns to baseline and there are occasional beats with a short R–R interval, which are likely to be ectopic beats.

Intracardiac electrograms

- Information similar to that obtained from the box plot can be gained by looking at the intervals on the recording (see Figure 4.9.9)
- The relative timings between the A and V lead can be determined
- The device can monitor an electrogram between the can of the generator and the RV shock coil. This can provide useful information about the morphology of the QRS complex (see Figure 4.9.10)

4.9.7 Complications and deactivation

Complications

- Complications can occur either early or late, with an estimated incidence of up to 30% in some series.
- Early complications:
  - Pneumothorax: 1%
  - Lead displacement: 1%
  - Pericardial effusion: rare
- Late complications:
  - Infection: 1%
  - Lead failure: up to 30% at 10 years although this was with older leads
  - Inappropriate shocks: more common than appropriate shocks

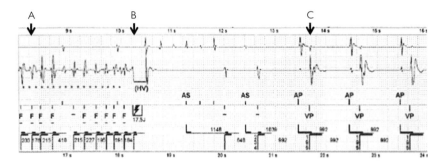

Figure 4.9.9 This recording has the atrial lead at the top, ventricular lead next, markers for the device sensing and then the intervals on the bottom line. **A.** At the beginning of the trace it can be seen that there is a regular relatively slow rate in the atrial lead but a fast irregular rate in the V lead. **B.** This has correctly been detected as VF and a shock is delivered (note the 'lightning' icon that documents the delivery of the shock). **C.** Following on from the shock there is some atrial and ventricular ectopy before settling to a paced rhythm in which the A lead is clearly paced first followed by a paced beat in the V. This is a successful shock for VF and has restored a normal-paced rhythm

Defibrillator de-activation

- The decision-making around defibrillator de-activation in the context of end-stage disease or palliative patients should be multi-disciplinary and the potential psychological impact on the patient should not be underplayed
- Ideally a senior cardiologist who the patient knows, and potentially a devices specialist, should be involved in the process, alongside palliative care representation. Most local trusts will have pathways/standard operating protocols in place for this process
- Note that de-activation of defibrillator function does not remove the device's pacing capacity—only the tachycardia therapies including ATP and shocks

4.9.8 ICD troubleshooting

Multiple *appropriate* shocks

- A 'VT storm' implies three or more sustained VT/VF episodes within 24 hours
- May be due to incessant VT, acute ischaemia, electrolyte abnormalities, drug proarrhythmia, or non-compliance with antiarrhythmics
- Acute treatment involves identifying the underlying cause
- If the problem relates to ineffective ATP then more aggressive ATP can be programmed (see Figure 4.9.11)
- Beta blockers are important in the acute setting to decrease sympathetic tone, which often drives incessant VT
- Intravenous amiodarone or lignocaine can be effective in an acute situation, with other options including over-drive pacing and sedation/general anaesthetic if unsuccessful
- High rate pacing from the atrium (or ventricle) can be effective in preventing recurrence
- Ablation of VT may be required

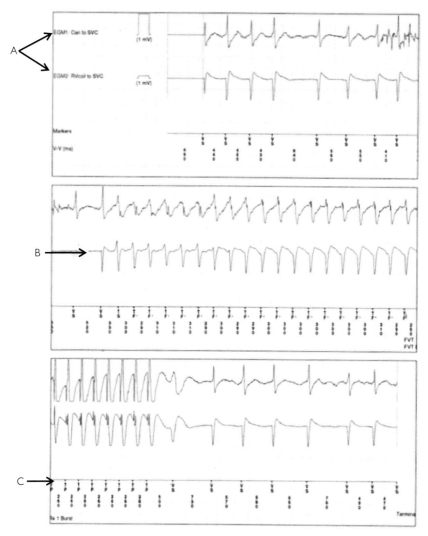

Figure 4.9.10 Intracardiac electrograms showing successful treatment of VT with ATP **A.** This recording comes from a single chamber but there are two traces which can cause confusion. The top trace is measured from the ICD can to the SVC coil and the lower trace is recorded from the RV coil to the SVC coil. The RR intervals are irregular, demonstrating AF. **B.** It can be seen that there is a sudden onset regular tachycardia with a clear change in morphology that is easiest to see in the can-to-SVC lead. The device marks the each event with a TF' to denote that they fall within the fast VT zone. **C.** After 18 consecutive events the device marks the diagnosis of fast VT and delivers a burst of 8 beats of ATP, marked as TP, which successfully terminates the VT and the rhythm returns to AF

Shock therapy fails to cardiovert arrhythmia

- The DFT should be re-evaluated
- The DFT can be increased by certain antiarrhythmics (amiodarone, flecainide, phenytoin), infarction, cardiac surgery, hyperkalaemia, or lead movement
- Can be altered by changing shocking vector or by placing a subcutaneous patch or electrode array lead

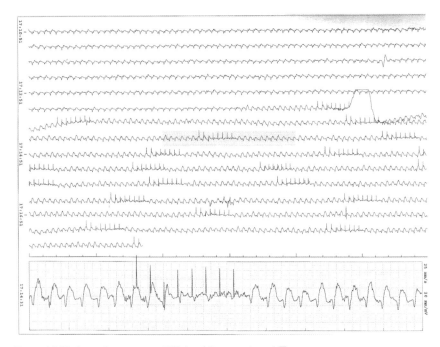

Figure 4.9.11 Several attempts at ATP that fail to terminate VT
Reproduced by kind permission of Richard Chambers of St Jude Medical Inc.

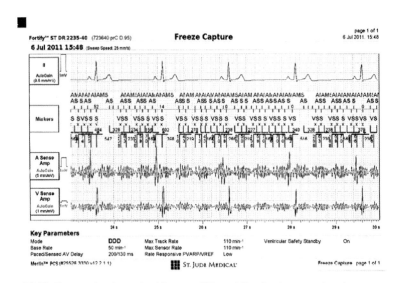

Figure 4.9.12 Oversensing due to lead fracture. This could lead to inappropriate therapy
Reproduced by kind permission of Richard Chambers of St Jude Medical Inc.

Inappropriate shocks

- In the situation of multiple inappropriate shocks the ICD should be deactivated, either with a magnet or programmer, and the patient should be placed on telemetry with external defibrillation pads placed
- Most commonly caused by atrial arrhythmias
- The atrial arrhythmias should be treated in the conventional manner and SVT discriminators re-programmed on the ICD
- Ablation of the arrhythmia or AV node can be useful
- Other causes for inappropriate therapy are over-sensing of T waves ('double counting') and lead fracture (see Figure 4.9.12)

Ventricular arrhythmias without therapy being delivered

- The most common cause for this scenario occurs when the tachyarrhythmia rate is less than the VT rate programmed on the device
- Slow VT can occur spontaneously or the VT may be slowed by antiarrhythmic medication
- Can be treated by external DCCV, internal DCCV, or ATP using the device
- The VT zones can be changed, VT ablation can be used or reduction/withdrawal of antiarrhythmic medications may be considered
- May also be due to magnet application, therapies not reprogrammed after being switched off, or no VT zone programmed at implant in a patient who has previously only had VF

Further reading

Boersma L, Barr C, Knops R, Theuns D, Eckardt L, Neuzil P, Scholten M, Hood M, Kuschyk J, Jones P, Duffy E, Husby M, Stein K, Lambiase PD; EFFORTLESS Investigator Group. Implant and Midterm Outcomes of the Subcutaneous Implantable Cardioverter-Defibrillator Registry: The EFFORTLESS Study. J Am Coll Cardiol. 2017 Aug 15;70(7):830–41. doi: 10.1016/j.jacc.2017.06.040. PMID: 28797351

Brignole M, Moya A, de Lange FJ, Deharo JC, Elliott PM, Fanciulli A, Fedorowski A, Furlan R, Kenny RA, Martín A, Probst V, Reed MJ, Rice CP, Sutton R, Ungar A, van Dijk JG; ESC Scientific Document Group. 2018 ESC Guidelines for the diagnosis and management of syncope. Eur Heart J. 2018 Jun 1;39(21):1883–1948. doi: 10.1093/eurheartj/ehy037. PMID: 29562304

Ellenbogen KA, Wood MA. *Cardiac Pacing and ICDs*. John Wiley & Sons, 31 Aug 2011.

Moss AJ, Zareba W, Hall WJ, Klein H, Wilber DJ, Cannom DS, Daubert JP, Higgins SL, Brown MW, Andrews ML; Multicenter Automatic Defibrillator Implantation Trial II Investigators. Prophylactic implantation of a defibrillator in patients with myocardial infarction and reduced ejection fraction. N Engl J Med. 2002 Mar 21;346(12):877–83. doi: 10.1056/NEJMoa013474. Epub 2002 Mar 19. PMID: 11907286

NICE guidelines: Implantable cardioverter defibrillators and cardiac resynchronisation therapy for arrhythmias and heart failure. Technology appraisal guidance [TA314] Published date: 25 June 2014.

Zeppenfeld K, Tfelt-Hansen J, de Riva M, Winkel BG, Behr ER, Blom NA, Charron P, Corrado D, Dagres N, de Chillou C, Eckardt L, Friede T, Haugaa KH, Hocini M, Lambiase PD, Marijon E, Merino JL, Peichl P, Priori SG, Reichlin T, Schulz-Menger J, Sticherling C, Tzeis S, Verstrael A, Volterrani M; ESC Scientific Document Group. 2022 ESC Guidelines for the management of patients with ventricular arrhythmias and the prevention of sudden cardiac death. Eur Heart J. 2022 Oct 21;43(40):3997–4126. doi: 10.1093/eurheartj/ehac262. PMID: 36017572.

4.10

Cardiac resynchronization therapy and His bundle pacing

Richard Bond and Howell Williams

TABLE OF CONTENTS

4.10.1 Cardiac resynchronization therapy (CRT) 409
    Landmark trials of CRT in heart failure 410
    Non-response to CRT 411
4.10.2 Conduction system pacing 412
4.10.3 Driving restrictions (UK) 414
    Driving restrictions 414

4.10.1 Cardiac resynchronization therapy (CRT)

- CRT was first described in 1994 and has now become a standard therapy for HFrEF.
- CRT helps to restore AV, inter- and intra-ventricular synchrony, which induces reverse LV remodelling. This increases LVEF, and reduces functional MR if present.
- Implant rate in the UK is below comparable European countries and is likely to increase in future.
- The device may be a pacemaker alone (CRT-P) or have both pacing and defibrillation capability (CRT-D).
- In Europe as a whole, ~70% of implants are CRT-D and ~30% CRT-P
- Both CRT-P and CRT-D reduce morbidity and mortality in HfrEF. Randomized clinical trials evidence in atrial fibrillation is absent, however cohort studies demonstrate a reduction in hospitalizations with CRT in this patient group.
- See Table 4.10.1 below for indications for CRT and primary prevention ICD therapy in systolic heart failure with LV EF ≤ 35%, despite optimal medical therapy (OMT) for heart failure, according to current NICE guidelines.
- It is however important to note that patients with RBBB appear to benefit less from CRT than patients with LBBB.
- The majority of patients in CRT trials had LBBB, with RBBB present in no higher than 17% of patients in any of the RCTs.
- Although CRT is currently approved in NICE and ESC guidelines in both RBBB (ESC class IIA) and LBBB (ESC class 1), most centres now offer an individualized approach to patients with RBBB and LVEF ≤ 35% that often does not involve offering CRT. Future guidelines are likely to reflect this.
- There are additional indications for CRT, in addition to those listed in the above table. These include:

Table 4.10.1 Current NICE guideline indications for CRT and primary prevention ICD therapy in systolic heart failure with LVEF ≤ 35%.

QRS Duration <120 milliseconds	NYHA			
	I	II	III	IV
	ICD if there is a high risk of sudden cardiac death			ICD and CRT not indicated
120–149 milliseconds without LBBB	ICD	ICD	ICD	CRT-P
120–149 milliseconds with LBBB	ICD	CRT-D	CRT-P or CRT-D	CRT-P
≥150 milliseconds with or without LBBB	CRT-D	CRT-D	CRT-P or CRT-D	CRT-P

CRT-D—CRT with defibrillator, CRT-P—CRT without defibrillator.
Reproduced from NICE guidelines – Technology appraisal guideline [TA314], June 2014.

- Patients with RV pacing who have heart failure with reduced ejection fraction (LVEF ≤ 35%) and a high percentage of RV pacing, who remain in NYHA III/IV despite OMT. Upgrade to CRT (ESC class I, level of evidence B)
- Patients with an indication for bradycardia pacing who have pre-existing reduced LVEF and expected high percentage of RV pacing (ESC class IIa, level of evidence B)
- A full summary listing the ESC guidelines for CRT in heart failure by level of evidence is listed in Box 4.10.1.

Landmark trials of CRT in heart failure

- *COMPANION*: CRT-P and CRT-D in patients with NYHA class III/IV with EF < 35% and a QRS > 120 ms already on optimal medical therapy versus optimal medical therapy alone. CRT-P/D reduced hospitalizations, CRT-P reduced all-cause mortality by 24%, and CRT-D reduced all-cause mortality by 36%
- *CARE-HF*: CRT-P with NYHA class III/IV heart failure and EF < 35%, QRS > 120 ms on optimal medical therapy against medical therapy alone. RRR of 36% in all-cause mortality in the CRT-P group
- MADIT-CRT and REVERSE showed benefit in NYHA class II with reduced morbidity. 18% in REVERSE and 15% in MADIT-CRT were in NYHA class I at baseline, although most of these patients had been previously symptomatic. Improvement was primarily seen in patients with QRS ≥ 150 ms and/or typical LBBB
- In NYHA class II and III heart failure, CRT-D reduced the risk of death or hospitalization by 25% compared with ICD alone in the RAFT study. 80% of the patients were in NYHA class II

At implant

- The threshold of the LV lead is usually higher than the RV lead. It will produce a RBBB morphology when tested; important to confirm a positive R wave in V1.
- The position of the lead can affect the response; poor responses seen in the great cardiac vein or very apical positions.

BOX 4.10.1 ESC INDICATIONS FOR CRT IN HEART FAILURE BY EVIDENCE LEVEL

Class I

- Recommended for symptomatic patients in SR with QRS ≥ 150 ms of LBBB morphology, with LVEF ≤ 35% despite OMT, to improve symptoms, morbidity, and mortality. For patients in AF this is a IIa indication
- Recommended over RV pacing for patients with HFrEF (EF ≤40% regardless of NYHA class) who have an indication for ventricular pacing and high degree AV block (who will therefore require a high burden of RV pacing) in order to reduce morbidity
- Recommended over RV pacing for patients with HFrEF in AF with uncontrolled heart rate who are undergoing AV node ablation

Class IIa

- Recommended for symptomatic patients in SR with a QRS of 130–149 ms, LBBB morphology and LVEF ≤ 35% despite OMT in order to improve symptoms and reduce morbidity and mortality
- Consider for symptomatic patients in SR with a QRS duration ≥ 150 ms, non-LBBB morphology and LVEF ≤ 35% despite OMT in order to improve symptoms and reduce morbidity and mortality
- Consider for patients with AF, a QRS duration ≥ 130 ms and an LVEF ≤ 35% in NYHA Class III/IV despite OMT in order to improve symptoms and reduce morbidity and mortality, provided a strategy to ensure bi-ventricular capture is in place or the patient is expected to return to SR
- Consider over RV pacing for patients with HFmrEF in AF with uncontrolled heart rate who are undergoing AV node ablation
- Consider upgrade to CRT in patients who have a conventional pacemaker or ICD who have a significant (> 20%) burden of RV pacing and who subsequently develop symptomatic HFrEF with LVEF ≤ 35% despite OMT

Class IIb

- Consider for symptomatic patients in SR with a QRS of 130–149 ms, non-LBBB morphology and LVEF ≤ 35% despite OMT in order to improve symptoms and reduce morbidity and mortality

Glikson M, Nielsen JC, Kronborg MB, et al; ESC Scientific Document Group. 2021 ESC Guidelines on cardiac pacing and cardiac resynchronization therapy. Eur Heart J. 2021 Sep 14;42(35):3427–3520. doi: 10.1093/eurheartj/ehab364. Erratum in: Eur Heart J. 2022 May 1;43(17):1651. © European Society of Cardiology. With permission from Oxford University Press

Non-response to CRT

- The natural history of cardiac failure is deterioration over time
- The majority of patients with CRT feel better but some do not notice an improvement. As a general rule one-third feel a lot better, one-third a little better, and one-third no better
- Factors that predict increased response are:
    - LBBB pattern
    - Wider QRS
    - Female patients
    - Non-ischaemic cause of LV impairment

- Lack of improvement may be due to
    - The underlying condition, especially widespread MI
    - Failure to receive biventricular pacing due to rapid atrial arrhythmias. The goal of CRT is to achieve biventricular pacing as close to 100% of the time as possible (the opposite approach to RV pacing)
    - Sinus tachycardia or atrial arrhythmias are common causes of reduced biventricular pacing
    - Increased biventricular pacing in this setting can be achieved with rate limiting drugs (typically increasing beta-blocker dose, or adding ivabradine if SR)
    - In atrial arrhythmia, consideration should routinely be given to restoring SR
        - This can be achieved with catheter ablation either of the arrhythmia or of the AV node
        - AV node ablation renders patients fully dependent on CRT pacing but will increase biV pacing to 100%
    - Technical failure to place the LV lead in an adequate vein (e.g. pacing too far towards the apex)—some patients may require LV lead revision.
    - Anodal stimulation: in a normal situation capture occurs at the cathode, but to improve pacing parameters CRT devices can be programmed to pace from LV tip (cathode) to RV ring (anode). Anodal stimulation occurs when the site of capture becomes the anode (RV lead) rather than the cathode (LV lead) and is an important cause of non-response. It can be difficult to detect unless considered, as the LV lead will appear to be capturing, but the ECG morphology of pacing will be exactly the same as RV pacing.
    - The AV interval can be altered to maximize LV filling whilst minimizing diastolic MR. The timings between the stimulation of the RV and LV lead can also be altered, and there are device-based algorithms that time intrinsic conduction through the AV node with biventricular or LV-only pacing. There is variable data on the efficacy of this 'CRT optimisation' programming but the overall weight of evidence does favour individualised programming of these parameters, using both device-based algorithms and 12-lead ECG assessment to achieve the narrowest possible QRS duration.

4.10.2 Conduction system pacing

His bundle pacing
- His bundle (HB) pacing was first described in 2000.
- It involves implanting an active fixation lead into the bundle of His (see Figure 4.10.1).
- This can lead to 'physiological' activation of the ventricles, through pacing stimulation of the intrinsic specialised conduction system.
- The His-SYNC trial (2019) demonstrated the feasibility and safety of HB pacing as an alternative to CRT. Other observational studies have provided promising initial data.
- HB pacing can be considered as an alternative to RV pacing for conventional bradycardia pacing indications. However, this technique is significantly limited by unpredictable and rapid changes in lead parameters including stimulation threshold that can cause loss of ventricular capture. Many centres therefore currently also implant an RV lead in patients with AV node disease (see Figure 4.10.1).
- HB pacing is also being further investigated as an alternative to CRT in patients with heart failure and reduced ejection fraction, with LBBB.
    - Observational data has demonstrated that His pacing can overcome LBBB

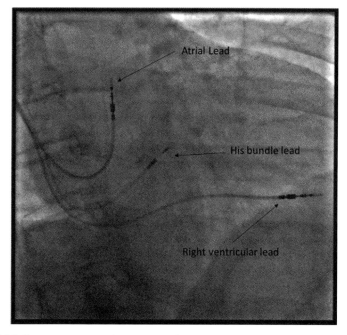

Figure 4.10.1 Fluoroscopic image demonstrating lead positions in His bundle pacing. Note right ventricular lead for backup pacing in case of His bundle pacing failure.

- This is presumed to result from implant of the His lead distal to the site of LBBB (i.e. the fibres that will create the left bundle are damaged within the His bundle, and so a lead in the distal His bundle is distal to the block) although other theories also exist
- Current ESC guidelines recommend His bundle pacing be considered as an option in CRT candidates in whom coronary sinus lead placement is not successful, alongside other techniques such as epicardial pacing (class IIa, level of evidence B).

Left bundle branch area pacing

- Left bundle branch area pacing (LBBAP) is an increasingly common technique. It involves implanting an active fixation lead deep into the proximal interventricular septum, aiming to stimulate the intrinsic conduction system by capturing the left bundle branch
- It was first described by Huang and colleagues in 2017
- It typically leads to a significantly narrower QRS duration than conventional RV septal or apical pacing. It is an attractive alternative to conventional RV pacing in patients with an anticipated high burden of RV pacing, as current observational data shows that RV-pacing-induced LV systolic impairment is markedly less common with LBBAP than conventional RV pacing
- As with His bundle pacing there is also some evidence that it can 'overcome' intrinsic left bundle branch block and improve LV systolic function in a way that is comparable to CRT
- It is important to note that this data comes from small trials and further evidence is needed. At present LBBAP is not used as an alternative to CRT unless there are technical reasons that CRT cannot be implanted

- Importantly the LBBAP lead parameters appear to more stable than His bundle pacing lead parameters. It is also technically easier to achieve than HPB.
- The role of conduction system pacing is likely to evolve and increase over the coming years. Long-term large RCT evidence is needed to confirm its role. This is particularly important when considering conduction system pacing as an alternative to CRT, given the very large body of RCT evidence supporting the role of CRT.

4.10.3 Driving restrictions (UK)

Driving restrictions

- Driving regulations vary internationally, and Cardiologists are recommended to familiarize themselves with their national guidance
- ESC guidelines are listed in section 4.2.7. The following relate to current UK DVLA guidance:

All arrhythmias

- Group 1 licence: must not drive if arrhythmia has caused or is likely to cause incapacity. Driving may resume without informing DVLA after cause of arrhythmia has been identified and arrhythmia controlled for at least 4 weeks
- Group 2 licence: must notify the DVLA. Must not drive if arrhythmia has caused or is likely to cause incapacity. Licence will be refused or revoked.
  - May be relicensed/licensed only after underlying cause has been identified, arrhythmia has been controlled for at least 3 months, and LV ejection fraction is at least 40%

Pacemaker implant including CRT-P and pacemaker box changes

- Group 1 licence: must not drive for 1 week and must notify DVLA
- Group 2 licence: must not drive for 6 weeks and must notify the DVLA Driving may resume after 6 weeks if LV EF is greater than or equal to 40% and symptoms in NYHA I or II

ICD implant—secondary prevention

- Group 1 licence: must not drive and must notify DVLA. Driving may resume after 6 months providing no therapy has been delivered and no revision to ICD leads or change in antiarrhythmic drug treatment has occurred
- Group 2 licence: permanently revoked

ICD implant—primary prevention

- Group 1 licence: must not drive for 1 month and must notify DVLA
- Group 2 licence: permanently revoked

Specific to Group 1 licence holders

- ICD box change
  - Must not drive for 1 week, no need to notify DVLA
- ICD therapy that is not associated with incapacity
  - Must not drive for 6 months, must notify DVLA
- ICD therapy that is associated with incapacity—must notify DVLA
  - Due to inappropriate therapy, e.g. AF or programming issue: 1 month only if the cause is completely controlled to the satisfaction of the cardiologist

- Due to appropriate therapy for VT/VF, with subsequent treatment to prevent recurrence (change of drugs, VT ablation): 6 months
    - If neither of the above categories apply, must not drive for 2 years
- Any revision to ICD device, or change of anti-arrhythmic drug treatment in patients with an ICD *in situ*
    - Must not drive for 1 month, no need to inform the DVLA

Further reading

Boersma L, Barr C, Knops R, Theuns D, Eckardt L, Neuzil P, Scholten M, Hood M, Kuschyk J, Jones P, Duffy E, Husby M, Stein K, Lambiase PD; EFFORTLESS Investigator Group. Implant and Midterm Outcomes of the Subcutaneous Implantable Cardioverter-Defibrillator Registry: The EFFORTLESS Study. *J Am Coll Cardiol*. 2017 Aug 15;70(7):830–41. doi: 10.1016/j.jacc.2017.06.040. PMID: 28797351

Brignole M, Moya A, de Lange FJ, Deharo JC, Elliott PM, Fanciulli A, Fedorowski A, Furlan R, Kenny RA, Martín A, Probst V, Reed MJ, Rice CP, Sutton R, Ungar A, van Dijk JG; ESC Scientific Document Group. 2018 ESC Guidelines for the diagnosis and management of syncope. *Eur Heart J*. 2018 Jun 1;39(21):1883–948. doi: 10.1093/eurheartj/ehy037. PMID: 29562304

Burri H, Jastrzebski M, Cano Ó, Čurila K, de Pooter J, Huang W, Israel C, Joza J, Romero J, Vernooy K, Vijayaraman P, Whinnett Z, Zanon F. EHRA clinical consensus statement on conduction system pacing implantation: endorsed by the Asia Pacific Heart Rhythm Society (APHRS), Canadian Heart Rhythm Society (CHRS), and Latin American Heart Rhythm Society (LAHRS). Europace. 2023 Apr 15;25(4):1208–36. doi: 10.1093/europace/euad043. PMID: 37061848; PMCID: PMC10105878.

Glikson M, Nielsen JC, Kronborg MB, Michowitz Y, Auricchio A, Barbash IM, Barrabés JA, Boriani G, Braunschweig F, Brignole M, Burri H, Coats AJS, Deharo JC, Delgado V, Diller GP, Israel CW, Keren A, Knops RE, Kotecha D, Leclercq C, Merkely B, Starck C, Thylén I, Tolosana JM; ESC Scientific Document Group. 2021 ESC Guidelines on cardiac pacing and cardiac resynchronization therapy. *Eur Heart J*. 2021 Sep 14;42(35):3427–520. doi: 10.1093/eurheartj/ehab364. PMID: 34455430

Huang W, Chen X, Su L, Wu S, Xia X, Vijayaraman P. A beginner's guide to permanent left bundle branch pacing. Heart Rhythm. 2019 Dec;16(12):1791–6. doi: 10.1016/j.hrthm.2019.06.016. Epub 2019 Jun 22. PMID: 31233818.

Moss AJ, Zareba W, Hall WJ, Klein H, Wilber DJ, Cannom DS, Daubert JP, Higgins SL, Brown MW, Andrews ML; Multicenter Automatic Defibrillator Implantation Trial II Investigators. Prophylactic implantation of a defibrillator in patients with myocardial infarction and reduced ejection fraction. *N Engl J Med*. 2002 Mar 21;346(12):877–83. doi: 10.1056/NEJMoa013474. Epub 2002 Mar 19. PMID: 11907286

NICE guidelines: Implantable cardioverter defibrillators and cardiac resynchronisation therapy for arrhythmias and heart failure. Technology appraisal guidance [TA314] Published date: 25 June 2014

Priori SG, Blomström-Lundqvist C, Mazzanti A, Blom N, Borggrefe M, Camm J, Elliott PM, Fitzsimons D, Hatala R, Hindricks G, Kirchhof P, Kjeldsen K, Kuck KH, Hernandez-Madrid A, Nikolaou N, Norekvål TM, Spaulding C, Van Veldhuisen DJ; ESC Scientific Document Group. 2015 ESC Guidelines for the management of patients with ventricular arrhythmias and the prevention of sudden cardiac death: The Task Force for the Management of Patients with Ventricular Arrhythmias and the Prevention of Sudden Cardiac Death of the European Society of Cardiology (ESC). Endorsed by: Association for European Paediatric and Congenital Cardiology (AEPC). *Eur Heart J*. 2015 Nov 1;36(41):2793–867. doi: 10.1093/eurheartj/ehv316. Epub 2015 Aug 29. PMID: 26320108

CHAPTER 5

HEART FAILURE

5.1

Heart failure syndromes

Abdul Hameed, Andrew Clark, Christopher N Floyd, and Alexander Carpenter

TABLE OF CONTENTS

5.1.1 Definition and clinical features 419
5.1.2 Epidemiology and prognosis 420
5.1.3 Classification and grading 421
5.1.4 Aetiology and pathophysiology 426
5.1.5 Investigations 429
5.1.6 Medical management 433
5.1.7 Arrhythmia, pacing and device therapy 445
 Atrial fibrillation 445
 Ventricular arrhythmias 446
 Devices 446
5.1.8 Surgical and transcatheter interventions in heart failure 448
5.1.9 Advanced heart failure therapies: mechanical circulatory support (MCS) and heart transplantation 450
5.1.10 Co-morbidities and multi-disciplinary care in HF 454
 Anaemia and iron deficiency 455
 Multidisciplinary team management recommendations 455
 Long-term follow-up and monitoring 455
5.1.11 Acute heart failure 456
 Causes and precipitants 456
 Assessment and investigations 456
 Acute management for the three modes of presentation 457
 Right heart failure and pulmonary hypertension 458
5.1.12 Palliative care in heart failure 458

5.1.1 Definition and clinical features

Several definitions have been coined to define heart failure over the decades but a sensible and pragmatic one is the Universal Definition in the 2021 International Consensus Statement (contributors included the Heart Failure Association of the European Society of Cardiology):

Heart failure is a clinical pathophysiological syndrome characterized by:

1) Typical symptoms (e.g. dyspnoea or fatigue on exertion, ankle swelling)
2) Clinical signs (e.g. elevated JVP, pulmonary crackles, dependent oedema)
3) Caused by a structural/functional cardiac abnormality
4) And corroborated by elevated natriuretic peptide levels and/or objective evidence of pulmonary or systemic congestion and/or reduced cardiac output and/or elevated intra-cardiac pressures at rest/stress

For a detailed list of symptoms and signs see Table 5.1.1

Table 5.1.1 Signs and symptoms of heart failure.

SYMPTOMS	SIGNS
Typical	**More specific**
Breathlessness, reduced exercise tolerance orthopnoea, paroxysmal nocturnal dyspnoea, fatigue, tiredness, delayed recovery post exercise Ankle swelling	Elevated jugular venous pulse Hepatojugular reflux Third heart sound (gallop rhythm) Laterally displaced apex beat
Less Typical	**Less specific**
Nocturnal cough, wheeze Palpitations, dizziness, syncope, Bendopnea (dyspnoea on bending/stooping) Abdominal bloating, right upper quadrant pain, loss of appetite Confusion (especially in elderly) Hoarse voice Depression, loss of libido	Weight gain (> 2 kg/week) Pulmonary crackles or signs of pleural effusions Peripheral oedema (ankle, scrotal, sacral) Hepatomegaly, ascites, Cardiac murmur Tachycardia, irregular pulse Cold extremities, oliguria, narrow pulse pressure Weight loss in advanced HF or wasting (cachexia)

McDonagh TA, Metra M, Adamo M, et al; ESC Scientific Document Group. 2021 ESC Guidelines for the diagnosis and treatment of acute and chronic heart failure. *Eur Heart J*. 2021 Sep 21;42(36):3599–3726. doi: 10.1093/eurheartj/ehab368. © European Society of Cardiology. With permission from Oxford University Press

5.1.2 Epidemiology and prognosis

- The incidence and prevalence of HF increases with age, with the average age at first diagnosis being 76
- Prevalence is approximately 1–2% in overall population of developed nations, and >10% in those over 70 years of age
- Lifetime risk of HF at age 55 is 33% for men and 28% for women
- Heart failure with a reduced ejection fraction (HFrEF) incidence appears to be decreasing, whereas prevalence is rising, mainly due to increasing survival from acute and chronic ischaemic heart disease
- Heart failure with preserved ejection fraction (HFpEF) accounts for approx. 30–70% depending on definition, population, and era studied
- In population studies using echo, approximately half of people with left ventricular systolic dysfunction (LVSD) are asymptomatic (i.e. do not meet definition of clinical HF)
- Prior to 1990, 5-year survival was 30–40% and has improved with 30–50% relative risk reduction in hospitalization
- Figures from the 2018–19 National Heart Failure Audit for England & Wales reported:
  - Age: mean 78 y (males 76.1 y females 80.4 y), median 81 y
  - Mortality: inpatient 9.1%, 30-day 16%, 1-year 32%
  - Specialist care linked to significantly reduced mortality and higher use of optimal medical therapy (OMT)
- Risk stratification in HF for an individual patient is challenging. All currently available multivariable scoring systems have modest predictive power (Area Under Curve < 0.7)
- Examples of prognostic scoring systems include
  HFSS: Heart failure Survival Score
  SHFM: Seattle Heart failure Model

MAGGIC: Meta-Analysis Global Group in Congestive Heart Failure
MECKI: Metabolic Exercise test data combined with Cardiac and Kidney Indexes.
- The HFSS and MECKI scores incorporate data from cardiopulmonary exercise testing (peak VO2 and VE/VCO2), which is known to carry its own prognostic data

5.1.3 Classification and Grading

- Historically LV ejection fraction (EF) has been used to subdivide patients with heart failure on the basis of presence of and severity of systolic dysfunction
- Ejection fraction (EF) is defined as:
  stroke volume (end diastolic volume − end systolic volume) / end diastolic volume
- Two principal categories: reduced EF (≤ 40%) and preserved/normal EF (≥5 0%)
- The term heart failure with mildly reduced EF (HFmrEF) has been introduced for those in between these two distinct entities (EF 41–49%), recognizing that studies have demonstrated patients in this group gain some benefit from therapies used to treat HFrEF. The three entities are outlined in Table 5.1.2
- Patients with a recovered EF who had previous overt LV systolic dysfunction should be considered to have HF with improved EF (HFimpEF) rather than HFpEF:

  = HF with a baseline LVEF of ≤ 40%, a 10-point increase from baseline LVEF, and a second measurement of LVEF of >40%

- Identifying the aetiology of heart failure is fundamental to its treatment, including considering and excluding other conditions with clinical features overlapping heart failure. These include, but are not limited to:
    - Valvular heart disease
    - Pericardial disease (may require right and left heart catheterization)
    - Pulmonary hypertension
    - Chronic pulmonary thrombo-embolic disease
    - Lung disease (COPD, parenchymal, etc.)
    - Primary renal/hepatic failure

Table 5.1.2 The ESC defined categories for diagnosing heart failure by ejection fraction.

Heart failure with reduced EF (HFrEF)	Heart failure with preserved EF (HFpEF)	Heart failure with mildly reduced EF (HFmrEF)
Symptoms +/− signs	Symptoms +/− signs	Symptoms +/− signs
LV ejection fraction ≤ 40%	LV ejection fraction ≥ 50%	LV ejection fraction 41–49%
	• Elevated natriuretic peptides • Relevant structural heart disease (e.g. LVH, LA enlargement and/or diastolic dysfunction)	

McDonagh TA, Metra M, Adamo M, et al; ESC Scientific Document Group. 2021 ESC Guidelines for the diagnosis and treatment of acute and chronic heart failure. *Eur Heart J*. 2021 Sep 21;42(36):3599–3726. doi: 10.1093/eurheartj/ehab368. © European Society of Cardiology. With permission from Oxford University Press

Table 5.1.3 Accepted upper limits of normal for natriuretic levels (PV = predictive value).

Marker	Community/outpatient setting	Acute setting
BNP	35 pg/ml	100 pg/ml
NT pro BNP	125 pg/ml	300 pg/ml
Mid regional pro ANP		120 pmol/L
Predictive values	Negative PV 0.94–0.98 Positive PV 0.44–0.57	Negative PV 0.94–0.98 Positive PV 0.66–0.67

McDonagh TA, Metra M, Adamo M, et al; ESC Scientific Document Group. 2021 ESC Guidelines for the diagnosis and treatment of acute and chronic heart failure. *Eur Heart J.* 2021 Sep 21;42(36):3599–3726. doi: 10.1093/eurheartj/ehab368. © European Society of Cardiology. With permission from Oxford University Press

Natriuretic peptides (NPs)

The types of NP:

- A-type NP is a 28 amino acid fragment of pro-ANP and is not routinely measured
- B-type NP is co-secreted with a 76-amino-acid fragment NT-proBNP in a 1:1 ratio
- NT-proBNP is biologically inactive with a longer half-life so values are higher than BNP
- BNP and NT-proBNP are mainly produced in the cardiac ventricles and serum levels rise in response to an increase in myocardial wall stress

NPs are:

- A useful initial diagnostic test, especially when echocardiography initially unavailable
- Primarily used for *ruling out* the diagnosis. When normal in the presence of a normal ECG, makes the diagnosis of HF very unlikely—they have a high negative predictive value and levels at which a diagnosis of HF is excluded are listed in Table 5.1.3
- Can be raised in a variety of pathologies (Box 5.1.1)
- Affected mainly by age, renal function, and AF (which all raise levels)

BOX 5.1.1 OTHER CAUSES OF ELEVATED NATRIURETIC PEPTIDES INCLUDE:

Cardiac
Heart failure
Acute coronary syndromes
Pulmonary embolism
Myocarditis
Left ventricular hypertrophy
Hypertrophic or restrictive cardiomyopathy
Valvular heart disease
Congenital heart disease
Atrial and ventricular tachyarrhythmias
Heart contusion
Cardioversion, ICD shock
Surgical procedures involving the heart
Pulmonary hypertension

Non-Cardiac
Advanced age
Ischaemic stroke
Subarachnoid haemorrhage
Renal dysfunction
Liver dysfunction (mainly liver cirrhosis with ascites)
Paraneoplastic syndrome
Chronic obstructive pulmonary disease
Severe infections (including pneumonia and sepsis)
Severe burns
Anaemia
Severe metabolic and hormone abnormalities (e.g. thyrotoxicosis, diabetic ketosis)

McDonagh TA, Metra M, Adamo M, et al; ESC Scientific Document Group. 2021 ESC Guidelines for the diagnosis and treatment of acute and chronic heart failure. *Eur Heart J.* 2021 Sep 21;42(36):3599–3726. doi: 10.1093/eurheartj/ehab368. © European Society of Cardiology. With permission from Oxford University Press

- Disproportionately low in obesity, constrictive pericarditis, or patients with LVSD on optimal medical therapy with few/no symptoms
- Unexpectedly low in some patients with acute right heart failure, decompensated end-stage HF and flash pulmonary oedema

Diagnosis of HFpEF

- HFpEF patients are a heterogenous group, making its diagnosis challenging
- Key features include the presence of clinical risk factors, abnormal natriuretic peptides, and features of diastolic dysfunction
- Strictly speaking, HFpEF includes patients with valvular heart disease, pericardial disease, restrictive cardiomyopathy or cor pulmonale in whom LVEF is > 50%: however, it should be used to refer to patients with structural LV and LA remodeling
- Compared to HFrEF, patients with HFpEF tend to be older, more often female and have a higher prevalence of hypertension, AF, diabetes, obesity, pulmonary hypertension, and renal dysfunction
- 10–15% cases of HFpEF have ATTR amyloidosis and so this should be excluded, particularly as an RCT has shown symptomatic and prognostic benefit for the ATTR stabilizing drug, tafamidis (ATTR-ACT Study)
    - Features suggestive of this include low normal BP in patients with a history of hypertension, intolerance to beta blockers/ACEi, bilateral carpal tunnel syndrome, low voltage ECG with echocardiographic features (e.g. hypertrophied septum, posterior wall or RV wall, enlarged atria, small pericardial effusion, or valve thickening)

Assessment of diastolic function

- Criteria are evolving and have not been adequately validated
- The detailed role of imaging in HF is covered in section 5.1.5, but the 2021 ESC guidelines highlight the following structural changes as features of probable diastolic dysfunction:
    1. Left atrial volume index (LAVi) > 34 mL/m^2 (or > 40 mL/m^2 in AF)
    2. Left ventricular mass index (LVMI) ≥ 115 g/m^2 for males and ≥95 g/m^2 for females, relative wall thickness > 0.42
    3. E/e' ratio > 9 (at rest), mean septal e' < 9 cm/s and mitral E velocity < 90 cm/s
    4. Pulmonary hypertension (from velocity of TR jet (> 2.8 m/s) or PASP > 35 mmHg)
    5. Reduced LV global longitudinal strain (≤16%) (sensitivity 54% specificity 85%)
- Consensus documents on the subject have been periodically updated over the past decade, and guidance published jointly by American and European cardiac imaging societies are defined in Figure 5.1.1
- The two most recent algorithms (scores) proposed for diagnosing HFpEF are refinements of previous and consist of clinical variables (age, BMI, AF), NP levels (adjusted for AF), and echocardiographic measures

i) H$_2$ FPEFF score (2018)

- Outlined in Table 5.1.4 below, with a score > 5 giving a > 90% probability for the presence of HFpEF

ii) HFA-PEFF Score (2019)

- The European Society of Heart Failure (HFA) have produced a similar scoring system, outlined in Table 5.1.5
- In the case of an intermediate score, the HFA proposes further evaluation with diastolic exercise stress echocardiography
    - Criteria for HFpEF are an average E/e' >15 (2 points) and/or TR velocity > 3.4 m/s (1 point)

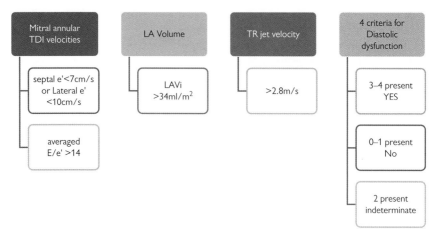

Figure 5.1.1 LV Diastolic dysfunction by ASE/EACVI criteria (2016)

Source data from Nagueh et al. Recommendations for the Evaluation of Left Ventricular Diastolic Function by Echocardiography: An Update from the American Society of Echocardiography and the European Association of Cardiovascular Imaging. *J Am Soc Echocardiogr*. 2016 Apr;29(4):277–314. doi: 10.1016/j.echo.2016.01.011

- If these are not met then invasive (right and left heart catheterization) haemodynamic measurements are advised (resting LVEDP ≥ 16 or PAWP ≥ 16 mmHg or with exercise PAWP ≥ 25 mmHg)
- It is also increasingly recognized that the HFpEF spectrum includes different 'phenogroups' with different disease trajectories and prognosis. This type of research uses machine learning and incorporates clinical, echocardiographic and ECG variables as well as biomarkers (plasma, metabolomic and genetic) but is still in its infancy.

Grading of heart failure severity

- The NYHA functional classification of symptom severity is subjective but nonetheless clinically useful and is routinely employed in clinical trials (see Table 5.1.6)
- The Weber–Janicki classification (see Table 5.1.7) classifies heart failure severity according to exercise capacity, as assessed by cardiopulmonary exercise testing

Table 5.1.4 H_2 FPEFF score—a simple, evidence-based approach to help guide diagnosis of heart failure with preserved ejection fraction.

	Variable	Value	Points
H_2	Heavy	BMI > 30	2
	Hypertensive	≥ 2 antihypertensive medications	1
F	Atrial Fibrillation	Paroxysmal or persistent	3
P	Pulmonary hypertension	Doppler Echo est PASP > 35	1
E	Elderly	Age > 60 y	1
F	Filling pressure	Doppler Echo E/e' > 9	1

Reproduced from Reddy YNV, Carter RE, Obokata M, Redfield MM, Borlaug BA. A Simple, Evidence-Based Approach to Help Guide Diagnosis of Heart Failure With Preserved Ejection Fraction. *Circulation*. 2018 Aug 28;138(9):861–870. doi: 10.1161/CIRCULATIONAHA.118.034646. with permission from Wolters Kluwer.

Table 5.1.5 HFA-PEFF Score—a consensus recommendation from the Heart Failure Association (HFA) of the European Society of Cardiology for the diagnosis of heart failure with preserved ejection fraction.

	Functional	Morphological	Biomarker (SR)	Biomarker (AF)
MAJOR	Septal e' < 7 cm/s or Lateral e' < 10cm/s or Average E/e' > 15 or TR vel > 2.8m/s (PASP > 35)	LAVI > 34 ml/m^2 or LVMI ≥ 149/ 122g/m^2 and RWT > 0.42	NTpBNP > 220 pg/ml or BNP > 80 pg/ml	NTpBNP > 600 pg/ml or BNP > 240
MINOR	Average E/e' 9–14 or GLS ≤ 16%		NTpBNP 125–220 pg/ml or BNP 35–80 pg/ml	NTpBNP 365–660 pg/ml or BNP 105–240 pg/ml

≥ 5 points: HFpEF diagnosed
2–4 points: Intermediate: Perform diastolic stress Echo +/− invasive haemodynamic assessment

Pieske B, Tschöpe C, de Boer RA, et al. How to diagnose heart failure with preserved ejection fraction: the HFA-PEFF diagnostic algorithm: a consensus recommendation from the Heart Failure Association (HFA) of the European Society of Cardiology (ESC). *Eur Heart J*. 2019 Oct 21;40(40):3297–3317. doi: 10.1093/eurheartj/ehz641. © European Society of Cardiology. With permission from Oxford University Press.

Table 5.1.6 Grading heart failure by ACC/AHA vs NYHA classification.

ACC/AHA stages of heart failure (2005)		NYHA functional classification (1994)	
Stage of heart failure based on structure and damage to heart muscle		Severity based on symptoms and physical activity	
Stage A	At high risk for developing heart failure. No identified structural or functional abnormality or raised HF biomarkers; no signs or symptoms	**Class I**	**No limitation** of physical activity. Ordinary physical activity does not cause undue fatigue, palpitation, or dyspnoea
Stage B	Developed structural heart disease or elevated biomarkers that are strongly associated with the development of heart failure, but without signs or symptoms **Asymptomatic Structural HD**	**Class II**	**Slight limitation** of physical activity. Comfortable at rest, but ordinary physical activity results in fatigue, palpitation, or dyspnoea
Stage C	Current or prior symptomatic heart failure associated with underlying structural or functional heart disease **Symptomatic HF**	**Class III**	**Marked limitation** of physical activity. Comfortable at rest, but less than ordinary activity results in fatigue, palpitation, or dyspnoea
Stage D	Advanced structural heart disease and marked symptoms of heart failure at rest despite maximal medical therapy **Advanced HF**	**Class IV**	**Symptoms at rest**. If any physical activity is undertaken, discomfort is increased. Unable to carry on any physical activity without discomfort

N.B. The 2021 Consensus Statement adjusted names to: Stage A = At-risk for HF; B = Pre-HF; C = HF, and D = Advanced HF. Stage D was defined as patients with severe symptoms and/or signs of HF at rest, recurrent hospitalizations despite guideline-directed management and therapy (GDMT), refractory or intolerant to GDMT, requiring advanced therapies such as consideration for transplant, mechanical circulatory support, or palliative care; though this was not covered in the 2021 ESC Heart Failure guidelines.

Table 5.1.7 Grading heart failure by the Weber–Janicki classification.

Grade	Severity	Peak VO2 (ml/kg/min)	Anaerobic Threshold
A	None-mild	> 20	> 14
B	Mild-moderate	16–20	11–14
C	Mod-severe	10–16	8–11
D	Severe	6–10	5–8
E	Very Severe	< 6	< 4

5.1.4 Aetiology and pathophysiology

- HF is a clinical syndrome and thus not a primary diagnosis
- The underlying cause(s) of HF should always be sought so as to direct the most appropriate therapies (e.g. valve repair/replacement, antihypertensive therapy, iron chelation therapy)
- Cardiac dysfunction can occur when abnormalities in either *one or more* of the following are present:
  1. Endo-myocardial disease: impaired contractility and/or relaxation of one or both ventricles
  2. Altered loading conditions:
     a. Increased afterload: systemic or pulmonary hypertension, valvular stenosis, outflow tract obstruction, aortic coarctation
     b. Altered preload: e.g. valvular regurgitation, high output states
     c. Intra/extra-cardiac shunts: e.g. patent ductus arteriosus (PDA), atrial or ventricular septal defects (ASD or VSD), anomalous pulmonary venous connections, fistulae (e.g. coronary, ruptured aneurysm of sinus of Valsalva)
     d. Hypovolaemia: e.g. bleeding or significant fluid/electrolyte losses
  3. Cardiac arrhythmias: e.g. AF
  4. Pericardial disease
- The commonest causes of heart failure in Europe are
  - Acute/chronic ischaemic heart disease
  - Dilated LV cardiomyopathy, usually idiopathic
  - Valvular heart disease—usually degenerative aortic/mitral valve disease
  - Atrial fibrillation—uncontrolled/persistent
  - Hypertensive heart disease—often in elderly females
- A detailed list of causes (based on 2021 ESC guidelines) is summarized in Table 5.1.8
- The clinical features of underlying conditions may be present and should be sought during clinical evaluation of the patient (see Table 5.1.1)

Potentially reversible causes of HFrEF and/or cardiomyopathies

- For some conditions, there is a 'window' in the natural history during which timely intervention (standard HFrEF therapies, specific corrective approaches, and even LV assist devices (LVAD)) might lead to recovery/reversal
- Examples include:
  - Timely correction of valve defects before irreversible reduction in LV function
  - Target driven management of hypertension

Table 5.1.8 Causes of cardiomyopathy.

Diseased Myocardium		
Ischaemic heart disease	Myocardial scar, stunning, hibernation, epicardial or microvascular coronary disease	Acute and chronic ischaemic heart disease (can be occult)
Toxic damage	Recreational substance abuse	Cocaine, amphetamines, alcohol, anabolic steroids
	Heavy metals	Copper, iron, lead, cobalt
	Radiation	Previous history of malignancy (e.g. lymphoma, lung, breast)
	Medications	Chemotherapy (e.g. anthracyclines,) Immunomodulating drugs (e.g. anti-TNFα, transtuzumab, immune checkpoint inhibitors), antiarrhythmics, NSAIDs, anaesthetic agents, anti-depressants
Immune/ inflammatory mediated	Related to infection	Bacteria, spirochaetes, fungi, protozoa, parasites (Chagas disease), rickettsia, viruses (HIV/AIDS), in setting of septic shock
	Not related to infection	Lymphocytic/giant cell myocarditis, autoimmune diseases (e.g. Graves' disease, rheumatoid arthritis, connective tissue disorders, mainly systemic lupus erythematosus), hypersensitivity, and eosinophilic myocarditis (Churg–Strauss).
Infiltrative disease	Related to malignancy	Direct infiltration or metastatic disease
	Not related to malignancy	Amyloidosis, sarcoidosis, haemochromatosis, (iron overload in transfusion dependency), glycogen storage diseases (e.g. Pompe disease), lysosomal storage diseases (e.g. Fabry disease)
Metabolic	Hormonal	Thyroid diseases, acromegaly, growth hormone deficiency, hypercortisolaemia, Conn's disease, Addison disease, diabetes, metabolic syndrome, obesity, phaeochromocytoma, Takotsubo CM, carcinoid syndrome, pathologies related to pregnancy and post-partum
	Nutritional	Deficiencies in thiamine, L-carnitine, selenium, Iron, phosphates, calcium, complex malnutrition (e.g. malignancy, AIDS, anorexia nervosa), obesity
Genetic disease	Various forms	HCM, DCM, LV non-compaction, ARVC, restrictive cardiomyopathy (for details see respective ESC expert documents), muscular dystrophies and laminopathies
Abnormal Loading Conditions		
Systemic hypertension		Primary or secondary causes
Valve and structural defects	Acquired	Mitral, aortic, tricuspid, pulmonary valve disease from their respective causes

(continued)

Table 5.1.8 Continued

	Congenital	Simple and complex lesions: ASD, PDA, VSD, aortic coarctation, transposition of the great arteries (TGA), systemic right ventricle
Pericardial & Endomyocardial diseases	Pericardial	Constrictive pericarditis, pericardial effusion
	Endomyocardial	Hypereosinophilic syndrome, endomyocardial fibrosis, endocardial fibroelastosis
Disturbances in Cardiac Rhythm		
Tachyarrhythmias		Atrial, ventricular arrhythmias; frequent ventricular ectopy
Bradyarrhythmias		Sinus node dysfunction, AV conduction disorders

McDonagh TA, Metra M, Adamo M, et al; ESC Scientific Document Group. 2021 ESC Guidelines for the diagnosis and treatment of acute and chronic heart failure. *Eur Heart J.* 2021 Sep 21;42(36):3599–3726. doi: 10.1093/eurheartj/ehab368. © European Society of Cardiology. With permission from Oxford University Press

- New/recent onset persistent AF/flutter ('tachycardiomyopathy' is often retrospectively confirmed)
- Revascularization of viable myocardium in patients with inducible ischaemia
- Thyroid disease, adrenal insufficiency, phaeochromocytoma
- Iron overload cardiomyopathy, e.g. transfusion dependence, haemochromatosis
- Enzyme replacement therapy, e.g. Fabry disease
- Alcoholic/recreational drug-induced cardiomyopathy following complete abstinence
- Approx. 25% of cases of idiopathic DCM with recent onset HF (usually post myocarditis) demonstrate spontaneous recovery
- Up to 50% of peri-partum cardiomyopathy cases
- LVAD patients may demonstrate significant recovery (EF > 40%) as judged by echo (approx. 10%) but only in 1% lead to device explant (excluding 'bridge-to-recovery' patients)
- In patients with LVSD in remission without a reversible cause. N.B. relapse is common if medical therapy (ACEi/BB/MRA) is withdrawn, therefore, patients in remission should be advised to continue optimal medical therapy and have long-term follow-up

Pathophysiology of heart failure

- This is more clearly defined for HFrEF, less so for HFpEF
- Initial insult(s) or triggers include abnormal genetics, toxins, ischaemia, arrhythmia, etc.
- Traditional teaching describes the pathophysiology of HF in terms of the Frank-Starling relation (see Figure 5.1.2)
- The grey dashed lines demonstrate the cardiac output required at rest or for mild or severe levels of exertion
- In the normal circulation, there is a straight-line relation between the load placed on the heart (pre-load) and the work done (solid grey line). With worsening severity of HF, the line moves down and to the right (solid black lines)
- The consequence is that to maintain a given cardiac output for a given activity, the patient with HF requires a higher and higher LV filling pressure. This is transmitted back to the pulmonary capillaries, increasing the hydrostatic pressure forcing fluid from the capillaries into the air spaces, causing pulmonary oedema

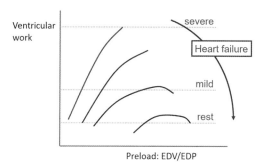

Figure 5.1.2 The Frank–Starling law represents the relationship between stroke volume (ventricular workload) and end diastolic volume (described in text below)

- The resulting sympathetic nervous system activation only makes matters worse by increasing afterload (the load against which the heart has to eject blood)
- This remains an accurate description of what happens in acute pulmonary oedema, in which an acute insult (e.g. myocardial infarction, arrhythmia) causes an acute decline in LV systolic function
- Much more commonly, HF leads to fluid retention and peripheral (rather than pulmonary) oedema. Here, the major problem is decreased renal perfusion resulting in avid sodium and water retention
- Chronic HF is in some sense an 'iatrogenic' disease: successful treatment of the acute state (with diuretics) should result in a patient with no congestion, but impaired cardiac function. Several changes happen in consequence, including:
  - Activation of renin-angiotensin-aldosterone system
  - Sympathetic activation
  - Both of these trigger adverse LV re-modelling apoptosis and fibrosis, with an increase in peripheral vascular resistance
  - The LV dilates, increasing wall tension
  - Change to skeletal muscle (loss of bulk, change to distribution of fibre types, increased fatiguability, altered biochemistry) associated with impaired nutritive flow causes symptoms of breathlessness and fatigue and cause further neurohormonal activation
  - There is also evidence of ventilatory inefficiency
  - These mechanisms are more pronounced with exertion and lead to effort intolerance

5.1.5 Investigations

- The initial patient assessment will include a thorough history and clinical assessment, assessing for the previously described symptoms, signs, and relevant co-morbidities
- These will not only help confirm or refute the diagnosis of HF, but also in the assessment of its type, cause, and severity
- This assessment is supplemented by the following series of investigations

ECG

- Should be performed in all patients with suspected HF
- If ECG and BNP are normal, HF is highly unlikely
- Examples of ECG abnormalities seen in HF are summarized in Table 5.1.9

Table 5.1.9 ECG abnormalities seen in heart failure and their associated potential causes.

ECG Abnormality	Causes
Sinus tachycardia	Decompensated HF, anaemia, fever, hyperthyroidism
Sinus bradycardia	Beta blocker, digoxin, hypothyroidism, sick sinus syndrome
Atrial tachycardia/fibrillation/flutter	Hyperthyroidism, infection, mitral valve diseases, decompensated HF, infarction, amyloidosis, lamin AC
Ventricular arrhythmias	Ischaemia, infarction, cardiomyopathy, myocarditis, hypokalaemia, hypomagnesaemia, digitalis overdose
Ischaemia/infarction	Coronary artery disease
Q waves	Infarction, HCM, LBBB, pre-excitation
LV hypertrophy	Hypertension, AV disease, HCM
AV block	Infarction, drug toxicity, myocarditis, sarcoidosis, Lyme disease, lamin A/C cardiomyopathy
Low voltage	Obesity, emphysema, pericardial effusion, amyloidosis
QRS >120ms	RBBB: in congenital HD, Pulmonary hypertension LBBB: seen in a variety of causes of LVSD

McDonagh TA, Metra M, Adamo M, et al; ESC Scientific Document Group. 2021 ESC Guidelines for the diagnosis and treatment of acute and chronic heart failure. *Eur Heart J.* 2021 Sep 21;42(36):3599–3726. doi: 10.1093/eurheartj/ehab368. © European Society of Cardiology. With permission from Oxford University Press.

Chest X-ray

- Limited value in the diagnostic work-up of patients with suspected chronic HF
- Significant LV systolic dysfunction is commonly present without cardiomegaly
- Useful for identifying other causes for dyspnoea, e.g. COPD, interstitial lung disease or malignancy (mass, unilateral pleural effusion, collapse, etc.)
- In acute situation can be indicative of elevated LV filling pressures showing:
  - Pulmonary oedema,
  - Bilateral pleural effusions,
  - Kerley B lines
  - Venous congestion

Routine blood laboratory testing

- Full blood count: anaemia, eosinophilia (endomyocardial fibrosis)
- Electrolytes and renal function: to exclude significant renal disease, monitor drug toxicity (hyponatraemia is a simple marker of poor prognosis)
- Bone profile: elevated calcium in myeloma (AL amyloid) or sarcoidosis (DCM)
- LFTs: rising bilirubin is an adverse marker, raised ALT suggests hepatic ischaemia
- Natriuretic peptides: as discussed above in section 5.1.3
- Troponin: elevated in ACS, myocarditis but often also elevated in acute HF
- Iron studies/ferritin: for suspected iron overload, haemochromatosis, detect iron deficiency (low transferrin saturation < 20%)
- TSH to exclude thyroid disease or amiodarone toxicity
- Lipid profile and glucose/HbA1C for targeting preventive strategies (as per ESC)
- PT and INR: rise with hepatic congestion and ischaemia, over-anticoagulation

Additional Lab tests may be indicated in specific clinical scenarios:

- CK: muscular dystrophies/mitochondrial disease associated cardiomyopathy
- Serum/urine electrophoresis/immunofixation and serum free light chain ratio: if AL amyloid suspected or in context of myeloma (TTR amyloid not associated with paraprotein)
- Urine protein:creatinine ratio: to quantify proteinuria in renal disease or amyloidosis
- Metabolic tests: α-galactosidase ↓ in Fabry disease (males) or IGF1 (acromegaly)
- Antibody testing for HIV or Lyme disease
- Vasculitis and autoimmune screen, e.g. ANCA, ANA/ENA
- Additional tests can be considered depending on the suspected underlying aetiology (as listed in Table 5.1.8)

Pulmonary function tests

- Useful in assessing lung disease as a cause for breathlessness and during surgical workup
- Transfer factor should be corrected for haemoglobin

Cardiopulmonary exercise testing

- Is recommended when assessing patient for transplantation (*Class I C*)
- Should be considered to investigate breathlessness of unclear cause or to optimize prescription of exercise training
- Particularly poor prognosis if:
    - Peak oxygen consumption (VO_2) < 14 ml/kg/min or < 12 ml/kg/min if on BB/CRT
    - Slope of relation between ventilation and carbon dioxide production ($VE/VCO2$) > 35
    - A maximal test is defined by attaining a respiratory exchange ratio (RER) > 1.05
- Covered in more detail in Chapter 7.1

Ambulatory ECG for detection/monitoring of:

- Bradyarrhythmias (to identify pacing indication)
- AF/flutter
- VT
- Frequent ventricular ectopy (if suspected as aetiology)

Genetic screening

- Formal referral to clinical genetics service for suspected inherited cardiomyopathies

99mTc-DPD scintigraphy (nuclear)

- Non-invasive diagnosis of TTR amyloid
- Tracers used include DPD, PYP, or HMDP
- Serum free light chains and immunofixation of urine *and* plasma must be normal before a positive test can be considered diagnostic of ATTR cardiac amyloidosis
- ATTR amyloid is usually associated with HFpEF but can also cause HFrEF

Endomyocardial biopsy

- Consider in patients with rapidly progressive HF despite standard therapies and suspected aetiology only diagnosable by myocardial biopsy with possible therapy, e.g. giant cell myocarditis
- May be used in suspected amyloidosis if non-invasive investigations are inconclusive

Imaging in HF
- Principle tests are transthoracic echocardiography (TTE) and MRI
- Selective role for TOE, invasive catheterization, CT, PET, and nuclear imaging
- TTE is the workhorse and most versatile initial imaging modality, with a combination of 2D, Doppler colour mapping (as well as strain and 3D imaging) addresses most clinical questions:
    - Assess LV systolic and diastolic function
    - Determine presence/severity of valve disease
    - Estimate pulmonary arterial pressure
    - Assess RV function
    - See section 5.1.3 on diastolic dysfunction and HFpEF
- TOE indicated to assess:
    - Valve disease and suitability for repair
    - Suspected congenital heart disease
    - Endocarditis (especially left sided, prosthetic valves or device related)

N.B. See Chapter 1.1 for a more detailed discussion of echocardiography

Indications for imaging modalities (all level of evidence (LoE) grade C unless stated otherwise)

Class I Indications (recommended)
TTE:
- Myocardial structure/function to diagnose HFrEF/pEF/mrEF
- Valve disease, RV function, and severity of pulmonary hypertension prior to corrective valve surgery
- Serial monitoring of LV function/EF in at-risk individuals (e.g. chemotherapy)

Cardiac MRI (CMR):
- Myocardial structure/function to diagnose HF in subjects with poor echo windows
- Patients with complex congenital HD
- Infiltrative myocardial diseases (myocarditis, amyloidosis, sarcoidosis, Chagas disease, Fabry disease, non-compaction cardiomyopathy, haemochromatosis) or suspected pericardial disease (CT also has *class I* role in constrictive pericarditis)

Cardiac catheterization:
- In patients with HF and with refractory angina despite optimal medical therapy, ventricular arrhythmias or aborted cardiac arrest to diagnose CAD; and to plan revasculariation in selelcted patients (*LoE B*)
- Right heart catheterization as part of the assessment for heart transplantation or MCS

Class IIa indications
- CMR with late gadolinium enhancement (LGE) in DCM, for determining aetiology when other tests equivocal
- Cardiac CT: low–intermediate risk of CAD risk or those with equivocal functional imaging
- Right heart catheterization in patients with suspected pulmonary hypertension or pericardial diseases with equivocal non invasive testing
- Strain/speckle echo for preclinical detection of disease in patients at risk of HF

Class IIb indications
- Non-invasive stress testing (CMR stress, stress echo, SPECT, PET) in those with HF and CAD to assess presence of ischaemia/viability prior to revascularization decisions (*LoE B*)
- Invasive coronary angiography: HF patients with intermediate–high risk CAD and positive stress ischaemia tests prior to considering revascularization in those deemed suitable (*LoE B*)

5.1.6 Medical Management

1. In patients *at risk* for developing HF
   ESC Class I recommendations (*LoE: level of evidence*)
   - Treatment of systemic hypertension (*LoE: A*)
   - Statin therapy in patients with or at high risk coronary disease (*LoE: A*)
   - Sodium-glucose cotransporter-2 (SGLT2) inhibitors for patients with diabetes at high risk of CV disease or with CV disease (*LoE: A*)
   - ACE inhibitors for asymptomatic LVSD (*LoE: A*)
   - Beta blockers for asymptomatic LVSD and prior MI (*LoE: B*)
   - Counselling/treatment for alcohol-intake reduction (in those drinking to excess), smoking cessation, and against sedentary lifestyle (*LoE: C*)
2. In patients with *established* HF, goals of management are to improve symptoms, functional capacity and quality of life, prevent hospitalization and reduce mortality

Pharmacological management of HFpEF
- Multiple phase II and III clinical trials with ACEi, ARB, MRA, digoxin, PDE5 inhibitors, angiotensin receptor and neprilysin inhibitors (ARNIs) in patients with HFpEF have been neutral
- Possible reasons include:
   - Incomplete understanding of complex pathophysiology
   - Hetrogenous phenotype with a range of CV and non-CV comorbidities
   - Hospitalization and deaths are more likely due to non-cardiovascular reasons
- However, recent studies have now shown SGLT2 inhibitors reduce the risk of HF hospitalization or cardiovascular death and are guideline recommended in patients with HFpEF and HFmrEF (*Class I A*)
- It is is essential before a diagnosis of HFpEF is established that conditions mimicking it are excluded (see section 5.1.3). However, inaddition to SGLT2 inhibitors:
   - Diuretics relieve congestion and improve symptoms (*Class I C*)
   - Candesartan and spironolactone may reduce hospitilizations
   - Nebivolol in older patients may reduce combined end-point of hospitalization and death
   - Optimal control of hypertension is recommended
- Recent reviews on the subject are listed in further reading

Main classes of pharmacological therapy for use in HFrEF (LV systolic dysfunction)
- In HF with reduced EF (HFrEF), neurohormonal anatagonists listed below should be used *in all patients* unless contrainidcated or not tolerated, and uptitrated to maximum tolerated doses:
   - Angiotensin receptor and neprilysin inhibitors (ARNI) or angiotensin coverting enzyme inhibitors (ACEi)

- Beta blockers (BB)
- Mineralocortocid receptor antagonists (MRA)
- In addition, SGLT2 inhibitors (e.g. dapagliflozin or empagliflozin) are now also recommended in all patients (regardless of whether they have diabetes) to reduce HF hospitalization and mortality, unless contraindicated or not tolerated
- In patients who remain symptomatic despite optimal doses of these medications there are additional medications available for HFrEF treatment, outlined below
- Table 5.1.10 lists the starting and target doses of the commonest drugs in each class, and for the key studies see Table 5.1.11

ACEi: Angiotensin converting enzyme inhibitors (e.g. enalapril, lisinopril, ramipril, captopril)

Indications:

- ACE inhibitors should be used in all patients with HF and EF ≤ 40%
- Also have a major role in treating hypertension and improve the long-term prognosis in patients following an acute coronary syndrome, likely via limiting adverse cardiac remodelling

Mechanism:

- Disordered function of the renin-angiotensin-aldosterone (RAAS) axis contributes to the pathophysiology of both hypertension and HF (see Figure 5.1.3)
- Inhibit angiotensin converting enzyme (ACE), which converts angiotensin I to angiotensin II. As well as acting as a direct vasoconstrictor, angiotensin II has multiple downstream effects which act to retain Na+ and water, primarily via the action of aldosterone on the kidney
- Because of this key function in body water homeostasis, ACE-inhibitors (as well as most drugs targeting the RAAS system) have a major role in treating hypertension

Contraindications:

- History of angioedema
- Bilateral renal artery stenosis (in such patients, renal autoregulation is dependent entirely on changes in post-glomerular arteriolar tone. ACE-inhibitors reduce post-glomerular arterial tone and can cause an excessive drop in glomerular perfusion and subsequent renal ischaemic injury. For this reason, monitoring of renal function and serum K^+ is recommended post-initiation)
- Pregnancy/risk of pregnancy
- Known allergy reaction/other adverse reaction

Use and monitoring (also applies to ARBs and MRAs):

- Before initiation
  - Seek specialist input if K^+ > 5 mmol/L and/or creatinine > 221 μmol/l (> 2.5 mg/dL) or eGFR < 30
- After initiation
  - Measure renal function and electrolytes before, 1–2 weeks after initiation, and 1–2 weeks after final dose titration; renal function should be checked every 4 months thereafter
  - An increase in creatinine of up to 50% *or* up to 266 μmol/l (3 mg/dL) *or* eGFR > 25 ml/min/1.73m², whichever is the smaller, is acceptable
    - Review other medications (e.g. NSAIDs/K^+-sparing diuretics) and reduce dose of diuretics if patient not congested. Exclude concomitant urinary tract infection and consider renal tract ultrasound

Table 5.1.10 List of doses of commonly used drugs in heart failure.

	Starting dose	Target dose or usual dose (diuretics)
ACE-i		
Enalapril	2.5 mg BD	10–20 mg BD
Ramipril	1.25 mg BD	5 mg BD
Lisinopril	2.5–5 mg OD	20–35 mg OD
BB		
Carvedilol	3.125 mg BD	25 mg BD
Bisoprolol	1.25 mg OD	10 mg OD
Metoprolol succinate (CR/XL preparation)	12.5–25 mg OD	200 mg OD
Nebivolol	1.25 mg OD	10 mg OD
MRAs		
Eplerenone	25 mg OD	50 mg OD
Spironolactone	25 mg OD	50 mg OD
ARNI		
Sacubitril/valsartan	49/51 mg BD	97/103 mg BD
SGLT2 Inhibitors		
Dapagliflozin & Empagliflozin	10 mg OD	10 mg OD
SGCSs		
Vericiguat	2.5 mg OD	10 mg OD
I$_f$ Channel blocker		
Ivabradine	2.5–5 mg BD	7.5 mg BD
ARBs		
Candesartan	4 mg OD	32 mg OD
Valsartan	40 mg BD	160 mg BD
Losartan	25 mg OD	150 mg OD
Loop Diuretics		
Furosemide	20–40 mg	40–240 mg (divided BD)
Bumetanide	1 mg	1–5 mg (divided BD)
Torasemide	5–10 mg	10–20 mg (divided)
Thiazide Diuretics		
Bendroflumethiazide	2.5 mg OD	2.5–10 mg OD
Metolazone	2.5 mg OD	2.5–10 mg OD

OD once a day, BD twice daily.

Table 5.1.11 Key randomized controlled trials in ACEi; BB, MRA, ARNI, and I$_f$ channel inhibition.

Trial/year	Drug	Main Population	Mean FU (years)	Results
RCTs with ACE inhibitors (ACEi)				
CONSENSUS, 1987, n = 253	Enalapril vs Placebo	CHF, NYHA IV, cardiomegaly CXR IHD 75%	6months	All cause Mortality 6m RRR 40% ARR18% 12m RRR 31% (52% v 36%)
SOLVD-T, 1991, n = 2569	Enalapril vs Placebo	LVEF≤35%, NYHA I-IV (90% class II-III) IHD 85%	3.5years	All cause mortality RRR 16%, (35 % v 40%) HF/death RRR 26%
ATLAS 1999 n = 3164	Lisinopril high dose vs low dose	LVEF≤30%, NYHA II-IV, IHD 65%	3.8 years	Death/HF hosp 15% RRR Mortality 43% vs 45% RRR 8% (p=NS 0.13)
SAVE 1992, n = 2231	Captopril vs placebo	Post MI (no HF)	3.5 years	Mortality RRR 19% (20% v 25%)
AIRE 1993, n = 2006	Ramipril vs Placebo	HF after an acute MI (3-10d onwards)	1.3 years	Mortality 27% RRR
TRACE 1995, n = 1749	Trandolopril	Post MI		Mortality RRR 18% (34.7% vs 42.3%)
RCTs with Beta Blockers (BB)				
CIBIS II, 1999, n = 2647	Bisoprolol vs placebo	Chronic HF, LVEF≤35%, NYHA III-IV, IHD 50%	1.3 years	All cause death RRR 34% (12% v 17%) CV Death/HF hosp RRR 21%
MERIT-HF, 1999, n = 3991	Metoprolol XL vs placebo	LVEF≤40%, NYHA II-IV, IHD 65%	1 year	All cause death RRR, 34% (7% vs 11%) RRR in HF death 49%, SCD 41%, CV death 38%
COPERNICUS 2002, n = 2289	Carvedilol vs Placebo	LVEF≤25%, NYHA IV, IHD 67%	0.9 years	All cause death RRR 35% (11% vs 17%)
COMET, 2003, n = 3029	Carvedilol vs Metoprolol	LVEF≤35%, NYHA II-IV,	4.8 years	All cause mortality RRR 15% (34% vs 40%)
SENIORS, 2005, n=2128	Nebivolol vs Placebo	>70y + HF Hosp / LVEF≤35%, IHD 69%	1.8 years	All cause death/CV hosp RRR 14% (31%vs 35%)
RCTs with Mineralocorticoid receptor anatgonists (MRA)				
RALES 1999, n = 1663	Spironolactone vs Placebo	LVEF ≤ 35%, NYHA III–IV (class IV within prior 6 m)	2 years	All cause death RRR 30% (35% v 46%) HF hosp RRR 35%

Trial	Intervention	Inclusion	Duration	Outcome
EPHESUS, 2003, n = 6642	Eplerenone vs Placebo	LVEF ≤ 40%, 3 d after acute MI with signs of HF or if diabetic	1.4 years	CV death/CV Hosp RRR 11% (26.7% vs 30%) CV death RRR 14% (14.4%vs 16.7%)
EMPHASIS-HF, 2011, n = 1737	Eplerenone vs placebo	NYHA II + LVEF ≤ 30% or LVEF 30–35% with QRS > 120 ms, recent HF hosp or NT-proBNP ≥ 500 ng/L	1.8 years	CV death/HF hosp RRR 37% (18% vs 26%) RRR in All caused death RRR 24%, CV death 24% and HF hosp 42%

RCTs with Angiotensin receptor antagonist and neprilysin inhibitors (ARNI)

Trial	Intervention	Inclusion	Duration	Outcome
PARADIGM HF, 2014, n = 8442	Sacubitril/Valsartan vs Enalapril	LVEF ≤ 35%, NYHA II–IV with raised BNP	2.3 years	All cause death/HF hosp RRR 20% (22% vs 27%) All cause death RRR 16%, CV death 20% HF hosp 21%

RCTs with Sodium glucose co-transporter 2 inhibitors (SGLT2i)

Trial	Intervention	Inclusion	Duration	Outcome
DAPA-HF, 2019, n = 4744	Dapagliflozin vs Placebo	LVEF ≤ 40%, NYHA II–IV 58% were not diabetic	1.5 years	HF hosp/CV death RRR 26% (16.3% vs 21.2%, NNT 21) All cause death RRR 17%
EMPEROR reduced, 2020 n = 3730	Empagliflozin vs placebo	LVEF ≤ 40%, NYHA II–IV 50% were not diabetic	16 months	Combined CV mortality or worsening HF reduced by 25% (19,4% vs 24,7%) primarily driven by 30% RRR in HF hospitalization
EMPORER-Preserved, 2021 n = 5988	Empagliflozin vs placebo	LVEF > 40%, NYHA II–IV, NT-proBNP > 300 pg/ml (SR)/ > 600 pg/ml (AF)	26 months	Combined CV mortality or HF hospitalization reduced by 21%, mainly driven by reduction in HF hospitalization
DELIVER, 2022 =6n263	Dapagliflozin vs Placebo	LVEF > 40% at recruitment, NYHA II–IV, NT-proBNP > 300 pg/ml (SR)/ >600 pg/ml	27 months	Combined CV mortality or HF hospitalization reduced by 18%, again mainly driven by reduction in HF hospitalization

RCT with sGC activators

Trial	Intervention	Inclusion	Duration	Outcome
VICTORIA, 2020 n = 5050	Vericiguat vs placebo	LVEF < 45% NYHA II–IV, high-risk patients with recent HF hospitalization (67% ≤ 3 m)	11 months	CV death/1st HF hospitalization RRR 10% (35.5% vs 38.5%, ARR 3% NNT 33)

If channel inhibition

Trial	Intervention	Inclusion	Duration	Outcome
SHIFT, 2010, n=6558	Ivabradine vs placebo	LVEF ≤ 35%, HF hosp < 12 m, SR > 70 bpm, NYHA II–IV	1.9 years	CV death/HF hosp RRR 18% (38% vs 42%)

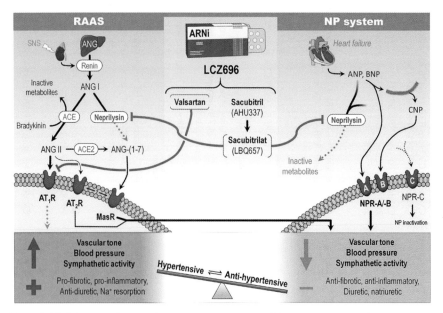

Figure 5.1.3 Schematic diagram showing renin-angiotensin-aldosterone system and its constituent pathways. Highlighted are the actions of ACE inhibitors, angiotensin II receptor blockers (ie. Valsartan) and the novel angiotensin receptor neprilysin inhibitor sacubitril-valsartan (brand name Entresto; known as LCZ696 during development). ANG, angiotensinogen; ANG I, Angiotensin I; ANG II, angiotensin II, ACE, angiotensin-converting enzyme; AT1R, angiotensin receptor 1; AT2R, angiotensin receptor 2; NP, natriuretic peptides; MasR, Mas receptor; NPR, natriuretic peptide receptor; RAAS, renin–angiotensin–aldosterone system; SNS, sympathetic nervous system

Reproduced from Nielsen PM, Grimm D, Wehland M, Simonsen U, Krüger M. The Combination of Valsartan and Sacubitril in the Treatment of Hypertension and Heart Failure-an Update. Basic Clin Pharmacol Toxicol. 2018 Jan;122(1):9–18. doi: 10.1111/bcpt.12912. with permission from John Wiley and Sons.

- If creatinine is 266 μmol/l–310 μmol/l or K^+ > 5.5, halve dose of ACEi and re-check renal biochemistry after 1–2 weeks; if abnormality persists stop drug and seek specialist input
- If creatinine increases > 100%, or to > 310 μmol/l or K^+ > 5.5 mmol/l, stop drug. Seek specialist input and monitor serial renal biochemistry until values have reached plateau
- If cough can be attributed to ACEi and is sufficiently intrusive then consider an ARB

BB: Beta blockers (carvedilol, bisoprolol, metoprolol succinate, nebivolol)

Indications: beta blockers should be used in **all** patients with HF and EF ≤ 40%, including:

- Clinically mild-moderate HFrEF (NYHA II–III)
- Asymptomatic LVSD post MI
- Patient clinically stabilized after an exacerbation (class IV) HF

Contraindications:

- Asthma is a relative contraindication (unless brittle asthma) whilst COPD is not
- Second- or third-degree heart block, sick sinus syndrome, sinus bradycardia (< 50 bpm) with no pacemaker back-up
- Critical limb ischaemia

Use and monitoring:

- Use with caution/care in severe class IV HF
- If persistent signs of fluid overload, hypotension (SBP < 90 mmHg), or marked peripheral oedema, try to relieve congestion and aim for euvolaemia before initiating
- Slow dose titration every 2 weeks
- Review other negative chronotropic medications if bradycardia (HR < 50) is a problem

MRA: Mineralocorticoid receptor antagonists (spironolactone, eplerenone)

HF indications:

- LVEF ≤ 40%
- NYHA II–IV
- Receiving optimal dose of ACEi and BB

Mechanism:

- MRAs inhibit the mineralocorticoid receptor (also known as aldosterone receptor) located in the distal convoluted tubule and collecting duct of the nephron, thus limiting the re-absorption of water in the kidney

Contraindications and side effects:

- Baseline potassium > 5.0 mmol/l and/or creatinine > 221 µmol/l (eGFR < 30)
- Concomitant potassium-sparing diuretic or potassium supplement
- Pregnancy/risk of pregnancy
- Spironolactone is associated with gynaecomastia in men due to its effects on oestrogen and testosterone; the incidence is significantly reduced with eplerenone
- Use with caution in acute porphyria as they may predispose to an acute attack

Use and monitoring:

- Consider dose titration after 4–8 weeks
- Check renal biochemistry 1–2 weeks after starting and any dose titration. Re-check after 2, 3, 6, 9, and 12 months respectively; thereafter check after every 4 months
- If potassium rises to > 5.5 mmol/l or creatinine > 220 µmol/l halve the dose of drug
- If potassium rises to > 6.0 mmol/l or creatinine > 310 µmol/l stop drug
- If breast tenderness/gynaecomastia switch spironolactone to eplerenone

ARNIs: Angiotensin receptor and neprilysin inhibitors (sacubitril-valsartan)

Indications:

- LVEF ≤ 40%
- NYHA class II–III
- Symptomatic HF despite optimal therapy with ACEi, BB, and MRA with modestly elevated NPs (N.B. it has not been formally tested yet in ACEi/ARB-naïve patients)

Mechanism:

- Neprilysin is a neutral endopeptidase predominantly in the kidney
- It breaks down vasoactive peptides (ANP, BNP, bradykinin, and adrenomedullin) as well as the vasoconstrictors angiotensin II and endothelin I

- When its inhibition (with sacubitril) is combined with an ARB, levels of endogenous NPs are augmented with beneficial effects believed to include natriuresis, vasodilation, and reverse-remodelling
- Valsartan blocks the angiotensin II receptor, responsible for aldosterone secretion and vascular smooth muscle contraction

Contraindications:

- Concomitant use of ACE inhibitor or ARB
- Prior history of angioedema
- Symptomatic hypotension or SBP < 95 mmHg
- K^+ > 5.4 mmol/L or eGFR < 30 ml/min/1.73m^2
- Pregnancy/risk of pregnancy

Use and monitoring:

- ACEi and ARB must be withdrawn at least 36 hours before initiating sacubitril valsartan
- Check renal biochemistry 1–2 weeks after starting and any dose titration. Thereafter check every 4 months. Renal dysfunction guidance is as detailed for ACEi above
- Symptomatic hypotension (SBP < 90 mmHg) was almost twice as common with ARNI than ACEi in the PARADIGM trial, whilst the PIONEER-HF trial showed a similar safety profile to enalapril in patients admitted with decompensated HFrEF
- BNP levels rise with therapy whilst NT-pro BNP levels fall

UK only: *NICE recommendations on sacubitril-valsartan (Technology appraisal TA388, April 2016)*

- Recommended as second line therapy for *symptomatic* HFrEF who fulfil all of the following:
    - NYHA class II–IV symptoms
    - LVEF < 35%
    - Already taking a stable dose of ACEi or ARB
- Started by a HF specialist with access to multidisciplinary HF team; Dose titration and monitoring to be performed by a competent team member

SGLT2 inhibitors: sodium-glucose co-transporter 2 inhibitors

- SGLT2 is present in the proximal renal tubule
- SGLT2 inhibitors are a class of oral hypoglycaemics that promote glycosuria and weight loss
- Serendipitously it was observed in RCTs of SGLT2i in high-risk diabetics that CV death and HF hospitalization were significantly reduced (but not MI or stroke)
- The DAPA-HF Trial was the first RCT demonstrating the prognostic benefit of dapagliflozin in HFrEF patients, and only 45% had type 2 diabetes at baseline
- Further published analyses indicate that the benefit of dapagliflozin was incremental to baseline use of neurohormonal antagonists (including ARNI), independent of loop diuretic dose and just as effective in non-diabetics
- Recent EMPORER-Preserved and DELIVER studies demonstrated reduction in hospitalization and CV death observed with SGLT2 inhibitors across all classes of LVEF
- A complete understanding of the mechanistic benefits are not fully established but proposed mechanisms include: enhanced natriuresis, vasodilation and cardiac energy metabolism, as well as a reduction in oxidative stress, inflammation, adverse cardiac remodeling, and renal protection
- In addition, empagliflozin met its primary endpoints (HF hospitalization and CV death) in the EMPEROR-reduced study (for HFrEF)

Use and monitoring:

- All classes of LVEF
- NYHA class II–IV
- Previous hospitalization for HF
- Monitoring of renal function if eGFR 30–60

Contraindications:

- eGFR < 30 ml/min/1.73m² or rapidly declining renal function
- Diabetic ketoacidosis (Type II diabetics can rarely develop euglycaemic ketoacidosis and thus should be advised of sick day rules and mandate monitoring blood ketone level in any unwell patient)
- Type 1 diabetics are at a much higher risk for DKA and so SGLT2i should be avoided or used with caution with routine monitoring of ketone levels
- Pregnancy/risk of pregnancy

ARB: Angiotensin receptor blockers (candesartan, valsartan, losartan)

- Angiotensin receptor blockers have not been shown to reduce mortality
- They should be used second line only if ACEi causes intractable and intolerable cough/side effects
- Renal side effects as for ACEi, so should not be used if ACEi withdrawn for renal dysfunction

Indications:

- LVEF ≤ 40%
- NYHA class II–IV
- Intolerance of ACEi
- ARB and ACEi are not routinely advised but can be used together under strict supervision if patient intolerant of MRA and remains symptomatic

Contraindications:

- Concomitant use of ACEi and MRA
- Renal dysfunction as detailed for ACEi above
- Pregnancy/risk of pregnancy

Key studies:

- Val-HEFT (valsartan) 24% RRR hospital admission for worsening HF, improved symptoms and quality of life
- CHARM-Alternative: in patients intolerant of an ACEi, candesartan reduced both primary end points of CV death and HF hospitalization (HR 0.7 (0.6–0.81) ARR 7%)
- CHARM-Added (candesartan) 17% RRR hospital admission for worsening HF, improved symptoms and quality of life

Ivabradine

- Ivabradine inhibits *If*, the so-called '*funny*' current (as the current behaved unusually compared with other known currents at the time of discovery)
- *If* is an important pacemaker current and heavily expressed within the conduction system and spontaneously active cells such as those of the sinoatrial (SA) node
- Selective blockade of If by ivabradine occurs in a dose-dependent manner and slows depolarization at the SA node
- Ivabradine is used in both HF and angina, where reduction of heart rate is thought to improve symptoms by enhancing diastolic filling time

Indications: for patients in sinus rhythm

- EF ≤ 35% and resting HR > 70 bpm with persisting symptoms (NYHA II–IV) despite optimal-dose BB, ACEi (or ARB), and MRA (or ARB)
- EF ≤ 35% and resting HR > 70 bpm with persisting symptoms (NYHA II–IV) on ACEi (or ARB) and MRA (or ARB) who are unable to tolerate BBs

Contraindications

- AF
- Sinus node or other conduction disease, or in those taking non-dihydropyridine calcium antagonists due to the risk of significant bradycardia
- Use in caution with other CYP3A4 inhibitors

Key studies:

- SHIFT (NYHA II–IV, EF ≤ 35%, bpm > 70) RRR CV death or hospitalization 18%
- BEAUTIFUL (CAD and EF < 40%)

Diuretics

- Relieve symptoms and signs of pulmonary and systemic venous congestion in patients with HF irrespective of EF
- Effects on mortality have not been directly studied
- Loop diuretic usually required in moderate or severe HF (examples include furosemide and bumetanide)
    - Loop diuretics act on the thick ascending limb of the renal Loop of Henle, inhibiting Na^+ and therefore water reabsorption; they also reduce K^+ and Cl^- reabsorption, which explains the tendency towards causing hypokalaemia
    - The bioavailability of frusemide can be impaired in decompensated heart failure due to gut oedema; in these patients, intravenous frusemide is likely to be more effective
- Thiazide diuretic may be used as adjunctive therapy in addition to loop diuretic for resistant oedema with caution when there is inadequate diuresis
    - Caution should be exercised to avoid over-vigorous diuresis and risk of resultant kidney injury
    - Their use can lead to gout and/or pseudo-gout
- After initial decongestion, diuretic dose should be adjusted after reviewing body weight, congestion, and renal function using the lowest dose to maintain euvolaemia
- Intravenous infusions are generally better tolerated haemodynamically and some evidence (DRAIN trial, 2020) indicates they promote a greater diuresis
- The DOSE study suggested that 24-hour furosemide infusion was equivalent to bolus dosing in acute HF; however, the study did suggest that higher doses overall are associated with more favourable outcomes

Hydralazine and isosorbide dinitrate (H-ISDN)

Indications:

- H-ISDN is an alternative to ACEi/ARB when neither tolerated if EF ≤ 45% and dilated LV (or EF ≤ 35%) on BB and MRA
- EF ≤ 45% and dilated LV (or EF ≤ 35%) and persisting symptoms despite treatment with BB and ACEi (or ARB) and MRA (or ARB)
- Evidence strongest in African-American patients

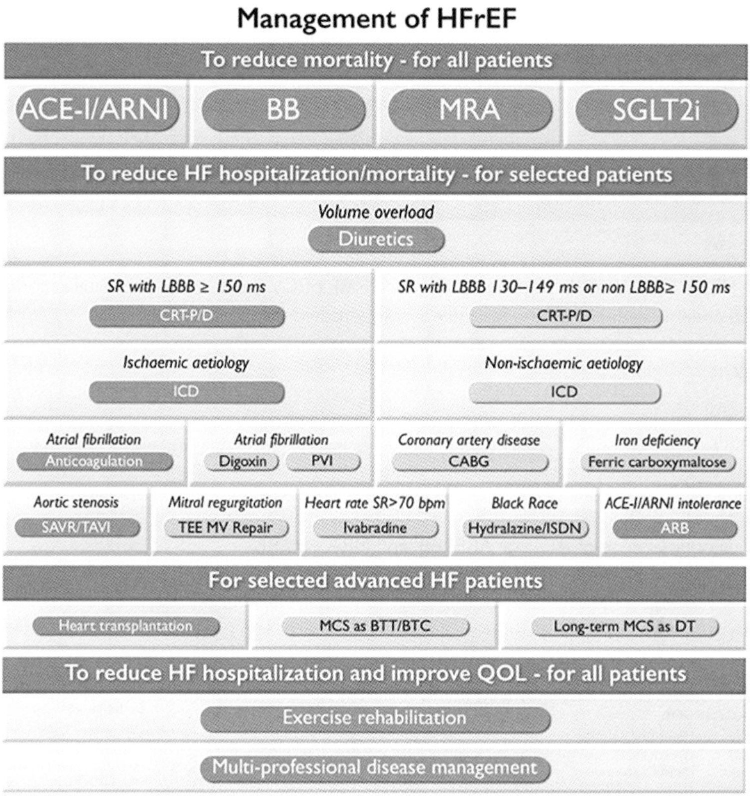

Management of HFrEF

To reduce mortality - for all patients

ACE-I/ARNI | BB | MRA | SGLT2i

To reduce HF hospitalization/mortality - for selected patients

Volume overload
- Diuretics

SR with LBBB ≥ 150 ms
- CRT-P/D

SR with LBBB 130–149 ms or non LBBB≥ 150 ms
- CRT-P/D

Ischaemic aetiology
- ICD

Non-ischaemic aetiology
- ICD

Atrial fibrillation — Anticoagulation
Atrial fibrillation — Digoxin | PVI
Coronary artery disease — CABG
Iron deficiency — Ferric carboxymaltose

Aortic stenosis — SAVR/TAVI
Mitral regurgitation — TEE MV Repair
Heart rate SR>70 bpm — Ivabradine
Black Race — Hydralazine/ISDN
ACE-I/ARNI intolerance — ARB

For selected advanced HF patients
- Heart transplantation
- MCS as BTT/BTC
- Long-term MCS as DT

To reduce HF hospitalization and improve QOL - for all patients
- Exercise rehabilitation
- Multi-professional disease management

Figure 5.1.4 Therapeutic algorithm for patients with symptomatic heart failure with reduced ejection fraction, showing the major medication classes and recommended alternative treatments to be considered, with the classes of recommendation indicated: Class I and Class IIa.

(ACE-I = angiotensin-converting, enzyme inhibitor; ARB = angiotensin receptor blocker; ARNI = angiotensin receptor-neprilysin inhibitor; BB = beta-blocker; b.p.m. = beats per minute; BTC = bridge to candidacy; BTT = bridge to transplantation; CABG = coronary artery bypass graft; CRT-D = cardiac resynchronization therapy with defibrillator;

CRT-P = cardiac resynchronization therapy with pacemaker; DT = destination therapy; HF = heart failure; HFrEF = heart failure with reduced ejection fraction; ICD = implantable cardioverter-defibrillator; ISDN = isosorbide dinitrate; LBBB = left bundle branch block; MCS = mechanical circulatory support; MRA = mineralocorticoid receptor antagonist; MV = mitral valve; PVI = pulmonary vein isolation; QOL = quality of life; SAVR = surgical aortic valve replacement; SGLT2i = sodium-glucose co-transporter 2 inhibitor; SR = sinus rhythm; TAVI = transcatheter aortic valve replacement; TEE = transcatheter edge to edge)

McDonagh TA, Metra M, Adamo M, et al; ESC Scientific Document Group. 2021 ESC Guidelines for the diagnosis and treatment of acute and chronic heart failure. *Eur Heart J*. 2021 Sep 21;42(36):3599–3726. doi: 10.1093/eurheartj/ehab368. © European Society of Cardiology. With permission from Oxford University Press

Contraindications:
- Symptomatic hypotension
- Systemic lupus erythematosus
- Severe renal failure

Key studies:
- V-HeFT (placebo, prazosin, or H-ISDN added to diuretic and digoxin); H-ISDN indicated
- A-HeFT (African-American in NYHA III–IV, randomized to placebo or H-ISDN added to diuretic, digoxin, ACEi/ARB, BB, and spironolactone) RRR mortality 43%

SGCSs: Soluble guanylate cyclase receptor stimulator (e.g. Vericiguat)

- Vericiguat is a novel oral soluble guanylate cyclase stimulator, which directly stimulates SGC and sensitizes it to endogenous nitric oxide

Indications:

- Consider if NYHA II–IV with worsening HF despite treatment with an ACE-I/ARNI, a beta blocker and an MRA

Key studies

- The VICTORIA study demonstrated a reduced risk of CV mortality and hospitalizations for HF in patients with HFrEF and recently decompensated HF

Digoxin

Indications:

In sinus rhythm

- LVEF < 40%
- NYHA class II–IV
- Taking optimal dose of ACEi or ARB, BB, and MRA or ARB

In atrial fibrillation

- Ventricular rate at rest > 80 bpm, during exercise > 110–120 bpm

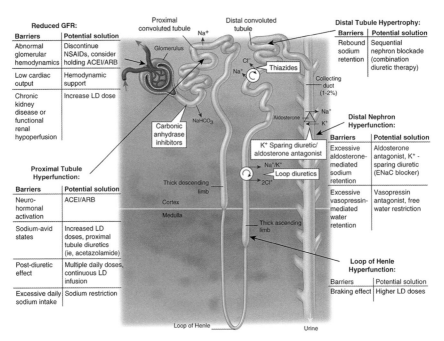

Figure 5.1.5 Diagram showing anatomy of nephron, drug activity at various sites as well as potential challenges in heart failure therapy

Reproduced with permission from Baliga R.R., & Abraham W.T.(Eds.), (2018). Color Atlas and Synopsis of Heart Failure. McGraw Hill. https://accesscardiology.mhmedical.com/content.aspx?bookid=2489&sectionid=198056303.

Key studies:

- DIG trial 28% RRR for hospital admission for worsening HF

Therapies which have little/no benefit or are harmful in HFrEF

- Warfarin or low-dose rivaroxaban did not reduce MACE in patients with HFrEF *and sinus rhythm*
- Rosuvastatin was safe but did not reduce MACE in patients with HFrEF
- Pharmacological rhythm control is not superior to a rate control strategy in HFrEF
- Dronedarone increased mortality in patients with HFrEF
- Diltiazem/nifedipine have been shown to worsen HF in patients with LVSD (amlodipine is safer and has been given an ESC class IA recommendation for controlling hypertension in patients with HF despite ACEi/BB/MRA
- Non-invasive ventilation (adaptive servo-ventilation) to treat *central* sleep apnoea increased mortality in patients with HF and LVEF < 45%
- Many non-cardiovascular medications (including some diabetic medications, chemotherapeutics, and anti-psychotics) can cause or worsen heart failure (see further reading)

HFmrEF

- Diuretics are recommended in patients with congestion to alleviate symptoms (I C)
- SGLT2 inhibitor is recommended to reduce risk of heart faulure hospitalization and CV death (I A)
- ESC Heart Failure Guidelines advise that treatment with ACEi/ARB/ARNI, beta blocker, and MRA may be considered on the basis of sub-group analyses for trials of each drug class (IIb-C recommendation)

5.1.7 Arrhythmia, pacing and device therapy

Atrial fibrillation

- Commonest arrhythmia in HF irrespective of LVEF
- New onset HF pecipitated by AF has a more favourable prognosis compared to new onset AF in patients with established HF; the latter often precipiates decompensation
- Exclude hyperthyroidism, electrolyte imbalance and precipitants (e.g. pneumonia, sepsis, pulmonary embolism)
- Assess stroke risk and anticoagulate as per ESC AF 2020 guidelines
- Rate control strategy:
    - Beta blockers are first line for rate control, though evidence for mortality or morbidity benefits of BB in HFrEF with AF are lacking
    - Optimization of ventricular rate control, target resting rate 70–90 bpm usually adequate (more stringent control is associated with adverse outcomes)
    - Add digoxin when inadequate rate control with beta blockers. Some evidence (AFFIRM, DIG trial) suggest that higher digoxin doses/levels are associated with excess mortality
- Rhythm control strategy:
    - Urgent electrical cardioversion is recommended in the presence of acute decompensated HF with rapid ventricular rates and haemodynamic instability
    - Cardioversion may be considered (*Class IIb B*) where AF is associated with worsening of HF symptoms despite OMT
    - Catheter ablation should be considered (*Class IIa B*) where a clear association between paroxysmal or persistent AF and worsening of HF symptoms is present despite OMT

- Amiodarone use for AF should generally be limited to 6 months and often to improve maintainance of SR after DC cardioversion
  - Dronaderone is contraindicated in HFrEF
- AV node ablation useful if inadequate rate control, persistence of HF and/or CRT indication with AF (see below)
- See Chapter 4.5 for further information on AF

Ventricular arrhythmias

- Ambulatory ECG detects premature ventricular complexes (PVCs) in virtually everyone and non-sustained VT (NSVT) in many with HFrEF but is not routinely indicated, unless there is history of presyncope, dizziness, or syncope
- LVEF < 35% remains the single most powerful marker of risk for sudden cardiac death
- OMT (particularly BB, MRA, and ARNI) reduces risk of sudden death and the importance of this cannot be overemphasized
- Routine use of amiodarone is not indicated in asymptomatic ventricular arrhythmia
- In symptomatic arrhythmias, serum magnesium/potassium/calcium should be corrected
- QT interval can be prolonged by concomitant medications as well as amiodarone/sotalol
- See Chapter 4.7 for further information on ventricular arrhythmias

Devices

- Ventricular arrhythmias, bradycardia and asystole are the commonest modes of sudden death in patients with HF, and implantable devices can potentially reduce the risk of all 3
- A standard pacemaker paces from the right ventricular apex/septum (and the right atrium in patients in sinus rhythm) and prevents bradycardia
- A CRT (cardiac re-synchronization therapy) pacemaker paces from the right and left ventricles simultaneously, perhaps improving co-ordination of ventricular contraction
- An inplantable cardioverter-defibrillator (ICD) detects and treats ventricular tachyarrhythmia
- It has become apparent that over time the rates of SCD in HFrEF have fallen due to increased background use of OMT
- Devices are covered in detail across Chapters 4.3, 4.9 and 4.10, however guidance specific to HF include:

Brady pacing

- In HFrEF, if pacing is required for high degree AV block then CRT rather than RV pacing recommended—including for patients in AF (*IA*)
- In HFrEF, patients who have a pre-existing conventional pacemaker or ICD that later develop worsening HF despite OMT alongside a significant proportion of RV pacing should be considered for 'upgrade' to CRT (*IIa B*)

ICD

Primary prevention

- Symptomatic HF (NYHA II–III), LVEF < 35%, on optimal medical therapy for > 3 months in whom life expectancy is > 1 year with good functional status with either
  - IHD (but only **after** 40 days an acute MI) (*IA*)
  - Dilated cardiomyopthy (*IIa A*)

Secondary prevention

- Survivors of VT/VF causing haemodynamic instability/ cardiac arrest in whom life expectancy is > 1 year with good functional status (*IA*)

Table 5.1.12 Indications for CRT in heart failure and the strength of associated evidence base (note cut-off for QRS duration is now 130 ms, not 120 as previously).

Indications for CRT	Class	Level
Symptomatic, SR, QRS > 150 ms, LBBB, LVEF < 35% on OMT	I	A
HFrEF and pacing indication for high degree AV Block (CRT to reduce morbidity)	I	A
Symptomatic, SR, QRS 130–149ms, LBBB, LVEF < 35% on OMT	IIa	B
Symptomatic, SR, QRS > 150 ms, non-LBBB, LVEF < 35% on OMT	IIa	B
Symptomatic, SR, QRS 130–149 ms, non-LBBB, LVEF < 35% on OMT	IIb	B
Worsening HF symptoms despite OMT, high frequency RV pacing, upgrade to CRT	IIa	B
Symptomatic, AF, QRS ≥ 130 ms, provided a strategy is in place to ensure biventricular capture	IIa	C
Symptomatic, AF with uncontrolled heart rate undergoing AV node ablation (irrespective of QRS duration)	I	B
In patients with symptomatic AF and an uncontrolled heart rate who are candidates for AV node ablation (irrespective of QRS duration), CRT rather than standard RV pacing should be considered in patients with HFmrEF.	IIa	C
If QRS < 130 ms then CRT is contraindicated	III	A

McDonagh TA, Metra M, Adamo M, et al; ESC Scientific Document Group. 2021 ESC Guidelines for the diagnosis and treatment of acute and chronic heart failure. *Eur Heart J.* 2021 Sep 21;42(36):3599–3726. doi: 10.1093/eurheartj/ehab368. © European Society of Cardiology. With permission from Oxford University Press

In addition

- ICD not recommended in patients with severe HF with symptoms refractory to medical therapy (NYHA Class IV) **unless** they are candidates for CRT, LVAD, or transplantation
- A wearable ICD may be considered in patients with HFrEF at risk of sudden cardiac death for a limited period or as a bridge to an implanted device

CRT

- CRT-P provides both symptomatic and prognostic benefit in HFrEF
- It is used in HFrEF paients who remain symptomatic despite OMT, or with a brady-pacing indication where a high degree of pacing (> 40%) is anticipated (see Table 5.1.12)
- There is no role for CRT in HFpEF
- In patients at high risk for ventricular tachyarrhythmias (see ICD above) the CRT should include a defibrillator (CRT-D)

Additional notes:

- Annual incidence of LBBB is approx 10% in ambulatory patients with HFrEF
- Despite findings of the COMPANION trial, it is still unclear whether CRT-D is superior to CRT-P as no adequately powered study has been performed
- Optimal medical therapy (OMT) requires a proactive approach in uptitrating doses of BB, ACEi and MRA (along with diuretics to relive congestion) with review after a minimum of 3 months
- Individual patient data meta-analyses suggest that QRS duration rather than morphology (LBBB vs non LBBB) should guide selection of patients for CRT
- There is no trial evidence that CRT confers benefit in patients in AF (although CRT is commonly implanted in such patients, sometimes with concommitant AV node ablation)

Key CRT studies
CRT-P compared with optimal medical therapy:
- CRT-P with optimal pharmacological therapy (CARE-HF, COMPANION, MIRACLE, and MUSTIC-SR) reduced all-cause mortality compared with optimal pharmacological therapy alone. All four RCTs showed consistent improvements in exercise capacity and health-related quality of life for CRT-P

CRT-D versus optimal medical therapy alone:
- COMPANION and CONTAK-CD: a meta-analysis demonstrated reduction in all-cause mortality for CRT-D compared with optimal pharmacological therapy alone (HR 0.65, 95% CI 0.49–0.85)
- COMPANION also reported reduction in death from HF (HR 0.73, 95% CI 0.47–1.11, p = 0.143), sudden cardiac death (HR 0.44, 95% CI 0.23–0.86, p = 0.02) and NYHA class (pooled RR 1.40, 95% CI 1.13–1.75, p < 0.0001)
- COMPANION reported reduction in hospitalization for HF with CRT-D (rate ratio 0.59, 95% CI 0.49–0.70, p < 0.0001)

CRT-D versus ICD:
- In patients with a QRS duration ≥ 150 ms, MADIT CRT (NYHA I/II, EF < 30%) showed a 41% reduction in the risk of heart failure events with CRT. There was no effect on risk of death, with a 3% annual mortality rate in each treatment group

CRT-ON versus CRT-OFF:
- REVERSE (NYHA I/II, QRS ≥ 120 ms, EF ≤ 40%) showed that CRT, in combination with optimal medical therapy (±defibrillator), reduces risk of HF hospitalization and improves ventricular structure and function in NYHA I/II patients with previous HF symptoms
- EchoCRT (2013) was stopped prematurely for futility in HFrEF patients with QRS < 130 ms and was associated with increased mortality

CRT-D versus CRT-P:
- COMPANION was the only RCT directly comparing CRT-P with CRT-D. Both CRT-D and CRT-P reduced the risk of death or hospitalization compared with optimal medical therapy alone, but CRT-D was associated with a statistically significant reduction in all-cause mortality (p = 0.003) whereas CRT-P was not (p = 0.059). There was no difference between CRT-P and CRT-D

Risks:
- Perioperative death with CRT (CRT-P/D pooled) in RCTs was 0.8% (95% CI 0.5–1.2%)
- CRT devices implanted successfully on average in 90.8% of patients (95% CI 89.6–92.0%)
- CRT device implanted successfully without an improvement in patient condition ranges from 11–46% (patient condition is assessed by NYHA class and echocardiographic variables)

5.1.8 Surgical and transcatheter interventions in heart failure

Revascularization in HFrEF with significant CAD
- The role for coronary revascularization in patients with HFrEF has remained controversial
- There is only one meaningful surgical RCT (STICH trial):
    - In 1212 patients with LVEF < 35% there was no statistically significant difference in all-cause mortality (primary EP) with CABG (36%) vs OMT (41% HR 0.86 95% CI 0.72–1.04 p = 0.12) over a median 4.7-y follow-up

- The trial excluded patients with LMS stenosis > 50% and severe angina (CCS III–IV), and 61% were classified as NYHA ≤ II whilst 52% had none/mild angina (CCS ≤ I)
- 30-day mortality was 4% in CABG patients (vs 1% OMT) and thereafter mortality rates remained similar up to 2.5 years
• The STICH extension study reported a small improvement in 10-year survival with CABG (58.9%) over OMT (66.1%) with a 16% RRR, 7.2% ARR, and NNT 14
• Several large registries suggested that PCI is associated with much higher MACE compared with CABG in patients with LVEF < 40%
• The REVIVED-BCIS2 RCT (NEJM 2022) in 700 patients with LVEF<35% and demonstrable myocardial viability, showed no advantage of PCI over OMT in reducing mortality or HF hospitalisation

The ESC guidelines on HF (2021) and revascularization (2018) stipulate:

• CABG should be the first-choice revascularization strategy in patients with acceptable surgical risk (as judged by STS or Euroscore II), especially in the presence of multi-vessel disease or diabetes
• Consider revascularization for:
  - Persistent symptoms despite OMT and anti-anginal therapy (*IIa C*)
  - Improving outcomes in patients with HFrEF, CCS, and coronary anatomy suitable for revascularization, after evaluation of the individual risk to benefit ratio, coronary anatomy, comorbidities, life expectancy, and patient's perspective (*IIb C*)
  - PCI may be considered as an alternative to CABG, based on Heart Team evaluation, considering coronary anatomy, comorbidities, and surgical risk (*IIb C*)

Role of surgery in functional (secondary) mitral valve regurgitation (FMR)

• In aortic valve disease (stenosis/regurgitation) and primary (organic) mitral regurgitation, timely valve intervention (repair/replacement/TAVR) should be undertaken as per the ESC guidelines in valvular heart disease (see Chapter 3)
• Unlike primary MR, FMR cannot be completely corrected by just restoring mitral valve competence
• FMR occurs in the setting of dilated cardiomyopathy (central MR), hypertrophic CM (due to SAM), AF (atrial FMR), but most commonly is due to chronic IHD
• Ischaemic FMR is related to inferior wall motion defects and can lead to posterior leaflet tethering and eccentric MR jets. However, ischaemic MR can also cause central MR if there are additional wall motion defects due to multi-vessel disease
• In patients undergoing CABG surgery with a *moderate* degree of ischaemic MR, simultaneous MV repair did not improve survival or LV function over 2 years (Michler et al., *NEJM* 2016)
• In patients with *severe* ischaemic MR, surgical repair or replacement were equivalent for survival and LV remodelling but MV repair was associated with greater residual MR and HF hospitalization (Goldstein et al. *NEJM* 2016)

Transcatheter intervention for secondary mitral regurgitation and HFrEF

• A role for transcatheter mitral valve edge–edge repair (MitraClip device) in patients with secondary MR and HFrEF was investigated in two RCTs (MITRA-FR and COAPT trials)
• MITRA-FR (*NEJM* Aug. 2018):
  1. $n = 304$, severe FMR, mean LVEF 33%, and EROA 31 mm^2
  2. MitraClip did not reduce HF hospitalization or mortality compared to OMT over 2 years

- COAPT (*NEJM* Sep. 2018):
    3. $n = 614$ medically optimized but persistent severe FMR (mean EROA 41 mm^2) and mean LVEF 31%
    4. MitraClip significantly reduced HF hospitalization (RRR 47% ARR 36%) and mortality (RRR 38% and ARR 16%) at 2 y
- The trials showed strikingly discordant findings that have stimulated significant discussion and the proposal of an appealing concept of 'disproportionate MR' (EROA/LVEDV ratio > 0.14) which is hypothesized to account for the findings in COAPT
- In essence the COAPT study predominantly performed MitraClip in patients that had been optimized (medical/CRT) in whom there was residual severe FMR but without marked LV dilatation
- Further studies are ongoing

Recommendations from the 2021 ESC guidelines on HF on FMR are:

- In patients with HF, severe secondary mitral regurgitation, and CAD requiring revascularization, CABG and mitral valve surgery should be considered (*IIa C*)
- Consider percutaneous edge-to-edge repair should be considered in carefully selected symptomatic patients on OMT with FMR who are not eligible for surgery and do not require revascularization, and:
    5. Fulfil the following criteria: (*IIa B*)
        - LVEF 20–50%
        - LVESD < 70 mm
        - Systolic pulmonary pressure < 70 mmHg
        - Absence of moderate or severe RV dysfunction or severe TR
        - Absence of haemodynamic instability
    6. Do not fill criteria (*IIa C*)

Inter-atrial shunt devices for HF

- Several small phase I and II trials have shown favourable effects on haemodynamics in patients with HF and LVEF > 40% using devices that shunt blood from the LA into the RA
- A large phase III RCT (REDUCE LAP-HF II, Lancet 2022), however was neutral in 626 patients with LVEF>40%.

5.1.9 Advanced heart failure therapies: mechanical circulatory support (MCS) and heart transplantation

The ESC/HFA (2018) guidelines define advanced HF in the presence of *ALL* of:

1. Severe and persistent symptoms of heart failure (NYHA class III (advanced) or IV).
2. Severe cardiac dysfunction defined by a reduced LVEF ≤ 30%, isolated RV failure (e.g. ARVC) or non-operable severe valve abnormalities or congenital abnormalities or persistently high (or increasing) BNP or NT-proBNP values and data suggesting severe diastolic dysfunction or LV structural abnormalities according to the ESC definition of HFpEF and HFmrEF.
3. Episodes of pulmonary or systemic congestion requiring high-dose intravenous diuretics (or diuretic combinations) or episodes of low output requiring inotropes or vasoactive drugs or malignant arrhythmias causing > 1 unplanned visit or hospitalization in the last 12 months.
4. Severe impairment of exercise capacity with inability to exercise or low 6-minute walk test distance (< 300 m) or peak VO2 (< 12–14 mL/kg/min), due to cardiac disease.

5.1.9 Advanced heart failure therapies: MCS and heart transplantation 451

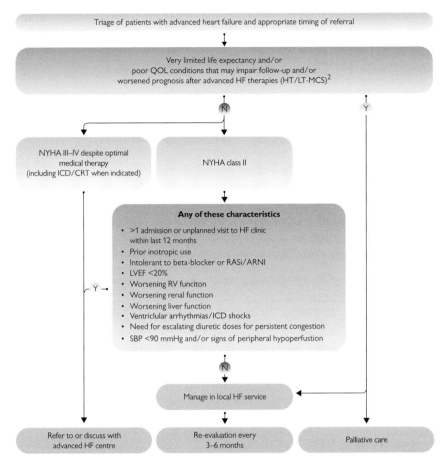

Figure 5.1.6 Appropriate triage and timing of referral for patients with advanced heart failure

McDonagh TA, Metra M, Adamo M, et al; ESC Scientific Document Group. 2021 ESC Guidelines for the diagnosis and treatment of acute and chronic heart failure. *Eur Heart J.* 2021 Sep 21;42(36):3599–3726. doi: 10.1093/eurheartj/ehab368. © European Society of Cardiology. With permission from Oxford University Press.

The ESC recommendations regarding the triage and referral of patients with advanced HF is presented in Figure 5.1.6. In general, advanced HF is present and a referral to a transplant centre should be considered with one or more of the following (adapted from *UK guidelines for referral & assessment of adults for heart transplantation*):

- ≥ 2 admissions for treatment of decompensated HF within 12 months (and no reversible precipitants)
- Persistent clinical evidence of overt heart failure after optimized medical treatment
- Calculated Seattle Heart Failure Model score suggesting ≥ 20% 1-year mortality
- Echocardiographic evidence of RV dysfunction or increasing pulmonary artery pressure on optimal treatment (aim to refer before PA systolic pressure > 50 mmHg)
- Anaemia, involuntary weight loss, liver dysfunction, or hyponatraemia attributable to HF
- Deteriorating renal function attributable to HF or inability to tolerate diuretic dosages sufficient to clear congestion without change in renal function (refer before creatinine clearance < 50 ml/min or eGFR < 40 ml/min/1.73m^2)

- Significant episodes of ventricular arrhythmia despite full drug and electrophysiology and/or device treatment
- Increasing plasma BNP or NT-proBNP levels despite adequate HF treatment

It is important that reversible causes are excluded or managed accordingly, including:

- Non-/poor compliance with medication and fluid balance
- Drug interactions (e.g. NSAIDs, glitazones)
- Anaemia or thyroid disturbance
- Arrhythmias e.g. atrial fibrillation/flutter, VT (interrogate device where present)
- Myocardial ischaemia
- Other causes of oedema, e.g. renal failure, nephrotic syndrome
- New/worsening valve disease (e.g. MR, AS)
- If flash pulmonary oedema consider renal artery stenosis
- Exclude constrictive pericarditis before transplant referral

Severe HF (both acute and chronic) is graded using the 2009 INTERMACS classification (Table 5.1.13) which guides the urgency of mechanical circulatory support or transplantation

Table 5.1.13 The 2009 INTERMACS classification for severe heart failure (both acute and chronic).

INTERMACS LEVEL	Description	NYHA class	Time frame for intervention
1 'Crashing and burning' Critical cardiogenic shock	Haemodynamic instability in spite of increasing doses of catecholamines and/or mechanical circulatory support with critical hypoperfusion of target organs (severe cardiogenic shock)	IV	Hours
2 'Sliding on inotropes' Progressive decline despite inotropic support	Intravenous inotropic support with acceptable blood pressure but rapid deterioration of renal function, nutritional state, or signs of congestion	IV	Days
3 'Dependant stability' Stable but inotrope dependent	Haemodynamic stability with low or intermediate doses of inotropes, but necessary due to hypotension, worsening of symptoms, or progressive renal failure	IV	Elective (weeks-months)
4 'Frequent flyer' Resting symptoms	Temporary cessation of inotropic treatment is possible, but patient presents with frequent symptom recurrences and typically with fluid overload	IV ambulatory	Elective (weeks-months)
5 'Housebound' Exertion intolerant	Severe limited tolerance for activity, comfortable at rest with some volume overload and often with some renal dysfunction	IV ambulatory	Variable
6 'Walking wounded' Exertion limited	Minor limitation on physical activity and absence of congestion while at rest. Easily fatigued by light activity	III	Variable
7 'Placeholder' Advanced NYHA III symptoms	Patient without current or recent unstable fluid balance, NYHA class II or III	III	Variable

McDonagh TA, Metra M, Adamo M, et al; ESC Scientific Document Group. 2021 ESC Guidelines for the diagnosis and treatment of acute and chronic heart failure. *Eur Heart J*. 2021 Sep 21;42(36):3599–3726. doi: 10.1093/eurheartj/ehab368. © European Society of Cardiology. With permission from Oxford University Press.

Left ventricular assist device (LVAD)

- Current devices propel blood via continuous flow rather than pulsatile flow and include:
    - Second-generation extra-pericardial Heartmate II
    - Third-generation centrifugal intra-pericardial Heartmate III and Heartware HVAD (The FDA placed a recall on this device in 2022)
- In patients with severe HF initially ineligible for transplantation, a continuous flow left ventricular assist device (CF-LVAD) used as bridge-to-decision (to allow recovery of, for example, renal dysfunction, or improvement in pulmonary haemodynamics) or as destination-treatment to reduce mortality in patients with severe symptoms (> 2 months) despite OMT with device therapy plus one of:
    - NYHA functional class III/IV; LVEF ≤ 25%; peak VO2 < 12 ml/kg/min
    - ≥ 3 HF hospitalizations in 3 months without an obvious precipitating cause
    - Dependence on i.v. inotropic therapy
    - Progressive end-organ dysfunction (worsening renal and/or hepatic function due to reduced perfusion in the absence of an adequate filling pressure (pulmonary capillary wedge pressure (PCWP) ≥ 20 mmHg and systolic blood pressure (SBP) ≤ 80–90 mmHg or cardiac index (CI) ≤ 2 L/min/m^2)
    - Deteriorating RV function but not when severe RV dysfunction/severe TR present

Complications of LVAD

- These depend on the generation of device and quality of anticoagulation, but include:
    - Pump thrombosis
    - Thromboembolism (stroke 10%)
    - Bleeding (10–15% gastrointestinal, cerebral, epistaxis, etc.)
    - Infection (10%, often the driveline in abdominal wall)
    - Early (20–30%) and late right heart failure
- Actuarial survival is 80% at 1 year and 70% at 2 years in predominantly non-transplant-eligible patients
- Different mechanical circulatory support devices are available to support patients with worsening HF and those in cardiogenic shock and their uses can be categorized as outlined in Figure 5.1.7

Cardiac transplantation

- Annual number of heart transplants worldwide is static (UK 125/yr, Europe approx. 1500/yr, North America approx. 2000/yr) and is thus an option for only a small number of patients with HF
- In appropriately selected patients, transplantation offers:
    - Improvements in survival, exercise capacity, and quality of life
    - Median survival 12 years (2004–08 vs 10.4 years for 1999–2001 cohort, ISHLT data)
    - If surviving first year, median survival 13.2 years (1999–2001 cohort)
- Table 5.1.14 outlines relevant patient factors and contraindications

Complications of heart transplantation

- Early to medium term: surgical, bleeding, graft failure, RV failure, acute rejection, infection, multiorgan failure, stroke
- Longer term: renal failure, graft failure, chronic allograft vasculopathy (CAV) malignancy (commonly lymphoproliferative disease and skin malignancy)

BTT Bridge to Transplant	• Use of MCS (LVAD or BiVAD) to keep patient alive who is otherwise at high risk of death before transplantation until a donor organ becomes available.
BTC Bridge to candidacy	• Use of MCS (usually LVAD) to improve end-organ function, improve RV function/reduce PH in order to make an ineligible patient eligible for heart transplantation
BTD Bridge to decision	• Use of short-term MCS (e.g. ECLS or ECMO) in patients with cardiogenic shock until haemodynamics and end-organ perfusion are stabilized, contra-indications for long-term MCS are excluded (brain damage after resuscitation) and additional therapeutic options including long-term VAD therapy or heart transplant can be evaluated
BTR Bridge to recovery	• Use of MCS (typically LVAD) to keep patient alive until cardiac function recovers sufficiently to remove MCS
DT Destination therapy	• Long-term use of MCS (LVAD) as an alternative to transplantation in patients with end-stage HF ineligible for transplantation or long-term waiting for heart transplantation

Figure 5.1.7 Categories of indication for mechanical circulatory support
McDonagh TA, Metra M, Adamo M, et al; ESC Scientific Document Group. 2021 ESC Guidelines for the diagnosis and treatment of acute and chronic heart failure. *Eur Heart J.* 2021 Sep 21;42(36):3599–3726. doi: 10.1093/eurheartj/ehab368. © European Society of Cardiology. With permission from Oxford University Press

5.1.10 Co-morbidities and multi-disciplinary care in HF

- Depression, diabetes, AF, fraility, sleep-disordered breathing, COPD, anaemia, renal dysfunction, and obesity commonly coexist with HF, especially with increasing age

Table 5.1.14 Relevant patient factors and contraindications to consider pre-cardiac transplant.

Patients to consider	Contraindications (some are relative)
• End-stage HF with severe symptoms, a poor prognosis, and no remaining alternative treatment options • Motivated, well informed, and emotionally stable • Capable of complying with the intensive treatment required postoperatively	• Active infection • Severe peripheral arterial or cerebrovascular disease • Pharmacologically irreversible pulmonary hypertension (LVAD should be considered with a subsequent re-evaluation to establish candidacy) • Cancer (a collaboration with oncology specialists should occur to stratify each patient as to their risk of tumour recurrence) • Irreversible renal dysfunction (e.g. creatinine clearance < 30 ml/min) • Systemic disease with multi-organ involvement • Other serious co-morbidity with poor prognosis • Pre-transplant BMI > 35 kg/m² (weight loss is recommended to achieve a BMI < 35 kg/m²) • Current alcohol or drug abuse • Any patient for whom social supports are deemed insufficient for compliance in the outpatient setting • History of prior non-compliance to treatment or follow-up (require psychological/psychiatric evaluation)

Adapted from 2021 ESC Guidelines for the diagnosis & treatment of acute and chronic heart failure.

- Can render the diagnosis/management of HF challenging
- May exacerbate HF symptoms and precipitate hospitilization
- Underlying conditions and treatments can exacerbate HF and cause adverse drug effects or toxicities (bleeding, due to concomitant use of anticoagulants, worsening renal function with NSAIDs)
- Involve relevant specialists where necessary
- A detailed review of comorbities is available in 2021 ESC HF guidelines

Anaemia and iron deficiency

- Iron deficiency (ID) is common in HF and can impair functional capacity with or without anaemia
- Diagnostic criteria for ID used in trials:
    - Low ferritin (< 100 ug/ml) or
    - Ferritin (100–299) and transferrin saturation (< 20%)
- i.v. iron (ferric carboxymaltose) improves HF symptoms, exercise capacity, and QoL, and may reduce HF hospitalization
    - Oral iron (IRONOUT trial) is ineffective whilst an erythropoetin stimulant (RED-HF trial) did not improve HF outcomes and increased risk of thromboembolism
- If anaemia and ID present: check B12, folate, TSH, and undertake GI investigations
- ESC recommends:
    - All HF patients be periodically screened for anaemia and ID with a full blood count, serum ferritin, and a transferrin saturation (*class I C*)
    - i.v. iron supplementation should be considered in symptomatic patients with ID and HFrEF or HFmrEF:
        - To alleviate HF symptoms and improve quality of life (*class I A*)
        - And may be considered ro reduce the risk of HF hospitalization (*IIa A*)

Multidisciplinary team management recommendations

- Patients with HF are managed using a multidisciplinary team approach to reduce HF hospitalization and mortality (*class IA*)
- In patients with HFrEF, regular aerobic exercise improves symptoms and exercise capacity and reduces HF hospitalization (*class IA*)
- Optimal long-term management of patients with HF involves the co-ordination of care between hospital, primary care, community HF team along with timely access to advanced HF, palliative care and cardiac rehabilitation services

Long-term follow-up and monitoring

- Patients benefit from regular follow up through a combination of hospital (HF and devices clinic), primary care and community HF team to ensure clinical stability and detect complications or disease progression.
- Optimal monitoring depends on local systems and resources but should include clinical/therapy review, ECG, bloods, and device interrogation (where applicable)
- Telemonitoring has not consistently been shown to improve outcomes but should be considered if a robust system is available locally.
- The use of NPs to guide chronic HF management has not been unequivocally proven but could be used as part of holistic patient assessment.
- Invasive PA pressure monitoring devices (e.g CardioMems device) may be considered in selected patients to prevent HF hospitalization and further studies are ongoing (*class IIb B*)

5.1.11 Acute heart failure

- Refers to rapid onset or worsening of HF; can be first presentation (*de novo*) or decompensation in those with chronic HF
- Often a life threatening medical emergency
- Two common presentations
    - Pulmonary oedema: abrupt onset, drammatic medical emergency; associated with sympathetic activation (palor, clamminess, swetating, hypertension). Usually an obvious precipitant (e.g. arrhythmia, ischaemia)
    - Fluid retention: much more common; often develops over weeks; fluid retention (and weight gain) can be gross (> 20 L excess fluid); no obvious precipitant; associated with hypotension and renal impairment
- Blood pressure (BP) during presentation dictates immediate management (diuretics, vasodilators, or inotropes) whilst the aetiology/precipitants guide more specific management, e.g. revascularization
- Cardiogenic shock (usually after acute MI or other mechanical catastrophe) is rare as a 'heart failure' presentation.
    - Definition: SBP < 90mmHg and/or hypoperfusion (agitation, narrow pulse pressure, cold peripheries, elevated lactate)
- Diagnostic workup, pharmacological and non pharmacological treatment should start promptly and often in parallel
- Unstable haemodynamics +/− respiratory failure mandates immediate clinical review with ECG, echocardiography, CXR, blood gas, laboratory bloods, and liaison with critical care team

Causes and precipitants

- Myocardial ischaemia (usually critical coronary disease)
- Acute mechanical complication: LV free wall/septal rupture, severe mitral regurgitation, acute valve dysfunction due to degeneration, infection, thrombosis, or aortic dissection
- Infection: pneumonia, sepsis, endocarditis, COPD
- Non-/poor compliance with medication and fluid balance
- Drug interactions (e.g. NSAIDs, glitazones, negative chronotropes)
- Uncontrolled hypertension (if flash pulmonary oedema consider renal artery stenosis)
- Thromboembolism: consider pulmonary embolus
- Metabolic: thyroid, phaeochromocytoma, diabetic ketosis, hypoadrenalism, Takotsubo
- Arrhythmia, e.g. AF/flutter, VT (interrogate device where present), complete heart block
- Exclude other causes of oedema, e.g. renal failure, nephrotic syndrome

Assessment and investigations

- Bedside clinical assessment: thorough history incorporating symptoms, prior CV history, potential causes/precipitants, and examination for vital signs, detect signs of underlying causes, evidence of congestion and hypoperfusion
- ECG, CXR and routine laboratory bloods
- Echocardiography: immediately when unstable haemodyanamics, otherwise within 48-hours when cardac structure/function unknown or may have changed since previous study
- CT if pulmonary embolism or aortic dissection suspected
- Routine use of central venous pressure (CVP) line, intra-arterial line or PA (pulmonary artery) catheter for diagnosis is not indicated

Acute management for the three modes of presentation

1. **Pulmonary oedema:** the patient is typically anxious, scared and in extremis
   - If BP permits, i.e. SBP > 90 mmHg and no symptomatic hypotension:
     - Consider IV diuretic (*class I C*), although patients often intravascularly depleted as fluid shifts to lungs
     - Consider IV nitrovasodilator (e.g. isosorbide dinitrate, nitroglycerine) to reduce LV end-diastolic pressure (LVEDP) quickly (*class IIaB*)
   - Consider ventilatory support (*class IIa B*)
     - C3PO study showed non-invasive positive pressure ventilation is safe
     - Oxygen if SpO2 < 90% or PaO2 8 < kPa (60 mmHg), but not routinely
     - Blood gas if pulmonary oedema, concerns with COPD, and type II respiratory failure
     - Consider invasive ventilation with type II respiratory (PaCO2 > 6.65kPa, PH < 7.35, PaO2 < 8kPa) not managed with non-invasive ventilation
   - If inadequate relief of congestion, consider renal replacement therapy, MCS, other devices or palliative care

2. **Cardiogenic shock**
   - Consider revascularization in patients with ischaemia +/− signs of HF, STEMI with cardiogenic shock, ischaemic MR +/− mechanical complications
   - Consider mechanical support (intra-aortic balloon pump, ventricular assist device, ECMO) where possible reversible cause (*class IIa*)
     - Recent RCTs demonstrate no mortality benefit in patienst with acute MI and cardiogenic shock and should not be routinley used (*III*)
   - Positive inotropic support associated with adverse outcomes
     - Consider short term i.v. inotropes or vasopressors (dobutamine, dopamine, phosphodiesterase III (PDE III) inhibitors) if persistent hypotension/hypoperfusion (*IIb C*), otherwise they are not recommended (*III*)
     - Consider vasopressors (noradrenaline, adrenaline, high-dose dopamine) if cardiogenic shock despite inotropes; arterial line required (*IIb B*)

3. **Fluid retention:** the key to patient management is to reduce fluid load
   - Bed rest
   - Monitor fluid input/output
   - Daily weights and urea and electrolytes
   - Thromboembolism prophylaxis (IA)
   - Stop any 'nephrotoxins' (e.g. NSAIDs) or redandant (e.g. calcium antagonists) drugs
   - IV loop diuretics (e.g. furosemide, bumetanide, torasemide) are recommended if evidence of congestion with regular clinical review monitoring urine output, electrolytes, and renal function (class IC):
     - Initial 20–40 mg IV furosemide (or equivalent) for diuretic naive patients, or 1–2 times the daily oral dose for those with chronic HF
     - Check urinary sodium after 2 hours (aiming for ≥ 50–70 mEq/l) and urine output after 6 hours (aiming for ≥ 100–150 ml/hour)
- If adequate urine sodium & urine output, continue dose 12 hourly until complete decongestion
- If inadequate response, double i.v. dose until adequate diuresis or maximum dose reached Combination diuretic therapy can be introduced with the addition of thiazides or spironolactone if inadequate response persists
- Diuretics often under-used or withheld (wrongly) for renal dysfunction. In CARRESS, a maximum of an 80 mg bolus of furosemide followed by 30 mg per hour by continuous

infusion *and* metolazone twice daily given specifically to patients recruited due to worsened renal function, demonstrated renal function improved with diuretic therapy
- As diuresis is achieved, aim to commence/re-start ACEi, BB, and MRA
- The STRONG-HF study showed a large and statistically signficant reduction in HF hospitalisation following aggressive uptitration of OMT (BB, ACEi, MRA) prior to and shortly after the index admission for acute heart failure

Right heart failure and pulmonary hypertension

- Right HF can be caused by one or more of: pressure overload, volume overload, or myocardial/pericardial disease—they are not mutually exclusive
  - Volume overload:
    - Tricuspid regurgitation, either primary (e.g. carcinoid, Ebstein's, rheumatic/myxomatous) or secondary (annular dilatation)
    - Congenital/acquired pre-tricuspid shunts (ASD, anomalous PVD, fistulae, etc.)
  - Pressure overload:
    - Most commonly due to left heart diseases (HFrEF, HFpEF, AF, or valvular HD), lung diseases, chronic PE, or less commonly due to group 1 PAH
    - Myocardial/pericardial causes of RHF include RV infarction, acute myocarditis, DCM, ARVC, infiltration (sarcoid/amyloid), and pericardial constriction
- Pulmonary hypertension is common in all forms of HF and is managed with OMT or correcting valve disease
- Available evidence does not support using pulmonary vasodilators (e.g. sildenafil, endothelin receptor antagonists, prostacyclin analogues) in PH due to left heart diseases.
- See relevant chapters on pulmonary hypertension, valve and pericardial disease

5.1.12 Palliative care in heart failure

Aims:
To prevent and relieve suffering and to promote the best quality of life for patients and their families/carers

- Although the last section in this chapter, palliative care should be part of standard care from diagnosis onward
- Palliative care services are often involved after management options are exhausted or failing to relieve symptoms
- However, they should be integrated and available much earlier and be 'problem based' rather than 'prognosis based', because patients with HF often are:
  - Complex with holistic care needs
  - Older with multiple comorbidties and progressive fraility
  - Affected by refractory symptoms
  - Not eligible for LVAD or transplantation
- Identifying the dying patient is difficult because disease trajectory is often interspersed with dips (decompensation/hospitilization) and plateau (recovery after hospitilization)
- Adverse clinical indicators include:
  - Persistent/progressive NYHA Class III/IV symptoms
  - Increasing fraility and care needs/dependance
  - Recurrent HF hospitilizations despite maximal/optimal tolerated treatment
  - Progressive decline in renal function, falling albumin/sodium
  - Persistent symptomatic hypotension requiring reduction/withdrawl of medication

- Chronic poor quality of life
- Weight loss (cachexia)
- Indicators of terminal stage include inability to take oral fluids/medications, bed bound, increasingly weak, withdrawn, or unresponsive
• Palliative care services should also be involved when:
  - There are persistent and/or complex symptoms
  - Wider support needed for family
  - 'Difficult' discussions regarding dying, prefered place of care/death, deactivation of ICD, etc.
  - Refractory symptoms develop: pain, breathlessness, persistent cough, fatigue, anxiety, depression, poor sleep, nausea, confusion, and constipation
• Resources and training by local palliative care services supporting heart failure should be explored and used, and a collaborative approach from the outset is vital

Further reading

Bhagra SK, Pettit S, Parameshwar J. Cardiac transplantation: indications, eligibility and current outcomes. *Heart*. 2019 Feb;105(3):252–60. doi: 10.1136/heartjnl-2018-313103. Epub 2018 Sep 12

Bozkurt B, Coats AJ, Tsutsui H, Abdelhamid M, Adamopoulos S, Albert N, Anker SD, Atherton J, Böhm M, Butler J, Drazner MH, Felker GM, Filippatos G, Fonarow GC, Fiuzat M, Gomez-Mesa JE, Heidenreich P, Imamura T, Januzzi J, Jankowska EA, Khazanie P, Kinugawa K, Lam CSP, Matsue Y, Metra M, Ohtani T, Francesco Piepoli M, Ponikowski P, Rosano GMC, Sakata Y, Seferović P, Starling RC, Teerlink JR, Vardeny O, Yamamoto K, Yancy C, Zhang J, Zieroth S. Universal Definition and Classification of Heart Failure: A Report of the Heart Failure Society of America, Heart Failure Association of the European Society of Cardiology, Japanese Heart Failure Society and Writing Committee of the Universal Definition of Heart Failure. *J Card Fail*. 2021 Mar 1;27(4):P387–413. doi: 10.1016/j.cardfail.2021.01.022. Epub ahead of print. PMID: 33663906

Crespo-Leiro MG, Metra M, Lund LH, Milicic D, Costanzo MR, Filippatos G, Gustafsson F, Tsui S, Barge-Caballero E, De Jonge N, Frigerio M, Hamdan R, Hasin T, Hülsmann M, Nalbantgil S, Potena L, Bauersachs J, Gkouziouta A, Ruhparwar A, Ristic AD, Straburzynska-Migaj E, McDonagh T, Seferovic P, Ruschitzka F. Advanced heart failure: a position statement of the Heart Failure Association of the European Society of Cardiology. *Eur J Heart Fail*. 2018 Nov;20(11):1505–35. doi: 10.1002/ejhf.1236. Epub 2018 Jul 17. PMID: 29806100

Clark AL, Gardner RS, McDonagh TA, (eds), *Oxford Textbook of Heart Failure*. Oxford: Oxford University Press, 2nd edition, 2022 ISBN: 9780198766223

McDonagh TA, Metra M, Adamo M, Gardner RS, Baumbach A, Böhm M, Burri H, Butler J, Čelutkienė J, Chioncel O, Cleland JGF, Crespo-Leiro MG, Farmakis D, Gilard M, Heymans S, Hoes AW, Jaarsma T, Jankowska EA, Lainscak M, Lam CSP, Lyon AR, McMurray JJV, Mebazaa A, Mindham R, Munaretto C, Francesco Piepoli M, Price S, Rosano GMC, Ruschitzka F, Skibelund AK; ESC Scientific Document Group. 2023 Focused Update of the 2021 ESC Guidelines for the diagnosis and treatment of acute and chronic heart failure. *Eur Heart J*. 2023 Oct 1;44(37):3627–39. doi: 10.1093/eurheartj/ehad195. PMID: 37622666.

McDonagh TA, Metra M, Adamo M, Gardner RS, Baumbach A, Böhm M, Burri H, Butler J, Čelutkienė J, Chioncel O, Cleland JGF, Coats AJS, Crespo-Leiro MG, Farmakis D, Gilard M, Heymans S, Hoes AW, Jaarsma T, Jankowska EA, Lainscak M, Lam CSP, Lyon AR, McMurray JJV, Mebazaa A, Mindham R, Munaretto C, Francesco Piepoli M, Price S, Rosano GMC, Ruschitzka F, Kathrine Skibelund A; ESC Scientific Document Group. 2021 ESC Guidelines for the diagnosis and treatment of acute and chronic heart failure. *Eur Heart J.* 2021 Sep 21;42(36):3599–726. doi: 10.1093/eurheartj/ehab368. PMID: 34447992

Mullens W, Damman K, Harjola VP, Mebazaa A, Brunner-La Rocca HP, Martens P, Testani JM, Tang WHW, Orso F, Rossignol P, Metra M, Filippatos G, Seferovic PM, Ruschitzka F, Coats AJ. The use of diuretics in heart failure with congestion - a position statement from the Heart Failure Association of the European Society of Cardiology. *Eur J Heart Fail.* 2019 Feb;21(2):137–55. doi: 10.1002/ejhf.1369. Epub 2019 Jan 1

Pieske B, Tschöpe C, de Boer RA, Fraser AG, Anker SD, Donal E, Edelmann F, Fu M, Guazzi M, Lam CSP, Lancellotti P, Melenovsky V, Morris DA, Nagel E, Pieske-Kraigher E, Ponikowski P, Solomon SD, Vasan RS, Rutten FH, Voors AA, Ruschitzka F, Paulus WJ, Seferovic P, Filippatos G. How to diagnose heart failure with preserved ejection fraction: the HFA-PEFF diagnostic algorithm: a consensus recommendation from the Heart Failure Association (HFA) of the European Society of Cardiology (ESC). *Eur J Heart Fail.* 2020 Mar;22(3):391–412. doi: 10.1002/ejhf.1741. Epub 2020

Seferović PM, Polovina M, Bauersachs J, Arad M, Gal TB, Lund LH, Felix SB, Arbustini E, Caforio ALP, Farmakis D, Filippatos GS, Gialafos E, Kanjuh V, Krljanac G, Limongelli G, Linhart A, Lyon AR, Maksimović R, Miličić D, Milinković I, Noutsias M, Oto A, Oto Ö, Pavlović SU, Piepoli MF, Ristić AD, Rosano GMC, Seggewiss H, Ašanin M, Seferović JP, Ruschitzka F, Čelutkiene J, Jaarsma T, Mueller C, Moura B, Hill L, Volterrani M, Lopatin Y, Metra M, Backs J, Mullens W, Chioncel O, de Boer RA, Anker S, Rapezzi C, Coats AJS, Tschöpe C. Heart failure in cardiomyopathies: a position paper from the Heart Failure Association of the European Society of Cardiology. *Eur J Heart Fail.* 2019 May;21(5):553–76. doi: 10.1002/ejhf.1461. Epub 2019 Apr 16. PMID: 30989768

The ESC-HFA website has a comprehensive series of consensus and position papers on all aspects of heart failure. https://www.escardio.org/Guidelines/Scientific-Documents/heart-failure

5.2

Cardiomyopathies

Angus Nightingale, Eva Sammut, Victoria McKay, Stewart Brown, and Rhian Richardson

TABLE OF CONTENTS

- 5.2.1 Classification of cardiomyopathies 461
- 5.2.2 Hypertrophic cardiomyopathy 462
- 5.2.3 Dilated cardiomyopathy 471
- 5.2.4 Non-dilated left ventricular cardiomyopathy 474
- 5.2.5 Arrhythmogenic right ventricular cardiomyopathy 475
- 5.2.6 Restrictive cardiomyopathy 479
  - Amyloid heart disease 481
  - Sarcoid heart disease 483
- 5.2.7 Storage diseases 485
- 5.2.8 Inflammatory myocardial disease 488
  - Pathophysiology 488
  - Clinical presentation 489
  - Management 489
  - Prognosis and outcome 490
  - HIV cardiomyopathy 490
  - Chagas disease 490
  - Lyme disease 491
- 5.2.9 Secondary myocardial diseases 491
  - Alcoholic cardiomyopathy 491
  - Metabolic cardiomyopathy 491
  - Tachycardia-related cardiomyopathy 492
  - Muscular dystrophy cardiomyopathy 492
  - Peripartum cardiomyopathy 492
  - Left ventricular hypertrabeculation/non-compaction 494
  - Takotsubo syndrome (stress-induced 'cardiomyopathy') 495
- 5.2.10 Cardiac transplantation 496

5.2.1 Classification of cardiomyopathies

- Patients with primary disorders of the myocardium tend to have a genetic component
- Five phenotypes are used to primarily classify cardiomyopathy and from there specific features of investigations can determine underlying aetiology
- Different cardiomyopathy phenotypes may coexist in the same family, and disease progression in an individual patient can include evolution from one cardiomyopathy phenotype to another
- The five phenotypes are as follows (Figure 5.2.1):
  - Hypertrophic cardiomyopathy (HCM)
  - Dilated cardiomyopathy (DCM)
  - Non-dilated left ventricular cardiomyopathy (NDLVC)
  - Arrhythmogenic right ventricular cardiomyopathy (ARVC)
  - Restrictive cardiomyopathy (RCM)
- An inflammatory cardiomyopathy may also exist and is defined as inflammation of the myocardium and its structures by infectious or non-infectious agents.

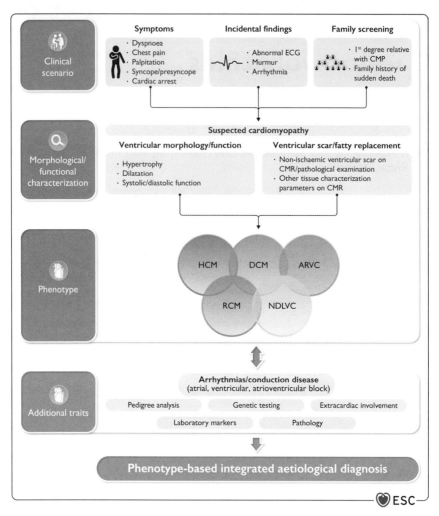

Figure 5.2.1 Clinical diagnostic workflow of cardiomyopathy. ARVC, arrhythmogenic right ventricular cardiomyopathy; CMP, cardiomyopathy; CMR, cardiac magnetic resonance; DCM, dilated cardiomyopathy; ECG, electrocardiogram; HCM, hypertrophic cardiomyopathy; NDLVC, non-dilated left ventricular cardiomyopathy; RCM, restrictive cardiomyopathy.

Arbelo E, Protonotarios A, Gimeno JR, et al; ESC Scientific Document Group. 2023 ESC Guidelines for the management of cardiomyopathies. *Eur Heart J.* 2023 Oct 1;44(37):3503–3626. doi: 10.1093/eurheartj/ehad194. © European Society of Cardiology. With permission from Oxford University Press

5.2.2 Hypertrophic cardiomyopathy

Four cardinal features are key to diagnosis:

1. **Unexplained hypertrophy of the left ventricle**
2. **Cardiac myocyte disarray**
3. **Familial occurrence**
4. **Association with sudden cardiac death.**
    - Concentric, asymmetric, and apical patterns of hypertrophy are all well recognized

> **BOX 5.2.1 SARCOMERIC PROTEIN MUTATIONS**
>
> β-myosin heavy chain (MYH7)
> Myosin-binding protein C (MYBPC3)
> Troponin I/Troponin T (TNNI3, TNNT2)
> Tropomyosin α1 chain (TPM1)
> Myosin light chain 3 (MYL3)

- The presence of left ventricular outflow tract obstruction (LVOTO), although not essential for diagnosis, occurs in around a 1/3 of patients at rest and 1/3 with provocation with clinical and prognostic implications.

Genetics

- Hypertrophic cardiomyopathy is an inherited disorder with mutation of the sarcomeric proteins
- Sarcomere is the contractile apparatus within the myocardial cells
- Mutation leads to myocyte disarray and fibrosis, myocardial hypertrophy, and small vessel coronary artery disease.
- Autosomal dominant mode of inheritance is most common, with increasing penetrance with age
- Most common mutation is the gene for β-myosin heavy chain but many other mutations have been implicated (see Box 5.2.1)
- Prevalence is estimated at 0.2%
- Only 55–75% are estimated to have a detectable mutation in sarcomeric genes
- 5–10% patients have phenocopies of HCM, i.e. a phenotype suggestive of HCM but an alternative underlying condition (e.g. Fabry's disease, glycogen storage disorder, disorders of metabolism)
- Phenocopies tend to have extra-cardiac manifestations and an increased incidence of conduction disease, cavity dilation, and heart failure.

Pathophysiology

Increased LV wall thickening in the absence of abnormal loading conditions

- In adults, wall thickness ≥ 15 mm in one or more LV myocardial segments (by any imaging modality)
- Concentric, asymmetric, and apical patterns of hypertrophy are all well recognized

Myocardial fibrosis

- Scar (identified by CMR) is present in 65% patients
- Typically, patchy mid-wall pattern in areas of hypertrophy and the anterior and posterior LV/RV insertion points
- May be seen in non-hypertrophied segments in association with wall thinning in late 'burnt out' stage of disease

Morphological abnormalities of mitral valve apparatus +/– LVOT obstruction

- Outflow tract obstruction occurs in 25% of patients (it can occur in the mid cavity and apex as well as at sub-aortic level)
- Reflects abnormal septal geometry, mitral leaflet elongation and abnormalities of sub-mitral apparatus

- Systolic anterior motion of the mitral valve caused by abnormal mitral apparatus and abnormal haemodynamics leads to further obstruction as well as a degree of mitral regurgitation.
- May be seen at rest or only on provocation (Valsalva, exercise)
- Over time can impair exercise tolerance, lead to atrial dilatation and consequent arrhythmia.

Diastolic dysfunction
- Normal calcium uptake, required in early diastole, is disrupted
- Hypertrophy and interstitial fibrosis decrease compliance and cause failure of passive relaxation
- In 5% progresses to burnt-out phase with systolic impairment

Microvascular ischaemia
- Changes occur in the microcirculation, with reduced arteriolar luminal size and capillary density
- There is also a reduction in coronary flow reserve

ECG changes +/– atrial fibrillation
- Variable—can include LVH, ST and T wave abnormalities and pathological Q waves

Clinical presentation
- Asymptomatic:
  - Screening due to family history or abnormal ECG
- Angina:
  - Microvascular dysfunction
  - Increased LV wall stress
  - LVOT obstruction
- Breathlessness:
  - Diastolic dysfunction due to left ventricular hypertrophy (LVH), systolic dysfunction
  - Mitral regurgitation
  - LVOT obstruction
- Raised pulmonary pressures:
  - Ischaemia ± mitral regurgitation
- Dizziness/syncope:
  - Left ventricular tract obstruction
  - Ventricular and atrial arrhythmias
  - Abnormal vascular reflexes

Physical signs include:

- Rapid upstroke to pulse
- Forceful left ventricle at apex ('double impulse')
- Mid-late systolic murmur (no carotid radiation), which can be provoked with exercise or Valsalva manoeuvre.

Diagnosis
Echocardiography
See Box 5.2.2.

- Caution should be used to distinguish HCM from athlete's heart in young, fit individuals and phenocopies of HCM

> **BOX 5.2.2 ECHOCARDIOGRAPHIC GUIDELINES FOR THE DIAGNOSIS OF HYPERTROPHIC CARDIOMYOPATHY**
>
> **Major criteria**
>
> LV wall thickness ≥ 13 mm in the anterior septum or ≥15 mm in the posterior septum or free wall.
>
> Severe SAM (septum–leaflet contact).
>
> **Minor criteria**
>
> LV wall thickness of 12 mm in the anterior septum or posterior wall or of 14 mm in the posterior septum or free wall.
>
> Moderate SAM (no septum–leaflet contact).
>
> Redundant mitral valve leaflets.
>
> Guidelines are applicable only to first-degree relatives of index cases with confirmed hypertrophic cardiomyopathy, all of whom have a 50% probability of carrying the mutation. Diagnosis is established in the presence of one major criterion, or two minor echocardiographic criteria, or one minor echocardiographic plus two minor electrocardiographic criteria. Other causes of left ventricular hypertrophy (e.g. athletic training and hypertension) may confound diagnosis.
>
> LV, left ventricular; SAM, systolic anterior motion of the mitral valve. Reproduced from the *ESC Textbook of Cardiovascular Medicine*, 2nd edn, ed. John Camm, Thomas Lüscher, and Patrick Serruys, copyright 2009 with permission of Oxford University Press.

- Athletes tend to have milder degrees of left ventricular hypertrophy (LVH) (septal thickness of 13–14 mm), the LV cavity tends to be enlarged, and diastolic parameters are normal or enhanced
- Measurements at rest and during Valsalva manoeuvre to detect LVOTO is recommended.

Electrocardiography
Resting ECG
- Can be normal at presentation
- Generally, shows combination of LVH, ST- and T-wave abnormalities and pathological Q waves
- AV block can sometimes be seen and should prompt consideration of amyloidosis as aetiology
- Should be done at time of initial referral and repeated whenever there is a change in symptoms

Ambulatory ECG monitoring
- Asymptomatic non-sustained VT (120–200 bpm) occurs in 25% patients with HCM
- Paroxysmal supraventricular tachycardia occurs in up to 38% patients
- Should be performed as part of risk stratification (see below) or after stroke

See Box 5.2.3.

Genetic testing
Genetic counselling and testing are recommended in HCM patients

> **BOX 5.2.3 ECG GUIDELINES FOR THE DIAGNOSIS OF HYPERTROPHIC CARDIOMYOPATHY**
>
> **Major criteria**
>
> Left ventricular hypertrophy and repolarization changes.
>
> T wave inversion in leads I and aVL ($\geq$ 3 mm) (with QRS–T wave axis difference $\geq$30°), V3–V6 ($\geq$ 3 mm) or II and III and aVF ($\geq$ 5 mm).
>
> Abnormal Q (>40 ms or >25% R wave) in at least two leads from II, III, aVF (in absence of left anterior hemiblock), V1–V4; or I, aVL, V5–V6.
>
> **Minor criteria**
>
> Complete bundle branch block or (minor) interventricular conduction defect (in LV leads).
>
> Minor repolarization changes in LV leads.
>
> Deep S V2 (> 25 mm).
>
> Reproduced from the *ESC Textbook of Cardiovascular Medicine*, 2nd edn, ed. John Camm, Thomas Lüscher, and Patrick Serruys, copyright 2009 with permission of Oxford University Press.

Cardiac magnetic resonance imaging

LV wall thickness

- CMR provides similar information on ventricular morphology and function in patients with good echocardiographic windows. CMR preferable where echocardiography image quality is suboptimal, particularly to visualize apical and anterolateral hypertrophy, and apical aneurysms (due to mid cavity systolic obliteration)
- Superior to echocardiography for measurement of LV mass—overall mass may be normal even in HCM depending on number of segments affected

LVOT obstruction

- Can measure flows through LVOT; however difficult to make accurate quantification and can only be measured at rest—echocardiography is superior

Diastolic function

- Can measure diastolic function; highly specialized and not routinely done

Systolic function

- CMR is reference method for calculation of volumes and ejection fraction

Fibrosis

- Gadolinium contrast agent detects expansion of myocardial interstitium caused by fibrosis
- Late gadolinium enhancement imaging permits direct visualization of areas of scar and replacement fibrosis and is present in 65% of HCM patients
- Newer T1 mapping techniques show promise for quantification of diffuse fibrosis (can be done pre-contrast)
- Fibrosis can be helpful in distinguishing HCM from other causes of LVH
    - Anderson–Fabry disease characterized by a reduction in T1 signal and the presence of posterolateral LGE
    - In cardiac amyloidosis there is often global, subendocardial, or segmental LGE

- Absence of LGE may also be helpful in differentiating HCM from athlete's heart, but may not be present in earlier stages of HCM

Screening investigations
- Patients screened for HCM with ECG and echocardiography if family history or symptoms:
    - Pre-pubescent children only if symptomatic, have a high-risk family history, undertake competitive sport, or there are high levels of parental anxiety
    - Adolescents: annual review from early adolescence, as clinical manifestations occur during puberty
    - In later life, 5-yearly screening of relatives due to incidence of late onset HCM
    - Diagnosis of HCM in a first-degree relative is made if LV wall thickness is ≥ 13 mm in 1 or more LV myocardial segments.

Prognosis and outcome
- Clinical course is variable—annual mortality estimated at 1% for asymptomatic patients; 5% for symptomatic (overall 2–3%). See Box 5.2.4
- Morbidity / mortality related to (overall annual risk of death 1–2%):
    - Thrombo-embolism
    - Sudden cardiac death
    - Heart failure

BOX 5.2.4 RISK FACTORS FOR SUDDEN CARDIAC DEATH IN HYPERTROPHIC CARDIOMYOPATHY

- Family history of premature death (first degree relative)
- Recurrent syncope (exercise related)
- Septal thickness > 30 mm
- A genetic phenotype associated with sudden cardiac death (SCD)
- Non-sustained ventricular tachycardia (VT) (especially if under 30 years old)
- Inadequate rise in blood pressure during exercise (defined as a failure to increase systolic pressure by ≥ 20 mmHg from rest to peak exercise, or a fall of > 20 mmHg from peak pressure)
- Resting LVOTO > 30 mmHg
- Younger age (but > 6 years old)
- Higher LGE on cardiac MRI (≥ 15%)

Risk stratification for patients with confirmed HCM
- Risk stratification should be performed every 1 to 3 years
- Echocardiography to assess LV thickness and LVOTO
- Exercise testing: inadequate BP response
- 24-h Holter monitor:
    - ≥ 3 beats of VT at rate of ≥ 120 bpm
    - Presence of AF (refer for formal anticoagulation)
    - Consider implantable loop recorder if suspicious history for malignant arrhythmia.

- Symptoms tend to be due to left ventricular outflow tract obstruction (LVOTO) and diastolic dysfunction due to LVH
- Left ventricular thinning also occurs secondary to abnormal haemodynamics, leading to myocyte loss and fibrosis.

Management
Aims of management
- Alleviate symptoms
- Prevent complications, e.g. atrial fibrillation
- Reduce risk of SCD.

Medical therapy
- Asymptomatic patients:
    - Mild LVH—no treatment
    - Severe LVH—verapamil to improve relaxation and diastolic dysfunction
- Symptomatic patients:
    - Beta blockers are first line with the addition of a calcium antagonist (verapamil or diltiazem) if still symptomatic; these act as negative inotropes and reduce systolic LVOT gradient
    - Diuretics should be used with caution as patients can be very volume sensitive
    - In patients with resting/provocable LVOTO ≥ 50 mmHg, Disopyramide can be used to alter calcium kinetics in the myocytes and is associated with reduced symptoms and reduced systolic pressure gradient. Mavacamten is an alternative.
    - Cautious use of nitrates and/or ranolazine for patients with angina-like chest pain without LVOTO, or confirmed obstructive CAD
    - Amiodarone to reduce the burden of atrial fibrillation; formal anticoagulation should be strongly considered.
    - Avoid vasodilators and digoxin in patients with LVOT obstruction

Additional therapy
LVOT obstruction
Invasive treatment should be considered in patients with LVOT gradient ≥ 50 mmHg, NYHA functional class III–IV, and or recurrent exertional syncope despite maximally tolerated medical therapy.
Special consideration for patients with mid-cavity obstruction (~10%) who tend to be very symptomatic and at increased risk of heart failure and SCD.

Ventricular septal myectomy:
- Morrow procedure—rectangular trough created in basal septum below aortic valve
- Abolishes or substantially reduces LVOT gradient in > 90% cases, reduces SAM-related MR and improves exercise capacity and symptoms.
- Long-term symptomatic benefit achieved in > 80% patients with long term survival comparable to general population (pre-operative determinants of good outcome—male, < 50 years, left atrial size < 46 mm, absence of AF)
- Good long-term results but remodelling and cavity dilation seen in 15–20%
- Complications include most commonly LBBB, and less commonly; AV block requiring pacemaker implantation (3%), aortic regurgitation and ventricular septal defect (VSD; 1%)

- Concomitant mitral valve surgery is required in 11–20% cases (replacement, realignment of papillary muscles, excision/mobilization papillary muscles, leaflet plication or extension)
- Concomitant surgical AF ablation and/or LAA occlusion procedures should be considered for HCM patients with symptomatic AF

Alcohol septal ablation:
- Selective injection of alcohol into a septal perforator artery to create localized septal scar
- Artery identified by myocardial contrast echocardiography
- Outcomes similar to surgery in terms of gradient reduction, symptom improvement, and exercise capacity.
- Main non-fatal complication is AV block requiring pacemaker implantation in 7–20%, with procedural mortality lower than isolated myomectomy.

Dual chamber pacing:
- Small randomized studies only
- Reported to result in reduction in LVOT gradients with variable response in terms of exercise capacity and symptoms
- Consider permanent AV sequential pacing in patients who are unsuitable or high risk for more invasive approaches and ideally those who also have a pacing indication—optimize to achieve maximum pre-excitation of the RV with minimal compromise to LV filling—may also facilitate use of beta blockers/calcium channel blockers

Heart failure
- In patients with normal EF and no resting or provable LVOTO, aim is to reduce LV diastolic pressure and improve LV filling
    - Use beta blockers or rate limiting calcium antagonists with cautious use of diuretics
    - Prompt restoration of sinus rhythm or ventricular rate control. Digoxin not recommended (positively ionotropic)
- In patients with reduced LVEF
    - Treat with diuretics, beta blockers, inhibition of RAAS system when LVEF < 50% (limited studies specifically in HCM)
    - Caution with diuretics and RAAS inhibitors due to small cavity size—may be poorly tolerated
    - Consider CRT according to normal guidelines—can be considered on an individual basis for symptomatic patients with LVEF < 50% but meeting ECG criteria for CRT
- Consider heart transplant in patients with moderate to severe drug refractory symptoms and no LVOTO who meet standard criteria.

Atrial tachyarrhythmias
Atrial fibrillation most common
- Prevalence 22.5%, annual incidence 3.1%
- Related to increased LA pressure and size, caused by diastolic dysfunction, LVOTO and MR
- Patients with HCM with left atrial diameter ≥ 45 mm should undergo 48-hour ambulatory ECG monitoring 6–12 monthly
- Recommended all patients with paroxysmal, persistent, or permanent AF are formally anticoagulated due to high risk of stroke, regardless of CHA_2DS_2-VASc score.
- Prompt restoration of sinus rhythm with antiarrhythmics, DCCV or ablation

Sudden cardiac death
Prevention of SCD
- Exercise restriction
    - General advice is no competitive or intense physical training, especially if risk factors for SCD or LVOTO, however latest ESC guidance state high-intensity exercise may be considered in asymptomatic adults without high-risk markers
- Implantable cardiac defibrillator implantation
    - Secondary prevention
        - Patients with HCM who survive a VF/ sustained VT arrest are at high risk of subsequent lethal arrhythmia and should receive an ICD
        - Patients with haemodynamically tolerated VT should be considered for ICD implantation
    - Primary prevention
        - Patients with HCM with no history of VF who are at high risk of SCD, remain a challenge to balance risk versus device complications and inappropriate therapy
        - HCM Risk-SCD risk prediction model should be used to guide decision-making—provides 5-year risk estimates—incorporates age, maximal wall thickness, left atrial diameter, maximal LVOT gradient, FH of SCD, NSVT, unexplained syncope. Not to be used for
            - Paediatric patients (< 16 years old)
            - Elite/competitive athletes
            - HCM associated with metabolic disease and syndromes
        - ICD implantation (see figure 5.2.2):
            - *Should* be considered if SCD risk is ≥ 6%
            Or
            - *Should* be considered if SCD risk is 4–6% and any of (i) significant LGE at CMR (usually ≥ 15% of LV mass), (ii) LVEF < 50%, (iii) abnormal BP response to exercise, (iv) LV apical aneurysm, or (v) presence of a sarcomeric pathogenic mutation
            Or
            - *May* be considered if SCD risk is 4–6%
            Or
            - *May* be considered if SCD risk is < 4% with (i) significant LGE at CMR (usually ≥ 15% of LV mass), or (ii) LVEF < 50%, or (iii) LV apical aneurysm
- No evidence that antiarrhythmic therapy reduces the risk of SCD, however ESC consensus opinion is that they should be considered in patients with recurrent ventricular arrhythmia

Special considerations
- Pregnancy:
    - Cardiomyopathy generally well tolerated with low maternal mortality if asymptomatic with no high-risk features
    - Joint cardiac and obstetric care is recommended
- Exercise:
    - Patients with symptomatic HCM should not undertake competitive sport and burst exertion (e.g. sprints) and isometric exercise (e.g. weight lifting) should be discouraged
    - However, high-intensity exercise may be considered in asymptomatic adults without high-risk markers
- Elderly patients:
    - Elderly patients with HCM should be distinguished from those with non-genetic hypertensive heart disease. Hypertrophy tends to be milder in hypertensive disease

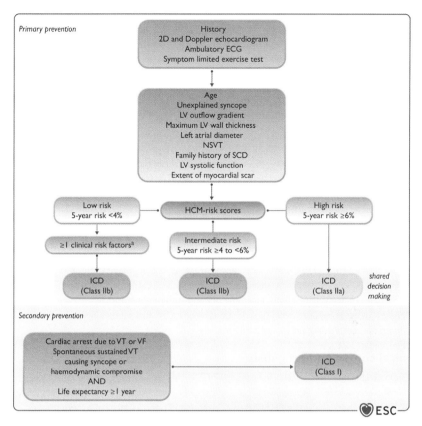

Figure 5.2.2 Flow chart for implantation of an implantable cardioverter defibrillator in patients with hypertrophic cardiomyopathy. 2D, two-dimensional; CMR, cardiac magnetic resonance; ECG, electrocardiogram; HCM, hypertrophic cardiomyopathy; ICD, implantable cardioverter defibrillator; LGE, late gadolinium enhancement; LV, left ventricular; LVEF, left ventricular ejection fraction; NSVT, non-sustained ventricular tachycardia; SCD, sudden cardiac death; VF, ventricular fibrillation; VT, ventricular tachycardia. aClinical risk factors: extensive LGE (>15%) on CMR; LVEF <50%.
Arbelo E, Protonotarios A, Gimeno JR, et al; ESC Scientific Document Group. 2023 ESC Guidelines for the management of cardiomyopathies. *Eur Heart J.* 2023 Oct 1;44(37):3503–3626. doi: 10.1093/eurheartj/ehad194. © European Society of Cardiology. With permission from Oxford University Press

- In the absence of a genotype, the presence of LVOTO, a disproportionate level of hypertrophy compared to the degree of hypertension, or an unusual pattern of hypertrophy, suggests HCM.

5.2.3 Dilated cardiomyopathy

- Dilated cardiomyopathy (DCM) is a chronic heart muscle disease with cavity enlargement and impaired systolic function of the left or both ventricles in the absence of abnormal loading conditions (hypertension or valve disease) or significant coronary artery disease.
- LV dilatation is defined by echo as LVEDD > 58 mm in males and > 52 mm in females, and an LVEDV index of ≥ 75 mL/m^2 in males and ≥ 62 mL/m^2 in females.

- The diagnosis is made once other specific cardiomyopathies have been excluded
- The causes are classified as genetic or non-genetic. Around 30–40% of cases are genetically transmitted
- Prevalence of familial DCM is likely underestimated due to poor disease expression and a variability of phenotype for the same genetic abnormality leading to a number of presentations, e.g. arrhythmia, stroke, conduction system disease, and sudden cardiac death
- Inheritance is commonly autosomal dominant but recessive, X-linked, and mitochondrial forms are recognised
- Main genes associated with predominant cardiac phenotype are titin (20–25% of familial DCM), lamin A/C, myosin heavy chain, troponin T, myosin binding protein C, RNA-binding Motif-20, myopalladin, sodium channel alpha unit, BaCl2-associated athanogene 3 and phospholamban
- Other genetic subtypes are neuromuscular disorders such as Duchenne muscular dystrophy, Becker muscular dystrophy, and myotonic dystrophy or Steinert
- Some environmental factors may unmask incomplete genetic penetrance, e.g. alcohol excess
- Other causative factors include toxins, cancer drugs, psychiatric medications, tachyarrhythmias, nutritional deficiency (selenium, thiamine, zinc, copper, and carnitine), electrolyte disturbance, endocrine syndromes, infections, inflammatory and autoimmune disease
- Peripartum cardiomyopathy is a specific sub-type of DCM. Risk factors include multiparity, African descent, familial DCM and autoimmunity

Clinical course and prognosis

- The course is heterogenous
- Better outcomes are associated with young age, shorter clinical history, improvement in LV function with medical therapy, a worse NYHA class on presentation, and a history of hypertension
- Demonstrable genetic mutations are associated with a worse prognosis

Diagnostic testing

Neurohormones:

- Elevated brain natriuretic peptide (BNP) relates to myocardial stretch

Electrocardiography:

- Atrial fibrillation and prolongation of QTc are associated with increased mortality and heart failure progression
- Prolongation of QRS duration (> 130) implies dyssynchrony and allows consideration for cardiac resynchronization therapy (CRT)
- Ventricular arrhythmias detected on Holter monitoring are associated with increased mortality and allow consideration of implantable defibrillator (ICD)

Genetic testing:

- Genetic testing can be beneficial in all patients with DCM, including children and those with alcohol-/chemotherapy-induced and peri-partum DCM

Cardiopulmonary exercise testing:

- Assessment of anaerobic threshold and ventilatory efficiency are reliable markers of mortality as well as part of the assessment for cardiac transplantation

Echocardiography:
- Confirms chamber sizes, global and regional LV anatomy, function (including estimated ejection fraction), and haemodynamics
- Advanced echocardiography including speckle tracking and contrast can allow early detection of subclinical myocardial dysfunction in some situations

Cardiac magnetic resonance imaging:
- Cardiac MRI is recommended to assess LV size, function, myocardial mass, and regional wall motion
- Late gadolinium enhancement imaging can be helpful to identify scar and other patterns of uptake indicative of specific aetiologies

Endomyocardial biopsy:
- Endomyocardial biopsy is usually non-specific in DCM.

Management
1. Treatment for heart failure:
   - ACE inhibitors/ARBs
   - Beta blockers (BBs)
   - Mineralo-corticoid Receptor Antagonists (MRA)
   - Angiotensin Receptor Neprilysin Inhibitors (ARNI)
   - Heart rate controlling drugs such as I_f channel blockers should be considered if HR > 70 bpm in sinus rhythm despite maximally tolerated beta-blockers
2. Discontinuation of cardiotoxics, e.g. alcohol, anthracyclines
3. Assessment for device therapy:
   - Risk assessment for SCD
   - QRS > 130 ms and NYHA > Class II for consideration of CRT
4. Exercise training/cardiac rehabilitation
5. Left ventricular assist device as bridge to transplant or to recovery
6. Cardiac transplantation

Risk assessment, screening, and prognosis
- First-degree relatives of patients with DCM should be screened with ECG and echocardiography for early detection
- Medical therapy with ACE inhibitors, BBs, MRAs, ARNIs improve pump function in 50% of patients; normalization occurs in 16%
- Late gadolinium enhancement on MRI is associated with increased risk of all-cause mortality, sudden death, and HF hospitalization.
- Death occurs in around one-fifth of cases probably secondary to SCD; the remainder have terminal heart failure
- Five-year survival is estimated at 30–35%
- Optimised medical therapy has improved LV ejection fraction, NYHA class, risk for SCD, and transplant-free survival
- Primary prevention ICD:
  - Should be considered in patients with symptomatic HF (NYHA class II–III) and LVEF ≤ 35% after ≥ 3 months of OMT, particularly in younger patients (*Class IIa A*)
  - Should be considered in patients with a high SCD-risk genotype (e.g. pathogenic mutation in LMNA gene) or additional risk factors (syncope, LGE on CMR

- Secondary prevention ICD:
  - Recommended in cardiac arrest survivors or VT with haemodynamic compromise

5.2.4 Non-dilated left ventricular cardiomyopathy

- Non-dilated left ventricular cardiomyopathy (NDLVC) is defined as the presence of non-ischaemic LV scarring, fatty replacement, or isolated global LV hypokinesia without scarring (as assessed by the presence of LGE on CMR), in the absence of LV dilatation, abnormal loading conditions (hypertension or valve disease), or significant coronary artery disease.
- This is the newest sub-category of cardiomyopathy, which encompasses the previously 'unclassified cardiomyopathy', DCM (but without LV dilatation), arrhythmogenic left ventricular cardiomyopathy (ALVC), left dominant ARVC, or arrhythmogenic DCM (but often without fulfilling diagnostic criteria for ARVC)
- Findings of NDLVC should prompt a multiparametric approach to diagnosis and establishing aetiology
- No specific epidemiological data are yet available given its novel classification as a subcategory of cardiomyopathy
- There are genetic variants recognized in NDLVC, as there are in DCM and ARVC
- Inheritance is commonly autosomal dominant but recessive forms are also recognized. Rarely presents in infants
- Most commonly found variants are that of the desmosomal protein genes including; DSP, FLNC, DES, LMNA, and PLN
- Diagnosis can be more difficult as patients can be less symptomatic or show fewer signs due to normal LV size. More commonly acute presentations are that of myocarditis but decompensated heart failure symptoms are also prevalent.

Clinical course and prognosis
- Largely asymptomatic but can present in various ways including acute or recurrent myocarditis, symptoms related to arrhythmia or diastolic dysfunction
- Prevalence of AF is ~40%
- Very few data regarding clinical course and prognosis for this cohort but data can be derived from patients with ARVC and DCM.

Diagnostic testing

Electrocardiography:
- Low QRS
- AV block and ectopy

Ambulatory monitoring:
- AV block, ectopy, NSVT or sustained ventricular arrhythmias as well as AF may be found, and can help (i) determine timing of surveillance intervals and (ii) risk stratify patients

Genetic testing:
- Is recommended in all patients with NDLVC as identification of a P/LP gene variant allows better prediction of disease outcome, progression, and determining need for preventative device implantation.
- Should be considered for first-degree relatives of an individual with established NDLVC and SCD, or for first-degree relatives who have LV dysfunction or electrocardiographic abnormalities.

Echocardiography:
- Confirms chamber sizes, global and regional LV anatomy, function (including estimated ejection fraction), and haemodynamics
- Advanced echocardiography including speckle tracking and contrast can allow early detection of subclinical myocardial dysfunction in some situations

Cardiac magnetic resonance imaging:
- CMR is particularly useful for diagnosing NDLVC as often echocardiographic findings can be subtle. CMR will be able to ascertain subtle regional or global hypokinesia as well as LGE often essential for diagnosis
- Late gadolinium enhancement imaging can be helpful to identify oedema, scar, or fatty replacement

Computed tomography:
- Recommended to rule out significant coronary artery disease as an alternative diagnosis or comorbidity affecting clinical manifestation and course. *(Class IIa C)*

Endomyocardial biopsy:
- Endomyocardial biopsy can be considered where investigations show myocardial inflammation, but only in specific situations where results may affect diagnosis and treatment.

Management
- Standard ESC guideline management of heart failure (as outlined in DCM chapter) and arrhythmias.

Risk assessment, screening, and prognosis
- Specific genotypes (PLN and LMNA variants) in NDLVC patients have been found to be a major determinant of SCD risk, irrespective of LVEF
- Recommendations for both primary and secondary prevention ICD implantation in NDLVC should be the same as those for DCM (see section 5.2.3)
- Ambulatory monitoring for NDLVC patients recommended annually or when there is a change in clinical status, to aid management and risk stratification
- Screening recommended for first-degree relatives of an individual with established NDLVC and SCD, or if a first-degree relative has sudden death at < 50 years of age and autopsy findings suggestive of the NDLVC phenotype
- Screening to be considered for first-degree relatives of an individual with NDLVC who have LV dysfunction or electrocardiographic abnormalities.

5.2.5 Arrhythmogenic right ventricular cardiomyopathy

- Characterized by a progressive myocardial atrophy with fibro-fatty replacement of the RV myocardium, which can lead to functional abnormalities. Lesions can also be present or even predominant in the LV myocardium
- Areas affected are the outflow tract, apex, and subtricuspid areas of the free wall, the septum is spared
- There is replacement of myocardial tissue with fibro-fatty infiltrates (mainly diffuse) with increase wall thickness
- Saccular aneurysms are present in 50% of cases

- Genetic predisposition plays a part—familial component in 60% of cases with several genes implicated (autosomal dominant and recessive).
- Men more affected than women, and usually manifests in the second to fourth decade of life.

Clinical presentation
- Exercise-induced symptomatic VT of RV origin (LBBB pattern)
- Palpitations/syncope/pre-syncope
- Myocarditis (often in younger patients)
- Sudden cardiac death—ARVC is widely regarded as one of the most common causes of SCD around the world
- Some patients present with heart failure and ventricular arrhythmia and misdiagnosed as DCM or NDLVC
- 10–30% prevalence of AF in patients with ARVC.

Diagnostic testing

Electrocardiography:
- is abnormal in 90% of cases
- suspicious changes are TWI V1–V3, atypical RBBB, or low RV voltages
- the presence of an epsilon wave was thought of being a distinct marker of disease, however, has shown poor sensitivity and specificity so should be interpreted with caution.

Ambulatory monitoring:
- Frequent VEs or NSVT (LBBB morphology)

Echocardiography:
- RV dilatation
- RV wall structural and/or functional abnormalities, e.g. bulging

CMR:
- First line for assessing RV dilatation, segmental or regional wall motion abnormality. and the presence of saccular aneurysms due to superior sensitivity
- Contrast-enhanced CMR used to detect LV involvement (often underestimated)

Genetic testing:
- Genetic testing recommended
- Desmosomal gene variants most common
- Severity of phenotype linked to number of variants
- Patients with DSP and DSG2 variants more prone to developing heart failure
- Definite diagnosis of ARVC fulfilled by either (i) two major criteria, (ii) one major plus two minor criteria, or (iii) four minor criteria (Box 5.2.5).

Endomyocardial biopsy:
- Can be useful to differentiate ARVC from myocarditis or sarcoidosis, but not routine procedure

Differentials
- Myocarditis
- Sarcoidosis
- RV outflow tract VT
- Athletic heart

BOX 5.2.5 DIAGNOSTIC FEATURES OF ARRHYTHMOGENIC RIGHT VENTRICULAR CARDIOMYOPATHY

Major criteria

I) *Global or regional dysfunction and structural alteration (ECHO, CMR or angiography)*
   Regional RV akinesia, dyskinesia or bulging
   +
   Global RV dilation (increase of RV EDV according to the imaging test specific normograms for age and sex)
   Or
   Global RV systolic dysfunction (reduction of RV EF according to the imaging test specific normograms for age and sex)

II) *Tissue characterization*
   Transmural LGE (stria pattern) of ≥ 1 RV region(s) (inlet, outlet, and apex in 2 orthogonal views). On CE-CMR
   Fibrous replacement of the myocardium in ≥ 1 sample, with or without fatty tissue. On EMB (limited indication)

III) *Repolarization abnormalities*
   Inverted T waves in right precordial leads (V1, V2, and V3) or beyond in individuals with complete pubertal development (in the absence of complete RBBB)

IV) *Depolarization and conduction abnormalities*

See minor criteria

V) *Arrhythmias*
   Frequent ventricular extrasystoles (> 500 per 24 h), non-sustained or sustained ventricular tachycardia of LBBB morphology

VI) *Family history/genetics*
   ACM confirmed in a first-degree relative who meets diagnostic criteria
   ACM confirmed pathologically at autopsy or surgery in a first-degree relative
   Identification of a pathogenic or likely pathogenetic ACM mutation in the patient under evaluation

Minor criteria

I) *Global or regional dysfunction and structural alteration (ECHO, CMR or angiography)*
   Regional RV akinesia, dyskinesia, or aneurysm of RV free wall

II) *Tissue characterization*

See major criteria

III) *Repolarization abnormalities*
   Inverted T waves in leads V1 and V2 in individuals with completed pubertal development (in the absence of complete RBBB)
   Inverted T waves in V1, V2, V3, and V4 in individuals with completed pubertal development in the presence of complete RBBB

IV) *Depolarization and conduction abnormalities*
   Epsilon wave (reproducible low-amplitude signals between end of QRS complex to onset of the T wave) in the right precordial leads (V1 to V3)

Terminal activation duration of QRS ≥ 55 ms measured from the nadir of the S wave to the end of the QRS, including R', in V1, V2, or V3 (in the absence of complete RBBB)

V) *Arrhythmias*

Frequent ventricular extrasystoles (> 500 per 24 h), non-sustained or sustained ventricular tachycardia of LBBB morphology with inferior axis ('RVOT pattern')

VI) *Family history/genetics*

History of ACM in a first-degree relative in whom it is not possible or practical to determine whether the family member meets diagnostic criteria

Premature sudden death (< 35 y of age) due to suspected ACM in a first-degree relative

ACM confirmed pathologically or by diagnostic criteria in second-degree relative.

ACM indicates arrhythmogenic cardiomyopathy; BSA, body surface area; CMR, cardiac magnetic resonance; EDV, end diastolic volume; EF, ejection fraction; EMB, endomyocardial biopsy; ITF, International Task Force; LBBB, left bundle-branch block; LGE, late gadolinium enhancement; LV, left ventricle; MRI, magnetic resonance imaging; PLAX, parasternal long axis; PSAX, parasternal short axis; RBBB, right bundle-branch block; SAECG, signal-averaged ECG; RV, right ventricle; and RVOT, right ventricular outflow tract.

*The morphology of 'Major' ventricular arrhythmias is LBBB with a QRS axis other than inferior (i.e. intermediate or superior).

Adapted from Corrado et al. Diagnosis of arrhythmogenic cardiomyopathy: the Padua criteria. *Int J Cardiol.* 2020; 319:106–14. DOI: 10.1016/j.ijcard.2020.06.005., copyright ©2020, Elsevier.

- DCM
- Chagas
- Pulmonary hypertension with volume overload

Management

- Use standard heart failure treatment with ACE inhibitors/ARBs, BBs, aldosterone antagonists, and digoxin (see Table 5.2.1)
- Beta blockers may help in patients with ventricular arrhythmia
- Amiodarone or flecainide are alternative options if beta-blockers are not tolerated or don't control arrhythmias
- Catheter ablation can be used but new foci arise in 30–50% of patients
- ICD use may be limited due to the abnormal RV myocardium giving low endocardial signals and increased pacing thresholds
- Primary prevention ICD should be considered in patients with:
    - Arrhythmic syncope
    - Severe LV or RV dysfunction
    - Symptomatic patients with moderate LV or RV dysfunction and NSVT or inducible VT at EP study

Table 5.2.1 Arrhythmia management.

Good systolic function Non-life-threatening arrhythmias	Medical therapy with amiodarone, beta blockers, or propafenone
Reduced systolic function	Amiodarone, beta blockers, or class I agents
Syncope, cardiac arrest, documented VT/VF and a family history of sudden cardiac death	Implantable defibrillator

- Secondary prevention ICD:
    - Is recommended in patients who have survived a cardiac arrest or haemodynamically unstable VT/VF
    - Should be considered in patient with haemodynamically stable VT
- Transplantation should be considered in those patients with refractory symptoms despite full standard therapy
- Sustained VT refractory to drug treatment may require transplantation.
- Discontinuation of strenuous physical activity proven to slow progression and reduce ventricular arrythmia burden.

Prognosis and outcome

- An ARVC calculator can be utilized to help offer patients an estimated risk of SCD, and aid decisions on ICD implantation on an individual basis
- Biventricular dysplastic involvement leading to a DCM is rare
- Progressive right ventricular failure occurs in some patients
- Untreated sustained or non-sustained VT may be well tolerated but can degenerate to VF in 1–2% of cases.

5.2.6 Restrictive cardiomyopathy

- In restrictive cardiomyopathy (RCM) there is abnormal diastolic function due to rigid or thickened ventricular walls leading to elevated right- and left-sided filling pressures
- This can be cause by abnormalities in the endocardium, myocardium, or pericardium
- Normal ventricular volumes, normal wall thickness, and bi-atrial enlargement
- Unlike constrictive cardiomyopathy, there is dissociation between the right and left chambers with respiration, i.e. there is ventricular discordance.
- There is a spectrum of underlying causes (see Figure 5.2.3)
- Precision diagnosis as to aetiology of RCM is key.

Clinical presentation

- Often present with features of heart failure/decompensation but HFpEF.
- Primary causes, including genetic variants, present in children and carry poor prognosis. Often the phenotype is mixed RCM/HCM
- Syndromes
- Hepatomegaly, ascites, peripheral oedema, and raised JVP

Diagnostic testing

Electrocardiography and ambulatory monitoring:
- AV block
- 45–50% prevalence of concomitant AF

Echocardiography:
- Diastolic dysfunction—can be mild and only truly restrictive in nature as disease progresses

Cardiac magnetic resolution imaging:
- Can differentiate between fibrotic, metabolic, or inflammatory diseases
- Can distinguish restrictive cardiomyopathy from constrictive pericarditis
- May show LGE at endocardial level

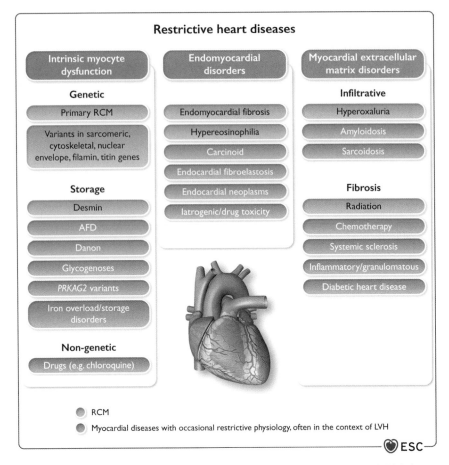

Figure 5.2.3 Spectrum of restrictive heart diseases. AFD, Anderson–Fabry disease; LVH, left ventricular hypertrophy; PRKAG2, Protein kinase AMP-activated non-catalytic subunit gamma 2; RCM, restrictive cardiomyopathy.

Arbelo E, Protonotarios A, Gimeno JR, et al; ESC Scientific Document Group. 2023 ESC Guidelines for the management of cardiomyopathies. *Eur Heart J.* 2023 Oct 1;44(37):3503–3626. doi: 10.1093/eurheartj/ehad194. © European Society of Cardiology. With permission from Oxford University Press

Genetic testing:
- Most commonly presents as an autosomal dominant disorder
- *TNNI3* gene implicated often (encodes thin filament troponin I)
- Associated with certain syndromes and metabolic disorders; such as Noonan's and RAS-opathies

Cardiac catheterization:
- Recommended in all children with RCM to measure pulmonary artery pressures and PVR at diagnosis and every 6–12 months to assess change in PVR
- Can be required to distinguish RCM from constrictive pericarditis

Endomyocardial biopsy:
- Syndromic and metabolic disease can be further subcategorized via EMB in certain cases
- Utilised for RCM phenotypes if aetiology in doubt, as can help guide urgency of management

Management
- RCM phenotype is associated with high risk of stroke therefore low threshold to anticoagulate patients
- Heart failure management as per guidelines
- ICD implantation decision made on an individual basis but follow basic criteria as discussed in earlier chapters.

Prognosis and outcome
- Carries the worst prognosis of all the cardiomyopathy phenotypes.
- > 50% children with RCM are at risk of death or early transplantation at diagnosis
- 75% of surviving patients either die or require heart transplant a few years after diagnosis
- Prognostic indicators include; heart failure symptoms, reduced LVSF, increased LA size, syncope, ischaemia, and impaired LV diastolic function

Primary RCM
1. Loffler's endocarditis (acute)
2. Endomyocardial fibrosis (chronic)
3. Idiopathic.
   - Pathophysiology is associated with inflammation (hypereosinophilia)
   - This is secondary to a chronic inflammatory process, e.g. parasitic infection, autoimmune disease, eosinophilic leukaemia
   - It is rare in the Western world but endemic in the tropics and is a frequent cause of death in Africa, India, South and Central America, and Asia.

Secondary RCM
This is due to specific material deposition within the myocardium by infiltrative disease, e.g. amyloid, storage disorders, diabetic cardiomyopathy, scleroderma, or replacement by other molecules.

Specific restrictive cardiomyopathy diseases
Amyloid heart disease
- Amyloid is deposition of a soluble extracellular protein as an insoluble fibril causing loss of tissue architecture and function:
   - **Acquired amyloid (AL or 1°)** is deposition of fibril proteins from immunoglobulin light chains produced by plasma cells. It is associated with myeloma or monoclonal gammopathies
   - **Secondary amyloid (AA)** is associated with chronic inflammatory conditions such as rheumatoid arthritis, ankylosing spondylitis, and familial Mediterranean fever. The amyloid fibrils consist of protein A. Nephrotic syndrome and renal failure are common at presentation
   - **Senile systemic amyloidosis (ATTRwt)** involves the deposition of a fibril precursor of the protein transthyretin. Heart failure, heart block, and atrial fibrillation are recognized manifestations. It is slowly progressive and has a better prognosis than acquired forms
   - **Hereditary amyloid (ATTRv)** is typically autosomal dominant. It is a mutation in any of the fibril precursor proteins for transthyretin, apolipoprotein AI or AII, lysozyme, fibrinogen Aa chain, gelsolin, and cystatin C

- Cardiac amyloid is mainly seen in primary, senile systemic (ATTRwt), and certain hereditary forms
- Cardiovascular involvement is seen in AA forms of the disease but is an unfavourable marker if present
- Amyloid fibrils deposit within the myocardium, papillary muscles, valves, conduction tissue, and in the vessels
- Suspicion of amyloid should be raised if there is
    - Cardiac disease in the presence of established AL amyloid ± plasma cell dyscrasia
    - Ventricular dysfunction/arrhythmia in patients with long-standing connective tissue disease or chronic inflammatory disorder
    - Any restrictive cardiomyopathy without explanation
    - Thickened ventricle on echocardiography but low-voltage ECG
    - Heart failure of unknown cause or refractory to treatment.

Investigations

See Table 5.2.2

Table 5.2.2 Investigations for cardiac amyloid.

12-lead ECG	Low voltage (though this is not always seen)
	Varying degrees of atrioventricular block Interventricular conduction delay/bundle branch block Left-axis deviation Poor R-wave progression*
Holter	Atrial fibrillation Other tachyarrhythmia or bradyarrhythmia
Two-dimensional echocardiography	Concentric or asymmetric thickening of the left ventricular wall Occasional thickening of the right ventricle Thickened interatrial septum* Sparkling/granular appearance of myocardium* Thickened valves and/or papillary muscles Left atrial or bi-atrial dilation Diastolic dysfunction in early disease (E/A reversal) Restrictive physiology (E >> A) Pericardial effusion Systolic impairment with normal end-diastolic volume
Histology	Apple-green birefringence under polarised light microscope after staining with Congo red* Immunoperoxidase stains to differentiate light chains/transthyretin/protein A, etc.
Cardiac catheterization	Raised filling pressures
Protein electrophoresis	Serum and urine electrophoresis for presence of monoclonal protein in patients with suspected AL amyloidosis
Genetic testing	Commercially available to detect common mutations

* Features considered relatively more specific for amyloidosis.
Reproduced from the *ESC Textbook of Cardiovascular Medicine*, 2nd edn, ed. John Camm, Thomas Lüscher, and Patrick Serruys, copyright 2009 with permission of Oxford University Press.

Diagnosis
- Invasive and non-invasive criteria, the former applies to all amyloid whereas non-invasive criteria only applies to ATTR.
- Invasive criteria involves demonstrating amyloid fibrils in cardiac tissue or amyloid deposits in extracardiac biopsy alongside classic features on echocardiogram/cMR
- Non-invasive criteria is based on typical echocardiogram/cMR findings accompanied by uptake on SPECT or DPD scan, and exclusion of clonal dyscrasia (using free light chain assay, urine and plasma electrophoresis and immunofixation)
- DPD and SPECT uptake cannot distinguish between ATTRv and ATTRwt and hence TTR genetic testing is recommended in patients of all ages.

Management
- Management aims at treatment of the underlying condition—hence identification of subtype is crucial
- Treatment of heart failure is mainly with diuretics
- ACE inhibitors/ARBs should be used with caution due to the frequency of hypotension
- Digoxin is relatively contraindicated as it binds to amyloid fibrils and increases susceptibility to digoxin toxicity.
- Conduction disease including high-grade AV blocks are common and there should be low threshold for PPM given progressive nature of the disease
- If AF occurs, consider cautious low-dose BB and careful digoxin
- BBs can promote AV blockade so should be used with caution
- Ventricular arrhythmias can predict SCD
- Cardiac transplantation is relatively contraindicated in AL amyloid.
- Amyloid cardiomyopathy is associated with a high risk of intracardiac thrombus. Anticoagulate if in AF. Uncertain benefit in SR
- In patients with transthyretin amyloid cardiomyopathy, tafamidis has been shown to reduce all-cause mortality, cardiovascular related hospitalizations and the decline in functional capacity and quality of life. Not available for routine use (NICE, UK recommendation July 2020)
- An ICD should be considered in patients with light-chain or transthyretin-associated cardiac amyloidosis and haemodynamically not-tolerated VT (*class IIa C*)

Prognosis
- AL amyloid is rapidly progressive with a very poor prognosis (median survival 4–6 months with heart failure), but improvements have been seen since introduction of newer effective therapies to reduce the production of cardiotoxic light chains
- Systemic senile amyloid is slowly progressive and requires no specific treatment
- Reactive AA amyloid may improve with anti-inflammatory treatments.

Sarcoid heart disease
- Sarcoid is a multisystem disorder characterized by deposition of non-caseating granuloma
- It most commonly affects the lungs and lymphatics
- Cardiac involvement is seen in around a quarter of cases, affecting mainly the LV free wall and septum but up to 70% of autopsy studies.
- Right-sided and atrial involvement is recognized

- Sarcoid should be considered in
    - Young people presenting with conduction disease
    - Patients with unexplained DCM and AV block and features of abnormal wall thickness, regional wall motion abnormality, or apical/septal perfusion defects that improve with stress nuclear imaging
    - Patients with sustained VT with no obvious cause
    - Patients with RCM of unknown cause
    - Presumed ARVC or AV block in patients with chronic respiratory disease.

Clinical presentation
- Arrhythmia/conduction abnormality
- Heart failure
- Pericardial effusions, constriction, and valvular disease recognized
- SCD can be first presentation
- Isolated cardiac involvement is rare—presentation usually follows systemic manifestation of the disease.

Diagnosis
- Investigations can include:
    - Serum ACE
    - 12-lead ECG
    - Holter monitoring
    - Chest X-ray
    - Echocardiography
    - Myocardial perfusion imaging
    - Cardiac MR
    - Cardiac catheterization
    - Endomyocardial biopsy
- See Table 5.2.3 for guidelines on diagnosis.

Management
- Early treatment with corticosteroids is first-line treatment
- Other treatments include chloroquine, hydroxychloroquine, cyclosporine, and methotrexate

Table 5.2.3 Guidelines for diagnosis based on study report on diffuse pulmonary disease for Japanese Ministry of Health and Welfare, 1993.

Histology	Endomyocardial biopsy demonstrating epitheloid granulomata without caseating granulomata
Clinical	Exclusion of other aetiologies and the presence of complete RBBB, LAD, AV block, VT, ventricular ectopy on ambulatory ECG plus one of the following: • Abnormal wall motion, regional wall thinning or dilatation of the left ventricle • Perfusion abnormality on perfusion imaging • Abnormal intracardiac pressure, low cardiac output, abnormal wall motion, or reduced left ventricular ejection fraction • Evidence of interstitial fibrosis or cellular inflammation

Adapted from Hiraga H, Yuwai K, Hiroe M. et al., 'Guideline for diagnosis of cardiac sarcoidosis', published in 'Cardiac sarcoidosis', Abdul R. Doughan, Byron R. Williams, *Heart* 92, 282–8, copyright 2006 with permission of BMJ Publishing.

- Resolution of arrhythmia and conduction disease can be seen, as well as some resolution in LV function
- Treatment should be started prior to standard heart failure treatment if possible
- In patients with high-grade AV block and a pacing indication, ICD implantation should be considered regardless of LVEF
- Primary prevention ICD:
    - Is recommended for patients with LVEF ≤ 35%
    - Should be considered in patients with LVEF > 35% but significant LGE at CMR after resolution of acute inflammation
    - An EP study may be considered in those with LVEF 35–50% and minor LGE at CMR, with ICD considered in patients with inducible VT
- Secondary prevention ICD is recommended in patients with documented sustained VT or aborted cardiac arrest
- Pacemaker/ICD implantation and steroid treatment improve prognosis
- Anti-arrhythmic drugs and catheter ablation can be used to treat recurrent VT
- Transplantation is rare.

5.2.7 Storage diseases

- Storage diseases are inborn errors of metabolism resulting in the abnormal accumulation of the substrate or byproduct in tissues (see Table 5.2.4)
- Intracellular deposition distinguishes them from infiltrative disease, where deposition is within the interstitium
- Within the myocytes, the presence of these metabolites is toxic, causing either concentric (HCM-like phenotype) or eccentric (DCM-like phenotype) changes

Anderson–Fabry's disease
- Fabry's disease is an X-linked genetic disorder causing a deficiency in α-galactosidase
- It leads to a deposition of glycosphingolipids (particularly globotriaosylceramide) in the skin, endothelium, kidneys, liver, pancreas, and central nervous system
- Patients may present with multi-system disease—obstructive airways disease, proteinuria, end-stage renal disease, or stroke
- Cardiovascular deposition is within the myocardium, conduction tissue, valves, and vascular endothelium.
- Although it mostly affects men, most heterogenous females are affected, albeit at an older age.
- 'Classical' Anderson–Fabry is a severe clinical phenotype that presents in childhood/adolescence and leads to progressive multiorgan failure
- 'Non-classical' is a later onset, incomplete systemic involvement phenotype.

Cardiovascular presentations
- Patients can present with heart failure, conduction disease, arrhythmia, and angina
- It is an incidental finding on echocardiography with unexplained LVH.
- Mitral and aortic regurgitation are often seen although mild.
- Endothelial involvement is associated with subendocardial ischaemia
- LVH and reduced coronary flow reserve may also be the cause of angina
- Renal involvement increases the incidence of hypertension and hypercholesterolaemia and leads to premature coronary artery disease
- Aortic root dilation is observed in 33%.

Table 5.2.4 Summary of cardiovascular manifestations of some inborn errors of metabolism.

	Mechanism	Genetics	Presentation	Diagnosis	Management
Haemachromatosis	Iron overload and deposition	Mutation on HFE gene encoding for transferrin receptor. AR inheritance with variable penetrance.	Liver, pancreas, joints and heart affected. Heart failure, SVTs, AV blockade, raised atrial pressures (restrictive filling)	Echo: normal LV thickness CMR Histology: stainable iron within the sarcoplasm	Regular phlebotomy Serial EMB ± CMR, FBC and iron studies to assess treatment. Standard heart failure and arrhythmia management Screening of first-degree relatives
GSD Type II (Pompe's Disease)	Acid α galactosidase (acid maltase) deficiency	AR inheritance	Within first few months—failure to thrive, hypotonia, macroglossia, hepatomegaly	CXR: cardiomegaly Raised cardiac enzymes ECG: short PR, LAD, high voltage QRS Enzyme assay of muscle or skin fibroblasts shows no acid maltase activity Echo: bilateral ventricular hypertrophy; HCM phenotype ± SAM	Previously poor prognosis with death. New treatment with recombinant acid maltase (acid α galactosidase) enzyme replacement now promising.
GSD Type III (Corbi or Farbe's disease)	Amylo-1,6,-glucosidase deficiency causing phosphorylase limit dextran accumulation	AR inheritance with variable phenotype	Fasting hypoglycaemia and hepatomegaly. Many patients asymptomatic but recurrent sustained VT and SCD seen	Echo: HCM-type phenotype ± SAM. CMR: late gadolinium suggestive of late fibrosis	
GSD Type IV	Amylo 1,4–1,6 transglucosidase deficiency with accumulation of polyglucosan bodies in the liver		Liver dysfunction, skeletal myopathy and heart failure		

GSD = glycogen storage disorders.

- Increased prevalence of smoking in this population also contributes to this higher risk of premature coronary artery disease
- Stroke is seen as a consequence of deposition within the cerebral endothelium.

Extra-cardiac features
- Cutaneous:
  - Angiokeratomas
  - Lymphoedema
- Neurological:
  - Tinnitus
  - Vertigo
  - Headache
  - TIA/stroke
  - Chronic arm and leg pain
  - Fabry crisis (severe acute pain precipitated by emotional or physical stress)
- Gastrointestinal:
  - Diarrhoea
  - Abdominal discomfort or vomiting
- Renal:
  - Proteinuria
  - Renal failure

Investigations
- Echocardiography reveals increased wall thickness (concentric and septal patterns)
- Systolic function is preserved whilst mild–moderate diastolic dysfunction is seen
- Restriction is rare
- Thickened papillary muscles and mitral valve leaflets occur in over 50% of patients
- ECG often shows LVH pattern
- Late enhancement with gadolinium is seen on MRI identifying fibrosis (more often in men)
- The diagnosis is made by demonstration of reduced α-galactosidase activity in the plasma or peripheral leukocytes
- 6% of patients with 'late-onset HCM' have Fabry's disease
- Women have relatively high levels of α-galactosidase which can limit the assay in its use (women express varying phenotypes due to random inactivation of an X-chromosome)
- Genetic testing can be helpful (and recommended in suspected female carriers)

Management
- Treatment is with enzyme replacement therapy, which can reduce the overall tissue and serum load of glycosphingolipids leading to a reduction in pain symptoms, renal complications, and improved quality of life. Early initiation is recommended
- There is currently limited evidence in the regression of cardiac disease
- Anginal symptoms should be treated with antiplatelet agents and calcium antagonists
- BBs are used with caution due to the incidence of conduction disease and bradycardia
- Heart failure is treated with standard treatments; transplant can be considered in severe cases.

Post-radiation disease
- Radiation damage can affect any part of the heart (see Table 5.2.5) and is seen after treatment for lymphoma as well as breast, lung, and testicular malignancy

Table 5.2.5 Summary of cardiac complications from radiation.

Structure	Mechanism	Clinical features
Myocardial	Damage occurs due to microcirculatory damage and free radical toxicity. Acute inflammation of small/medium sized arteries is followed by latent phase of thrombosis and ischaemia. Myocyte death and fibrosis follows.	Clinically overt cardiomyopathy (restrictive CM) is uncommon. Anthrocycline-induced DCM-like phenotype does occur with more frequency when associated with radiation exposure.
Pericardial	Early complications are associated with radiation-induced necrosis of tumour masses adjacent to the heart. Treatment is usually continued with no long-term sequelae. Late presentation is due to a chronic constrictive pericarditis and presence of a chronic pleural effusion	Acute symptoms of pericarditis—fever, chest pain. Chronic constriction leads to right-sided heart failure. Pericardectomy is treatment of choice in intractable cases.
Conduction disease		Sick sinus syndrome and AV block have been reported
Valve disease		Around a third of patients have demonstrable valve disease (mainly aortic) post radiation therapy
Coronary artery disease		Ostial left main stem and left anterior descending disease can be seen in patients who have had mediastinal radiotherapy. Often, other risk factors for CAD are present

Reproduced from the *ESC Textbook of Cardiovascular Medicine*, 2nd edn, ed. John Camm, Thomas Lüscher, and Patrick Serruys, copyright 2009 with permission of Oxford University Press.

- Symptoms are associated with the area affected
- Regular assessment with 12-lead ECG, echocardiography, exercise testing, Holter monitoring, and cardiac MR is useful for occult disease
- Newer radiotherapy techniques involve smaller doses as well as shielding
- Cardiovascular risk assessment and aggressive treatment can reduce the risk of coronary disease
- The use of cardiotoxic chemotherapy with radiotherapy should be avoided.

5.2.8 Inflammatory myocardial disease

- Inflammatory cardiomyopathy is characterized by myocarditis in association with cardiac dysfunction
- The underlying cause may be idiopathic, autoimmune, or infectious (Box 5.2.6).

Pathophysiology

- There are various hypotheses regarding the mechanism of myocarditis
- It may be secondary to a virus triggered inflammation in those patients with a genetic predisposition to myocardial inflammation

> **BOX 5.2.6 CARDIOTROPIC VIRUSES INVOLVED IN MYOCARDITIS AND INFLAMMATORY CARDIOMYOPATHY**
>
> | Coxsackie virus | Adenovirus | Parvovirus B19 |
> |---|---|---|
> | Human herpesvirus type 6 | Epstein–Barr virus | Cytomegalovirus |
> | Echovirus | Mumps virus | Influenza A and B viruses |
> | Flavovirus | Human immunodeficiency virus | Measles virus |
> | Polio virus | Hepatitis C virus | Rabies virus |
> | Rubella virus | Variola virus | Varicella-zoster virus |
> | *Borrelia burgdorferi* | Parasitic infection | |
>
> Reproduced from the *ESC Textbook of Cardiovascular Medicine*, 2nd edn, ed. John Camm, Thomas Lüscher, and Patrick Serruys, copyright 2009 with permission of Oxford University Press.

- The virus can cause a direct toxic effect or cause a secondary immune response, which can persist despite elimination of the virus
- Alternatively, there may also be persistent chronic infection driving a continued inflammatory response. This could be in the form of antibodies cross-reacting with myocardial antibodies or the release of cardiodepressive cytokines causing myocardial dysfunction.

Clinical presentation

- Patients present with heart failure, chest discomfort, palpitations, syncope, or SCD
- There can be a temporal relationship with a viral infection, although this is quite often subclinical
- Acute fulminant myocarditis: acute and rapid onset with severe LV dysfunction which may need inotropic or mechanical support
- Acute non-fulminant myocarditis: usually presents with chest pain, non-specific ECG changes, and a rise in serum troponin and C reactive protein
- The coronary arteries are normal
- Echo shows preserved systolic function but may demonstrate regional wall motion abnormality
- Pericardial effusion and wall oedema is seen on echo and cardiac MR
- In both clinical scenarios, arrhythmias can be seen. Patients can present with SCD.

Management

- Secondary causes of heart failure should be excluded
- Standard heart failure treatment including ICD and LVAD, either as bridge to recovery or transplantation
- If patients improve they should be closely monitored with serial echo, ECG, and Holter monitoring
- If there is progressive LV dysfunction, immunomodulatory treatment and transplantation should be considered
- Endomyocardial biopsy and immunohistology may be necessary to help with aetiology (Figure 5.2.4)
- Immunomodulatory treatment strategies are dependent on the absence of viral persistence by immunohistology
- Persistent inflammation due to an autoimmune response in the absence of any virus may respond to immunosuppression

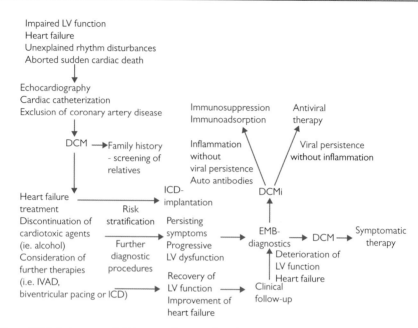

Figure 5.2.4 Endomyocardial biopsy and immunohistology may help with aetiology.
Reproduced from Camm, A. John, Thomas F. Lüscher, and Patrick W. Serruys (eds), The ESC Textbook of Cardiovascular Medicine, 2 edn, The European Society of Cardiology (Oxford, 2009), https://doi.org/10.1093/med/9780199566990.001.0001.

- ICD implantation is recommended for patients with haemodynamically not tolerated VT in the chronic phase of myocarditis, and should be considered before discharged if this occurs in the acute phase
- Amiodarone or beta-blockers are the preferred antiarrhythmic drugs for patients with symptomatic ventricular arrhythmias in the acute phase, whilst ablation may be considered in the chronic phase

Prognosis and outcome

- No clinical parameter predicts outcome
- The presence of viral persistence and chronic inflammation is associated with an adverse prognosis
- 5-year survival is estimated at around 35%; initial presentation of fulminant myocarditis and heart failure is associated with a better outcome.

HIV cardiomyopathy

- Cardiac involvement can be seen in 50% of HIV positive patients (usually sub-clinical)
- The pathogenesis is felt to be a result of either continued infection by HIV-1 of the myocardial cells, further opportunistic infection of the myocardium by other organisms, or as a result of nucleoside analogue treatment
- Management is with standard heart failure treatment, but caution should be used given the interactions with protease inhibitors.

Chagas disease

- Chagas disease is a protozoal myocarditis after infection with *Trypanosoma cruzi*
- It is endemic in south and central America and is transmitted by realuvid bug, but can be from animal reservoirs, blood transfusion, and vertical transmission

- Patients present with fatigue, fluid retention, conduction disease, progressive left ventricular dysfunction, ventricular arrhythmia, sudden cardiac death, and thrombo-embolic disease
- Investigations include the Machado–Guerreiro complement fixation test, indirect immunofluorescence or ELISA, 12-lead ECG, and echocardiography
- Echo can demonstrate global LV systolic dysfunction but can show septal sparing, posterior wall hypokinesia, and apical aneurysm formation.

Treatment

1. Antiparasitics, e.g. benznidazole, which reduces but does not eradicate the organism
2. Heart failure treatment
3. Antiarrhythmics, e.g. amiodarone
4. Anticoagulation.
5. Ablation and/or ICD implantation in patients with recurrent VT where antiarrhythmic drugs (amiodarone and beta blockers) have been ineffective or not tolerated

Lyme disease

- Lyme disease is an infection with a tick borne spirochete, *Borrelia burgdorferi*
- Patients present with erythema migrans and general malaise
- Cardiac and neurological features occur after weeks and months
- It is more common in females, but men tend to suffer more complications
- Cardiac sequelae include conduction disease, myo-pericarditis, and a self-limiting cardiomyopathy
- Other complications include cranial nerve palsies and a migratory polyarthritis
- Diagnosis is made on the basis of the history of tick bite, clinical findings, and serological studies
- Treatment should be in an expert centre
- The antibiotic of choice is doxycycline
- Intravenous ceftriaxone is used for 2–4 weeks if there are cardiac or neurological signs.

5.2.9 Secondary myocardial diseases

These specific diseases can slot into the 5 cardiomyopathy phenotypes as outlined above, but this chapter goes into some more detail about important aetiologies.

Alcoholic cardiomyopathy

- Ethanol at a level of > 90 g daily for > 5 years is felt to unmask a genetic predisposition to dilated cardiomyopathy via a direct toxic effect on myocytes and function
- Two phases of the disease are recognized:
  i. Initial asymptomatic phase with isolated LV cavity enlargement and diastolic dysfunction
  ii. Clinically overt phase with signs and symptoms of heart failure and LV systolic dysfunction
- Incidence of arrhythmia such as AF and non-sustained VT are similar to those patients with DCM
- SCD rates are also comparable but this figure can be attenuated by abstinence
- Standard heart failure treatment improves ventricular function
- Therapy is more effective when the patient abstains from alcohol.

Metabolic cardiomyopathy

- Metabolic cardiomyopathy is myocardial dysfunction secondary to a derangement in metabolism

- It includes nutritional disorders such as thiamine deficiency, which is a cause of cardiomyopathy worldwide
- The most common metabolic disorder is diabetes.

Tachycardia-related cardiomyopathy

- Incessant arrhythmia, such as SVT or AF (heart rates 180–200 bpm), can lead to LV dysfunction
- The restoration of sinus rhythm improves left ventricular function
- Heart rate reduction: BBs and ivabradine have demonstrated prognostic benefit in patients with heart failure
- Catheter ablation to restore sinus rhythm has been beneficial in restoring LV function in patients with incessant tachycardia.

Muscular dystrophy cardiomyopathy

- Primary disorders of skeletal muscle may affect cardiomyocytes
- There are many disorders associated with myocardial disease (Table 5.2.6)
- Skeletal deformity of the chest also leads to raised pulmonary pressures, leading to secondary cardiomyopathy
- Patients with muscular dystrophy should be periodically monitored with ECG, Holter monitoring, and echocardiography
- See Chapter 9.2 for further discussion.

Peripartum cardiomyopathy

- Peripartum cardiomyopathy occurs in around 1/3000–1/10,000 pregnancies
- It is defined as left ventricular systolic impairment with the following:
    1. Development of heart failure towards the end of pregnancy or in the months following delivery
    2. Absence of pre-existing cardiac disease
    3. No other cause for cardiac dysfunction
- Aetiology is unclear, with hypotheses including an inflammatory component, malnutrition, or a familial DCM that is unmasked by the cardiovascular burden of pregnancy
- There are some features that predispose patients to developing the disease (Box 5.2.7)
- Physical examination can be difficult as third heart sound and systolic murmurs can be heard as part of normal pregnancy
- ECG: sinus tachycardia and left axis deviation are normal for pregnancy
- Echocardiography is the investigation of choice. The definition of LV systolic dysfunction is LVEF < 45% or fractional shortening of < 30% with an end-diastolic diameter of 2.7 cm/m^2 body surface area.

Management

- Standard heart failure therapy is used, e.g. diuretics and supportive measures including intra-aortic balloon pumps for cardiogenic shock
- ACE inhibitors/ARBs/mineralo-corticoid receptor antagonists are contraindicated in the first trimester—they cause oligohydramnios
- Thrombo-prophylaxis: increased risk from prolonged bed rest, diuretic use, and impaired left ventricular function.
- Mechanical circulatory support and transplantation may be required
- Limited evidence for bromocriptine in small studies.

Table 5.2.6 Cardiac manifestations in muscular dystrophies.

Type	Inheritance	Mechanism of disease expression	Extracardiac manifestations	Cardiac manifestations
Duchenne	X-linked	Absence of dystrophin leads to disruption of the mechanical link between the sarcolemma and the extracellular matrix	Childhood onset Progressive proximal myopathy	Dilated cardiomyopathy
Becker	X-linked	Dystrophin present but at reduced levels	Onset age > 12 years with slowly progressive proximal myopathy	Dilated cardiomyopathy
Emery-Dreifuss	X-linked AD, rarely AR	Loss of emerin (inner nuclear protein) Lamins A and C (nuclear envelope proteins)	Ankle, elbow, and neck contractures Slowly progressive myopathy	Absent/reduced p waves refractory to atrial pacing; require V pacing AF/A flutter Massive atrial dilatation requiring anticoagulation Dilated cardiomyopathy SCD
Myotonic (Type A)	AD	Abnormal expansion of trinucleotide repeat sequence on myotonin protein kinase gene (DMPK) which modifies actin cytoskeleton. Demonstrates genetic anticipation	Myotinia Facial, pharyngeal and distal limb muscles Diabetes and thyroid dysfunction Cataracts	Conduction disease—may require pacing AF/flutter Ventricular arrhythmia SCD LV dilatation ± systolic impairment Mitral valve prolapse Left ventricular hypertrophy

Adapted from the *ESC Textbook of Cardiovascular Medicine*, 2nd edn, ed. John Camm, Thomas Lüscher, and Patrick Serruys, copyright 2009 with permission of Oxford University Press.

BOX 5.2.7 RISK FACTORS FOR DEVELOPING PERI-PARTUM CARDIOMYOPATHY

Increasing maternal age
Multiple pregnancy
Gestational hypertension
Familial occurrence
Cocaine use by mother
Selenium deficiency
Enterovirus infection

Multiparity
Pre-eclampsia
Afro-Caribbean
Malnutrition
Long-term tocolytic therapy
Chlamydia infection

Data from 'Peripartum cardiomyopathy: a condition intensivists should be aware of', E. de Beus, W. N. van Mook, G. Ramsay et al., *Intensive Care Med.*, 29, 167–74, copyright 2003 with kind permission from Springer Science and Business Media; and 'A review of peripartum cardiomyopathy', P. R. James, *Int. J. Clin. Pract.* 58, 363–5, copyright 2004 with permission from John Wiley and Sons.

Prognosis and outcome
- Mortality and transplant rates are around 7%.
- Death is usually from pump failure
- Counselling is important after the event:
    - Subclinical LV systolic dysfunction exists, and another pregnancy is likely to cause decompensation thus risk of recurrence must be emphasized
    - Incidence of complication is higher, e.g. maternal death, foetal prematurity, and loss
    - Women with completely normalized LV function are at low risk but heart failure will occur in 20% of those patients with residual LV impairment
- All patients with previous peripartum cardiomyopathy need close monitoring in the event of subsequent pregnancies.

Left ventricular hypertrabeculation/non-compaction
- Is characterized by is a 2-layer myocardium: a thin compacted layer adjacent to the epicardium and a thicker non-compacted layer adjacent to the endocardium. This results in the presence of deep recesses which are in continuity with the left ventricular cavity
- It may be sporadic or familial and there is an overlap with other types of cardiomyopathy
- Diagnosis can be difficult in athletes, especially black individuals
- Not considered a cardiomyopathy, but seen as a phenotypic trait.

Aetiology on LV non-compaction cardiomyopathy
- The myocardium is a loose network of fibres separated by deep recesses during embryogenesis
- At weeks 5–8, these fibres compact down, with the intratrabecular recesses becoming capillary networks
- LVNC is the arrest of normal myocardial maturation by unknown mechanisms
- Isolated LVNC usually shows autosomal dominant inheritance although X-linked and autosomal recessive inheritance are seen
- Over 10 genes have been linked to LVNC. These include mutations in the Tafazzin gene, alpha-dystrobrevin and several sarcomeric proteins.

Pathophysiology
- Subendocardial ischaemia due to compression of intramural coronary vessels may cause areas of ischaemia and fibrosis
- It can lead to remodelling and dilatation causing systolic impairment and heart failure, as well as acting as a substrate for arrhythmia
- Excess trabeculation limits myocardial compliance and causes diastolic dysfunction
- Thromboembolism (cerebral, mesenteric, or pulmonary) is seen due to stagnation of blood within the trabeculae.

Clinical presentation
- Patients present at any age with heart failure, arrhythmia, or thromboembolic complications
- Can be transiently seen in athletes, pregnancy, or vigorous exercise
- It can also be an incidental finding or be observed as part of family screening for SCD
- ECG can show high-voltage QRS and repolarization abnormality and shifts in QRS axis
- High-quality transthoracic echo, with or without the use of contrast, or cardiac MR is used to confirm the diagnosis.

Diagnostic criteria
- There is no single agreed criteria for diagnosis.
- The ratio of N/C ≥ 2 in adults (N/C ≥ 1.4 in children) where N and C are the maximal end-systolic thickness of the non-compacted and compacted layer respectively
- Colour doppler shows evidence of flow deep within the recesses.
- The ratio of the depth of the intratrabecular recesses and overall wall thickness is also significantly high
- Other features include:
  1. Prominent and excessive trabeculation in the non-compacted layer
  2. Deep intratrabecular recesses that fill completely with blood
  3. Localization of the non-compacted regions at the apex, lateral, and inferior walls
- Although left ventricular dilatation and systolic impairment is seen, it is not essential for diagnosis
- Can be misdiagnosed as apical HCM, DCM, apical thrombus, or apical infarction.

Management
1. Standard heart failure treatment is used for LV dysfunction
2. Arrythmia management: ICD implantation should follow DCM recommendations
3. Thromboprophylaxis: formal anticoagulation in patients with ventricular dilatation and systolic impairment, or previous embolic event
4. Cardiac transplantation in patients refractory to treatment.
5. Screening and counselling of family members

Prognosis and outcome
- Initially felt to have high mortality but increase in diagnosis rates has demonstrated patients at lower risk
- Timely detection, appropriate treatment, and ICD implantation may also improve prognosis.

Takotsubo syndrome (stress-induced 'cardiomyopathy')
- Initially described in Japan as the LV cavity resembles a Japanese octopus pot.
- Stress-induced phenomenon, also known as apical ballooning syndrome, Takotsubo cardiomyopathy and broken heart syndrome.
- Characterised by transient regional wall motion abnormalities, typically at the apex, unexplained by a coronary artery distribution
- Given its transient nature it is no longer regarded as a 'cardiomyopathy' as such
- The 3 most common patterns of LV dysfunction are:
  - Apical (with or without mid LV involvement) 75–80%
  - Mid LV 10–15%
  - Inverted or basal 5%
- Prevalence of 1–2% in patients presenting with troponin-positive ACS
- More common in post-menopausal women
- Often there is a history of extreme emotional or physical stress prior to presentation
- Possible pathophysiological explanations are coronary artery spasm, catecholamine excess, and microvascular dysfunction.
- Diagnosis is made by combination of:
  - typical pattern of transient LV dysfunction on cardiac imaging (echo or MRI),
  - coronary angiography showing no significant coronary artery disease (or plaque event),

- new ECG changes and
  - absence of other identified cause (especially myocarditis and phaeochromocytoma).
- In-hospital mortality is around 2–5% mainly due to refractory cardiogenic shock or ventricular fibrillation.
- Recurrence rates up to 22% have been reported over 5-year follow-up
- Most patients recover fully with no long-term symptoms.
- Patients should be risk stratified into high- or low-risk categories using the Heart Failure Association of the ESC recommendations.
- Supportive treatment and observation in a coronary care unit are recommended.
- Beta blocker may be used if EF < 40%
- In high-risk cases, avoid inotropes and use mechanical support if required. If not available, levosimendan may be considered as a catecholamine-sparing inotrope.
- Thromboembolism occurs in around 4%. If LV thrombus is detected, anticoagulation is recommended (in absence of high bleeding risk).
- P2Y12 antiplatelet agents can be stopped when MI has been excluded.
- Repeat cardiac imaging should be performed at between 3 and 6 months after discharge.

5.2.10 Cardiac transplantation

- Cardiac transplantation is the final option for those patients with progressive heart failure despite optimal medical and device therapy
- Patients considered for transplantation should not only have severe disease, but should have no significant co-morbidity
- As well as major surgery, physical and psychological suitability for long-term immunosuppression should be considered
- Primary indication worldwide is split equally between cardiomyopathy of ischemic and non-ischaemic origin
- The most commonly performed procedure is orthotopic transplant where the heart is replaced by the donors.

Indications for cardiac transplantation

- Advanced heart failure refractory to maximum tolerated medical/device or surgical treatment with
- Expected mortality of > 25%
- Limiting symptoms attributable to heart failure
- Life-threatening acute heart failure unresponsive to treatment
- Refractory life-threatening arrhythmia
- Intractable angina not amenable to revascularization.

Contraindications to transplantation

- Irreversible pulmonary hypertension (raised pulmonary pressures, raised transpulmonary gradient)
- Irreversible hepatic or lung dysfunction (FEV1 < 50% predicted)
- Cerebrovascular disease
- Active infection
- Systemic disease, e.g. amyloid, vasculitis, sarcoid
- Inability to comply with drug therapy
- Continued alcohol/substance misuse.

Relative contraindications

- Age > 70 years
- Irreversible renal dysfunction with eGFR < 30 ml/min
- Diabetes with end-organ damage
- Peripheral vascular disease not amenable to revascularization
- Malignancy
- Learning difficulties/dementia
- Hep B/C or HIV
- BMI > 30
- Recent pulmonary embolism (within three months)
- Active peptic ulcer disease
- Osteoporosis
- Current smoker
- Inadequate social support likely to prevent compliance with care

Further reading

Arbelo E, Protonotarios A, Gimeno JR, Arbustini E, Barriales-Villa R, Basso C, Bezzina CR, Biagini E, Blom NA, de Boer RA, De Winter T, Elliott PM, Flather M, Garcia-Pavia P, Haugaa KH, Ingles J, Jurcut RO, Klaassen S, Limongelli G, Loeys B, Mogensen J, Olivotto I, Pantazis A, Sharma S, Van Tintelen JP, Ware JS, Kaski JP; ESC Scientific Document Group. 2023 ESC Guidelines for the management of cardiomyopathies. *Eur Heart J*. 2023 Oct 1;44(37):3503–626. doi: 10.1093/eurheartj/ehad194

Authors/Task Force members, Elliott PM, Anastasakis A, Borger MA, Borggrefe M, Cecchi F, Charron P, Hagege AA, Lafont A, Limongelli G, Mahrholdt H, McKenna WJ, Mogensen J, Nihoyannopoulos P, Nistri S, Pieper PG, Pieske B, Rapezzi C, Rutten FH, Tillmanns C, Watkins H. 2014 ESC Guidelines on diagnosis and management of hypertrophic cardiomyopathy: the Task Force for the Diagnosis and Management of Hypertrophic Cardiomyopathy of the European Society of Cardiology (ESC). *Eur Heart J*. 2014 Oct 14;35(39):2733–79. doi: 10.1093/eurheartj/ehu284

Camm AJ, Lüscher TF, Serruys PW (eds). The European Society of Cardiology Textbook of Cardiovascular Medicine. Oxford University Press, 2009

Corrado D, van Tintelen PJ, McKenna WJ, Hauer RNW, Anastastakis A, Asimaki A, Basso C, Bauce B, Brunckhorst C, Bucciarelli-Ducci C, Duru F, Elliott P, Hamilton RM, Haugaa KH, James CA, Judge D, Link MS, Marchlinski FE, Mazzanti A, Mestroni L, Pantazis A, Pelliccia A, Marra MP, Pilichou K, Platonov PGA, Protonotarios A, Rampazzo A, Saffitz JE, Saguner AM, Schmied C, Sharma S, Tandri H, Te Riele ASJM, Thiene G, Tsatsopoulou A, Zareba W, Zorzi A, Wichter T, Marcus FI, Calkins H; International Experts. Arrhythmogenic right ventricular cardiomyopathy: evaluation of the current diagnostic criteria and differential diagnosis. *Eur Heart J*. 2020 Apr 7;41(14):1414–29. doi: 10.1093/eurheartj/ehz669

Dubrey SW, Hawkins PN, Falk RH. Amyloid diseases of the heart: assessment, diagnosis, and referral. *Heart*. 2011 Jan;97(1):75–84. doi: 10.1136/hrt.2009.190405

Merlo M, Cannatà A, Gobbo M, Stolfo D, Elliott PM, Sinagra G. Evolving concepts in dilated cardiomyopathy. *Eur J Heart Fail*. 2018 Feb;20(2):228–39. doi: 10.1002/ejhf.1103

Ponikowski P, Voors AA, Anker SD, Bueno H, Cleland JGF, Coats AJS, Falk V, González-Juanatey JR, Harjola VP, Jankowska EA, Jessup M, Linde C, Nihoyannopoulos P, Parissis JT, Pieske B, Riley JP, Rosano GMC, Ruilope LM, Ruschitzka F, Rutten FH, van der Meer P; ESC Scientific Document Group. 2016 ESC Guidelines for the diagnosis and treatment of acute and chronic heart failure: The Task Force for the diagnosis and treatment of acute and chronic heart failure of the European Society of Cardiology (ESC)Developed with the special contribution of the Heart Failure Association (HFA) of the ESC. *Eur Heart J*. 2016 Jul 14;37(27):2129–200. doi: 10.1093/eurheartj/ehw128. Epub 2016 May 20. Erratum in: *Eur Heart J*. 2016 Dec 30

Zeppenfeld K, Tfelt-Hansen J, de Riva M, Winkel BG, Behr ER, Blom NA, Charron P, Corrado D, Dagres N, de Chillou C, Eckardt L, Friede T, Haugaa KH, Hocini M, Lambiase PD, Marijon E, Merino JL, Peichl P, Priori SG, Reichlin T, Schulz-Menger J, Sticherling C, Tzeis S, Verstrael A, Volterrani M; ESC Scientific Document Group. 2022 ESC Guidelines for the management of patients with ventricular arrhythmias and the prevention of sudden cardiac death. *Eur Heart J*. 2022 Oct 21;43(40):3997–4126. doi: 10.1093/eurheartj/ehac262

5.3

Pericardial disease

Nav Masani and Abbas Zaidi

TABLE OF CONTENTS

5.3.1 Anatomy of the pericardium 499
5.3.2 Physiology of the pericardium 500
Ventricular interdependence 501
5.3.3 Acute pericarditis 502
Recurrent and chronic pericarditis 506
5.3.4 Pericardial effusion 507
5.3.5 Tamponade 508
5.3.6 Constrictive pericardial disease 510
5.3.7 Rare causes of pericardial disease 515
Primary pericardial tumours 515
Congenital abnormalities 515
5.3.8 Special circumstances 515
Pregnancy and lactation 515
The elderly 516

5.3.1 Anatomy of the pericardium

- The pericardium is a thin, predominantly fibrous layer of tissue encapsulating the heart and roots of the great vessels
- It is attached via ligaments to the sternum and vertebrae, anchoring it in place
- It covers the entire heart other than a small posterior part of the left atrium
- It extends upwards to cover the proximal parts of the great vessels.

The components of the pericardium are as follows:

Visceral pericardium

- Monolayer of ciliated mesothelial (serosal) cells adherent to the surface of the epicardium. It is of microscopic thickness.

Parietal pericardium

- Collagen and elastin layer lined with mesothelial (serosal) cells
- Contains both elastic and collagenous matrices, which result in the physical properties of compliance and stiffness
- Anatomically, the parietal layer of pericardium is only 1 mm thick (although current imaging modalities detect it at 2 mm thick).

Pericardial space and fluid

- The continuity of the mesothelial visceral and parietal pericardial layers establishes the pericardial space, completely lined by a layer of serosal cells
- 15–50 ml of a high phospholipid ultrafiltrate fluid acts as a lubricant between these 2 layers
- The visceral and parietal layers can move up to 1.5 cm over each other per cardiac cycle
- There is continuous production and absorption of pericardial fluid
- Pericardial fluid usually drains via the thoracic and right lymphatic ducts.

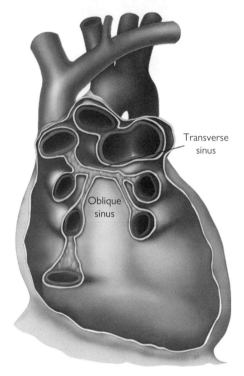

Figure 5.3.1 Posterior parietal pericardial anatomy.
Reprinted from 'Pericardial diseases: clinical diagnostic imaging atlas', Stuart J. Hutchison, copyright 2008 with permission from Elsevier.

The pericardial sac forms a complex shape as it envelopes the chambers of the heart and forms sleeves around the roots of the great vessels. See Figure 5.3.1.

5.3.2 Physiology of the pericardium

The functions of the pericardium and pericardial fluid include the following:

- It is predominantly made of collagen, which results in a tough physical barrier to the spread of infection and malignancy from adjacent organs
- It is attached via ligaments to the sternum and vertebrae, anchoring the heart, preventing excessive cardiac movement, and protecting it from acceleration/deceleration forces
- It reduces friction between the heart and adjacent tissues
- It has limited ability to stretch, thereby preventing acute volume distension and myocardial stretch, preserving sarcomere architecture, and maintaining myocardial systolic function
- It acts to distribute hydrostatic forces over the heart.

Intrapericardial pressure
- Intrapericardial pressure is usually slightly negative and is an important determinant of the filling pressure of the cardiac chambers

> The true (transmural) filling pressure of the cardiac chambers is diastolic pressure less intrapericardial pressure.

- As the intrapericardial pressure elevates over 0 mmHg, the true (transmural) filling pressure of the chamber reduces—the chamber will underfill during diastole
- When the intrapericardial pressure exceeds the diastolic pressure of a cardiac chamber, the chamber wall will compress inwards and collapse during diastole
- Once the pericardial reserve volume is exceeded pressure rise is rapid
- Equally (in these situations) removal of a small volume of fluid results in a rapid drop in pressure
- The transition from compliance to non-compliance happens more gradually in a chronically volume-overloaded pericardium
- Figure 5.3.2 shows pressure/volume relations in an animal with no previous pericardial effusion (closed circle) and an animal with a chronically volume overloaded pericardium (open circle).

Ventricular interdependence

- The parietal pericardium is compliant within the range of usual cardiac filling but can only stretch a limited amount further beyond this
- Overfilling of one ventricle will result in reduced filling of the other: ventricular interdependence
- In physiological states, during inspiration, RV filling increases with a parallel reduction in filling of the LV; during expiration this is reversed
- When the pericardium reaches its maximum 'stretch' and intrapericardial pressures begin to elevate, the phenomenon of ventricular interdependence becomes pathological
- The increased filling of one ventricle results in underfilling of the other. This is seen in the following disease states:
    - Constrictive pericarditis (non-compliant pericardium)
    - Effuso-constrictive pericarditis (non-compliant pericardium and fluid)
    - Pericardial tamponade
    - Right ventricular infarction with acute severe dilatation of the RV
    - Tumour encasement of the heart (non-compliant tumour mass).

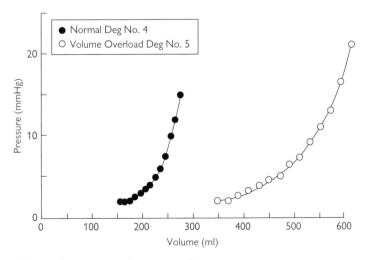

Figure 5.3.2 Pericardial pressure/volume relationship.
Reproduced from GL Freeman, M M LeWinter, 'Pericardial adaptations during chronic cardiac dilatation in dogs', *Circulation Research* 54 (3):294 (1984), with permission from Wolters Kluwer Health.

5.3.3 Acute pericarditis

- Pericarditis is a clinical syndrome caused by inflammation of the pericardium
- It encompasses a vast spectrum from mild, clinically silent disease to fulminant purulent inflammation
- In acute pericarditis, there is a thickening of both the parietal and serosal pericardium with rough irregularity of the surfaces
- The approach to patients with suspected acute pericarditis involves:
    - Establishing the clinical diagnosis of acute pericarditis
    - Establishing the aetiology of the acute pericarditis
    - Assessing for complications (such as pericardial effusion and tamponade)
    - Treatment

Establishing a clinical diagnosis

Acute pericarditis is characterized by:

- Chest pain (seen in more than 85–90% of cases)
- Pericardial friction rub (seen in ≤ 33%)
- Typical ECG repolarization changes (seen in up to 60%)
- Pericardial effusion (generally mild, seen in up to 60%)

The diagnosis of acute pericarditis requires at least two of these four elements.

- Acute pericarditis usually presents with subretrosternal chest pain (may be pleuritic), exacerbated by lying flat, or twisting
- A minority of patients experience a more visceral type of pain, which is readily confused with ischaemic pain
- Other symptoms depend on the aetiology of the pericarditis but often include prodromal fever, malaise, and myalgia.
- Physical signs are shown in Table 5.3.1.
- The ECG is abnormal in 85–90% of patients with acute pericarditis; characteristic ECG findings are outlined in Table 5.3.2
- All four ECG stages are only seen in up to 60% of cases and only if the underlying ECG is normal
- Baseline abnormalities render changes much less sensitive and specific for acute pericarditis
- Pericarditis is a clinical diagnosis and cannot be made echocardiographically
- Most cases of pericarditis do not develop a significant pericardial effusion
- The role of an echocardiogram is to: identify pericardial effusion, identify pericardial thickening, and assess LV function
- Routine blood analyses usually only provide non-specific information of raised inflammatory markers
- Small troponin elevation is seen in 35–50% of patients indicating myocardial involvement
- Additional blood tests should be tailored to identifying the aetiology of the suspected pericarditis depending on the nature of patient's presentation
- A CXR will show cardiomegaly when effusions exceed 250 ml
- The classic features of pericardial effusion are described as a 'water bottle' or 'globular' heart shadow
- Evidence of left pleural effusion should be sought and the CXR is useful in identifying additional pulmonary/mediastinal pathology, which may point towards aetiology.

Table 5.3.1 Physical signs in pericarditis.

Physical sign	Characteristic features
Pericardial rub (Described in some texts as being pathognomic of acute pericarditis). Found in less than 33% of cases of acute pericarditis. Optimal positioning may be required to increase detection (supine, left lateral position with arms above head or sitting and leaning forward. Listening at end-expiration with the diaphragm). Note: pericardial rubs are often transient, therefore repeated examination may be required to detect them.	Typically made up of three components related to the motion of the heart: • systolic motion • early diastolic filling • late diastolic atrial contraction when in sinus rhythm. If only 2 or 1 component audible then may be confused with cardiac murmur. Note: pericardial rub can be audible even in the presence of a pericardial effusion.
Pericardial effusion (May be absent in 40% of cases) or tamponade	See section 5.3.4
Pleural effusion	Particularly of the left side in patients with pleuropericarditis
Ewart's sign	Bronchial breathing at the left base caused by compression of the left lower lobe of the lung.

Table 5.3.2 ECG changes found in pericarditis.

ECG in pericarditis	Characteristic findings	ECG example
Stage I May be confused with acute MI or early repolarization (normal variant of repolarization)	Anterior and inferior concave ST segment elevation (usually less than 5 mm) with positive T waves in several leads. PR segment depression (indicating atrial injury).	
Early stage II **Late stage II**	ST segments return to baseline. PR remains deviated. T waves progressively flatten and invert.	
Stage III (an ECG at this stage on its own cannot be reliably differentiated from diffuse myocardial injury, biventricular strain or myocarditis.)	Generalized T wave inversion	
Stage IV (occasionally this stage does not occur and there are permanent T wave changes on the ECG.)	ECG returns to pre-pericarditis state.	

Typical lead involvement includes I, II, aVL, aVF, and V3–V6. The ST segment is always depressed in aVR, frequently in V1, and occasionally in V2. Pericarditis is likely if in V6 the J point is > 25% of the height of the T wave apex (using the PR segment as baseline). Reproduced with permission from ECGpedia.org.

Establish the aetiology of acute pericarditis

Acute pericarditis is usually either associated with an obvious clinical condition—making a cause–effect relationship likely—or is idiopathic (routine diagnostic tests fail to uncover the aetiology—the majority of these cases are likely to be viral). Figure 5.3.3 outlines the aetiological classification of acute pericarditis.

Idiopathic and viral

- In the Western world (immunologically competent patients with no predisposing diseases) 90% of cases of acute pericarditis are idiopathic (presumed viral)
- If the clinical features of acute pericarditis fade over a few days, then the likelihood of the aetiology being idiopathic approaches 100%
- The most common specific viral causes include coxsackievirus, echovirus, adenovirus, mumps virus, varicella zoster virus, and Epstein–Barr virus
- A diagnosis can be made by comparing acute and convalescent neutralizing antibodies
- Because viral pericarditis is usually a self-limiting disease, viral serology and invasive pericardial procedures to clarify the exact aetiology are not usually undertaken.

Bacterial

- Purulent bacterial pericarditis is most commonly caused by streptococci, staphylococci, pneumococci, Gram-negative rods, *Haemophilus influenza*, *Mycoplasma*, and *Legionella*
- Patients more likely to develop bacterial pericarditis include those with pneumonia, empyema, those recently having undergone chest surgery, and the immunocompromised
- Patients with bacterial pericarditis are more likely to develop tamponade
- TB pericarditis is rare in the western world. Its incidence is increased in immunocompromised patients, especially those with HIV infection.

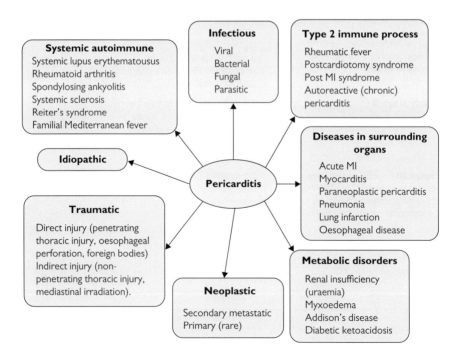

Figure 5.3.3 Aetiological classification of pericarditis.

Systemic disease

- In patients who are known to suffer from a disease predisposing them to pericarditis (renal failure, recent MI, autoimmune disease, widespread neoplasia) it is very likely that acute pericarditis is caused by that disease
- Of patients with autoimmune disease, up to 30% with SLE, 30% with rheumatoid arthritis, and over 50% with systemic sclerosis have evidence of episodes of pericarditis
- Pericarditis caused by systemic autoimmune disease is often clinically mild or silent
- Some form of pericardial inflammation in patients with uraemia is common and up to 30% of myxedematous patients develop pericarditis
- Other metabolic causes of pericarditis are rare.

Post myocardial infarction and myocarditis

- Early post-infarction pericarditis develops in approximately 10% of patients 2 to 3 days after a transmural infarction
- Delayed post-infarction pericarditis (Dressler's syndrome) occurs 2 weeks or so after MI
- Up to 30% of patients with myocarditis develop an associated pericarditis, a syndrome termed 'perimyocarditis'. Where the clinical picture is predominantly that of pericarditis with concomitant cardiac biomarker elevation without significant ventricular dysfunction, the term 'myopericarditis' is applicable. Angiography is recommended in combined myocardial–pericardial syndromes to rule out acute coronary syndromes, and cardiac MRI is recommended to confirm myocardial involvement.

Diagnostic pathway in acute pericarditis

Figure 5.3.4 is a pragmatic diagnostic pathway.

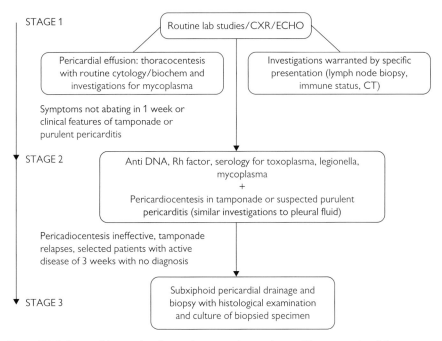

Figure 5.3.4 Protocol for routine diagnostic approach to patients with acute pericarditis.

Table 5.3.3 Features recommending a patient for inpatient investigation and treatment.

Major predictors of poor prognosis:
Fever > 38°C
Subacute onset over days
- Pericardial effusion > 2 cm
- Cardiac tamponade
- Lack of response to aspirin or NSAIDs after at least 1 week of therapy

Minor predictors of poor prognosis:
- History of anticoagulation use
  Myopericarditis
- Chest trauma
- Immunosuppression

Management of acute pericarditis

Inpatient versus outpatient management

Consider the risk of an immediate complication, adverse aetiology, and long-term sequlae when considering which patients need inpatient care (see Table 5.3.3).

- Patients with acute idiopathic or viral pericarditis should rest until the symptoms abate and CRP has normalized. Athletes should not return to competitive sports for a minimum of 3 months, and until symptoms, CRP and echocardiographic findings have normalized.
- Pain and fever should be managed with paracetamol and either aspirin (750–1000 mg every 8 h) or NSAIDs such as ibuprofen (600 mg every 8 h).
- Treatment with aspirin or NSAIDs should continue whilst pain and fever are present and should be tapered gradually over 1–2 weeks in uncomplicated cases. Typical treatment duration is 1–2 weeks for uncomplicated cases.
- Colchicine is also recommended as first-line therapy in addition to aspirin or NSAIDs, in order to improve clinical response and prevent recurrences. The recommended dose is 0.5 mg once daily (< 70 kg) or 0.5 mg twice daily (≥ 70 kg). Colchicine should be continued for 3 months. Tapering is not mandatory.
- Systemic corticosteroid therapy should be avoided—it is probably associated with an increased risk of relapse. Its use should be restricted to connective tissue diseases, autoreactive, or uremic pericarditis (intrapericardial administration of corticosteroids is highly effective and avoids systemic side effects). To avoid rebound pericarditis as steroids are tapered, NSAIDS or colchicine should be introduced early.
- Corticosteroids should be considered as a second option in patients with contraindications and failure of aspirin and NSAIDs.
- Despite the widely held perception that anticoagulant therapy is associated with an increased risk of tamponade in pericarditis, recent meta-analyses have not found in support of this.

Recurrent and chronic pericarditis

- Recurrent pericarditis occurs after a documented first episode of pericarditis, with at least a 4–6 week symptom-free interval, followed by a recurrence of signs and symptoms.
- Incessant pericarditis is defined as pericarditis lasting > 4–6 weeks, but less than 3 months, without remission.
- Pericarditis lasting > 3 months is termed chronic.
- The recurrence rate after an acute episode of pericarditis is between 15–30%, although this may be as high as 50% in cases not treated with colchicine, or if corticosteroids have been used.
- Relapses may be accounted for by inadequate courses of anti-inflammatories as well as the use of corticosteroids.

- There is no definitive treatment for the prevention of relapses
- Long-term colchicine may be advantageous (≥ 6 months)
- Oral corticosteroids with slow tapering may be used as adjunctive therapy in addition to aspirin or NSAIDs and colchicine
- Immunomodulatory drugs such as azathioprine, intravenous immunoglobulin, and the recombinant IL-1β antagonist anakinra may be considered as steroid-sparing agents
- Pericardectomy may be considered as a last resort
- Serious complications, such as the development of constrictive pericarditis, are rare.

5.3.4 Pericardial effusion

Many pericardial effusions are incidental findings on echo and CT. They consist of increased pericardial fluid, pus, or blood. The causes of pericardial effusions are:

- Any cause of acute pericarditis; most commonly idiopathic due to high incidence
- Malignancy: pericardial tumour involvement
- Iatrogenic: post cardiac surgery or perforation of coronary artery post PCI
- Acute bleed into pericardium from cardiac rupture or dissection of ascending aorta
- Hydrostatic forces: heart failure, lymphatic obstruction, raised central pressure.

Pericardial effusions are qualified as small (< 10 mm depth in diastole), moderate (10–20 mm), or large (> 20 mm).

- Sizing of the pericardial effusion may be misleading, as often effusions are not uniformly distributed
- Importantly, the size of an effusion often has a poor association with its haemodynamic consequences and is more of a marker of its chronicity.

Diagnostic evaluation

- History, examination, and investigations should be focused on elucidating the cause of the pericardial effusion and identifying any haemodynamic consequence
- In the majority of patients presenting with a moderate or large pericardial effusion, an obvious causal disease will be present
- Inflammatory features associated with pericardial effusion are highly suggestive of acute idiopathic pericarditis
- Moderate–large pericardial effusions persisting for longer than 3 months are considered chronic. In most cases, the cause is unknown
- A large pericardial effusion without tamponade is likely to be an idiopathic, chronic pericardial effusion
- Even in asymptomatic patients, intrapericardial pressures are usually elevated and patients are at an increased risk of developing unexpected tamponade
- In patients presenting with tamponade and no inflammatory features, the effusion is likely to be neoplastic
- Echocardiography is the diagnostic test of choice for evaluating pericardial effusions
- Echocardiography can establish the presence of pericardial fluid, identify important underlying causes (MI, masses, aortic dissection), evaluate haemodynamic consequence of the pericardial effusion, evaluate optimal drainage method if needed, and guide drainage.

Minimum assessment of a pericardial effusion should include the following (see Table 5.3.4):

- Analysis of pericardial fluid has a low aetiological detection rate when undertaken in the absence of features of tamponade (5%)
- In the context of tamponade aetiological detection rates may be up to 40%.

Table 5.3.4 Assessment of patients with pericardial effusion.

Assessment	Comments
History and physical examination	Focused on elucidating the cause and haemodynamic consequence
ECG	Assess for evidence of low voltage, electrical alternans, pericarditis, recent MI
CXR	Assess for associated pleural or parenchymal lung disease, abnormal hilar, or abnormal aortic contours
Serum biochemistry	Renal function, thyroid function
Serum haematology	FBC
Blood cultures	If infection suspected
Troponin	If recent MI is suspected
Immunological testing	If autoimmune disease suspected, e.g. SLE, RA
PPD skin testing	If TB is suspected
CT	If malignancy is suspected

The haemodynamic consequence of a pericardial effusion is far more important than its size. Only a small subset of pericardial effusions result in tamponade.

Management

- In the case of cardiac tamponade, or if there is suspected bacterial or neoplastic aetiology, pericardiocentesis and aetiology search should be performed
- If inflammatory markers are elevated, treatment as for acute pericarditis should be commenced (empiric anti-inflammatory therapy)
- If there is a known associated disease, this should be considered to be the likely aetiology of the effusion and should be treated accordingly
- If none of the above features is present, pericardiocentesis and drainage of large idiopathic effusions persisting > 3 months should be considered, in view of a 30–35% likelihood of progressing to tamponade. Chronic effusions between 10–20 mm in size should be followed up with 3–6 monthly echocardiography.

5.3.5 Tamponade

- Tamponade is a clinical syndrome with an eventual low-output, high venous state
- The diagnosis is made using bedside clinical signs and objective testing (echocardiography).

In a patient presenting with cardiac tamponade, the clinical goals are to:

- Establish the diagnosis
- Establish the aetiology
- Stabilize the patient.

Establish the diagnosis

Clinical features may include:

- Chest discomfort, pericardial rub, quiet heart sounds, dyspnoea, tachycardia
- Raised JVP with loss of y descent

- **Kussmaul's sign** (elevation of JVP during inspiration)
- **Pulsus paradoxus** (detected as a fall in systolic BP and pulse pressure of > 10 mmHg occurring during inspiration); total pulsus paradoxus is where no pulse can be felt during inspiration
- Falling BP (once the elevation in heart rate and vasoconstriction fail to compensate for the low stroke volume)
- **Beck's triad** (hypotension, quiet heart sounds, raised JVP with absent y descent).

Investigations

See Table 5.3.5. Echocardiographic features may include:

- Loss of cardiac transmural distension pressure, which results in inward displacement of chamber walls (RA and RV) and eventual compression
- RA collapse, which only has a 30% positive predictive value for tamponade
- RA and RV collapse, which is more specific, with a positive predictive value of 74%
- Increase in RV volumes during inspiration and leftward movement of the septum during diastole (exaggeration of normal)
- IVC distension with < 50% reduction on inspiration.
- In large pericardial effusion there may be marked swinging of the heart beat to beat
- Increased tricuspid and pulmonary flow velocities (> 50%) with decreased mitral and aortic flow velocities (> 25%) during inspiration (exaggeration of normal). See Figure 5.3.5.

Stabilize the patient

- The definitive management of patients with features of cardiac tamponade associated with life-threatening haemodynamic changes is pericardiocentesis (see Box 5.3.1)
- Pericardiocentesis and drainage in the context of tamponade is life saving
- The diagnostic yield of both pericardiocentesis and drainage with biopsy is significantly higher when done in the context of tamponade rather than purely for diagnostic purposes (35% vs 6%)
- It is important to recognize intrapericardial thrombus vs fresh blood, as pericardiocentesis cannot be used to drain thrombus and can result in chamber perforation during attempts
- Surgical pericardial drainage is the preferred method of stabilization in cardiac tamponade caused by thrombus
- Thrombus may be caused by the following:
    - Open cardiac surgery
    - Trauma (penetrating, blunt, iatrogenic)

Table 5.3.5 Indications of cardiac tamponade.

Imaging modality	Features indicating tamponade
ECG	Low voltage if there is significantly sized pericardial effusion. Electrical alternans (specific but insensitive sign—only seen in 20% of tamponade—only seen in large effusions where the heart responds to tamponade with dynamic contraction resulting in swinging in the fluid—seen in large malignant effusions).
CXR	200–250 ml fluid accumulation is required before the CXR starts to show signs of effusion. Useful to look for adjacent lung and mediastinal disease.
Echo	TTE is usually adequate. Echo should be used to confirm tamponade, determine cause (if possible), and determine the safest and most logical method of drainage.

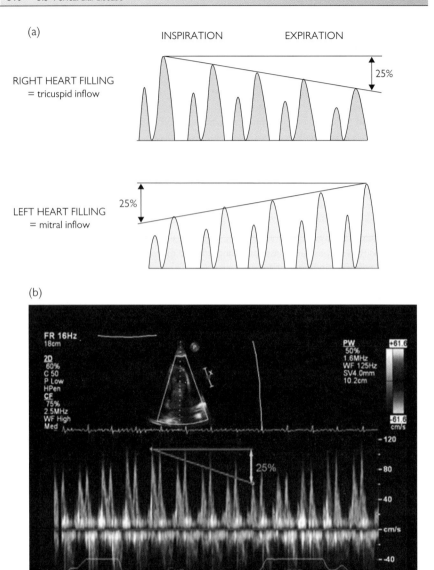

Figure 5.3.5 Tricuspid and mitral inflow Doppler velocities.
Reproduced from 'Echocardiography in ICU', with kind permission from The Stanford School of Medicine. Available online at https://www.stanford.edu/group/ccm_echocardio/cgi-bin/mediawiki/index.php/Main_Page

- Myocardial rupture post infarct
- Aortic dissection with intrapericardial rupture.

5.3.6 Constrictive pericardial disease

Constrictive pericardial disease refers to the syndrome of pathophysiological compression of the heart caused by rigid, thickened, and often fused pericardial membranes.

BOX 5.3.1 PROCEDURE FOR PERICARDIOCENTESIS

The following information is not intended to outline step by step the practical skill of performing pericardiocentesis. Rather, it is intended to summarize key points for consideration before, during, and after undertaking this practical procedure.

Pericardial fluid drainage can be achieved by:

- Pericardiocentesis tap (with needle)
- Pericardiocentesis catheter drainage (Seldinger techniques or chest tube techniques via surgical approaches)
- Percutaneous balloon pericardiostomy
- Pericardial window
- Surgical pericardiectomy.

Considerations pre-procedure

- Avoid positive pressure ventilation (invasive or non-invasive) as this will reduce cardiac output
- If tamponade occurs in the context of trauma then surgical drainage is required
- Where possible, formal consent should be sought from the patient before undertaking pericardiocentesis. The risk of the procedure in experienced hands is as follows:
  - 1% major complications (death, cardiac arrest, vascular or cardiac cavity laceration requiring surgery, pneumothorax requiring chest drain)
  - 4% minor complications (sepsis, vasovagal reflex, pneumothorax not requiring chest drain, non-sustained VT, pleuropericardial fistulae).

Considerations during the procedure

- Whenever possible, pericardiocentesis should be performed with imaging support. However, in the context of circulatory collapse, pericardiocentesis should not be delayed and should be done immediately
  - Echocardiography should be used to establish the safest and easiest access site. Agitated saline can be used to confirm position within the pericardial space
  - Fluoroscopy can be used to visualize the guide wire to ensure it is within the pericardium. The guide wire should be seen wrapping around the inside of the pericardial space and not advancing into the SCV or pulmonary trunk
- Position the patient at 30° to allow maximum fluid accumulation posteriorly
- As with all invasive procedures, it is essential to use sterile technique.

Considerations post procedure

- It is important for further management that the cause of pericardial fluid accumulation is identified. Pericardial fluid should be sent to the labs for analysis; including cytology, microbiology, and biochemistry for glucose, amylase, protein, and haemoglobin if relevant.

- The stiff, non-compliant pericardium resists deformation outwards resulting in increased diastolic pressures with reduced diastolic filling
- Eventually the cardiac chamber diastolic pressures become equal to each other
- The reduced diastolic filling initially limits stroke volume, and then reduces stroke volume

- The stroke volume becomes fixed and thus the cardiac output is reliant on heart rate (tachycardia).
- The stiffened pericardium also resists deformation inwards resulting in exaggerated ventricular recoil outward in early diastole on cessation of ventricular contraction.
- Due to the phenomena of ventricular interdependence, inspiration results in increased right ventricular diastolic pressures with the consequence of a fall in left ventricular venous return and pressure.
- Specific sub-forms are now recognized, including transient constriction which may develop after acute pericarditis, effusive-constrictive pericarditis in which there are clinical features of constriction as well as tamponade, and chronic constriction persisting more than 3–6 months.

The approach to a patient with suspected pericardial constriction is:

- Establish the diagnosis
- Establish the aetiology
- Treatment.

Establish the diagnosis

Patients usually present with:

- Symptoms secondary to right-sided heart failure
- Symptoms secondary to low cardiac output.

There is often a delay in diagnosis (typically 1–2 years) due to the insidious onset of symptoms. Physical signs are shown in Table 5.3.6.

Diagnostic approach

See Table 5.3.7.

Establish the aetiology

Idiopathic pericardial constriction is the most common aetiology. Other causes of pericardial constriction include the following:

- Trauma
    - Post open heart surgery
    - Post trauma
    - Post radiation

Table 5.3.6 Physical signs of constrictive pericarditis.

Physical signs	Features associated with physical signs
Features of right-sided heart failure	• Enlarged liver • Ascites • Peripheral oedema • Pleural effusions
JVP	• Increased V wave (due to increased RA diastolic filling pressures) • Prominent y descent (due to brisk early diastolic recoil) • Kussmaul's sign (failure of JVP to fall during inspiration or increase in JVP during inspiration indicating severe non-compliance of right sided cardiac chambers)
Proto-diastolic pericardial knock	• As the ventricles relax and 'knock' against the stiffened pericardium (may be confused clinically with the opening snap heard in mitral stenosis)

Table 5.3.7 Diagnostic approach in constrictive pericarditis.

Diagnostic tool	Possible findings in constrictive pericarditis
ECG	May be normal • Atrial arrhythmias common (incidence 25%) • P wave abnormalities (due to atrial enlargement) • Low voltage complexes (if pericardium is thickened impairing surface reading of ECG) • Pseudo-infarction pattern (rare—associated with penetration of fibrotic process into myocardium
CXR	May be normal • Mild cardiac silhouette enlargement with LA enlargement is common • Pericardial calcification • Pleural plaques • Pleural effusions common
Echocardiography • Echo measurements should be taken with concurrent respirometry tracings • Echo features will be compounded by concurrent AF, abnormal breathing effort as well as valvular/myocardial disease • TTE is not a good imaging tool for measuring pericardial thickening. Although TOE can be used to assess pericardial thickening, CMR and CT are the preferred tests	*Mitral inflow* • Exaggerated interventricular interdependence with > 25% reduction in mitral inflow during inspiration *Tricuspid regurgitation velocity* • Exaggeration of interventricular interdependence with > 25% reduction in tricuspid inflow velocities during expiration *Elevated central pressure* • Dilated IVC • Failure of IVC collapse during inspiration • Spontaneous contrast in IVC *Interventricular septum* Classically the septum appears to flutter during diastole • Early diastolic motion towards the left ventricle (due to early diastolic pressure dip). Best appreciated using M mode • Septal flattening during inspiration (ventricular interdependence) *Tissue Doppler* • Lateral mitral annulus E prime > 8 cm/sec • Features of diastolic dysfunction as myocardial relaxation is inhibited by the stiffened pericardium—E/A ratio exaggeration with shortening of deceleration time
Cardiac CT and cardiac MRI • Cardiac CT and MRI are not used to assess the complex haemodynamics found in constrictive pericarditis • Not all patients with pericardial constriction have pericardial thickening and not all patients with pericardial thickening have pericardial constriction	• Useful in measuring pericardial thickness and assessing for calcification • Tube like configuration of one or both ventricles • Enlargement of one or both atria • Narrowing of AV grooves and congestion of the caval veins • Useful if assessing underlying myocardial fibrosis (a poor prognosticator for pericardiectomy) • Septal flattening during inspiration, assessed during real-time free-breathing cine MRI (ventricular interdependence)

(continued)

Table 5.3.7 Continued

Diagnostic tool	Possible findings in constrictive pericarditis
Right and left cardiac catheterization • Measurements should be taken with simultaneous respirometer • Pacing may be needed to overcome R–R interval variability in patients in AF	• Interdependence of filling. Simultaneous increase in RV systolic pressure and decrease of LV systolic pressure during the first or second beats of inspiration • Pulmonary capillary wedge pressure/LV diastolic pressure gradient increase of > 5% during inspiration. • Elevated RV diastolic pressure > 1/3 of RV systolic pressure • Pulmonary artery pressure <50 mmHg • LV end diastolic pressure: RV end diastolic pressure equalization within a pressure range difference of < 5 mmHg • Kussmaul's sign on RA pressure recording • Early diastolic dip followed by plateau in pressure curve of RV and LV (see Figure 5.3.6)

- Inflammation
    - Post pericarditis
    - Post uraemia
    - Post Dressler's
    - Associated with inflammatory disease
    - Associated with infiltrative disease
- Infection
    - Tuberculous
    - Fungal

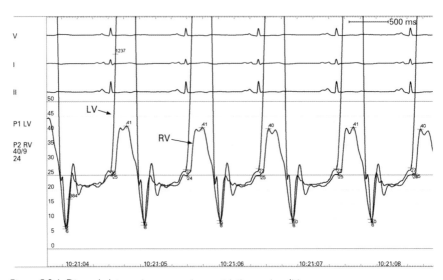

Figure 5.3.6 Dip and plateau sign as seen in constrictive pericarditis.
Reproduced from The BMJ Case Reports, Imran Patanwala, Jenifer Crilley, Peter N Trewby, copyright 2009 with permission from BMJ Publishing Group Ltd.

Management

- Widespread pericardiectomy is the only effective treatment
- Involves resection of the parietal pericardium as well as visceral pericardium if it is found to be thickened
- Once severe constrictive pericarditis has been diagnosed, surgery should not be delayed as mortality and poor outcome increase with age and advanced functional class
- Surgery in these patients carries a higher risk of incomplete success or significant damage to the myocardium
- Mortality in patients undergoing pericardiectomy for constrictive pericarditis ranges between 6% and 12%
- Major operative complications include perioperative heart failure (low output syndrome as a consequence of right ventricular dilatation) and ventricular wall rupture
- Normalization of haemodynamics occurs in 60% of patients
- Patients who fail to improve post pericardiectomy often have underlying myocardial atrophy or fibrosis.

Factors predicting worse prognosis include:

- Radiotherapy (there is often concurrent fibrosis in the underlying myocardium)
- Renal failure
- Pulmonary hypertension
- Left ventricular systolic impairment
- Hyponatraemia
- Hepatic impairment (Child–Pugh score ≥ 7)
- Increasing age.

5.3.7 Rare causes of pericardial disease

Primary pericardial tumours

Primary pericardial tumours are exceptionally rare. They are often detected when presenting with pericardial effusions. Surgery is indicated in benign neoplasms (lipomas, fibromas).

Congenital abnormalities

Congenital abnormalities include the following:

- Absence of the pericardium
    - Complete absence—requires no treatment; it may present with atypical chest pain but is usually asymptomatic
    - Partial absence—may require surgery; it increases the risk of cardiac herniation presenting with severe, non-exertional chest pain
- Pericardial cysts
    - Usually benign and asymptomatic malformations located in the right costophrenic angle. No treatment is required.

5.3.8 Special circumstances

Pregnancy and lactation

- A benign, self-limiting, mild pericardial effusion (hydropericardium) is found in up to 40% of pregnant women by the third trimester.

- Acute pericarditis is the most common pericardial syndrome requiring treatment during pregnancy and breastfeeding.
- High-dose aspirin is the treatment of choice during the first trimester. All NSAIDs other than aspirin ≤ 100 mg/day may impair foetal renal perfusion after 20 weeks of gestation.
- Low-dose corticosteroids can be used throughout pregnancy and lactation.
- Ibuprofen, indomethacin, and naproxen can be safely used during breastfeeding
- Colchicine is contraindicated during pregnancy and breastfeeding.

The elderly

- Pericardial diseases in the elderly have not been specifically assessed in any trials. Recommendations are therefore based on consensus agreement. Indomethacin should be avoided. Colchicine dose should be halved. Particular care should be taken to monitor renal function and avoid drug interactions.

Further reading

Adler Y, Charron P, Imazio M, Badano L, Barón-Esquivias G, Bogaert J, Brucato A, Gueret P, Klingel K, Lionis C, Maisch B, Mayosi B, Pavie A, Ristic AD, Sabaté Tenas M, Seferovic P, Swedberg K, Tomkowski W; ESC Scientific Document Group. 2015 ESC Guidelines for the diagnosis and management of pericardial diseases: The Task Force for the Diagnosis and Management of Pericardial Diseases of the European Society of Cardiology (ESC)Endorsed by: The European Association for Cardio-Thoracic Surgery (EACTS). *Eur Heart J*. 2015 Nov 7;36(42):2921–64. doi: 10.1093/eurheartj/ehv318

Cosyns B, Plein S, Nihoyanopoulos P, Smiseth O, Achenbach S, Andrade MJ, Pepi M, Ristic A, Imazio M, Paelinck B, Lancellotti P; European Association of Cardiovascular Imaging (EACVI); European Society of Cardiology Working Group (ESC WG) on Myocardial and Pericardial diseases. European Association of Cardiovascular Imaging (EACVI) position paper: Multimodality imaging in pericardial disease. *Eur Heart J Cardiovasc Imaging*. 2015 Jan;16(1):12–31. doi: 10.1093/ehjci/jeu128

5.4

Cardiac tumours

Arjun Ghosh

TABLE OF CONTENTS

5.4.1 Overview 517
5.4.2 Clinical features 517
5.4.3 Diagnosis 518
    Echocardiography 518
    Computed tomography 518
    Magnetic resonance 518
5.4.4 Benign tumours 518
    Myxoma 519
    Lipoma 520
    Papillary fibroelastoma 520

Haemangioma 521
Rhabdomyoma 522
Fibroma 522
Cystic tumour of the AV node 523
5.4.5 Malignant tumours 523
    Angiosarcoma 523
    Rhabdomyosarcoma 524
    Fibrosarcoma 524
    Cardiac lymphoma 524
    Cardiac metastases 524

5.4.1 Overview

- Primary cardiac tumours are uncommon; prevalence 0.05% at autopsy
- Most common: myxoma in adults and the rhabdomyoma in children
- Secondary tumours are more common; around 1% of autopsies
- 10% of primary cardiac tumours are malignant (majority sarcomas)

5.4.2 Clinical features

Obstruction

- Atrial tumours can become very large and exert mass effect—ventricular inflow or pulmonary venous obstruction
- Ventricular tumours may outflow tract obstruction resulting in syncope, dyspnoea, or chest pain
- Superior vena cava (SVC) syndrome:
    - The obstruction of blood flow through the SVC often due to lung cancer (70% of cases).
    - Dyspnoea, facial swelling, chest pain, and hoarseness can be seen.
    - CT imaging is diagnostic, and radiotherapy is a standard treatment for most patients.
    - Chemotherapy may have a role in SVC syndrome secondary to non-Hodgkin lymphoma.
    - Surgery and SVC stenting have a role in the palliative setting

Embolization

- Tumour mass or associated thrombus—systemic or pulmonary

Arrhythmia

- Re-entrant circuits and other arrhythmias are common, with both intracavity and intramural tumours
- Some infiltrate the conductive tissue resulting in heart block or, occasionally sudden cardiac death

5.4.3 Diagnosis

- Histology is the definitive test
- Quality of the report depends on a reasonable mass of tissue being obtained and percutaneous tissue biopsy samples may occasionally be insufficient
- The percutaneous approach may sometimes be technically challenging
- Imaging techniques attempt to make the diagnosis non-invasively and a combination of modalities may be used

Echocardiography

See chapter 1.1.10.

- Mainstay of imaging: real-time images and haemodynamic data
- Management is often surgical; definition of location and boundaries essential to differentiate tumour from other structures (may avoid unnecessary surgery)
- Some masses have classic echo appearances but, ultimately, tissue diagnosis is gold standard

Computed tomography

- Gated CT with intravenous contrast can help characterize a tumour (size, shape, site) and define the borders to assess infiltration into local structures
- Particularly useful in patients with poor echocardiographic windows
- Allows concomitant evaluation of the coronary arteries prior to surgical intervention

Magnetic resonance

See section 1.2.13 in Chapter 1.2.

- High spatial and temporal resolution imaging in any anatomical plane. Can help in tissue characterization
- Thrombus can be differentiated from other masses due to its poor uptake of gadolinium (low signal on T1/T2-weighted images)
- Lipomas have an almost identical T2 signal to subcutaneous fat
- Malignant tumours are usually isointense to the myocardium on T1-wi imaging, have high signal on T2-wi, and most commonly heterogenous enhancement on LGE imaging.

5.4.4 Benign tumours

Majority are myxomas, lipomas, and papillary fibroelastomas.

Myxoma

- Atrial myxoma is by far the most common cardiac tumour, with a slight female predominance
- Can occur from paediatric age to the elderly—peak prevalence in the sixth decade
- 90% are located in the left atrium and 90% are solitary
- Carney complex is an autosomal dominant syndrome of endocrine adenoma, facial freckling, and multiple atrial myxomas
- Presentation is variable:
  - Constitutional symptoms 30% (due to interleukin-6)
  - Obstruction 60%: syncope, dyspnoea, and congestive cardiac failure
  - Embolism 16%
  - Clubbing and rash may be present
  - Signs of pulmonary hypertension (right-sided tumours that have embolized or obstructive left-sided tumours) possible

There are some imaging characteristics which help to distinguish myxomas from thrombus:

- Presence of a peduncle should be sought and its relationship with the intra-atrial septum and coronary sinus is carefully delineated (see Figure 5.4.1)
- Atrial myxoma diagnosis is almost assured if attachment to the intra-atrial septum is identified.
- Typically heterogenous but may be homogeneous or have central areas of hyperlucency representing haemorrhage and necrosis, together with patches of calcification
- May appear villous (35% more prone to embolization) or smooth (65%)
- Usually large—mean size of 5–6 cm at time of detection
- In contrast, thrombus is homogenous and usually arises from the left atrial appendage but may exist as large free-floating circular shape

When a suspected atrial myxoma is identified urgent surgery is considered mandatory especially for large left-sided tumours near the mitral valve. Some advocate a more conservative approach in the elderly with small tumours not causing haemodynamic compromise.

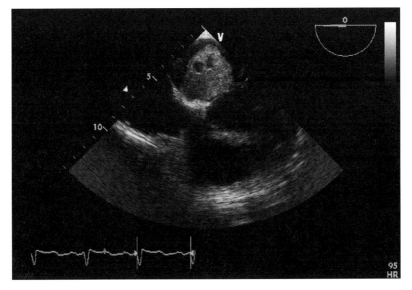

Figure 5.4.1 Transoesophageal echocardiography image of large heterogenous atrial myxoma. A broad-based peduncle is seen originating from the intra-atrial septum.

Lipoma

There are two main variants of lipoma, which are distinct entities:

Capsulated masses

- Usually subepicardial but may arise from any location in the heart
- Can occur from the endothelium of the valves
- Often have a broad peduncle
- Rarely symptomatic but may present with embolic phenomena, arrhythmias, obstruction of valves, or compression of epicardial vessels
- Require surgical resection if symptomatic

Lipoma of the intra-atrial septum

- Non-capsulated
- Common in obese, elderly patients
- Extension of the subepicardial fat through the right AV sulcus
- May present with palpitations due to atrial arrhythmia or AV block
- Very rarely, lipomatous hypertrophy of the intra-atrial septum can be so extreme as to occlude vena caval inflow

Echo appearance depends on location:

- In pericardium they range from being hypoechoic to hyperechoic
- In cavities they tend to be homogenous and hyperechoic

Despite often being pedunculated not usually as mobile as myxomas. Both true lipoma and lipoma of the intra-atrial septum are easily detected on CMR due to non-enhancing high fat signal (see Figure 5.4.2).

Papillary fibroelastoma

- Second most common primary cardiac tumour (excluding lipomatous hypertrophy of intra-atrial septum)

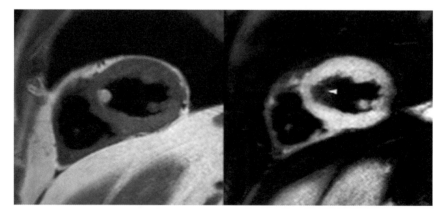

Figure 5.4.2 T1 weighted MRI shows a hyperintense spherical mass, which becomes hypointense with fat-suppression sequencing (arrowed).

Reproduced from Ganame J, Wright J, Bogaert J. Cardiac lipoma diagnosed by cardiac magnetic resonance imaging. *Eur Heart J.* 2008 Mar;29(6):697. doi: 10.1093/eurheartj/ehm476. with permission from Oxford University Press.

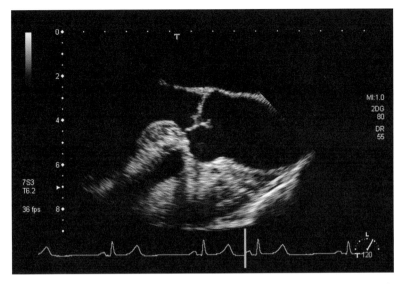

Figure 5.4.3 Papillary fibroelastoma seen on the tips of the aortic valve at transoesophageal echo.
Reproduced from Truscelli G, Torromeo C, Miraldi F, Vittori C, Silenzi PF, Caso A, Gallo P, Gaudio C, Tritapepe L. The role of intraoperative transoesophageal echocardiography in the diagnosis and management of a rare multiple fibroelastoma of aortic valve: a case report and review of literature. *Eur J Echocardiogr.* 2009 Oct;10(7):884–6. doi: 10.1093/ejechocard/jep087 with permission from Oxford University Press.

- Majority are incidental findings at autopsy
- When symptomatic, usually present with embolic phenomena (typically too small to cause obstruction) in the fourth to eighth decade
- Slightly more common in males
- May grow to 1–2 cm in diameter
- Majority arise from the aortic or mitral valves but may originate from any endomyocardial tissue
- Sometimes mistaken for a giant Lambl excrescence
- Histologically composed of a non-vascular fibroelastic axis surrounded by myxoid tissue and an endothelial cover
- Described as having a shimmering edge on echocardiography, which may help distinguish from thrombus (see Figure 5.4.3)
- Left-sided tumours should always be treated surgically in view of embolic risk whereas right-sided tumours may be treated conservatively

Haemangioma

- A very rare tumour; can occur in adult and paediatric populations
- Principally comprised of neoplastic vessel proliferation
- There are three well described types—arteriovenous haemangioma (infiltrative), capillary haemangioma (capsulated), and cavernous haemangioma (infiltrative)
- Exist as subendocardial nodules, which can grow up to 4 cm in diameter
- 75% are intramural, which may result in arrhythmia and pericardial effusions
- 25% extend into cavities and may mimic myxoma, with obstructive symptoms
- The most common site is the left ventricle (Figure 5.4.4)
- Despite often containing fat, haemangiomas are readily distinguishable from lipomas on CMR as they appear heterogenous, with marked enhancement

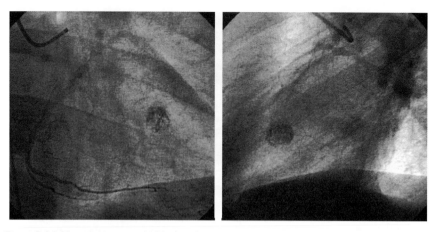

Figure 5.4.4 Haemangioma are highly vascular structures seen on angiography. Although highly suggestive of the haemangioma, myxoma and angiosarcoma may have similar appearances.
Reproduced from Serri K, Schraub P, Lafitte S, Roudaut R. Cardiac hemangioma presenting as atypical chest pain. *Eur J Echocardiogr.* 2007 Jan;8(1):17–8. doi: 10.1016/j.euje.2006.01.002 with permission from Oxford University Press.

- Natural history is variable; some tumours regress over time and others continue to proliferate
- Management is dependent on the site, size, history, and complications
- Mainstay of treatment is surgical
- Follow-up is considered mandatory, with echo to detect tumour recurrence.

Rhabdomyoma

- Most common cardiac tumour in the paediatric population
- 50–80% of cases associated with tuberous sclerosis (neurofibromatous lesions causing seizures, mental slowing, and cutaneous adenoma sebaceum lesions)
- Consists of a non-proliferative hamartomatous lesion
- Commonly multiple
- Usually located within the ventricular myocardium
- Rarely arises from the subendocardium; pedunculated mass invading the cavity (can result in obstruction)
- Presents in the prenatal or neonatal group with hydrops, arrhythmia, heart block, and retarded growth
- Natural history is of spontaneous regression; possibly due to resorption of glycogen stores and as such management is usually conservative with surgical resection being reserved for obstructive lesions

Fibroma

- Benign, low-grade, non-capsulated connective tissue tumours
- Account for around 20% of cardiac tumours in the paediatric population
- Usually present before the age of 15 with obstructive symptoms such as heart failure or re-entrant arrhythmia
- Firm, greyish tumours that can grow up to 10 cm in diameter
- Characteristic finding both to the naked eye and on echocardiography is the multiple foci of calcification

- Unlike many primary cardiac tumours, they have no evidence of cystic change, areas of haemorrhage or necrosis
- Seen as large, solid, non-contractive masses on echocardiography and as a homogenous mass with soft tissue attenuation on CT
- Usually intramural within the interventricular septum or ventricular free wall
- Commonly interfere with the conductive system causing AV block or SCD
- Fibromas with medically refractory arrhythmias or haemodynamically significant obstruction require surgery

Cystic tumour of the AV node
- Located in the triangle of Koch and can grow up to 2 cm in diameter
- Comprise multiple cysts filled with mucoid substance
- Through infiltration of the AV node, heart block and SCD can occur

Pericardial cyst
- Congenital pericardial cysts are uncommon
- Both unilocular and multilocular forms and a diameter up to 5 cm
- Most patients are asymptomatic when cysts are detected incidentally on chest radiographs usually at the right cardiophrenic angle
- When symptomatic, pericardial cysts can cause chest discomfort, dyspnoea, cough, or palpitations due to compression of cardiac chambers
- Diagnosis is through echocardiography, CT, or CMR
- Percutaneous aspiration and ethanol sclerosis may be performed
- Video-assisted thoracotomy or surgical resection may be necessary

5.4.5 Malignant tumours

Ten percent of primary cardiac tumours can be considered malignant, of which around 95% are sarcomas and 5% are lymphomas.

Angiosarcoma
- One-third of primary cardiac malignancies
- More common in men
- Peak incidence third to fifth decade
- Found almost exclusively in the right atrium, near the AV groove
- Asymptomatic until advanced
- Commonly present with complications of lung metastasis
- Other symptoms include fever, chest pain, weight loss, and haemorrhagic pericardial effusion
- Like its benign cousin, the angioma, appears as a highly vascular mass on angiography
- Appearance on CT and CMR is of an irregular, heterogenous mass with areas of haemorrhage and necrosis
- Gross appearance is a lobulated brown neoplasm
- Invades local structures: commonly the right atrial wall, pericardium, and IVC
- Two thirds are moderately well differentiated
- One third are poorly differentiated and appear as anaplastic spindle cells on histology
- Mean survival is 4 months without surgical resection. The benefit from adjuvant chemotherapy and/or radiotherapy is unclear

Rhabdomyosarcoma

- Second most common primary cardiac malignancy; still very rare
- Arise from and infiltrate the myocardium
- Rarely invade further than the parietal pericardium
- Usually of the embryological subtype comprising of mesenchymal cells with striated muscle differentiation
- Unlike other sarcomas, rhabdomyosarcoma usually present before the age of 20 with a male predominance
- Complete surgical resection is challenging. Chemotherapy may help in delaying tumour progression and radiotherapy may be useful pre and post-surgery

Fibrosarcoma

- Malignant proliferation of mesenchymal cells showing fibroblastic features
- Accounts for 5% of primary cardiac malignancies
- Usually left sided
- Can be mural or protrude into cavities
- Median survival is 5 months
- Complete surgical removal is challenging. Chemotherapy and radiotherapy may have a role in incomplete surgical resection

Cardiac lymphoma

- 10% of primary cardiac malignant tumours
- Can occur at any age; median age of presentation around 60 years
- Three times more common in males
- Presents abruptly with heart failure, arrhythmia, heart block, chest pain, superior vena caval obstruction, and pericardial effusion
- Most common location is the right atrial wall (two out of three cases); any chamber can be affected
- In 75% of cases more than one cavity wall is affected, including the pericardium
- 80% are B-cell with CD20-positive cells and 20% are T-cell with CD3-positive cells
- Gross appearance is of multiple firm, white nodular masses
- On CT and CMR can have a variable non-diagnostic morphology presenting as a mass or as infiltrative disease
- Biopsy is often required to confirm diagnosis, as pericardial fluid cytology is often negative
- Chemotherapy can lead to significant tumour regression although prognosis remains poor
- Significant mortality may be related to massive pulmonary emboli, refractory heart failure, and cardiac arrhythmias

Cardiac metastases

- Cardiac metastases were found in up to 25% of cases of metastatic disease in autopsy series
- Metastatic spread to the heart can be via four possible routes:
    - haematic spread
    - lymphatic spread
    - direct infiltration
    - transvenous extension
- Due to their incidence and location lung and breast carcinoma are the most common
- Primaries leading to cardiac metastases

- Around half the cases of metastatic melanoma involve the heart
- Solitary cardiac metastases are rare; usually small and multiple
- Myocardial involvement is usually a result of haematic spread
- Lymphatic spread typically results in pericardial disease and may result in large effusions and/or pericarditis
- A constrictive picture may persist following draining of an effusion due to thickening and reduced compliance of the pericardium
- Majority of cases clinically asymptomatic and are only discovered at autopsy
- Pericardial effusions, heart failure, or rhythm disturbances in known cases of metastatic disease suggest cardiac spread
- Treatment of cardiac metastases is focused on management of the primary cancer usually with a mix of chemotherapy and radiotherapy

5.5

Cardio-oncology

Arjun Ghosh

TABLE OF CONTENTS

5.5.1 Overview of cancer treatment cardiac side effects 527
　Anthracyclines 527
　Monoclonal antibodies 527
　Vascular endothelial growth factor (VEGF) signalling pathway inhibition 528
　Proteasome inhibitors 528
　Immune checkpoint inhibitors 528
　Fluoropyrimidines 530
5.5.2 Arrhythmias with cancer therapies 531
5.5.3 Cardiac side effects of radiotherapy 531
5.5.4 Pericardial effusions in cancer patients 532
5.5.5 Thrombotic and anticoagulation issues in cancer patients 532
　Central venous catheter associated complications 532
5.5.6 Cardiac assessment prior to the initiation of cardiotoxic treatment 533
5.5.7 Monitoring during cardiotoxic treatment 533
　Imaging in cardio-oncology 533
　Definitions of cardiotoxicity by echocardiography in patients receiving anthracyclines and/or trastuzumab 534
　Cardioprotection 534
　Late effects 535
5.5.8 The cardio-oncology multidisciplinary team (MDT) approach 535
　The ideal cardio-oncology service 535

5.5.1 Overview of cancer treatment cardiac side effects

Anthracyclines

See Box 5.5.1.

- Commonly used in treating solid tumours and in haematological malignancies
- Dose-related risk of left ventricular systolic dysfunction (LVSD) especially when lifetime dose exceeds 400 mg/m^2
- Acute toxicity (< 1% of patients) usually reversible on stopping infusion
- Early effects within first year
- Late effects at a median of 7 years
- If detected early and treated some potential for functional recovery

Monoclonal antibodies

- Trastuzumab, pertuzumab, and trastuzumab-emtansine (TDM1) have improved outcomes of breast cancer patients by inhibiting the human epidermal growth factor receptor 2 (HER2)
- High rate of cardiotoxicity when trastuzumab given concomitantly with anthracyclines; less LVSD when trastuzumab given after anthracyclines or when using an anthracycline-free regime
- Typically manifests during treatment

> **BOX 5.5.1 CANCER TREATMENT CARDIAC SIDE EFFECTS**
>
> **Chemotherapy and immunotherapy:**
>
> Heart failure, ischaemia, arrhythmias, myocarditis, pericardial effusions
>
> **Radiotherapy:**
>
> Coronary artery disease, valve disease, pericarditis, arrhythmias

- Usually reversible (potentially as cell death usually does not happen) on stopping treatment and initiating cardiac medications (ACE inhibition and beta blockade)
- Risk factors for cardiotoxicity include previous exposure to anthracyclines, short interval between anthracycline and trastuzumab therapy, hypertension, pre-existing LVSD, older age, obesity, and previous radiotherapy

Vascular endothelial growth factor (VEGF) signalling pathway inhibition

- VEGF inhibition used to treat many solid cancers
- Use after conventional chemotherapy increases risk (LVSD in 2% of patients exposed to bevacizumab after conventional chemotherapy)
- Risk of congestive heart failure increased nearly threefold with the use of VEGF receptor tyrosine kinase inhibitor (TKI) drugs like sunitinib, sorafenib, and ponatinib
- Off-target effects can lead to significant arterial hypertension which should be managed as per standard hypertension guidelines
- LVSD and hypertension can both be reversible if intensively treated

Proteasome inhibitors

- Significant risk of developing heart failure (HF) with irreversible proteasome inhibitor carfilzomib (up to 25%) which can manifest as acute pulmonary oedema
- 3% mortality in patients developing high-grade toxicity
- Increased risk of cardiotoxicity with increased duration of therapy and in those with previous cardiac disease
- Management is as per routine acute HF guidelines

Immune checkpoint inhibitors

- Have dramatically improved prognosis in cancers like melanoma
- Include Cytotoxic T-Lymphocyte Associated Protein 4 (CTLA-4) inhibitor ipilimumab and Programmed Cell Death Protein 1 (PD-1) and Programmed Death Ligand 1 (PD-L1) inhibitors nivolumab and pembrolizumab
- Associated with multiple cardiotoxicities—atrioventricular block, myocarditis, pericarditis, acute myocardial infarction, and non-inflammatory LVSD
- Risk of myocarditis is low as per registries (~1%) but may be fatal in up to 50% of cases
- CMR is diagnostic in 50% of cases and thus cardiac biopsy may be required in some cases
- Management involves anti- immune therapy, e.g. steroids, abatacept, mycophenolate mofetil, ruxolitinib, immunophoresis along with traditional HF therapy if LVSD present
- Normalization of troponin levels can take more than 1 year

Table 5.5.1 Mechanism of action, uses and cardiac side effects of common chemotherapeutic and immunotherapeutic agents.

Drug class	Mechanism of Action	Therapy area	Cardiac side effects
Cytotoxic agents			
Anthracyclines: doxorubicin, epirubicin, daunorubicin	Impair topoisomerase 2 beta, intercalate into nuclear DNA	Leukaemia, sarcoma, breast cancer	Dose dependent risk of left ventricular systolic dysfunction LVSD (1–48% depending upon agent, dose, and formulation)
Antimicrotubule agents (Taxanes): Paclitaxel, docetaxel	Polymerize tubulin impairing cell division	Breast and ovarian cancer	Up to 13% risk of LVSD
Antimetabolites (Fluoropyrimidines): 5-fluorouracil, capecitabine, gemcitabine	Bind to DNA and RNA causing apoptosis	Gastrointestinal cancers	Up to 20% risk of myocardial ischaemia
Platinum agents: cisplatin, carboplatin	Cross link to purine bases in DNA leading to apoptosis	Testicular, ovarian, and lung cancers	8% absolute risk over 20 years of myocardial ischaemia 2% risk of arterial thrombosis
Alkylating agents: cyclophosphamide, ifosfamide	Attachment of alkyl groups to DNA bases causing DNA fragmentation	Lymphoma, myeloma, sarcoma, breast, and lung cancers	Up to 28% risk of LVSD with cyclophosphamide and 17% with ifosfamide
Arsenic trioxide	Direct mitochondrial toxicity leading to apoptosis	Leukaemia	QT prolongation
Molecular-targeted therapy			
Monoclonal antibodies: trastuzumab, pertuzumab, TDM1	Humanized monoclonal antibody directed against HER2 protein	Breast cancer	Up to 20% risk of LVSD
Vascular endothelial growth factor (VEGF) inhibitors: • antibodies bevacizumab, ramucirumab • tyrosine kinase inhibitors sunitinib, pazopanib, sorafenib, dasatanib	Inhibit VEGF mediated tumour angiogenesis and stop protein activation by blocking signal transduction cascades	Breast, gastrointestinal, stromal, renal cancers, leukaemia, non-Hodgkin lymphoma	Arterial hypertension, thromboembolism, LVSD
Other tyrosine kinase inhibitors: Ibrutinib, nilotinib, lapatinib, imatinib	Inhibit B Cell Receptor (BCR) pathway signalling preventing overexpression of protein tyrosine kinases, e.g. BCR-ABL	Leukaemia, gastrointestinal stromal tumour	Atrial fibrillation, QT prolongation, hypertension

(continued)

Table 5.5.1 Continued

Drug class	Mechanism of Action	Therapy area	Cardiac side effects
Proteasome inhibitors: carfilzomib and bortezomib	Inhibit proteasome-mediated protein degradation resulting in inhibition of tumour growth	Myeloma	Up to 25% risk of LVSD with carfilzomib and up to 5% risk with bortezomib
Immune checkpoint inhibitor therapy: ipilimumab, nivolumab, pembrolizumab	Removes regulatory inhibition to body's T cells to allow an effective anti-tumour response	Melanoma, renal and lung cancers	Up to 2% risk of myocarditis
Other agents			
Anti-androgen therapy: goserelin, degarelix, abiraterone, bicalutamide	Modify effect of gonadotropin-releasing hormone or affect androgen receptor directly	Prostate cancer	Obesity, lipid profile abnormalities, metabolic syndrome, LVSD with abiraterone

Fluoropyrimidines

- Commonly used in the management of gastrointestinal cancers and in bladder, breast and head and neck cancers either as intravenous 5-fluorouracil (5-FU) or the oral prodrug capecitabine
- Cardiac toxicities manifest as chest pain (coronary spasm and myocardial infarction)
- Histopathological studies have demonstrated arterial cytolysis and denudation of the elastic lamina. Haemorrhagic infarction and fibrosis of the myocardium also seen
- Normal functional imaging, e.g. stress cardiac magnetic resonance (CMR) and coronary angiography do not indicate that patient will not have chest pain/coronary spasm/myocardial infarction
- Role of prophylactic vasodilators (nitrates, diltiazem) is unclear; no clear evidence that risk of cardiovascular events is diminished in this context
- In patients with high cardiovascular risk, e.g. known coronary artery disease with angina, alternative cancer treatment may be used such as raltitrexed

BOX 5.5.2 RISK FACTORS FOR POST-ANTHRACYCLINE CARDIOTOXICITY

- Cumulative dose
- Age (< 18 y and > 65 y)
- Female sex
- Concomitant or previous radiotherapy to a field including the heart
- Concomitant chemotherapy with monoclonal antibodies, targeted therapies, alkylating and antimicrotubule agents
- Pre-existing cardiac disease
- Hypertension
- Genetic predisposition

5.5.2 Arrhythmias with cancer therapies

Table 5.5.2 Arrhythmias with cancer therapies.

Class	ST	SB	AVB	AF	SVT	VT	TdP	SCD
Anthracyclines	+++	++	cr	+++	++	++	cr	+
Cyclophosphamide	+++	cr	cr	++	++	cr	-	-
Melphalan	cr	-	-	+++	++	cr	-	-
Arsenic trioxide	+++	-	cr	cr	-	+++	++	++
Antimetabolites								
Capectiabine	+++	++	cr	++	cr	cr	cr	+
5FU	cr	+++	cr	++	cr	++	cr	++
HER2 inhibitors								
Trastuzumab	cr	cr	-	-	-	cr	-	cr
Immune check point inhibitors								
Ipilimumab	-	-	-	cr	-	cr	-	cr
Tyrosine kinase inhibitors								
Ibrutinib	-	-	cr	++	-	cr	-	cr
Ponatinib	-	+	+	++	+	-	-	-
VEGF inhibitors								
Sunitinib	cr	cr	-	cr	-	-	+	cr

Key: – no data, + <1 %, ++ 1%–10%, +++ > 10%, 5-FU—5 fluorouracil, AF—atrial fibrillation, AVB—atrioventricular block, cr—case reports; HER2—human epidermal receptor 2, SB—sinus bradycardia, ST—sinus tachycardia, SVT—supraventricular tachycardia, TdP—Torsades de Pointes, VEGF—vascular endothelial growth factor, VT—ventricular tachycardia.

5.5.3 Cardiac side effects of radiotherapy

- Acute toxicity can manifest as an acute pericarditis
- More commonly effects are seen several years later
- Macrovascular injury accelerates age-related atherosclerosis leading to premature coronary artery disease (CAD)
- Microvascular injury causes myocardial ischaemia resulting in progressive myocardial fibrosis
- Microvascular injury also increases capillary permeability of the pericardium causing pericardial effusions and constriction
- Direct valvular injury (potentially due to endothelial injury) leading to leaflet thickening and fibrosis causing valvular regurgitation and/or stenosis
- Ultimately can result in HF from any of the above mechanisms
- Consider prior exposure to radiotherapy in patients presenting with premature CAD or valve disease

5.5.4 Pericardial effusions in cancer patients

- 5–15% of cancer patients have a malignant pericardial effusion and up to 7% have a non-malignant effusion
- Cancer metastasizing to the pericardium (e.g. breast, lung, Hodgkin lymphoma) can commonly cause pericardial effusion as can primary cardiac cancers (mesothelioma, sarcoma, and lymphoma)
- May present acutely following pericarditis or chronically
- Tamponade mandates urgent drainage
- Nonacute cases can be managed medically as they may respond to intensive chemotherapy and/or steroids
- Surgical drainage is preferred through the creation of a pericardial window and cancer-related effusions often recur and a surgical approach allows direct pericardial tissue biopsy for histology
- Pericardial sclerosis (using talc, bleomycin, etc.) is a painful procedure and can lead to pericardial constriction which can be very challenging to treat, and is thus not commonly undertaken

5.5.5 Thrombotic and anticoagulation issues in cancer patients

- Cancer itself is a pro-thrombotic state increasing the risk of arterial and venous thromboembolism (VTE)
- Increased risk of bleeding events due to low blood counts and cancer-related coagulopathy
- A number of drugs are associated with increased risk of atrial arrhythmias (see Table 5.5.2)
- Traditional risk scores (CHA$_2$DS$_2$-VASc) should be applied to determine individual stroke risk in cancer patients with AF together with cancer and therapy-specific factors
- Cancer treatments also increase arterial and venous thromboembolic risk, e.g. platinum agents, hormonal therapy, anti-VEGF therapy, proteasome inhibitors, and immunomodulators (thalidomide and lenalidomide)
- Several clinical trials are ongoing directly comparing the efficacy of direct oral anticoagulants (DOACs) with low molecular weight heparin (LMWH) in the management of VTE in cancer patients
- Currently LMWH remains the standard of care in treating cancer-associated VTE
- Thrombocytopaenia can be a concern in cancer patients presenting with acute coronary syndromes.
- An individualized approach needs to be taken when deciding on choice of intervention (balloon angioplasty versus bare metal stent versus drug-eluting stent). Some newer generation stents allow shorter durations of dual antiplatelet therapy (DAPT)
- Cancer surgery for patients on warfarin for metal valves is challenging. An individualized approach in a multidisciplinary team (MDT) setting is required to bring together the views of the Surgeon, Oncologist, Cardiologist, Thrombosis Specialist and patient.

Central venous catheter associated complications

- Central venous catheters (CVCs) account for 70% of cancer-associated upper extremity deep vein thromboses (DVTs)
- Current guidelines for CVC-associated DVTs in cancer patients recommend treatment with LMWH bridged to warfarin or LMWH monotherapy for ≥ 12 weeks without removal of the catheter (unless defective, non-functional, or infective)

- Randomized controlled trials (RCTs) assessing the role of inferior vena cava filter placement are lacking
- Thrombus on the tip of a CVC may require prolonged anticoagulation and may not resolve without line removal

5.5.6 Cardiac assessment prior to the initiation of cardiotoxic treatment

- Assess cardiac risk factors at baseline (structural heart disease, CAD, arrhythmias, extreme of age, family history of premature CAD, hypertension, diabetes mellitus, hypercholesterolaemia, smoking status, obesity, alcohol excess, sedentary lifestyle)
- Different risk scores exist for oncology cohorts, but none has been prospectively validated
- Baseline echocardiography and biomarkers e.g. troponin and NT-pro brain natriuretic peptide (NT-pro BNP) may be useful if serial monitoring will be performed (usually in high-risk individuals)
- Identify patients with high risk of development of cardiotoxicity with anthracyclines or anti-HER2 receptor therapy based on presence of risk factors as detailed in Box 5.5.2 and in 'monoclonal antibody' section

5.5.7 Monitoring during cardiotoxic treatment

- Imaging and biomarker assessments are currently the main methods used to monitor patients on cardiotoxic treatment
- Echocardiographic assessment is ideally recommended at baseline in all patients proposed to have cardiotoxic chemotherapy
- If left ventricular ejection fraction (LVEF; ideally measured by the reproducible 3-dimensional assessment) is impaired and/or the global longitudinal strain (GLS) is less than the lower limit of normal for the institution (GLS values are machine and analysis software dependent) and/or troponin is elevated cardiology review (ideally by a cardio-oncologist) is recommended
- If the tests are normal follow-up assessments are recommended at completion of therapy and 6 months later for doses < 240 mg/m^2 of doxorubicin. If this dose is exceeded, measurements are recommended before each additional 50 mg/m^2
- All patients on trastuzumab are recommended to have similar assessments at baseline and at every 3 months during therapy
- The role of other biomarkers (NT-pro BNP, C-reactive protein, myeloperoxidase) is unclear in terms of timing of assessment and as yet there is no consensus on the appropriate modification of therapy in response to abnormal results

Imaging in cardio-oncology

- Echocardiography is the mainstay due to easy accessibility, portability, and cost. Echocardiography also has the ability to fully assess cardiac function (systolic and diastolic), regional wall motion abnormalities, valvular heart disease, and pericardial abnormalities
- LVEF is insufficient as a single measure of LVSD as it is a 'late' change
- LVEF is a composite measure produced by the contraction or circumferential, radial, and longitudinal cardiac muscle fibres. Abnormal contraction is often seen first in longitudinal fibres

as they are most distant from their blood supply. Abnormal contraction in longitudinal fibres can be compensated for by increased contraction in circumferential and radial cardiac fibres providing false reassurance due to a 'stable' LVEF on serial imaging
- GLS can identify this 'early' abnormality in longitudinal fibre function even while LVEF remains 'stable'
- Abnormal GLS is a marker of early cardiotoxicity and may be able to identify an optimal time to intervene with cardioprotection
- CMR can be useful if echocardiographic windows are poor. CMR can additionally identify other cardiotoxicities, e.g. myocarditis, pericardial complications, etc.
- Cardiac computed tomography (CT) can be used to image the coronary arteries in patients with previous radiotherapy or in patients with chest pain on fluoropyridine therapy. Cardiac CT can also be diagnostic in cancer treatment-related pericardial complications
- Nuclear multigated acquisition (MUGA) scans can be used to quantify LVEF. They however expose the patient to further radiation (especially if serial measures of LVEF required) and do not provide ancillary evidence

Definitions of cardiotoxicity by echocardiography in patients receiving anthracyclines and/or trastuzumab

- ASE/EACVI: ≥ 10% drop in LVEF to a value < 53%; > 15% fall in global longitudinal strain (GLS)
- BSE/BCOS (Table 5.5.3)

Cardioprotection

- There are some emerging RCT data regarding the cardioprotective role of angiotensin converting enzyme (ACE) inhibitors, angiotensin receptor blockers (ARBs), and beta blockers (BBs) on preventing systolic and diastolic LV dysfunction prophylactically in cancer patients proposed for cardiotoxic therapies
- Currently the evidence base is not compelling enough to recommend universal cardioprotection with ACE inhibitors/ARBs and BBs
- An individualized approach is required to identify those at highest risk of cardiotoxicity to follow them closely and identify subclinical toxicity (i.e. abnormal GLS and fall in LVEF but to a value above normal ranges without symptoms or signs of HF) at the earliest stage
- The use of prophylactic cardioprotection on the identification of subclinical disease is less well established and is currently the focus of RCTs. An individualized approach in an MDT setting is strongly recommended

Table 5.5.3 BSE/ BCOS echocardiographic definitions of cardiotoxicity.

Definition of cardiotoxicity
LVEF: A decrease in LVEF by > 10 percentage points to a value < 50%
Definition of potential cardiotoxicity by echocardiography
LVEF: A decrease in LVEF by > 10 percentage points to a value ≥ 50% with an accompanying fall in GLS > 15% (where GLS measurement available)
LVEF: A decrease in LVEF by < 10 percentage points to a value < 50%
LV GLS: When LVEF ≥ 50%, a *relative* percentage reduction in GLS by > 15%

- Dexrazoxane may be considered in those exposed to significant anthracycline doses to decrease risk of cardiotoxicity and is often used in the management of children and young adults with sarcoma

Late effects
- A variety of cardiac complications of cancer therapies are seen many years after completion of cancer treatment
- Anthracycline cardiotoxicity is seen at a median of 7 years after completion of treatment
- Radiotherapy-related side effects are usually seen many years after treatment and can be seen even 30 years after treatment
- Survivors of childhood cancer are often lost to follow-up once they reach adulthood or have no suitable local service at which they can be followed up
- Teenage and Young Adult (TYA) cancer patients present a unique group as their post-treatment follow up can vary widely depending upon geography and links between paediatric and adult services
- The timing, duration, and components of late effects reviews remain unclear

5.5.8 The cardio-oncology multidisciplinary team (MDT) approach

- The MDT approach is well established in cardiology
- The MDT meeting is an essential component of any cardio-oncology service given the lack of consensus/guidelines for many cardiac issues affecting cancer patients and the developing evidence base
- An individualized approach is needed for many patients best obtained in an MDT setting
- The MDT involves Oncologists (medical, clinical, and haemato-oncologists), specialist nurses, physiologists, and ideally patient advocates. A variety of Cardiologists are required for optimal decision-making (i.e. imaging, interventional, heart failure, and electrophysiology specialists) due to the multifaceted cardiac manifestations of cardiotoxicity

The ideal cardio-oncology service
- Clinics should be rapidly accessible to minimize delays to the initiation of cancer treatment and to minimize suspensions of cancer treatment
- Cancer patients have to attend hospital frequently for a variety of cancer investigation and treatment appointments. Minimizing hospital visits by combining cardiology and oncology reviews can greatly help in this very difficult time
- A one-stop approach with clinical assessment, advanced imaging (advanced echocardiography and CMR), blood tests etc. on the day allows rapid formulation of the management plan
- Clinical and research database creation is essential to develop a better understanding of different cardiotoxicities
- Excellent lines of communication with oncology colleagues required
- Education and research are key components of this new and rapidly expanding subspecialty in cardiology

---
CHAPTER 6

ACUTE CARDIOVASCULAR CARE

6.1 Acute cardiovascular care

Ben Gibbison and Ursula McHugh

TABLE OF CONTENTS
- 6.1.1 Introduction 539
- 6.1.2 Assessment 540
  - Laboratory investigations 541
  - Recognizing the deteriorating patient 541
- 6.1.3 Post cardiac surgery management 541
  - Temperature management and warming 541
- 6.1.4 Respiratory issues 542
  - Respiratory failure 542
  - Oxygenation and ventilatory support 542
  - Ventilation 543
  - Following extubation 545
- 6.1.5 Cardiovascular issues 546
  - Haemodynamics 546
  - Left ventricular dysfunction 547
  - Right ventricular dysfunction 548
  - Hypotension 549
  - Tamponade 551
- Hypertension 552
- Pacing in the cardiac surgical population 552
- 6.1.6 Renal issues 553
- 6.1.7 Neurological issues 555
  - Delirium 555
  - Post cardiac arrest brain injury 556
  - Post-operative cognitive dysfunction 557
  - Stroke 557
- 6.1.8 Analgesia 558
- 6.1.9 Haematological issues 559
- 6.1.10 Gastrointestinal issues 562
- 6.1.11 Infective issues 564
  - Surgical site infection 564
- 6.1.12 Discharge from intensive care 565
- 6.1.13 Communication, palliation, and end-of-life care 566

6.1.1 Introduction

- Acute cardiovascular care represents the interface of cardiology, cardiac surgery, and critical care medicine. Two distinct groups of patients should be considered—acutely ill patients with cardiac pathology who have decompensated and require intensive care management and patients who require intensive care management following cardiac procedures.

Medical patients
- A broad range of illnesses are treated, but the majority of these patients are post acute coronary syndrome, post cardiac arrest, or have been identified in a peri-arrest situation and require organ support with ongoing management of the underlying cause.
- While this group of patients may appear to be heterogeneous, the treatment goals are similar and the supportive interventions required are often common to many. A systematic approach can improve survival and decrease morbidity.

Surgical patients
- A wide range of procedures are performed, however again the needs of the majority of cardiac surgical patients are similar and the aims of management are universal.

- Consequently, it is possible to implement protocols that can allow streamlined management under the care of cardiac intensive care nursing staff, guided by doctors.
- The critical care destination of surgical patients varies between centres and may be:
    - A dedicated cardiac intensive care unit
    - A general intensive care unit with capability to manage cardiac patients
    - An intermediate high acuity recovery unit designed for fast-track recovery of uncomplicated patients with good ventricular function

Management

- This section will discuss the specific aspects of management of medical and surgical patients and the organ support mechanisms common to both groups.

6.1.2 Assessment

- Cardiac critical care patients should be assessed and managed in a similar way to all critical care patients. A systematic, organ-based approach is appropriate. (Table 6.1.1)
- Outcomes in intensive care have improved through the use of 'care bundles'. These are lists designed to make sure that vital aspects of routine ICU care are addressed. The 'FAST HUG' mnemonic is a useful tool to ensure that several important factors are not forgotten:
    - Feeding
    - Analgesia
    - Sedation
    - Thromboprophylaxis
    - Head-of-bed angle sitting up at 30°
    - Ulcer prophylaxis
    - Glucose control

Table 6.1.1 Assessment of cardiac critical care patients.

SYSTEM	ISSUES
Airway	Patient's own/endotracheal tube/tracheostomy
Respiratory	Mode of ventilation/blood gases/chest examination/*in situ* drains
Cardiovascular	Cardiovascular observations/inotropes/vasopressors/cardiac output measurements/echocardiography examinations
Renal	Serum creatinine/fluid balance/electrolytes
Neurology	Neurological function/analgesia
Gastrointestinal	Abdominal examination/gastrointestinal tract function/feeding mode/glucose control
Haematology	Haemoglobin/clotting tests
Infection	Temperature/inflammatory markers/antimicrobials
Drugs	Drug review/reconciliation
Laboratory results	Latest results
Imaging	Recent imaging results

Laboratory investigations

- On arrival in the intensive care unit (ICU), all patients should have baseline investigations performed:
  - Full blood count
  - Renal profile
  - Coagulation profile
  - Arterial blood gas
  - 12-lead ECG
- In addition, any specific investigations indicated by the underlying pathology should be considered.

Recognizing the deteriorating patient

- A gradual decline in physiological parameters occurs prior to cardiac arrest and recognizing deterioration in the clinical condition of a patient is key to ensuring early intervention, which can improve survival and reduce morbidity.
- The parameters which are most useful are:
  - Level of consciousness
  - Heart rate
  - Respiratory rate
  - Systolic blood pressure
  - Oxygen saturation
  - Temperature
  - Urine output
  - Biochemical analysis
- Early Warning Scores (EWS) are used internationally as part of track and trigger systems designed to identify patients who are becoming critically unwell. These highlight patients who require more senior medical input and may require escalation to intensive care management.

6.1.3 Post cardiac surgery management

- The majority of patients will follow a predictable pattern of events post-operatively.
- At all stages in this process there should be ongoing intensive care nursing and regular review by medical staff (Table 6.1.2).

Temperature management and warming

- Hypothermia is often employed in the operating theatre to facilitate organ protection whilst on cardiopulmonary bypass (CPB). The level to which the body is cooled to depends on the operative procedure and the surgical approach required. Most cases require a temperature of 32–36°C, but in true circulatory arrest this may be as low as 18°C.
- Complications of hypothermia include:
  - Coagulopathy
  - Myocardial infarction
  - Impaired wound healing
  - Hypokalaemia
  - Pain
  - Altered drug pharmacology

Table 6.1.2 Time course.

Time	Events
0 hrs	Admit to intensive care unit Full set of laboratory investigations and ABG
Within 3 hrs	Warm to 36.5°C
Within 6 hrs	Ensure adequate analgesia Wean ventilatory support Extubate
Overnight	Wean vasoactive and inotropic drugs Trial of oral intake as tolerated
Day 1 post-op morning	Multidisciplinary team ward round Review and remove drains Remove pulmonary artery catheter Remove arterial line
Day 1 post-op afternoon	Transfer to ward or high-dependency unit Review by physiotherapy

- These are clearly undesirable in a post-operative patient. Although care is taken to actively warm patients, maintenance of normothermia in the operating theatre can be challenging. If the temperature is low on arrival in ICU, this must be returned to normal prior to waking and extubation.
- Patients can be actively warmed in ICU using a variety of methods, including:
  - Warmed intravenous fluids
  - Warming mattresses
  - Forced air warming blanket
  - Warmed and humidified ventilator gases
- Rewarming may cause significant vasodilatation. This may require vasopressor support in the early post-operative period.

6.1.4 Respiratory issues

Respiratory failure

- The most common causes of respiratory failure in acute cardiac and cardiac surgical patients are:
  - Atelectasis
  - Pneumonia
  - Pneumothorax
  - Bronchospasm
  - Pulmonary embolism
  - Acute Respiratory Distress Syndrome
- Treatment required and the ventilation strategies used vary with the pathology and thus a diagnosis is needed to ensure an individualized management plan can be formulated for each patient.

Oxygenation and ventilatory support

- When respiratory failure occurs, management is aimed at ensuring adequate oxygenation and carbon dioxide removal.

- Patients are often started on supplemental oxygen therapy via nasal prongs or facemask.
- If this is not sufficient, increased support is provided in a stepwise fashion.

Non-invasive ventilation
- Non-invasive ventilation (NIV) is used to treat atelectasis and respiratory failure.
- It may be employed either as Continuous Positive Airway Pressure (CPAP) or BiLevel Positive Airway Pressure (BiPAP), depending on the ventilatory needs of the patient.
- NIV improves lung volumes by opening areas of atelectasis, increases alveolar ventilation, and reduces the work of breathing.
- It also has positive effects on the cardiovascular system, as it reduces left ventricular afterload and thus improves cardiac output.
- It is contraindicated in those with pneumothoraces and broncho-pleural fistula.

High-flow nasal oxygen
- High-flow nasal oxygen therapy has been demonstrated as non-inferior to non-invasive ventilation in cardiac patients post-operatively and should be considered as a useful alternative treatment modality.
- High flow rates of oxygen applied through the nose result in low levels (< 5 cmH2O PEEP) of positive pressure in the upper airways.
- In addition, it is postulated that the high flow rates cause a reduction in physiological dead space by forcing expired carbon dioxide out from the upper airways and thus contribute to a reduction in the work of breathing.
- Often the use of this device is more comfortable for patients and may result in improved compliance.

Mechanical ventilation
- If non-invasive measures fail, mechanical ventilation may be necessary.
- This will require intubation and management of the underlying cause.
- Of note, the majority of patients undergoing cardiac surgery return to the ICU intubated and ventilated.

Extra-corporeal membrane oxygenation (ECMO)
- This is an advanced technique used to manage patients with respiratory failure refractory to usual interventions and is undertaken in specialist centres.
- There are two modalities:
    - VV–ECMO—Veno-venous ECMO provides oxygenation only
    - VA–ECMO—Veno-arterial ECMO provides mechanical circulatory support

Ventilation
- Lung protective ventilation should be employed if possible. This comprises:
    1. Limiting tidal volumes (5–7 mls/kg of ideal body weight)
    2. Limiting end-inspiratory plateau pressure (< 35 cmH2O)
    3. Ensuring adequate positive end expiratory pressure (PEEP)
    4. Limiting FiO2
- While the benefit to patients without lung pathology remains uncertain, multiple studies suggest that high tidal volumes may have negative effects on all patients and therefore should be avoided. The negative effects include organ failure, multiple organ failure, and prolonged intensive care unit stay.

- Women and obese patients are at higher risk of receiving high tidal volumes, therefore great caution should be taken with higher tidal volumes in these groups.

Ventilator settings
- Ideal body weight should be used for all calculations.
- Any ventilator mode may be used. There is there is no convincing evidence that any mode is superior, however this remains under investigation.
- Aim for a tidal volume of 5–7 mls/kg.
- Set a respiratory rate to achieve optimal minute ventilation (not > 30/min).
- Aim for oxygen saturations in the pre-operative range for the patient.
- Many of the lung-protective ventilation strategies were developed for use in a cohort of patients with acute respiratory distress syndrome (ARDS). These may not be appropriate for patients with significant cardiac dysfunction or those with normal function in the immediate post cardiac surgery period.
- Causes of hypoxia in cardiac patients are more likely to be poor cardiac output, right ventricular dysfunction and intra-cardiac shunts. High PEEP, low FiO2 and permissive hypercapnia may therefore not be appropriate. The key is to make a diagnosis and respond with appropriate ventilator settings.

Weaning and assessing for extubation
- Appropriately timed extubation is important to avoid the potential complications of prolonged tracheal intubation and ventilation. The major concern is infection from bypassing the normal protective mechanisms of the respiratory tract—nasal hairs, respiratory cilia and mucus escalator, and adequate cough.
- Successful extubation necessitates that both the cardiovascular and respiratory systems are functioning adequately. The change from assisted to self-ventilation may raise cardiac output demand by 30%.
- Early extubation also has cost benefits and improves resource utilization.

Spontaneous breathing trial
- When the following parameters have been achieved it is appropriate to perform a spontaneous breathing trial:
    - Temperature > 36.5°C
    - All neuromuscular blockade ceased and sedation off
    - Adequate analgesia given
    - Minimal vasopressor or inotropic support
    - Electrolyte and metabolic data normal
    - Chest drain output < 100 ml/hr for two consecutive hours
    - FiO2 ≤ 0.40 and PEEP ≤ 8 OR FiO2 ≤ 0.50 and PEEP ≤ 5
    - Patient has acceptable spontaneous breathing effort
- A spontaneous breathing trial is performed in the following manner:
    1. Place on a T-piece or CPAP/PS mode with PEEP ≤ 5 cmH2O with PS < 10 cmH2O
    2. Assess for tolerance, which is indicated by the following:
        - SpO2 maintained at appropriate level for patient
        - Spontaneous VT ≥ 4 ml/kg
        - RR ≤ 35/min
        - ABG acceptable with pH ≥ 7.35, paO2 ≥ 90 mmHg, paCO 35–40 mmHg, BE –3–3
        - No respiratory distress

3. If tolerated for at least 30 minutes, consider extubation
4. If not tolerated resume pre-weaning settings

Rapid Shallow Breathing Index
- The rapid shallow breathing index (RSBI) may also be used to determine suitability for extubation and has been found to aid early extubation in cardiac surgery patients.
- This is defined as the ratio of respiratory frequency to tidal volume in litres (f/VT) when breathing with no support.
- A value of > 105 breaths/min/L is highly predictive of weaning failure, while a value of < 105 breaths/min/L is associated with weaning success.
- For example, in a patient with a RR 30 and VT 300 mls, the RSBI = 30 bpm/0.3L = 100

Following extubation
- Patients should be continued on supplemental humidified oxygen therapy via a facemask and titrated to oxygenation.
- Oxygen should be continued for 24–48 hrs post-operatively to ensure desaturation does not occur. In patients with normal pre-operative oxygenation saturation levels, a target of ≥ 94% should be set. For patients with respiratory co-morbidities or intra-cardiac shunts, this target should be individualized.
- There is some evidence that in patients with a high risk of re-intubation, extubation to mask CPAP can reduce this risk, thus it is a useful tool to aid weaning from invasive ventilation.
- Physiotherapy is invaluable in ensuring patients adequately recover respiratory function and should be instituted early in any patient who has known respiratory pathology or who appears to be developing compromise.

Prolonged ventilation
- While the majority of cardiac surgery patients are successfully extubated along a fast-track route, some require a longer period of ventilation.
- Predictors of the need for prolonged ventilation (> 48 hrs) in the cardiac surgical population are:
    - Female patients
    - Hypertension
    - Chronic obstructive pulmonary disease
    - Chronic kidney disease
    - History of endocarditis
    - Valve surgery
    - Prolonged surgical or cardiopulmonary bypass time
    - Need for transfusion
    - Post-operative bleeding
    - Need for inotropes

Failed extubation
- Reintubation (or 'failed extubation') is associated with a significant increase in morbidity—a significant component of this is likely to be correlation rather than causation. This prolongs the length of mechanical ventilation and is associated with prolonged ICU and hospital stays.
- Factors which predict failed extubation are:
    - Patient factors:
        - Age over 65 years
        - Being an inpatient pre-operatively

- Arterial vascular disease
- Congestive heart failure
- Procedural factors:
  - Redo surgery
  - Procedures on thoracic aorta
  - Massive transfusion of > 10 units of red blood cells
  - Prolonged cardiopulmonary bypass time (> 120 mins)
- Respiratory factors:
  - Chronic obstructive pulmonary disease and severity of this
- Cardiac factors:
  - Severe left ventricular dysfunction, with lower pre-operative and post-operative ejection fraction
  - Valvular disease
  - Arrhythmia
  - Post-operative intra-aortic balloon pump requirement
  - Post-operative inotrope requirement
- Laboratory values:
  - Haematocrit < 35
  - Serum albumin concentration of < 40.0 g/L
- Other:
  - Renal failure
  - Positive fluid balance at 24 hrs

6.1.5 Cardiovascular issues

Haemodynamics

- Following a large cardiac insult (ACS, cardiopulmonary arrest, or cardiac surgery), cardiovascular management is focused on optimizing organ perfusion, thereby enabling oxygen delivery to the essential tissues, particularly the heart and brain.

Haemodynamic assessment

CARDIAC OUTPUT = HEART RATE × STROKE VOLUME

- left ventricular (LV) function
  - Pre-load
  - Contractility
  - Afterload
- right ventricular (RV) function
- heart rate and rhythm
- oxygen-carrying capacity of the blood
- vasoactive/inotropic medications

Peri-operative considerations

- Myocardial function (systolic and diastolic) is a critical factor in determining the success of recovery post cardiac surgery.
- In patients undergoing cardiac surgery there is a temporary decline in left ventricular function post-operatively.

- In those with normal pre-operative function, this reaches its lowest point at 24 hours post-operatively and returns to its pre-operative level by 1 week.
- In patients with pre-operative ventricular dysfunction, this decline is more pronounced, occurs later in the post-operative course and takes longer to recover, sometimes not returning to the pre-operative status.

Left ventricular dysfunction
Pre-load
- Pre-load is the mechanical state of the heart at the end of diastole—the degree of myocardial distension prior to shortening.
- Volume status can be optimized by ensuring adequate intra-vascular filling.
- Volume status in acute cardiac patients is difficult to determine using single haemodynamic parameters and a global assessment should be made of the patient. Measurements such as blood pressure, heart rate, central venous pressure, cardiac output, pulmonary capillary wedge pressure, pulse contour analysis, and urine output should be considered.
- In non-surgical patients the picture is complicated. Factors such as dehydration, poor nutritional status, intravenous fluid resuscitation, cardiac failure, oedema development, and diuretic therapy all mean that intravascular volume status is difficult to ascertain.
- In surgical patients an awareness of the peri-operative fluid balance is important but can also often be difficult to assess as fluid alterations in theatre can be challenging to determine.
- The use of dynamic assessments such as a passive leg raise test is beneficial.
- Echocardiography is also useful in this circumstance.

Contractility
- Contractility is the intrinsic ability of the myocardium to contract.
- Cardiac arrest will inevitably impact on contractility.
- In the context of cardiac surgery, patients with impaired contractility pre-operatively are at higher risk of post-operative impairment.
- Causes of impaired contractility post-operatively include:
  - Long cardiopulmonary bypass time
  - Tamponade
  - Arrhythmia
  - Graft occlusion
  - Graft spasm
- Again echocardiography is a valuable assessment tool.
- Treatment strategies for poor contractility include:
  - Reversing the precipitating cause if possible, e.g. ischaemia
  - Inotropes
  - Mechanical circulatory support
    - Intra-aortic balloon pump
    - Ventricular assist device
    - Extra-corporeal membrane oxygenation
- Heart transplantation

Afterload
- Afterload is the work done by the heart after the aortic valve has opened.

- In the cardiac population there are other causes rather than just raised systemic vascular resistance:
  - Vasoconstriction
  - Patient-prosthesis mismatch
  - Residual aortic stenosis
  - Repairing or replacing a previously incompetent valve
  - Systolic anterior motion (SAM) of the mitral valve
  - Excessive vasopressor use
  - Hypertension

Right ventricular dysfunction
Causes
- RV dysfunction may occur directly because of RV infarction or secondary to either volume or pressure overloading. The thin-walled RV is tolerant of volume loading, but very intolerant of pressure loading.

Volume overload
- Excess fluid administration or excess transfusion
- Tricuspid regurgitation
- Pulmonary regurgitation
- Atrial septal defect

Pressure overload
- Pulmonary hypertension
- Pulmonary embolus
- Left ventricular failure
- Excessive vasoconstrictor use
- Pulmonary stenosis
- Intrinsic pulmonary pathology
- Raised pulmonary vascular resistance (hypoxia, hypercarbia, acidosis, excess PEEP)

Diagnosis
- Cardiogenic shock develops, with hypotension and reduced cardiac output, and the central venous pressure (CVP) usually rises.
- Echocardiography is useful to confirm the diagnosis

Management
- Identify and treat any reversible causes.
- Management principles are mainly supportive.
- Aim for sinus rhythm and AV synchrony, with a rate of 80–100 bpm.
- Optimize RV pre-load by ensuring optimal fluid resuscitation. Echocardiography is invaluable, however remember that a non-functioning RV will not deliver volume to the LV and the LV can often look 'empty'. Excessive fluid loading is poorly tolerated.
- Maintain RV perfusion pressure. The higher wall tension requires higher systemic blood pressure to maintain right coronary artery perfusion. Noradrenaline and vasopressin are the mainstays of treatment. An intra-aortic balloon pump is useful, although not specifically indicated for the treatment of RV dysfunction.

- Maintain RV contractility. There is little extra contractility to be gained by augmenting contractility per se as the RV wall is thin with smaller amounts of contractile fibres. Inodilators, particularly the phosphodiesterase inhibitors enoximone and milrinone, provide contractility and pulmonary vasodilation.
- Reduce RV afterload. Avoid factors which trigger raised pulmonary vascular resistance, such as hypoxia, hypercarbia, and acidosis. Ventilator settings should be altered to reduce PEEP and avoid over inflation.
- Specific therapies to reduce RV afterload are nitric oxide, prostacyclin, and sildenafil. Inhaled preparations may avoid systemic effects.
- Acute right ventricular dysfunction following cardiac surgery is a major contributor to morbidity and mortality and is a difficult clinical situation to manage.

Hypotension

- Hypotension is a common problem in acute cardiac patients and should be managed as dictated by the findings of a thorough clinical assessment considering all the factors outlined above.
- Often the cause is a combination of:
- Reduced pre-load
- Reduced contractility
- Vasodilatation due to reduced vasomotor tone
- The target MAP is generally 65–70 mmHg, taking into consideration renal and cerebral auto-regulatory limits. In some patients a higher or lower limit may be considered.

Fluid management

- The choice of resuscitation fluid remains a subject of ongoing debate.
- Crystalloid is generally the first choice unless there is a specific indication for colloid, in which case blood and human albumin solution are the only choices. Synthetic colloid use has reduced in recent years due to concerns over renal toxicity.

Vasoactive medications

- The term 'vasoactive medications' is used to describe drugs which have variable effects on cardiac contractility and peripheral vasculature. These are often separated into inotropes and vasopressors and are commonly used in the management of in cardiac intensive care and cardiac surgery patients.
- The evidence for the use of one medication above the others is not satisfactory and despite significant investigation, relatively few conclusions or guidelines have been drawn.
- In practice the drugs are often used in combination in order to maximize effect and offset unwanted side effects.

Inotropes

- Inotropes (Table 6.1.3) alter the force of contraction of cardiac muscle without changing pre-load or afterload and should be considered where there is impaired contractility.
- Common drugs in use are:
    - Adrenergic agonists: dobutamine, dopamine, adrenaline
    - Phosphodiesterase inhibitors: enoximone, milrinone
    - Calcium sensitisers: levosimendan

Vasopressors

Table 6.1.3 Inotropes.

Drug	Dose	Mechanism of Action	Clinical Effects	Side Effects
Dobutamine	Infusion 5–10 mcg/kg/min	Direct stimulation of β receptors ($\beta_1 > \beta_2$)	Increased contractility Increased cardiac output Increased heart rate Decreased systemic vascular resistance 'Inodilator'	Arrhythmias Hypoglycaemia
Dopamine	Infusion Low dose 0.5–3 mcg/kg/min Intermediate dose 3–10 mcg/kg/min High dose 10–20 mcg/kg/min	Direct stimulation of dopaminergic D1 and D2 receptors Weak stimulation of β_1 receptors Stimulation of α_1 receptors	Increased renal blood flow Increased contractility Increased cardiac output Increased heart rate Increased coronary artery blood flow Increased systemic vascular resistance	Arrhythmias Nausea Vomiting Dyskinesia
Adrenaline	Infusion 0.1–0.5 mcg/kg/min	Stimulation of α and β receptors	Increased contractility Increased cardiac output Coronary artery vasodilatation Increased systemic vascular resistance	Increased blood glucose Increased lactate Increased coagulability
Enoximone	Loading infusion 0.5–1.0 mg/kg (over 10–30 mins) Infusion 5–20 mcg/kg/min	Phosphodiesterase inhibitor - PDE IV - PDE III	Increased contractility Decreased systemic vascular resistance	Requires dedicated infusion line
Milrinone	Loading infusion 50 mcg/kg (over 30 mins) Infusion 0.5 mcg/kg/min	Phosphodiesterase inhibitor - PDE III	Increased contractility Increased cardiac index Decreased pulmonary vascular resistance Decreased systemic vascular resistance No increase in oxygen consumption	Ventricular ectopics Angina
Levosimendan	Loading infusion 6–12 mcg/kg (over 10 mins) Infusion 0.05–0.2 mcg/kg/min Given for 24 hrs only	Calcium sensitization	Increased contractility Increased cardiac index Decreased pulmonary vascular resistance Decreased systemic vascular resistance No increase in oxygen consumption	Arrhythmias Headache

Table 6.1.4 Vasopressors.

Drug	Dose	Mechanism of Action	Clinical Effects	Side Effects
Noradrenaline	Infusion 0.1–0.5 mcg/kg/min	Stimulation of α and β receptors	Increased systemic vascular resistance Increased myocardial oxygen consumption Coronary artery vasodilatation	Peripheral vasoconstriction Increased pulmonary vascular resistance Bradycardia
Vasopressin	Infusion 0.01–0.1 Units/min	Stimulation of V1, V2 and V3 receptors	Increased systemic vascular resistance	Increased pulmonary artery pressure Increased coagulability
Adrenaline	See above			

- Vasopressors (Table 6.1.4) cause vasoconstriction and should be considered where decreased vascular tone is a concern. They may also be required to counteract the vasodilatory effect of some inotropes.
- The main drugs in use are:
  - Noradrenaline
  - Vasopressin
  - Adrenaline

Other interventions

- In situations of severe hypotension secondary to cardiogenic shock unresponsive to the above management, an intra-aortic balloon may be considered to provide mechanical assistance.
- Mechanical circulatory support using ventricular assist devices and VA-ECMO can also be considered.

Tamponade

- The incidence of pericardial tamponade after cardiac surgery varies greatly depending on the surgical procedure performed, with coronary artery bypass graft having the lowest (0.2%) and heart transplant the highest (8.4%).
- It most commonly occurs rapidly in the first 24 hours post-op but can develop sub-acutely in the first seven days. Beyond 7 days it is described as late tamponade.

Clinical features

- Haemodynamic instability—hypotension and tachycardia
- Raised CVP
- Muffled heart sounds
- Chest pain
- Dyspnoea
- Orthopnoea

Diagnosis

- A high degree of clinical suspicion is needed in all cardiac surgery patients. Small volumes of blood on low pressure chambers can prevent cardiac filling and lead to tamponade physiology.
- Echocardiography is useful. However, a negative study should not prevent re-exploration.

Management

- Surgical management is the definitive treatment.
- The overall aims are maintenance of cardiac output until the source of the bleeding is identified and controlled.
- Fluid resuscitation, blood product transfusion, vasopressor and inotropic support are likely to be necessary to control the situation.
- Percutaneous drainage is not indicated due to the localized, clotted nature of the blood. In addition, sources of bleeding cannot be controlled using percutaneous devices.

Hypertension

- Patients are often hypertensive after cardiac surgery due to a combination of factors including pain, inotropic support, and the release of a flow restricting lesion. In the immediate post-operative period this may put tension on surgical suture lines, therefore blood pressure is often controlled to reduce this risk. The blood pressure value targeted should consider the risk of organ dysfunction in those with pre-operative hypertension.
- Investigation and treatment of underlying causes is imperative.
- Infusions of nitrates and beta blockers are used for the first 24 hours until oral therapy can be started.

Pacing in the cardiac surgical population

- Many cardiac surgical patients will have epicardial pacing wires sited intra-operatively, particularly for valve surgery or more complex procedures. In many circumstances these are not attached to a pacing box unless the need for pacing arises.

Indications

- Cardiac surgery may result in direct injury to the AV node and cardiac conducting system, or the development of myocardial oedema in the post-operative period can result in delayed effects on these.
- Most patients can be successfully weaned from cardiopulmonary bypass without the need for pacing, but it is difficult to predict those who will require the intervention in the days following surgery.
- In addition, there is evidence that prophylactic pacing may reduce the incidence of atrial fibrillation post-op.

Positioning

- Pacing wires are most commonly located only on the right ventricle, which allows for ventricular stimulation. This is not co-ordinated with atrial contraction but is often sufficient.
- However, some patients are highly dependent on the atrial contraction component of ventricular filling and therefore benefit from the addition of pacing leads sited on the right atrium also, to allow for A-V sequential pacing.
- Epicardial wires should be colour coded or clearly labelled to highlight which are atrial and which are ventricular.
- Epicardial wires may be unipolar or bipolar, but in practice the management of both follows the same principles.

Complications

- Cardiac:
  - Myocardial damage
  - Perforation
  - Tamponade
  - Infection
  - Arrhythmia induced by micro-shocks
  - Disruption of coronary anastomoses
- Pacing:
  - Failure to capture
  - Output failure
  - Under-sensing
  - Over-sensing
  - Pacemaker-mediated tachycardia

Routine checks

- Underlying rhythm should be assessed daily to determine if ongoing pacing is still required.
- Inflammation develops around the pacing wires and this limits the lifespan of epicardial wires. Initially increasing the energy output will overcome this, but this further contributes to inflammation and cannot be sustained indefinitely.

Removal

- If pacing is not required, the epicardial wires are usually removed on day 3–6 post-operatively.
- Patients with an ongoing requirement for pacing on day 3 should be considered for permanent pacemaker insertion.
- Risk factors for requiring permanent pacing post cardiac surgery are: increasing age, pre-existing bundle branch block, prolonged cardiopulmonary bypass time, and inadequate intra-operative myocardial protection.
- Therapeutic heparin should be discontinued four hours prior to wire removal.
- INR should be less than 2.5 for patients receiving warfarin.
- Pacing wires should be removed prior to restarting DOACs and at least 12 hours should elapse after removal before taking the first dose.
- Wires are removed by constant gentle traction. If excessive resistance is felt, it may be necessary to cut the wires at the skin surface, allowing the cut ends to retract.
- Patients should be closely monitored for four hours after wire removal, as there is a risk of tamponade developing.

6.1.6 Renal issues

- All cardiac patients in the critical care unit should have a urinary catheter sited. After cardiac surgery, this should remain in place for at least 48 hours post-operatively.

Acute kidney injury

- Acute kidney injury is highly prevalent among intensive care patients, although the incidence has fallen over the years due to increased understanding of contributing causes.
- Acute kidney injury occurs commonly following cardiac surgery and is a poor prognostic feature, associated with increased morbidity and mortality. 1–2% of patients will require dialysis and this is associated with an even higher mortality (60%).

- The underlying mechanism of kidney injury in cardiac surgical patients is usually ischaemic injury, which is caused by a number of factors:
    - Hypotension and resulting renal hypoperfusion impairs the autoregulatory function of the kidney.
    - Many of these patients have conditions which contribute to pre-existing impaired autoregulation and in these patients, injury can occur even in the absence of hypoperfusion.
    - The systemic inflammatory response induced by surgery contributes to ischaemic injury.
    - Haemolysis caused by cardiopulmonary bypass results in products which may cause kidney ischaemia.
    - The use of nephrotoxic agents such as intravenous contrast.
- Kidney injury may be defined using the RIFLE criteria (Table 6.1.5) or AKIN criteria (Table 6.1.6), both are commonly used. The RIFLE criteria are defined as changes within 7 days, while the AKIN criteria are within 48 hours

Management
Prevention
- All efforts should be made to reduce the insult sustained by the kidneys in critically ill patients and peri-operatively.
- Renal perfusion is a combination of adequate *flow* AND *pressure*. Maintaining an adequate circulating volume, cardiac output and blood pressure should be prioritized.
- Avoid nephrotoxic drugs where possible.

Treatment
- Loop diuretics are often used to maintain a negative fluid balance but have no effect on renal function.
- No intervention (except adequate renal perfusion) has been shown to have an effect on the severity or time course of acute kidney injury.
- Renal replacement therapy (RRT) takes over the function of the kidneys until recovery.

Indications for renal replacement
- Anuria or oliguria (urine output < 200 ml/12 h)

Table 6.1.5 RIFLE Criteria.

STAGE	SERUM CREATININE	eGFR	URINE OUTPUT
RISK	↑ ×1.5	↓ > 25%	< 0.5 mL/kg/h × 6 h
INJURY	↑ ×2	↓ > 50%	< 0.5 mL/kg/h × 12 h
FAILURE	↑×3 If baseline ≥ 353.6 μmol/L ↑ SCr > 44.2 μmol/L (> 0.5 mg/dL)	↓ GFR > 75%	< 0.3 mL/kg/h × 24 h or anuria × 12 h
LOSS OF KIDNEY FUNCTION	Complete loss of	kidney function	> 4 weeks
END-STAGE KIDNEY DISEASE	Complete loss of	kidney function	> 3 months

Table 6.1.6 AKIN Classification.

AKIN STAGE	SERUM CREATININE	URINE OUTPUT
STAGE 1	↑ ≥ 26.5 μmol/l (≥ 0.3 mg/dl) OR ↑ ×1.5–2	< 0.5 ml/kg/h × 6 h
STAGE 2	↑ ×2–3	< 0.5 ml/kg/h × 12 h
STAGE 3	↑ ×3 OR serum creatinine ≥ 354 μmol/l (≥ 4.0 mg/dl) with an acute increase of at least 44 μmol/l (0.5 mg/dl) OR need for RRT	< 0.3 ml/kg/h ×. 24 h OR anuria for 12 h OR need for RRT

- pH < 7.1
- Urea > 30 mmol/l
- Potassium > 6.5 mmol/l refractory to treatment
- Clinically significant oedema
- Symptomatic uraemia—pericarditis, neuropathy, myopathy, encephalopathy, bleeding
- Na > 160 or < 115 mmol/l refractory to treatment
- Mg > 4 mmol with absent tendon reflexes
- Hyperthermia
- Overdose with a dialysable substance

Methods of renal replacement

- There are three main mechanisms:
    - Haemofiltration (convection)
    - Haemodialysis (diffusion)
    - Haemodialafiltration (combination of both)
- The mechanism used depends on a number of factors, including the purpose of the therapy (solute clearance or fluid removal), haemodynamic stability of the patient, and cost.

6.1.7 Neurological issues

Delirium

- Delirium is an acute, reversible state of mental confusion with disorders of attention and cognitive function and has a fluctuating course. It is classified into three subtypes:
    - Hyperactive—presents as agitation and acute confusion
    - Hypoactive—presents as passivity, with inattention and disinterest
    - Mixed—the most common form, with features of both hyperactive and hypoactive
- Delirium is the most common organ disorder in patients treated with mechanical ventilation in intensive care.
- After cardiac arrest, delirium may result from hypoxic-ischaemic injury.
- After cardiac surgery, the incidence of delirium is high, ranging from 26–52%.
- It is important to prevent, recognize, and treat delirium as it is associated with decreased functional status, cognitive decline, increased morbidity, and increased long-term mortality. It is difficult to tell whether this is correlation or causation.

- Delirium is difficult to diagnose, however the Confusion Assessment Method for ICU (CAM-ICU) tool has been designed for intensive care use and is both sensitive and specific in identifying patients with delirium.
- There is limited evidence for strategies that prevent and manage delirium specifically in cardiac patients. There have been robust studies in general critical care and these principles are applied.
- Non-pharmacological methods:
  - Early mobilization
  - Appropriate environment
  - Sleep promotion
  - Use of visual and hearing aids
  - Optimal hydration
- Pharmacological methods:
  - Antipsychotic medications are the mainstay of treatment although the evidence is mixed in relation to the efficacy
  - Haloperidol should be used as required only as there is evidence that prophylaxis has no effect on the incidence of delirium
  - Quetiapine
  - Risperidone (sublingual)
  - Benzodiazepines should be avoided except in patients with alcohol withdrawal

Post cardiac arrest brain injury

- Cardiac arrest often results in significant injury to the brain. The mechanism is complex and involves a combination of hypoxia and reperfusion and may continue to develop for several days after the initial insult.
- Perhaps the most difficult patients to manage are those who do not recover consciousness or are unable to follow verbal commands following cardiac arrest. It is vital to have an investigation and management strategy to quantify the extent of the injury and thus enable prognostication and further treatment planning or redirection.

Investigation

- Exclude factors which may hinder an accurate neurological examination, including paralytic agents, sedative medications, electrolyte derangements, metabolic abnormalities, and ongoing subclinical seizures.
- Assess conscious level using the Glasgow Coma Scale: https://www.glasgowcomascale.org/
- Imaging should be considered early in the course, including computerized tomography and magnetic resonance imaging.
- Diagnostic tests considered include electroencephalography (EEG) and median nerve somatosensory evoked potentials (SSEPs).
- If specified criteria are met, it may be appropriate to perform brainstem testing.

Management

- Management will vary widely depending on the pathology found and potential for recovery anticipated.
- Local guidelines should be consulted at all stages of the investigation process as the findings will have different implications depending on the legal framework of the country.

Post-operative cognitive dysfunction
- Post-operative cognitive dysfunction (POCD) is a well-recognized but not well-defined clinical syndrome. It is the most common neurological complication following cardiac surgery.

Risk factors
- POCD is thought to be multi-factorial, but the actual contribution made by the following risk factors is unclear.
- Patient
    - Increasing age
    - Cerebrovascular disease risk factors: hypertension, hypercholesterolaemia
    - Pre-operative cognitive decline
    - Genetic factors
- Pre-operative ejection fraction < 30%
- Anaesthetic
    - Use of propofol > volatile anaesthesia
    - Cerebral desaturation
    - Prolonged deep hypnotic time
- Surgery
    - Duration of procedure
    - Low intra-operative MAP
    - Hyperglycaemia
    - Aortic calcification
    - Hypothermia and rewarming
    - Alterations in pH balance
    - Haemodilution
- Post-operative
    - Hypoxia
    - Infection

Prevention and management
- It is important to identify patients who will be at higher risk of POCD and this should be discussed with the patient and the team as part of the pre-operative work-up.
- Any modifiable risk factors should be addressed.

Stroke
- The incidence of stroke after cardiac surgery varies depending on the surgical procedure performed. The overall incidence appears to be increasing as the age and complexity of patients presenting for cardiac surgery increases.
- Post-operative stroke is associated with a significant increase in mortality.

Risk factors
- The risk factors are similar to those identified for POCD above, with the added risk factor of a previous stroke indicating a high risk for a further peri-operative event.
- In addition, the development of atrial fibrillation (AF) may be associated with delayed post-operative stroke. Therefore, strategies to avoid and robustly treat of AF should be implemented.

Prevention and management
- The majority of strokes are ischaemic in nature.
- Identification of patients at high risk should occur pre-operatively and the risk should be discussed with the patient.
- Minimizing the impact of the known risk factors is the mainstay of preventative treatment.
- Management requires input from specialist stroke services and may be complicated by the post-operative status of the patient.

6.1.8 Analgesia

- Ensuring adequate analgesia is particularly important as untreated pain can have significant consequences on the recovery course of a patient. Patients who received chest compressions may have sustained significant mechanical damage including rib fractures. The traditional approach for cardiac surgery is via sternotomy, which is a large incision. Newer approaches to cardiac procedures are less invasive but may still cause significant tissue trauma and resulting pain.
- Excessive pain can result in haemodynamic instability which can have implications for any surgical repair and increase myocardial stress.
- In addition, pain can impair ventilation and increase the risk of respiratory tract infection.
- Furthermore, excessive pain can hinder mobilization and so increase the risk of infection, myopathy, and thromboembolism.
- A multimodal approach is best when constructing an analgesia regime.

Simple analgesics
- All patients should receive regular paracetamol, unless contraindicated.
- Non-steroidal anti-inflammatory drugs are avoided in the critically ill due to their effect on platelet function and renal perfusion.

Opiates
- The mainstay of post-operative pain control is the use of opiates. In the initial period, these are often given via continuous intravenous infusion and the drugs used have a short context-sensitive half time. As patients wake and become more responsive longer acting opiates are introduced and the use of patient-controlled analgesia is common. As pain scores decrease, this can be de-escalated to oral opiates and less potent opiates.
- Short-acting opiates are often used as part of the sedation regime for intubated and mechanically ventilated patients.

Adjuvant analgesics
- In patients with pain uncontrolled by opiates, adjuvant medications can be considered.
    - Tramadol
    - Gabapentin and pregabalin
    - Clonidine

Nerve blocks
- Intercostal, interpleural or paravertebral blocks may be useful for thoracotomy incisions.

Neuraxial techniques
- The use of neuraxial analgesia in cardiac surgery is an ongoing discussion, however most centres do not use it routinely.

6.1.9 Haematological Issues

Bleeding
- Bleeding is a complex issue in the cardiac intensive care unit. Most problems occur after cardiac surgery, but they can also occur in non-surgical patients due to the use of anti-coagulants.
- The causes of postoperative bleeding are:
    - Pre-operative drug induced platelet dysfunction
    - Pre-operative coagulopathy from any other cause
    - Residual heparinization
    - Cardiopulmonary bypass induced coagulopathy or fibrinolysis
    - 'Surgical bleeding'—sternal wires, anastomoses, graft side branches
- Following cardiac surgery, mediastinal drains are usually left in place to allow for drainage of any residual bleeding from the operative site.
- Drainage must be carefully monitored in the early post-operative period to ensure it does not become excessive and thus warrant further intervention.
- Levels of drainage that should prompt return to theatre are:
    - 400 ml in first hour
    - 200 ml in 2 consecutive hours
    - 100 ml in 4 consecutive hours

Risk factors
- Redo surgery
- Surgery using cardiopulmonary bypass (CPB)
- Prolonged cardiopulmonary bypass time
- Severity of hypothermia
- Pre-operative clotting disorders
- Pre-operative antiplatelet or anticoagulant therapy

Prevention
- Tranexamic acid is an anti-fibrinolytic agent commonly administered intra-operatively to reduce bleeding and decrease the requirement for blood products. The main side effect is seizure activity, but this is reduced with lower doses.
- Aprotinin is used in selected cases. This serine protease inhibitor was removed from practice between 2007 and 2012 following safety concerns, however following a re-analysis of the evidence it has been deemed that the benefits outweigh its risks in selected patients undergoing isolated coronary artery bypass graft surgery who are at high risk of major blood loss.

Management
- Bleeding should be aggressively investigated and treated.
- Investigations:
    - Full blood count
    - Activated clotting time

- Coagulation screen: APTT, PT, INR
- Fibrinogen
- Thromboelastography (TEG) or ROTEM (near patient testing devices that provide a dynamic assessment of clot strength)
- Red blood cell transfusion:
  - This should be targeted to maintain appropriate haemoglobin and haematocrit levels.
  - The transfusion trigger for cardiac patients (80 g/dL) is usually higher than general intensive care patients. In the bleeding patient it is prudent to maintain an even higher haemoglobin level (100 g/dL) as this is optimal for clotting.
  - It should be noted that most patients undergoing uncomplicated cardiac surgery will not receive a blood transfusion during their peri-operative course.
- Blood products:
  - Platelets are the most common blood product used due to CPB induced dysfunction.
  - Fresh frozen plasma is useful after long bypass times and in those with pre-existing coagulopathy (warfarin, liver disease).
  - Cryoprecipitate or fibrinogen concentrate should be given to target a fibrinogen level > 200 mg/dl.
  - Activated Factor VII is used off licence for patients with life-threatening bleeding refractory to other treatments.
- Administration of drugs:
  - Protamine: the half-life of heparin is significantly longer than that of protamine and therefore there can often be a degree of residual heparinization, particularly if the 'pump blood' (blood salvaged from the CPB circuit) is given back to the patient.
  - Vitamin K: may be considered.
- Surgical re-exploration for bleeding:
  - Required in approximately 2–5% of patients.
  - This is associated with a significant increase in morbidity and mortality.
- Other factors to consider:
  - Systolic BP target 100–120 mmHg
  - Restoration of normothermia
  - Addition of PEEP—may reduce bleeding by increasing mechanical intrathoracic pressure but may also reduce venous return and thus cardiac output in those who are hypovolaemic.
  - A chest X-ray or ECHO may show large pleural/pericardial collections which necessitate immediate return to theatre regardless of coagulation status.

Thromboprophylaxis

- Patients in intensive care are at a high risk for thromboembolic disease.
- The incidence of deep vein thrombosis (DVT) in critically ill patients ranges from 5–31% depending on the clinical case-mix. Pulmonary embolism (PE) is frequently undiagnosed, with autopsy studies demonstrating PE in 7–27 % of intensive care patients, of which only one-third had been clinically suspected or diagnosed.
- Following cardiac surgery, the incidence of DVT is 3.2% and pulmonary embolism is 0.6%.

Thromboprophylaxis in ICU patients
- Mechanical venous thromboembolism (VTE) prophylaxis should be considered:
  - When pharmacological thromboprophylaxis is contraindicated.

- In combination with pharmacological therapy in patients at very high risk of thrombosis.
- Pharmacological prophylaxis:
  - Thromboprophylaxis with low molecular weight heparin (LMWH) is indicated in all patients admitted to ICU, unless there is a specific contraindication.
  - Unfractionated heparin is effective for thromboprophylaxis in the critically ill, but should only be used when LMWHs are contraindicated.

Thromboprophylaxis in cardiac surgery patients

- The use of thromboprophylaxis after cardiac surgery is associated with a decreased risk (c 50%) of pulmonary embolus or symptomatic venous thromboembolism, however the optimal schedule has been difficult to determine.
- Mechanical venous thromboembolism (VTE) prophylaxis should be started at admission, either:
  - Anti-embolism stockings
  - Foot impulse devices
  - Intermittent pneumatic compression devices
- Pharmacological prophylaxis should be added pre-operatively:
  - Low molecular weight heparin
  - Unfractionated heparin (in patients with significant renal impairment)
- Patients returning from theatre are deemed to have an element of residual coagulopathy following the use of heparin intra-operatively.
- Usual practice is to re-introduce pharmacological thromboprophylaxis on the first post-operative day.
- These measures should be continued for 5–7 days, until the patient has returned to an acceptable level of mobility.

Anti-platelets

- Guidelines for antiplatelet and anticoagulant therapy for cardiac conditions should be considered elsewhere. The following discussion is in relation to cardiac surgery patients.
- Aspirin should not be routinely stopped prior to surgery.
- Clopidogrel should be stopped prior to surgery in elective patients but is often continued in those with recent cardiac events or stents.

Warfarin

- Patients who present for cardiac surgery who are already receiving warfarin should be risk stratified depending on the indication for anticoagulation.
- In patients with a low risk of thrombosis, warfarin should be stopped 2–3 days before surgery to allow the INR to fall below 1.5 and heparin is not required.
- In patients with a high risk of thrombosis, 'bridging' therapy with therapeutic intravenous heparin should be started when the INR falls below 2.0. This should then be stopped 4–6 h before surgery and restarted as early possible post-operatively, once bleeding stability is achieved. It should be continued until Warfarin has been reintroduced and the INR is again therapeutic.

Direct Acting-Oral Anticoagulants (DOACs)

- The most common DOACs in use in clinical practice are dabigatran, rivaroxaban and apixaban.
  - Stop dabigatran 2–3 days before surgery.
  - Stop rivaroxaban 2 days before surgery.
  - Stop apixaban 2 days before surgery.

> **BOX 6.1.1 GI COMPLICATIONS IN ICU**
>
> Abdominal compartment syndrome
> Gastrointestinal haemorrhage
> Mesenteric ischaemia
> Diarrhoea
> Paralytic ileus
> Abdominal sepsis
> Liver failure

- In patients with renal impairment, consideration should be made to stopping these drugs for longer (1 further day).
- If there is no indication to change to warfarin and the pre-operative DOAC is to continue, this is usually restarted on post-operative day four.

6.1.10 Gastrointestinal issues

- Gastrointestinal complications in acutely ill cardiac patients are often associated with catastrophic consequences (Box 6.1.1). The recognition and treatment of such complications may be difficult due to pre-existing co-morbidities, the post-arrest or post-operative status of the patient.
- As with all critical care patients, early feeding, appropriate stress ulcer prophylaxis and a high degree of clinical suspicion are the cornerstones of appropriate management.

Post-operative

- The incidence of gastrointestinal complications after cardiac surgery is relatively low (0.4–3.7%), however their occurrence is associated with significant morbidity and high mortality rates (11–85%) (Box 6.1.2).
- Many patients report dysphagia post-operatively, with the cause thought to be multifactorial, however a major contributing factor is the performance of intra-operative trans-oesophageal echocardiography.

> **BOX 6.1.2 GI COMPLICATIONS POST CARDIAC SURGERY**
>
> Dysphagia
> Gastrointestinal haemorrhage
> Colonic pseudo-obstruction
> Mesenteric ischaemia (low flow or embolic)
> Paralytic ileus
> Acalculous cholecystitis
> Acute pancreatitis
> Liver failure

- Gastrointestinal haemorrhage is the most common severe GI complication. A combination of anti-coagulation therapy, antiplatelet medication, TOE use, ventilation, and altered feeding are likely to contribute.

Feeding

- Malnutrition has been identified as an independent risk factor for morbidity among critical care patients.
- Many cardiac patients will begin oral intake shortly after extubation and the total fasting time will be relatively short.
- If it is anticipated that there will be a longer delay in extubation (> 36 hours), a naso-gastric tube should be sited and enteral feeding initiated.
- Parenteral feeding should be reserved for those with prolonged failure of enteral intake (> 1 week).

Stress ulcer prophylaxis

- Stress ulcers are gastric erosions which can develop in critically ill patients. They can evolve into deeper penetrating ulcers and consequently result in significant gastrointestinal haemorrhage.
- Risk factors for the development are:
    - Mechanical ventilation for > 48 hours
    - Coagulopathy (INR > 1.5, platelets < 50, activated partial thromboplastin time (aPTT) > 2 times the control value)
- The use of pharmacological prophylactic therapy is well established in critical care patients and a recent review of the evidence suggests that there is a marginal benefit in cardiac surgery patients also, although the practice is associated with an increased incidence of pneumonia.
- Given the high mortality from GI haemorrhage in this patient population, routine administration of a proton pump inhibitor (PPI) is often used.
- Previously there were concerns regarding interaction between clopidogrel and PPIs resulting in reduced efficacy of clopidogrel. However, routine use of PPIs has not been shown to increase complications.

Blood glucose management

- Hyperglycaemia commonly occurs in critical illness due to hormonal alterations and catabolism. This occurs in cardiac surgery patients also due to the stress response to surgery.
- The mainstay of treatment is the use of intravenous insulin infusion (IVI), although the optimal glucose targets for this have not been determined.
- While hyperglycaemia is undesirable, at the other end of the spectrum strict glycaemic control has been shown to be associated with increased periods of hypoglycaemia and provides no outcome benefit.
- International guidelines vary, but most agree that moderate glucose control gives the compromise of controlled blood sugar with fewer incidences of unrecognized hypoglycaemia. The recommended blood glucose range is from 140 to 180 mg/dL (7.8–10 mmol/l).
- Diabetic patients on insulin therapy should continue long-acting insulin throughout the peri-operative period, but with dose alterations recommended on the day before and day of surgery in various specific guidelines. Short-acting insulin should be temporarily replaced by an IV infusion. Particular care must be taken with rapidly falling renal function and impaired clearance.

- Patients who are normally on insulin therapy are best started on an insulin infusion from the beginning of surgery, even before a hyperglycaemic reading is detected.
- Diabetic patients often benefit from specialist review in relation to withholding and restarting usual medications and insulin.

6.1.11 Infective issues

- Infective complications occur post cardiac surgery in 5–21% of cases and can have devastating consequences as they herald a large increase in mortality.
- Sites of infection include:
  - Respiratory
  - Devices and monitoring
  - Surgical site infection

Surgical site infection

- Sternal wound infections are the most concerning surgical site infections and may be classified as:
  - Superficial—skin, subcutaneous tissue, pectoralis fascia
  - Deep—sternal bone, substernal space, mediastinum
- Deep sternal wound infection is difficult to manage and results in a twofold increase in mortality.

Prevention

- A number of interventions have demonstrated an impact on reducing surgical site infection.
- Nasal muprocin for *staphylococcus sp.* decontamination.
- 2% chlorhexidine gluconate/70% isopropyl alcohol skin preparation.
- Antibiotic prophylaxis:
  - Choice of agent will depend on the patient population.
  - Should be delivered in a timely fashion to ensure that peak plasma concentration occurs at the time of skin incision.
  - Duration of treatment is unclear, but routine antimicrobials should not be continued for longer than 48 hours.
- Meticulous intra-operative sterility.
- Glucose control, particularly in diabetic patients.
- Avoidance of steroids.
- Avoidance of blood transfusion.
- Smoking cessation.

Presentation

- Presentation will vary depending on the severity of the infection.
- Systemic signs of sepsis occur.
- Raised inflammatory markers may be detected.
- Blood cultures may have a positive growth.
- On examination of the sternum, discharge may be seen or there may be instability detected.
- Computerized tomography is useful in investigating the extent of the infection beneath the sternum.

Table 6.1.7 Intensive care level of care.

Level of Care	Details
Level 3	Patient needing support of two or more organs Patient needing advanced respiratory support (mechanical ventilation) Managed in Intensive Care Unit Requires continuous observation
Level 2	Patient stepping down from level 3 care Patient needing single organ support Managed in High Dependency Unit Requires observations at least every hour
Level 1	Patient recently discharged from a higher level of care Requires observations at least every 4 hours May be managed on normal ward Requires additional clinical intervention
Level 0	Patient requires hospitalization Managed on normal ward Observations monitored less frequently than every 4 hours

Treatment

- Treatment will also vary depending on the severity of the clinical features and the radiological findings.
- Antimicrobial therapy is the foundation of management.
- For deeper infections, surgical debridement, primary closure, and ongoing irrigation may be necessary.
- The use of vacuum-assisted closure (VAC) may be considered with delayed closure.
- Reconstructive procedures may be considered at a later stage.

6.1.12 Discharge from intensive care

- Patients in intensive care are classified according to the intensity of therapy they require, both in terms of monitoring and treatment (Table 6.1.7).
- Level 3 care is generally considered as intensive care and level 2 care as high dependency care, although often patients are managed in the same physical environment.
- In general when patients require level 2 care they can be discharged from ICU to HDU.
- When they require level 1 or level 0 care they can return to the ward.
- Again a systematic approach is used to determine how appropriate it is to step down the level of care a patient requires. The situation is often dynamic and if the clinical status deteriorates the patient may move up through the level of care required.
- When a patient is discharged to the ward, monitoring and medications should be rationalized and instructions given for appropriate targets or triggers which should prompt escalation of the level of care.

6.1.13 Communication, palliation, and end-of-life care

Discussion with family

- Communication is the key to good ICU management. Perhaps the most vital communication is that which occurs between medical practitioners and critically unwell patients and their families.
- Poorly chosen words, badly delivered, in the wrong circumstance can leave psychological and emotional problems which may have more profound repercussions than the physical illness.
- If the patient is awake and cognitively intact, all discussions should directly involve them and their wishes should be used to guide management.
- If the patient is sedated or critically unwell it may be necessary to consult with the next of kin, who may be family or friends. This situation is more difficult and it is important to be aware of the legal framework of the country and take account of the patient's wishes (if known) before undertaking any discussions.

Palliation and end-of-life care

- The importance of palliative care within the intensive care environment should not be underestimated.
- In situations where treatment of the organ dysfunction of critical illness is no longer effective or the goals of care cannot be achieved, the focus of patient care should shift towards ensuring that the patient dies in the mot dignified way possible. The patient's comfort and wishes are the most vital aspects of treatment.
- The ABCD checklist of things to consider to ensure this occurs is:
    - Attitudes
    - Behaviours
    - Compassion
    - Dialogue
- Decisions regarding end-of-life care are difficult and should be made by medical practitioners following discussion and consideration with the family and colleagues.

Further reading

Carmona P, Mateo E, Casanovas I, Peña JJ, Llagunes J, Aguar F, De Andrés J, Errando C. Management of cardiac tamponade after cardiac surgery. J Cardiothorac Vasc Anesth. 2012 Apr;26(2):302–11. doi: 10.1053/j.jvca.2011.06.007.

Chochinov HM. Dignity and the essence of medicine: the A, B, C, and D of dignity conserving care. BMJ. 2007 Jul 28;335(7612):184–7. doi: 10.1136/bmj.39244.650926.47. PMID: 17656543; PMCID: PMC1934489.

Karangelis D, Oikonomou K, Koufakis T, Tagarakis GI. Gastrointestinal Complications Following Heart Surgery: An Updated Review. Eur J Cardiovasc Nurs Med. 2011 Sep 1;1.

Miskovic A, Lumb AB. Postoperative pulmonary complications. Br J Anaesth. 2017 Mar 1;118(3):317–34. doi: 10.1093/bja/aex002. PMID: 28186222.

Tan A, Amoako D. Postoperative cognitive dysfunction after: Cardiac surgery. Continuing Education in Anaesthesia. Crit Care Pain. 2013;13:218–23. doi: 10.1093/bjaceaccp/mkt022.

Vincent JL. Give your patient a fast hug (at least) once a day. Crit Care Med. 2005 Jun;33(6):1225–9. doi: 10.1097/01.ccm.0000165962.16682.46. PMID: 15942334.

6.2

Cardiac arrest and resuscitation

Richard Bond and Ahmed Merghani

TABLE OF CONTENTS

6.2.1 Introduction and advanced life support 567
    Basic life support 567
    Advanced life support 568
    Defibrillation 568
    Peri-arrest arrhythmias 569
    Tachycardias: guideline management 569
    Bradyarrhythmias: guideline management 569
6.2.2 Drugs used in resuscitation 570
6.2.3 Post-resuscitation care 570
6.2.4 Ethics of resuscitation 572

6.2.1 Introduction and advanced life support

- Cardiac arrest is defined by abrupt loss of cardiac output, respiration, and consciousness
- Successful resuscitation following a cardiac arrest is dependent on four factors which make up the 'chain of survival':
  1) Early recognition and call for help
  2) Early bystander cardiopulmonary resuscitation (CPR)
  3) Early defibrillation
  4) Post-resuscitation care

Basic life support

- The median time for arrival of emergency services in the community is 5–8 minutes and therefore survival is dependent on bystander CPR by trained or lay members of the public who have knowledge of basic life support
- The basic life support algorithm:
  1) Safety: make sure you, the victim and any bystanders are safe
  2) Recognition of cardiac arrest:
     a. Unresponsive
     b. Not breathing: open the airway using the head tilt and chin lift; look listen and feel for normal breathing for 10 seconds
  3) Call emergency services
  4) Give 30 chest compressions
  5) Give 2 rescue breaths
  6) Continue CPR 30:2
  7) If an automated defibrillator device is available, switch it on and follow instructions
- The ESC recommends automated external defibrillators be established in crowded public areas and places where there are no other access to defibrillation (e.g. trains, planes, and cruise ships) and at sites where cardiac arrest is more likely to occur — *Class I recommendation*

Effective chest compressions:

- Centre of the chest
- Depth of 5–6 cm
- Rate at 100–120 per minute
- Allowing chest recoil immediately after each compression

Advanced life support

- The 2021 European resuscitation council algorithm for advanced life support is summarized in Figure 6.2.1
- The algorithm divides heart rhythms causing cardiac arrest into two groups:
    - Shockable rhythms = pulseless VT and VF
    - Non-shockable rhythms = asystole and pulseless electrical activity
- The former group requires defibrillation and use of amiodarone but other interventions are common in both groups including chest compressions, airway management, venous access, and administration of adrenaline
- Considerable attention is given to correcting reversible causes termed the '4Ts and 4Hs', as summarized in Figure 6.2.1

Defibrillation

- The shock energy should be based on the manufactures guidance but an initial shock for a biphasic waveform should be at least 150 J and subsequent shocks at 150–360 J

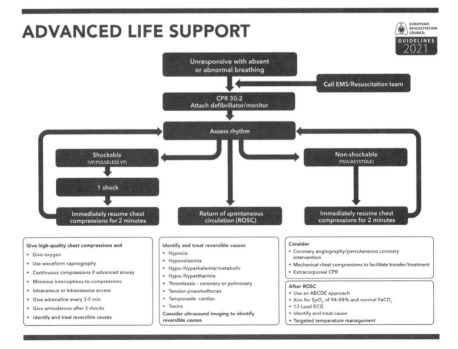

Figure 6.2.1 Advanced Life Support guidelines, including the "4 H's and 4 T's" of reversible causes

Taken from 2021 European resuscitation council algorithm for advanced life support

Reproduced from Soar et al. European Resuscitation Council Guidelines 2021: Adult advanced life support. *Resuscitation.* 2021 Apr; 161: 115–151. doi: 10.1016/j.resuscitation.2021.02.010 with permission from Elsevier.

- It is important to minimize interruption to CPR by limiting the time taken for defibrillation, continuing CPR during charging, and recommencing CPR promptly after defibrillation
  - Anticipatory charging of the defibrillator in the lead-up to a pulse check may reduce time to shock delivery
- In the case of a shockable witnessed monitored arrest, three stacked shocks may be considered

Peri-arrest arrhythmias

- In patients presenting with tachyarrhythmias or bradyarrhythmia's, the initial assessment using the ABCDE approach, should ascertain whether there is evidence of adverse signs:
  - Shock
  - Syncope
  - Myocardial ischaemia
  - Heart failure

Tachycardias: guideline management

1) If there is evidence of adverse signs, give:
   a. A synchronized DC shock (up to 3 attempts)
   b. IV amiodarone, 300 mg bolus (generally followed by an infusion of 900 mg over 24 hours) or procainamide 10–15 mg/kg over 20 minutes
2) In the absence of adverse signs, assess QRS duration:
   a. Broad (> 0.12 sec)
      i. Regular
         1. VT: Give IV amiodarone or procainamide
         2. SVT with aberrancy: Give IV adenosine
      ii. Irregular
         1. Polymorphic VT: Magnesium 2 g over 10 minutes
         2. Atrial fibrillation (AF) with aberrancy: see below
   b. Narrow (< 0.12 sec)
      i. Regular:
         1. SVT: Use vagal manoeuvres and if unsuccessful adenosine IV at a dose of 6 mg, 12 mg, and 18 mg at each failed attempt
         2. Atrial flutter: beta blockers or other rate limiting drugs
      ii. Irregular: likely AF. Beta blocker or calcium channel blocker, use digoxin or amiodarone if evidence of heart failure

Bradyarrhythmias: guideline management

- A patient is considered at increased risk of asystole in the presence of any of:
  - Recent asystole
  - Mobitz II AV block
  - Complete AV block with broad QRS
  - Ventricular pause > 3 seconds
- In those with adverse signs (shock, syncope, myocardial ischaemia, or severe heart failure), or if evidence of increased risk of asystole:
  a. Give atropine 500 mcg IV and repeat up to a maximum of 3 mg
  b. Consider isoprenaline 5 mcg/min, adrenaline 2–10 mcg/min or alternative drugs (aminophylline, dopamine, glucagon if suspected beta-blocker overdose, and glycopyrrolate)

c. Consider transcutaneous pacing and temporary transvenous pacing if resources and expertise allows

N.B. Atropine should not be used in transplant patients as it can cause high-degree AV block or even sinus arrest—use aminophylline

6.2.2 Drugs used in resuscitation

See Table 6.2.1.

6.2.3 Post-resuscitation care

- Following return of spontaneous circulation (ROSC), effective post-resuscitation care is instrumental in survival
- This should be delivered in an intensive care setting with input from other specialists
- The following factors require consideration
    1) Airway and breathing:
        - Insert advanced airway
        - Utilization of waveform capnography is recommended
        - Ventilate lungs to normocapnia
    2) Circulation:
        - 12-lead ECG
        - Obtain reliable IV access
        - Restore normovolaemia
        - Arterial blood pressure monitoring
        - Vasopressors and inotropes to maintain blood pressure as required
    3) Obtain and treat underlying cause:
        - If cardiac cause is suspected, even in absence of ST elevation, coronary angiography ± percutaneous intervention should be considered
        - Consider CT brain, and/or CTPA and treat non-cardiac causes of arrest
    4) Management in intensive care
        - Temperature control: increasing focus on prevention of hyperthermia to < 37°C rather than inducing active hypothermia, as previously sought (helps reduce tissue damage and preserve neurological function; improves survival and neurological function)
        - Maintain normoxia and normocapnia
        - Optimize haemodynamics
        - Echocardiography
        - Maintain normoglycaemia
        - Diagnose/treat seizures
        - Evaluate prognostication after 72 hours
    5) Secondary prevention:
        - Consideration of an ICD
        - Screening for inherited disorders
        - Risk factor modification
    6) Rehabilitation

Table 6.2.1 Drugs relevant to resuscitation.

Drug	Mechanism of action	Indications	Dose/Route	Caution/contra-indications
Adrenaline	Alpha-1 receptor agonist Vasopressor Increases HR Positive inotrope	Cardiac arrest Bradycardia Post arrest hypotension	1 mg stat IV/IO 2–10 mcg/min IV 0.1–0.5 mcg/kg/min IV	Use cautiously in myocardial infarction as the increase in HR and BP increases myocardial oxygen demand
Amiodarone	Class III antiarrhythmic agent	Ventricular and supraventricular arrhythmias	300 mg IV/IO (cardiac arrest) 300 mg IV loading followed by 900 mg/24 hours (peri-arrest)	Potentially harmful in Long QT and polymorphic VT Hypotension
Lidocaine	Class Ib antiarrhythmic drug	VT/VF arrest If amiodarone unavailable Stable VT	1–1.5 mg/kg IV/IO 30–50 mcg/kg/min IV	Can cause arrhythmias Lidocaine toxicity
Procainamide	Class Ia antiarrhythmic drug	VT/VF arrest If amiodarone unavailable Stable VT	10–15 mg/kg IV over 20 min	Can cause arrhythmias and hypotension
Atropine	Anticholinergic drug, Acetylcholine receptor antagonist	Bradycardia with adverse clinical signs	0.6–3 mg IV	Anticholinergic with high doses
Magnesium	Cofactor for myocardial sodium/potassium ATPase pump Calcium channel blocker	Polymorphic VT	2 g IV over 10 minutes	No benefit from routine use during cardiac arrest
Adenosine	Slows AV node conduction	SVT SVT with aberrancy	6 mg and subsequent doses of 12 mg, and 12 mg IV	Causes severe but transient side effects including chest tightness and flushing

6.2.4 Ethics of resuscitation

- End of life decisions can be emotionally difficult and challenging for both patient and physician, and should be undertaken in a multidisciplinary setting with consultation with the patient, relatives, and other medical staff
- The responsibility to make decisions about withholding resuscitation may vary from country to country, but generally rests with the most senior doctor acting in the patient's best interests and after consultation with the patient
- Where patients lack capacity, relatives should be consulted to obtain evidence of the patient's previously expressed wishes, beliefs, and views
- Any decisions or discussions regarding end of life care should be clearly documented in the medical notes
- Do not attempt resuscitation (DNAR) orders can be made on several grounds, including:
  - Patient autonomy in patients who have mental capacity
  - An advance directive
  - Medical futility
  - Resuscitation is likely to cause more harm than good
- Healthcare professionals should consider withdrawing CPR when:
  - The safety of the provider cannot be assured
  - There is obvious mortal injury or irreversible death
  - A valid advance directive becomes available
  - Strong evidence that further CPR would be against patient's values and preferences or is considered futile
  - Asystole for more than 20 min despite ongoing ALS

Further reading

Soar J, Böttiger BW, Carli P, Couper K, Deakin CD, Djärv T, Lott C, Olasveengen T, Paal P, Pellis T, Perkins GD, Sandroni C, Nolan JP. European Resuscitation Council Guidelines 2021: Adult advanced life support. *Resuscitation*. 2021 Apr;161:115–51. doi: 10.1016/j.resuscitation.2021.02.010. Epub 2021 Mar 24. PMID: 33773825.

6.3

Sudden cardiac death

Richard Bond and Ahmed Merghani

TABLE OF CONTENTS

6.3.1 Definitions of sudden death 573
6.3.2 Epidemiology of sudden cardiac death (SCD) 573
6.3.3 Aetiology of SCD 574
6.3.4 Pre-disposing conditions to SCD 574
  Coronary artery disease (CAD) 574
  Hypertrophic cardiomyopathy (HCM) 576
  Arrhythmogenic right ventricular cardiomyopathy (ARVC) 577
  Coronary artery anomalies 579
  Brugada syndrome 579
  Long QT Syndrome (LQTS) 580
  Catecholaminergic Polymorphic Ventricular Tachycardia (CPVT) 580
6.3.5 Diagnostic work-up and risk stratification of survivors and family members 581
  Autopsy and molecular autopsy 581
  Assessment of cardiac arrest survivors 581
  Familial screening 582
  ICD therapy 582

6.3.1 Definitions of sudden death

See Table 6.3.1.

6.3.2 Epidemiology of sudden cardiac death (SCD)

- SCD accounts for approximately 100,000 deaths per year in the UK alone and globally the incidence is between 50 and 100 per 100,000

Table 6.3.1 Useful definitions.

Sudden Death	Non-traumatic, unexpected fatal event occurring within 1 hour of the onset of symptoms in an apparently healthy subject
Sudden Cardiac Death (SCD)	Sudden natural death presumed due a congenital, genetic or acquired cardiac condition that occurs within 1 hour of symptom onset if witnessed, or within 24 hours of when last seen alive if unwitnessed
Sudden unexplained death syndrome (SUDS)	Sudden death without an apparent cause and in which an autopsy has not been performed
Sudden Arrhythmic death syndrome (SADS)	Sudden cardiac death where no cause can be found on autopsy
Aborted cardiac arrest	Unexpected circulatory arrest, occurring within 1 hour of onset of acute symptoms, which is reversed by successful resuscitation manoeuvres

- Coronary artery disease (CAD) is the leading cause (responsible for 75-80%) and SCD accounts for 50% of all CAD deaths
- The risk of SCD is fourfold more in men than women, which may be partially explained by the protection from CAD seen in premenopausal women
- The incidence increases from 1/100,000 for those < 35 years to 1/1000 in individuals ≥ 35 years old reflecting the higher burden of CAD with age
- Risk also varies according to ethnicity with black individuals being more susceptible to SCD

6.3.3 Aetiology of SCD

- The aetiology of SCD is age dependent
- In patients aged ≥ 35 years the commonest aetiologies are CAD, heart failure, and valvular heart disease
- In those < 35 years the commonest aetiology is an inherited cardiac disorder:
    - Morphologically ABNORMAL heart
        - Hypertrophic cardiomyopathy (HCM)
        - Arrhythmogenic right ventricular cardiomyopathy (ARVC)
        - Familial dilated cardiomyopathy (DCM)
        - Bicuspid aortic stenosis
        - Aortic dissection
        - Myocarditis
    - Morphologically NORMAL heart on post mortem (classified as SADS)
        - Ion channel disease (channelopathies) such as Brugada Syndrome, long QT syndrome (LQTS), catecholaminergic polymorphic ventricular tachycardia (CPVT), short QT syndrome
        - Congenital accessory pathways such as Wolff–Parkinson–White (WPW) syndrome

6.3.4 Pre-disposing conditions to SCD

- The following constitutes a list of conditions with an associated increased risk of SCD
- A short summary on each condition here is presented with the focus on the assessment and management of SCD risk
- Further information on these conditions is provided in Chapters 2.1, 2.2, 4.8, 5.2 and 8.6.

Coronary artery disease (CAD)
Key facts
- Despite a decline in CAD-related SCD due to better primary and secondary prevention measures, SCD accounts for > 50% of all CAD deaths
- A significant number occur in the pre-hospital setting and factors which are associated with better outcomes before attendance to hospital include:
    - Early basic life support and defibrillation
    - Reduction in symptom onset to reperfusion (call to balloon times)
    - Admission to expert centres offering primary coronary intervention

6.3.4 Pre-disposing conditions to SCD

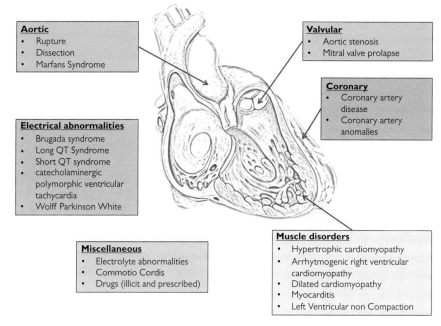

Figure 6.3.1 Aetiology of sudden cardiac death

Prevention of sudden cardiac death
- Early (< 40 days) implantation of an ICD following an acute coronary syndrome (ACS) is not recommended (*Class III recommendation*) except in specific conditions such as:
  - Pre-existing LV impairment
  - Incomplete revascularization
  - Arrhythmia occurring > 48 h after the onset of ACS
- However a wearable cardiac defibrillator may be considered in the early phase after MI in selected patients (*Class IIb*)
- Initial aim is optimal revascularization and medical therapy in particular with dual antiplatelet therapy, beta blockers, ACE inhibitors, and statins
- Such measures improve mortality risk and are associated with a 5–6% increase in left ventricular ejection fraction (LVEF) in up to a third of patients
- LVEF should be assessed at the time of admission and 6–12 weeks after coronary revascularization
- Primary prevention ICD:
  - Is recommended in patients with symptomatic heart failure (NYHA class II–III), and LVEF ≤ 35% 6 weeks following optimal medical treatment (OMT) for an MI who are expected to survive ≥ 1 year with good functional status (*Class I recommendation*)
  - Should be considered in patients with CAD, NYHA class I and LVEF ≤30% despite ≥3 months of OMT (*Class IIa*)
  - Should be considered in patients with CAD, LVEF ≤40% despite ≥3 months of OMT, and NSVT if they have inducible sustained monomorphic VT by EP study (*Class IIa*)

Management after aborted SCD
- Survivors of a sudden cardiac arrest who have ST elevation on a pre or post resuscitation ECG should undergo urgent revascularization (*Class I recommendation*)
- However 25–58% of patients may have absent ST elevation but harbour a culprit coronary lesion and the ECG is often difficult to interpret after a cardiac arrest; it is therefore recommended that all survivors of an out of hospital cardiac arrest with ongoing electrical instability suspicious for myocardial ischaemia should undergo coronary angiography (*Class I recommendation*)
- Administration of beta blockers and amiodarone can help prevent further arrhythmias, as well as correcting any electrolyte disturbances
- Catheter ablation is reserved for recurrent VT and fibrillation despite complete revascularization and optimum anti-arrhythmic treatment
- ICD implantation is recommended in patients without ongoing ischaemia with documented VF or haemodynamically not-tolerated VT occurring later than 48 hours after MI (*Class Ia*)

Hypertrophic cardiomyopathy (HCM)
Key facts
- Characterized by LVH and histological evidence of myocardial disarray and fibrosis with a predilection for potentially fatal arrhythmias, HCM is the most common cause of SCD in young adults and athletes
- It has a prevalence of 1 in 500 and is caused by mutations in sarcomeric contractile proteins, and patients with sarcomeric variants present earlier and are more likely to have a family history of HCM and SCD. They also tend to have more severe hypertrophy, microvascular dysfunction, and myocardial fibrosis
- Frequently transmitted as an autosomal dominant genetic trait, and due to the high probability of a genetic cause, testing should be considered in most patients with HCM
- Although symptoms of syncope, palpitations, chest pain, and dyspnoea are recognized, a significant proportion of patients may be asymptomatic
- SCD may be the initial presentation, especially in young adults and adolescents, and particularly those participating in vigorous physical exercise
- However, the overall prognosis is relatively good and the annual mortality risk is only between 0.5% and 3%

Risk of SCD in HCM
- The major clinical risk factors for sudden cardiac death in HCM (as per the 2014 ESC HCM guidelines) are detailed in Table 6.3.2
- HCMRisk-SCD study, a multicentre, retrospective, longitudinal cohort study of 3675 patients, developed and validated a new SCD risk prediction model. The model includes the risk factors detailed below, with the exception of BP response, and provides individualized 5-year risk estimates for SCD

Managing the risk of SCD in HCM
- No evidence that medical therapy reduces risk of SCD in HCM—risk stratification to decide which patients will benefit from ICD implant is therefore essential, using the 5-year HCM Risk-SCD score
- A prophylactic primary prevention ICD should be offered to patients with a high risk of SCD defined as a 5-year HCM Risk-SCD score ≥ 6% (*Class IIa B*)
- Individuals with an intermediate risk of SCD (HCM Risk-SCD score 4–6%) should be considered for a primary prevention ICD if any of (i) significant scar on cardiac MRI, (ii) LVEF

6.3.4 Pre-disposing conditions to SCD

Table 6.3.2 Risk factors for SCD in HCM.

Risk Factor	Comment
Age	Younger patients have an increased risk
Non-sustained VT	Defined as ≥ 3 consecutive ventricular beats at ≥ 120 BPM lasting <30 seconds
Maximum LV wall thickness	Greatest risk of SCD in patients with a maximum wall thickness of ≥ 30 mm
Family history of SCD	One or more first degree relatives have died suddenly aged < 40 years with or without a diagnosis of HCM or when SCD has a occurred in a first degree relative at any age with HCM
Syncope	Unexplained syncope is associated with increased risk of SCD
Left atrial diameter	Positive association between left atrial size and SCD
LVOT obstruction	A number of studies have reported a significant association with LVOT obstruction and SCD
Exercise blood pressure response	Failure to increase systolic pressure by at least 20 mmHg from rest to peak exercise or a fall of > 20 mmHg from peak pressure—*though this does not form part of the HCM Risk-SCD calculator*

<50%, (iii) abnormal BP response to exercise, (iv) LV apical aneurysm, or (v) presence of a sarcomeric pathogenic mutation (*Class IIa B*)
- All others in this intermediate risk category may be considered for primary prevention ICD after consultation with the patient, which takes into account lifelong risk factors of complications and the impact of ICD on lifestyle and socioeconomic status (*Class IIb B*)
- Primary prevention ICD is generally considered to not be indicated in individuals with a risk score < 4%
- A secondary prevention ICD is recommended in survivors of cardiac arrest or haemodynamically unstable sustained VT (*Class I B*)
- SCD may also be prevented in all HCM patients by simple lifestyle advice, such as cessation of intense athletic activity

N.B. *American ACC/AHA guidelines do not recommend the above % risk calculator—they recommend ICD implant can be considered based on presence of a single risk factor for SCD*

Arrhythmogenic right ventricular cardiomyopathy (ARVC)
Key facts
- Arrhythmogenic ventricular cardiomyopathy (AVC) is an arrhythmogenic disorder of the myocardium that is not secondary to ischaemic, hypertensive, or valvular heart disease and incorporates genetic and non-genetic causes (systemic, infectious, and inflammatory)
- It is an umbrella term that encompasses arrhythmogenic right ventricular cardiomyopathy (ARVC), arrhythmogenic left ventricular cardiomyopathy (ALVC), and DCM with an arrhythmic component. Whilst the RV is most frequently affected, LV involvement occurs in > 50% of cases and carries a worse prognosis
- It has a prevalence of between 1/1000 and 1/5000 and is an important cause of SCD in athletes and young adults

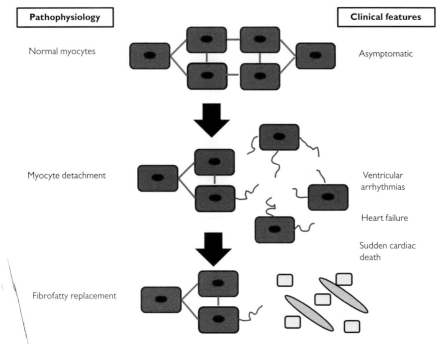

Figure 6.3.2 Pathophysiology and clinical features of ARVC

- It is an autosomal dominant trait caused by mutations within genes encoding cardiac desmosome proteins—thought to lead to myocyte detachment and an abnormal repair process, resulting in fibro-fatty replacement of the myocardium which has a predilection to fatal ventricular arrhythmias particularly during vigorous exercise (see Figure 6.3.2)
- Most causative variants are in desmosomal genes, and 3–6% of patients have more than one pathogenic variant which results in a more severe phenotype
- Family screening is important to identify relatives with sub-clinical disease. Typically, relatives identified on family screening have a milder phenotype and are older when overt clinical features are detectable
- Patients can be asymptomatic or present with palpitations, AF, syncope, heart failure, thromboembolic events, or, in some cases, SCD
- The ECG can be normal, especially in the early phase of the disease but often displays anterior T wave inversion and in some cases epsilon waves
- Arrhythmic events in family members usually occur in the presence of structural or ECG changes

Managing the risk of SCD in ARVC

- The annual risk of SCD is approximately 1%, and risk factors include the following:
    - Aborted SCD
    - Documented VT
    - Syncope
    - Family history of premature SCD
    - Severe RV dilatation and dysfunction
    - Marked QRS prolongation

          - Late gadolinium enhancement on CMR
          - LV dysfunction
          - Ventricular arrhythmias induction on electrophysiology studies
- Avoidance of high-intensity exercise is recommended (*Class I B*), and treatment with beta-blockers may be considered (*Class IIb C*) in patients with a definite diagnosis
- SCD can be reduced by primary prevention ICD implantation in patients with high-risk features and cessation of vigorous exercise/competitive sports (*Class IIa C*)
    - Data and firm recommendations are lacking and decisions should be individualized and must account for patient preference
- Patients with aborted SCD or haemodynamically unstable VT should be offered a secondary prevention ICD (*Class I C*)
- Antiarrhythmic drugs and catheter ablation of VT have not been shown to improve prognosis but may be considered
- Patients with progressive disease should be considered for transplantation

N.B. ICD implant carries an increased risk of RV perforation during the procedure, and difficulty finding an acceptable R wave due to the abnormal RV tissue, there may be a role for sub-cutaneous ICD

Coronary artery anomalies
Key facts
- Coronary artery anomalies are a relatively common finding, occurring in just under 1% of the general population
- The vast majority of cases are benign and cause no clinical sequelae, however individuals with anomalous coronary origins may be at risk of SCD, e.g. anomalous origin of the left coronary artery from the right sinus of Valsalva and coursing between the aorta and pulmonary arteries
- Individuals are often asymptomatic but can present with exertional chest pain or syncope
- Exercise testing seldom shows myocardial ischaemia and CT coronary angiography is the most preferred diagnostic test
- When present, cardiac stress imaging during physical exercise is recommended in addition to cardiopulmonary exercise test (*Class Ic*)

Managing the risk of SCD in coronary artery anomalies
- Patients with a high-risk variant or evidence of myocardial ischaemia should be offered surgical correction (*Class IIa*), and is recommended in patients with aborted cardiac arrest, syncope due to ventricular arrhythmia, or angina when other causes have been excluded (*Class I*)

Brugada syndrome
Key facts
- A disorder of the sodium ion channels of cardiac myocytes and is inherited as an autosomal dominant trait
- Prevalence ranges from 1 in 10,000 in Western countries to 1 in 1000 in South East Asia
- Mutations in the *SCN5A* gene are the most commonly recognized but at least 12 others have been described
- Patients are often asymptomatic and typically die during rest or sleep due to VF
- The typical Type 1 ECG pattern exhibits 'coved' ST elevation in leads V1–V3 (see Chapters 4.1 and 4.8)
- In suspected individuals with a normal ECG, a diagnosis can be made by drug provocation tests using ajmaline or flecainide

Risk stratification and ICD implantation in Brugada syndrome
- ICD offers the only proven option to reduce SCD and are reserved for individuals with high-risk features:
  - Aborted SCD
  - Documented sustained ventricular arrhythmias
  - Unheralded arrhythmic syncope
- Quinidine should be used as an adjunct for patients who qualify for an ICD but have a contraindication, decline or have recurrent ICD shocks
- Lifestyle advice is recommended in all patients with Brugada syndrome:
  - Abstaining from heavy meals prior to sleep
  - Avoidance of excessive alcohol intake
  - Avoidance of certain drugs (www.brugadadrugs.org)
  - Prompt treatment of any fever with antipyretic drugs

Long QT Syndrome (LQTS)
Key facts
- Congenital LQTS is an inherited group of potassium, sodium, or calcium ion channel disorders within cardiac myocytes that manifest as a prolonged corrected QT (QTc)
- Mutations in 13 culprit genes have been discovered with multiple modes of inheritance but the commonest subtypes are LQTS-1, LQTS-2, and LQTS-3 which account for 95% of all cases
- SCD is caused by polymorphic VT which degenerates into VF in the setting of adrenergic surges by well identified triggers
- Different triggers for SCD have been linked to each subtype:
  - Exercise and especially swimming in LQTS-1
  - Auditory stimuli in LQTS-2
  - Rest/sleep in LQTS-3

Risk stratification and reducing SCD
- Patients are initiated on beta adrenoreceptor blocking drugs
- Lifestyle advice includes avoiding genotype specific triggers (i.e. swimming, loud noises) and advised to avoid medications that prolong the QT interval (see www.qtdrugs.org)
- ICD insertion is reserved for high-risk cases:
  - QTc > 500 msecs
  - Syncope despite beta blockers
  - Aborted SCD

Catecholaminergic Polymorphic Ventricular Tachycardia (CPVT)
Key facts
- CPVT is a rare hereditary disorder characterized by adrenergic-induced bidirectional and polymorphic VT
- Two types of CPVT have been described:
  - CPVT1: an autosomal dominant form caused by mutations encoding the cardiac ryanodine receptor (RyR2)
  - CPVT2: less common autosomal recessive form caused by mutations in the gene encoding cardiac calsequestrin (CASQ2)

- CPVT typically presents in childhood with palpitations or syncope induced by exercise or psychological stress
- The resting ECG is often unremarkable and diagnosis is via an exercise test inducing the characteristic ECG changes

Risk of SCD can be negated with:
- Avoidance of strenuous exercise (*Class I C*)
- Beta blockers (*Class I C*)
- Left cardiac sympathetic denervation (LCSD) has been shown to reduce arrhythmic events and should be considered when the combination of beta-blockers and flecainide are either not effective, not tolerated, or contraindicated (*Class IIa C*)
- ICD is reserved for the following:
  - Aborted cardiac arrest
  - Recurrent syncope despite anti-arrhythmic therapy
  - Polymorphic/bidirectional VT despite optimal medical management, and/or LCSD

6.3.5 Diagnostic work-up and risk stratification of survivors and family members

Autopsy and molecular autopsy
- An autopsy is recommended in all victims of SCD with the aim of addressing the following questions:
  1) What is the nature of the cardiac disease if present?
  2) Is the cardiac disease inheritable and thus require screening of relatives?
  3) Have toxins, drugs, and unnatural deaths been excluded?
  4) Is the heart morphologically and histologically normal and therefore the death is the result of sudden arrhythmic death syndrome (SADS)?
- An autopsy may be inconclusive in around 2–54% of sudden deaths which likely reflects the heterogeneity of autopsy protocols and expertise
- It is recommended that in all cases of SCD the heart should be examined by an expert cardiac pathologist
- In cases where the heart is morphologically and histologically normal and toxicology and unnatural death is excluded, a diagnosis of SADS is made and the pathologist should recommend familial screening (Class I)
- In cases of SADS, molecular autopsy is an important addition to the standard autopsy and involves genetic testing of tissue of the deceased to diagnose the presence of a channelopathy; the yield of molecular autopsy is 15–25%

Assessment of cardiac arrest survivors
- The commonest cause of sudden cardiac death is CAD and ACS can readily be diagnosed from the history, ECG, serum cardiac biomarkers and coronary angiography (Figure 6.3.3)
- LVEF is the most important parameter in considering an ICD in CAD
- Assessment of a young (< 35 years) patient following an aborted SCD requires recognition of important red-flag symptoms in the personal and family history and a comprehensive array of investigations

Personal History	Family
• Exertional Chest pain • Exertional dizziness • Unheralded syncope • Excessive breathlessness • Palpitations • Siezures	• Known heritable discorder • Premature CAD (< 50 yrs) • Sudden cardiac death • Epilepsy • Unexplained drowning • Unexplained road traffic accidents

Figure 6.3.3 Red Flag symptoms to be considered in the assessment sudden cardiac arrest survivors and their family members

- Survivors of an unexplained sudden cardiac arrest where there is a suspicion of an inherited cardiac disease should be referred to a specialist inherited cardiac disease clinic where the following tests are routinely performed:
    - ECG: assessing for QT interval, Brugada pattern, Epsilon waves in ARVC, lateral T-Wave inversion in HCM
    - High lead ECG (at the level of the first and second intercostal spaces): has a higher yield of capturing Brugada pattern
    - Signal averaged ECG: assessing for late potentials in ARVC
    - 24-hour Holter monitor: assess for ventricular arrhythmias
    - Exercise ECG: documenting exercise induced ventricular arrhythmias, diagnosing CPVT, assessing for paradoxical prolongation of the QTc in LQT syndromes
    - Echocardiogram: assess for cardiomyopathy, risk stratification in HCM, excluding congenital and valvular heart disease, aortic root dimensions in Marfans syndromes and other inherited aortopathies
- Further tests may be deemed necessary in the following cases:
    - Cardiac MRI: provides superior resolution to diagnose subtle or early cardiomyopathic changes; late gadolinium enhancement present in HCM, ARVC, dilated cardiomyopathy, and left ventricular non-compaction
    - Ajmaline or flecainide test: diagnosis of Brugada syndrome when no abnormal cardiac morphology observed on echocardiography or MRI
    - Genetic testing: if there is a suspicion of an inheritable arrhythmogenic disease, and a positive result will enable cascade familial screening

Familial screening

- All first-degree blood relatives of patients with inherited cardiac diseases or victims of SADS should be investigated in an expert cardiac setting
- The ESC algorithm for familial screening is presented in Figure 6.3.4

ICD therapy

Full details provided in Chapter 4.9.

6.3.5 Diagnostic work-up and risk stratification of survivors and family members 583

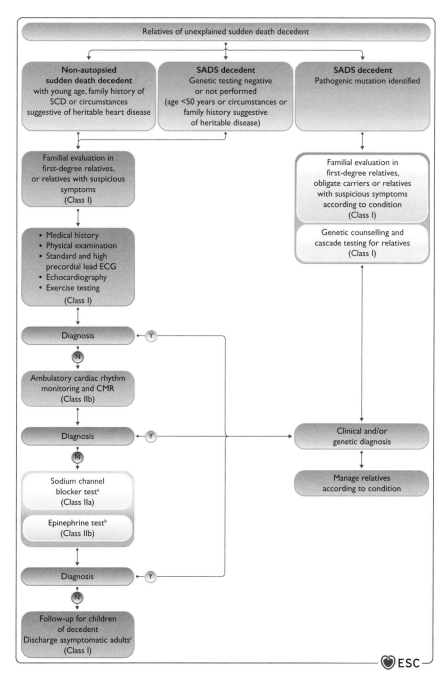

Figure 6.3.4 Zeppenfeld K, Tfelt-Hansen J, de Riva M, et al; ESC Scientific Document Group. 2022 ESC Guidelines for the management of patients with ventricular arrhythmias and the prevention of sudden cardiac death. *Eur Heart J.* 2022 Oct 21;43(40):3997–4126. doi: 10.1093/eurheartj/ehac262. © European Society of Cardiology. With permission from Oxford University Press

Further reading

Authors/Task Force members, Elliott PM, Anastasakis A, Borger MA, Borggrefe M, Cecchi F, Charron P, Hagege AA, Lafont A, Limongelli G, Mahrholdt H, McKenna WJ, Mogensen J, Nihoyannopoulos P, Nistri S, Pieper PG, Pieske B, Rapezzi C, Rutten FH, Tillmanns C, Watkins H. 2014 ESC Guidelines on diagnosis and management of hypertrophic cardiomyopathy: the Task Force for the Diagnosis and Management of Hypertrophic Cardiomyopathy of the European Society of Cardiology (ESC). *Eur Heart J*. 2014 Oct 14;35(39):2733–79. doi: 10.1093/eurheartj/ehu284. Epub 2014 Aug 29. PMID: 25173338

Corrado D, van Tintelen PJ, McKenna WJ, Hauer RNW, Anastastakis A, Asimaki A, Basso C, Bauce B, Brunckhorst C, Bucciarelli-Ducci C, Duru F, Elliott P, Hamilton RM, Haugaa KH, James CA, Judge D, Link MS, Marchlinski FE, Mazzanti A, Mestroni L, Pantazis A, Pelliccia A, Marra MP, Pilichou K, Platonov PGA, Protonotarios A, Rampazzo A, Saffitz JE, Saguner AM, Schmied C, Sharma S, Tandri H, Te Riele ASJM, Thiene G, Tsatsopoulou A, Zareba W, Zorzi A, Wichter T, Marcus FI, Calkins H; International Experts. Arrhythmogenic right ventricular cardiomyopathy: evaluation of the current diagnostic criteria and differential diagnosis. *Eur Heart J*. 2020 Apr 7;41(14):1414–29. doi: 10.1093/eurheartj/ehz669. PMID: 31637441; PMCID: PMC7138528

Deo R, Albert CM. Epidemiology and genetics of sudden cardiac death. *Circulation*. 2012 Jan 31;125(4):620–37. doi: 10.1161/CIRCULATIONAHA.111.023838. PMID: 22294707; PMCID: PMC3399522

Priori SG, Wilde AA, Horie M, Cho Y, Behr ER, Berul C, Blom N, Brugada J, Chiang CE, Huikuri H, Kannankeril P, Krahn A, Leenhardt A, Moss A, Schwartz PJ, Shimizu W, Tomaselli G, Tracy C. HRS/EHRA/APHRS expert consensus statement on the diagnosis and management of patients with inherited primary arrhythmia syndromes: document endorsed by HRS, EHRA, and APHRS in May 2013 and by ACCF, AHA, PACES, and AEPC in June 2013. *Heart Rhythm*. 2013 Dec;10(12):1932–63. doi: 10.1016/j.hrthm.2013.05.014. Epub 2013 Aug 30. PMID: 24011539

2022 ESC Guidelines for the management of patients with ventricular arrhythmias and the prevention of sudden cardiac death: Developed by the task force for the management of patients with ventricular arrhythmias and the prevention of sudden cardiac death of the European Society of Cardiology (ESC) Endorsed by the Association for European Paediatric and Congenital Cardiology (AEPC), *European Heart Journal*, 2022; ehac262, https://doi.org/10.1093/eurheartj/ehac262

CHAPTER 7

PREVENTION, REHABILITATION AND SPORT

7.1

Sports cardiology

Joyee Basu, Jamie O'Driscoll, and Daniel X Augustine

TABLE OF CONTENTS

- 7.1.1 Benefits of exercise on the body 587
- 7.1.2 Exercise physiology 588
- 7.1.3 The athlete's heart 589
  - Structural changes in the athlete's heart 594
  - Assessment of athlete's left ventricle 594
  - Assessment of the athlete's right ventricle 594
- 7.1.4 Sudden cardiac death in athletes 594
- 7.1.5 Causes of sudden cardiac death 596
  - Concealed ischaemic heart disease 596
  - Anomalous coronary arteries 597
  - Coronary artery dissection 597
  - Hypertrophic cardiomyopathy 597
  - Arrhythmogenic cardiomyopathy 597
  - Dilated cardiomyopathy 597
  - Myocarditis 597
  - Valvular heart disease 598
  - Aortic dissection 598
  - Long QT syndrome 598
  - Short QT syndrome 598
  - Brugada syndrome 598
  - Wolf–Parkinson–White 598
  - Catecholaminergic polymorphic ventricular tachycardia 598
  - Drugs 598
  - Commotio cordis 598
- 7.1.6 Prevention of sudden cardiac death in athletes 599
  - Primary prevention 599
  - Secondary prevention 599
- 7.1.7 Differentiating physiological adaptation from cardiomyopathy 599
  - Hypertrophic cardiomyopathy 599
  - Arrhythmogenic cardiomyopathy 600
  - Dilated cardiomyopathy 600
  - Left ventricular non compaction 600
- 7.1.8 Recommendation for professional and recreational sports participation 601
  - Recommendations for competitive sports participation in athletes with cardiomyopathies 601
  - Recommendations for competitive sports participation in athletes with arrhythmias 603
  - Recommendations for exercise in individuals with pacemakers and ICDs 604
  - Recommendations for competitive participation in athletes with ischaemic heart disease 605
  - Recommendation for sports participation in those with hypertension 605
  - Recommendations for sports participation in those with valve disease 606
  - Recommendation for sports participation in those with aortic root dilatation 608
- 7.1.9 Cardiopulmonary exercise testing 609
  - Anaerobic threshold 610
  - Ventilatory equivalents 611
  - Aerobic capacity 611
  - Minute ventilation/carbon dioxide ($\dot{V}E/\dot{V}CO_2$) slope 612
  - Differentiation between cardiovascular and pulmonary aetiology of exercise intolerance 613
  - Interpreting CPET data 613
  - Evaluation of patients with cardiovascular diseases 615

7.1.1 Benefits of exercise on the body

- The benefits of exercise are well established. Exercise leads to a reduction in weight and blood pressure and improves lipid profiles.
- It reduces the risk of developing conditions such as diabetes and exercising individuals demonstrate a 30–50% reduction in the risk of developing coronary artery disease (CAD).

- Exercise has also been shown to improve overall well-being, preventing conditions such as cancer, osteoporosis, depression, and dementia.
- Exercise has been associated with many multi system benefits including:
  - Neurological: reduced/dementia/stroke frequency; improved cognitive function
  - Cardiovascular: reduced mortality/CAD/hypertension
  - Endocrine: reduced weight/diabetes; LDL
  - Musculoskeletal: reduced osteoporosis/falls
  - Oncology: reduced cancer (prostate/breast/bowel)

7.1.2 Exercise physiology

- At the onset of exercise heart rate (HR) and stroke volume (SV) increase in order to increase cardiac output (CO). This is accompanied by changes in arterial blood pressure and peripheral vascular resistance. These changes are controlled by the autonomic nervous system.
- The HR increases as a direct result of the withdrawal of parasympathetic drive in favour of sympathetic stimulation. This leads to increased HR and contractility. Although SV increases secondary to increased contractility, it is influenced more greatly by venous return in the early stages of exercise.
- The increase in venous return causes an increase in left ventricular end diastolic volume, this in turn causes the myocardium to stretch leading to a stronger contraction (Frank Starling mechanism). A normal SV is 50–60 ml/beat and 70–90 ml/beat in an athlete. CO is a product of HR and SV. The usual cardiac output is between 5-l/minute which can increase to up to 25–30 L/minute in an athlete.
- Within muscle, some capillaries have little to no blood flow at rest. During exercise these capillaries vasodilate. Vasodilation improves blood flow to the muscles necessary for oxygen delivery and is triggered by oxygen depletion. This is controlled by vasoactive compounds.
- Noradrenaline is released from vasoconstrictor nerves stimulated by sympathetic nervous activation. In addition, adrenaline and noradrenaline are released from the adrenal medulla leading to peripheral vasoconstriction (sparing active muscles). This increases blood flow by 2L/minute.
- The most profound vasoconstrictor effect is in the venous system, which contains two-thirds of the total blood volume. This increases systemic venous filling pressure and the return of blood to the heart.
- During exercise the systolic blood pressure (SBP) increases but the diastolic blood pressure (DBP) remains relatively stable and does not tend to increase by more than 10 mmHg. The net effect is that mean arterial pressure (MAP) increases. MAP is defined as one-third (SBP – DBP) + DBP. In order to sustain blood supply, the blood flow rate is increased, this is supported by the higher SBP, which also stretches the vessel walls and further increases blood flow.
- In addition, oxygen delivery and carbon dioxide removal is facilitated by an increase in the rate and depth of respiration.
- Lactic acid generated is initially buffered by bicarbonate and leads to an increase in carbon dioxide. This in turn stimulates carotid body chemoreceptors which signals to the respiratory centre in the medulla and leads to a resultant increase in respiratory rate. Once the buffering capacity is exceeded the pH falls. This acts as a further signal to drive hyperventilation.
- The ability of the cardiovascular system to supply muscles with oxygen during exercise is measured by the VO_2 max. This is the point at which there is a plateau in oxygen uptake despite an increase in workload.
- The increase in CO and ventilation together with alterations in afterload enable the body to meet the necessary metabolic requirements.

7.1.3 The athlete's heart

- The athlete's heart refers to structural and electrical changes that occur in response to intensive exercise (minimum 4 hours per week).
- These changes may be evident on a routine ECG. This reflects chamber dilatation, hypertrophy and increased vagal tone.

Electrical changes in the athlete's heart

Normal and abnormal ECG findings in athletes are described in Table 7.1.1.

Table 7.1.1 International Consensus Standards for Electrocardiographic Interpretation in Athletes: Definition of ECG criteria

Abnormal ECG findings in athletes
These ECG findings are unrelated to regular training or expected physiologic adaptation to exercise, may suggest the presence of pathologic cardiovascular disease, and require further diagnostic investigation.

ECG abnormality	Definition
T wave inversion	≥ 1 mm in depth in two or more contiguous leads; excludes leads aVR, III, and V_1
• Anterior	• V_2-V_4 • excludes: black athletes with J-point elevation and convex ST segment elevation followed by TWI in V_2-V_4; athletes < age 16 with TWI in V_1-V_3; and biphasic T waves in only V_3
• Lateral	I and AVL, V_5 and/or V_6 (only one lead of TWI required in V_5 or V_6)
• Inferolateral	II and aVF, V_5-V_6, I and AVL
• Inferior	II and aVF
ST segment depression	≥ 0.5 mm in depth in two or more contiguous leads
Pathologic Q waves	Q/R ratio ≥ 0.25 or ≥ 40 ms in duration in two or more leads (excluding III and aVR)
Complete left bundle branch block	QRS ≥ 120 ms, predominantly negative QRS complex in lead V_1 (QS or rS), and upright notched or slurred R wave in leads I and V_6
Profound nonspecific intraventricular conduction delay	Any QRS duration ≥ 140 ms
Epsilon wave	Distinct low amplitude signal (small positive deflection or notch) between the end of the QRS complex and onset of the T wave in leads V_1-V_3
Ventricular pre-excitation	PR interval < 120 ms with a delta wave (slurred upstroke in the QRS complex) and wide QRS (≥ 120 ms)
Prolonged QT interval*	QTc ≥ 470 ms (male) QTc ≥ 480 ms (female) QTc ≥ 500 ms (marked QT prolongation)
Brugada Type 1 pattern	Coved pattern: initial ST elevation ≥ 2 mm (high take-off) with downsloping ST segment elevation followed by a negative symmetric T wave in ≥ 1 leads in V_1-V_3
Profound sinus bradycardia	< 30 BPM or sinus pauses ≥ 3 s

(continued)

Table 7.1.1 Continued

Abnormal ECG findings in athletes

These ECG findings are unrelated to regular training or expected physiologic adaptation to exercise, may suggest the presence of pathologic cardiovascular disease, and require further diagnostic investigation.

ECG abnormality	Definition
Profound 1° AV block	≥ 400 ms
Mobitz type II 2° AV block	Intermittently non-conducted P waves with a fixed PR interval
3° AV block	Complete heart block
Atrial tachyarrhythmias	Supraventricular tachycardia, atrial fibrillation, atrial flutter
Premature ventricular contractions	≥ 2 PVCs per 10 s tracing
Ventricular arrhythmias	Couplets, triplets, and non-sustained ventricular tachycardia

Borderline ECG findings in athletes

These ECG findings in isolation likely do not represent pathologic cardiovascular disease in athletes, but the presence of two or more borderline findings may warrant additional investigation until further data become available.

ECG abnormality	Definition
Left axis deviation	−30° to −90°
Left atrial enlargement	Prolonged P wave duration of > 120 ms in leads I or II with negative portion of the P wave ≥ 1 mm in depth and ≥ 40 ms in duration in lead V1
Right axis deviation	> 120°
Right atrial enlargement	P wave ≥ 2.5 mm in II, III, or aVF
Complete right bundle branch block	rSR′ pattern in lead V1 and a S wave wider than R wave in lead V6 with QRS duration ≥ 120 ms

Normal ECG findings in athletes

These training-related ECG alterations are physiologic adaptations to regular exercise, considered normal variants in athletes, and do not require further evaluation in asymptomatic athletes with no significant family history.

Normal ECG finding	Definition
Increased QRS voltage	Isolated QRS voltage criteria for left (SV1 + RV5 or RV6 > 3.5 mV) or right ventricular hypertrophy (RV1 + SV5 or SV6 > 1.1 mV)
Incomplete RBBB	rSR′ pattern in lead V1 and a qRS pattern in lead V6 with QRS duration < 120 ms
Early repolarization	J point elevation, ST elevation, J waves, or terminal QRS slurring
Black athlete repolarization variant	J-point elevation and convex ("domed") ST segment elevation followed by T wave inversion in leads V1-V4 in black athletes
Juvenile T wave pattern	T wave inversion V_1-V_3 in athletes < age 16 yrs
Sinus bradycardia	≥ 30 bpm
Sinus arrhythmia	Heart rate variation with respiration: rate increases during inspiration and decreases during expiration
Ectopic atrial rhythm	P waves are a different morphology compared to the sinus P wave, such as negative P waves in the inferior leads ("low atrial rhythm")
Junctional escape rhythm	QRS rate is faster than the resting P wave or sinus rate and typically <100 beats/minute with narrow QRS complex unless the baseline QRS is conducted with aberrancy

Table 7.1.1 Continued

Normal ECG findings in athletes
These training-related ECG alterations are physiologic adaptations to regular exercise, considered normal variants in athletes, and do not require further evaluation in asymptomatic athletes with no significant family history.

Normal ECG finding	Definition
1° AV block	PR interval 200–400 ms
Mobitz Type I (Wenckebach) 2° AV block	PR interval progressively lengthens until there is a nonconducted P wave with no QRS complex; the first PR interval after the dropped beat is shorter than the last conducted PR interval

* The QT interval corrected for heart rate is ideally measured using Bazett's formula with heart rates between 60 and 90 bpm; preferably performed manually in lead II or V5 using the teach-the-tangent method1 to avoid inclusion of a U wave (please see text for more details). Consider repeating the ECG after mild aerobic activity for a heart rate < 50 bpm, or repeating the ECG after a longer resting period for a heart rate > 100 bpm, if the QTc value is borderline or abnormal.
AV = atrioventricular block; ECG = electrocardiogram; PVC = premature ventricular complex; RBBB = right bundle branch block.
Reproduced from Sharma S et al. International Recommendations for Electrocardiographic Interpretation in Athletes. J Am Coll Cardiol. 2017 Feb 28;69(8):1057–1075. doi: 10.1016/j.jacc.2017.01.015 with permission from Elsevier.

Criteria for the interpretation of the athlete's ECG

- A small number of athletes may demonstrate ECG changes which may overlap with phenotypes of ECGs seen in individuals at risk of sudden cardiac death (SCD). Therefore, it is of vital importance to correctly differentiate physiology from pathology.
- The most up-to-date international recommendations for electrocardiographic interpretation in athletes were published in 2017. This clearly sets out the circumstances under which an athlete requires further investigation (Figure 7.1.1) and borderline ECG findings.

Investigations to consider where further investigation is recommended are listed in Table 7.1.2.

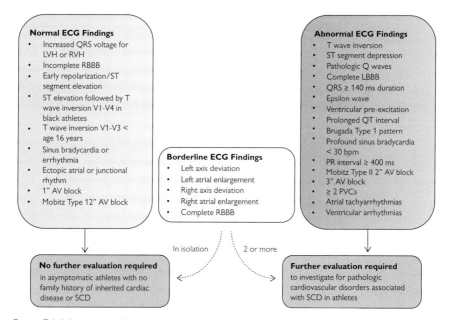

Figure 7.1.1 International consensus standards for electrographic interpretation in athletes.
Reproduced from Sharma S et al. International Recommendations for Electrocardiographic Interpretation in Athletes. J Am Coll Cardiol. 2017 Feb 28;69(8):1057–1075. doi: 10.1016/j.jacc.2017.01.015 with permission from Elsevier.

Table 7.1.2 Further investigations based on ECG abnormalities.

Pathology	Recommendations
Sinus bradycardia ≤ 30 bpm	Exercise the athlete (running on the spot/climbing stairs) and repeat ECG If no increase in HR further evaluation required with exercise stress testing and 24-hr Holter monitor
Profound first-degree AV block ≥ 400 ms	Exercise the athlete (running on the spot/climbing stairs) and repeat ECG If no increase in HR further evaluation required with exercise stress testing and 24-hr Holter monitor
Second-degree (Mobitz type II), third-degree heart block	Echocardiography Exercise stress testing 24-hr Holter monitor
Atrial arrhythmias	Echocardiography Exercise stress testing 24-hr Holter monitor
Ventricular arrhythmias	Echocardiography Exercise stress testing 24-hr Holter monitor CMR
Brugada Type 1 pattern	Referral to an electrophysiologist
Long QTc (measured using Bazett's formula in lead II and V5 using the teach the tangent rule). If the manual measurement of the QT interval is within 10 ms of the calculated QTc then the computer derived measurement is most likely accurate. N.B. Bazett's formula may underestimate the QTc at heart rates of < 50 bpm and overestimate the QTc at heart rates > 90 bpm	If > 470 ms in male and > 480 ms in female athletes; Repeat ECG on a separate occasion If still prolonged exercise stress testing (assessment of whether QTc shortens to < 480 ms in the 4th minute), 24-hr Holter monitor Drug history for evidence of QT prolonging drugs Family history for sudden cardiac death, unexplained road traffic accidents, unexplained drownings Consider family screening with an ECG +/− genetic testing if suspicion is high If the QTc is ≥ 500 ms direct referral to an electrophysiologist should be considered
Short QT	QRS ≤ 320 ms. 24-hr Holter monitor, echocardiogram, electrophysiology referral
Ventricular pre-excitation	Exercise ECG (early disappearance of the preexcitation on exercise is a sign of a low risk pathway) Echocardiography (due to the association of an accessory pathway and cardiomyopathy) Consider electrophysiological testing
Pathological Q waves (Q to R ratio of 0.25 or ≥ 40 ms in duration in 2 or more contiguous leads excluding III and aVR)	Repeat ECG if septal Q waves, with further investigation if persistent Echocardiography CMR If suspicion of coronary disease based on risk factors consider CTCA/ functional stress testing
ST segment depression ≥ 0.5 mm in ≥ 2 contiguous leads	Echocardiography Consider MRI based on the clinical suspicion
Complete LBBB	Echocardiography CMR +/− stress perfusion
Non-specific intraventricular delay ≥ 140 ms	Echocardiography with additional testing as governed by the results of echocardiography

(continued)

Table 7.1.2 Continued

Pathology	Recommendations
Multiple PVEs (≥ 2 on a resting 12 lead ECG)**	Echocardiography Exercise stress testing 24-hr Holter monitor MRI if evidence of > 2000 PVEs or NSVT Consider signal averaged ECG Cessation of exercise if ectopy thought to be caused by myocarditis
Epsilon wave (major criterion for ARVC)	Echocardiography Exercise stress testing 24-hr Holter monitor MRI Consider Signal averaged ECG depending on results of above investigations
TWI in the anterior leads (≥ 1 mm in 2 or more contiguous leads beyond V2 in Caucasians and V4 in black athletes)	Echocardiography Exercise stress testing 24-hr Holter monitor CMR Signal averaged ECG
TWI in the lateral/inferolateral leads (≥ 1 mm in 2 or more contiguous leads, I, aVL, V5/V6 (lateral) +/− II, and aVF (inferior) excluding III)	Echocardiography Exercise stress testing 24-hr Holter monitor CMR
TWI in the inferior leads (≥ 1 mm in 2 or more contiguous leads II, aVF excluding III)	Echocardiography Exercise stress testing 24-hr Holter monitor Consider MRI based on the clinical suspicion
Flat or biphasic T waves	Although there is no data regarding the significance of this in athletes, most physicians would agree that biphasic T waves where the negative part is ≥ 1 mm in 2 contiguous leads should be further evaluated.
QRS fragmentation	Although there is no data regarding the significance of isolated QRS fragmentation in athletes where there is a QRS duration of > 110 ms further evaluation should be considered.
LAE (biphasic P wave V1, negative portion ≥ 40 ms in duration and ≥ 1 mm deep) RAE (amplitude > 2.5 mm in II, III, aVF) LAD ≥ −30 degrees RAD ≥ 120 degrees RBBB	Whereas each of these in isolation is not deemed to indicate pathology. The presence of >/= 2 or more of these findings further evaluation should be considered.

*CTCA—Computed tomography coronary angiogram, MRI—magnetic resonance imaging, LBBB—left bundle branch block, PVE— premature ventricular ectopics, RVOT—right ventricular outflow tract, LAE—left atrial enlargement, RAE—right atrial enlargement, LAD—left axis deviation, RAD—right axis deviation, RBBB—right bundle branch block.
**Characteristics of ectopics
  Infundibular
- LBBB with late precordial transition (where the QRS becomes predominantly positive) R/S = 1 after V3 and inferior axis: right ventricular outflow tract (usually benign)
- LBBB with early precordial transition R/S = 1 by V2/V3 and inferior axis: left ventricular outflow tract (usually benign)

  Fascicular
- RBBB with superior axis and QRS < 130 ms: left posterior fascicle (usually benign)
- RBBB with inferior axis and QRS < 130 m: right posterior fascicle (usually benign)

  Abnormal
- RBBB and QRS ≥ 130 ms: mitral valve, papillary muscles, or left ventricle (may be associated with disease)
- LBBB with superior axis: septum or right ventricular wall (may be associated with disease)

Structural changes in the athlete's heart

- Structural changes observed depend on age, sex, ethnicity, and sporting discipline.
- Different sporting disciplines may lead to different degrees of cardiac remodelling.
  - Power sports (high static component) can lead to an increase in left ventricular (LV) wall thickness and modest increase in cavity size.
  - Mixed sports (dynamic and static components) can lead to an increase in cavity size and a modest increase in wall thickness.
  - Endurance sports (high dynamic component) can lead to an increase in LV cavity size.
- Athletes can have a low LV ejection fraction (LVEF), particularly in endurance athletes where there is a ventricular enlargement. Here, they are able to generate the required SV at lower heart rates. The diastolic function in an athlete should be normal.

Assessment of athlete's left ventricle

- Relative wall thickness (RWT) can be calculated by adding together the posterior and septal wall thickness in diastole and dividing it by the LV diastolic cavity size. This allows differentiation between normality and concentric remodelling (increased RWT > 0.42 and normal mass), concentric hypertrophy (increased RWT and mass) and eccentric hypertrophy (normal RWT and increased mass (Figure 7.1.2). An algorithm to differentiate physiology from pathology if left-sided parameters suggest abnormal geometry is shown in Figure 7.1.3.

Assessment of the athlete's right ventricle

- The right ventricle (RV) adapts to dynamic sports. The algorithm below may help to differentiate between pathology and physiology (Figure 7.1.4).

7.1.4 Sudden cardiac death in athletes

- Cardiovascular disease accounts for 17 million deaths worldwide and SCD accounts for 25% of these.
- SCD is defined as a 'non-traumatic, unexpected fatal event occurring within 1 hour of the onset of symptoms in an apparently healthy subject'. If the death was not witnessed the definition applies when the victim was in good health 24 hours before the event.

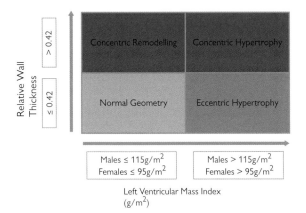

Figure 7.1.2 Defining left ventricular geometry.
Reproduced with permission from Oxborough, D., Augustine, D., Gati, S. et al. A guideline update for the practice of echocardiography in the cardiac screening of sports participants: a joint policy statement from the British Society of Echocardiography and Cardiac Risk in the Young. *Echo Res Pract* 5, G1–G10 (2018). https://doi.org/10.1530/ERP-17-0075. under a Creative Commons Attribution 4.0 International (CC BY 4.0).

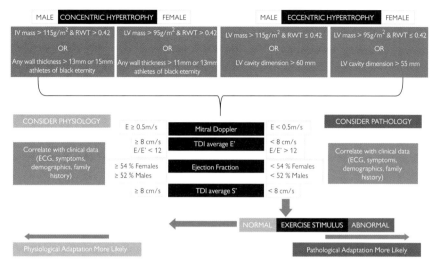

Figure 7.1.3 Algorithm when left-sided parameters suggest abnormal geometry.
Reproduced with permission from Oxborough, D., Augustine, D., Gati, S. et al. A guideline update for the practice of echocardiography in the cardiac screening of sports participants: a joint policy statement from the British Society of Echocardiography and Cardiac Risk in the Young. *Echo Res Pract* 5, G1–G10 (2018). https://doi.org/10.1530/ERP-17-0075. under a Creative Commons Attribution 4.0 International (CC BY 4.0).

- The cause of SCD varies by age with a predominance of cardiomyopathies and channelopathies below the age of 35 years and CAD over the age of 35 years.
- SCD is the leading cause of death in athletes and a large proportion of these deaths are associated with undiagnosed cardiovascular disease. The rate of SCD ranges from 1 in 23,000 to 1 in a million. A generally accepted prevalence is 1 in 50,000 in college aged athletes. The discrepancy in rates is due to methodological inconsistencies and population heterogeneity. In younger athletes the rates may be higher.

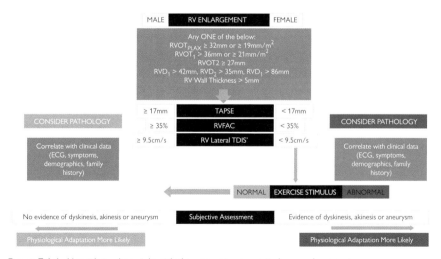

Figure 7.1.4 Algorithm when right-sided parameters suggest abnormal geometry.
Reproduced with permission from Oxborough, D., Augustine, D., Gati, S. et al. A guideline update for the practice of echocardiography in the cardiac screening of sports participants: a joint policy statement from the British Society of Echocardiography and Cardiac Risk in the Young. *Echo Res Pract* 5, G1–G10 (2018). https://doi.org/10.1530/ERP-17-0075. under a Creative Commons Attribution 4.0 International (CC BY 4.0).

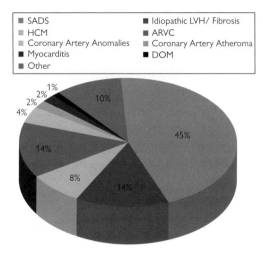

Figure 7.1.5 Causes of sudden cardiac death in athletes.
Reproduced with permission from Oxborough, D., Augustine, D., Gati, S. et al. A guideline update for the practice of echocardiography in the cardiac screening of sports participants: a joint policy statement from the British Society of Echocardiography and Cardiac Risk in the Young. *Echo Res Pract* 5, G1–G10 (2018). https://doi.org/10.1530/ERP-17-0075. under a Creative Commons Attribution 4.0 International (CC BY 4.0).

- Athletes demonstrate a 2.8-fold increased risk of SCD compared to sedentary individuals. This suggests that sporting activity may be a trigger for life-threatening arrhythmias in those with an underlying cardiac condition. The prevalence of underlying cardiac conditions capable of causing SCD in athletes is estimated to be 1 in 300.
- Men are at higher risk of SCD than women. Black athletes and in particular those playing sports such as basketball are also at higher risk.
- The leading cause of death in athletes is sudden arrhythmic death syndrome (SADS) (Figure 7.1.5).
- Individuals with suspected SCD should undergo autopsy in order to determine the cause of death.
    - The heart should be examined histologically, and labelled blocks of myocardium taken from both ventricles.
    - The heart should ideally be examined in a specialized centre.
    - It is also essential to analyze bloods/bodily fluids for molecular pathology and toxicology.
    - The spleen should be retained for genetic analysis of potential pathological genes.
    - All living first-degree relatives of the affected individual should be referred to a cardiologist with a specialist interest in inherited cardiac conditions for further investigations in order to assess for a potentially heritable phenotype.

7.1.5 Causes of sudden cardiac death

Concealed ischaemic heart disease

- This accounts for the majority of SCD in the older individuals and is most likely to be secondary to stress-related plaque rupture and thrombosis formation.
- Risk factors for IHD include family history, hypercholesterolemia, diabetes, hypertension, smoking, and a high BMI.
- In the young CAD occurs secondary to accelerated atherosclerosis. Unlike older individuals SCD is usually caused by temporary myocardial ischaemia secondary to plaque obstruction

to blood flow, which may trigger fatal arrhythmias. Risk factors may include a family history of dyslipidaemias, cocaine, or steroid use.

Anomalous coronary arteries
- This is usually caused by an anomalous left coronary system originating from the right coronary sinus. The blood flow is impeded either at the ostium of the anomalous artery, by compression of the anomalous artery between the pulmonary trunk and the aorta or coronary vasospasm. The ischaemia during exercise can precipitate a fatal arrhythmia.

Coronary artery dissection
- Coronary artery dissection leads to formation of an intramural haematoma which externally compresses the vessel leading to myocardial ischaemia.

Hypertrophic cardiomyopathy
- Hypertrophic cardiomyopathy (HCM) is characterized by asymmetric ventricular hypertrophy (> 15 mm) in the absence of other abnormal loading conditions.
- Histologically there is evidence of fibrosis and myocardial disarray.
- Deaths commonly occur during start-stop sports such as basketball and football. This may be secondary to arrhythmia or mechanical obstruction secondary to left ventricular outflow tract obstruction.
- The risk of SCD is calculated using the HCM Risk-SCD which estimates the 5-year risk of SCD. Variables include age, maximum wall thickness, left atrial size, left ventricular outflow tract gradient, non-sustained ventricular tachycardia (NSVT), history of syncope, and family history of SCD. However, this score is less applicable to an athletic population (who were not included in cohort studies).

Arrhythmogenic cardiomyopathy
- Arrhythmogenic cardiomyopathy (AC) is characterized by fibrofatty replacement of the myocardium. This leads to ventricular dilatation, regional wall abnormalities, and arrhythmias.
- Although this typically affects the RV the LV can be affected simultaneously or in isolation.
- The risk of SCD is highest in those who have poorly tolerated ventricular tachycardia, syncope, and aborted cardiac arrest.

Dilated cardiomyopathy
- Dilated cardiomyopathy (DCM) may predispose to ventricular arrhythmias.
- The risk is greater in those who are: symptomatic; have a left ventricular ejection fraction (LVEF) < 40%; extensive late gadolinium enhancement (LGE) on MRI; unexplained syncope and ventricular arrhythmias.
- In those with a known lamin A/C mutation, there is an increased risk of malignant ventricular arrhythmias in those who have with two out of the following risk factors: NSVT on ambulatory ECG monitoring; left ventricular ejection fraction of ≤ 45%; male sex; non-missense mutations (mutations affecting splicing, insertion-deletion/truncating).

Myocarditis
- Inflammation of the myocardium is caused most commonly by viral infections. Individuals may present with a prodrome of a viral illness and may develop arrhythmias and heart failure. SCD may occur in the active phase or post myocarditis secondary to arrhythmias. The risk of SCD is greater in those with reduced LVEF, arrhythmias on exercise testing or ambulatory monitoring. Residual LGE on MRI may also increase risk.

Valvular heart disease
- Aortic stenosis and mitral valve prolapse may be associated with SCD in athletes.

Aortic dissection
- This usually occurs in those with a genetic or congenital predisposition. This may be due to familial thoracic aortic disease, bicuspid aortic valve, Marfan, Ehlers–Danlos and Loeys–Dietz syndrome.
- Dissection usually occurs at times of intense physical exertion due to a rapid rise in blood pressure.

Long QT syndrome
- In athletes, long QT syndrome (LQTS) is defined as a QTc interval of > 470 ms in men and > 480 ms in women.
- The risk of SCD is highest in the following groups: those with syncope and aborted cardiac arrest; women with LQT type 2 and QTc > 500 ms; those with a QTc of > 500 ms with electrical instability; those who have high-risk genetics (two mutations).

Short QT syndrome
- Short QT syndrome (SQTS) is defined as a QT interval of < 320 ms.
- The risk of SCD is highest in those with an aborted cardiac arrest and spontaneous sustained VT.

Brugada syndrome
- The risk of SCD is highest in those in the following groups: those with an aborted cardiac arrest; documented VT; spontaneous type I pattern (J point elevation, coved ST segment, and T wave inversion in V1 and V2) with a history of syncope.

Wolf–Parkinson–White
- This is characterized by a short PR interval, delta wave, and widened QRS complex.
- SCD is usually caused by 1:1 conduction of atrial fibrillation (AF) through an accessory pathway with a short refractory period causing ventricular fibrillation (VF).
- The heart is morphologically normal unless associated with HCM.

Catecholaminergic polymorphic ventricular tachycardia
- Arrhythmias typically occur during exercise or during periods of emotional stress.
- The risk of SCD is highest in those with an aborted cardiac arrest; recurrent syncope; polymorphic or bidirectional VT despite optimal therapy.

Drugs
- Anabolic steroids can cause adverse events by several methods: alteration of lipoprotein concentrations; thrombosis; vasospasm; direct injury to the myocardium.
- 3% of SCD can be attributed to cocaine use. This can cause left ventricular hypertrophy (LVH), premature atheroma (with or without thrombosis), and small vessel disease.
- Cannabis can also cause thrombosis of the coronary arteries.

Commotio cordis
- A blow to the chest can cause VF due to alteration of the electrical stability when it occurs on the upstroke of the T wave.
- At post mortem there is usually bruising to the chest and a morphologically normal heart.

7.1.6 Prevention of sudden cardiac death in athletes

Primary prevention

- An athlete is defined as 'one who participates in an organized team or individual sport requiring systematic training and regular competition against others, while placing a high premium on athletic excellence and achievement'.
- The sudden death of an athlete is a tragic event which is often highly publicized, particularly as athletes represent the healthiest individuals within society.
- Screening enables early detection of underlying cardiovascular disease, as well as enabling lifestyle modification and therapeutic intervention.
- A pre-participation screening programme comprising of history, physical examination, and 12-lead ECG has been in practice in Italy for over 30 years. This has led to an 89% reduction in SCD, primarily due to improved identification of cardiomyopathies through cessation of ongoing competitive physical activity. Most individuals at risk will not be identified from their history and examination alone, given that 80% are asymptomatic with SCD often the first presentation of underlying cardiovascular pathology.
- Use of ECG screening improves the detection of early electrical changes which precede phenotypic expression. In addition, the ECG is essential to detect electrical conditions such as LQTS, Brugada syndrome, and Wolff–Parkinson–White syndrome.
- Prompt referral of affected individuals and first-degree relatives to a cardiologist with a specialist interest in inherited cardiac conditions enables appropriate assessment and follow-up.

Secondary prevention

- Most cardiac arrests occur out of hospital and therefore emergency response measures are crucial. A combination of cardiopulmonary resuscitation together with defibrillation compared to cardiopulmonary resuscitation alone has been shown to be the most effective in terms of survival outcomes.
- Public AEDs should be available and suitably stored wherever a cardiac arrest may arise (e.g. schools, stations, sports stadiums) or where access to defibrillation devices is unavailable (planes, trains, ships). This however does not prevent the 70% of cardiac arrests that occur in the home which are frequently unwitnessed and therefore cannot be prevented with home AEDs.

7.1.7 Differentiating physiological adaptation from cardiomyopathy

- The overlap between physiology and early pathology can make diagnosis difficult.
- The next section identifies aspects of the history, physical examination, and investigations that may point towards pathology.

Hypertrophic cardiomyopathy

- LVH can be seen in athletes and can vary with age, gender, and ethnicity. A 'grey' zone increase in wall thickness can be seen that overlaps with potential pathological processes. The following features may help to identify pathological features:
    1. Abnormal symptoms (shortness of breath, palpitations, syncope, pre-syncope, and chest pain).

2. Up to 95% of individuals with HCM have an abnormal ECG (large QRS voltages, Q waves, ST segment depression, inferior and/or lateral TWI, non-specific intraventricular delay (≥ 140 ms), complete LBBB, LAE, LAD, and PVEs.
3. The pattern of pathological hypertrophy is usually asymmetrical, septal, or apical.
4. Low peak VO2, NSVT on exercise testing.
5. NSVT/VT on Holter monitoring.
6. Myocardial crypts, LGE on MRI.
7. Positive family history/positive genetics.
8. Detraining for 3 months leading to regression of LVH is more suggestive of physiological hypertrophy in the absence of a family history.

Arrhythmogenic cardiomyopathy

- Differentiation between physiological RV enlargement and anterior TWI from pathological changes is particularly difficult in endurance athletes who may demonstrate both of these findings. The following features may help to identify pathological features:
  1. Abnormal symptoms.
  2. Up to 80% of individuals with AC have an abnormal ECG (ST segment depression, inferior and/or lateral TWI (left ventricular predominance), TWI in the anterior leads (right ventricular predominance), epsilon wave, RAD, PVEs.
  3. Late potentials on signal averaged ECG.
  4. Abnormal echocardiographic parameters (dilatation accompanied by wall motion abnormalities or aneurysms).
  5. NSVT/VT on Holter monitoring.
  6. LGE on MRI.
  7. Positive family history/positive genetics.

Dilated cardiomyopathy

- 15% of elite male athletes demonstrate LV end diastolic dimensions of > 60 mm which overlaps with pathological dilatation. The following features may help to differentiate physiology from pathology:
  1. Abnormal symptoms.
  2. Abnormal ECG (Q waves, ST segment depression, TWI, non-specific intraventricular delay, complete LBBB, atrial enlargement, axis deviation, PVEs).
  3. Low peak VO2, NSVT on exercise testing.
  4. NSVT/VT on Holter monitoring.
  5. LGE on MRI.
  6. Inability to augment LVEF by > 11% on exercise echocardiography
  7. Positive family history/positive genetics.

Left ventricular non compaction

- Athletes frequently demonstrate trabeculations within the LV cavity. 8% of athletes may even fulfil criteria for left ventricular non compaction (LVNC). The following features may help to differentiate physiology from pathology:
  1. Abnormal symptoms.
  2. Abnormal ECG (ST depression, inferolateral TWI, LBBB).
  3. Abnormal echocardiographic parameters (increased trabeculations).
  4. Low peak VO2, NSVT on exercise testing.
  5. NSVT/VT on Holter monitoring.
  6. Late gadolinium enhancement on MRI.
  7. Positive family history.

7.1.8 Recommendation for professional and recreational sports participation

- Individuals with underlying cardiovascular disease should as a minimum undergo a full history, including assessment of symptomatic status, physical examination, ECG, echocardiogram, exercise testing.
- Further investigations should be guided by the underlying pathology including prolonged ECG monitoring, functional stress testing and MRI. Athletes with an underlying pathology should be reassessed regularly.
- The following section addresses the exercise restrictions in those conditions most likely to be encountered in a clinical setting.

Recommendations for competitive sports participation in athletes with cardiomyopathies

Hypertrophic cardiomyopathy

- Markers of increased risk:
    - Cardiac symptoms
    - Prior cardiac arrest or unexplained syncope
    - ESC risk score of 4% or more
    - Exercise induced ventricular arrhythmias
    - LV outflow tract gradient of > 30 mmHg
    - Abnormal BP response to exercise
- Exercise recommendations:
    - If no markers of increased risk high-intensity/competitive sports acceptable (with the exception of sports where syncope may lead to harm/death)
    - If markers of increased risk:
        - low or moderate intensity recreational exercise following expert assessment
        - high intensity exercise not recommended
    - No restrictions in genotype positive/phenotype negative
- Follow-up:
    - Annual follow up for those who exercise regularly
    - 6-monthly follow up for adolescents/young adults who are more vulnerable to exercise induced SCD
    - Consider annual follow up for genotype positive/phenotype negative

Arrhythmogenic cardiomyopathy

- Markers of increased risk:
    - Prior cardiac arrest or ventricular arrhythmia (at rest or on exertion)
    - Unexplained syncope
    - Structural cardiac abnormalities
    - > 500 PVCs / 24 hrs
- Exercise recommendations:
    - 150 min low-intensity exercise per week
    - Consider low–moderate intensity recreational sports if no increased risk markers
    - High intensity exercise or any competitive sports not recommended (including those who are genotype positive/phenotype negative)

- Follow-up:
    - Annual follow-up for those who exercise regularly
    - 6-monthly follow-up for adolescents/young adults who are more vulnerable to exercise-induced SCD
    - Consider annual follow-up for genotype positive/phenotype negative
    - Consider 6-month follow-up for those with high-risk genotypes

Dilated cardiomyopathy

- Markers of increased risk:
    - Symptoms or prior cardiac arrest or unexplained syncope.
    - LVEF < 45%.
    - Frequent or complex ventricular arrhythmia (at rest or on exertion).
    - Extensive LGE on CMR (> 20%).
    - High-risk genotypes
- Exercise recommendations:
    - Low- to moderate-intensity recreational exercise in all irrespective of EF (unless symptoms or ventricular arrhythmia on exertion).
    - High intensity exercise or any competitive sports not recommended if any high-risk markers.
    - High-intensity/competitive sports (with the exception of sports where syncope may lead to harm/death) acceptable if:
        - EF > 44%
        - No frequent or complex ventricular arrhythmia (at rest or on exertion).
        - No LGE on CMR.
        - Ability to increase EF by 10–15% during exercise.
        - No high-risk genotype
    - No restrictions in genotype positive/phenotype negative (unless high-risk mutations, e.g. lamin A/C).
- Follow-up:
    - Annual follow-up for those who exercise regularly.
    - 6-monthly follow-up in high-risk mutations or adolescents/young adults, those with evolving phenotype.
    - Consider annual follow-up for genotype positive/phenotype negative.

Myocarditis

- Return to all forms of sport after 3–6 months in asymptomatic individuals and with:
    - Normal troponin/inflammatory biomarkers
    - Normal LV systolic function
    - No ongoing inflammation/fibrosis on CMR
    - Good functional capacity
    - No frequent or complex ventricular arrhythmia (at rest or on exertion).
- High-intensity or competitive sport not recommended in those with residual LV dysfunction and myocardial scar.

Pericarditis

- Sports participation not recommended if there is evidence of active inflammation.
- Return to exercise following pericarditis after a period of 30 days to 3 months acceptable depending on clinical scenario.

Recommendations for competitive sports participation in athletes with arrhythmias

Atrial fibrillation/flutter
- Evaluation: To assess for structural heart disease and primary causes of AF.
- Consider ablation in those with:
    - Recurrent symptomatic AF
    - Those who do not want drug therapy due to potential impact on athletic performance.
- Assessment of ventricular rate during exercise,
- If AF well tolerated without antiarrhythmic therapy and no structural heart disease then continue sports participation.
- Consider cavo-tricuspid isthmus ablation in those with documented flutter who would like to engage in intensive exercise (to prevent potential for 1:1 AV conduction).
- Consider cavo-tricuspid isthmus ablation to prevent flutter in those with AF and on class I drug therapy if they who would like to engage in intensive exercise.
- With a 'pill in the pocket' strategy participation in intensive sports is not recommended until two half-lives of the antiarrhythmic drug have elapsed
- In those who are anticoagulated sports with direct bodily contact/prone to trauma are not recommended.
- After successful ablation, if no reoccurrence of symptoms then competitive sports can be resumed after 1 month.

Paroxysmal SVT without pre-excitation
- PSVT without structural heart disease is usually not life threatening.
- May cause presyncope/exhaustion during exercise. Syncope is uncommon.
- Advice should be given on how to perform vagal manoeuvres.
- Prophylactic drug therapy can be considered.
- Consider ablation in those undertaking competitive sports.
- If PSVT symptoms are sporadic and not associated with haemodynamic consequences continue sports activity (unless increased risk of fatality from potential loss of consciousness—e.g. parachute jumpers).
- Following successful ablation, in most cases training can be resumed after 1 week and competitive activity after 1 month.

Paroxysmal SVT with pre-excitation
- Ablation of the accessory pathway is recommended in competitive and recreational athletes with preexcitation and documented arrhythmias.
- In competitive athletes with asymptomatic preexcitation an EP study is recommended to evaluate the risk for sudden death
- Following ablation resumption of competitive sports after 1–3 months is possible when the likelihood of accessory pathway recurrence and risk are negligible
- In those with asymptomatic pre-excitation:
    - An EP study recommended in those ≥ 12 years.

Premature ventricular contractions or non-sustained ventricular tachycardia
- If ≥ 2 PVC is seen on a resting ECG thorough evaluation to exclude structural abnormality is recommended
- In those with frequent PVCs/NSVT recommend Holter monitor, exercise test; imaging

Long QT syndrome
- Exercising individuals with LQTS or prolonged QTc recommended beta blockers.
- Exercising individuals with LQTS should avoid QT-prolonging drugs and electrolyte imbalance (e.g. hypokalaemia).
- Shared decision-making in patients with genotype positive/phenotype negative (i.e. QTc < 470/480 ms in men/women).
- Participation in high intensity recreational/competitive sport not recommended in those with a QTc > 500 ms or genetically confirmed LQTS with a QTc ≥ 470 ms in men or ≥ 480 ms in women.
- Recommend avoidance of competitive sport in those with LQTS and prior cardiac arrest or arrhythmic syncope.
- Reasonable to allow low- to moderate-intensity sports for asymptomatic athletes on beta blocker with LQT1 but QTc < 470/480 ms. Team sports and high intensity sports are discouraged.
- Reasonable to allow all types of sports participation for aymptomatic athletes on beta blocker with LQT2 or LQT3 with QTC < 470/480 ms.

Brugada syndrome (BrS)
- Recommend ICD in those with BrS and have had arrhythmic syncope/aborted SCD.
- Following ICD implantation consider resumption of leisure or competitive sport in those who have not experienced arrhythmia for 3 months.
- In those with asymptomatic BrS, asymptomatic mutation carriers and asymptomatic athletes with only an inducible ECG pattern participation in sports that are not associated with an increase of core temperature of > 39°C (e.g. endurance events under hot conditions) may be considered.

Catecholaminergic polymorphic ventricular tachycardia (CPVT)
- Competitive and intensive leisure-time sports not recommended
- Following appropriate treatment, if negative stress test and asymptomatic for at least 3 months then low- to moderate-intensity leisure time sports may be considered.
- Genotype positive/phenotype negative—manage as per phenotype +ve. Consider beta blocker.
- Recommend follow up to include ECG, Holter monitoring during low-intensity sport to ensure control of exercise-induced ventricular arrhythmias.
- Recommend avoidance of stressful/emotional situations/electrolyte disturbances and hyperthermia.

Recommendations for exercise in individuals with pacemakers and ICDs
- If no resynchronization therapy and no underlying disease then follow guidance as per disease process.
- Sports and exercise should be considered in all with a pacemaker who do not have pathological substrate for fatal arrhythmia.
- Avoid direct impact to the implanted device.
- Shared decision-making during decisions pertaining to continuation of intensive or competitive sports participation in individuals with an ICD.
- Remote monitoring recommended.

Recommendations for competitive participation in athletes with ischaemic heart disease

- IHD is the most common cause of SCD during exercise in those over the age of 35 years. This is thought to be caused by plaque rupture or high-intensity exercise exceeding the threshold of ischaemia.
- Physical inactivity is a risk factor for CAD and therefore it is essential to provide appropriate recommendations to athletes with IHD.
- Asymptomatic athletes should undergo exercise testing if they have a high-risk factor profile:
    - If this is normal there should be no restriction for competitive sport.
    - If the exercise test is borderline, an additional stress test is recommended (exercise echocardiography, stress echocardiography, CMR perfusion, SPECT/PET). If there is no evidence of inducible ischaemia the athlete should not be restricted from participation in competitive sports.
    - If the exercise test is positive then a CT coronary angiogram (CTCA) or coronary angiogram should be performed. Individuals with significant coronary disease should undergo percutaneous coronary intervention (PCI). In the case of non-significant coronary disease, as long as they are low risk then they should be advised that they may participate in competitive sports, however restrictions may apply to the sports with highest cardiovascular demands. In those with high-risk features competitive sports are not advised.
- Individuals who undergo PCI may be risk-stratified at 3 months and if low risk may compete in most competitive sports with the exception of those with high cardiovascular demand. High-risk individuals should not participate in competitive sports.
- Recommendations for competitive sports in individuals with IHD are listed in the Table 7.1.3 and Figure 7.1.6 below.

Recommendation for sports participation in those with hypertension

- Athletes with hypertension should be treated as per existing guidelines.
- Low, moderate, high, and very high risk equate to a 10-year risk of cardiovascular mortality of < 1%, 1–4%, 5–10%, and > 10% respectively according to the European SCORE system.
- In athletes with low to moderate cardiovascular risk no restrictions apply.

Table 7.1.3 Recommendations for competitive sports participation in athletes with coronary artery disease.

Condition	Eligibility criteria	Recommendations	Follow up
Athletes with IHD and high risk of cardiac events	Symptoms, LV function < 50%, ischaemia on exercise, arrhythmias on exercise, > 50% stenosis of the left main stem (LMS) or > 70% of the major coronary arteries)	No competitive sports	Annually
Athletes with IHD and low risk of cardiac events	No symptoms, LV function > 50%, no ischaemia on exercise, no ventricular arrhythmias on exercise or rest, < 50% stenosis of the LMS and < 70% stenosis of the major coronary arteries	Most competitive sports Restriction limited to sports with highest cardiovascular demands	Annually

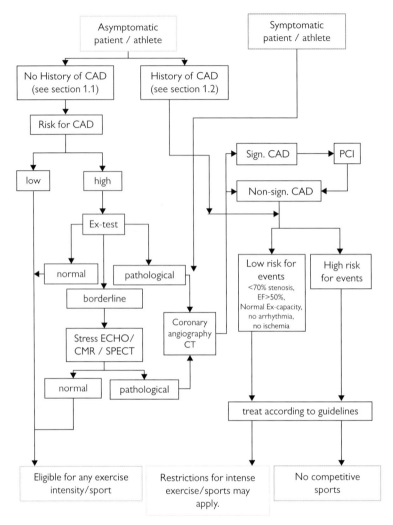

Figure 7.1.6 Clinical evaluation and recommendations of eligibility in athletes with coronary artery disease or risk of coronary artery disease.

Reproduced from Borjesson M, Dellborg M, Niebauer J et al. Recommendations for participation in leisure time or competitive sports in athletes-patients with coronary artery disease: a position statement from the Sports Cardiology Section of the European Association of Preventive Cardiology (EAPC). Eur Heart J. 2019 Jan 1;40(1):13–18. doi: 10.1093/eurheartj/ehy408 with permission from Oxford University Press.

- In athletes with high or very high risk where BP control is achieved competitive sports participation is allowed (with the exception of those with high static components). If the BP is not well controlled temporary restriction from competitive sport is recommended.
- Recommendations for competitive sports participation in athletes with hypertension is listed in Table 7.1.4.

Recommendations for sports participation in those with valve disease

- Recommendations for competitive sports in individuals with valvular heart disease are described below:
- Multivalvular diseases should be managed as per the predominant lesion.

Table 7.1.4 Recommendations for competitive sports participation in athletes with hypertension

Eligibility criteria	Recommendations	Follow-up
BP well controlled No other RF No TOD No ACC	All competitive sports	Annually
BP well controlled RF well controlled No TOD No ACC	All competitive sports	6–12 monthly
BP well controlled RF well controlled TOD present No ACC	All competitive sports apart from those with a high dynamic component e.g. power sports	6 monthly
BP well controlled RF well controlled TOD not present/present ACC present	All competitive sports apart from those with a high dynamic component e.g. power sports	6 monthly

*RF—risk factors, TOD—target organ damage, ACC—Associated clinical condition
**Target organ damage includes LVH, ultrasound confirmation of plaque or arterial wall thickening, micro albuminuria, and increase in creatinine.
***Clinical conditions include retinopathy, cerebrovascular disease, heart failure, IHD, impaired renal function, proteinuria, and peripheral vascular disease.

Adapted from Niebauer J, Borjesson M, Carre F et al. Recommendations for participation in competitive sports of athletes with arterial hypertension: a position statement from the sports cardiology section of the European Association of Preventive Cardiology (EAPC). *Eur Heart J.* 39:3664–71, 2018

- Post valvuloplasty lesions should be managed as per the degree of residual stenosis and/or regurgitation.

Asymptomatic aortic stenosis

- Mild: No restriction
- Moderate: Low–moderate intensity: No restriction if normal LV function; good functional capacity and normal exercise test.
- Severe:
  - Low intensity: No restriction if normal LVEF > 50%; good functional capacity and normal exercise test.
  - Competitive sport or moderate–high intensity not recommended.

Symptomatic aortic stenosis

- Mild: No restriction
- Moderate: Low–moderate intensity: No restriction if LVEF > 50%; good functional capacity and normal exercise test/normal BP response during exercise test.
- Severe:
  - Low intensity: No restriction if LVEF > 50%.
  - Competitive sport or moderate– high intensity not recommended.

Asymptomatic aortic regurgitation

- Mild: No restriction
- Moderate: No restriction if normal LV size and EF> 50%; and normal exercise test.

- Severe:
  - Low–moderate intensity: No restriction if no more than mild-moderate. LV dilatation; LVEF > 50% and normal exercise test.
  - Competitive sport or moderate–high intensity not recommended if LVEF < 50% and/or exercise induced arrhythmias.

Symptomatic aortic regurgitation
- Mild: No restriction
- Moderate: No restriction if normal LV size and EF > 50%; and normal exercise test.
- Severe:
  - Low–moderate intensity: No restriction if no more than mild-moderate LV dilatation; LVEF > 50% and normal exercise test.
  - Competitive sport or moderate–high intensity not recommended if LVEF < 50% and/or exercise-induced arrhythmias.

Asymptomatic mitral regurgitation
- Mild: No restriction
- Moderate: No restriction if no high-risk markers:
  - LVEDd < 60 mm (or < 35.3 mm/m^2 in men and < 40 mm/m^2 in women).
  - LVEF > 60%
  - Resting sPAP < 50 mmHg
  - Normal exercise test
- Severe: Low–moderate intensity if no high-risk markers.

Symptomatic mitral regurgitation
- Mild: No restriction
- Moderate: No restriction if no high-risk markers.
- Severe: Low–moderate intensity if no high-risk markers. Competitive sport not recommended if LVEF < 60%.

Asymptomatic mitral stenosis
- Mild: No restriction if systolic pulmonary artery pressure (sPAP) < 40 mmHg and normal exercise test.
- Moderate: Low–moderate intensity if sPAP < 40 mmHg and normal exercise test.
- Severe: Moderate–high intensity not recommended.

Symptomatic mitral stenosis
- Mild: No restriction if sPAP < 40 mmHg and normal exercise test.
- Moderate: Low intensity if sPAP < 40 mmHg and normal exercise test.
- Severe: Low intensity if sPAP < 40 mmHg and normal exercise test. Moderate–high intensity and competitive sports not recommended.

Recommendation for sports participation in those with aortic root dilatation
- Low risk (aorta < 40 mm in BAV or tricuspid valve); Turner syndrome without aortic dilatation:
  - No restriction
  - Follow-up 2–3 years
- Low–intermediate risk (Marfan syndrome; hereditary aortic disease without dilatation; aorta 40–45 mm in BAV or tricuspid valve); after successful surgery for BAV:
  - Avoid high-intensity sport; contact sport and power sports.

- Follow up 1–2 years
- Intermediate risk (aorta 40–45 mm in Marfan syndrome (MFS) or other hereditary aortic disease; aorta 45–50 mm in BAV or tricuspid valve); Turner syndrome aortic size index 20–25 mm/m^2; Tetralogy of Fallot < 50 mm; after successful surgery for MFS or other hereditary aortic disease:
    - Recommend low-intensity sports (skill sports/mixed or endurance).
- High risk (aorta > 45 mm in Marfan syndrome (MFS) or other hereditary aortic disease; aorta > 50 mm in BAV or tricuspid valve); Turner syndrome aortic size index > 25 mm/m^2; Tetralogy of Fallot > 50 mm; after surgery with sequalae.
    - Sports temporarily contraindicated. Re-evaluate after treatment.

7.1.9 Cardiopulmonary exercise testing

- Cardiopulmonary exercise testing (CPET) is a non-invasive simultaneous functional assessment of the cardiovascular and respiratory system during exercise to assess an individual's exercise tolerance (cardiopulmonary reserve).
- CPET involves the measurement of gas exchange (volume of oxygen uptake ($\dot{V}O_2$) and volume of carbon dioxide production ($\dot{V}CO_2$) at the airway, as well as ventilatory parameters (respiratory rate, tidal volume, and minute ventilation ($\dot{V}_E$)).
- Accompanied with an electrocardiogram, heart rate, blood pressure, and pulse oximetry measurements, a comprehensive assessment of the cardiovascular and respiratory system during a symptom limited exercise test can be performed.
- The main function of the cardiovascular and respiratory system is to support cellular respiration.
- As detailed in Figure 7.1.7, the lungs, heart, and muscles function independently, but are coupled in the process of delivering oxygen (O_2) from the external environment (pulmonary respiration) to support cellular (internal) respiration.
- At rest, O_2 supply and demand are equal. Under steady state conditions $\dot{V}O_2$ should reflect O_2 consumption of all tissue. However, dynamic aerobic exercise increases cellular demand (predominantly skeletal muscle) for oxygen and removal of metabolic waste products (carbon dioxide (CO_2)).

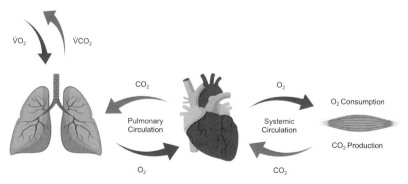

Figure 7.1.7 Oxygen (O_2) and carbon dioxide (CO_2) transport from external to internal respiration. An increase in O_2 requirements of skeletal muscle in response to exercise is achieved by an increase in O_2 extraction (increasing arterial-venous O_2 difference) and selected vasodilation of vessels supplying blood flow to working muscle and vasoconstriction in non-active areas. There is a concomitant increase in cardiac output (increased stroke volume and heart rate) to the pulmonary and systemic circulation to increase O_2 uptake and delivery, increase skeletal muscle perfusion and increase the rate of metabolic waste removal. The rise in CO_2 increases ventilation in order to maintain arterial CO_2 gas tension and hydrogen ion homeostasis.

- In order to support the increased demand, physiological control mechanisms interact to enable the cardiovascular and respiratory system to couple and coordinate their response to increase the delivery of O_2 and removal of metabolic CO_2.
- If O_2 delivery fails to adequately meet the increased O_2 demands of the skeletal muscles in response to exercise, metabolic acidosis and subsequently fatigue will result.

Anaerobic threshold

- During low-intensity steady-state exercise, aerobic metabolism is the predominant metabolic pathway for the oxidative phosphorylation of adenosine triphosphate (ATP) resynthesis.
- During low intensity exercise metabolic waste products are produced; however, levels remain stable due to effective physiological responses and buffering mechanisms. As such, exercise at a low intensity can be sustained for prolonged periods.
- As exercise intensity begins to increase, there becomes a point where aerobic and anaerobic energy metabolism is required to provide adequate resynthesis of ATP to continue work. Assessment of exercise using gas exchange can allow distinction between these two domains of exercise intensity and is termed the anaerobic threshold.
- The most popular and reliable method of identifying the anaerobic threshold is by plotting $\dot{V}CO_2$ against $\dot{V}O_2$, which is also widely known as the V-slope method. As demonstrated in Figure 7.1.8A, there is a lower slope (S1), which represents predominant aerobic metabolism, where CO_2 production is proportional to O_2 consumption.
- As the intensity of exercise increases and anaerobic metabolism is required to sustain work, blood lactate and free hydrogen ion concentrations increase, which is buffered by bicarbonate ions (enzyme carbonic anhydrase in red blood cells) and converted to CO_2 and water.

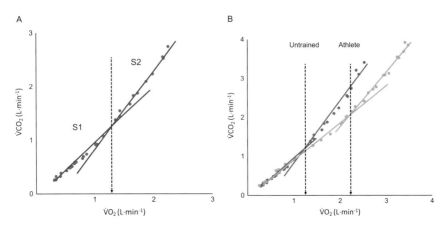

Figure 7.1.8 The relationship between $\dot{V}CO_2$ against $\dot{V}O_2$ during an incremental work rate exercise test. (A) is a normal response and the intersection of the lower slope (S1) and upper slope (S2) determines the anaerobic threshold. (B) is a comparison of the $\dot{V}CO_2$ against $\dot{V}O_2$ response between a normal untrained (blue) and endurance trained athlete (green). The figure illustrates the greater aerobic capacity of the athlete compared to an untrained individual, which is due to physiological adaptations (increased maximal stroke volume and therefore maximal cardiac output, improved O_2 transport through greater haemoglobin and therefore O_2 carrying capacity, greater plasma volume, capillarisation at muscle tissue to increase surface area and improved O_2 uptake due to an increase in the size and number of mitochondria and therefore number of aerobic enzymes). Importantly, it is clear to see that the anaerobic threshold (S1 and S2 intersect) occurs at a greater oxygen uptake in the athlete compared to the untrained individual.

- The increase in CO_2 derived from bicarbonate buffering increases ventilation ($\dot{V}_E$), known as isocapnic buffering, and the $\dot{V}CO_2$ and $\dot{V}O_2$ relationship exhibits a steeper slope (S2).
- Where the lower and upper slope intercept is the anaerobic threshold and should be reported as a percentage of predicted peak aerobic capacity ($\dot{V}O_{2peak}$).
- In untrained individuals the anaerobic threshold typically occurs at approximately 50% to 60% of $\dot{V}O_{2peak}$, while it can be 70% to 80% of $\dot{V}O_{2peak}$ in endurance trained athletes, as illustrated in Figure 7.1.8B.

Ventilatory equivalents

- Determination of the anaerobic threshold can be checked using the ventilatory equivalents for $\dot{V}O_2$ ($\dot{V}_E/\dot{V}O_2$) and $\dot{V}CO_2$ ($\dot{V}_E/\dot{V}CO_2$).
- Ventilatory equivalents are a measure of breathing efficiency and relates instantaneous $\dot{V}_E$ to the metabolic rate of $\dot{V}O_2$ uptake and $\dot{V}CO_2$ output. Resting values are generally between 30–60 and fall during exercise.
- The point of departure from the plateau (Figure 7.1.9) can identify the anaerobic threshold. $\dot{V}_E/\dot{V}CO_2$ does not increase from the plateau until $\dot{V}_E$ becomes dissociated from $\dot{V}CO_2$, when buffering mechanisms can no longer prevent a fall in blood pH and $\dot{V}_E$ responds to carotid body stimulation.
- This threshold is the ventilatory or respiratory compensation point and is usually attained at around 70–80% $\dot{V}O_{2peak}$ (Figure 7.1.9).

Aerobic capacity

- Aerobic capacity or maximal oxygen uptake ($\dot{V}O_{2max}$), is defined as the maximum amount of O_2 that can be taken up at the lung (pulmonary diffusion capacity), transported (via blood and maximal cardiac output) to skeletal muscle tissue, and the maximal skeletal muscle oxidative capacity (size and number of mitochondria).

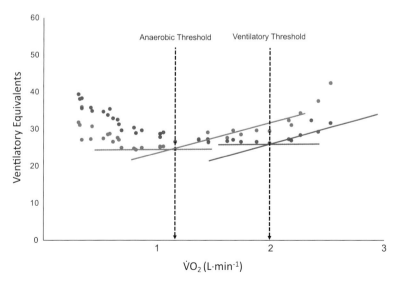

Figure 7.1.9 Alternative method for the determination of anaerobic threshold (blue) and ventilatory or respiratory compensation point (red) using the ventilatory equivalents (V_E/VO_2 and V_E/VCO_2) and VO_2.

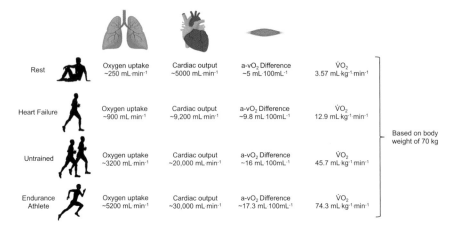

Figure 7.1.10 Differences in relative $\dot{V}O_2$, cardiac output and a-vO_2 difference at rest and peak exercise in heart failure, healthy untrained and endurance trained athlete (all calculated with the same body mass of 70 kg).

- Aerobic capacity is widely regarded as the best single measure of cardiorespiratory fitness.
- $\dot{V}O_{2max}$ is defined as a plateau in O_2 uptake, despite a continued increase in exercise intensity.
- However, in many exercise settings and clinical laboratories, individuals reach volitional fatigue before a plateau occurs in O_2 uptake and in such cases, the highest O_2 uptake should be reported as $\dot{V}O_{2peak}$. $\dot{V}O_2$ is usually reported in absolute (L·min^{-1} or ml·min^{-1}) and relative (ml·kg^{-1}·min^{-1}) to body mass.
- As detailed in Figure 7.1.7, the Fick principle reminds us that $\dot{V}O_{2max}$ = maximal cardiac output X maximal arterial-venous O_2 difference (a-vO_2 difference).
- Figure 7.1.10 highlights this principle further and demonstrates the differences in relative $\dot{V}O_2$, cardiac output and a-vO_2 difference at rest and peak exercise in heart failure, healthy untrained and endurance-trained athlete.
- Regular exercise training produces numerous physiological adaptations (central and peripheral), which overall produces a greater maximal cardiac output and greater O_2 uptake at the muscle (increased a-vO_2 difference).
- Deconditioning and clinical conditions impact the ability to transport and utilize O_2, which reduces aerobic capacity.

Minute ventilation/carbon dioxide ($\dot{V}E/\dot{V}CO_2$) slope

- The $\dot{V}_E/\dot{V}CO_2$ relationship is a measure of ventilatory efficiency and provides important information on cardiopulmonary function.
- $\dot{V}_E/\dot{V}CO_2$ is determined by dead space ventilation relative to tidal volume ($\dot{V}_D/\dot{V}_T$) and the partial pressure of arterial CO_2 (PaCO_2).
- Excessive increases in $\dot{V}_E$ during exercise is an important independent prognostic marker in clinical patients, such as those with chronic heart failure.
- $\dot{V}CO_2$ increases linearly during exercise with work rate for the tight regulation of PaCO_2.
- Once anaerobic metabolism is required to maintain work $\dot{V}_E$ becomes dissociated from $\dot{V}O_2$; however, $\dot{V}_E$ responds to additional CO_2 from metabolic buffering mechanisms and the linear relationship remains (isocapnic buffering).
- As exercise continues, hyperventilation in response to metabolic acidosis increases and $\dot{V}_E$ becomes dissociated from $\dot{V}CO_2$ (ventilatory threshold) (see Figure 7.1.11A). The normal

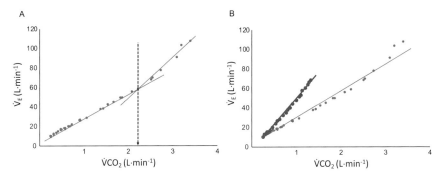

Figure 7.1.11 (A) Relationship between V_E and VCO_2 during an incremental work rate exercise test. The intersection of the blue slopes determines the ventilatory or respiratory compensation point. (B) Illustrates the difference between a normal $\dot{V}_E/\dot{V}CO_2$ slope (blue) and representative patient with chronic heart failure (red).

$\dot{V}_E/\dot{V}CO_2$ slope is < 30 and Figure 7.1.11B illustrates the difference between a normal $\dot{V}_E/\dot{V}CO_2$ slope and representative patient with chronic heart failure.

Differentiation between cardiovascular and pulmonary aetiology of exercise intolerance

- The key objective of cardiopulmonary exercise testing is to identify the cause of exercise intolerance.
- The cardiopulmonary responses to exercise in normal individuals are predictable and diseases affect the cardiac and pulmonary system responses in specific ways.
- In healthy, untrained individuals, the majority of evidence indicates that aerobic capacity is limited by the supply of O_2 delivered to working muscles (maximal cardiac output) as opposed to skeletal muscle oxidative capacity.
- The healthy pulmonary system is usually adequate at all levels of exercise intensity as PaO_2 is maintained at resting levels.
- As such, healthy untrained to moderately trained individuals should not exhibit respiratory limitation to exercise.

Interpreting CPET data

1. Was the test was maximal (i.e. sufficient effort).
   a. In addition to patient exhaustion, achievement of ≥ 85% of age predicted maximal heart rate (routinely calculated as 220-age) is a recognized indicator of sufficient participant effort.
   b. However, due to high variability and medication effects (e.g. beta-blocker therapy), it is important to gauge effort with additional parameters.
   c. The respiratory exchange ratio (RER), calculated as the ratio of instantaneous $\dot{V}CO_2/\dot{V}O_2$, is the strongest non-invasive marker of participant effort and obtained exclusively from expired gas analysis. A RER peak ratio > 1.1 is considered an indication of excellent effort.
   d. Rating of perceived exertion (RPE) is an additional tool to gauge exercise effort, with a score of 16–18 on a 6–20 Borg scale indicative of maximal effort.
2. Is the $\dot{V}O_{2peak}$ normal (> 80% of predicted/reference $\dot{V}O_2$) or reduced
3. Is the anaerobic threshold normal or reduced (< 40% of predicted/reference $\dot{V}O_2$ pathology is expected).
   - In general, a normal CPET test is highlighted by:
     - Normal $\dot{V}O_{2peak}$

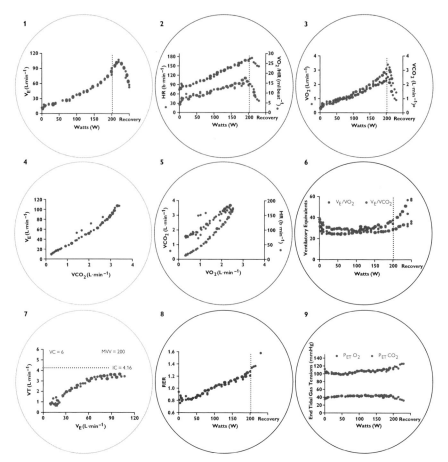

Figure 7.1.12 Nine panel plot, which is the standard layout for the graphical representation of data produced by a cardiopulmonary exercise test. Green circles (plots 1, 4 and 7) represent the ventilatory response; blue circles (plots 2 and 3) represent the cardiovascular response; red circle (plot 3) represents the metabolic response; black circles (plots 6, 8 and 9) represent the gas exchange response.

- Normal anaerobic threshold
- Heart rate reaches ≥ 85% predicted (low heart rate reserve)
- RER is > 1.1
- No ECG changes (ischaemic and/or significant arrhythmias)
- O_2 pulse is normal (instantaneous O_2 uptake divided by heart rate and is intricately related to stroke volume)
- $\dot{V}_E/\dot{V}CO_2$ is normal
- No evidence of ventilatory limitation (high breathing reserve, which is calculated from maximal voluntary ventilation or forced expiratory volume in 1-second (FEV_1) × 40)
- O_2 saturation is normal throughout exercise.

In this case, the test is limited by the cardiovascular system and considered normal. Figure 7.1.12 illustrates the 9-panel plot, which is the standard layout for the graphical representation of data produced by a cardiopulmonary exercise test.

Table 7.1.5 Weber classification for grading the severity of heart failure based on CPET.

Functional class classification	$\dot{V}O_{2peak}$ (ml·kg⁻¹·min⁻¹)	Anaerobic threshold (ml·kg⁻¹·min⁻¹)
A	> 20	> 14
B	16–20	11–14
C	10–16	8–11
D	< 10	< 8

Reproduced from Weber KT, Kinasewitz GT, Janicki JS, Fishman AP. Oxygen utilization and ventilation during exercise in patients with chronic cardiac failure. *Circulation.* 1982 Jun;65(6):1213–23. doi: 10.1161/01.cir.65.6.1213 with permission from Wolters Kluwer.

- Respiratory limitation is considered when $\dot{V}O_{2peak}$ is reduced, the anaerobic threshold is normal or reduced, breathing reserve is low (< 20%), which suggests a high $\dot{V}_E$ and ventilatory mechanical limitation, the $\dot{V}O_2$/work rate slope is normal, a drop in O_2 saturation of > 4% and overall < 90% (hypoxic response and suggests diffusion limitation) and high $\dot{V}_E/\dot{V}CO_2$ in the absence of heart disease, which suggests dead space ventilation.

Evaluation of patients with cardiovascular diseases

Functional evaluation and prognosis in patients with heart failure

- $\dot{V}O_{2peak}$ is a strong predictor for adverse outcomes in heart failure patients with reduced (LVEF < 39%), mid-range (LVEF 40×49%), and preserved ejection fraction (LVEF > 50%).
- O_{2peak} also carries an important role in selecting patients for advancing interventions, such as left ventricular assist devices and heart transplantation procedures.
- CPET interpretation should begin with ascertaining if the test was of sufficient effort (maximum volitional fatigue).
- Maximum heart rate is often not achieved in heart failure patients due to the effects of medication/chronotropic incompetence. This means attainment of 85% predicted heart rate is often not achieved. Instead, an RER of > 1 to 1.1 should be used. A $\dot{V}O_{2peak}$ < 14 ml·kg⁻¹·min⁻¹ (< 12 ml·kg⁻¹·min⁻¹ in patients taking beta-blocker therapy) and in young heart failure patients and those with high or low body mass index, a $\dot{V}O_{2peak}$ ≤ 50% of predicted $\dot{V}O_2$ is associated with poor prognosis.
- In patients unable to achieve sufficient physical exertion, an anaerobic threshold < 9 ml·kg⁻¹·min⁻¹ and an oxygen uptake efficiency slope of < 1.4 ($\dot{V}O_2$ uptake vs $\dot{V}_E$) indicates poor prognosis.
- A $\dot{V}_E/\dot{V}CO_2$ slope > 34/36 is also associated with poor prognosis.
- A peak systolic blood pressure < 120 mmHg and slow heart rate recovery (< 6 b·min⁻¹) are associated with poor prognosis.
- Poor O_2 uptake, inefficient ventilatory and haemodynamic response to exercise is associated with a > 20% risk of 1-year mortality and these data can be used to inform patient selection for left ventricular assist devices and heart transplantation.
- Heart failure patients with a $\dot{V}O_{2peak}$ > 20 ml·kg⁻¹·min⁻¹, anaerobic threshold > 11 ml·kg⁻¹·min⁻¹, and $\dot{V}_E/\dot{V}CO_2$ slope < 30, have a 95% event-free survival at 1-year.

The Weber functional classification for chronic heart failure patients can also be used to grade the severity of functional impairment in heart failure (Table 7.1.5).

Selection for cardiac transplantation

- In patients with a $\dot{V}O_{2peak}$ > 14 ml·kg⁻¹·min⁻¹, 1- and 2-year survival was similar to patients following heart transplant (94% and 84%, respectively), suggesting that transplantation could be safely deferred. However, those with a $\dot{V}O_{2peak}$ ≤ 14 ml·kg⁻¹·min⁻¹, 1- and 2-year survival rates were 47% and 32%, respectively.

The following CPET recommendations to guide heart transplantation listing are:

- In patients intolerant of a beta blocker, a cut-off for $\dot{V}O_{2peak}$ of ≤ 14 ml·kg^{-1}·min^{-1} should be used to guide listing (Class I, Level of Evidence: B).
- In the presence of a beta blocker, a cut-off for $\dot{V}O_{2peak}$ of ≤ 12 ml·kg^{-1}·min^{-1} should be used to guide listing (Class I, Level of Evidence: B).
- A maximal cardiopulmonary exercise test is defined as one with a RER > 1.05 and achievement of an anaerobic threshold on optimal pharmacologic therapy (Class I, Level of Evidence: B).
- In young patients (< 50 years) and women, it is reasonable to consider using alternate standards in conjunction with $\dot{V}O_{2peak}$ to guide listing, including percent of predicted ($\leq 50\%$) $\dot{V}O_{2peak}$ (Class IIa, Level of Evidence: B).
- In the presence of a sub-maximal CPET (RER < 1.05), use of the $\dot{V}_E/\dot{V}CO_2$ slope of >35 as a determinant in listing for transplantation may be considered (Class IIb, Level of Evidence: C).
- In obese (body mass index (BMI) > 30 kg·m^2) patients, adjusting $\dot{V}O_{2peak}$ to lean body mass may be considered. A lean body mass adjusted $\dot{V}O_{2peak}$ of < 19 ml·kg^{-1}·min^{-1} can serve as an optimal threshold to guide prognosis (Class IIb, Level of Evidence: B).
- Listing patients based solely on the criterion of a $\dot{V}O_{2peak}$ measurement should not be performed (Class III, Level of Evidence: C).
- In circumstances of ambiguity (e.g. $\dot{V}O_{2peak}$ >12 and < 14 ml·kg^{-1}·min^{-1}) a Heart Failure Survival Score (HFSS) may be considered, and it may add discriminatory value to determining prognosis and guide listing for transplantation for ambulatory patients (Class IIb, Level of Evidence: C).

Further reading

Ackerman MJ, Zipes D P, Kovacs RJ et al. Eligibility and disqualification recommendations for competitive athletes with cardiovascular abnormalities: Task force 10: The channelopathies. A scientific statement from the American Heart Association and American College of Cardiology. *Circulation*. 2015;132:e326–9.

Borjesson M, Dellborg M, Niebauer J et al. Recommendations for participation in leisure time or competitive sports in athletes-patients with coronary artery disease: a position statement from the Sports Cardiology Section of the European Association of Preventive Cardiology (EAPC). *Eur Heart J*. 2019 Jan 1;40(1):13–18. doi: 10.1093/eurheartj/ehy408.

Niebauer J, Borjesson M, Carre F et al. Recommendations for participation in competitive sports of athletes with arterial hypertension: a position statement from the sports cardiology section of the European Association of Preventive Cardiology (EAPC). *Eur Heart J*. 2018;39:3664–71.

Pellicia A, Fagard R, Halvor Bjornstad H et al. Recommendations for competitive sports participation in athletes with cardiovascular disease. *Eur Heart J*. 2005;26: 1422–45.

Pellicia A, Solberg EE, Papadakis M et al. Recommendations for participation in competitive and leisure time sport in athletes with cardiomyopathies, myocarditis, and pericarditis: position statement of the Sport Cardiology Section of the European Association of Preventive Cardiology (EAPC). *Eur Heart J*. 2019;40:19–33.

Priori SG, Blomstrom-Lundqvist C, Mazzanti A et al. ESC Guidelines for the management of patients with ventricular arrhythmias and the prevention of sudden cardiac death. The task Force for the management of patients with ventricular arrhythmias and the prevention of sudden cardiac death. *Eur Heart J*. 2015;36:2793–867.

Sharma S et al. International recommendations for electrocardiographic interpretation in athletes. *J Am Coll Cardiol*. 2017 Feb 28;69(8):1057–75. doi: 10.1016/j.jacc.2017.01.015.

7.2

Primary prevention

Scott Murray and David Murphy

TABLE OF CONTENTS
7.2.1 Overview 617
7.2.2 Cardiovascular risk 617
7.2.3 Risk estimation tools 618
7.2.4 Other risk factors 621
7.2.5 Management of risk profile 622
   Lifestyle 622
   Pharmacotherapy 624
Aggressive Management of relevant co-morbidities 625
7.2.6 Specific populations 626
   The young 626
   Older adults 626
   Women 627

7.2.1 Overview

- Cardiovascular disease (CVD) is the most common cause of death in Europe, resulting in 49% of deaths in women and 41% in men (> 4 million deaths/year)
- There is significant associated morbidity, economic, and social costs
- A growing number of cardiovascular risk factors have been identified since the original Framingham Heart Study, and in addition, the prevalence of some risk factors, notably diabetes mellitus (DM) and obesity, is increasing
- Modification of reversible risk factors (rather than interventional procedures) has been largely responsible for the decline in age-adjusted cardiovascular mortality in the Western world, and large global geographical variations in cardiovascular disease (CVD)
- *Prevention* is defined as a co-ordinated set of actions either at a population or individual level aimed at eliminating or minimizing the impact of CVD and their related disabilities
- The importance of CVD prevention is undisputed and should be delivered both at the general population level (promoting healthy lifestyle behaviour), and at the individual level by tackling unhealthy lifestyles and by reducing increased levels of causal CV risk factors discussed in detail in the following sections

7.2.2 Cardiovascular risk

- Prevention requires the assessment of a patient's future cardiovascular risk
- This can be done via a population approach or more relevant to the practising Cardiologist, an individual approach
- Identification of those at higher risk allows for the appropriate use of resources but there is no definite cut-off point as risk is a continuum—risk assessment tools exist to help with clinical decision-making

- Prevention of atherosclerotic CVD in a given person should relate to his or her total CV risk: the higher the risk, the more intense the action should be
- Of note, persons with documented atherosclerotic CVD, diabetes mellitus (Type 1 or 2), very high levels of individual risk factors, genetic dyslipidaemia (e.g. familial hypercholesterolaemia), or chronic kidney disease (CKD) are generally at *very high* or *high* total CV risk, and no risk estimation models are needed for such persons; they need active management of all risk factors

7.2.3 Risk estimation tools

- Many multivariable risk-scoring systems exist, as outlined in Table 7.2.1
- Comparator studies of the various systems have shown differences but failed to demonstrate a single system as superior
- ESC guidelines recommend an individual patient's risk should be assessed and a stepwise management plan instituted relative to their individual risk level
- Risk tools are based on a combined global risk and risk continuum (concepts central to the underlying multifactorial atherosclerotic process) where individual risk factors are multiplicative, rather than additive, interacting and amplifying harm when present in combination (as outlined in Figure 7.2.1 and Table 7.2.2)
- For example, a given blood pressure will be more damaging to an individual with Type 2 diabetes mellitus (T2DM) than equivalent pressures in a non-diabetic person
- A number of moderately raised risk factors constitute a higher risk than a single very elevated risk factor (as seen in patients with metabolic syndrome)
- Risk scoring systems tend to overestimate absolute risk and under appreciate relative risk
- The relatively short time frame (10 year) of risk estimation may underestimate lifetime risk. For example in the Framingham study 90% of individuals who were normotensive at the start of the study developed hypertension during the 20 years of follow-up
- Ideally, risk charts should be based on country-specific cohort data, but these are not available for every country
- ESC recommend a total CV risk estimation using a system such as SCORE2 (Systematic Coronary Risk Evaluation) for adults 40–69 years of age (unless they are automatically categorized as being at *high risk* or *very high risk*) as this was derived from a large pool of European cohort studies and may therefore be more relevant to northern European populations than Framingham data
- In patients ≥ 70 years of age then SCORE2-OP is recommended
- The SCORE2 risk estimates are outlined in three charts, for '*high-*', '*moderate-*', or '*low-risk*' regions in Europe, with the 10-year risk of fatal or non-fatal CVD that demarcates risk group varying according to age (recognizing the increased lifetime risk in younger patients)
- The original version of SCORE was specific for fatal events, rather than all CV events, however the now recommended SCORE2 encompasses fatal and non-fatal CV events
- In current guidelines those *automatically* categorized as very high risk are:
    - Documented CVD, clinical or unequivocal on imaging, which includes previous acute coronary syndrome (ACS), coronary revascularization and other arterial revascularization procedures, stroke and transient ischaemic attack (TIA), aortic aneurysm, and peripheral arterial disease (PAD)
    - Unequivocally documented CVD on imaging, including significant plaque on coronary angiography, carotid ultrasound, or CTCA

Table 7.2.1 An outline of cardiovascular risk assessment tools.

	Framingham	SCORE	QRISK 1 and 2	PROCAM	SCORE2
Data	Framingham Heart Study and Framingham offspring study	12 pooled prospective studies	QRESEARCH database	Prospective study	Combined prospective cohort across Europe
Sample Size	3969 men and 4522 women	117,098 men and 88,080 women	1.28 million (QRISK1) 2.29 million (QRISK2)	18,460 men and 8515 women	Developed with ~680,000, re-calibrated to region with ~10.8 million, validated with ~1.1 million
Age range	30–75	40–65	35–74	20–75	40–69
Variables	Sex, age, total cholesterol, HDL-C, SBP, smoking status, DM, Hypertensive treatment	Sex, age, total cholesterol/ HDL-C ratio, SBP, smoking status	QRISK1—sex, age, total cholesterol to HDL-C ratio, SBP, smoking cessation, DM, area based index of deprivation, family history, BMI, hypertensive treatment, ethnicity, and chronic diseases	Age, sex, LDL-C, HDL-C, DM, smoking, SBP	Age, sex smoking status, blood pressure, diabetes mellitus, total cholesterol, HDL-C
Calculates	10-year risk of CVD event	10-year risk of CVD mortality	10-year risk of CVD event	10-year risk of major coronary events and cerebral ischaemic events	10-year risk of *fatal and non-fatal* CVD
Recommended by guidelines	NCEP guideline, Canadian CV guideline	Now outdated	NICE, JBS (JBS 3rd iteration uses a lifetime CVD risk)	International Task force for the prevention of Coronary Disease Guidelines	European Guidelines on CVD prevention

SCORE and SCORE2—Systematic Coronary Risk Evaluation, SBP—systolic blood pressure, NCEP ATP—National Cholesterol Education Program Adult Treatment Panel, NICE—National Institute of Clinical Excellent, JBS—Joint British Societies.

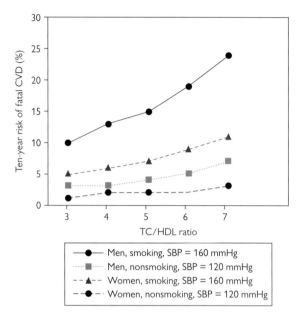

Figure 7.2.1 Graphical representation of the multiplicative actions of risk factors on total CVD risk. The relationship of total cholesterol (TC):HDL cholesterol ratio to 10-year fatal CVD events in men and women aged 60 years with and without risk factors, based on a risk function derived from the SCORE project; SBP = systolic blood pressure

Graham I, Atar D, Borch-Johnsen K, et al; European Society of Cardiology (ESC) Committee for Practice Guidelines (CPG). European guidelines on cardiovascular disease prevention in clinical practice: executive summary: Fourth Joint Task Force of the European Society of Cardiology and Other Societies on Cardiovascular Disease Prevention in Clinical Practice (Constituted by representatives of nine societies and by invited experts). *Eur Heart J.* 2007 Oct;28(19):2375–414. doi: 10.1093/eurheartj/ehm316. © European Society of Cardiology. With permission from Oxford University Press

- Diabetes mellitus (Type 2 or those with Type 1 and are > 40 years of age) with evidence of target organ damage, e.g. an eGFR <4 5 ml/min/1.73 m² OR eGFR 45–59 with an ACR of 30–300 mg/g OR ACR > 300 mg/g OR the presence of microvascular disease at ≥ 3 sites
- CKD with an eGFR < 30 ml/min/1.73 m² OR eGFR 30-44 ml/min/1.73 m² and ACR > 30 mg/g

Table 7.2.2 Table demonstrating the interaction between cholesterol, blood pressure and smoking in amplifying combined risk.

Sex	Age (years)	Cholesterol (mmol/l)	BP (mmHg)	Smoker	Risk (%)
F	60	8	120	No	2
F	60	7	140	Yes	5
M	60	6	160	No	8
M	60	5	180	Yes	21

Graham I, Atar D, Borch-Johnsen K, et al; European Society of Cardiology (ESC) Committee for Practice Guidelines (CPG). European guidelines on cardiovascular disease prevention in clinical practice: executive summary: Fourth Joint Task Force of the European Society of Cardiology and Other Societies on Cardiovascular Disease Prevention in Clinical Practice (Constituted by representatives of nine societies and by invited experts). *Eur Heart J.* 2007 Oct;28(19):2375–414. doi: 10.1093/eurheartj/ehm316. © European Society of Cardiology. With permission from Oxford University Press

- Those *automatically categorized* as *high risk*:
    - Markedly elevated cholesterol levels
    - Diabetes mellitus (Type 2 or those with Type 1 and are > 40 years of age) who do not have criteria for being very high risk but have long standing DM (> 10 years) or poorly controlled diabetes
    - Moderate CKD (eGFR 30–44 ml/min/1.73m² and ACR < 30 mg/g OR eGFR 45–59 ml/min/1.73m² and ACR 30–300 mg/g OR eGFR ≥ 60 ml/min/1.73m² and ACR > 300 mg/g)
- In addition, a SCORE2 CVD risk estimation at the following age-specific level for patients > 40 years of age without established CVD, DM, CKD, or FH puts them at *very high risk*:
    - < 50 years of age with a 10-year risk > 7.5%
    - 50–69 with a 10-year risk ≥ 10%
    - ≥ 70 with a 10-year risk ≥ 15%
- In the UK, NICE recommends treating anyone over 85 years of age as high risk
- It is worth noting that although > 200 CVD risk factors have now been identified, scoring systems remain focused on addressing 3 'classical' risk factors: cholesterol, diabetes, and hypertension—therefore significant under- and over-estimation of risk may result from ethnic and socio-economic variations, and other parameters excluded from charts

Additional risk screening options

Imaging:

- Total CV risk will be higher than indicated in the SCORE charts in asymptomatic persons with abnormal markers of subclinical atherosclerotic vascular damage
- Reclassification is of value in people identified as being at low-moderate CV risk by using markers such as coronary artery calcium score (CACS) of > 100 Agatston units, CTCA, or the presence of plaques at carotid ultrasonography
- In studies comparing these markers, CACS had the best reclassification ability

N.B. i) *Note that CACS is often very low in patients < 45 years with severe familial hypercholesterolaemia and has low specificity in this population*

ii) *CACS increases with statins and so should be interpreted with caution in this population*

Apolipoprotein B

- Provides an accurate estimate of the total concentration of atherogenic molecules under all circumstances, though adds little information above measuring LDL

7.2.4 Other risk factors

- Apart from the conventional risk factors of hypertension, elevated levels of apolipoprotein-B-containing lipoproteins, cigarette smoking, diabetes mellitus, and adiposity there are a number of other risk factors, risk modifiers, and clinical conditions which increase the CV disease risk
- *Family history of premature CVD*—fatal or non-fatal CVD event in first degree male relative < 55 years of age and < 65 in females
- *Ethnicity*—highest risk in South Asians and sub-Saharan Africans
- *Low socio-economic status*—relative risk (RR) of coronary artery disease (CAD) mortality is 1.5–2
- *Mental health* including depression (RR 1.6), schizophrenia (RR 1.2), chronic stress (RR 1.2–1.5)

- *Chronic kidney disease* (CKD) is associated with an increased risk of CVD independent of conventional risk factors. Not only does this increase the risk profile relative to the degree of renal impairment and proteinuria, but it also modifies its clinical presentation and cardinal symptoms (see Chapter 9.3)
- Some *chemotherapeutic* agents and *radiotherapy* can cause premature atherosclerosis and can increase the likelihood of developing hypertension. These affects can be seen many years from the initial treatment
- *Chronic immune-mediated inflammatory disorder* (e.g. rheumatoid arthritis with RR 1.5)
- *Obesity*, and in particular *central obesity* and *non-alcoholic fatty liver disease*
- *Obstructive sleep apnoea* syndrome has a RR of about 1.7 for cardiovascular morbidity and mortality
- *Human Immunodeficiency Virus* (RR 1.6)

7.2.5 Management of risk profile

Lifestyle

- Guidelines recommend all patients, independent of their risk profile, should receive lifestyle advice in both primary and secondary prevention of CVD
- This includes low-risk individuals to help them maintain this status
- Thus, the intensity of preventive actions should be tailored to the patient's total CV risk
- Appropriate advice, support, and follow-up should be provided to assist individuals in achieving and maintaining these goals
- This may require behavioural change, including cognitive behavioural strategies
- Lifestyle factors include:

Sedentary behaviour and physical activity

- Regular physical activity reduces CV mortality by about 20%
    - Light exercise—walking, light house work
    - Moderate—brisk walk, gardening, dancing
    - Vigorous—jogging, running, swimming
- There is a dose-response curve in someone going from a sedentary lifestyle to light or moderate physical activity with a smaller gain for more intense exercise
- Guidelines recommend 150–300 min a week of moderate intensity or 75–150 min a week of vigorous intensity aerobic physical activity per week (*Class 1A*)

> **TIP**
>
> *Physical Activity* = defined as any bodily movement produced by the skeletal muscle that results in energy expenditure
>
> *Exercise* = is physical activity that is structured, repetitive, and purposeful to improve or maintain one or more components of physical fitness
>
> *Sport* = involves physical activity and exercise but differs in that each sport also has a set of rules, or goals to train and excel in specific athletic skills

Body weight

- Body Mass Index (BMI) —weight (kg)/height (m^2)
    - Healthy weight—BMI of 18.5–24.9 kg/m^2

- Overweight—BMI of 25–29.9 kg/m^2
- Obesity I—BMI of 30–34.9 kg/m^2
- Obesity II—BMI of 35–39.9 kg/m^2
- Obesity III—BMI of 40 kg/m^2 or more
• CV mortality is lowest for a BMI of 20–25 kg/m^2 (in those < 60 years of age)
• In the presence of excess weight, even modest weight reduction (5–10%) improves lipid abnormalities and favourably affects the other CV risk factors often present in dyslipidaemic individuals
• Any intervention should include diet and exercise to enable the greatest improvement in physical performance and quality of life, and mitigates reductions in muscle and bone mass (especially in older people)
• Consider using waist circumference in addition to BMI when BMI is < 35 kg/m^2
    - For men a waist circumference > 94 cm and for women > 80 cm indicates an increased risk

Smoking cessation

- Significant effect on risk profile so cessation is vital
- Professional support either group or individual, supplemented with opportunistic advice
- Nicotine replacement therapy (NRT), varenicline. or bupropion should be offered
    - NRT—patches 16-hour (off overnight) or 24-hour patches, with lozenge or mouth spray for break-through cravings
    - Varenicline (12/52 course) or bupropion (7/52 course) need to be started 7–14 days prior to quit date

Nutrition

Discussed further in section 7.2.5.

- A healthy diet should be seen as an absolute essential ingredient in optimizing CV risk
- Dietary patterns with the most focus in research have been the *Dietary Approaches to Stop Hypertension (DASH) diet* (particularly in relation to BP control), and the *Mediterranean diet*; both have proved to be effective in reducing CV risk factors and, may contribute to CVD prevention
- Consistent epidemiological data reveal a CV benefit with increased consumption of fruit, non-starchy vegetables, nuts, legumes, fish, vegetable oils, yoghurt, and wholegrains, along with a lower intake of red and processed meats, foods higher in refined carbohydrates, and salt
- Replacement of animal/dairy fats with vegetable fats or polyunsaturated fatty acids (PUFAs) may also decrease CVD risk
- High-carbohydrate diets negatively affect triglycerides, particularly with refined carbohydrates, whilst they are less important if the diet is rich in fibre and low-glycaemic index foods (this is particularly important in diabetic and metabolic syndrome patients)
- Saturated fats should be < 10% of total energy intake. Fats should be substituted for Omega-3 sources and monounsaturated fatty acids (MUFAs) where possible
- Other recommendations include:
    - < 5 g of salt
    - 30–45 g of fibre/day
    - > 200 g of fruit/day
    - > 200 g of vegetables/day
    - 1–2 servings of fish/week
    - 30 g of nuts/day (unsalted)

Alcohol

- Reduce alcohol intake in accordance with recommended daily limits

Pharmacotherapy
Antiplatelet therapy

- The role of aspirin in primary prevention remains contentious
- Antiplatelet therapy is not recommended in individuals free from CVD for primary prevention purposes, though guidance differs in the presence of other co-morbidities, as discussed in the following sections

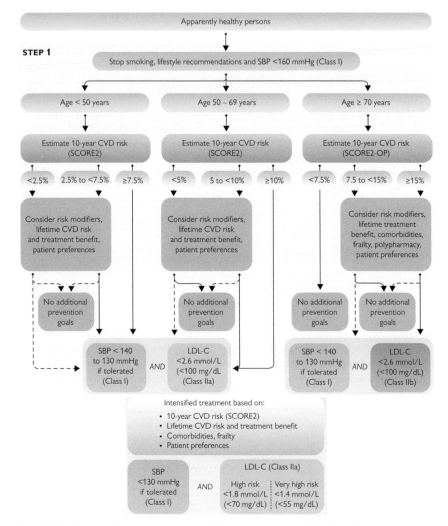

Figure 7.2.2 Proposed primary prevention risk factor management flowchart for apparently healthy individuals (blood pressure and lipid targets are reviewed in upcoming sections)

Visseren FLJ, Mach F, Smulders YM, et al; ESC National Cardiac Societies; ESC Scientific Document Group. 2021 ESC Guidelines on cardiovascular disease prevention in clinical practice. Eur Heart J. 2021 Sep 7;42(34):3227–3337. doi: 10.1093/eurheartj/ehab484. © European Society of Cardiology. With permission from Oxford University Press

Lipid-modifying therapy
- Statin and other lipid modifying therapies, alongside their indications and treatment targets, are discussed in detail in section 7.2.4
- Of note, statin therapy should be considered in all *high-risk* or *very high-risk* patients, or in patients where risk remains high despite attempts at lifestyle changes.

Aggressive management of relevant co-morbidities
- Hypertension (see Chapter 7.3)
- Dyslipidaemia (see Chapter 7.4)
- Diabetes mellitus (see Chapter 7.5)
- Metabolic syndrome (MetS)
    - Describes a cluster of risk factors which predict and promote atherosclerotic CVD and T2DM
    - Associated with a significant lifetime risk of and higher prevalence of CVD, with a worse prognosis when present, but may have disproportionately low 10-year risk estimates
    - There are various definitions but all are based on the combination of atherogenic dyslipidaemia, elevated blood pressure, and pre-diabetes
    - Different definitions have been proposed, with varying degrees of emphasis on insulin resistance and obesity as the predominant underlying abnormalities driving further disease (see Table 7.2.3)
    - First-line therapy for individuals with MetS is directed towards improving its constituent components of lipid profile, hypertension, and preventing diabetes (or controlling if already present)
    - Prime emphasis is on lifestyle changes to target obesity, sedentary lifestyle, and atherogenic diet, improvements of which can result in significant benefit of all the metabolic factors involved
- Lifestyle measures should be implemented, with specific aims to reduce weight and decrease calorie intake by approximately 500–1000 calories per day, aiming for 7–10% weight loss in 6–12 months to achieve a BMI ≤ 25 kg/m^2 and waist circumference < 94 and < 80 cm in men and women respectively
- If the absolute risk remains high (as calculated using risk estimation scores), drug therapy can be initiated for relevant components

Table 7.2.3 Metabolic syndrome is diagnosed if any three of the five criteria listed to be present according to the joint interim statement of the International Diabetes Federation Task Force on Epidemiology and Prevention.

Parameter	Criteria
Elevated waist circumference	≥ 102 cm men
	≥ 88 cm women
Elevated Tg	≥ 1.7 mmol/l or requiring treatment
Reduced HDL-C	≤ 0.9 mmol/l men
	< 1.1 mmol/l women or requiring treatment
Elevated blood pressure	≥ 130/85 or requiring treatment
Elevated FPG	≥ 100 mg/dl or requiring treatment

Tg—triglycerides, FPG—fasting plasma glucose.
Reproduced from Alberti KGMM, Eckel RH, Grundy SM, et al. Harmonizing the metabolic syndrome: A joint interim statement of the international diabetes federation task force on epidemiology and prevention; *Circulation*. 2009;120(16):1640–1645 with permission from Wolters Kluwer.

7.2.6 Specific populations

The young
- As outlined above, in risk prediction charts such as SCORE2, age is the most important factor in estimating absolute risk of CVD
- All young individuals will therefore be at low absolute risk, irrespective of risk factor levels and potentially a high lifetime and relative risk (up to 12 times higher than those of the same age with 'optimal' risk factors)
- Some European guidelines have suggested extrapolating risk to age 60 years, to demonstrate to younger individuals that without modification, they would become high risk by 60 years of age
- New scoring systems have been introduced, which calculate heart age and CVD risk age (expressed as life-years lost or gained for individuals' actual age)—to communicate and quantify future risk to younger patients
- NICE hypertension guidelines recommend considering a referral for specialist evaluation and consideration of secondary causes in individuals < 40 years of age with hypertension, regardless of presence of target organ damage

Older adults
- The proportion of older people is increasing, therefore > 80% of individuals who die from CVD are > 65 years of age
- Meta-analysis of observational studies has shown that higher total cholesterol is associated with increased CAD mortality at all ages
- A large meta-analysis of studies with patients aged > 75 years at randomization demonstrated statin therapy reduces major vascular events (RR 0.79) per 1 mmol/L reduction in LDL-C, with direct evidence of benefit aged > 75 years
- Benefit was similar irrespective of age among patients with pre-existing vascular disease, but appeared smaller among older individuals not known to have vascular disease
- Therefore, current evidence indicates statin therapy produces significant reductions in major vascular events irrespective of age, but that this evidence is weaker if aged > 75 without known occlusive vascular disease
- Risk factors do continue to apply to elderly individuals, although with different relative risks
- Current ESC lipid management recommendations for patients aged > 65 include:
    - Primary prevention with statin therapy is recommended according to the level of risk if aged ≤ 70 years *(Class IA)*
    - Statin therapy may be considered for primary prevention purposes in those aged > 70 years if at high risk or above *(Class IIb B)*
    - Treat atherosclerotic CVD with statins in the same way as for younger patients *(Class IA)*
    - If commencing statin therapy, start at a low dose if there is significant renal impairment and/or the potential for drug interactions, and then titrate upwards to achieve LDL-C treatment goals *(Class IC)*
- Studies have shown that calcium channel blockers may reduce progression to dementia in hypertensive elderly patients over 70 years and may help in stroke prevention through stabilizing blood pressure variability
- Non-morning dipping and orthostatic hypotension (OH) have been observed in a quarter of an unselected cohort of ambulatory older patients without CVD, and this was associated with a 2.4× increased risk of major cardiovascular event (CVE)

- Blood pressure measurements should be repeated while standing to identify OH, as a measure of autonomic dysregulation and risk for CVD
- Target blood pressure in those ≥ 70 years of age is < 140/80 mmHg and < 130/80 mmHg if tolerated
- Reversible factors should be sought in the first instance and non-pharmacological therapies tested prior to initiating medications
- Consideration should be made for polypharmacy, quality of life, and cognitive function when considering pharmacotherapy in older individuals

Women

- Risk estimates are lower in women than in men. However, risk is only deferred in women; the risk of a 60-year-old woman is similar to that of a 50-year-old man and ultimately, more women die from CVD than men
- Few statin RCTs have reported independently significant CV benefits in women, predominantly due to under-representation of female patients
- However, serial meta-analyses have demonstrated a reduction in all-cause mortality, vascular events, and revascularization in primary prevention with the impact similar in male and female patients
- The same is true of non-statin therapies, including ezetimibe and PCSK9 inhibitors
- The metabolic insult which pregnancy confers provides an insight to future risk and women with pre-eclampsia should therefore be referred to a cardiologist post partum
- As previously highlighted, systemic inflammatory states such as SLE have also been shown to be associated with significant CV risk and should therefore be taken into consideration in risk stratification
- The Euro Heart study showed similar risks for acute MI in women and men for lipid profile, current smoking, abdominal obesity, high-risk diet, and psychosocial stress factors, but an increased risk associated with hypertension, diabetes, and low physical activity
- Specific ESC recommendations include:
  - Statin treatment is recommended for primary prevention of atherosclerotic CVD in high-risk women
  - Statins are recommended for secondary prevention in women with the same indications and goals as in men
  - Lipid-lowering drugs should not be administered during pregnancy and the period of breast-feeding because data on possible adverse effects are lacking. However, bile acid sequestrants may be considered
  - Care should be taken to consider pregnancy in women of childbearing age when choosing anti-hypertensive medications and appropriate counselling regarding birth control if required

Further reading

Arnett DK, Blumenthal RS, Albert MA, Buroker AB, Goldberger ZD, Hahn EJ, Himmelfarb CD, Khera A, Lloyd-Jones D, McEvoy JW, Michos ED, Miedema MD, Muñoz D, Smith SC Jr, Virani SS, Williams KA Sr, Yeboah J, Ziaeian B. 2019 ACC/AHA Guideline on the Primary Prevention of Cardiovascular Disease: A Report of the American College of Cardiology/American Heart Association Task Force on Clinical Practice Guidelines. *Circulation*. 2019 Sep 10;140(11):e596–e646. doi: 10.1161/CIR.0000000000000678. Epub 2019 Mar 17. Erratum in: Circulation. 2019 Sep

10;140(11):e649–e650. Erratum in: *Circulation*. 2020 Jan 28;141(4):e60. Erratum in: *Circulation*. 2020 Apr 21;141(16):e774. PMID: 30879355; PMCID: PMC7734661

Cardiovascular disease: risk assessment and reduction, including lipid modification. London: *National Institute for Health and Care Excellence (NICE)*; 2023 May 24. PMID: 32200592.

SCORE2 working group and ESC Cardiovascular risk collaboration. SCORE2 risk prediction algorithms: new models to estimate 10-year risk of cardiovascular disease in Europe. *Eur Heart J*. 2021 Jul 1;42(25):2439–54. doi: 10.1093/eurheartj/ehab309. PMID: 34120177; PMCID: PMC8248998

Visseren FLJ, Mach F, Smulders YM, Carballo D, Koskinas KC, Bäck M, Benetos A, Biffi A, Boavida JM, Capodanno D, Cosyns B, Crawford C, Davos CH, Desormais I, Di Angelantonio E, Franco OH, Halvorsen S, Hobbs FDR, Hollander M, Jankowska EA, Michal M, Sacco S, Sattar N, Tokgozoglu L, Tonstad S, Tsioufis KP, van Dis I, van Gelder IC, Wanner C, Williams B; ESC Scientific Document Group; ESC National Cardiac Societies. 2021 ESC Guidelines on cardiovascular disease prevention in clinical practice. *Eur Heart J*. 2021 Sep 7;42(34):3227–337. doi: 10.1093/eurheartj/ehab484. PMID: 34458905.

7.3

Arterial hypertension

Tim Fairbairn and James Redfern

TABLE OF CONTENTS

7.3.1 Definition and classification 629
7.3.2 Assessing cardiovascular risk 629
  NICE Guidelines 630
  Joint British Societies recommendations on the prevention of cardiovascular disease (JBS3) 630
  Europe 630
7.3.3 Blood pressure measurement 630
  Ambulatory Blood Pressure Monitoring (ABPM) 631
  Home blood pressure monitoring 631
7.3.4 Patient assessment 632
  Clinical and family history, examination, and laboratory investigations 632
  Risk stratification according to blood pressure and level of HMOD according to ESC 2018 632
7.3.5 Secondary causes of hypertension 633
  Renal parenchymal disease (5% all HTN) 633
  Renovascular disease (1–2%) 633
  Aortic coarctation 633
  Cushings syndrome 633
  Conns disease (< 1%) 633
  Phaeochromocytoma (0.1%) 633
7.3.6 Hypertension-mediated organ damage (HMOD) 633
7.3.7 Anti-hypertensive treatment 634
  When to treat 634
  Treatment targets (ESC 2018) 634
  Lifestyle changes 635
  Pharmacological therapy (ESC 2018) 635
  Specific considerations 635
  The evidence for medication 636
7.3.8 Special considerations 638
  Elderly 638
  Young (age < 50 years) 638
  Diabetes 638
  Renal disease 639
  Stroke 639
  Pregnancy 639
7.3.9 Resistant hypertension 639
  Definition 639
  Management 640
  Interventional and surgical treatment options 640
7.3.10 Malignant hypertension 640
  Definition 640
  Management of malignant hypertension and hypertensive emergencies 641

7.3.1 Definition and classification

The 2018 ESC Hypertension Guideline classification of blood pressure is shown in Table 7.3.1.

7.3.2 Assessing cardiovascular risk

- Risk of adverse cardiovascular events (stroke, coronary heart disease (CHD), sudden death, heart failure, peripheral arterial disease, end stage renal failure) show a continuous relationship with BP. Every 2 mmHg rise in systolic BP is associated with a 7% increased risk of mortality from CHD.

Table 7.3.1 Classification of office blood pressure[a] and definitions of hypertension grade[b].

Category	Systolic (mmHg)		Diastolic (mmHg)
Optimal	< 120	and	< 80
Normal	120–129	and/or	80–84
High normal	130–139	and/or	85–89
Grade 1 hypertension	140–159	and/or	90–99
Grade 2 hypertension	160–179	and/or	100–109
Grade 3 hypertension	≥ 180	and/or	≥ 110
Isolated systolic hypertension[b]	≥ 140	and	< 90

BP—blood pressure; SBP—systolic blood pressure.
a BP category is defined according to seated clinic BP and by the highest level of BP, whether systolic or diastolic.
b Isolated systolic hypertension is graded 1, 2, or 3 according to SBP values in the ranges indicated.
Williams B, Mancia G, Spiering W, et al; ESC Scientific Document Group. 2018 ESC/ESH Guidelines for the management of arterial hypertension. *Eur Heart J.* 2018 Sep 1;39(33):3021–3104. doi: 10.1093/eurheartj/ehy339. © European Society of Cardiology. With permission from Oxford University Press.

- There is increasing evidence linking hypertension (HTN) with atrial fibrillation (AF) and dementia
- HTN is one of the most correctable risk factors
- HTN should not be treated in isolation, but on the basis of the total CVD risk.

NICE Guidelines

QRISK3 estimates 10-year risk of developing a heart attack or stroke

- Excludes patients with: Type 1 diabetes; CVD; age > 85; familial hyperlipidaemia.
- Is based upon age, sex, BMI, BP, lipids, ethnicity, post code, smoking status, family history, CKD and certain past medical history.

Joint British Societies recommendations on the prevention of cardiovascular disease (JBS3)

- JBS3 can be used to estimate lifetime CVD risk. This may be more applicable in younger individuals who have a low 10-year risk but significant modifiable risk factors.
- JBS is based on the British population and is now preferable to using Framingham risk functions that are developed based on American population data.

Europe

The SCORE model uses similar risk factors based on a population of 250,000 and calculates 10-year risk of **death** from CVD.

ESC 10-year cardiovascular risk categories (Systemic COronary Risk Evaluation) (see Table 7.3.2).

7.3.3 Blood pressure measurement

- NICE recommend 5-yearly BP measurements for all adults. Annually if previous high recording
- When considering the diagnosis measure blood pressure in both arms
- If BP is more than 140/90 mmHg offer ABPM (see below) to confirm the diagnosis
- If ABPM is not tolerated, home blood pressure monitoring (HBPM) is a suitable alternative

Table 7.3.2 ESC Ten-year cardiovascular risk categories (SCORE).

Very high risk	**People with any of the following:** **Documented CVD, either clinical or unequivocal on imaging.**<ul><li>**Clinical CVD** includes acute myocardial infarction, acute coronary syndrome, coronary or other arterial revascularization, stroke, TIA, aortic aneurysm, and PAD</li><li>**Unequivocal documented CVD on imaging** includes significant plaque (i.e. $\geq$ 50% stenosis) on angiography or ultrasound; it does not include increase in carotid intima-media thickness</li><li>**Diabetes mellitus with target organ damage**, e.g. proteinuria or a with a major risk factor such as grade 3 hypertension or hypercholesterolaemia</li><li>**Severe CKD** (eGFR < 30 ml/min/1.73 m²)</li><li>**A calculated 10 year SCORE of $\geq$ 10%**</li></ul>
High risk	**People with any of the following:**<ul><li>**Marked elevation of a single risk factor**, particularly cholesterol > 8 mmol/L (> 310 mg/dL), e.g. familial hypercholesterolaemia or grade 3 hypertension (BP $\geq$ 180/110 mmHg)</li><li>**Most other people with diabetes mellitus** (except some young people with type 1 diabetes mellitus and without major risk factors, who may be at moderate risk)</li></ul>**Hypertensive LVH** **Moderate CKD eGFR 30–59 ml/min/1.73 m²)** **A calculated 10 year SCORE of 5–10%**
Moderate risk	**People with:**<ul><li>**A calculated 10-year SCORE of $\geq$ 1 to < 5%**</li><li>**Grade 2 hypertension**</li><li>**Many middle-aged people belong to this category**</li></ul>
Low risk	**People with:**<ul><li>**A calculated 10 year SCORE of < 1%**</li></ul>

SCORE2 working group and ESC Cardiovascular risk collaboration. SCORE2 risk prediction algorithms: new models to estimate 10-year risk of cardiovascular disease in Europe. *Eur Heart J.* 2021 Jul 1;42(25):2439–2454. doi: 10.1093/eurheartj/ehab309. © European Society of Cardiology. With permission from Oxford University Press.

- While awaiting confirmation of the diagnosis carry out investigations for target organ damage

Ambulatory Blood Pressure Monitoring (ABPM)

- Gives mean daytime and night-time measurements and variability in BP
- When making a diagnosis ensure at least 2 measurements per hour during patients usual waking hours. Use the average value of at least 14 measurements
- Diagnosis of grade I hypertension = 135/85 mmHg

Can also be used in:

- Variable BP
- Suspected white coat hypertension
- Assessment of drug efficacy or resistance
- Pregnancy-related hypertension
- Symptomatic hypotension

Home blood pressure monitoring

- Ensure that for each reading, 2 consecutive measurements are taken, at least 1 minute apart
- That recordings are taken at least twice daily (ideally morning and evening)

- That monitoring continues for at least 4, and ideally 7 days
- Discard measurements taken on the first day. Take the average of the remaining days

7.3.4 Patient assessment

The clinical assessment of a patient should include the four Cs:

- **C**ontributory and risk factors
- **C**auses, i.e. secondary causes
- **C**omplications—Hypertension Mediated Organ Damage (HMOD)
- **C**ontraindications to drugs

Clinical and family history, examination, and laboratory investigations
Routine investigations
Urinary albumin:creatinine ratio, test for haematuria, creatinine, and electrolytes, eGFR, LFTs, plasma glucose and HBA1c, serum total cholesterol and HDL cholesterol, examine the fundi for hypertensive retinopathy, and arrange a 12-lead ECG.

Risk stratification according to blood pressure and level of HMOD according to ESC 2018
See Table 7.3.3.

Table 7.3.3 Risk stratification according to blood pressure and level of HMOD according to ESC Guidelines 2018.

Hypertension disease staging	Other risk factors, HMOD, or disease	BP (mmHg) grading			
		High normal SBP 130–139 DBP 85–89	Grade 1 SBP 140–159 DBP 90–99	Grade 2 SBP 160–179 DBP 100–109	Grade 3 SBP ≥ 180 or DBP ≥ 110
Stage 1 (uncomplicated)	No other risk factors	Low risk	Low risk	Moderate risk	High risk
	1 or 2 risk factors	Low risk	Moderate risk	Moderate to high risk	High risk
	≥ 3 risk factors	Low to Moderate risk	Moderate to high risk	High Risk	High risk
Stage 2 (asymptomatic disease)	HMOD, CKD grade 3, or diabetes mellitus without organ damage	Moderate to high risk	High risk	High risk	High to very high risk
Stage 3 (established disease)	Established CVD, CKD grade ≥ 4, or diabetes mellitus with organ damage	Very high risk	Very high risk	Very high risk	Very high risk

Williams B, Mancia G, Spiering W, et al; ESC Scientific Document Group. 2018 ESC/ESH Guidelines for the management of arterial hypertension. *Eur Heart J*. 2018 Sep 1;39(33):3021–3104. doi: 10.1093/eurheartj/ehy339. © European Society of Cardiology. With permission from Oxford University Press.

7.3.5 Secondary causes of hypertension

More likely if young age (< 40), severe hypertension, rapid onset, and unresponsive to medication.

Renal parenchymal disease (5% all HTN)
- Normal urinalysis and creatinine usually exclude renal parenchymal disease.
- Blood and protein could suggest either glomerulonephritides or polycystic kidney disease (PKD).
- Renal USS and specialist referral would be appropriate next steps.

Renovascular disease (1–2%)
- Renal USS (difference of > 1.5 cm between kidney length) or contrast MRA for diagnosis with selective X-ray renal angiography for certainty.

Aortic coarctation
- Post ductal stenosis of thoracic aorta.
- Associated Bicuspid Aortic Valve (BAV) and aortopathy.
- Murmur of mid-systole- anterior chest to interscapular area.
- Cardiac MRI allows non-invasive, non-ionizing assessment of anatomy, severity, and routine follow-up (including post-operative complications).

Cushings syndrome
- Obese, diabetic, striae, cushingoid facies, and hypertension.
- Hypercortisolaemia diagnosed by 24-hour urine collection (> 40 mcg).
- Low-dose dexamethasone suppression test can confirm Cushing's syndrome and a high-dose test may differentiate pituitary and adrenal cause.
- Pseudocushings is associated with alcohol excess, obese and depressed individuals.

Conns disease (< 1%)
- Muscle fatigue, hypokalaemia.
- Low renin activity (< 1 ng/ml/hr), raised aldosterone and a renin:aldosterone ratio of > 50 (a ratio driven by high aldosterone is more meaningful than one dependent on low renin).
- Drugs that affect renin activity ideally should be withdrawn (4 weeks) prior to testing.

Phaeochromocytoma (0.1%)
- Tumour with raised urinary and plasma catecholamines.
- Diagnosed with MRI, CT, USS, or MIBA.
- The 10% tumour (10% bilateral, 10% extra adrenal, 10% malignant).
- Up to 10% are familial and these are usually bilateral.
- Malignancy can only be confirmed by secondary spread, not histology.
- The currently favoured diagnostic test is excess urinary secretion of the metabolites of catecholamines (normetadrenaline/normetanephrine or metadrenaline/metanephrine) over a 24-hour period

7.3.6 Hypertension-mediated organ damage (HMOD)

When assessing patients with HTN it is important to assess for evidence and degree of HMOD as this will influence cardiovascular risk and subsequent treatment.

Basic screening for all cases:

- ECG to assess for LVH ($S_{v1} + R_{v5} > 35$ mm—Sokolow–Lyon criteria) and document rhythm
- Urinary ACR—to detect elevations in albumin secretion (30–300 mg/24 hr) suggestive of renal disease
- Creatinine and eGFR—to quantify renal disease
- Fundoscopy—to detect hypertensive retinopathy (especially in patients with grade 2 or 3 HTN)

Consider:
Echocardiography, carotid ultrasound, abdominal ultrasound, pulse wave velocity (> 12 m/s), ankle–brachial index (< 0.9), cognitive function testing and brain imaging in specific cases.

7.3.7 Anti-hypertensive treatment

Irrespective of the region, across the world ~40% of people with HTN are treated and of these only ~35% achieve a target BP of < 140/90 mmHg. There are a number of contributory factors to this which need consideration:

1. Efficacy of pharmacological treatment—only 5–10% of patients in trials exhibit resistance to medical therapy
2. Physician treatment inertia
3. Patient adherence to treatment—population studies suggest that < 50% of patients consistently adhere to therapy
4. Insufficient use of combination therapy—combination therapy utilizing multiple pharmacological mechanisms is required in *most* patients to adequately control BP
5. Complexity of treatment strategies

Current ESC guidance therefore encourages early use of combination therapy (usually as single pill combination (SPC)) to improve compliance and reduce the complexity of treatment algorithms.

When to treat

Treatment of HTN in the ESC, BHS, and NICE guidelines all focus on cardiovascular risk and grade of hypertension:

- Drug treatment is not recommended in patients with high-normal blood pressure
- Patients with Grade 1 HTN at low–moderate risk should be treated with lifestyle advice for 3–6 months before considering drug treatment
- Patients with Grade 1 HTN at high/very high risk, plus all patients with Grade II/III HTN should be initiated on drug therapy and given lifestyle advice simultaneously.
- Patients > 80 years old should be treated with drug therapy if BP > 160 mmHg systolic.

ESC 2018 Guidance on when to initiate pharmacological therapy in HTN.

Treatment targets (ESC 2018)

- Initially aim for office BP < 140/90 in all patient groups.
- In patients < 65 years old, if treatment is well tolerated the target should be lowered to < 130/80 mmHg.
- Treated SBP should not be targeted to < 120 mmHg.
- In diabetic patients the target should be office SBP < 130 mmHg.

7.3.7 Anti-hypertensive treatment

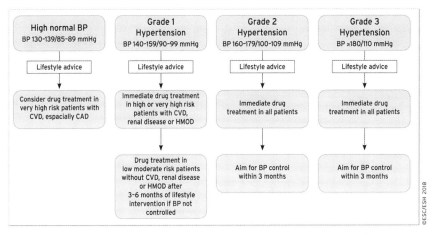

Figure 7.3.1 ESC 2018 Guidance on when to initiate pharmacological therapy in HTN

Williams B, Mancia G, Spiering W, et al; ESC Scientific Document Group. 2018 ESC/ESH Guidelines for the management of arterial hypertension. *Eur Heart J.* 2018 Sep 1;39(33):3021–3104. doi: 10.1093/eurheartj/ehy339. © European Society of Cardiology. With permission from Oxford University Press.

Lifestyle changes

- Salt restriction
- Moderation of alcohol intake (men < 14 units, women < 8 units)
- High consumption of fruit and vegetables
- Weight loss and maintenance of normal BMI
- Regular physical activity (30 minutes of moderate intensity exercise 5–7 times/week)

Pharmacological therapy (ESC 2018)

General principles

- Initiate treatment in most patients with an SPC of a RAS blocking agent plus a CCB or diuretic
- Use monotherapy for low-risk patients with stage 1 HTN or very high-risk patients with high–normal BP
- Use a 3-drug SPC (RAS blocker + CCB + diuretic) if BP not controlled with a 2-drug SPC.
- Add spironolactone for resistant hypertension

Specific considerations

- RAS blocking agents reduce albuminuria more than other anti-hypertensive medications and are effective at delaying progression of diabetic and non-diabetic CKD.
- CCBs have a greater effect on stroke reduction than expected for the BP reduction achieved.
- Diuretics appear to be more effective at preventing the onset of heart failure but are associated with a less favourable side-effect profile than RAS blocking agents.
- Beta blockers are particularly useful in hypertensive patients with angina, HFREF and post-MI.
- Doxazosin is an effective third-line agent, but is less effective than spironolactone.

The 2019 NICE guidance recommends initial monotherapy with a RAS blocking agent (ACE/ARB) to people age < 55 and those with Type 2 Diabetes. Monotherapy with a CCB is recommended to those age 55 or over and people of Black African or African-Caribbean origin of any age.

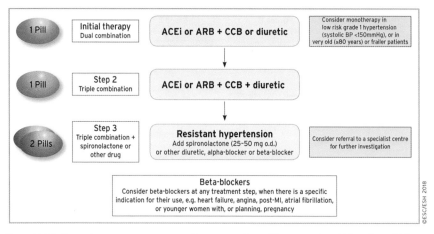

Figure 7.3.2 Core drug treatment strategy for uncomplicated hypertension (Taken from ESC Guidelines)

Williams B, Mancia G, Spiering W, et al; ESC Scientific Document Group. 2018 ESC/ESH Guidelines for the management of arterial hypertension. *Eur Heart J.* 2018 Sep 1;39(33):3021–3104. doi: 10.1093/eurheartj/ehy339. © European Society of Cardiology. With permission from Oxford University Press.

The evidence for medication

Most trials are CVD outcome trials rather than specific hypertension endpoints.

Anti-hypertensives vs placebo

The Blood Pressure Lowering Treatment Trialists Collaboration (BPLTT) is a meta-analysis of 21 trials comprising > 194,000 patients comparing various treatment regimens against placebo:

- ACE Inhibitors:
    - Heart Outcomes prevention Evaluation (HOPE)—reduction in risk of stroke (32%), MI (20%), and CVD (26%) with ramipril.
    - Perindopril Protection Against Recurrent Stroke Study (PROGRESS)—28% reduction in stroke with perindopril, increased to 43% reduction with addition of indapamide.
    - Efficacy of perindopril in reduction of cardiovascular events among patients with stable coronary artery disease: randomized, double-blind, placebo-controlled, multicentre trial (EUROPA)—20% reduction in cardiovascular events with perindopril.
- Angiotensin receptor blockers:
    - Reduction of Endpoints in NIDDM with the Angiotensin II Antagonist Losartan (RENAAL)—losartan achieved a 16% reduction in the rate of ESRF or doubling of creatinine.
    - The Study on Cognition and Prognosis in the Elderly (SCOPE)—28% reduction in non-fatal stroke and 11% reduction in stroke, MI, and CV death in patients aged 70–89 years with candesartan.
    - Irbesartan Diabetic Nephropathy Trial (IDNT)—irbesartan is associated with a 20% reduction in the progression of nephropathy related to T2DM than placebo.
- Calcium channel blockers:
    - BPLTT examined 2 trials showing a risk reduction in stroke (39%) and major cardiovascular events (28%).

- Diuretics (thiazide-like):
  - Good evidence for reducing risk of stroke (RR 0.66), CHD (RR 0.72), heart failure (RR 0.58), and mortality (RR 0.9).
  - Most patients will require combination therapy to achieve BP within target range.
- Beta blockers:
  - Majority of evidence based on atenolol
  - Reduces risk of stroke (RR 0.71) and heart failure (RR 0.58) but not CHD (RR 0.93) or mortality (RR 0.95).
  - Given the evidence of BB benefit in CHD patients regardless of their BP, the lack of reduced CHD evidence in hypertension is confusing:
    - One explanation is the use of atenolol; as in CHD studies mortality benefit with metoprolol (RR 0.8), propranolol (RR 0.71), and timolol (RR 0.59) were far superior to atenolol (RR 1.02).

Comparison trials

Several trials have tried to answer the question of whether one drug is superior to another.

- Anti-hypertensive and Lipid Lowering Treatment to prevent Heart Attack Trial (ALLHAT) compared amlodipine, lisinopril, and doxazosin with chlorthalidone (control):
- Limitations in study design favouring chlorthalidone, but remains important due to large size (42,000 patients):
  - Doxazosin stopped at 3 years due to inferiority
  - Other 3 arms showed no significant difference in non-fatal MI and fatal CHD.
  - Lisinopril was inferior for heart failure (vs chlorthalidone) and stroke (vs amlodipine) but this was attributed to lower BP response.
- Australian National Blood Pressure Study (ANBP2): Hydrochlorthiazide vs ACE inhibitor:
  - Equivocal findings with borderline superiority of ACE inhibitors, but several limitations.
- Losartan Intervention For Endpoint reduction in hypertension (LIFE) trial examined losartan vs atenolol:
  - ARB had reduced cardiovascular events due to reduced risk of stroke with similar BP levels.
- Outcomes in hypertensive patients at high cardiovascular risk treated with regimens based on valsartan or amlodipine (VALUE):
  - Heart failure was included in the primary outcome with a RR of 1.04.
- International Verapamil Trandolapril Study (INVEST) compared verapamil with atenolol.
  - Found no difference in all-cause mortality, MI, and stroke.
- Anglo-Scandinavian Cardiac Outcomes—Blood Pressure Lowering Arm (ASCOT-BPLA) compared amlodipine with atenolol in patients with high cardiovascular risk:
  - Stopped early as end-points favoured amlodipine, however BB group was under treated in 45% and primary outcome (death and non-fatal MI) did not include heart failure.
- Ongoing Telmisartan Alone and in Combination with Ramipril Global Endpoint Trial (ONTARGET) compared telmisartan with ramipril and a combination of both:
  - No difference between telmisartan and ramipril arms but less angioedema with telmisartan
  - Combination group had significantly greater side effects with no increase in efficacy

Comparisons of 2-drug combinations

Very few trials have directly compared two different two-drug combinations of first-line anti-hypertensive therapies:

- Avoiding Cardiovascular Events Through Combination Therapy in Patient Living With Systolic Hypertension (ACCOMPLISH) compared benazepril and amlodipine with benazepril and hydrochlorothiazide:

- The benazepril–amlodipine group had significantly lower rates of the primary outcome (composite of cardiovascular events or death from cardiovascular causes) driven by reduction in MI.
- Combination of OLMesartan and a calcium channel blocker or diuretic in Japanese elderly hypertensive patients (COLM) compared olmesartan with a long-acting dihydropyridine CCB (ARB/CCB group) or with a low-dose diuretic (ARB/diuretic group):
  - The 2 groups had similar efficacy but a better safety profile was observed in the ARB/CCB group.

Summary of evidence

- Cardiovascular outcomes are more dependent upon total BP lowering than the class of drug used.
- Individual response to treatment is however variable, with all classes of drug having similar effects except in the instance of age and ethnicity.
- Monotherapy has been shown to rarely achieve target BP which is reflected in the latest ESC guidelines.
- Single pill combinations of 2 antihypertensive drugs are preferred as reducing the number of pills increases adherence and rate of BP control.
- The preferred 2 drug combination is a RAS blocker with a CCB or diuretic.
- A beta blocker in combination with a diuretic or any drug from the other major classes is preferred when there is a primary indication for BB.

7.3.8 Special considerations

Various situations will affect the treatment strategy

Elderly

- Increasing prevalence with age—~75% over the age of 75.
- Diastolic BP plateaus with age due to a loss of arterial compliance causing increased pulse pressure in the elderly.
- Antihypertensive treatment significantly reduces CV morbidity and all-cause mortality in those > 80 (Hypertension in the Very Elderly Trial, SPRINT Trial).
- Treatment is generally well tolerated.
- In very old patients (> 80 year of age) it may be appropriate to initiate treatment with monotherapy.
- In all older patients treatment is more likely to cause hypotensive episodes and symptoms of possible postural hypotension should be investigated with ABPM
- Treated SBP of < 130 mmHg should be avoided.

Young (age < 50 years)

- Greater likelihood of detecting a secondary cause (up to 10%).
- Difficult to conduct outcome trials to demonstrate benefit of treating Grade 1 hypertension in younger patients as the outcome measures only occur after many years.
- However, long-term epidemiological studies have demonstrated relationship between hypertension and longer-term risk of cardiovascular events and mortality in young adults.

Diabetes

- BP reduction in people with diabetes reduces macro- and microvascular complications as well as mortality and reduces the rate of retinopathy, end-stage nephropathy, albuminuria, and neuropathy.

- Antihypertensive treatment is advised if BP > 140/> 90 mmHg and should include an ACEi or ARB.
- The target should be a SBP < 130 mmHg.

Renal disease

- Hypertension is the most common cause of end-stage renal disease. Lowering BP reduces the progression of nephropathy and all-cause mortality.
- In addition to lifestyle advice and sodium restriction medical therapy should be initiated when BP > 140/90 mmHg.
- In patients with albuminuria > 1 g/day BP target may be 110–119 mmHg.
- A 10–20% drop in eGFR should be expected in renal patients being commenced on antihypertensive therapy.

Stroke

- Hypertension is a major risk factor for ischaemic and haemorrhagic stroke.
- Treatment of hypertension in the acute setting (< 48 hours) of haemorrhagic stroke has not be demonstrated to reduce disability or death and is thus not recommended.
- Secondary outcome data from one RCT suggested a possible benefit in functional recovery in patients with SBP > 220 mmHg and so careful lowering via infusion may be considered.
- In patients receiving thrombolysis SBP should be maintained below 180/105 mmHg.
- Treatment of hypertension in patients with prior TIA or stroke to a target < 140/90 mmHg has been shown to reduce recurrence.

Pregnancy

- Hypertension affects 5–10% of pregnancies worldwide and increases risk of placental abruption, stroke, DIC, IUGR, prematurity, and foetal death.
- The types of hypertension and the thresholds for treatment are:
  - Pre-existing hypertension—develops before 20-weeks gestation. Treatment at 150/90 mmHg in the absence of subclinical organ damage.
  - Gestational hypertension—develops after 20 weeks and resolves by 6 weeks post partum. Treatment at 140/90 mmHg.
  - Pre-eclampsia is hypertension with significant proteinuria (> 0.3 g/24 hr). Treatment at 140/90 mmHg.
- SBP > 170 mmHg or DBP > 110 mmHg in pregnancy is considered an emergency and admission is recommended.
- Methyldopa, labetalol, and CCBs are the most commonly used medications.
- ACE inhibitors, angiotensin II antagonists, and renin inhibitors are absolutely contraindicated.
- All anti-hypertensive agents are excreted into breast milk. Labetalol, nifedipine, enalapril, captopril, atenolol, and metoprolol are considered safe.

7.3.9 Resistant hypertension

Definition

Resistant hypertension is defined by office blood pressures of > 140/> 90 mmHg despite recommended therapy and confirmed on either ABPM or HBPM in patients with proven adherence. In this context recommended therapy is defined as:

- Lifestyle modification
- Maximal tolerated doses of ≥ 3 drugs (ideally including a diuretic, ACEi/ARB, and CCB)

The prevalence of true resistant hypertension according to the above definition is likely to be < 10% and is more commonly found in older, male patients (aged ≥ 75), of Black African origin with higher initial BP at diagnosis and past medical history including obesity, diabetes, atherosclerotic disease, and CKD. Before making a diagnosis of resistant hypertension it is important to consider the possibility of pseudo-hypertension. This may be caused or contributed to by the following factors:

- Poor adherence to medications
- White-coat phenomenon (elevated office BP with normal ABPM/HBPM)
- Poor office BP measurement technique (e.g. incorrectly sized BP cuff)
- Brachial artery calcification (particularly in elderly patients)
- Clinician inertia.

Management

There is a stepwise escalation strategy in the management of resistant hypertension:

1. Further education and re-enforcement of lifestyle measures, particularly salt restriction.
2. Escalation of diuretic therapy: Consider the use of more potent thiazide-like diuretics (indapamide, chlorthalidone).
3. Most patients will also require the addition of a fourth agent. The PATHWAY-2 study supports the role of MRAs, although the antiandrogenic side effects may limit their tolerability.
4. When compared to placebo in the PATHWAY-2 study, both bisoprolol 5–10 mg or doxazosin 4–8 mg significantly reduced BP in patients with resistant hypertension. They were however found to be inferior to spironolactone.

Interventional and surgical treatment options

Device-based therapy for resistant hypertension is a fast-growing field with growing evidence, however they are not currently recommended for use outside of clinical trials.

- Renal denervation as a method to reduce BP by reducing sympathetic tone to the kidney. It has been an area of significant interest since the publication of the open label study SIMPLICITY-HTN1 in 2009 which demonstrated a significant reduction in BP. Several subsequent trials including SIMPLICITY-HTN2, PRAGUE-15, and SIMPLICITY-HTN3 published conflicting results. Most recently the SPYRAL HTN-OFF MED study employed a more aggressive approach and demonstrated a significant reduction in BP at 3 months.
- Carotid baroreceptor stimulation aims to reduce blood pressure by applying pressure to the carotid bulb thereby inhibiting the sympathetic nervous system. First- and second-generation surgically implanted devices have proven efficacy with improving safety profiles but remain expensive. Most recently stent-like devices have been developed, but data from randomized trials are awaited.
- Arteriovenous fistula formation is another surgical method to reduce BP in resistant hypertension. In the ROX CONTROL HTN trial patients randomized to receive an arteriovenous coupler demonstrated a significant drop in BP, although there were important safety concerns as 29% developed ipsilateral venous stenosis requiring intervention.

7.3.10 Malignant hypertension

Definition

Hypertensive emergency is defined by severe hypertension (stage 3) in association with acute HMOD and may be life-threatening. It is important to be mindful that the rate and magnitude of the rise in BP may be as important as the absolute level of BP.

Malignant hypertension is defined as severe hypertension that is associated with any or all of the following:

- fundoscopic changes (papilloedema and/or flame haemorrhages);
- Disseminated intravascular coagulopathy
- Encephalopathy
- Acute heart failure
- Acute kidney injury

Symptoms are dependent on the affected organs but may include headache, visual disturbance, breathlessness, chest pain, and dizziness. The prognosis is extremely poor if left untreated.

Severe hypertension is also considered an emergency in situations where urgent BP control is required such as acute aortic dissection, myocardial ischaemia, phaeochromocytoma associated with organ damage, and pre-eclampsia.

Management of malignant hypertension and hypertensive emergencies

RCTs evaluating different treatment strategies are lacking, but it is recommended that consideration is given to the underlying cause and affected organs as well as the timescale and magnitude of BP lowering that is required.

Recommended treatments for specific situations are suggested in Table 7.3.4.

These patients remain at high risk and should be closely followed up following discharge until optimal target BP is achieve and screened for secondary hypertension.

Table 7.3.4 Hypertensive emergencies requiring immediate blood pressure lowering with intravenous drug therapy (ESC Guidelines 2018).

Clinical presentation	Timeline and target for BP reduction	First-line treatment	Alternative
Malignant hypertension with or without acute renal failure	Several hours Reduce MAP by 20–25%	Labetalol, nicardipine	Nitroprussiden urapidil
Hypertensive encephalopathy	Immediately reduce MAP by 20–25%	Labetalol, nicardipine	Nitroprusside
Acute coronary event	Immediately reduce SBP to <140 mmHg	Nitroglycerine, labetalol	Urapidil
Acute cardiogenic pulmonary oedema	Immediately reduce SBP to < 140 mmHg	Nitroprusside or nitroglycerine (with loop diuretic)	Urapidil (with loop diuretic)
Acute aortic dissection	Immediately reduce SBP to < 120 mmHg AND heart rate to <60 bpm	Esmolol and nitroprusside or nitroglycerine or nicardipine	Labetalol OR metoprolol
Eclampsia and severe pre-eclampsia/HELLP	Immediately reduce SBP to < 160 mmHg AND DBP to <105 mmHg	Labetalol or nicardipine and magnesium sulfate	Consider delivery

Williams B, Mancia G, Spiering W, et al; ESC Scientific Document Group. 2018 ESC/ESH Guidelines for the management of arterial hypertension. *Eur Heart J.* 2018 Sep 1;39(33):3021–3104. doi: 10.1093/eurheartj/ehy339. © European Society of Cardiology. With permission from Oxford University Press.

Further reading

Camm AJ, Lüscher TF, Serruys PW (eds). *The European Society of Cardiology Textbook of Cardiovascular Medicine*. Oxford: Oxford University Press, 2018

Carey RM, Calhoun DA, Bakris GL, Brook RD, Daugherty SL, Dennison-Himmelfarb CR, Egan BM, Flack JM, Gidding SS, Judd E, Lackland DT, Laffer CL, Newton-Cheh C, Smith SM, Taler SJ, Textor SC, Turan TN, White WB; American Heart Association Professional/Public Education and Publications Committee of the Council on Hypertension; Council on Cardiovascular and Stroke Nursing; Council on Clinical Cardiology; Council on Genomic and Precision Medicine; Council on Peripheral Vascular Disease; Council on Quality of Care and Outcomes Research; and Stroke Council. Resistant Hypertension: Detection, Evaluation, and Management: A Scientific Statement From the American Heart Association. *Hypertension*. 2018 Nov;72(5):e53–e90. doi: 10.1161/HYP.0000000000000084

NICE Guidelines (2019), available at https:// www.nice.org.uk/guidance/ng136

Whelton PK, Carey RM, Aronow WS, Casey DE Jr, Collins KJ, Dennison Himmelfarb C, DePalma SM, Gidding S, Jamerson KA, Jones DW, MacLaughlin EJ, Muntner P, Ovbiagele B, Smith SC Jr, Spencer CC, Stafford RS, Taler SJ, Thomas RJ, Williams KA Sr, Williamson JD, Wright JT Jr. 2017 ACC/AHA/AAPA/ABC/ACPM/AGS/APhA/ASH/ASPC/NMA/PCNA Guideline for the Prevention, Detection, Evaluation, and Management of High Blood Pressure in Adults: A Report of the American College of Cardiology/American Heart Association Task Force on Clinical Practice Guidelines. *Hypertension*. 2018 Jun;71(6):e13–e115. doi: 10.1161/HYP.0000000000000065. Epub 2017 Nov 13. Erratum in: *Hypertension*. 2018 Jun;71(6):e140–e144

Williams B, Mancia G, Spiering W, Agabiti Rosei E, Azizi M, Burnier M, Clement DL, Coca A, de Simone G, Dominiczak A, Kahan T, Mahfoud F, Redon J, Ruilope L, Zanchetti A, Kerins M, Kjeldsen SE, Kreutz R, Laurent S, Lip GYH, McManus R, Narkiewicz K, Ruschitzka F, Schmieder RE, Shlyakhto E, Tsioufis C, Aboyans V, Desormais I; ESC Scientific Document Group. 2018 ESC/ESH Guidelines for the management of arterial hypertension. *Eur Heart J*. 2018 Sep 1;39(33):3021–104. doi: 10.1093/eurheartj/ehy339. Erratum in: *Eur Heart J*. 2019 Feb 1;40(5):475

7.4

Dyslipidaemia

Scott Murray, David Murphy, Christopher N. Floyd, and Alexander Carpenter

TABLE OF CONTENTS

7.4.1 Overview of lipid molecules and metabolism 643
7.4.2 Cardiovascular risk associated with dyslipidaemia 646
7.4.3 Treatment goals 647
7.4.4 Pharmacological treatment 650
    Statin therapy 650
    Fibrates 652
    Bile acid sequestrants 653
    Selective cholesterol absorption inhibitors 654
    Pro-protein convertase subtilisin/kexin type 9 inhibitors (PCSK9 inhibitors) 655
    Omega-3 (n-3) fatty acids 655
    Cholesterol synthesis inhibitors 656
    Pharmacological strategy 656
7.4.5 Classifying dyslipidaemias 658
    Primary disorders of LDL 659

7.4.1 Overview of lipid molecules and metabolism

- Main classes of lipids:
  - Fatty acids
  - Triglycerides
  - Phospholipids
  - Cholesterol
- Lipids provide fat and muscle with a steady source of fatty acids for storage and energy utilization respectively
- They provide cholesterol for synthesis of bile acids, cell membranes, and steroid hormones

Cholesterol and cholesterol esters

- Cholesterol and cholesterol esters are carried by all lipoproteins but predominantly by low-density lipoprotein (LDL) (see below)
- Cellular cholesterol demands are met through:
  - Uptake of cholesterol esters from LDL via the LDL receptor *or*
  - Intracellular synthesis pathway that involves HMG-CoA (3-hydroxy-3-methyl-glutaryl-coenzyme A) reductase as its rate-limiting step

Triglycerides

- Hydrolysed to free fatty acids, providing an important energy source
- Triglyceride demands are met through:
  - Intestinal uptake
  - Endogenous hepatic synthesis

- Stored as adipose tissue
- Carried by all lipoproteins but predominantly by very low-density lipoproteins (VLDL) and chylomicrons

Plasma lipoproteins and apolipoproteins

- Lipids are hydrophobic and therefore require a transport medium for circulation (Figure 7.4.1)
- They are composed of a shell of phospholipids and protein components, known as apolipoproteins, surrounding a core of lipids (triglycerides and cholesteryl esters)
- The apolipoproteins act as structural components, enzyme activators/inhibitors, and cellular receptors
- Six major groups of lipoproteins exist—separated on the basis of their density—chylomicrons, VLDL (very low density lipoprotein), IDL (intermediate low density lipoproteins), LDL (low density lipoproteins), Lp(a) (lipoprotein a), and HDL (high-density lipoproteins) (Figure 7.4.2)
- This forms the basis of the Fredrickson classification of dyslipidaemias discussed later
- The key initiation of the atherosclerotic inflammatory process is the retention and accumulation of cholesterol rich lipoproteins
- Apolipoprotein B (Apo-B) containing lipoproteins in particular provoke a complex inflammatory process that leads to the initiation of atherosclerosis
- This is not limited to the coronary circulation and includes the cerebrovascular circulation, peripheral vascular circulation, as well as the renovascular circulation
- A persons total atherosclerotic plaque burden is directly proportional to the cumulative exposure to these Apo-B containing lipoproteins (both its concentration and duration of exposure)
- LDL is by far the most numerous of the Apo-B containing lipoproteins (but also IDL, VLDL), with apolipoprotein A forming HDL
- Consistent evidence from numerous and multiple types of clinical and genetic studies unequivocally establishes that, in specific circumstances, LDL is implicated as one of the multi-factorial causes of CVD
- The risk of experiencing an acute CV event rises with increasing Apo B-containing lipoproteins, thus explaining the need to encourage and target low levels of Apo B-containing lipoproteins throughout life to achieve the primary prevention of CVD

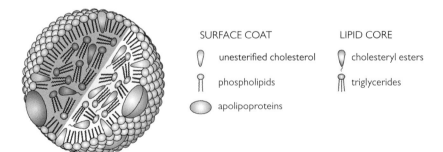

Figure 7.4.1 Lipoprotein structure

Reproduced from Kronenberg, H., Memed, S., and Polonsky, K., The Williams Textbook of Endocrinology, © 2011 with permission from Elsevier.

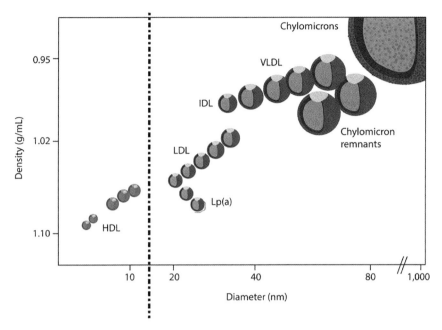

Figure 7.4.2 Relative size of lipoprotein fractions
Reproduced with permission from Kjellmo CA, Hovland A, Lappegård KT. CVD Risk Stratification in the PCSK9 Era: Is There a Role for LDL Subfractions? *Diseases*. 2018 May 27;6(2):45. doi: 10.3390/diseases6020045 under a Creative Commons Attribution 4.0 International (CC BY 4.0).

HDL

- HDL is anti-atherogenic via multiple mechanisms including:
  - Reverse cholesterol transport: transfer of peripheral cholesterol to the liver for breakdown and excretion in bile
  - Inhibition of thrombosis and LDL oxidation

LDL

- The main carrier of cholesterol
- LDL receptor mutations result in the familial hypercholesterolaemia phenotype
- Oxidized LDL can be internalized by macrophages leading to the formation of foam cells and plaque development
- Oxidized LDL plays a pivotal role in atherogenesis via a number of mechanisms including:
  - Endothelial damage
  - Macrophage recruitment
  - Increased platelet aggregation
- Triglyceride levels affect LDL composition and measurement
- When triglyceride levels are high, the triglyceride content of LDL can increase and becomes more atherogenic
- This qualitative difference in LDL to a degree explains the increased likelihood of atherosclerotic disease for any given LDL concentration in individuals with metabolic syndrome
- At high triglyceride concentrations (> 5 mmol/L), LDL measurements may be inaccurate

VLDL and chylomicrons

- VLDL and chylomicrons are the largest lipoproteins and contain proportionally the most triglyceride

- Both chylomicrons and VLDL may undergo metabolism to become smaller lipoproteins, including LDL

Lipoprotein(a)

- Lp(a) is an LDL particle with an Apo(a) moiety
- Demonstrates a pro-inflammatory effect within the vascular endothelial wall, which it can freely cross into
- Higher plasma levels are associated with an increased risk of atherosclerotic disease
- This risk appears to be proportional to the absolute change in the plasma levels but those with very high levels have a lifetime risk similar to those with heterozygous FH (discussed later)
- 90% of a person's Lp(a) is inherited thus there is potential for a significant disease process to be familial

7.4.2 Cardiovascular risk associated with dyslipidaemia

- There is a strong linear relation between elevated total cholesterol (TC) and CV death with TC > 4 mmol/L
- Every 1 mmol/L (38.7 mg/dL) reduction in LDL-C is associated with a 12% reduction in all-cause mortality, 19% reduction in coronary mortality, and 21% reduction in any major vascular event
- Management therefore is focused on comprehensive cardiovascular risk assessment and treatment and lowering lipid levels should be viewed as aiming to lower cardiovascular risk rather than lipid levels per se
- Even patients without particularly high lipid indices should be treated with lipid-lowering therapy

LDL and cardiovascular risk

- There is a strongly positive continuous and independent relationship between LDL-C (the amount of cholesterol contained in LDL) concentrations with the risk of major adverse cardiovascular events (MACE)
- This relationship is apparent over a wide range of concentrations (with no apparent threshold) and patient ages, and is present in both sexes
- Statin therapy is associated with a linear relationship between the absolute LDL cholesterol reduction achieved and the proportional reduction in MACE
- A sustained reduction of LDL-C concentration of 1 mmol/l produces a proportional reduction in major vascular events of almost a quarter
- Currently the lowering of LDL-C concentrations is the primary target of lipid-lowering interventions recommended by all consensus guidelines

HDL and cardiovascular risk

- HDL-C concentrations have a strong continuous and independent inverse relationship with cardiovascular risk, which displays no apparent threshold
- An increase of 0.03 mmol/L in HDL-C levels is associated with a 6% reduction in coronary mortality
- Low HDL is often associated with other lipid profile abnormalities, such as increased LDL and triglyceride concentrations, as is found in the metabolic syndrome
- HDL's relationship with CAD risk is independent and present throughout a range of LDL concentrations

- Low HDL-C levels (< 1.03 mmol/L for men and < 1.3 mmol/L for women) are found in almost half of patients with known CVD
- Most interventions that increase HDL-C also decrease triglycerides and LDL-C, which complicates the assessment of the impact of pharmacologically mediated HDL increases on MACE
- Indirect evidence suggests therapeutic increases in HDL levels may reduce MACE but there have been no large-scale trials that have been designed to show that increasing HDL will result in lower event rates
- Therefore, LDL-C reduction remains the primary target of lipid-lowering strategies in primary and secondary prevention of CVD

Non-HDL cholesterol, apolipoprotein B, and cardiovascular risk

- All the atherogenic lipoproteins (LDL mainly, but also IDL and VLDL) are associated with apolipoprotein B
- Apolipoprotein B levels represent all cholesterol present in serum that is not bound as HDL-C and therefore it conveys the full atherogenic potential of a given lipid profile
- Non-HDL-C concentrations carry similar prognostic information to apolipoprotein, with the added advantage of being easily calculated from the standard lipid profile:

$$\text{Non-HDL cholesterol concentration} = \text{total cholesterol} - \text{HDL-C}$$

Triglycerides and cardiovascular risk

- High triglyceride levels are often found with other disorders of lipid metabolism producing either increased LDL/VLDL/IDL or decreased HDL
- The decision to treat an elevated triglyceride level should be guided by the likely aetiology
- After adjustment for lipid and non-lipid factors, elevated triglycerides do not confer additional risk for the development of CAD
- Severe elevations in triglyceride level (> 10 mmol/L) may mandate treatment to reduce the risk of pancreatitis, which is itself a condition with a high mortality (Figure 7.4.3)

7.4.3 Treatment goals

- Lipid treatment goals should be part of a comprehensive CV risk reduction strategy and should be individualized to the patient
- Depending on patient risk and preference, it is reasonable to attempt lifestyle measures for between 6 months and 1 year prior to pharmacological intervention (in the primary prevention setting) (Table 7.4.1)
- The decision to initiate therapy is based on overall global cardiovascular risk, particularly as there are no 'normal' values in lipid indices but rather a continuum of risk associated with rising values
- Specific treatment goals include:

Smoking
- No exposure

Diet
- Specific measures recommended in ESC guidance include:
    - Reduction in saturated fat intake (increase LDL-C)—should be < 10% of total calorie intake (or < 7% if raised cholesterol)

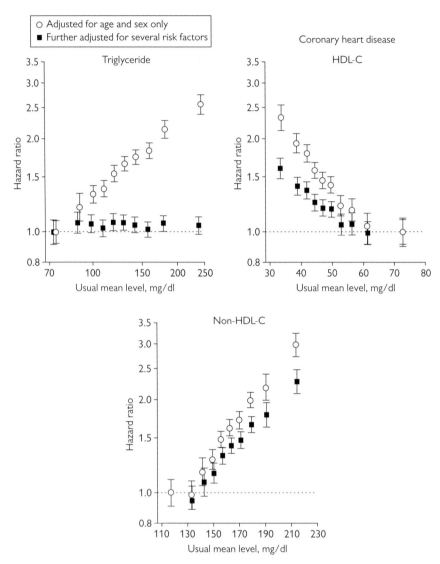

Figure 7.4.3 Hazard ratios for CHD or ischaemic stroke across quantiles of usual triglyceride, HDL-C, and non-HDL-C levels

Source data from Emerging Risk Factors Collaboration; Di Angelantonio E, Sarwar N, Perry P, Kaptoge S, Ray KK, Thompson A, Wood AM, Lewington S, Sattar N, Packard CJ, Collins R, Thompson SG, Danesh J. Major lipids, apolipoproteins, and risk of vascular disease. *JAMA*. 2009 Nov 11;302(18):1993–2000. doi: 10.1001/jama.2009.1619.

- Avoid trans fats (increase LDL-C and decrease HDL-C)
- Reduce dietary cholesterol intake (< 300 mg/day)
- Complex carbohydrate intake should account for about 45–55% of energy intake
- Increase in whole grain products, as dietary fibre (particularly of the soluble type, e.g. legumes, fruits, vegetables, etc.) has a hypocholesterolaemic effect and represents a good dietary substitute for saturated fat to maximize the effects of the diet on LDL-C levels

Table 7.4.1 Impact of specific lifestyle changes on lipid levels.

	Magnitude of the effect	Level
Lifestyle interventions to reduce TC and LDL-C levels		
Avoid dietary trans fats	++	A
Reduce dietary saturated fats	++	A
Increase dietary fibre	++	A
Use functional foods enriched with phytosterols	++	A
Use red yeast rice nutraceuticals	++	A
Reduce excessive body weight	++	A
Reduce dietary cholesterol	+	B
Increase habitual physical activity	+	B
Lifestyle interventions to reduce TG-rich lipoprotein levels		
Reduce excessive body weight	+	A
Reduce alcohol intake	+++	A
Increase habitual physical activity	++	A
Reduce total amount of dietary carbohydrates	++	A
Use supplements of n-3 polyunsaturated fats	++	A
Reduce intake of mono- and disaccharides	++	B
Replace saturated fats with mono- or polyunsaturated fats	+	B
Lifestyle interventions to increase HDL-C levels		
Avoid dietary trans fats	++	A
Increase habitual physical activity	+++	A
Reduce excessive body weight	++	A
Reduce dietary carbohydrates and replace them with unsaturated fats	++	A
Modest consumption in those who take alcohol may be continued	++	B
Quit smoking	+	B

Mach F, Baigent C, Catapano AL, et al; ESC Scientific Document Group. 2019 ESC/EAS Guidelines for the management of dyslipidaemias: lipid modification to reduce cardiovascular risk. *Eur Heart J*. 2020 Jan 1;41(1):111–188. doi: 10.1093/eurheartj/ehz455. © European Society of Cardiology. With permission from Oxford University Press.

- ▪ Added sugars should not exceed 10% of total energy consumption (though more restrictive advice concerning sugars may be useful for those needing to lose weight or with high plasma TG values, metabolic syndrome, or DM)
- ▪ Reduce alcohol intake (significant effect on TG levels)
- Dietary modification and weight loss:
  - ▪ Mild decease in LDL
  - ▪ Significant decrease in TG
  - ▪ HDL levels inversely proportional to BMI (increase in 0.01 mmol/L per 1 kg lost)
  - ▪ Low carbohydrate diet increases HDL

Physical activity
- 3.5–7 hours of moderately vigorous activity per week or 30–60 minutes most days
    - Small decrease in LDL
    - Small decrease in TG
    - Significant increase in HDL

Body weight
Discussed in section 7.2.
- Target = BMI 18.5–25 kg/m² and waist circumference < 94 cm (men) and < 80 cm (women)

LDL-C
- No level of LDL-C below which benefit ceases or harm occurs has been defined and recommended treatment targets are based on risk stratification (i.e. very high risk, high risk, etc.) in the primary prevention setting:
    - In patients (< 70) at *very high risk* an LDL-C reduction > 50% from baseline and LDL goal < 1.4 mmol/L is recommended
    - In patients (< 70) with *high risk* an LDL-C reduction of > 50% from baseline and an LDL-C goal of < 1.8 mmol/L should be considered
    - For patients in lower risk categories an LDL-C < 2.6 mmol/L should be considered
    - The highest intensity statin at the highest tolerated dose is recommended to achieve these goals—if this is not achieved then ezetimibe should be added in
    - Statin therapy for those ≥ 70 may be considered for primary prevention purposes if at high risk or above
    - In patients failing to achieve their LDL targets addition of PCSK9 inhibitors may be considered for primary prevention purposes and is recommended for secondary prevention

Triglycerides
- No specific goal, but < 1.7 mmol/L indicates lower risk

Blood pressure
- For patients aged 18–69 with:
    - Hypertension only = 120–130/< 80 mmHg
    - CAD and/or stroke/TIA and/or diabetes = 120–130/< 80 mmHg
    - CKD = 130–139/< 80 mmHg
- For patients aged ≥ 70 the target is 130–139 mmHg/< 80 mmHg regardless of comorbidity (though lower SBP is acceptable if tolerated)

Diabetes
- < 7% (< 53 mmol/mol)

N.B. Target and choice of therapy can vary in high-risk patients, and are discussed in detail in their relevant sections (e.g. diabetes and chronic kidney disease)

7.4.4 Pharmacological treatment

Statin therapy
Mechanism of action
- Statins reduce the *de novo* hepatic synthesis of cholesterol

- They act as competitive inhibitors of HMG-CoA reductase, the rate-limiting enzyme responsible for cholesterol biosynthesis, achieving:
  - Decrease in intracellular cholesterol concentration
  - Upregulation of LDL-receptor expression
  - Increased clearance from the bloodstream of VLDL and LDL
  - Also reduce apolipoprotein B and triglyceride-rich lipoprotein synthesis (modest), and enhance lipoprotein lipase activity
- Possible additional benefit through plaque stabilization, improved endothelial function, as well as reducing thrombogenicity and systemic inflammation (so-called *pleiotropic* effects)

Efficacy

- Major effect is the reduction of LDL levels—most potent agents available for routine prescription, and the degree of benefit conferred appears to be proportional to the degree of LDL lowering achieved
- There is a dose-dependent reduction, and significant inter-individual variation (with the same dose)
- By definition a high-intensity statin regime results in (on average) a reduction in LDL of > 50% vs moderate intensity, which produces a reduction of 30–50%
- Overall moderate effect in lowering triglyceride levels (~10–20% reduction). The degree of reduction in triglyceride levels is variable and proportional to the baseline level and potency of the statin
- Exert only mild effects on HDL and plasma Lp(a) levels, with an approximately 1–10% increase in HDL
- The various statins have differing comparative efficacies with regards to the reduction of LDL concentrations:
  - Where the goal is moderate LDL reduction—equivalent dosages of various statins may be utilized
  - For intensive reduction in LDL it can be seen from the dose-response curve in Figure 7.4.4 that even the maximum dose of older statins (such as pravastatin and simvastatin) will not achieve the degree of LDL-lowering achievable with newer generation potent agents (such as atorvastatin and rosuvastatin)

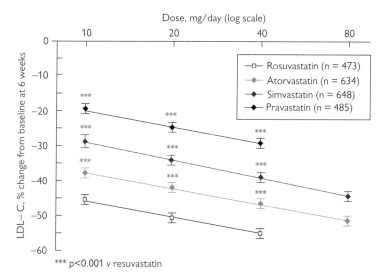

Figure 7.4.4 Comparative LDL lowering efficacy of commonly prescribed statins
Reproduced from Thompson GR. Management of dyslipidaemia. *Heart*. 2004 Aug;90(8):949–55. doi: 10.1136/hrt.2003.021287 with permission from BMJ Publishing.

- There is no convincing evidence to suggest the superiority of any specific agent in the reduction of clinical endpoints by mechanisms other than through the lowering of LDL
- Additional benefits are thought to arise from pleiotropic anti-inflammatory effects and a stabilizing effect on coronary atherosclerotic plaques (or even the promotion of plaque regression)
- Impact on reduction in CVEs well documented across multiple well known RCTs (WOSCOPS, ASCOT-LLA, JUPITER)
- Statins are not effective in a few specific groups, including heart failure or patients receiving haemodialysis
- Most statins undergo significant hepatic CYP450 cytochrome metabolism, with the exception of rosuvastatin, pravastatin, and pitavastatin

Potential side effects

- Mild elevation in transaminases (< 2–3 × upper limit of normal (ULN) is common, is dose related, and can be transient)
    - ESC described common definition of clinically relevant transaminase elevation is an increase of 3× ULN on 2 consecutive occasions
    - In the UK, NICE recommends LFT's prior to initiation and again at 3 months
    - Usually resolves with dose reduction or cessation
- Muscle pain and cramps are associated with statin therapy, though a nocebo effect is well recognized
    - In several blinded RCTs of statin vs placebo there was no, or only a slight, increased frequency of cramps in statin-allocated groups (ASCOT-LLA trial)
- Risk of myopathy is low, and risk of rhabdomyolysis is very rare
    - CK levels of < 10 × ULN without symptoms may simply be monitored +/− dose reduction (repeat in 2–6 weeks)—see Figure 7.4.5 for ESC recommendation on approach
- Associated with increased haemorrhagic CVA in observational studies, however overall benefit on other stroke subtypes greatly outweighs this small (and uncertain) hazard
- Event rate plots from TIMI 22 PROVE IT trial of intensive statin therapy after an ACS showed a significant reduction in event frequency after just 30 days of intensive therapy. This time frame is much shorter than would be expected from plaque regression alone (hence proposed pleiotropic effects)
- In the UK, NICE recommends the use of atorvastatin therapy (10 mg) as a primary prevention measure in those who are estimated to have a 10% or greater 10-year risk of developing CVD using the QRISK2 calculator (ESC guidance is outlined later)

Fibrates

- Bezafibrate and fenofibrate (most common)
- Mechanism:
    - Agonists of peroxisome proliferator-activated receptor-a (PPAR-a), acting via transcription factors regulating steps in lipid and lipoprotein metabolism
    - Increases breakdown of TG-rich particles, reduces hepatic secretion of VLDL (the most TG rich lipoprotein), increases HDL synthesis, and increases LDL removal
- Efficacy:
    - Quite variable but those with high TG and low HDL derive the most benefit
    - Have good efficacy in lowering fasting and post-prandial TG levels (~50%)
    - ~20% reduction in LDL-C and < 20% increase in HDL-C
    - Trials for primary prevention have not demonstrated reductions in CV or all-cause mortality despite reductions in coronary events and major adverse CVEs, which has been confirmed in meta-analyses
- The benefits that have been demonstrated appear to be in specific subsets of patients with features of the metabolic syndrome, such as elevated triglycerides and low HDL

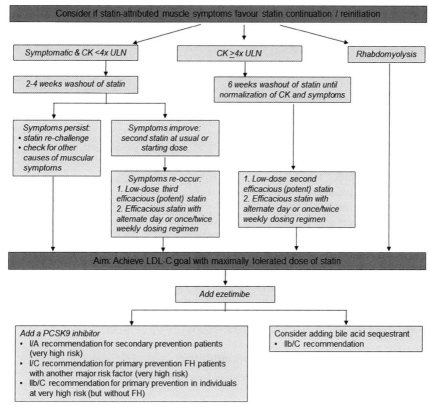

Figure 7.4.5 Suggested algorithm for management of patients with muscular symptoms secondary to statin use

Mach F, Baigent C, Catapano AL, et al; ESC Scientific Document Group. 2019 ESC/EAS Guidelines for the management of dyslipidaemias: lipid modification to reduce cardiovascular risk. *Eur Heart J*. 2020 Jan 1;41(1):111–188. doi: 10.1093/eurheartj/ehz455. © European Society of Cardiology. With permission from Oxford University Press.

- In the UK, NICE does not recommend the routine use of fibrate monotherapy as a primary or secondary prevention agent, but it may be considered in those intolerant to statins
- NICE does not recommend the use of fibrate in combination therapy with statins for primary prevention
- In moderate-to-severe hypertriglyceridemia fibrates are highly effective in lowering the risk of pancreatitis
- Side effects:
    - Generally well tolerated with mild adverse effects, typically GI disturbances, skin rashes, myopathy, liver enzyme elevations, and cholelithiasis

Bile acid sequestrants

- Examples include cholestyramine, colestipol, and colesevelam
- Mechanism:
    - Bile acids are synthesized in the liver from cholesterol and released into the intestinal lumen, but most of the bile acid is returned to the liver from the terminal ileum via active absorption
    - Bile acid sequestrants act as bile acid-binding exchange resins, are not systemically absorbed or altered by digestive enzymes, and by binding the bile acids, the drugs

prevent the reabsorption of both the drug and cholesterol into the blood, and thereby remove a large portion of the bile acids from the enterohepatic circulation
  - The liver, depleted of bile, synthesizes more from hepatic cholesterol, therefore increasing the hepatic demand for cholesterol and increasing LDLR expression, which results in a decrease of circulating LDL
- Efficacy:
  - At top daily doses, reduction in LDL-C of 18–25% has been observed
  - No major effect on HDL-C has been reported, while TGs may increase in some predisposed patients
  - There is some evidence to indicate a reduction in coronary events with the use of bile acid sequestrants
- The Lipid Research Clinics Coronary Primary Prevention trial examined cholestyramine as a primary prevention agent. There was a statistically significant reduction in the composite primary end point of coronary mortality and non-fatal coronary events of almost a fifth, but all-cause mortality was not reduced
- Side effects:
  - GI side effects predominantly
  - TG may go up in certain patients
  - Major drug interactions with several commonly prescribed drugs, and must therefore be administered either 4 hours before or 1 hour after other drugs
- Due to problems with tolerability and drug interactions they are not commonly prescribed but may have a role as adjunctive therapy and in those who are statin intolerant

Selective cholesterol absorption inhibitors

- Ezetimibe was the first member of this class of lipid-lowering agents
- Mechanism:
  - It inhibits intestinal uptake of dietary and biliary cholesterol at the level of the brush border of the intestine without affecting the absorption of fat-soluble nutrients
  - By inhibiting cholesterol absorption, ezetimibe reduces the amount of cholesterol delivered to the liver. In response to reduced cholesterol delivery, the liver reacts by upregulating LDLR expression, which in turn leads to increased clearance of LDL from the blood
- Efficacy:
  - In monotherapy trials it reduces LDL-C in hypercholesterolaemic patients by 15–22%, though relatively high inter-individual variation
  - A meta-analysis of RCTs that included over 2700 people showed an 18.5% reduction in LDL-C as compared with placebo. In addition, there was a significant 3% increase in HDL-C, a significant 8% reduction in TGs, and a 13% reduction in TC with ezetimibe as compared with placebo
  - Added to statin therapy, reduces LDL-C levels by additional 21–27% compared with placebo in patients with hypercholesterolaemia
  - In statin-naïve patients, ezetimibe and statin combination therapy has resulted in around a 15% greater reduction in LDL-C when compared with the same statins and doses in monotherapy
  - In other studies, this combination has also significantly improved reductions in LDL-C levels when compared with doubling of the statin dose (13–20%), and after switching from statin monotherapy to ezetimibe and statin combination therapy (11–15%)

- Co-administration with bile acid sequestrants and PCSK9 inhibitors has also been shown to have an additional effect
- Side effects:
  - Well tolerated, though gastrointestinal side effects include diarrhoea or cramping
- Guidance:
  - Ezetimibe should be used as second-line therapy in association with statins when the therapeutic goal is not achieved at the maximal tolerated statin dose, or in cases where a statin cannot be prescribed

Pro-protein convertase subtilisin/kexin type 9 inhibitors (PCSK9 inhibitors)

- PCSK9 inhibitors are a novel drug class
- Mechanism:
  - PCSK9 is a protein involved in the control of LDL receptor expression
  - High levels cause reduction in LDL-R expression and an associated increase in plasma LDL concentrations, and vice versa for lower concentration or function of PCSK9
  - Monoclonal antibodies (mAbs), e.g. alirocumab and evolocumab, target the PCSK9 proteins and the inhibition of this leads to enhanced clearance of circulating LDL-C
  - Statin treatment increases circulating PCSK9 serum levels, and thus the best effect of these mAbs has been demonstrated in combination with statins
- Efficacy:
  - Approximately 60% reduction in LDL (dose dependent), and estimated 25% reduction in TG (requires confirmation) and small increases in HDL and apo A
  - Also shown to reduce Lp(a) levels ~30–40%
- FOURIER trial—significant reduction in cardiovascular death, MI, stroke, hospitalization for unstable angina, or coronary revascularization using evolocumab (secondary prevention purposes)
- ODYSSEY trial—significant reduction in CHD death, MI, stroke, unstable angina using alirocumab in those who suffered an MI in the preceding 1–12 months (secondary prevention)
- No evidence for primary prevention purposes
- Can be used in combination with statin or ezetimibe therapy
- Side effects
  - Side effects include itching at injection site (administration is subcutaneous on a fortnightly or monthly basis), and possible flu-like symptoms
  - No potential for interaction with orally absorbed drugs

Omega-3 (n-3) fatty acids

- Examples include eicosapentaenoic acid (EPA)
- They affect serum lipids and lipoproteins, in particular VLDL concentrations
- The underlying mechanism is poorly understood, although it may be related, at least in part, to their ability to interact with PPARs and to decreased secretion of apo B
- Reduces TGs, but effects on other lipoproteins are trivial, and more detailed data on clinical outcomes are needed to justify wide use
- No evidence of benefit in primary prevention, with a Cochrane meta-analysis reporting no overall effect on total mortality (RR 0.98), or CV events (RR 0.99), and only a suggestion of reduced CHD events

Cholesterol synthesis inhibitiors
- Bempedoic acid is a first-in-class cholesterol synthesis inhibitor
- Mechanism:
    - Inhibits adenosine triphosphate-citrate lyase (ACL) and consequently cholesterol biosynthesis, leading to increased expression of LDL receptors and increasing LDL clearence
- Efficacy:
    - Reduces LDL-C levels by ~30% (monotherapy) and ~50% when combined with ezetimibe
- Key outcome studies have been published since the last ESC guidance so no current role, but should be considered for patients who are statin intolerant in whom it has been shown to lower risk of MACE

N.B. Other specific drugs are available for familial hypercholesterolaemia patients, but are typically prescribed by lipid specialists and will not be covered in this text

Pharmacological strategy

The following is considered a reasonable approach to primary prevention outlined in ESC guidance:

- Evaluate the total CV risk of the individual and establish if pharmacotherapy is indicated
- Determine treatment targets relative to individual risk
- Involve the patient in decision-making
- Choose a statin regimen +/− additional treatments as needed, to meet the treatment targets
- Response to statin treatment is variable, therefore dose up-titration is sensible prior to additional LDL-lowering treatments

LDL-C

- Intervention strategies (as suggested in Figure 7.4.6) should be planned as a function of both total CV risk and LDL-C level, with a graded approach addressing the graded reduction in CVD risk achieved in response to reductions in TC and LDL-C levels
- Where pharmacotherapy is indicated, statin monotherapy is recommended at the highest intensity required to achieve the goal set based on the specific level of risk for LDL-C *(Class IA)*
- The absolute LDL-C reduction achieved (relative to the pre-treatment LDL-C) dictates the relative risk reduction, which in turn defines the associated absolute CV risk reduction in individual patients
- Due to inter-individual variation in response to therapy, side effects and compliance, patients should have follow-up to track response to therapy
- A significant proportion of patients at high-risk or with very high LDL-C levels will need additional treatment:
    - If the goal is not achieved then ezetimibe should be added *(Class IB)*
    - For primary prevention purposes, if the goal is not reached in *very high-risk* individuals (excluding FH patients) with a statin and ezetimibe combination then a PCSK9 inhibitor may be considered *(Class IIbC)*
    - For *very high-risk* FH patients (i.e. with confirmed CVD or another major risk factor) who do not achieve their goal on a maximum tolerated dose of a statin and ezetimibe, a combination with a PCSK9 inhibitor is recommended *(Class IC)*
    - In all individuals, if the goal is not achieved, statin combination with a bile acid sequestrant may be considered *(Class IIbC)*
- Strategies for intolerance to statin therapy:

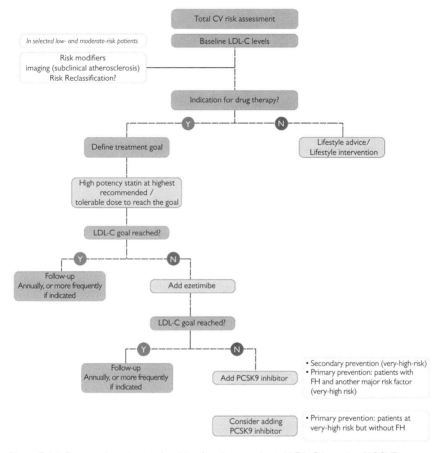

Figure 7.4.6 Proposed treatment algorithm for pharmacological LDL-C lowering (ASCVD = atherosclerotic cardiovascular disease)

Mach F, Baigent C, Catapano AL, et al; ESC Scientific Document Group. 2019 ESC/EAS Guidelines for the management of dyslipidaemias: lipid modification to reduce cardiovascular risk. Eur Heart J. 2020 Jan 1;41(1):111–188. doi: 10.1093/eurheartj/ehz455. © European Society of Cardiology. With permission from Oxford University Press.

- Studies demonstrated considerable LDL-C-lowering effect of alternative dosing, such as every other day or twice a week and this strategy should be considered in *high-risk* patients in whom statin treatment with daily doses is not possible
- If a statin-based regimen not tolerated at any dosage (even after re-challenge), ezetimibe should be considered *(Class IIaC)*
- If a statin-based regimen is not tolerated at any dosage (even after re-challenge), a PCSK9 inhibitor added to ezetimibe may also be considered *(Class IIbC)*
- See Figure 7.4.6 for a proposed summary of treatment strategy for LDL-C

(N.B. Specific guidance regarding PCSK9 indication will vary nationally in light of associated costs)

Triglycerides:

- For *high-risk* individuals with hypertriglyceridaemia (TG > 2.3 mmol/L) statin therapy is recommended first-line *(Class IB)*
- In *high-risk* (or above) patients with TG levels 1.5–5.6 mmol/L despite statin therapy, omega-3 PUFAs (e.g. icosapent ethyl) should be considered in combination with a statin *(Class IIaB)*

- In primary prevention patients who are at LDL-C goal with TG levels > 2.3 mmol/L, co-treatment with a fibrate may be considered in combination with statins *(Class IIbB)*
- In *high-risk* patients who are at LDL-C goal with TG levels > 2.3 mmol/L, co-treatment with a fibrate may be considered in combination with statins *(Class IIbC)*

7.4.5 Classifying dyslipidaemias

- Traditionally the Frederickson classification system has been used to sub-classify lipid profile abnormalities (see Table 7.4.2)
- This has largely been replaced by a simpler focus on primary/secondary and isolated/combined dyslipidaemia
    - Primary refers to a genetic origin and secondary refers to acquisition through environmental factors/other disease processes, e.g. hypothyroidism, though this is an oversimplification as those with a genetic predisposition towards dyslipidaemia may only manifest it in the presence of secondary causes
    - Isolated dyslipidaemias affect one component of plasma lipids and combined affects multiple components
- Laboratory assessments generally do not measure lipoproteins but do estimate them by measuring their cholesterol content

Table 7.4.2 Fredrickson classification system of lipid profile abnormalities.

Type	Lipoprotein abnormality	Biochemical feature	Prevalence	Association with premature CAD	Comments
I	Familial chylomicronaemia	Elevated TG	Rare	No	Lipoprotein lipase deficiency, autosomal recessive, often leads to pancreatitis
IIa	Hypercholesterolaemia	Elevated LDL	Common	Yes	Absence/deficiency of LDL receptor. Autosomal dominant
IIb	Combined Hypercholesterolaemia	Elevated TG/cholesterol	Common	Strong	
III	Dysbetalipoproteinaemia	Elevated TG/cholesterol	Uncommon	Strong	
IV	Hypertriglyceridaemia	Elevated TG +/− cholesterol	Common	Weak	Often reduced HDL
V	Mixed Hypertriglyceridaemia	Elevated TG and cholesterol (mild)	Rare	Weak	

- The difference is small between fasting and non-fasting samples for most lipid parameters and unlikely to be of clinical significance
- A standard profile measures total cholesterol (TC) and HDL-C. LDL-C is estimated using Friedewald formula:

  LDL-C = TC − HDL-C − (TG/2.2) in mmol/L

  or

  LDL-C = TC − HDL-C − (TG/5) in mg/dL
- Apo-B analysis, if available, is recommended for risk assessment particularly, for patients with high TG, diabetes, obesity, or very low levels of LDL
- Lp(a) measurement should be considered at least once in each person's lifetime to identify those with very high Lp(a) levels who may have a risk profile similar to those with heterozygous familial hypercholesterolaemia (FH)

Primary disorders of LDL

- Elevated LDL cholesterol may results from one or both of:
  - Increased lipoprotein synthesis
  - Decreased clearance due to:
    - Abnormal lipoprotein
    - Abnormal lipoprotein receptors

Familial hypercholesterolaemia

- The most common of the autosomal dominant hypercholesterolaemias, with a significant risk of premature CAD
- Heterozygous FH occurs in 1 in 500 individuals of European descent and is the most common monogenic cause of CAD
- Mutation in the LDL-receptor gene (LDLR 19p 13.3) is most common—encodes for LDL receptor which removes LDL from the circulation
- Phenotype is determined by how active the receptor is (depends on how many defective copies of the LDLR gene are inherited), i.e. homozygotes have more severe disease
- Excess LDL is deposited around the body, resulting in:
  - Skin—xanthalesma
  - Tendons—xanthoma
  - Aortic valve—calcification
  - Eyes—arcus cornealis
  - Arteries—atheroma
- Overall cardiovascular risk can be stratified using the Montreal-FH Score, which incorporates simple clinical risk factors alongside lipid results
- In men the risk of coronary disease is > 50% by the age of 50 if untreated and 30% in women by the age of 60
- Diagnosis is often made using Simon Broome criteria (see Table 7.4.3)
- Should ideally be confirmed by genetic testing, and once an index case is confirmed, cascade screening is recommended (see Chapter 10.1 for further details on genetic screening)
- Other diagnostic criteria are the Dutch Lipid Clinic Network and the WHO criteria
- Children at risk of FH should be assessed by the age of 10 years
- It is recommended that FH patients with confirmed CVD or who have another major risk factor are treated as *very high risk*, and that those with no prior atherosclerotic CVD or other risk factors are treated as *high risk*

Table 7.4.3 Simon Broome Register diagnostic criteria for familial hypercholesterolaemia (recognized causative genes include defective LDL receptor, apo B, or PCSK9 mutation).

Definite familial hypercholesterolaemia

< 16 years Total cholesterol > 6.7 mmol/L or LDL > 4.0 mmol/L **Adult** Total cholesterol > 7.5 mmol/L or LDL > 4.9 mmol/L	plus	Tendon xanthomas in patient or first- or second-degree relative or Mutation in a recognized causative gene

Possible familial hypercholesterolaemia

< 16 years Total cholesterol > 6.7 mmol/L or LDL > 4.0 mmol/L **Adult** Total cholesterol > 7.5 mmol/L or LDL > 4.9 mmol/L	plus	Myocardial infarct at < 50 in second-degree relative or < 60 in first-degree relative or Total cholesterol in first- or second-degree relative as in lipid criteria

Reproduced from 'Risk of fatal coronary heart disease in familial hypercholesterolaemia', Scientific Steering Committee on behalf of the Simon Broome Register Group, *BMJ* 303 (6807), 893–6

- There is no recommended safe level of LDL but a reduction by > 50% is recommended and an LDL of < 1.8 mmol/L or < 1.4 mmol/L if at *very high risk*
- Pharmacological treatment is with statins as first-line therapy
  - High-intensity statins recommended (i.e. those that produce a 40% reduction in LDL—atorvastatin > 20 mg/day or rosuvastatin > 10 mg/day)
- Ezetimibe is recommended if statin therapy is contraindicated/not tolerated or as an additional medication if there is a failure to reduce LDL > 50% despite optimally tolerated doses of statin
- Treatment with a PCSK9 inhibitor is recommended in *very high-risk* FH patients if the treatment goal is not achieved on maximal tolerated statin plus ezetimibe
- Intolerance to both may require the use of a bile acid sequestrant or a fibrate
- For difficult to control homozygous FH (and for some rare heterozygous individuals) LDL apheresis may be an option

Familial combined hyperlipidaemia (FCH)

- Common—estimated prevalence of 1–2% and 10–20% of survivors of an MI
- Lipid profile:
  - Elevated TG and apo B present in more than one family member and evidence of premature CAD
  - LDL may be normal or elevated, and an LDL:apo B ratio of < 1.2 is suggestive of the condition
  - HDL may be low
  - In cases where the predominant abnormality is hypertriglyceridemia it can be difficult to distinguish from FH. Elevated apolipoprotein B levels (a marker of the total number of atherogenic particles including LDL, VLDL, and IDL) supports a diagnosis of FCH
- Treatment is based on which lipid rises—LDL targeted with statins and TG with fibrates

Polygenic hypercholesterolaemia
- Moderate hypercholesterolaemia in family members with the exclusion of FH
- No xanthomata are seen
- Primarily a diagnosis of exclusion
- TG levels remain relatively normal
- Treatment is with statin therapy

Primary disorders of HDL
- There is an inverse relationship between HDL and the risk of CVD. Despite this, trials that produced an elevation in HDL whilst the other lipid constituents were kept constant failed to show a reduction in CV events
- Low HDL levels are frequently found in CAD patients, particularly in those who develop the disease prematurely
- Low HDL levels may be caused by impaired apo A1 synthesis or increased breakdown of HDL. Disorders causing isolated low HDL levels are rare

Familial primary hypoalphalipoproteinemia
- Autosomal dominant condition
- Decreased apo A1 production
- Associated with premature CAD
- Low HDL, relatively normal VLDL and LDL with no secondary causes identified and a similar lipid profile in a first-degree relative

Secondary disorders of HDL
- Secondary causes of low HDL are more common and include:
    - Metabolic syndrome
    - Smoking
    - Elevated TG
    - Elevated carbohydrate intake
    - Medications (e.g. progestins, anabolic steroids)
    - Hypothyroidism

Disorders of triglyceride metabolism
- TG are mainly carried by VLDL and chylomicrons therefore there is a rise in these lipoproteins, typically as a result of increased synthesis (most commonly) and/or decreased catabolism
- Severe elevations in TG levels are most frequently due to heritable genetic disorder acting in concert with secondary causes
- Risk of pancreatitis is clinically significant if TGs are > 10 mmol/L, and actions to prevent acute pancreatitis are mandatory:
    - Restriction of calories and fat content (10–15% recommended)
    - Alcohol abstinence
    - Fibrate therapy +/− omega-3 fatty acids as adjunct therapy
- Common causes of hypertriglyceridaemia are outlined in Table 7.4.4
- The two main reasons to treat elevated triglyceride levels are:
    - Prevention of CAD
    - Prevention of pancreatitis

Table 7.4.4 Causes of hypertriglyceridaemia.

Common primary disorders of triglyceride metabolism that are associated with premature CAD	Common causes of elevated triglycerides encountered in clinical practice	Other common causes of elevated triglycerides
Familial combined hyperlipidaemia Residual dyslipidaemia in well controlled type II DM Familial hypoalphalipoproteinaemia	Increased caloric intake Obesity Diabetes Alcohol	Metabolic syndrome/obesity Uncontrolled or untreated DM Medications and alcohol Hypothyroidism ESRF Nephrotic syndrome HIV
These are mixed dyslipidaemias that each affect 1–5% of the population and together are thought to be responsible for half of all premature CAD.	*Most of the patients will also have an abnormality of another component of the lipid profile*	

- Dietary modification and reduction/cessation of alcohol can have a profound impact on TG levels

Secondary causes of dyslipidaemias

- Reversible secondary causes should always be sought and treated before any lipid lowering medication (Table 7.4.5)
- Approximately 90% of patients with hypothyroidism will have an abnormality of TG or LDL levels
  - Hypothyroid patients are more likely to suffer from statin induced myopathy
  - In general, appropriate thyroxine replacement corrects the dyslipidaemia
- Overall insulin resistance (associated with metabolic syndrome) produces a lipid phenotype that is particularly atherogenic
- As discussed previously, insulin resistance changes all aspects of a patients lipid profile
  - Elevated TG
  - Elevated VLDL
  - Elevated LDL
  - Decreased HDL

Table 7.4.5 Secondary causes of dyslipidaemia.

Endocrine	Hepatic	Renal	Miscellaneous
Type 2 diabetes Hypothyroidism Cushing's syndrome Obesity	Cholestatic liver disease Primary biliary cirrhosis	Nephrotic syndrome Chronic renal failure	Cigarette smoking SLE Medications

Further reading

Cardiovascular disease: risk assessment and reduction, including lipid modification. London: National Institute for Health and Care Excellence (NICE); 2023 May 24. PMID: 32200592.

Cholesterol Treatment Trialists' (CTT) Collaboration, Baigent C, Blackwell L, Emberson J, Holland LE, Reith C, Bhala N, Peto R, Barnes EH, Keech A, Simes J, Collins R. Efficacy and safety of more intensive lowering of LDL cholesterol: a meta-analysis of data from 170,000 participants in 26 randomised trials. *Lancet.* 2010 Nov 13;376(9753):1670–81. doi: 10.1016/S0140-6736(10)61350-5. Epub 2010 Nov 8. PMID: 21067804; PMCID: PMC2988224

Mach F, Baigent C, Catapano AL, Koskinas KC, Casula M, Badimon L, Chapman MJ, De Backer GG, Delgado V, Ference BA, Graham IM, Halliday A, Landmesser U, Mihaylova B, Pedersen TR, Riccardi G, Richter DJ, Sabatine MS, Taskinen MR, Tokgozoglu L, Wiklund O; ESC Scientific Document Group. 2019 ESC/EAS Guidelines for the management of dyslipidaemias: lipid modification to reduce cardiovascular risk. *Eur Heart J.* 2020 Jan 1;41(1):111–88. doi: 10.1093/eurheartj/ehz455. PMID: 31504418

Visseren FLJ, Mach F, Smulders YM, Carballo D, Koskinas KC, Bäck M, Benetos A, Biffi A, Boavida JM, Capodanno D, Cosyns B, Crawford C, Davos CH, Desormais I, Di Angelantonio E, Franco OH, Halvorsen S, Hobbs FDR, Hollander M, Jankowska EA, Michal M, Sacco S, Sattar N, Tokgozoglu L, Tonstad S, Tsioufis KP, van Dis I, van Gelder IC, Wanner C, Williams B; ESC Scientific Document Group; ESC National Cardiac Societies. 2021 ESC Guidelines on cardiovascular disease prevention in clinical practice. *Eur Heart J.* 2021 Sep 7;42(34):3227–337. doi: 10.1093/eurheartj/ehab484. PMID: 34458905

7.5

Diabetes

Mimi Z. Chen and Konstantinos Gkastaris

TABLE OF CONTENTS

7.5.1 Definition 665
7.5.2 Classification, pathophysiology, and diagnosis 665
  Type 1 diabetes (T1DM) 666
  Type 2 diabetes (T2DM) 667
  Gestational diabetes (GDM) 667
  Other specific types of diabetes 667
7.5.3 Epidemiology 668
7.5.4 Complications 668
  Microvascular complications 668
  Macrovascular complications 670
7.5.5 Prevention and management of cardiovascular disease in diabetes 671
  Specific aspects of management 672

7.5.1 Definition

- Diabetes mellitus (DM) describes a spectrum of diseases of abnormal carbohydrate metabolism that are characterized by hyperglycaemia
- It is associated with a relative or absolute impairment in insulin secretion, along with varying degrees of peripheral resistance to the action of insulin
- The chronic hyperglycaemia of DM is associated with long-term damage, dysfunction and failure of various organs, especially the eyes, kidneys, nerves, heart, and blood vessels

7.5.2 Classification, pathophysiology, and diagnosis

- The classification and diagnosis of DM are defined by guidelines from the World Health Organization (WHO) and American Diabetes Association (ADA)
- Glycated haemoglobin A1c (HbA1c) has been recommended as a diagnostic test for DM, but there are concerns over its sensitivity in accurately predicting DM
  - An HbA1C value of < 48 mmol/mol does not always exclude DM therefore fasting plasma glucose (FPG) levels and/or a 2-hour 75 g standard oral glucose tolerance test (OGTT) are sometimes used to confirm the diagnosis in unclear cases (Table 7.5.1)
- DM is diagnosed if any one of the following criteria is met:
  - HbA1c > 48 mmol/mol
  - FPG ≥ 7 mmol/L (2 tests usually recommended in the absence of symptoms)
  - Random elevated glucose value ≥ 11.1 mmol/L with symptoms
  - Positive OGTT
- OGTT remains the gold-standard test for the diagnosis of DM, however HbA1c is now used widely for population screening and monitoring due to its low cost and convenience

Table 7.5.1 Criteria for the diagnosis of diabetes mellitus.

Glycaemic marker	WHO criteria (2011, 2019)[5,6]	ADA criteria (2021)[7]
	Diabetes	
FPG	≥ 7.0 mmol/L (≥ 126 mg/dL)	
2hPG (OGTT)	≥ 11.1 mmol/L (≥ 200 mg/dL)	
HbA1c	≥ 6.5% (≥ 48 mmol/mol)	
RPG	≥ 11.1 mmol/L (≥ 200 mg/dL)	
	Pre-diabetes	
FPG	6.1–6.9 mmol/L (110–125 mg/dL)	5.6–6.9 mmol/L (100–125 mg/dL)
2hPG (OGTT)	7.8–11.0 mmol/L (140–199 mg/dL)	
HbA1c	6.0–6.4% (42–47 mmol/mol)	5.7–6.4% (39–47 mmol/mol)

ADA—American Diabetes Association, 2hPG—2 h plasma glucose, FPG—fasting plasma glucose, HbA1c—glycated haemoglobin, RPG—random plasma glucose, OGTT—oral glucose tolerance test, WHO—World Health Organization. Marx N, Federici M, Schütt K, et al; ESC Scientific Document Group. 2023 ESC Guidelines for the management of cardiovascular disease in patients with diabetes. *Eur Heart J.* 2023 Oct 14;44(39):4043–4140. doi: 10.1093/eurheartj/ehad192. © European Society of Cardiology. With permission from Oxford University Press.

- Patients with impaired fasting glucose (IFG) and/or impaired glucose tolerance (IGT) have an increased risk for DM:
    - IFG is characterized by fasting venous plasma glucose levels of 6.1–7.0 mmol/L
    - IGT can only be diagnosed following an OGTT: 2-hour post-load plasma glucose ≥ 7.8 and < 11.1 mmol/L
- N.B. In June 2011, unit of HbA1c reporting changed from a percentage to a measurement in mmol/mol in the UK; the former is known as the DCCT (Diabetes Control and Complications Trial) units, whereas the latter is known as the IFCC (International Federation of Clinical Chemistry) units, and this has been adopted by UK to allow easier comparisons to European reporting
- Four main aetiological types of DM have been identified

Type 1 diabetes (T1DM)

- Characterized by deficiency of insulin due to destruction of pancreatic beta-cells, progressing to absolute insulin deficiency
- It is a non-reversible, auto-immune process and requires lifelong treatment with insulin
- Typically occurs in younger individuals (peak diagnosis in the UK is between 9 and 14 years of age) presenting with polyuria, polydipsia, and weight loss with a tendency to ketosis. However T1DM can occur at any age, occasionally with slow progression where insulin dependence develops over years (e.g. Latent Auto-immune Diabetes in Adults: LADA)
- It affects all races, but its prevalence is higher in Northern European populations. In the UK, approximately 400,000 adults and children have Type 1 diabetes (prevalence 0.41%) representing approximately 10% of the total population of people who have diabetes
- Auto-antibodies targeting pancreatic beta-cells, such as glutamic acid decarboxylase (GAD), insulin, or zinc-transported protein can be useful in differentiating those of autoimmune in origin such as in T1DM and other types of diabetes in cases where the clinical diagnosis is difficult to reach

Type 2 diabetes (T2DM)

- Is characterized by a combination of insulin resistance (IR) and various degrees of beta-cell failure in association with obesity and sedentary lifestyle, often as part of the metabolic syndrome
- Insulin secretion is biphasic:
    - First-phase insulin is released from granules of a 'readily releasable pool' triggered by increased blood glucose levels, and lasts about 10 minutes
    - The second phase is a sustained, slow release of insulin from the 'reserve pool', which requires mobilization before release triggered independently of glucose, progressing to a steady state at 2–3 hours
    - Reduced first-phase insulin release may be the earliest detectable beta-cell defect predicting onset of Type 2 diabetes and its main clinical manifestation is post-prandial hyperglycaemia
    - This is followed by persistent hyperglycaemia in the fasting stage as the disease progresses due to a deteriorating second-phase insulin response
- Historically, T2DM affected adults over the age of 40. However, with increasing obesity in the young and non-Caucasian populations, there is a steady trend towards an onset at much younger age
- Approximately 60 million people have diabetes within the European Region, or ~10.3% of men and ~9.6% of women aged ≥ 25 years
- In the UK, approximately 3.6–3.8 million people have T2DM (diagnosed or undiagnosed) which represents 6% of the UK population or 1 in every 16, and T2DM accounts for 90% of all diabetes
- Obesity is the most potent risk factor for T2DM. It accounts for 80–85% of the overall risk of developing T2DM and underlies the current global spread of the condition

Gestational diabetes (GDM)

- Develops during pregnancy and key risk factors are:
    - BMI > 30 kg/m^2
    - Previous macrosomic baby weighing ≥ 4.5 kg
    - Previous gestational diabetes
    - Family history of diabetes (first-degree relative with diabetes)
    - Minority ethnic family origin with a high prevalence of diabetes
- The diagnosis is made following a standard OGTT if the woman has either a fasting plasma glucose level of ≥ 5.6 mmol/L, or a 2-hour plasma glucose level of ≥ 7.8 mmol/L
- This is usually performed at 24–28 weeks of gestation or as soon as possible at booking if previous GDM with confirmation at 24-28 weeks if first OGTT normal
- Post-partum, most individuals return to a euglycaemic state, but they are at significantly increased risk for overt T2DM and subsequent gestational diabetes
- Normal fasting glucose or HbA1c by 13 weeks post partum excludes frank DM

Other specific types of diabetes

- Mature-onset diabetes of the young (MODY), a form of monogenic diabetes, characterized by single genetic mutations
- Secondary diabetes: DM due to other pathological conditions or diseases either of the pancreas (pancreatitis, pancreatic malignancy, trauma or surgery to the pancreas) or other endocrine systems (acromegaly, Cushing's etc.)
- Medication-induced DM (glucocorticoids, beta blockers, thiazides, etc.)

7.5.3 Epidemiology

- The International Diabetes Federation's global estimates for 2011 and 2030 suggest a clear increase in the number of people having DM or IGT (see Figure 7.5.1)
- A total of 281 million men and 317 million women worldwide died with DM in 2011, most from cardiovascular disease
- The healthcare expenditure for DM in Europe and in the UK was about 75 billion Euros and 23 billion pounds (direct and indirect cost) respectively in 2011 and is projected to increase to 90 billion Euros and 39 billion pounds respectively by 2030
- Screening is recommended in all individuals with CVD with fasting glucose and/or HbA1c (*Class IA recommendation*)

7.5.4 Complications

- Diabetes is associated with increased microvascular and macrovascular complications
- The clustering of vascular risks seen in association with insulin resistance (IR), described by some as metabolic syndrome, has led to the conclusion that there is early development of CV complications prior to the diagnosis of T2DM
- The strong relationship between hyperglycaemia and microvascular disease indicates that this risk may not be apparent until frank hyperglycaemia appears; this is a reflection of the progressive nature of DM (Figure 7.5.2)

Microvascular complications

- The microvascular triad of retinopathy, nephropathy, and neuropathy is unique to DM
- Landmark clinical trials such as the UK Prospective Diabetes Study (UKPDS) and Diabetes Control of Complications Trial (DCCT) have established a clear relationship between microvascular disease and glucose control
- The development of disease is a combination of direct glucose-mediated endothelial damage, oxidative stress, and altered blood flow and changes in endothelial permeability, extravascular protein deposition, and coagulation resulting in organ dysfunction

Diabetic retinopathy

- One of the commonest causes of visual loss in working-age adults in the UK and the developed world
- It occurs following hyperglycaemia-mediated damage within the retinal microvasculature, resulting in ischaemia, neovascularization, retinal bleeds, and macular oedema

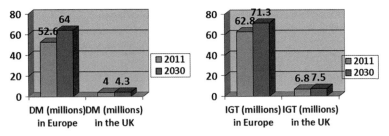

Figure 7.5.1 The International Diabetes Federation's global estimates for people having DM or IGT in 2011 vs 2030

Source data from Whiting et al. IDF diabetes atlas: global estimates of the prevalence of diabetes for 2011 and 2030. *Diabetes Res Clin Pract*. 2011 Dec;94(3):311–21. doi: 10.1016/j.diabres.2011.10.029

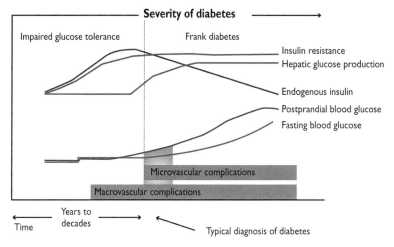

Figure 7.5.2 Glycaemic continuum, complications and cardiovascular disease
Rydén L, Grant PJ, Anker SD, et al. ESC Guidelines on diabetes, pre-diabetes, and cardiovascular diseases developed in collaboration with the EASD: the Task Force on diabetes, pre-diabetes, and cardiovascular diseases of the European Society of Cardiology (ESC) and developed in collaboration with the European Association for the Study of Diabetes (EASD). *Eur Heart J.* 2013 Oct;34(39):3035–87. doi: 10.1093/eurheartj/eht108. © European Society of Cardiology. With permission from Oxford University Press.

- DM duration, glycaemic control, blood pressure and lipid management, and smoking are the strongest risk factors for its development and progression
- Good glycaemic control delays the presentation and slows down the progression of diabetic retinopathy
- In the UK, screening for diabetic retinopathy is part of the standard of care for people with diabetes
- There are different stages of the disease: background (non-proliferative) retinopathy, maculopathy, and proliferative retinopathy
- The existing treatments are successful in slowing or stopping further vision loss, however they do not cure diabetic retinopathy. They include, depending on the stage of the disease, laser photocoagulation, pan-retinal photocoagulation, intravitreal anti-VEGF drugs, intravitreal steroids, or vitrectomy

Diabetic nephropathy

- Arises from the combination of hyperglycaemia and hypertension leading to glomerular damage
- The underlying pathological changes involve thickening of basement membrane, atrophy, interstitial fibrosis, and arteriosclerosis
- Increased glomerular filtration pressures result in albuminuria, a driver for ongoing renal damage
- Risk of CVD increases progressively with reducing eGFR. The presence of microalbuminuria reflects general atherosclerotic process and represents an independent risk factor for stroke, MI, and CCF; the identification of microalbuminuria should prompt clinicians to manage all CV risk factors aggressively
- Treatment to delay diabetic nephropathy progression involves good control of metabolic and haemodynamic abnormalities; in practical terms, this means blood glucose lowering and control of hypertension
- Patients receiving intensive glucose treatment are less likely to develop renal failure or to progress to end-stage renal disease

- ACE inhibitors and angiotensin receptor blockers are preferred based on studies that have demonstrated reductions in proteinuria or preservation of glomerular filtration rate (GFR), or both

Increasing evidence-base recommends the following treatments in patients with diabetes and CKD to reduce the risk of CV and/or kidney failure risk:
  - ACEi or ARB (maximum tolerated dose)
  - SGLT2 inhibitor (if eGFR ≥ 20 ml/min/1.73 m^2)
  - Finerenone (in addition to ACEi/ARB)

Diabetic neuropathy

- Refers to a spectrum of neurological disorders associated with diabetes mellitus
- The most common form is a distal, symmetrical sensorimotor neuropathy, which may be asymptomatic in up to 50%
- The spectrum can include a wide range of clinical syndromes including cranial nerve palsies, mononeuropathies, and autonomic dysfunction
- The main sequel of neuropathy includes neuropathic pain, which is extremely common and difficult to treat, paraesthesia, ulceration, foot deformity, and Charcot's arthropathy
- The combination of neuropathy, arteriopathy, and infection, in addition to delayed diagnosis and treatment, are the driving factors behind most diabetic foot amputations

In summary, the management of the microvascular diseases in diabetes consists of good glycaemic control, effective blood pressure, lipid and proteinuria management, and regular monitoring and multidisciplinary input from Diabetologists, Ophthalmologists, Nephrologists, and Podiatrists, Vascular and Orthopaedic Surgeons

Macrovascular complications

Macrovascular complications and DM as a CV risk factor

- Epidemiologic analyses suggest a correlation between chronic hyperglycaemia and higher rates of cardiovascular disease (CVD)
- In the Framingham Heart Study, the presence of DM doubled the age-adjusted risk for CVD in men and tripled it in women, with similar observations noted in subsequent trials and meta-analyses
- Most studies have found that DM is associated with an increased risk of MI and the extent of the disease in the coronary arteries is greater among DM patients
- Additionally, more than half the mortality and a vast amount of morbidity in people with DM is related to CVD
- Hyperglycaemia, insulin resistance, and CVD are closely linked through various pathophysiological mechanisms (Figure 7.5.3):
  - About 80–90% of patients with T2DM are either overweight or obese, and the release of free fatty acids (FFAs) and cytokines from adipose tissue impairs insulin sensitivity resulting in hyperinsulinaemia and hyperglycaemia
  - FFA-induced impairment of the PI3K pathway results in decreased production of nitric oxide (NO), endothelial dysfunction, vascular inflammation, and vascular remodelling, which are important predictors of CVD development
  - Macrophage dysfunction also plays a key role in metabolic inflammation and insulin resistance
  - Atherogenic dyslipidaemia in DM is an independent predictor of CV risk due to a lipid profile characterized by high triglycerides (TGs), low high-density lipoprotein cholesterol (HDL-C), increased remnant lipoproteins, apolipoprotein B (apo B) synthesis and small, dense LDL particles
  - In T2DM patients, IR and hyperglycaemia participate in the pathogenesis of a pro-thrombotic state characterized by increased plasminogen activator inhibitor-1 (PAI-1), factor VII and XII, fibrinogen and reduced tissue plasminogen activator (tPA) levels

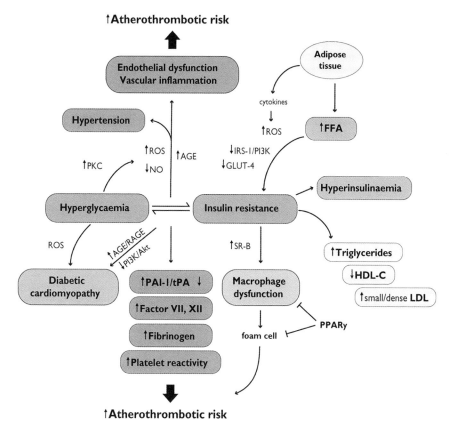

Figure 7.5.3 The links between hyperglycaemia, insulin resistance and cardiovascular disease through various pathophysiological mechanisms

Rydén L, Grant PJ, Anker SD, et al. ESC Guidelines on diabetes, pre-diabetes, and cardiovascular diseases developed in collaboration with the EASD: the Task Force on diabetes, pre-diabetes, and cardiovascular diseases of the European Society of Cardiology (ESC) and developed in collaboration with the European Association for the Study of Diabetes (EASD). *Eur Heart J.* 2013 Oct;34(39):3035–87. doi: 10.1093/eurheartj/eht108. © European Society of Cardiology. With permission from Oxford University Press.

Diabetic cardiomyopathy

- A clinical condition diagnosed when ventricular dysfunction occurs in the absence of coronary atherosclerosis and hypertension
- In patients with DM, insulin resistance impairs myocardial contractility via reduced Ca^{2+} influx through L-type Ca^{2+} channels and reverse mode Na^+/Ca^{2+} exchange
- Impairment of phosphatidylinositol 3-kinases (PI3K)/Akt pathway is critically involved in cardiac dysfunction in T2DM
- Additionally, hyperglycaemia directly contributes to cardiac and structural abnormalities leading to myocardial hypertrophy and fibrinolysis with ventricular stiffness and chamber dysfunction

7.5.5 Prevention and management of cardiovascular disease in diabetes

- Diabetes optimization, i.e. normalizing blood glucose readings, reduces CV risks, prevents micro- and macro-vascular complications and slows progression of these complications

- The fundamental approach is the assessment for and reduction of risk factors, including better glycaemic control, lifestyle modification including weight control, increased physical activity, smoking cessation, aggressive BP control, optimizing lipid profile, and secondary prevention in those with established atherosclerotic CVD

Specific aspects of management
Assess CVD risk in all patients with DM
- Screen all patients with T2DM for presence of severe target organ damage, defined as:
    - eGFR < 45 ml/min/1.73 m^2, irrespective of albuminuria;
    - OR eGFR 45–59 ml/min/1.73 m^2 and microalbuminuria (UACR 30–300 mg/g; stage A2);
    - OR proteinuria (UACR > 300 mg/g; stage A3);
    - OR presence of microvascular disease in ≥ 3 sites (e.g. microalbuminuria, retinopathy, neuropathy).
- Estimate 10-year CVD risk via SCORE2-Diabetes algorithm for patients with T2DM without symptomatic atherosclerotic CVD (ASCVD) or severe TOD
- CV risk should be graded as outlined in Figure 7.5.4, which dictates subsequent risk factor targets for blood pressure and lipid control

Glycaemic control
- DCCT and UKPDS showed that in T1DM and T2DM:
    a) Tight glycaemic control is important for reducing long-term macrovascular complications
    b) A very long follow-up period is required to demonstrate an effect
    c) Early glucose control is important (metabolic memory)

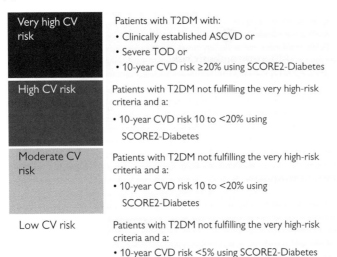

Very high CV risk	Patients with T2DM with: • Clinically established ASCVD or • Severe TOD or • 10-year CVD risk ≥20% using SCORE2-Diabetes
High CV risk	Patients with T2DM not fulfilling the very high-risk criteria and a: • 10-year CVD risk 10 to <20% using SCORE2-Diabetes
Moderate CV risk	Patients with T2DM not fulfilling the very high-risk criteria and a: • 10-year CVD risk 10 to <20% using SCORE2-Diabetes
Low CV risk	Patients with T2DM not fulfilling the very high-risk criteria and a: • 10-year CVD risk <5% using SCORE2-Diabetes

ASCVD, atherosclerotic cardiovascular disease; CV, cardiovascular; CVD, cardiovascular disease; eGFR, estimated glomerular filtration rate; SCORE2-Diabetes, type 2 diabetes-specific 10-year CVD risk score; T2DM, type 2 diabetes mellitus; TOD, target-organ damage; UACR, urinary albumin-to-creatinine ratio.
Severe TOD defined as eGFR <45 mL/min/1.73 m^2 irrespective of albuminuria; or eGFR 45–59mL/min/1.73 m^2 and microalbuminuria (UACR 30–300 mg/g; stage A2; or proteinuria (UACR >300 mg/g; stage A3); or presence of microvascular disease in at least three different sites [e.g. microalbuminuria (stage A2) plus retinopathy plus neurophay].[43–45]

Figure 7.5.4 Cardiovascular risk categories in type 2 diabetes
Marx N, Federici M, Schütt K, et al; ESC Scientific Document Group. 2023 ESC Guidelines for the management of cardiovascular disease in patients with diabetes. *Eur Heart J.* 2023 Oct 14;44(39):4043–4140. doi: 10.1093/eurheartj/ehad192. © European Society of Cardiology. With permission from Oxford University Press.

- The aim of the treatment is to either improve different phases of insulin secretion or improve insulin resistance
- The treatment for patients with T2DM can be intensified (Table 7.5.2 and Figure 7.5.5) aiming for an HbA1c of 53 mmols/mol or less (< 7%) (*Class IA*)
    - If ASCVD present, SGLT2 inhibitors and GLP1 agonists are recommended first line (*Class I*) independent of baseline or target HbA1c
    - Metformin (*Class IIa*) and/or pioglitazone (*Class IIb*) as additional glucose-lowering agents if needed
- An individualized approach should be adopted with involvement of the patient in the decision-making about their individual HbA1c targets and consideration of CV risk
- Preferential selection of anti-glycaemic agents with effective glycaemic reduction as well as superior cardiovascular and/or renal outcomes
- Hypoglycaemia avoidance

Blood pressure control

- Drug treatment is recommended in any patient with DM and office BP ≥ 140/90 mmHg (*Class IA*)
- Target SBP 120–129 mmHg, unless > 65 years old in which case aim 130–139 mmHg (*Class IA*)
- Treat with combination therapy of inhibitor of the renin-angiotensin-aldosterone system (ACEi/ARB) with a calcium channel blocker and/or thiazide/thiazide-like diuretic (*Class IA*)

Management of dyslipidaemia

- Dyslipidaemia is a major risk factor and independent risk predictor for CVD due to a cluster of lipid and lipoprotein abnormalities
- As previously discussed, grade CV risk in people with T2DM (Figure 7.5.5), using SCORE2-Diabetes (ESC) and QRISK3 (NICE guidelines), to set personalized lipid targets
    - N.B. The QRISK3 tool should not be used in patients with T1DM, patients with established CVD or those at high risk of developing CVD because of familial hypercholesterolaemia or other inherited disorders of lipid metabolism
- LDL targets:
    - < 2.6 mmol/L in patients at moderate or lower risk
    - < 1.8 mmol/L with a ≥ 50% LDL cholesterol reduction from baseline in high-risk patients
    - < 1.4 mmol/L with a ≥ 50% LDL cholesterol reduction in very high-risk patients
- Statin therapy is the recommended first line medication (*Class IA*)
- If LDL target not met, intensification of statin therapy followed by combination therapy with the addition of ezetimibe is recommended (*Class IB*)
- In very high-risk patients, a PCSK9 inhibitor should be considered if LDL target not reached despite maximum tolerated dose of statin in combination with ezetimibe, or if statin not tolerated (*Class IA*)
- In any individual statin intolerant not at LDL target, a PCSK9 inhibitor in combination with ezetimibe should be considered (*Class IIaB*)

Platelet stabilization

- Platelet activation plays a key role in the initiation and progression of atherothrombosis
- Both post-prandial and persistent hyperglycaemia have been shown to cause platelet activation in the early and late phases of the progression of T2DM
- Low-dose aspirin may be considered as primary prevention for individuals with T2DM and no history of ASCVD if no clear contraindication (*Class IIbA*)

Table 7.5.2 Summary of actions and effects of anti-diabetes drugs.

Drug	Function	Effect on weight	Hypoglycaemia	CV effect	Comments
Biguanides • Metformin	Improve insulin sensitivity	– / ↓ (0.6–2.9 kg)	No	Significant reduction in CV events Reduces BP and LDL Increases HDL levels	• GI side effects • Lactic acidosis • B12 deficiency • Low eGFR
Sulfonylureas • Gliclazide • Tolbutamide • Glimepride	Increase insulin secretion	↑ (2 kg)	Yes	First generation showed increased CV risk Recent studies have shown newer agents may slow progression of atherosclerosis leading to CV benefit	
Meglitinides • Repaglinide • Nateglinide	Increase insulin secretion	↑ (1.77 kg)	Yes	No effect on reducing CV outcomes	
Thiazolidinediones • Pioglitazone • Rosiglitazone	Improve insulin sensitivity	↑ (2.08 kg)	No	Risk–benefit data uncertain Caution with pioglitazone in patients with/at risk of HF Rosiglitazone not recommended	• HF • Oedema • Fractures • Low bone density
DPP-4 inhibitors • Saxagliptin • Sitagliptin • Linagliptin • Alogliptin	Inhibit glucagon release and increase insulin secretion	– / ↓ (saxagliptin)	No	Increased risk of HF with DPP-4 inhibitors as a class effect even in those without pre-existing HF	• Pancreatitis
GLP-1 agonists • Exenatide • Liraglutide • Dulaglutide • Albiglutide	Increase insulin secretion	↓ (3–5 kg)	No	Significant reduction in composite CV disease especially in those where it is already established Reduction in CV death and hospitalization in HF Reduction in BP/lipids	• GI side effects • Injectable • Pancreatitis • Uncommon, but may be associated with tachycardia

Drug class	Mechanism	Weight effect	Hypoglycaemia risk	Benefits	Side effects/cautions
SGLT-2 inhibitors • Empagliflozin • Dapagliflozin • Canagliflozin • Ertugliflozin	Inhibit SGLT2 in proximal tubule to increase renal excretion of urine glucose	↓ (2–3 kg)	No	Significant recent evidence of CV benefits in recent CV outcome trials • Improvement in MACE especially in those with established CVD (*Empa-Reg* and *CANVAS*) • Reduced mortality from HF across all EF (*DELIVER, EMPORER-preserved*) • BP lowering	• UTIs • Dehydration • Risk of euglycaemic ketoacidosis • Should be temporarily omitted when sick day rule incurs and peri-operatively where fasting is necessary
Alpha-glucosidase inhibitor • Acarbose	Glucose absorption inhibitor	– / ↓	No	Reduction in BP and CV effects	GI side effects
Insulin	Increase insulin	↑	Yes		Injectable

HF—heart failure, CV—cardiovascular, MACE—major adverse cardiovascular event, BP—blood pressure, GI—gastrointestinal, UTI—urinary tract infection, LDL—low-density lipoprotein, HFrEF—heart failure with reduced ejection fraction, HFpEF—heart failure with preserved ejection fraction.

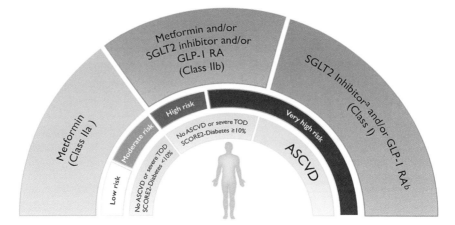

Figure 7.5.5 Risk assessment for patients with type 2 diabetes based on presence of ASCVD, severe target organ damage and 10-year CVD risk estimation via the SCORE2-Diabetes algorithm
Marx N, Federici M, Schütt K, et al; ESC Scientific Document Group. 2023 ESC Guidelines for the management of cardiovascular disease in patients with diabetes. *Eur Heart J*. 2023 Oct 14;44(39):4043–4140. doi: 10.1093/eurheartj/ehad192. © European Society of Cardiology. With permission from Oxford University Press.

- Aspirin 75 mg once daily should be used in patients with CVD and DM (*Class IA*)
- Drug regimen post ACS is considered in Chapter 2.1, however:
    - Extended DAPT to > 12 months post-ACS should be considered for up to 3 years in diabetic patients who tolerated DAPT without major bleeding (*Class IIaA*)
    - Adding very low-dose rivaroxaban to low-dose aspirin should be considered for long-term prevention of serious CV events in diabetic patients with chronic coronary syndrome or peripheral vascular disease and no high bleeding risk (*Class IIaB*)
    - Proton pump inhibitors are recommended in diabetic patients taking combination antithrombotic therapy

Smoking

- Cessation is strongly recommended
- Nicotine replacement therapy, medications such as varenicline and bupropion, and counselling should be considered (*Class IIaB*)

Physical activity

- 150 minutes moderate intensity or 75 minutes vigorous intensity exercise is recommended per week (*Class IA*)
- For additional health benefits or weight loss, adults should increase their moderate-intensity aerobic physical activity to 300 minutes per week
- In addition, resistance exercise at least twice weekly is recommended (*Class IB*)

Weight loss and dietary habits

- Weight reduction with intensive lifestyle intervention has been shown to reduce the incidence of diabetes in high-risk patients, for example those with IGT
- Modest weight loss of approximately 5% of body weight is clinically significant as it associated with a 0.5% point reduction in HbA1c, a 5 mmHg decrease in systolic and diastolic BP, a 0.13 mmol/L increase in HDL cholesterol, and a 0.45 mmol/L decrease in triglycerides
- The Mediterranean or a plant-based diet with high unsaturated fat content is recommended in T2DM (*Class IA*)

Table 7.5.3 Summary of treatment targets for patients with diabetes mellitus and coronary artery disease.

Glycaemic control HbA1c (mmol/mol)	• General target < 53 mmol/mol (<7%) • Individualized target: 48–52 mmol/mol • Individualized approach and patient involvement
Blood pressure (mmHg)	• Aim SBP 120–129 if < 65, 130–139 if > 65 years old
Lipid profile (mmol/L)	• Aim for LDL < 2.5 mmol/L • Aim for LDL < 1.8 mmol/L and 50% reduction in high risk patients • Aim for LDL < 1.4 mmol/L and 50% reduction in very high risk patients
Platelet stabilization	• Aspirin 75 mg once daily in patients with CVD and DM
Smoking	• Cessation
Weight	• Aim for weight reduction of 5–10% of body weight
Physical activity	• Moderate to vigorous 150 mins/week • Moderate to vigorous 300 mins/week for additional health benefits
Dietary habits	• Fat intake should represent < 35% of total daily energy intake with < 10% saturated and > 10% monounsaturated fatty acids

- Glucose-lowering medications with weight loss effects (e.g. GLP-1 RAs) should be considered in overweight or obese patients (*Class IIaB*)
- Bariatric surgery is effective at improving glycaemic control and can lead to diabetes resolution in a high percentage of patients with significant weight loss being maintained at 10 years, and sustained glycaemic control up to 16 years and a reduction in mortality in patients with diabetes
    - Consider bariatric surgery for 'high-' and 'very high" risk patients with BMI ≥ 35 kg/m^2 when lifestyle change interventions combined with weight-loss medications do not achieve sustained weight loss (*Class IIaB*)

Acute coronary syndromes and diabetes

- Glycaemic status should be assessed in all patients with ACS
- Clinical trials, such as DIAGAMI, DIAGAMI2, HI-5, and observational studies have not shown robust evidence to support definitive improvements in morbidity or mortality in the intensively treated patients
- As such the general consensus is that anti-diabetes medications should be started for glucose optimization aiming to keep random glucose < 10 mmol/L and avoid hypoglycaemia

Heart failure and diabetes

- SGLT2 inhibitors recommended in all patients with heart failure regardless of ejection fraction
- GLP1 agonists, metformin, insulin (glargine and degludec), and sitagliptin/linagliptin have neutral effects on risk of heart failure development and may be considered in addition to SGLT2 inhibitors for glycaemic control
- Pioglitazone and the DPP-4 inhibitor saxagliptin are associated with increased risk of heart failure in diabetic patients and are not recommended in patients at risk of heart failure
- Optimal medical therapy (e.g. sacubitril/valsartan or an ACE-inhibitor, beta blockers, etc.) and device therapy should be recommended to patients with diabetes as in the general population (see Chapter 5.1)

Further reading

Arnett DK, Blumenthal RS, Albert MA, Buroker AB, Goldberger ZD, Hahn EJ, Himmelfarb CD, Khera A, Lloyd-Jones D, McEvoy JW, Michos ED, Miedema MD, Muñoz D, Smith SC Jr, Virani SS, Williams KA Sr, Yeboah J, Ziaeian B. 2019 ACC/AHA Guideline on the Primary Prevention of Cardiovascular Disease: A Report of the American College of Cardiology/American Heart Association Task Force on Clinical Practice Guidelines. *Circulation*. 2019 Sep 10;140(11):e596–e646. doi: 10.1161/CIR.0000000000000678. Epub 2019 Mar 17. Erratum in: Circulation. 2019 Sep 10;140(11):e649–e650. Erratum in: Circulation. 2020 Jan 28;141(4):e60. Erratum in: Circulation. 2020 Apr 21;141(16):e774. PMID: 30879355

Cosentino F, Grant PJ, Aboyans V, Bailey CJ, Ceriello A, Delgado V, Federici M, Filippatos G, Grobbee DE, Hansen TB, Huikuri HV, Johansson I, Jüni P, Lettino M, Marx N, Mellbin LG, Östgren CJ, Rocca B, Roffi M, Sattar N, Seferović PM, Sousa-Uva M, Valensi P, Wheeler DC; ESC Scientific Document Group. 2019 ESC Guidelines on diabetes, pre-diabetes, and cardiovascular diseases developed in collaboration with the EASD. *Eur Heart J*. 2020 Jan 7;41(2):255–323. doi: 10.1093/eurheartj/ehz486. Erratum in: Eur Heart J. 2020 Dec 1;41(45):4317. PMID: 31497854.

Grant PJ, Cosentino F. The 2019 ESC Guidelines on diabetes, pre-diabetes, and cardiovascular diseases developed in collaboration with the EASD: New features and the 'Ten Commandments' of the 2019 Guidelines are discussed by Professor Peter J. Grant and Professor Francesco Cosentino, the Task Force chairmen. *Eur Heart J*. 2019 Oct 14;40(39):3215–17. doi: 10.1093/eurheartj/ehz687. PMID: 31608951

Marx N, Federici M, Schütt K, Müller-Wieland D, Ajjan RA, Antunes MJ, Christodorescu RM, Crawford C, Di Angelantonio E, Eliasson B, Espinola-Klein C, Fauchier L, Halle M, Herrington WG, Kautzky-Willer A, Lambrinou E, Lesiak M, Lettino M, McGuire DK, Mullens W, Rocca B, Sattar N; ESC Scientific Document Group. 2023 ESC Guidelines for the management of cardiovascular disease in patients with diabetes. *Eur Heart J*. 2023 Oct 14;44(39):4043–140. doi: 10.1093/eurheartj/ehad192. PMID: 37622663.

Type 2 diabetes in adults: management, NICE guideline (NG28) Published date: December 2015. Last updated: 28 Aug 2019

7.6

Cardiac rehabilitation

Dimitra Nikoletou

TABLE OF CONTENTS

7.6.1	What is cardiac rehabilitation? 679		Evidence for the benefits of exercise training 682
7.6.2	The structure of cardiac rehabilitation 680		Exercise recommendations 683
7.6.3	Access to cardiac rehabilitation 680	7.6.6	Education 685
	Accessibility 681	7.6.7	Dietary advice and weight management 686
	Staffing 681	7.6.8	Smoking cessation 687
	Partner/carer involvement 681	7.6.9	Psychological status and quality of life 687
7.6.4	Core components of cardiac rehabilitation programmes 681	7.6.10	Vocational rehabilitation 688
		7.6.11	Long-term CR management 688
7.6.5	Physical activity and exercise 682	7.6.12	Audit and evaluation of CR programmes 688

7.6.1 What is cardiac rehabilitation?

- Cardiac rehabilitation (CR) is a multi-disciplinary, complex intervention which aims to optimize functional capacity, quality of life, and reduce cardiovascular risk in patients with cardiovascular disease.
- Cardiac rehabilitation is defined by the British Association of Cardiovascular Prevention and Rehabilitation (BACPR, 2017) as:

   The coordinated sum of activities required to influence favourably the underlying cause of cardiovascular disease, as well as to provide the best possible physical, mental and social conditions, so that the patients may, by their own efforts, preserve or resume optimal functioning in their community and through improved health behaviour, slow or reverse progression of disease

- The range of interventions in CR include:
    - tailored physical activity and exercise
    - education
    - psychological support
    - diet and nutritional advice
    - smoking cessation
    - vocational rehabilitation.
- The main effects and benefits of CR are:
    - reduction in cardiovascular mortality
    - reduction in unplanned hospital admissions

- reduction in healthcare costs
- improvement in physical function and exercise capacity
- improvement in quality of life
- improvement in self-management of cardiovascular disease.
- High priority for CR should be given to patients with acute coronary syndrome, coronary revascularization (PCI, CABG), and heart failure (BACPR, 2023).
- Other groups that benefit from CR are patients with stable angina, peripheral artery disease, post-cerebrovascular event, post-implantation of cardiac defibrillators and resynchronization devices, post-heart valve repair/replacement, post-heart transplantation and ventricular assist devices, and patients with Adult Congenital Heart Disease (ACHD).
- NICE guidelines recognize CR as an essential part of cardiac care.
- The updated NICE 'Guidelines for Chronic Heart Failure' (2018) include exercise-based CR as an essential part of management.
- The NICE guidelines on MI (NICE 2013) position CR as an important element for rehabilitation and prevention of further episodes.
- The recent NHS long-term plan (NHS England, 2019), called for an ambitious increase in access and uptake of CR programmes amongst those eligible to 85% by 2028.

7.6.2 The structure of cardiac rehabilitation

- Comprehensive CR programmes should aim to integrate CR with secondary prevention.
- Historically, the division of CR into 'phases' was based on the UK National Service Framework for CHD (2000) that aimed to represent the stages of a patient's journey to long-term management. The original phases were:
    - Phase I—before discharge from hospital
    - Phase II—from hospital discharge up to the start of a structured exercise-based CR programme (usually up to 4 weeks duration)
    - Phase III—the period during a structured exercise-based CR programme (6–12 weeks)
    - Phase IV—long-term maintenance of changed behaviour
- A Phase 0 or Pre-operative rehabilitation, the 'Prehabilitation' phase, was added more recently to represent the preparatory period for patients undergoing elective surgery.
- Prehabilitation usually last 4–6 weeks and aims to prompt behavioural and lifestyle changes to support recovery from surgery. Sessions include education on diet modifications, advice on alcohol intake and smoking cessation, and optimization of fitness and physical function through structured exercise programmes. Prehabilitation often includes psychological support and more specific information about the upcoming surgical procedures and recovery plan.
- There is strong evidence that prehabilitation reduces post-operative complications

7.6.3 Access to cardiac rehabilitation

- Despite the strong evidence for the efficacy of CR, uptake remains low.
- In Europe, only 45% of coronary patients are advised to participate in CR and in the US the several registries and databases show that participation is even lower, even though referral is improving.
- One of the clear barriers to CR uptake is low referral from acute cardiology services.
- Patients should have automatic referral that is supported by a cardiologist, stressing the importance of CR.

- Referral to CR should be made early. Patients should begin cardiac rehabilitation as soon as possible after admission and before discharge from hospital.
- There is a relationship between early appointments and subsequent adherence to CR, which has been estimated to be 1% decreased for every day of delay between hospital discharge and CR enrolment.

Accessibility

- Patients should be offered the choice of hospital-based or home-based programmes.
- CR sessions should be held in more accessible community venues or transport provided whenever possible.
- CR services should be able to adapt to an individual patient's gender, age, ethnicity, and mental and physical co-morbidities.
- CR programmes should be culturally sensitive with bilingual team members and resources for the visually and hearing impaired.
- Home-based CR programmes may be a better option for low- to moderate-risk patients to encourage participation from subgroups who have been identified as low attenders.
- A number of strategies have been identified to improve uptake such as structured telephone calls, visits by a nurse or therapist, early appointments to CR, women-only CR programmes, and intermediate phase programmes for older people.

Staffing

- CR should be provided by an appropriately trained multidisciplinary team consisting of Cardiologists, GPs, specialist nurses, Physiotherapists and exercise specialists, Psychologists, Dieticians, Occupational Therapists, Pharmacists, and with a designated team leader.
- Staff should be trained to respond to emergency situations including basic life support and the use of a cardiac defibrillator where appropriate.

Partner/carer involvement

- CR programmes should consider participation of partners, family members, and carers to strengthen a patient's support system post-cardiac event.
- Consider specific support groups to focus on issues of partners and carers.
- Equality and diversity issues should also be considered for carers and partners to increase involvement.

7.6.4 Core components of cardiac rehabilitation programmes

The British Association for Cardiovascular Prevention and Rehabilitation (BACPR, 2023) recommends the following five core components for a CR programme

1. Health behaviour change and education
2. Lifestyle risk factor management
    - Physical activity and exercise training
    - Healthy eating and body composition
    - Tobacco cessation and relapse prevention

3. Psychosocial health
4. Medical risk management
5. Long-term management
    - Patient education and long-term management are key themes of the pathway
    - The CR provider should offer choice and inform the patient of the available types of cardiac rehabilitation intervention (e.g. individual or group sessions or a combination) and locations (e.g. hospital, community, or home)
    - The CR provider should agree with the patient that they are ready and willing to commence cardiac rehabilitation in accordance with the care plan developed.

Guidance from the Department of Health (2010) suggests the measurement of baseline trends to inform patient agreed goals, which are then assessed for change post rehabilitation. The recommended measures include:

- Psychological well-being (HADs)
- Functional capacity (fitness) 6MWT, SWT, SMWT, etc.
- BMI and waist circumference
- Quality of life (Dartmouth or MLWHF)
- Smoking cessation
- Compliance with medication
- Compliance with healthy eating plan.

Ongoing secondary risk factor measures should also be reported, e.g. BP and cholesterol.

7.6.5 Physical activity and exercise

Evidence for the benefits of exercise training
Clinical evidence

- There is strong evidence that exercise-based CR increases PA and improves cardiovascular risk and outcomes.
- Evidence from a systematic review and meta-analysis shows that 'education-only programmes' do not reduce all-cause mortality, recurrent MI, revascularization, and hospitalization 1 year later
- RCT studies of exercise-based CR in patients with heart failure, demonstrated reduction in the risk of overall hospital admissions in the short term and some improvement in all-cause mortality in trials with an over 12-month follow-up.
- Although CR improves PA levels, it does not appear to have an effect on reducing sedentary time in highly sedentary, physically inactive patients (Biswas et al., 2018). Since physical inactivity is a major risk factor for CVD, reducing sitting time as well as increasing PA should be included as strategies of exercise-based CR programmes.

Physiological evidence

- In patients with CHD there are multiple suggested mechanisms for the clinical benefits seen from CR.
- These partly relate to the modification of established risk factors, with evidence that exercise training can result in a reduced BP, weight loss, reduced insulin resistance, and an improved lipid profile.
- Exercise also has strong anti-inflammatory effects and several neurohormonal effects.

- The anti-inflammatory effects of exercise in CVD are:
  - Increased release of cytokines that stimulate lipolysis (IL-6 and IL-10) and inhibition of the pro-inflammatory cytokine TNF-a
  - Prevention of accumulation of visceral fat and reduction of abdominal fat
- The neurohormonal effects of exercise are:
  - Changes in the autonomic nervous system reduce the resting sympathicoadrenergic tone, and modifications within the renin–angiotensin–aldosterone system result in reduced plasma renin activity.
  - On a microvascular level there is improved endothelium-dependent vasodilation, with increased expression and activity of endothelial NO synthase, as well as increased angiogenesis and collateralization.
- In patients with heart failure, as well as the benefits of exercise training, studies have shown a reduction in circulating levels of angiotensin II, aldosterone, and atrial natriuretic peptide.
- These patients also benefit from better respiratory function and improved skeletal muscle metabolism and function.

Exercise recommendations
General for health and prevention
- General recommendations for prevention of CVD should aim for increase of physical activity (PA) as well as reduce of sitting or sedentary time.
- Regular PA needs to be lifelong and be at least 150 min/week of moderate activity (such as cycling or brisk walking) or at least 75 min/week vigorous activity (such as running) or an equivalent combination.
- There is evidence of a dose-response relationship between PA and CVD prevention and the most recent update from the UK Chief Medical Officers for Physical Activity (2019) recommendation states that more exercise is better than some.

Tailored CR programmes
- Aim to tailored exercise prescribed for patients post-cardiac event and in specific populations, such as frail older people.
- Patients should be assessed and risk stratified prior to commencing exercise training:
  - Low-risk patients can be assessed via a history, examination, resting ECG, and functional testing (e.g. shuttle walk test or 6-min walk test)
  - High-risk patients should be assessed with a clinical history and examination, resting ECG, echocardiogram, and formal exercise testing
  - High-risk patients should participate in exercise sessions with appropriate staff-to-patient ratios (often) based in a hospital environment with access to a defibrillator and staff trained in advanced life support
  - High-risk patients include those with:
    - MI complicated by heart failure, cardiogenic shock, and/or complex ventricular arrhythmias.
    - Angina or breathlessness occurring at a low level of exercise, e.g. inability to complete the first 4-min of the shuttle walking test.
    - ST segment depression ≥ 1 mm on resting ECG
    - Exercise testing with marked ST depression ≥ 2 mm or angina at <5 METS (see Box 7.6.1), e.g. 3 min of a Bruce protocol
  - Patients unsuitable for exercise training include those with:
    - Decompensated heart failure
    - Severe valvular stenosis or regurgitation

BOX 7.6.1 METABOLIC EQUIVALENTS (METS) FOR SPECIFIC PHYSICAL ACTIVITIES

- A metabolic equivalent is a way of expressing the metabolic energy requirements of a task as multiples of the resting metabolic rate (RMR)
- 1 MET is equivalent to the RMR when sitting quietly and has a conventional reference value of 3.5 ml $O_2 \cdot kg^{-1} \cdot min^{-1}$, which is equal to 1 $kcal \cdot kg^{-1} \cdot h^{-1}$.

Physical activities	METS
Sleeping	0.9
Light-intensity activities (e.g. gentle stroll)	< 3
Moderate-intensity activities (e.g. moderate paced to brisk walking, gentle cycling and swimming)	3–6
Moderate- to high-intensity activities (e.g. hill walking, jogging, skipping, swimming at pace)	6–8
High-intensity activities (e.g. running, fast cycling)	>8

- Refractory arrhythmias
- Other clinical conditions that worsen with exertion

Risk categories for 'a cardiovascular event on exertion' based on levels of aerobic fitness are:

- Poor or low fitness; high risk: VO2max < 21 ml/kg/min (< 6 METs)
- Poor to average fitness; moderate risk: VO2max 21–29 ml/kg/min (6–8 METs)
- Average to good fitness; low risk: VO2max 30–40 ml.kg/min (8.5–11 METs)

(ACSM guidelines for exercise testing and prescription)

Early activity after cardiac surgery

- After surgery, whilst awaiting CR, patients are advised to be physically active for 20–30 min per day to the point of slight breathlessness.
- Patients who are not achieving this should be advised to increase their activity in a gradual, step-by-step way.
- All physical activity and exercise sessions should start with a graded warm-up to enable physiological adjustments, and on completion of the main exercise there should be a graded cool-down period.
- Coronary artery bypass graft (CABG) patients should be advised to avoid heavy lifting for 3 months.
- Patients should be advised to avoid short, sharp, strenuous activity.

CR exercise-based programmes

- Exercise sessions:
    - Aerobic activity at least 2 times a week for a minimum of 8 weeks
    - Intensity of training should be prescribed in an individualized exercise regime and adapted in respect of associated co-morbidity, e.g. arthritis, COPD, stroke, etc.
    - Low-to-moderate risk patients can undertake resistance training
    - Exercise sessions usually last 1 h including:
- 10 to 15 min warm up
- Aerobic phase for 20–30 min

Table 7.6.1 Commonly used perceived exertion scales.

Exercise training level	Rate of perceived exertion (Borg)	Borg CR 10 scale	% maxima heart rate from symptom limited exercise test
	6 No exertion at all	0	
	7 Very, very light	0.5	
	8	1	
	9 Very light	2	
	10	3	
LOW	11 Fairly light	4	50–60
	12		
MODERATE	13 Somewhat hard	5	60–75
	14	6	
HIGH	15 Hard (heavy)	7	75–85
	16		
	17 Very hard	8	
	18		
	19 Very, very hard	9	
	20 Maximal exertion	10	

- 10-min cool down
- Period of relative rest, often in sitting position
    - Monitor exercise intensity as a percentage of acquired maximal heart rate or maximal age predicated heart rate or based on the heart rate reserve method using a pulse monitor, or as a perceived level of exertion on the Borg scale (see Table 7.6.1)
    - The heart rate reserve method is regarded more accurate, especially for patients on beta blockers and older people as it does not underestimate training intensity.
- Technology-based interventions, such as pedometers should be considered for patients participating in CR.
- Neuromotor training involving balance, agility and coordination exercise are recommended in specific indications.

Long-term advice/maintenance

- Long-term advice should be given to continue with at least 150 min of moderate aerobic exercise per week, ideally spread over 3–5 days per week.
- Aim to incorporate activity into everyday life for long-term adherence and risk management.

7.6.6 Education

- Education refers to information shared with patients and carers throughout the cardiac rehabilitation pathway to improve knowledge and empower individuals to gain confidence and self-manage their cardiac disease.

- Provision of information should be given using a variety of formats—written and verbally using face-to-face conversation, by telephone or online methods—and should be offered in a timely manner.
- Online methods can also be used for group sessions, especially for patients living in remote areas.
- Initial assessment of existing knowledge and learning needs is advised to design education sessions based on individual patient/carer needs.
- It is advised that all patients are offered a contact number for ongoing advice and support if and when needed.
- Patients should be given information about:
  - Their diagnosis, pathophysiology, symptoms, and plan of action should these symptoms occur (e.g. symptoms of angina)
  - Common misconceptions about cardiac illness
  - Cardiac risk factors, including blood pressure, lipids, and glucose
  - Physical activity, exercise, and appropriate daily activities to support and maintain recovery at any setting
  - Diet and weight management
  - Smoking cessation and relapse prevention
  - Psychological and emotional self-management
  - Social support and contextual factors
  - Vocational factors
  - Medication, purpose, instructions for use, potential side effects, and ways to encourage concordance
  - Resuming and maintaining sexual relations and dealing with sexual dysfunction
  - Details of any cardiac investigations, interventions, devices, or surgery that may be required
- Training for the patient and family members in basic cardiopulmonary resuscitation.

7.6.7 Dietary advice and weight management

- Dietary advice and weight management are important for primary and secondary prevention of CVD and key components in any CR programme.
- Baseline assessment should include measurement of weight and body mass index (BMI), waist circumference and calculation of the waist-to-hip ratio, investigation of dietary habits, alcohol consumption, and information on cultural or other individual needs that could help formulate a tailored dietary programme.
- Dietary advice should revolve around establishing long-term healthy eating habits. Modify diet by avoiding certain categories of food and/or replacing them with alternative healthier options.
- A Mediterranean diet is considered cardio protective. A Mediterranean-style diet is based on reduced saturated fat (main sources of fat are olive oil or other vegetable and plant oils), low intake of red meat, higher intake of fish, poultry, and legumes, and it is rich in fruit and vegetables.
- Advise reduction of salt intake
- Omega-3 fatty acid supplements should not be routinely recommended for the prevention or reduction of CVD (Aung et al., 2018; AHA Science Advisory, 2018).
- There is no evidence to support recommendation of any single or multi-vitamin, b-carotene, or folic acid supplementation for the prevention or treatment of CVD.

- Reduce alcohol consumption and advise avoiding binge drinking. The recommended limit for men and women is 14 units per week but it is advised that this is spread evenly over 3 or more days
- Offer information and examples of what is a unit of alcohol or how many units of alcohol are contained in common drink measures.
- Weight management may include advice to:
  - Reduce weight and cholesterol levels
  - Gain weight (such as in older, frail patients)
  - Maintain same weight (such as after quitting smoking)
- Overweight and obese patients should be prioritized for weight reduction using various strategies which may include referral for bariatric surgery. Priority should also be given at improving cardiorespiratory fitness levels to reduce all-cause mortality risk.
- Consider using a range of strategies to enhance adherence to dietary advice, including telephone follow-ups, educational tools, contracts, nutritional tools, and feedback.
- Patients with more complex needs should be referred to a specialized dietitian.

7.6.8 Smoking cessation

- Smoking cessation advice and support should be offered to all patients who smoke.
- Assessment of current and past tobacco use should include frequency and quantity of use (for e.g. 'pack years'= (number of cigarettes per day/20 × number of years smoked), exposure to second-hand smoke (at home, social or work environment), motivation and readiness to quit and number of past quit attempts.
- Smoking cessation interventions may include pharmacological interventions such as nicotine replacement therapy (NRT), varenicline or sustained-release bupropion, non-pharmacological interventions such as behavioural therapy, telephone support, self-help materials, or a combination of these methods.
- According to the 2017 Public Health England statistics (Public Health England, 2017), referral to a local 'stop smoking' service was the most effective way to give up smoking and electronic cigarettes (e-cigarettes) the most popular. Smokers who combined both methods had the highest success rates.

7.6.9 Psychological status and quality of life

- CHD risk has been related to 5 specific psychosocial factors: anxiety, depression, personality factors and character traits, social isolation, and chronic life stress
- As part of a comprehensive CR programme these issues should be identified and appropriate help and support offered
- Psychological interventions include individual and group counselling, stress management and relaxation, cognitive-behavioural approaches, and goal setting.

Further support should incorporate the following:

- Assessment with the Hospital Anxiety and Depression Scale (HADS)
  - Treatment of anxiety and depression if identified, including specialist referral if appropriate
- Assessment of quality of life using the Dartmouth Coop Scales
- Identification and addressing of economic, welfare rights, housing, or social support issues
- Stress awareness and stress management approaches

7.6.10 Vocational rehabilitation

- CR services should be flexible in terms of time and location to enable working-age cardiac patients to return to employment while attending CR programmes.
- CR exercise programmes should train patients in activities anticipated at their work place (SIGN, 150).
- Explore patients' health beliefs and perceptions about their ability to return to work and consider support and empowerment when needed.

7.6.11 Long-term CR management

- CR programmes should aim to enhance self-management to enable better long-term management.
- Aim to establish lifelong adherence to exercise and control of CVD risk factors.
- There are two aspects to long-term management: Patient self-management and GP-supported management.

Patient self-management could include:

- Community-based programmes such as Phase IV exercise groups.
- Leisure centre and gym memberships.
- Continuing diet and weight management support with specialized community initiatives.
- Contact with voluntary groups/resources and self-help groups such as coronary support groups.
- Online applications or tools and self-monitoring resources to promote ongoing self-management strategies.

GP supported management should include:

- Patients entered onto GP practice CHD/CVD registers for structured follow up in primary care.
- Continuation of smoking cessation services.
- Risk factor management: blood pressure, lipids, glucose, and weight management.
- Shared care for more complex patients or those awaiting intervention or surgery.
- On completion of a structured CR programme patients should be encouraged to maintain a healthy lifestyle.
- Patients should be advised to continue with at least 150 min of moderate aerobic exercise per week.

7.6.12 Audit and evaluation of CR programmes

- All cardiac rehabilitation programmes should be audited and evaluated against local, regional, and national or international standards to ensure quality in service delivery.
- Similarities and differences between all available CR registries across the world has been examined recently by a systematic review which recommended the need for inclusion of questions in registries to link and refer clinicians to national standards.
- In the UK, CR standards are audited yearly by the National Audit for Cardiac Rehabilitation (NACR) against BACPR standards. The NACR forms part of the NHS Quality accounts and data input is mandatory (since 2017).

- A European CR registry (EuroCaReD), collects data on CR programmes from 12 European countries
- A UK CR National Certification Programme (NCP_CR) has been established. CR programmes are assessed against 7 key performance indicators that are based on the BACPR standards (http://www.cardiacrehabilitation.org.uk/NCP-CR.htm).

Further reading

Ambrosetti M, Abreu A, Corrà U, Davos CH, Hansen D, Frederix I, Iliou MC, Pedretti RFE, Schmid J-P, Vigorito C, Voller H, Wilhelm M, Piepoli MF, Bjarnason-Wehrens B, Berger T, Cohen-Solal A, Cornelissen V, Dendale P, Doehner W, Gaita D, Gevaert AB, Kemps H, Kraenkel N, Laukkanen J, Mendes M, Niebauer J, Simonenko M, Swisler A-DO. Secondary prevention through comprehensive cardiovascular rehabilitation: From knowledge to implementation. 2020 update. A position paper from the Secondary Prevention and Rehabilitation Section of the European Association of Preventive Cardiology. *Eur J Prev Cardiol*. 2021 May 14;28(5):460–495. doi: 10.1177/2047487320913379.

British association for cardiovascular prevention and rehabilitation (BACPR) 2023. The BACPR standards and core components for cardiovascular disease prevention and rehabilitation. London: BACPR, 2023. https://www.bacpr.org/resources/publications

CHAPTER 8

CARDIAC PATIENTS IN OTHER SETTINGS

8.1

Aortic disease

David Wilson

TABLE OF CONTENTS

8.1.1 The normal aorta 693
8.1.2 Pathology 693
8.1.3 Non-invasive and invasive investigations 695
8.1.4 Aortic aneurysms 697
    Aetiology of aortic aneurysms 697
    Thoracic aortic aneurysms (TAA) 698
    Surgical and endovascular management 701
    Thoracoabdominal aneurysms (TAAA) 704
    Abdominal aortic aneurysm 705
8.1.5 Acute thoracic aortic syndromes 708
    Diagnostic work-up for acute aortic syndromes 709
    Acute aortic dissection 709
    Intramural haematoma 716
    Penetrating aortic ulcer 716
    Aortic pseudoaneurysm 716
    Contained rupture of aortic aneurysm 717
8.1.6 Genetic diseases affecting the aorta 717
    Non-syndromic familial thoracic aortic aneurysms and dissection 717
    Bicuspid aortic valve 717
    Other conditions associated with aortopathy 718
8.1.7 Aortitis 719
8.1.8 Aortic atheromatous disease: thrombotic or cholesterol emboli 720

8.1.1 The normal aorta

Role of the aorta

- Conduit of blood from the heart to the organs
- Control in systemic vascular resistance and heart rate via pressure-responsive receptors in ascending aorta and aortic arch
- Windkessel function—aortic elasticity allows it to act as a second pump during diastole

Normal size

- Normal aortic diameters < 40 mm
- Diameter diminishes downstream
- Diameter influence by age, gender, body size, and blood pressure
- Rate of expansion is < 1.0 mm per year

8.1.2 Pathology

Aortic wall—up to 4 mm thick and made up of the intima, media, and adventitia
    Vessel weakness typically due to abnormal composition of medial layer

- Cystic medical degeneration—present in bicuspid aortic valve (BAV) and Marfan syndrome

- Matrix metalloproteinases (MMP). MMP-2 and MMP-9 have been found in higher levels in Marfan patients. Thought to result in breakdown in elastin within the medial layer and results in aneurysm formation.
- Loss of vascular smooth muscle
- Loss of elastic fibres
- Inflammatory response with T-cell clonal expansion, increased cytokine activity, and subsequent granuloma formation seen only in aortitis

This leads to reduced wall strength and vessel dilatation.

The Law of Laplace can be used to calculate circumferential wall stress (W):

$$W = Pr/2h \quad P - \text{pulse pressure}, r - \text{radius}, h - \text{wall thickness}$$

Important factors increasing wall stress and leading to dissection or rupture (Figure 8.1.1):

- Hypertension
- Wall thinning
- Aortic enlargement

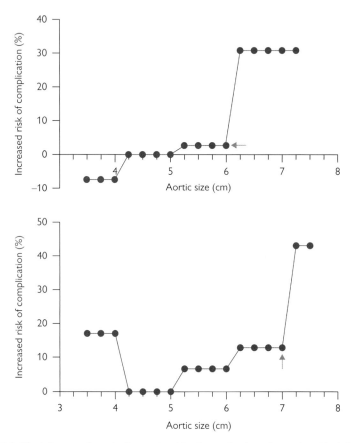

Figure 8.1.1 The influence of aortic size on the risk of complications. Beyond a critical diameter of 6cm in the ascending aorta and 7 cm in the descending aorta, the risk of future complications increases significantly.

Reproduced from Elefteriades JA. Natural history of thoracic aortic aneurysms: indications for surgery, and surgical versus nonsurgical risks. *Ann Thorac Surg.* 2002 Nov;74(5):S1877–80; discussion S1892-8. © 2002 The Society of Thoracic Surgeons. doi: 10.1016/s0003-4975(02)04147-4 with permission from Elsevier.

- Aortic diameter (although not always, especially in connective tissue diseases)
    i. 6 cm—Critical diameter of ascending aorta (30% rupture/dissection rate/annum)
    ii. 7 cm—Critical diameter of descending aorta (40% rupture/dissection rate/annum)

8.1.3 Non-invasive and invasive investigations

Aim of investigations:

1. Confirm the presence of thoracic aortic disease
2. Identify the anatomical extent of the diseased segment
3. Identify the underlying pathological process
4. Provide supplementary information potentially of value in treatment planning i.e. aortic valve competence/entry tear, side branch involvement.

No single imaging modality can do all the above. An average of 1.8 modalities are needed for the diagnosis of aortic dissection.

Modalities available—Computed Tomography (CT), Magnetic Resonance Imaging (MRI), positron emission tomography (PET), transthoracic echocardiography (TTE), and transoesophageal echocardiography (TOE). Aortography is available but rarely used.

Choice depends on local availability, urgency, safety, relative and absolute contraindications and the question that needs answering. These are presented in Table 8.1.1, with ESC recommendations in Table 8.1.2.

CXR

- Helps exclude other causes of acute chest pain, e.g. pneumothorax
- Lacks specificity
    - Pooled analysis of predictive sensitivity of a widened mediastinum/abnormal cardiac contour with significant thoracic aortic disease of 64% and 71% respectively
- Helpful in very low-risk patients
    - A completely normal CXR is unlikely to be associated with significant thoracic disease

Table 8.1.1 Strengths and weaknesses of the commonly used imaging modalities in the assessment of aortic disease.

Modality	CXR	TTE	TOE	CT	MRI	PET
Emergency use	+++	+++	++	+++	+	-
Accuracy	+	+	++	+++	+++	++
Image quality of aorta	-	+	++	+++	+++	+++
3D images	-	-	-	+++	+++	-
Image entire length of aorta	-	-	-	+++	+++	++
Radiation	+	-	-	++	-	++
Supplementary data on cardiac status	-	++	++	++	++	--
Long term follow-up use	-	-	-	++	+++	-
Expense	+++	+++	++	++	+	---

+++ = strength - = weakness

Table 8.1.2 European Society of Cardiology recommendations on imaging of the aorta 2014.

Recommendation	Class	Level of evidence
Aortic diameters should be measured at pre-specified anatomical landmarks, perpendicular to the longitudinal axis	I	C
When repetitive imaging is required, use of a modality with the lowest iatrogenic risk is recommended	I	C
When repetitive imaging over time is required, use of the same modality with a similar method of measurement is recommended	I	C
It is recommended that all relevant aortic diameters and abnormalities be reported according to the aortic segmentation	I	C
It is recommended that renal function, pregnancy status and history of contrast allergy be check prior to selecting the optimal imaging modality with the exception of emergency cases	I	C
The risk of radiation exposure should be assessed, especially in younger adults and in those undergoing repetitive imaging	IIa	B
Aortic diameters may be indexed to the body surface area especially for outliers in body size	IIb	B

Erbel R, Aboyans V, Boileau C, et al; ESC Committee for Practice Guidelines. 2014 ESC Guidelines on the diagnosis and treatment of aortic diseases: Document covering acute and chronic aortic diseases of the thoracic and abdominal aorta of the adult. The Task Force for the Diagnosis and Treatment of Aortic Diseases of the European Society of Cardiology (ESC). *Eur Heart J.* 2014 Nov 1;35(41):2873–926. doi: 10.1093/eurheartj/ehu281. © European Society of Cardiology. With permission from Oxford University Press.

TTE

- Artefacts may mimic dissection flap (need to scan in 2 orthogonal views, use colour and presence of independent motion to help exclude artefact)
- Relatively low sensitivity and specificity 77–80% and 93–96% for TTE in proximal aortic dissection and less for distal dissection
- Limited by patient factors, e.g. habitus and acoustic windows
- Distal ascending and proximal aortic arch not well seen

Abdominal ultrasound

- Most common imaging modality for abdominal aortic disease
- In aortic dissection, colour Doppler is useful to detect flow in the true and false lumen and to assess perfusion of side branches
- There is an inter-operator reproducibility error of approximately ± 5 mm

Transoesophageal echocardiography

- Sensitivity and specificity with TOE 88–98% and 90–95% in proximal aortic dissection
- Can be performed intraoperatively
- TOE often requires sedation
- Distal ascending and proximal aortic arch not well seen
- Artefacts may mimic dissection flap (need to scan in 2 orthogonal views, use colour and presence of independent motion)

Computed tomography

- Able to distinguish between causes of acute aortic syndromes
- ECG gating has improved sensitivity and specificity and should be used when motion artefact are likely to occur, e.g. proximal aorta and coronary arteries

- Sensitivity and specificity of 100% and 98–99% respectively
- Good in trauma with sensitivity, specificity and accuracy of 96%, 99%, and 99% respectively
- Excellent negative predictive value for trauma, 100%
- Can image proximal coronary arteries
- Drawback of requiring contrast and exposing the patient to radiation. Not ideal for multiple follow-up scans

Computed tomography/positron emission tomography

- Useful for investigation for the presence of inflammation within the aorta by assessing the degree of take up of ^{18}F-fluorodeoxyglucose (FDG)
- Useful in the assessment of aortic involvement in Takayasau arteritis and Giant cell arteritis
- Can be used to track inflammation over time

Magnetic resonance imaging

- Highly sensitive and specific for thoracic aortic disease
- Prolonged duration of acquisition—limits use in emergencies
- Unable to use gadolinium in patients with renal impairment
- Claustrophobia and presence of metal implants/devices can limit its use
- Not widely available out of hours

8.1.4 Aortic aneurysms

After atherosclerosis, aneurysm formation is the second most common pathology affecting the aorta. Aneurysm formation can occur anywhere along the aorta. When an aneurysm is identified, the entire aorta be should be assessed for the presence of other aneurysms.

If an abdominal aortic aneurysm is identified, a duplex ultrasound of the peripheral arteries should be undertaken to detect for the presence of peripheral artery disease and peripheral aneurysms. In patients with aortic aneurysms, cardiovascular preventative strategies should be considered as these patients have elevated cardiovascular risk.

Aetiology of aortic aneurysms
Risk factors

1. Atherosclerosis
    a. Smoking
    b. Dyslipidaemia
    c. Hypertension
2. Bicuspid aortic valve (BAV)
3. Genetic defects
    a. Marfan syndrome
    b. Ehlers–Danlos syndromes
    c. Familial connective tissue diseases ('overlap' syndromes). Familial clustering occurs in about 20%
4. Aortitis/inflammatory
    a. Microbial disease
        i. Syphilis
        ii. Staphylococcus aureus
    b. Multisystem vasculitis

i. Kawasaki's syndrome
ii. Behçet's disease
iii. Giant cell arteritis
5. Drugs
    a. Cocaine
    b. Amphetamines
6. Aortic stenosis
7. Previous surgery
8. Trauma

Thoracic aortic aneurysms (TAA)
Definition and classification
Normal values of aortic diameters are presented in Table 8.1.3. Localized aneurysm is defined as > 50% dilatation compared to the diameter of the adjacent normal vessel.
Ascending aortas measuring > 5.5 cm is therefore generally considered aneurysmal (Figure 8.1.2). Indexing the aortic size to body surface area is recommended:

- Normal vessel: Ascending 2.1 cm/m^2
- Descending 1.6 cm/m^2

Normal growth of 1 mm/decade during adulthood.
True aneurysm: enlargement of the inner lumen due to vessel wall expansion.
False/pseudoaneurysm: due to a defect in the vessel wall with the resultant extravasation of blood. The pseudoaneurysm is not lined by vascular endothelium (Figure 8.1.3). The management of pseudoaneurysm is discussed in more detail in a later section of this chapter.

Epidemiology
Mean age 65 years for men and 77 years for women. 55% ascending, 11% arch, descending 38%. Death from aneurysms and dissection—1.5/100 00 per year. 22% don't reach hospital and rupture occurs in 74% with mortality rate of 94.3%.
Male:female 1:1 unlike AAA which is more common in males.
Concomitant aneurysmal disease—25% infrarenal aneurysm. Up to 13% had multiple aneurysms (Table 8.1.4).

Natural history
Rate of growth and risk of dissection/rupture depends upon aetiology and location of aneurysm. Mean growth rate for TAA is significantly less than AAA (1–4 mm/yr vs 2–5 mm/yr respectively). 5-year survival of symptomatic TAA is 27% vs 58% in asymptomatic patients.

Table 8.1.3 Normal diameters of the aorta.

	Male (cm)	Female (cm)
Aortic annulus (TTE)	2.6 (+/- 0.3)	2.3 +/- 0.2
Sinus of valsalva (TTE)	3.4 (+/- 0.3)	3.4 (+/- 0.3)
Aortic root (TTE)	<3.7	<3.7
Ascending aorta (TTE)	<3.7	<3.7
Descending aorta (CT)	<2.8	<2.8

8.1.4 Aortic aneurysms 699

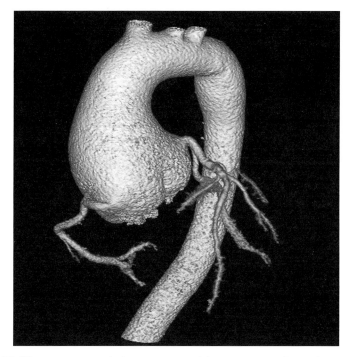

Figure 8.1.2 3D reconstruction of a huge aneurysm of the aortic root and ascending aorta with normal coronary arteries. Used with permission from Dr N Manghat, Consultant Radiologist Bristol Heart Institute

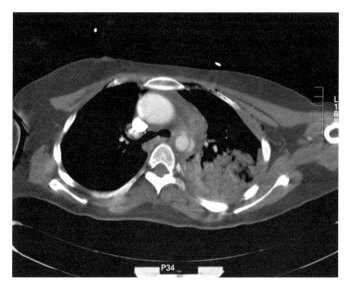

Figure 8.1.3 Post traumatic pseudoaneurysm of the descending aorta (arrow) with associated hydropneumothorax of the left lung in a 41 year old construction worker following a 10 meter fall.
Reproduced from Ballesta Moratalla M. Aortic post-traumatic pseudoaneurysm. *Emergency Medicine Journal*, 2008 Aug;25(8):533. © 2008. doi: 10.1136/emj.2007.056895 with permission from BMJ Publishing Group Ltd.

Table 8.1.4 Variables associated with increased rate of aneurysmal growth.

Location	Descending aorta
Wall integrity	Dissected aorta
Initial size	< 5 cm (2%)
	5–5.9 cm (3%)
	> 6 cm (7%)
	(Annual rate of rupture)
Genetic	Marfan
Hormonal	Pregnancy

In 63 untreated patients with arteriosclerotic TAA 40% died of rupture and 27% died of unrelated cardiovascular conditions.

Clinical features
Normally asymptomatic
Possible consequences due to compression/erosion/distortion of various structures:

1. Vascular—superior vena cava obstruction, aortic regurgitation, thromboembolic sequelae
2. Neural—phrenic, vagus, or recurrent laryngeal nerve
3. Airway compression and dysphagia

Diagnostic procedures
See section 8.1.3 for details.

Medical management
Generally reserved for asymptomatic aneurysms.
Aortic size index (aortic diameter/m^2) may be useful to predict increasing rates of rupture, dissection, or death.

- < 2.75 cm/m^2—low risk (4%/year)
- 2.75–4.24 cm/m^2—moderate risk (8%/year)
- > 4.25 cm/m^2—high-risk (20%/year)

Reducing the aortic *dp/dt* (the rate of aortic pressure change over time) is the goal of medical management.

- Aggressive blood pressure control
    - < 140/90 mmHg
    - < 130/80 mmHg for patients with diabetes or chronic kidney disease
- Smoking cessation
- Beta blockers are first line—reduce rate of aortic dilatation in the young and in Marfan syndrome. Data from retrospective reviews or open label, randomized trial of 70 patients with Marfan syndrome using propanolol
- Evidence for Angiotensin Converting Enzyme inhibitors (ACEi) from randomized, double blind placebo controlled trial of 17 patients with Marfan syndrome using perindopril followed up for 24 weeks

- Angiotensin receptor blockers (ARBs) evidence supports valsartan (open label trial of 3081 adults) and losartan/irbesartan (18 Marfan syndrome paediatric patients). There is also evidence to suggest ARBs have Tissue Granulating Factor blocking properties and result in regression of aortic dilatation in Loeys–Dietz syndrome.
- Statins shown to reduce mortality after endovascular repair in AAA repair but not in TAA
- Surveillance—important, either CT/MRI generally annually
- Lifestyle—avoidance of manoeuvres that result in increased intra-thoracic pressure, e.g. weightlifting
- Screening—family screening in those with heritable conditions

Surgical and endovascular management

Generally, intervention (surgery/endovascular) reserved for symptomatic or expanding aneurysms. As the risk of rupture increases significantly in ascending aortas > 60 mm (Figure 8.1.1), surgery is recommended in when the size reaches > 55 mm. However, importantly in higher risk populations the threshold is lower.

Features requiring consideration for intervention

- Increasing size—> 0.5 cm/year
- Aneurysm causing symptoms
- Size > 5.5 cm in ascending aneurysm

Operative mortality in ascending aneurysms

- 1.5% for elective
- 2.6% for urgent
- 11.7% for emergency

ESC recommendation 2014 for threshold of thoracic aortic aneurysm for intervention

Surgery is indicated in aortic root aneurysm with maximal aortic diameter

- Aortic diameter > 50 mm for Marfan syndrome

Surgery should be considered in root aneurysm with maximal aortic diameters

- Root aneurysm > 45 mm Marfan syndrome with risk factors[1] (Class IIa Level C)
- Root > 5.0 cm bicuspid with risk factors[2] (Class IIa Level C)
- Root > 5.5 cm for patients with no elastopathy (Class IIa Level C)

Surgery may be considered at lower thresholds if:

- Small stature (index aortic size using body surface area) (Class IIb Level C)
- Rapid progression of aneurysm (Class IIb Level C)
- Presence of aortic valve incompetence (Class IIb Level C)
- Planned pregnancy (Class IIb Level C)
- Patient preference (Class IIb Level C)

---

1. Family history of aortic dissection and/or aortic size increase > 3 mm/year, severe aortic or mitral regurgitation or desire for pregnancy.
2. Coarctation of the aorta, systemic hypertension, family history of aortic dissection, increase in aortic diameter > 3 mm/year

ESC recommendation 2014 for intervention on aortic arch aneurysm

Surgery should be considered

- Isolated aortic arch aneurysm > 55 mm (Class IIa Level C)
- If there is an indication for surgery at an adjacent aneurysm (Class IIb Level C)

ESC recommendation 2014 for intervention on descending aortic aneurysm

TEVAR should be considered

- When anatomy is suitable (Class IIa Level C)
- Descending aorta > 55 mm (Class IIa Level C)

Surgery should be considered

- If TEVAR is not technically possible in patients who have a maximal descending diameter > 60 mm (Class IIa Level C)
- In the presence of Marfan Syndrome or other elastopathies if indicated (Class IIa Level C)

Composite mechanical valve conduits (essentially tube with valve attached) preferred especially if the aneurysm involves the aortic root or the sinus of valsalva.
Valve sparing operation (Tirone David Operation).
Localized aneurysms can be successfully resected, graft replacements and coronary buttons can be reimplanted whilst keeping native valve. Advantage of avoiding anticoagulation, disadvantage of having a higher rate of residual regurgitation and are not always technically possible (Figure 8.1.4). Re-operation—more common in valve-preserving operations (16% vs 5%) and needed in 10–20% of all patients by 10–20 years. Indications same as above.

Risk factors for re-operation

- Annulus diameter > 2.5 cm
- Marfan syndrome

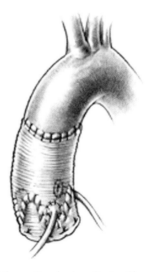

Figure 8.1.4 Reimplantation of the aortic valve in patients with annuloaortic ectasia and aortic root aneurysm, commonly called the Tirone David operation.

Reproduced from David TE, Feindel CM, Bos J. Repair of the aortic valve in patients with aortic insufficiency and aortic root aneurysm. J Thorac Cardiovasc Surg. 1995 Feb;109(2):345–51; discussion 351-2. doi: 10.1016/S0022-5223(95)70396-9 with permission from Elsevier.

- Mitral valve prolapse
- AF
- Valve-preserving operation
- Concomitant procedures performed

Predictors of late death
- Female sex
- Older age
- Untreated with beta blockers
- Significant mitral regurgitation at presentation
- Mitral ring calcification
- Post-operative dysrhythmias
- Post-operative inotropes

20-year survival rate 50%.

Endovascular repair

Graft-stent technology is developing fast and this is a rapidly changing field. Open surgical repair carries significant risk of mortality and morbidity and therefore patients not fit for surgical repair may be candidates for endovascular repair.

There is an increasing amount of data to show that the risk of endovascular approaches is lower and the morbidity is less but the reintervention rate is higher than with open repairs. The long-term durability of the stent graft is currently unknown, though data up to now are promising.

In general, the following should be considered when assessing a patient for endovascular repair both for aneurysms and dissection:

- What is the patient's surgical risk?
- Is the anatomy suitable for endovascular repair?
    - Do they have adequate vascular access—sheaths can be up to 20–25F
    - Is there an adequate 'landing zone' for the stent?
- Is there a risk of side branch occlusion and organ hypoperfusion as a result of the stent?
    - Will this require a debranching (the sequential ligation of the supra-aortic vessels to allow a stent placement without risk of side branch compromise) procedure before deployment of the stent?
    - Will this require placement of a fenestrated graft in order to preserve organ function?

Technique
- Mostly under general anaesthesia
- Peripheral access requires a surgical cut down for 22–24F sheaths
- Common femoral artery used most, though iliac and even retroperitoneal exposure to the abdominal aorta has been used in frail elderly women
- Graft stent advanced using a stiff wire and positioning is confirmed with TOE. The blood pressure can be lowered either by rapid pacing of the right ventricle or pharmacologically if the BP is very high allowing the stent to be deployed
- Endoleaks are secured with further balloon inflations

Complications of endograft procedures
- Related to access
    - Use of iliac or aorta is required in 15%

- Bleeding
    - Mean blood loss 371 ml and blood transfusion required in 3%
- Thromboembolic complication
• Related to device
    - Major adverse event in 10–12%
        - Stroke in 2.5–3.6%
        - Paraplegia 1.3–3%
        - MI 2–4%
        - Acute renal failure requiring dialysis 1.3%
        - Infection—very rare when performed electively
        - Endoleaks—classified I–V according to cause of perigraft blood flow
        - Aortic perforations/dissection—more common in uncovered or bare proximal attachment
        - Beaking of the endograft, or partial collapse/infolding of the endograft can occur due to graft oversizing and can result in collapse of the endograft and vessel occlusion.
        - Conversion of a Type B dissection into a retrograde Type A dissection hence a surgical emergency
• Post-operative
    - Pneumonia < 5%
    - Endoleaks
    - Endograft failure, migration
    - Infection
    - Perforation and oesophageal fistula
    - Need for repeat interventions—6–7%
    - Conversion to open operation—1–2%

Cost of endograft procedures has yet to be shown to be less than open procedures.
Given all these factors patients should be carefully assessed and counselled with regard to pros and cons of both surgical and endovascular procedures and care individualized to them.

Aortic arch

Surgical repair has historically been the norm, but due to complex anatomy with the head and neck vessels involved mortality and significant morbidity are high (mortality 2–9%, paraplegia and stroke 4–13%). Conventional surgical techniques either employ deep hypothermic circulatory arrest (15–18C) or a range of antegrade cerebral perfusion techniques.

Thoracoabdominal aneurysms (TAAA)

Various surgical techniques including permissive hypothermia in the repair of descending aneurysms and thoraco-abdominal aortic aneurysms have reduced the frequency of ischaemic complications such as paraplegia and renal failure over the last 15 years. 5-year survival of 1773 patients in one series is 75%.

Hybrid arch procedures (HAP) are a combination of debranching bypass (supra-aortic vessel transposition) to establish cerebral perfusion and subsequent endovascular repair are increasingly used. This technique could be used in older patients with severe co-morbidities and redo surgery ineligible for open intervention. The key to success is the quality of the unaffected ascending aorta as the site of the debranching bypass and landing site for the endograft (Figure 8.1.5).

Mortality rate—usually dependent upon premorbid condition of patient—5% in hospital mortality, follow-up mortality 8.5%, persistent endoleak 15.2%, 1-year survival 92.5%.

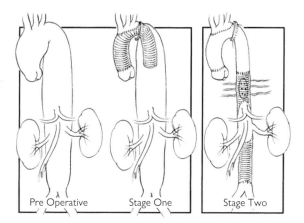

Figure 8.1.5 Artist's impression of the staged elephant's trunk technique
Reproduced from Safi HJ, Miller CC 3rd, Estrera AL, Huynh TT, Rubenstein FS, Subramaniam MH, Buja LM. Staged repair of extensive aortic aneurysms: morbidity and mortality in the elephant trunk technique. *Circulation*. 2001 Dec 11;104(24):2938–42. © 2001 American Heart Association, Inc. doi: 10.1161/hc4901.100362 with permission from Wolters Kluwer.

Abdominal aortic aneurysm
Definition
- Mostly infrarenal
- > 30 mm or > 50% increase in diameter from reference disease free segment

Risk factors
- Age
- Male gender
- Previous atherosclerotic vascular disease
- Smoking
- Hypertension
- Family history

Natural history
- Prevalence in screening programs 5.5%, though this may be reducing in some countries as rates of smoking diminish
- Long subclinical phase
- Estimated growth rate of < 1–6 mm/year
- Growth rate proportional to aortic diameter
- Rupture of AAA occurs at smaller diameters in women

Diagnosis
- Diagnosis is usually incidental
- Symptoms may include abdominal pain or back pain
- AAA rupture presents with an acute abdomen

Imaging
Ultrasonography is the mainstay of imaging modes due to cost and ease of access
CT and MRI are considered the 'gold-standard' imaging modality especially in the peri-operative period.

Screening
- Mass population screening for AAA for patients at risk has been trialled in over 125,000 participants in 4 randomized trials
- A 45% reduced risk of AAA-related mortality at 10 years and a non-significant 2% all-cause mortality reduction
- No benefit in women
- The uptake of national screening programmes has not been universal

ESC recommendations
Screening for AAA with ultrasound

i) Is recommended for all men > 65 years of age (Class 1 Level A)
ii) May be considered in women > 65 years of age with a history of current/past smoking (Class IIb Level C)
iii) Is not recommend in female non-smokers without familial history (Class III Level C)
iv) May be considered in first-degree siblings of a patients with AAA (Class IIa Level B)

Opportunistic screening for AAA during TTE

i) Should be considered in all men > 65 years (Class IIa Level B)
ii) May be considered in women > 65 years of age with a history of current/past smoking (Class IIb Level C)

Management—small AAA
Small AAA defined as 30–49 mm or 30–54 mm
Generally, the risks of intervention are greater than not intervening
Medical therapy in order to

- Prevent cardiovascular events
- Limit AAA growth
- Prepare the patient in anticipation of future vascular intervention in order to reduce operative risk

Medical therapy includes

- Smoking cessation advice to reduce rate of AAA growth
- Diet and exercise prescription
- Beta blocker first line for hypertension in the presence of AAA
- Some evidence supports the use of ACE inhibitors
- Some evidence supports the use of Statin therapy
- Data on the use of aspirin in order to reduce thrombus burden and hence rate of AAA growth is contradictory, however, given the presence of other cardiovascular risk factors associated with AAA, the use of aspirin is may be considered.

Follow-up
For men

- Aortic diameter < 25 mm—follow up in 10 years
- Aortic diameter 26–29 mm—follow up in 4 years
- Aortic diameter 30–39 mm—follow up in 3 years
- Aortic diameter 40–44 mm—follow up in 2 years
- Aortic diameter 45–49 mm—follow up in 1 year

For women
AAA rupture occurs at small aortic diameters than compared to men. For instance, the rate of AAA rupture in women with an aortic diameter of 45 mm is equivalent to that of men with an aortic diameter of 55 mm, therefore the threshold for follow-up should be lower in women.

AAA repair
Pre-operative evaluation
This is dependent on the risk of the interventional strategy (open repair versus endovascular repair) and the patient-specific risk factors.

- Coronary artery disease (CAD) is the main cause of post-operative mortality.
- The prevalence of CAD in patients with AAA is high, approximately 66%
- Risk of peri-operative cardiovascular complication is
    i) High (> 5%) with open repair
    ii) Lower (1–5%) with endovascular repair

Repair in asymptomatic AAA
Management depends on the diameter of the aorta and the need to balance the risk of any intervention with the risk of rupture if no intervention is undertaken.
Consider intervention once aneurysm

i) > 55 mm in diameter
ii) Becomes symptomatic
iii) Increases in size rapidly (> 10 mm/year).

Lower thresholds for intervention in women (see above).

Open repair
- Traditionally, this has been the standard of care
- Operative mortality vary between centres and countries (1–8%)
- Predictors of mortality include the presence of cardiovascular, pulmonary, and renal co-morbidity
- Operative mortality is higher in emergency versus elective surgery and varies between centres and countries
- Open repair preferred in more complex anatomy

Endovascular repair
This is an evolving field.

- Lower initial mortality rates (1–2%) compared to open repair, with a 66% relative reduction in operative mortality
- Initial survival advantage decreases over time with risk of late rupture and re-intervention rate with endovascular repair, though this has been improving over time
- Lifelong imaging surveillance is required to monitor for sac enlargement
- Endovascular repair suitable in between 15–68% of AAA

Contained rupture of AAA
Presentation
- Abdominal pain
- Hypotension

- Pulsatile abdominal mass
- Back pain
- May mimic other abdominal emergencies

Imaging
- Ultrasound sonography
- Computed tomography—imaging of choice

Treatment
At present, there is no consensus as to whether open repair or endovascular repair is preferable.

ESC guidelines 2014 for management of patients with symptomatic abdominal aortic aneurysm
In patients with:

- Suspected rupture of AAA, immediate abdominal ultrasound of CT is recommended (Class I Level C)
- Ruptured AAA, emergency repair is recommended (Class I Level C)
- Symptomatic but non-ruptured AAA, urgent repair is recommended (Class I Level C)
- Symptomatic AAA anatomically suitable for EVAR, with open repair or endovascular aortic repair is recommended. (Class I Level A)

Long-term prognosis and follow-up following repair
After open repair, a 3-month recovery time is usually needed before patients return to their baseline. The rate of graft-related complications is low for open repair (approximately 6% at 10 years). These include anastomotic pseudoaneurysm, graft limb thrombosis, and graft infection.

8.1.5 Acute thoracic aortic syndromes

Acute aortic syndromes (AAS) (Figure 8.1.6) is an umbrella term that cover a range of emergency conditions with similar clinical characteristics which affect the aorta. They occur when the blood breaches the endothelial lining of the aorta either as a result from a tear or an ulcer or when a penetrating blood vessel (vasa vasorum) ruptures and blood enters the tunica media. They comprise acute aortic dissection, intramural haematoma, penetrating aortic ulceration, and aortic rupture. The following illustrates their relationships.

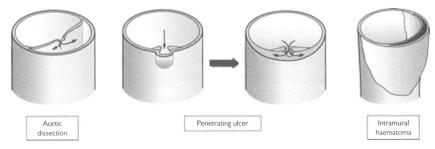

Figure 8.1.6 Representation of the 8.
Reproduced from Nienaber, Christoph A., 'Diseases of the Aorta and Trauma to the Aorta and the Heart', in A. John Camm, Thomas F. Lüscher, and Patrick W. Serruys (eds), The ESC Textbook of Cardiovascular Medicine, 2 edn, The European Society of Cardiology (Oxford, 2009), https://doi.org/10.1093/med/9780199566990.003.031

Diagnostic work-up for acute aortic syndromes

The diagnostic tests undertaken are dependent upon the pre-test probability that the patient has this condition (Figure 8.1.7). A diagnostic algorithm proposed in 2014 ESC Guidelines on the diagnosis and treatment of aortic diseases is based on clinical data, laboratory and imaging tests, as should be done in patients presenting with chest pain in whom an acute aortic syndrome is suspected. Table 8.1.6 outlines ESC recommendations.

Acute aortic dissection

Definition

Dissection is defined as disruption and separation of the media layer of the aortic wall with bleeding along and within the wall resulting in separation of the layers.

1. Acute dissection—within 2 weeks of onset of symptoms
2. Subacute—15–90 days
3. Chronic dissection—> 90 days

One-third of patients have chronic dissection.
Acute aortic syndromes have been defined by the American Heart Association and American College of Cardiology as acute aortic dissection, intramural haematoma, and penetrating atherosclerotic ulcer.

Classification

Classified according to pathology or anatomy. The latter is more frequently used (Figure 8.1.8).
   Pathological Class I–V

1. Class I—classic aortic dissection subdivided into the DeBakey and Stanford classifications.
2. Class II—intramural haemorrhage/haematoma

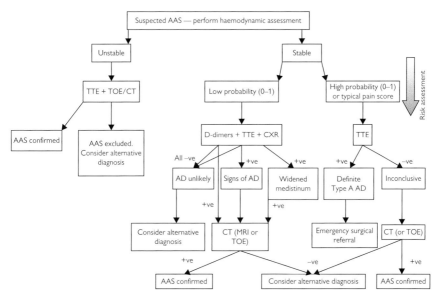

Figure 8.1.7 Flow chart of decision making aid in the case of suspected acute aortic syndrome using the risk assessment in table 8.1.5.
Erbel R, Aboyans V, Boileau C, et al; ESC Committee for Practice Guidelines. 2014 ESC Guidelines on the diagnosis and treatment of aortic diseases: Document covering acute and chronic aortic diseases of the thoracic and abdominal aorta of the adult. The Task Force for the Diagnosis and Treatment of Aortic Diseases of the European Society of Cardiology (ESC). *Eur Heart J.* 2014 Nov 1;35(41):2873–926. doi: 10.1093/eurheartj/ehu281. © European Society of Cardiology. With permission from Oxford University Press.

Table 8.1.5 High-risk clinical characteristics in acute aortic syndromes.

High-risk conditions	High-risk pain features	High-risk examination features

• Marfan syndrome (or other connective tissue disease)
• Family history of aortic disease
• Known aortic valve disease
• Known thoracic aortic aneurysm
• Previous artic manipulation
	• Chest, back, or abdominal pain described as any of the following:
	• Abrupt onset
	• Severe intensity
	• Ripping or tearing
		• Evidence of perfusion deficit:
		  • Pulse deficit
		  • Systolic blood pressure difference
		  • Focal neurological deficit (with pain)
		• Aortic diastolic murmur (new and with pain)
		• Hypotension or shock

Table 8.1.6 European Society of Cardiology recommendations (2014) for the diagnostic work-up of acute aortic syndromes.

Recommendation	Class	Level of evidence
History and clinical assessment		
It is recommended that all patients with suspected AAS should have a pre-test probability assessment performed according to the patient's condition, symptoms, and clinical features.	I	B
Laboratory testing		
In the case of suspected AAS, the interpretation of biomarkers should always be considered along with the clinical pre-test probability.	IIa	C
In the case of a low clinical probability of AAS, a negative D-dimer should be considered a rule out of the diagnosis.	IIa	B
In the case of an intermediate clinical probability of AAS with positive D-dimer, further imaging should be considered.	IIa	B
In patients with high probability risk scores (2 or 3) of AD, testing of D-dimers is not recommended.	III	C
Imaging		
TTE is recommended as an initial imaging investigation	I	C
In unstable patients with suspected AAS, TOE and CT are recommended according to local availability and expertise.	I	C
In stable patients with suspected AAS, CT, MRI and TOE are recommended according to local availability and expertise.	I (IIa for TOE)	C
It is recommended that repeat imaging be performed if symptoms persists if initial imaging was negative	I	C
Chest X-ray may be considered in cases with low clinical probability of AAS	IIb	C
In cases of uncomplicated Type B AAS treated medically, repeated imaging (CT or MRI) during the first days is recommended.	I	C

Erbel R, Aboyans V, Boileau C, et al; ESC Committee for Practice Guidelines. 2014 ESC Guidelines on the diagnosis and treatment of aortic diseases: Document covering acute and chronic aortic diseases of the thoracic and abdominal aorta of the adult. The Task Force for the Diagnosis and Treatment of Aortic Diseases of the European Society of Cardiology (ESC). *Eur Heart J.* 2014 Nov 1;35(41):2873–926. doi: 10.1093/eurheartj/ehu281. © European Society of Cardiology. With permission from Oxford University Press.

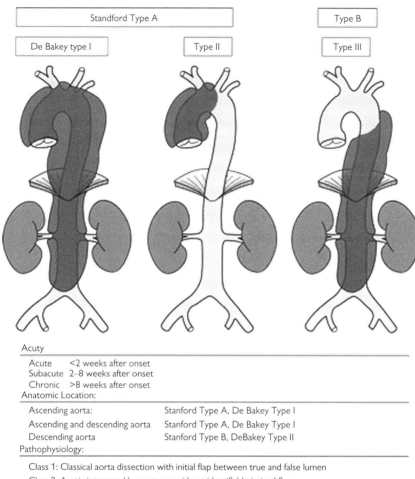

Figure 8.1.8 Classification of aortic dissection.
Reproduced from Nienaber, Christoph A., 'Diseases of the Aorta and Trauma to the Aorta and the Heart', in A. John Camm, Thomas F. Lüscher, and Patrick W. Serruys (eds), The ESC Textbook of Cardiovascular Medicine, 2 edn, The European Society of Cardiology (Oxford, 2009), https://doi.org/10.1093/med/9780199566990.003.031

3. Class III—ulcerating aortic plaque
4. Class IV—subtle/discrete aortic bulge. Difficult to diagnose—typically seen in Marfan syndrome
5. Class V—Iatrogenic/traumatic, e.g. post cardiac catheter manipulation

Anatomical

1. Proximal—involving aortic root or ascending aorta
2. Distal—beyond left subclavian artery

Stanford Classification

1. Type A—involves ascending aorta
2. Type B—does not involve ascending aorta

Surgery recommended for Type A dissections.
Note that a Type B dissection that involves the aortic arch remains a Type B dissection.
DeBakey Classification (based on origin of the intimal tear)

1. Type I—starts in the ascending aorta and extends distally, typically involving entire aorta
2. Type II—starts in the ascending aorta and remains confined to the ascending aorta
3. Type III—starts in the descending aorta and extends distally
    a. Type IIIa—limited to descending aorta
    b. Type IIIb—extends below diaphragm

Surgery recommended in DeBakey Type I and Type II

Pathology

Aortic dissection results from separation of aortic wall layers in the context of elevated blood pressure and degenerative changes in the aortic media.
The proximal aorta is at highest risk of dissection as it is subject to the steepest fluctuations in pressure.

Epidemiology

Rare

- Incidence—2.6–3.5 cases per 100,000 person/year
- High prevalence in Italy 4.04/100,000/year
- 0.5% of admissions to A&E with chest/back pain are due to aortic dissection.
- Two-thirds male
- Mean age 65 years
- Hypertension most common risk factor—seen in up to 72%

Causes in the < 40-year-old category tend to be due to connective tissue diseases.
Risk factors—as for aneurysm formation plus previous aortic/valvular surgery.

Clinical features

Characterized by rapid development of an intimal flap separating the true and false lumen which in 90% is the site of communication between true and false lumen. Anterograde or retrograde spread can occur. Propagation of the dissection anterogradely or retrogradely can causes significant morbidity. Can involve side branches and result in malperfusion syndrome from obstruction of aortic flow, cardiac tamponade, and aortic regurgitation.

Typical features

1. Onset—acute (most specific feature)
2. Location—chest (73% (anterior 61%, posterior 36%)), back pain (53%), abdomen (30)
3. Sharp, ripping, tearing, or knife like in nature
4. Syncope (20%) from tamponade, severe hypotension, and carotid obstruction

Signs

Patients usually present in acute cardiac decompensation and shock. Other signs include:

- Hypertension
- Hypotension in 25% due to haemopericardium and pericardial tamponade
- Mediastinal bleeding

- Acute aortic insufficiency in 50% of ascending dissections
- Aortic rupture
- Lactic acidosis
- Spinal shock
- Connective tissue disorder may be present
- Malperfusion syndrome related to side branch obstruction with signs and symptoms secondary to organ involvement in one-third, e.g.
- Cardiovascular—ischaemia
- Cerebrovascular manifestations—paraplegia or stroke
- Limb ischaemia
- Renal failure
- Visceral ischaemia
- Pulse differentials in 38% and most specific sign of dissection
- Aortic regurgitation (second most common cause of death)

Natural history

28–55% die without a correct diagnosis.
Predictors of in-hospital mortality:

- Tamponade
- Coronary artery involvement
- Malperfusion of the brain or intestine
- Age > 70 years
- Hypotension
- Renal failure
- Pulse deficits.

Risk of fatal rupture in untreated proximal aortic dissection is 90%.
Mortality with surgery is as follows: 10% day 1, 12% day 2, 20% week 2.
Acute dissection of descending aorta is less lethal.
Mortality with no treatment in type B dissection is 11% 1 month, 16% 1 year, 20% 5 year.

Diagnostic work-up

Use the risk assessment tool described above.

Management

There is a lack of randomized controlled trials with long-term follow-up and randomized trials comparing medical to surgical techniques. However, it is clear that rapid decompression of the false lumen followed by complete thrombosis of the false lumen is beneficial (Table 8.1.7).

Medical management

Admit to intensive care unit
Target systolic BP of 110 mmHg

1. i.v. beta blockers (metoprolol, esmolol, or labetalol)
2. Sodium nitroprusside 0.3 mcg/kg/min
3. Angiotensin converting enzyme inhibitors
4. i.v. verapamil, diltiazem if beta blocker contraindicated

Occasionally dual therapy with beta blocker and sodium nitroprusside needed.
Normotensive patients need evaluating for potential blood loss/pericardial effusion/heart failure prior to volume administration. Intubation and ventilation is required if there is profound

Table 8.1.7 Management.

Surgical management	Medical management	Interventional management
Type A aortic dissection	Uncomplicated, acute type B dissection	Unstable, acute type B dissection **
Type B dissection complicated by • Retrograde extension • Dissection in fibrillinopathies *	Stable, isolated aortic arch dissection	Stable type B dissection (under evaluation)
	Chronic type B dissection	Type B dissection with retrograde extension to ascending aorta
		Hybrid procedure for extended type A dissection

* e.g. Marfan syndrome, Ehlers–Danlos syndrome
** Malperfusion, rapid expansion (> 1 cm/yr), critical diameter (≥ 5.5 cm), refractory pain
Source data from Akin I, Kische S, Ince H, Nienaber CA. Indication, timing and results of endovascular treatment of type B dissection. *Eur J Vasc Endovasc Surg.* 2009 Mar;37(3):289–96. doi: 10.1016/j.ejvs.2008.12.004.

haemodynamic instability. Urgent imaging to characterize nature of the dissection with TOE/TTE/CT. Pericardiocentesis as a temporizing measure often fails and can accelerate bleeding and shock so it is generally contraindicated.

Surgical management

The key to success is rapid surgery prior to any haemodynamic instability or deterioration.
Type A dissection (ESC class I indication)

- Emergency to avoid tamponade/rupture
- Valve-preserving surgery—tubular graft *if* normal sized aortic root and no pathological changes of valve cusps
- Replacement of aorta and aortic valve (composite graft) *if* ectatic proximal aorta and/or pathological changes of valve/aortic wall

Type A dissection (ESC class II indication)

- Valve-sparing operations with aortic root remodelling for abnormal valves
- Valve preservation and aortic root remodelling in Marfan patients

Type B dissection (ESC class I indication)

- Only in persistent pain and other complications

If dissecting and non-dissecting aneurysms extend to the descending aorta, an elephant trunk extension of the aortic graft can be used. This free-floating section of the graft can be connected to the distal descending aorta either surgically or using endovascular stent-graft techniques.

Involvement of aortic arch

Management is more complicated as either resecting of or leaving unrecognized intimal tears predisposes to later distal re-operation which carries a substantial operative mortality (15–35%). Arch tears occur in approximately 30% of patients with acute dissection.

Management of aortic arch involvement

- Consensus suggests that a dissected arch should be explored during hypothermic circulatory arrest.

- When extensive tears are found, subtotal or total arch replacement may be required with reattachment of the supra-aortic vessels with anterograde cerebral perfusion
- In the absence of a tear, an open distal anastomosis of the graft and the conjoined aortic layers at the junction of the ascending and arch portions is justified.

Endovascular therapy in aortic dissection

Currently the treatment of choice in complicated type B dissection. Use in type A dissection still experimental.

Principles and considerations:

- To cover the entry site of the false lumen
- Consider whether organs are perfused by the false lumen
    i. Will occlusion of the false lumen result in hypoperfusion of an organ/limb?
    ii. Will stenting the 'at-risk' vessel or creating a fenestration (window) improve perfusion to the organ?

Endovascular repair in type B aortic dissection may be considered in the following scenarios:

- Stenting of obstructed branch origin for static obstruction of branch artery
- Balloon fenestration of dissecting membrane plus stenting of aortic true lumen
- For dynamic obstruction
- Stenting to keep fenestration open
- Fenestration to provide re-entry tear for dead-end false lumen
- Stenting of true lumen
    i. To enlarge compressed true lumen
    ii. To seal entry (covered stent).

Other possible indications:

- Aortic aneurysms (with suitable morphology for repair)
- Rupture
- Type B dissections (acute and chronic)
- Giant penetrating ulcer
- Traumatic aortic tear
- Aorto-pulmonary fistulae.

Patient co-morbidities increase open surgical repair risk. Combined surgical/endovascular repair is often required when arch is involved and stent is used to seal distal end.

Follow-up

Data from the International Registry of Acute Aortic Dissection (IRAD) shows that the 3-year survival of patients discharged alive after acute Type A dissection is approximately 90%. For type B dissection 3-year mortality is 77.6 +/− 6.6% (treated medically), 82.8 +/− 18.9% (treated surgically), 76.2 +/− 25.2% (with endovascular therapy). Higher-risk patients are those with hypertension, the elderly, large aortic size, presence of patent false lumen, previous aortic aneurysm, female gender and Marfan syndrome.

- Aggressive treatment of hypertension with beta blockade is the cornerstone of medical therapy.
- Up to 40% develop resistant hypertension requiring up to 6 antihypertensive agents.
- Target of < 135/80 mmHg (< 130/80 in patients with Marfan syndrome) and heart rate of < 60/min.

- Serial imaging is mandatory and has previously been recommended at 1, 3, 6, 9, and 12 months and then yearly thereafter. Choice of modality is dependent on local availability and expertise.
- Repair is recommended if ascending aorta > 5.5–6.0 cm (4.5–5.5 cm if Marfan syndrome present) and > 6.0 cm in distal aorta.
- Rate of change and risk factors should be taken into consideration when considering repair.

Intramural haematoma

Precursor of classic dissection with 30-day mortality of 20% and early death in 16%. May be due to ruptured vasa vasorum in medial layers leading to secondary communication with the lumen. See Figure 8.1.6 for a representation of acute aortic syndromes. Can be initiated by aortic wall infarction.

Outcome

- Progress to dissection in 21–47%
- Regress in 10%
- Resorption

Therapeutic options

Type A →Surgery
Type B →Medical management
Beta blocker use associated with improved outcome.
Age > 55 years at diagnosis associated with improved outcomes possibly due to more focal scars in the aortic wall therefore limiting spread of haematoma.
Watchful waiting/graft stent placement appropriate if distal aorta affected (i.e. Type B intramural haematoma) and if patient > 65 years.

Penetrating aortic ulcer

Occurs mostly in the descending thoracic and abdominal aorta in association with intramural haematoma. Result from progressive erosion of mural plaque penetrating the elastic lamina leading the separation of media layers. Can lead to intramural haematoma, penetration, and dissection. Repeat imaging may be required in uncomplicated Type B lesions.
Symptomatic penetrating atherosclerotic ulcers imply impending complications and should prompt detailed imaging.
Aim of treatment is to prevent progression to acute dissection and to prevent aortic rupture. Medical therapy under careful surveillance including pain relief and blood pressure control is usually indicated for uncomplicated Type B lesions (Class I Level C).
If a penetrating aortic ulcer occurs in the ascending aorta, surgery should be considered. (Class IIa Level C).
Treatment is usually offered (surgery/graft/stent) if width > 2 cm and depth > 1 cm.

Aortic pseudoaneurysm

Defined as a dilatation of the aorta due to disruption of *all* of the layers of the aortic wall with the resultant defect only being contained by the periaortic tissues.

Causes

Thoracic aorta—blunt trauma, rapid deceleration, iatrogenic (surgery, catheter-related interventions) and infections, e.g. mycotic aneurysms (rare).

Complications
- Aortic rupture—this occurs when the pressure within the pseudoaneurysm exceeds the pressure that is exerted by periaortic tissues
- Fistula formation
- Erosion of surrounding structures

Treatment
Surgery or catheter intervention if feasible.

Contained rupture of aortic aneurysm
Clinical suspicion in a patient with thoracic aortic aneurysm—acute onset chest/back pain, new or worsening pleural effusions with possible respiratory compromise, haemoptysis (aortobronchial fistula—rare), haematemesis (aorto-oesophageal fistula—rare).
Contained vs free rupture:

- Patients with a contained rupture are haemodynamically stable
- Patients with free rupture have disruption to all the layers of the aortic wall and massive haematoma formation. Unrestrained, death occurs rapidly.

Diagnosis
CT with a non-contrast phase to detect intramural haematoma followed by a contrast phase to identify the site and severity of leak.

Treatment
Urgent repair is recommended with endovascular repair (TEVAR) prioritized over open repair.

8.1.6 Genetic diseases affecting the aorta

General considerations
- Usually, autosomal dominant
- Either syndromic or non-syndromic
- Usually have more extensive involvement of the arterial tree than just the thoracic aorta
- Variable penetrance within families
- Cystic medial necrosis is a common pathological finding
- The common syndromic genetic conditions that are associated with thoraco-abdominal aortic dissection are presented in Table 8.1.8.

Non-syndromic familial thoracic aortic aneurysms and dissection
- Familial clustering seen in up to 19% of cases
- May be associated with BAV +/− persistent ductus arteriosus
- Usually autosomal dominant inheritance
- Various genetic mutations have been identified though it is rare to have overlap with the mutations found in syndromic forms of thoraco-abdominal aortic dissection.

Bicuspid aortic valve
- Common affecting 1–2% of the population.
- 9% of these have an affected first-degree relative and can be inherited in an autosomal dominant fashion
- In these families, some have thoracic aortic disease without BAV

Table 8.1.8 Genetic syndromes associated with thoracic aortic aneurysm and dissection.

Genetic syndrome	Common clinical features	Genetic defect	Diagnostic test
Marfan syndrome	Facial, skeletal, eye, cardiac, skin, spinal features	FBN1 mutations	Ghent oncology DNA sequencing
Loeys–Dietz syndrome	Clinical triad • Bifid uvula/cleft palate • Arterial tortuosity • Hypertelorism Other features • Skeletal features • Craniosynostosis • Aneurysms and dissections of other arteries	TGFBR1 TGFBR2	DNA for sequencing
Ehlers–Danlos Type (IV vascular form)	• Thin, fragile, and translucent skin • Typical facies (pinched and thin nose, thin lips, prominent ears, hollow cheeks, and tightness of the skin over the face). • Gastrointestinal rupture • Rupture of the gravid uterus • Rupture of medium to large sized vessels • Short stature • Primary amenorrhoea • BAV • Aortic coarctation	COL3A1	DNA for sequencing
Turner syndrome	• Webbed neck • Low-set ears • Low hairline • Broad chest • Wide carrying angle • Short stature • Congenital cardiac defects • Aortic abnormalities (coarctation of the aorta 12%, bicuspid aortic valve 30%) • Metabolic abnormalities (dyslipidaemia, glucose intolerance) • Hormonal abnormalities (ovarian failure)	45,X karyotype	Clinical findings and cytogenic analysis

Reproduced from Hiratzka LF, Bakris GL, Beckman JA, et al; American College of Cardiology Foundation/American Heart Association Task Force on Practice Guidelines; American Association for Thoracic Surgery; American College of Radiology; American Stroke Association; Society of Cardiovascular Anesthesiologists; Society for Cardiovascular Angiography and Interventions; Society of Interventional Radiology; Society of Thoracic Surgeons; Society for Vascular Medicine. 2010 ACCF/AHA/AATS/ACR/ASA/SCA/SCAI/SIR/STS/SVM guidelines for the diagnosis and management of patients with Thoracic Aortic Disease: a report of the American College of Cardiology Foundation/American Heart Association Task Force on Practice Guidelines, American Association for Thoracic Surgery, American College of Radiology, American Stroke Association, Society of Cardiovascular Anesthesiologists, Society for Cardiovascular Angiography and Interventions, Society of Interventional Radiology, Society of Thoracic Surgeons, and Society for Vascular Medicine. *Circulation*. 2010 Apr 6;121(13):e266–369. doi: 10.1161/CIR.0b013e3181d4739e with permission from Wolters Kluwer.

- 20% who underwent BAV at the Cleveland Clinic also had ascending aortic aneurysm repair
- 15% of patients with dissection have BAV

Other conditions associated with aortopathy

- Aberrant right subclavian artery
  i. Courses behind oesophagus and causes dysphagia as the artery enlarges (Kommerell diverticulum)
  ii. Aorta prone to aneurysm formation and dissection

- Coarctation of the aorta—associated with aortic dissection
- Right sided aortic arch—can cause either oesophageal or tracheal obstruction and Kommerell diverticulum may form

8.1.7 Aortitis

Definition
Inflammation of the aorta categorized by underlying aetiology:

- Infective syphilitic
- Infective non-syphilitic (bacterial/fungal)
- Non-infective—due to large vessel vasculitis or atherosclerosis

Determining the aetiology is critical as immunosuppressive therapy can worsen active infective processes.

Epidemiology
Incidence of giant cell arteritis 18.8/100,000/year with male: female 2:1 mean age 75 years.
Incidence of Takayasu arteritis much rarer, 0.4–1.0/1,000,000/year.
Non-infective large vessel vasculitis is the most common cause of aortitis.

Pathogenesis
Infective aortitis—microorganisms gain entry via a number of mechanisms:

- Haematogenous spread
- Direct invasion of the aortic wall
- Spread from nearby structures
- Secondary infection following trauma
- Septic emboli.

Bacterial and fungal infections can result in non-infectious vasculitis by generating immune complexes or cross-reactivity. This tends to occur in atherosclerotic lesions or aneurysms.
Tertiary syphilis is now rare but may be seen in immunocompromised patients. Can present with aortitis.
S. aureus is the most common gram positive species. Gram negative bacilli are less common but include Salmonella, Proteus, and E. coli. Autoimmune disorders can affect the blood supply to the vasa vasorum. The causes of aortitis in Takayasu's and Giant cell arteritis are unknown.

Clinical features
Non-specific features such as fatigue, malaise, arthralgia, low-grade fever, and raised inflammatory markers. Thoracic pain may be present in 60%.

- Look ill with mild fever
- Carotidynia suggests vascular inflammation
- Reduced/absent pulses, ocular disturbance, neurological deficits, claudication resulting in gangrene or myocardial infarction as a result of ostial involvement of a coronary artery
- Bruits over major arteries
- New AR due to aortitis related aneurysms of the ascending aorta

Therefore, picture may mimic infective endocarditis.

Diagnosis

- Suspect it basis on clinical presentation and imaging.
- Blood cultures important if infective causes as guide antibiotic choice.
- Inflammatory markers usually raised.
- CXR—can demonstrate opacities of different sizes.
- Angiography—used to be the gold standard.
- CT/MRI/TOE can all be used and have various advantages/disadvantages as already discussed.

Therapeutic management

- Prognosis related to aetiology and thus to potential complications.
- Worst scenario is aneurysm formation with resultant rupture.
- Treat according to cause with antibiotics or immunosuppressive therapy.
- Optimal management of infective non-syphilitic is early surgical intervention with a prolonged course of antibiotics.
- Mortality for infected aneurysms treated with antibiotics alone is approximately 90%.
- Endovascular repair has yet to be used widely for non-infective vasculitic causes

8.1.8 Aortic atheromatous disease: thrombotic or cholesterol emboli

Tend to affect the aortic arch and descending aorta.
Aortic intimal atheroma can be classified as follows:

- Grade I: normal
- Grade II: increased intimal echo-density without lumen irregularity
- Grade III: increased intimal echo-density with single or multiple well-defined atheromatous plaque of 3 mm
- Grade IV: atheroma > 3 mm or mobile or ulcerated plaque.

Reduced aortic compliance is thought to be an early expression of atheromatous disease.
Spontaneous emboli generally results from Grade IV intima.
Iatrogenic emboli with wires and catheters or during surgery can loosen mobile plaque and result in cholesterol crystal showers in 1–2% of cardiac catheterization cases with cutaneous signs or renal insufficiency.
Risk factors are same as for coronary heart disease.
Aortic plaque of 4 mm (measured as aortic wall thickness) is thought to be a major risk factor for stroke with an annual occurrence of 12%.

Diagnosis

TOE is usually the first modality. CT and MRI can be used thereafter.

Management

Risk factor modification and antiplatelet medication.
Anticoagulation is controversial.
Statins are superior to anticoagulation and antiplatelets in those with atheromatous disease in the aorta and at high-risk of emboli.

Further reading

Erbel R, Aboyans V, Boileau C, Bossone E, Bartolomeo RD, Eggebrecht H, Evangelista A, Falk V, Frank H, Gaemperli O, Grabenwöger M, Haverich A, Iung B, Manolis AJ, Meijboom F, Nienaber CA, Roffi M, Rousseau H, Sechtem U, Sirnes PA, Allmen RS, Vrints CJ; ESC Committee for Practice Guidelines. 2014 ESC Guidelines on the diagnosis and treatment of aortic diseases: Document covering acute and chronic aortic diseases of the thoracic and abdominal aorta of the adult. The Task Force for the Diagnosis and Treatment of Aortic Diseases of the European Society of Cardiology (ESC). *Eur Heart J*. 2014 Nov 1;35(41):2873–926. doi: 10.1093/eurheartj/ehu281. Epub 2014 Aug 29. Erratum in: Eur Heart J. 2015 Nov 1;36(41):2779.

Hiratzka LF, Bakris GL, Beckman JA, Bersin RM, Carr VF, Casey DE Jr, Eagle KA, Hermann LK, Isselbacher EM, Kazerooni EA, Kouchoukos NT, Lytle BW, Milewicz DM, Reich DL, Sen S, Shinn JA, Svensson LG, Williams DM; American College of Cardiology Foundation/American Heart Association Task Force on Practice Guidelines; American Association for Thoracic Surgery; American College of Radiology; American Stroke Association; Society of Cardiovascular Anesthesiologists; Society for Cardiovascular Angiography and Interventions; Society of Interventional Radiology; Society of Thoracic Surgeons; Society for Vascular Medicine. 2010 ACCF/AHA/AATS/ACR/ASA/SCA/SCAI/SIR/STS/SVM guidelines for the diagnosis and management of patients with Thoracic Aortic Disease: a report of the American College of Cardiology Foundation/American Heart Association Task Force on Practice Guidelines, American Association for Thoracic Surgery, American College of Radiology, American Stroke Association, Society of Cardiovascular Anesthesiologists, Society for Cardiovascular Angiography and Interventions, Society of Interventional Radiology, Society of Thoracic Surgeons, and Society for Vascular Medicine. *Circulation*. 2010 Apr 6;121(13):e266–369. doi: 10.1161/CIR.0b013e3181d4739e. Epub 2010 Mar 16. Erratum in: Circulation. 2010 Jul 27;122(4):e410.

Nienaber CA, Akin I, Erbel,R, Haverich A. Diseases of the Aorta and Trauma to the Aorta and the Heart. In A John Camm, TF Lüscher, PW Serruys (Eds.), *The ESC Textbook of Cardiovascular Medicine, 2 edn, The European Society of Cardiology*. Oxford, 2009; online edn, Oxford Academic, 1 Aug. 2009.

8.2

Trauma to the aorta or heart

David Wilson

TABLE OF CONTENTS

8.2.1 Traumatic rupture of the aorta 723
  Aetiology 723
  Pathogenesis 723
  Clinical presentation 723
  Diagnosis 723
  Management 723

8.2.2 Trauma to the heart 724
  Aetiology 724
  Pathology 724
  Penetrating trauma 724
  Blunt trauma 725

8.2.1 Traumatic rupture of the aorta

Aetiology

21% mortality due to aortic rupture in 613 fatalities of road traffic accidents. 8000 victims per year in the USA.

Pathogenesis

Any deceleration injury, e.g. fall from height, road collision etc., can result in traumatic aortic rupture. Airbags and seatbelts do not protect against lateral impact and this mechanism typically results in partial laceration of the lesser curve of the distal part of the aortic arch just above the isthmus, the most common site of rupture (80–95%).

Clinical presentation

Signs may be non-specific and there are often other significant injuries which may require attention.
Symptoms: dyspnoea and chest pain, syncope, dysphagia, hoarseness.
Signs: hypotension, hypertension (17%), paraplegia, pulse differences, 'pseudo-coarctation'—results from a flap which acts as a ball valve resulting in partial obstruction and upper limb hypertension. Hypertension can also be due to stretching/stimulation of the cardiac plexus.
Normal physical findings are seen in 5–14% of cases.

Diagnosis

Early diagnosis important as aortic rupture has an unpredictable and unfavourable outcome.
CT is the accepted cornerstone in contemporary practice.

Management

Almost all patients with traumatic aortic rupture are candidates for surgical repair.
Early surgery carries high mortality (15–20%) and morbidity risk, the most significant of which is paraplegia.

There are 2 groups of populations with traumatic aortic rupture:

- Unstable with signs of active bleeding
- Stable

Survival in the first group is low 17.7% and is much higher in the second group (fatal rupture 4.5% in first 72 hours) and therefore major intervention can be put on hold.

After diagnosis, therapeutic hypotension with vasodilators and beta blockers is mandatory.

In selected patients with pseudo-aneurysm or haematoma the risk of rupture is low (same as a 'normal' pseudo-aneurysm) as fibrous tissue will develop. Blood pressure should be maintained at 90 mmHg and fluid replacement should be limited to prevent extension and rupture. Patients are often intubated. Surgical repair of the aorta electively improves outcomes.

Operative measures include either a primary suture repair or Dacron graft repair.

Endovascular repair is another option which avoids thoracotomy and heparin and risk of destabilizing other traumatic lesions in the lungs, brain, and abdomen. This has rapidly become the treatment of choice in traumatic aortic rupture.

8.2.2 Trauma to the heart

Aetiology

Most common cause of death for men < 40 years.

Common causes of penetrating injuries include knives, ice picks, stilettos, screwdrivers, and shot gun wounds etc.

Most common cause of blunt cardiac injury is high speed deceleration injury.

Pathology

As a result of:

- Penetrating trauma—i.e. stab wound to right ventricle resulting in haemopericardium
- Blunt trauma—compression between sternum and vertebrae resulting in possible rupture of free wall, malignant arrhythmias, damage to epicardial coronary vessels.

Penetrating trauma

Clinical signs

Varies from very mild to severe and depends on:

- Site of injury
- Signs of cardiac tamponade
- Signs of shock (hypovolaemic/cardiogenic).

1–20% of asymptomatic patients may develop complications of blunt cardiac trauma that require treatment.

Investigations

Screening asymptomatic patients

- Cardiac enzymes—no rise in levels is reassuring.
- ECG—a normal ECG has a very good negative predictive value for complications. If present further investigations are not necessary.
- Echocardiography.

Symptomatic patients for diagnosis of tamponade:

- Subxiphoid access with TTE is standard
- Sternotomy/thoracotomy should be used if patients present with penetrating thoracic injury and diagnostic tools unable to show definitive evidence of cardiac penetration, e.g. in presence of haemopneumothorax.

Management

- Life-threatening condition—may need thoracotomy in the emergency department
- Left anterolateral lateral thoracotomy incision of choice
- If mechanism due to stabbing and knife *in situ* it must only be removed in theatre
- Digital occlusion of haemorrhage if possible
- Simple closure if possible
- Transfer to operating room if injuries more complex, i.e. require CABG etc.

Classification—Scale I–VI according to American Association of Surgery of Trauma and its Organ Injury Scaling Committee. Uncertainties remain of its use in an emergency setting.

Prognosis

Dependent upon premorbid condition and nature of injury.

- Missile injury more severe than stab wounds 16 vs 65% 2-year survival
- In penetrating trauma, patients who are alive in the emergency department have 80% survival
- Myocardial contusion—benign
- Poor prognosis if thoracotomy required for blunt trauma

Blunt trauma

Clinical signs

Vary depending of nature and force of injury.

Investigations

As per penetrating trauma.

Management—medical

- Early mobilization and rehabilitation after monitoring if young and normal/slightly abnormal ECGs
- Anticoagulants/fibrinolytics are contraindicated due to increased risk of bleeding
- Arrhythmias, e.g. atrial fibrillation, treated with digoxin
- Analgesia—avoid NSAIDs
- Corticosteroids—only in Dressler's
- Angiotensin converting enzyme inhibitors/beta blockers—no evidence of use.

Further reading

Erbel R, Aboyans V, Boileau C, Bossone E, Bartolomeo RD, Eggebrecht H, Evangelista A, Falk V, Frank H, Gaemperli O, Grabenwöger M, Haverich A, Iung B, Manolis AJ, Meijboom F, Nienaber CA, Roffi M, Rousseau H, Sechtem U, Sirnes PA, Allmen RS, Vrints CJ; ESC Committee for Practice Guidelines. 2014 ESC Guidelines on the diagnosis and treatment of aortic diseases: Document covering acute and chronic aortic diseases of the thoracic and abdominal aorta of the adult.

The Task Force for the Diagnosis and Treatment of Aortic Diseases of the European Society of Cardiology (ESC). *Eur Heart J*. 2014 Nov 1;35(41):2873–926. doi: 10.1093/eurheartj/ehu281. Epub 2014 Aug 29. Erratum in: Eur Heart J. 2015 Nov 1;36(41):2779.

Nienaber CA, Akin I, Erbel, R, Haverich A. Diseases of the Aorta and Trauma to the Aorta and the Heart. In A John Camm, TF Lüscher, PW Serruys (Eds.), *The ESC Textbook of Cardiovascular Medicine, 2 edn, The European Society of Cardiology*. Oxford, 2009; online edn, Oxford Academic, 1 Aug. 2009.

8.3

Peripheral artery disease

Marcus Brooks and Fjalar Elvarsson

TABLE OF CONTENTS

8.3.1 Peripheral arterial disease 728
    Epidemiology 728
    Pathophysiology 728
    Symptoms 728
    Assessment 728
    Classification 728
    Imaging 728
    Lifestyle and support 729
    Medication 730
    Coronary angiography, intervention, and
        CABG in patients with LEAD 730
8.3.2 Diabetic foot disease 730
8.3.3 Intermittent claudication 730
    Diagnosis 730
    Supervised exercise programme 731
    Other interventions 731
    Prognosis 731
8.3.4 Critical limb threatening ischaemia 731
    Diagnosis 731
    Intervention 732
    Prognosis 732
8.3.5 Acute limb ischaemia 732
    Pathophysiology 732
    Diagnosis 732
    Intervention 733
    Prognosis 733
8.3.6 Upper limb ischaemia 733
    Epidemiology and pathophysiology 733
    Assessment 733
    Imaging 734
    Intervention 734
8.3.7 Extra-cranial carotid artery disease 734
    Definitions 734
    Epidemiology and pathophysiology 734
    Assessment 734
    Imaging 734

    Lifestyle and medication 735
    Asymptomatic carotid stenosis 735
8.3.8 Carotid artery stenting (CAS) 736
    Symptomatic carotid stenosis 736
8.3.9 Carotid intervention prior to cardiac
       surgery 737
    Prognosis 737
8.3.10 Vertebral artery disease 737
8.3.11 Abdominal aortic aneurysm 737
    Definition 737
    Epidemiology and pathophysiology 737
    Assessment 738
    Imaging 738
    Lifestyle and support 738
    Medication 738
    Population based screening 738
    Genetic testing 738
    Surveillance 738
    Intervention 738
    Ruptured AAA 739
    Prognosis 739
8.3.12 Mesenteric artery disease 739
    Definitions 739
    Epidemiology and pathophysiology 739
    Diagnosis 740
    Assessment and imaging 740
    Lifestyle, support, and medication 740
    Intervention 740
    Prognosis 740
8.3.13 Renal artery stenosis 740
    Epidemiology and pathophysiology 740
    Diagnosis 741
    Imaging 741
    Lifestyle, support, and medication 741
    Intervention 741
    Prognosis 741

8.3.1 Peripheral arterial disease

Epidemiology
- Advancing age, smoking, and Type II diabetes mellitus important risk factors
- Common cause of reduced walking distance and can lead to limb loss
- 25–33% of people with peripheral arterial disease are asymptomatic

Pathophysiology
- Majority atherosclerotic associated with cerebral, cardiac and/or renal arterial disease
- Other causes; embolus, popliteal artery aneurysm, aortic dissection, or vasculitis
- Diabetes and renal failure are associated with arterial wall stiffening and calcification, both affect the below knee (crural) arteries

Symptoms
- Assess a patient for peripheral arterial disease when
    - Symptoms of intermittent claudication (IC) or critical limb threatening ischaemia (CLTI)
    - Aged over 50 years old with diabetes
    - Non-healing ulcer or wound
    - Unexplained leg pain
- Patients with CLTI may have
    - Rest pain severe enough to stop them sleeping at night
    - Lower limb tissue loss, ulceration, or necrosis

Assessment
- Abdominal aorta palpated for an abdominal aortic aneurysm
- Presence or absence of femoral, popliteal, and foot pulses recorded
- Feet examined for ulceration or necrosis
- Patients with CLTI may demonstrate Buerger's sign; white limb (pallor) on elevation and redness (rubor) on dependency
- Listen for bruits over abdominal aorta and femoral arteries
- Ankle-Brachial Index (ABI) measurement (Figure 8.3.1) for the diagnosis of PAD: Positive predictive value of ABI < 0.8 is > = 95%. Negative predictive value ABI > 1.1 is > 99%
- ABI may be falsely elevated with diabetes, end-stage renal failure or in the elderly
- In patients with incompressible ankle arteries or ABI > 1.4, alternative methods such as the toe–brachial pressure index, Doppler waveform analysis or pulse volume recording are indicated
- Undertake treadmill test if normal resting ABI with history highly suggestive of PAD

Classification
- The two classification systems for CLTI are those of Fontaine and Rutherford (Table 8.3.1)

Imaging
- Duplex ultrasound provides both anatomical and physiological (velocity) information
- Duplex may be performed in outpatient clinic, but interpretation is operator dependent
- MR angiography avoids ionizing radiation and is useful when the arteries are calcified
- CT angiography is alternative and is best for imaging the aorta and iliac arteries

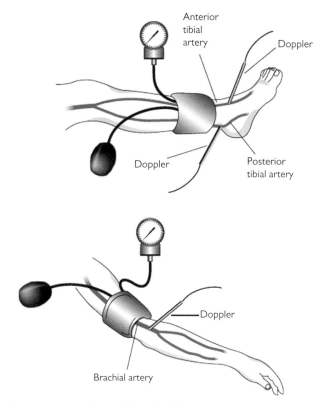

Figure 8.3.1 How to measure the Ankle-Brachial Index

Aboyans V, Ricco JB, Bartelink MEL, et al; ESC Scientific Document Group. 2017 ESC Guidelines on the Diagnosis and Treatment of Peripheral Arterial Diseases, in collaboration with the European Society for Vascular Surgery (ESVS): Document covering atherosclerotic disease of extracranial carotid and vertebral, mesenteric, renal, upper and lower extremity arteriesEndorsed by: the European Stroke Organization (ESO)The Task Force for the Diagnosis and Treatment of Peripheral Arterial Diseases of the European Society of Cardiology (ESC) and of the European Society for Vascular Surgery (ESVS). *Eur Heart J.* 2018 Mar 1;39(9):763–816. doi: 10.1093/eurheartj/ehx095. © European Society of Cardiology. With permission from Oxford University Press.

Lifestyle and support

- Offer patients written information about diagnosis and steps they can take to reduce:
    - Cardiovascular events (stroke and MI)
    - Progression to worsening intermittent claudication or limb loss
- Explain modifiable risk factors; cigarette smoking, diabetes, and cholesterol
- Explain benefit of regular walking

Table 8.3.1 Classification of severity of peripheral arterial disease (PAD).

Fontaine		Rutherford	
I	Asymptomatic	0	Asymptomatic
IIa	Mild claudication (> 200 m)	1	Mild claudication (> 200 m)
IIb	Moderate-severe claudication	2	Moderate claudication
III	Ischaemic rest pain	3	Severe claudication (< 50 m)
IV	Ulceration or gangrene (necrosis)	4	Ischaemic rest pain Minor tissue loss
		5	Ulceration or gangrene
		6	

Medication

- Intervention to reduce future cardiovascular events
  - Lipid modification with statin therapy
  - Clopidogrel is first-line antiplatelet treatment (24% lower risk of CV events than aspirin in patients with peripheral arterial disease; CAPRIE, *Lancet* 1996)
  - Low dose (75 mg) aspirin is recommended is patients unable to take clopidogrel
  - No additional benefit has been shown for dual therapy (CHARISMA, *NEJM* 2006) or mono therapy with ticagrelor (EUCLID, *NEJM* 2017)
  - Antiplatelet therapy is not routinely indicated in patients with asymptomatic lower extremity arterial disease (LEAD)
  - In patients with PAD and AF, OAC is recommended when the CHA_2DS_2-VASc score is ≥ 2
- For patient with ischaemic rest pain, analgesia, usually opioids, is key
- No contraindication to the use of beta blockers
- The COMPASS-PAD trial showed that compared with aspirin alone, low-dose rivaroxaban 2.5 mg bd + aspirin 100 mg od was associated with a reduction in major adverse cardiac events (7–5%) and major adverse limb events (2.6–1.5%) but with an increase in major bleeding (2–3%).
- The VOYAGER PAD trial showed that in patients with PAD who had undergone revascularization rivaroxaban 2.5 mg BD plus aspirin, as compared to aspirin alone, was associated with better composite cardio-vascular outcomes (including reduced acute limb ischaemia) but with as increased bleeding risk on one of two definitions used.

Coronary angiography, intervention, and CABG in patients with LEAD

- Radial artery access recommended for coronary angiography
- In patients undergoing CABG, screening for LEAD with an ABI (or TBI) should be considered—in advanced LEAD, the great saphenous vein should be spared where possible (may be required for autologous bypass, associated with delayed wound healing)
- Screening for lower and upper extremity arterial disease is indicated in patients undergoing TAVI or other structural interventions requiring an arterial approach

8.3.2 Diabetic foot disease

- Diabetic patients are at high risk of limb loss due to the combination of ischaemia, neuropathy, and/or infection
- A new foot ulcer in a patient with diabetes should be seen in a multidisciplinary foot clinic within 24 hours as deterioration can be rapid
- Specialist multidisciplinary foot team ideally includes Diabetologist, Specialist nurse, Podiatrist, Vascular Surgeon, Orthopaedic Surgeon, Orthotist, and Microbiologist

8.3.3 Intermittent claudication

Diagnosis

- Typical symptoms
  - Reproducible cramp-like pain in calves, thighs, or hips/buttocks brought on by walking and relieved by rest
  - Predictable walking distance, usually shorter if walking up incline
- Aorto-iliac disease may be associated with impotence (LeRiche's syndrome)
- Edinburgh claudication questionnaire is a specific and sensitive assessment tool
- Differential diagnoses; sciatica, spinal canal stenosis, venous claudication, entrapment syndromes, chronic compartment syndrome, and musculoskeletal problems

Supervised exercise programme
- Participation in a supervised exercise programme, i.e. 2 hours of supervised exercise a week for 3 months, should ideally be offered to patients with intermittent claudication
- Randomized controlled trials report 50–200% 2-year improvement in walking distance; a benefit similar to that following angioplasty or stenting, and at lower cost
- Exercise should be to the point of maximal pain and include stretching exercises

Other interventions
- Cardiovascular risk reduction and walking advice in asymptomatic patients
- Referral for revascularization, in symptomatic patient when
    - Received lifestyle modification advice and information
    - Risk factors addressed and on appropriate antiplatelet and statin therapy
    - Failed to improve their walking distance with supervised exercise (if available)
    - Impaired quality of life due to reduced mobility
    - Suitable target lesion for durable treatment
- Revascularization of aorto-iliac occlusive lesions
    - An endovascular-first strategy is recommended for short (i.e. < 5 cm) lesions
    - Aorto-iliac occlusions: aorto-(bi)femoral bypass should be considered if fit for surgery (consider endovascular surgery if severe co-morbidities)
    - Ilio-femoral occlusions: hybrid procedure (iliac stenting + femoral endarterectomy/bypass) should be considered
    - Open surgery should be considered in fit patients with an aortic occlusion extending up to the renal arteries
- Revascularization of femoro-popliteal occlusive lesions
    - An endovascular-first strategy with primary stent implantation is recommended in short (i.e. < 25 cm) lesions
    - In patients not at high risk for surgery, bypass surgery is indicated for long (i.e. > 25 cm) superficial femoral artery lesions when an autologous vein is available (great saphenous vein conduit of choice) and life expectancy is > 2 years
- Naftidofuryl oxalate or cilostazol moderately increase walking distance. Consider if no revascularization option, and stop after 3-6 months if no improvement
- Benefit of intermittent pneumatic compression devices are under investigation

Prognosis
- Patients with intermittent claudication have increased mortality from CV disease
- In respect of their legs, over a 5-year period
    - 10–20 % develop worsening symptoms
    - 5–10 % develop critical limb ischaemia
    - Only 1–2% will have amputation, this increases to 5% in people with diabetes
- Worse outcome for both angina and acute coronary syndrome

8.3.4 Critical limb threatening ischaemia

Diagnosis
- Ischaemic rest pain and/or tissue loss with ulceration or gangrene and severely reduced ankle (or toe) pressure (Ankle pressure < 55 mmHg, Toe pressure < 30 mmHg)
- Rest pain is typically relieved only by opiate analgesia or dependency

Intervention
- Intervention should be planned by a multidisciplinary team including Vascular Surgeon, Anaesthetist, Radiologist, specialist nurses, and ideally a Rehabilitation physician
- Urgent revascularization is needed, with better outcomes if performed within 2 weeks
- Decision between angioplasty and bypass is based on patient specific factors
  - Pattern of disease
  - Fitness for procedure; bypass carries greater peri-procedural risk of MI or death
  - Patient choice, early morbidity/mortality vs durability of intervention
  - Availability of vein; BASIL I (*Lancet* 2005) showed patency of bypass using vein best option, with vein graft patency reported as high as 90% at 4 years.
  - BASIL II (Lancet, 2023) reported that for infra-popliteal revascularisation, a best endovascular first revascularisation strategy was associated with a better amputation-free survival, largely driven by fewer deaths in endovascular than surgery treatment group.
- Iloprost (prostaglandin) infusion may be of benefit in reducing pain and achieving ulcer healing in patients unsuitable for revascularization
- Trials of gene therapy have failed to show benefit in preventing limb loss or death
- Percutaneous atherectomy, lumbar chemical sympathectomy and spinal cord stimulation are currently under investigation in clinical trials

Prognosis
- Approximately 1 in 3 patients will require amputation within one year
- 5–20% of patients presenting with CLTI undergo primary amputation
  - Unsuitable for revascularization
  - Neurological impairment
  - Do not walk
- Three-fold excess risk of heart attack, stroke, or CV death
- Mortality after lower-limb bypass is 3% by 30 days and up to 20% by 1 year
- 15% of patients undergoing below-knee amputation will have undergone contra-lateral major amputation by 2 years

8.3.5 Acute limb ischaemia

Pathophysiology
- Sudden onset of limb ischaemia due either to *in situ* thrombus or embolus
- Causes *in situ* thrombosis
  - Progression of peripheral arterial disease
  - *In situ* thrombosis of an arterial stent or lower limb bypass graft
- Causes of embolus
  - Atrial fibrillation
  - Recent MI with mural LV thrombus

Diagnosis
- Sudden onset of painful, pale, pulseless, and perishing cold limb
- Limb may appear pale (white) or mottled (purple/white)
- Sensation and movement may be lost

Table 8.3.2 Modified from Rutherford classification of acute limb ischaemia.

Grade	Category	Sensory loss	Motor loss	Prognosis
I	Viable	None	None	No immediate threat
IIA	Marginally threatened	None or minimal (toes)	None	Salvageable, revascularize 1–2 weeks
IIB	Immediately threatened	More than toes	Mild/Moderate	Salvageable, revascularize immediately
III	Irreversible	Profound, anaesthetic	Profound paralysis	Major tissue loss or amputation, Irreversible nerve damage

- Calf tenderness indicates possible muscle necrosis
- Table 8.3.2 shows grades of acute limb ischaemia modified from Rutherford classification

Intervention

- Heparin and analgesics are indicated as soon as possible
- Urgent revascularization indicated if there is neurological deficit
- Embolus; surgical embolectomy, percutaneous clot retrieval, or catheter-directed thrombolysis
- *In-situ* thrombus; surgical bypass or catheter-directed thrombolysis. Angioplasty is best avoided acutely because of the high risk of distal embolization
- Primary amputation when significant irreversible tissue (delayed presentation)
- When limb viable but severely ischaemic for ≥ 6 hours then fasciotomies performed

Prognosis

- Amputation may be necessary in up to 40% of cases
- 30-day mortality as high as 30%

8.3.6 Upper limb ischaemia

Epidemiology and pathophysiology

- Upper limb ischaemia is less common than lower limb ischaemia
- Most common cause is steal syndrome from dialysis access fistula
- Atherosclerosis most common in origins of subclavian and brachiocephalic arteries
- Other causes
    - Thoracic outlet syndrome; compression of subclavian artery by cervical or first rib
    - 'Steal syndrome' due to subclavian artery origin stenosis or occlusion
    - Buerger's disease in younger smokers
    - Takayasu's vasculitis; vasculitis affecting aortic arch and head vessels
    - Connective tissue disease (i.e. scleroderma)

Assessment

- History of symptoms of exertional cramp-like muscle pain, ulceration, or digital gangrene
- Subclavian steal symptoms; dizziness, vertigo, blurred vision, confusion, or syncope on arm exertion
- Examination of upper limb pulses and auscultation for supra-clavicular bruits
- Blood pressure in arms at rest; a difference of ≥ 15 mmHg suggests significant stenosis

Imaging

- Arterial Duplex; whilst subclavian artery origin cannot be imaged directly damped distal flow patterns will indicate if proximal stenosis
- MR angiography or CT angiography (as for peripheral arterial disease)
- Diagnosis of arterial thoracic outlet syndrome needs imaging in both resting (arm by side) and provocation (abducted and externally rotated) positions
- Catheter angiography is useful in distal disease (i.e. Buerger's disease)

Intervention

- Lifestyle modification and CV medication first line
- Smoking cessation is essential for patient with Buerger's disease
- Thoracic outlet syndrome and subclavian artery stenosis managed conservatively unless
    - Upper limb ischaemia—ulceration or severe symptoms
    - Internal mammary artery coronary graft
    - Bilateral stenosis, to allow accurate blood pressure measurement
- Thoracic outlet surgery requires resection of the first and/or cervical ribs
- Angioplasty or surgical bypass alternatives depending on distribution of disease
- Iloprost (prostaglandin) infusion can be effective for relief of distal ischaemia and pain

8.3.7 Extra-cranial carotid artery disease

Definitions

- Symptom duration ≤ 24 hours with no imaging evidence of an ischaemic lesion on diffusion weighted MRI imaging is termed a transient ischaemic attack (TIA)
- Imaging evidence of an ischaemic lesion or symptoms of > 24 hours duration are termed a stroke.
- A minor stroke is defined by a National Institute of Health Stroke Scale (NIHSS) score of 5 or less.
- Carotid artery disease is considered symptomatic if TIA or stroke within preceding 6 months (Rothwell et al., *Lancet* 2005)

Epidemiology and pathophysiology

- Approximately two-thirds of patients with an ischaemic stroke have mild deficits
- Of all strokes, 10–15% follow thromboembolism from a 50–99% internal carotid artery stenosis
- Other causes of extra-cranial disease; post-radiation, vasculitis, dissection, and fibro-muscular dysplasia (FMD)
- Stroke/TIA resulting from embolization and low flow symptoms are rare

Assessment

- Patients presenting with focal hemispheric symptoms (facial weakness, dysphasia, or limb weakness) or amaurosis fugax (transient visual loss) should be assessed by a Neurologist or Stroke Physician or Ophthalmologist to assess if carotid territory event
- The modified Rankin scale is a useful tool for recording the severity of a stroke (Table 8.3.3)
- The presence of a carotid bruit is poor predictor of the severity of carotid artery stenosis
- Other causes of stroke (i.e. atrial fibrillation) must also be considered

Imaging

- The gold-standard assessment to grade carotid artery stenosis is Duplex ultrasound
- Care should be taken and degree of stenosis reported using two different classification systems; ECST and NASCET (Figure 8.3.2)

Table 8.3.3 Modified Rankin Scale.

Modified Rankin Scale	
0	No symptoms
1	No significant disability despite symptoms; able to carry out all usual duties and activities
2	Slight disability: unable to carry out all previous activities, but able to look after own affairs without assistance
3	Moderate disability: requiring some help, but able to walk without assistance
4	Moderately severe disability: unable to walk without assistance and unable to attend to own bodily needs without assistance
5	Severe disability: bedridden, incontinent, and requiring constant nursing care
6	Dead

Bonita R, Beaglehole R. 'Modification of Rankin Scale: Recovery of motor function after stroke'. *Stroke* 1988 Dec;19(12):1497–500

- When Duplex not available, or when difficult to interpret due to heavy calcification, then MR angiography or CT angiography should be obtained
- Intra-arterial angiography is rarely used as invasive and carries a small risk of stroke

Lifestyle and medication

- Cardiovascular risk reduction
- Clopidogrel is first-line antiplatelet agent
- SPARCL showed Atorvastatin 80 mg vs placebo reduced 5-year stroke relative risk of stroke by 33% (*NEJM* 2006)
- Tight blood pressure control is essential

Asymptomatic carotid stenosis

- Asymptomatic stenosis may be discovered incidentally, i.e. work up for cardiac surgery or contra-lateral side when carotids imaged for symptoms

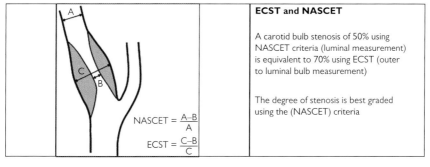

Figure 8.3.2 Definition of carotid bulb stenosis as defined by European Carotid Surgery Trial (ECST, 1998) and North American Symptomatic Carotid Endarterectomy Trial (NASCET, 1999)

Source data from Randomised trial of endarterectomy for recently symptomatic carotid stenosis: final results of the MRC European Carotid Surgery Trial (ECST). *Lancet*. 1998 May 9;351(9113):1379–87.

AND

Ferguson GG, Eliasziw M, Barr HW, et al. The North American Symptomatic Carotid Endarterectomy Trial : surgical results in 1415 patients. *Stroke*. 1999 Sep;30(9):1751–8. doi: 10.1161/01.str.30.9.1751.

- Two large RCTs, ACAS (1995) and ACST (2004, 2010), have shown benefit for intervention in asymptomatic patients with carotid stenosis of ≥ 60%, provided peri-operative stroke risk is < 3% and patient has at least 5 years life expectancy to gain benefit
    - **ACAS**: Aggregate 5-year ipsilateral stroke and any perioperative stroke or death estimated at 5.1% for endarterectomy and 11.0% for controls (risk reduction 53%)
    - **ACST**: Aggregate 5-year ipsilateral stroke and any peri-operative stroke or death 6.9% vs 10.9% at 5 years and 13.4% vs 17.9% at 10 years
- Absolute benefit in both trials was less in women than in men
- Contemporary data on TIA/minor stroke suggests that the risk of an event in a patient with asymptomatic carotid disease is now less than 2% per annum (by 2010 in the ACST control group the annual stroke risk was 1.4%)
- There is therefore uncertainty regarding the number of patients with asymptomatic disease to treat to prevent one stroke; some vascular surgeons no longer routinely offer carotid endarterectomy (CEA) for asymptomatic disease. Patients should be fully involved in treatment decisions.
- Current ESC guidelines: In 'average surgical risk' patients with asymptomatic 60–99% stenosis, CEA should be considered in the presence of clinical and/or more imaging characteristics that may be associated with an increased risk of late ipsilateral stroke, provided documented peri-operative stroke/death rates are < 3% and the patient's life expectancy is > 5 years (Class IIa, A). Consider CAS if high risk for CEA
- Two RCTs are currently recruiting asymptomatic patients;
    - **ASCT 2**; randomizing to CEA vs CAS
    - **ECST 2;** randomising both asymptomatic and low risk patients to medical therapy vs CEA vs CAS

8.3.8 Carotid artery stenting (CAS)

- Outcomes for CAS are broadly similar to carotid endarterectomy (CEA)
    - in symptomatic patients rate of minor stroke is greater (Relative risk, 1.48)
    - in symptomatic patients rate of myocardial infarction is lower (RRR, 0.43)
    - No difference in rates of ipsilateral major stroke in symptomatic or symptomatic patients in most recent trails either at 30 days or during follow-up
- CAS preferable in patients with a 'hostile neck' (i.e. previous radiation, recurrent stenosis). Appropriate attention to access vessels and the status of the aortic arch is required for optimal results
- Dual antiplatelet therapy (aspirin/clopidogrel) is mandatory for at least 1 month after CAS
- CAS is associated with larger cerebral emboli with MRI changes. This has been associated with cognitive impairment post CAS
- The use of embolic protection devices should be considered (Class IIa, C)

Symptomatic carotid stenosis

- Thrombolysis and mechanical thrombectomy are increasingly used acutely in stroke
- TIA and amaurosis fugax; clopidogrel 75 mg with or without aspirin 75 mg
- Stroke; aspirin 300 mg prescribed for 2 weeks and converted to clopidogrel long term
- Blood pressure control; Aggressive control should be avoided in the first 2–3 weeks following stroke to maximize cerebral perfusion
- 70–99% stenosis: CEA recommended (ESC guidelines, Class I, A), provide documented procedural death/stroke rate is < 6%

- 50–69% stenosis: CEA should be considered (Class IIa, A), provided the documented procedural death/stroke rate is < 6%. If there are adverse anatomical features or medical co-morbidities CAS should be considered
- Revascularization of should be performed as soon as possible, preferably within 14 days of symptom onset

8.3.9 Carotid intervention prior to cardiac surgery

- Incidence of significant carotid stenosis varies between 3% and 22%
- Peri-operative strokes are multi-factorial. Potential causes include emboli from the aortic arch, atrial fibrillation, reduced cardiac output, or hypercoagulability
- Recent (< 6 month history of TIA/stroke)
    - Duplex ultrasound screening is recommended
    - Carotid revascularization should be considered in patients with 50–99% stenosis with CEA as the first choice (ESC guidelines, Class IIa, B)
- Carotid revascularization is not recommended in neurologically asymptomatic patients with 70–99% stenosis

Prognosis

- In symptomatic disease, with significant stenosis, the risk of recurrent TIA or stoke within 30 days can be as high as 10–30%
- In asymptomatic disease, with significant stenosis, annual stroke risk in patient on optimal medical therapy is 1–1.5% per annum
- CARS score (Carotid Stenosis Risk Reduction Tool, Rothwell et al., *Lancet* 2013) can be used to predict risk in individual symptomatic patients

8.3.10 Vertebral artery disease

- Clinically significant vertebral arterial disease uncommon
- Imaging of the vertebral artery is technically challenging (fine-cut CTA or MRA)
- First-line management is with antiplatelet agent and statin therapy
- Indications for intervention, via an endovascular approach,
    - Recurrent posterior circulation events with significant vertebral artery stenosis
    - Refractory vertebra-basilar ischaemia

8.3.11 Abdominal aortic aneurysm

Definition

- AAA is defined as dilatation greater or equal to 30 mm in either anterior-posterior or transverse planes
- Aortic diameters of 2.5–2.9 cm are described as sub-aneurysmal

Epidemiology and pathophysiology

- Disease of aging, more common in men
- Men with sub-aneurysmal dilatation are at increased risk of future AAA
- Active smoking is an independent risk factor for both AAA growth and rupture

- Rarer causes; infection (mycotic), chronic dissection and connective tissue disease (Marfans, Ehlers–Danlos, or Loeys–Dietz)

Assessment
- General assessment includes lifestyle and history of co-morbid conditions
- May be palpable in epigastrium on abdominal palpation
- Tenderness is an indication for imaging and intervention
- Lower limb pulses, checking specifically for occlusive disease and popliteal aneurysm
- Rarely, athero-emboli are seen in the feet

Imaging
- Ultrasound is the preferred imaging modality for asymptomatic patients
    - Note: maximum diameter may be reported as inner-inner wall or outer-outer wall
- CT angiography used to assess symptomatic patients, or when intervention planned
- Assessment of the entire aorta is recommended at baseline and during follow-up
    - Detection of thoracic aortic aneurysm or atheroma
    - Detection of coexisting malignancy (e.g. lung cancer in smokers)

Lifestyle and support
- Patients with aortic aneurysm are at increased risk of CV disease
- Smoking cessation

Medication
- Statins and ACE-inhibitor likely to be of benefit
- Aspirin, or alternate antiplatelet agent should be prescribed

Population-based screening
- Has been shown to reduce aneurysm related mortality by half in men aged > 65 years invited for ultrasound scan (MASS Trial, 2002)
- Not cost effective in women (SWAN trial, 2017)
- ESC guidelines recommend screening all men > 65 years with ultrasound (Class 1, A), may be considered in women > 65 years with a history of current/past smoking (Class IIb, C)

Genetic testing
- Genetic testing should be considered for first-degree relatives of patients presenting at a young age (< 50 years old), with healthy 'at risk' individuals surveyed every 5 years

Surveillance
- Surveillance is safe in asymptomatic patient with AAA diameter of < 55 mm and slow (< 10 mm/year) growth (UKSAT, 2007)
- Recommended surveillance intervals are shown in Table 8.3.4.

Intervention
- Surgical repair is indicated when AAA symptomatic, expands to 5.5 cm or grows rapidly (> 10 mm/year)
- ESVS guidelines recommend a threshold for repair of 5.0 cm in women
- If anatomically suitable for EVAR, either open or endovascular repair is recommended in patients with acceptable surgical risk

Table 8.3.4 Surveillance intervals for abdominal aortic aneurysm.

ESC guidelines	UK AAA Screening Programme
Every 3 years for AAA 30–39 mm	Annually for AAA 30–44 mm
Every 2 years for AAA 40–44 mm	
Annually for AAA 45–54 mm	3 monthly for AAA 45–54 mm

- If AAA is anatomically unsuitable for EVAR, open aortic repair is indicated
- In patients with asymptomatic AAA who are unfit for open repair, EVAR along with best medical therapy may be considered (8 year follow-up from EVAR 2 trial showed that intervention reduced AAA related but not all-cause mortality)

Ruptured AAA

- Immediate abdominal CTA is recommended to confirm diagnosis and plan treatment
- If anatomically suitable for EVAR, either open repair or EVAR recommended; the IMPROVE trial showed no difference in early survival but better medium-term quality of life for patients treated with EVAR.
- For EVAR, local anaesthesia is preferred if the patient will tolerate (IMPROVE trial)

Prognosis

- Median diameter at which AAA rupture occurs is 8 cm maximum diameter
- Female gender and advanced age increase both the risk of rupture, for any aneurysm size, and the risk associated with operative repair
- Endovascular repair requires long-term surveillance because of risk of
  - Loss of seal between graft and aortic wall (Type I endoleak)
  - Side branch sac perfusion (Type II endoleak)
  - Loss of graft integrity due to component separation or fatigue (Type III endoleak)
  - Progressive sac expansion without cause (Type IV endoleak)

8.3.12 Mesenteric artery disease

Definitions

- Acute mesenteric ischaemia (AMI) is defined as abrupt cessation of mesenteric blood flow with symptoms that vary onset from minutes (embolus) to hours (atherosclerosis)
- Chronic mesenteric ischaemia (CMI) is defined by a duration of at least 3 months
- Non-occlusive mesenteric ischaemia (NOMI) develops in the context of unwell patient; causes include hypovolaemia, cardiac failure, vasoconstrictive inotropes, and raised abdominal compartment pressure

Epidemiology and pathophysiology

- Acute mesenteric ischaemia is the cause of approximately 1% of acute abdominal presentations; incidence is higher in an older population
- Stenosis of the coeliac axis, superior mesenteric artery, inferior mesenteric artery, or renal arteries is most commonly due to atherosclerotic disease (95%)

- Arterial dissection and arterial embolism, usually to superior mesenteric artery (SMA), are other important causes
- The median arcuate ligament of the diaphragm can cause extrinsic compression of the coeliac axis; this is rarely physiologically important but can rarely cause pain and weight loss in young patients (MALS, Median Arcuate Ligament Syndrome)
- Vasculitis is a rare cause
- Mesenteric aneurysm can result from trauma, pancreatitis, and connective tissue disorder

Diagnosis
- The typical presentation of CMI includes postprandial pain, fear of eating, nausea or vomiting, or unexplained diarrhoea due to malabsorption (ischaemic gastropathy)
- Weight loss may be severe, but is not always present
- AMI presents as an acute abdomen, is typical to have pain of greater severity than would be expected from the abdominal signs
- Biomarkers (lactate, D-dimer) are neither specific nor sensitive

Assessment and imaging
- CT angiography using fine cuts ($<=1$ mm) and ideally including a portal venous phase to assess bowel viability
- Duplex ultrasound can be used in CMI and for surveillance post intervention
- Angiography with selective mesenteric vessel catheterization, is the gold standard for diagnosis of NOMI; reflux of contrast (suggestive of distal infarction) predicts mortality

Lifestyle, support, and medication
- Cardiovascular risk factor modification
- Aspirin and lipid modifying medication prescribed

Intervention
- The superior mesenteric artery is the most important artery to revascularize
    - Angioplasty with or without stenting is first-line management
    - Mesenteric bypass if angioplasty unsuccessful or not technically feasible
- In the acute setting in patients with signs of peritonitis laparotomy is mandatory; this should be repeated if viability of bowel is questionable, usually after 18–24 hours

Prognosis
- Mesenteric ischaemia has a poor prognosis, only 50% of patients survive 5 years
- Prognosis is worse when all 3 mesenteric vessels are diseased

8.3.13 Renal artery stenosis

Epidemiology and pathophysiology
- Up to 20% of patients undergoing coronary angiography have renal artery stenosis (RAS)
- RAS is most commonly due to atherosclerotic disease over 50 years of age
- Fibro-muscular dysplasia (FMD) is alternative cause in younger, typically female, patients
- Systemic vasculitis or aortic dissection may also affect the renal arteries

Diagnosis

- The signs and symptoms related to renal artery stenosis are
  - Flash pulmonary oedema
  - Worsening of previously controlled hypertension
  - Early onset hypertension (age < 30 years or severe hypertension aged < 55 years)
  - Refractory hypertension (despite three anti-hypertensive medications)
  - Progressive deterioration in renal function, particularly related to ACE inhibitor/ARB
- An abdominal bruit may be audible

Imaging

- Duplex ultrasound is the first-line test
- CT angiogram or MR angiogram used to plan intervention

Lifestyle, support, and medication

- Beta blockers, ACE-I, ARB, diuretics, and calcium channel blockers are effective for hypertension except ACE inhibitors and ARBs contraindicated in bilateral RAS or solitary kidney with RAS
- Aspirin and lipid-modifying medication should be prescribed if atherosclerosis

Intervention

- The aim of treatment is to preserve renal function and control hypertension
- The ASTRAL (*NEJM* 2009), STAR (*Ann Int Med* 2009) and CORAL (*NEJM* 2014) trials failed to show benefit of angioplasty as compared to controls
- Renal revascularization does not generally improve blood pressure, renal or CV outcomes in patients with atherosclerotic renal artery disease—routine revascularization is not recommended
- Consider balloon angioplasty with bailout stenting in renal arterial FMD causing hypertension and/or renal impairment (ESC Guidelines Class IIa, B)
- Consider balloon angioplasty with bailout stenting in selected patients with RAS and unexplained recurrent congestive heart failure or sudden pulmonary oedema (ESC Guidelines Class IIb, C)
- Surgical revascularization should be considered for patients with complex anatomy, after a failed endovascular procedure or during open aortic surgery

Prognosis

- Renal artery stenosis is associated with risk of renal failure and need for dialysis
- Patients with RAS on dialysis have particularly poor long-term survival

Further reading

Aboyans V, Ricco JB, Bartelink MEL, Björck M, Brodmann M, Cohnert T, Collet JP, Czerny M, De Carlo M, Debus S, Espinola-Klein C, Kahan T, Kownator S, Mazzolai L, Naylor AR, Roffi M, Röther J, Sprynger M, Tendera M, Tepe G, Venermo M, Vlachopoulos C, Desormais I; ESC Scientific Document Group. 2017 ESC Guidelines on the Diagnosis and Treatment of Peripheral Arterial Diseases, in collaboration with the European Society for Vascular Surgery (ESVS): Document covering atherosclerotic disease of extracranial carotid and vertebral, mesenteric, renal, upper and lower extremity arteries. Endorsed by: the European Stroke Organization (ESO)The Task Force for the Diagnosis and Treatment of Peripheral Arterial Diseases of the European Society of Cardiology (ESC) and of the European Society for Vascular Surgery (ESVS). *Eur Heart J.* 2018 Mar 1;39(9):763–816. doi: 10.1093/eurheartj/ehx095

Becquemin JP. Management of the Diseases of Mesenteric Arteries and Veins: Clinical Practice Guidelines of the European Society for Vascular Surgery (ESVS) [corrected]. *Eur J Vasc Endovasc Surg.* 2017 Apr;53(4):455–7. doi: 10.1016/j.ejvs.2017.03.009. Erratum in: Eur J Vasc Endovasc Surg. 2018 Dec;56(6):920.

Erbel R, Aboyans V, Boileau C, Bossone E, Bartolomeo RD, Eggebrecht H, Evangelista A, Falk V, Frank H, Gaemperli O, Grabenwöger M, Haverich A, Iung B, Manolis AJ, Meijboom F, Nienaber CA, Roffi M, Rousseau H, Sechtem U, Sirnes PA, Allmen RS, Vrints CJ; ESC Committee for Practice Guidelines. 2014 ESC Guidelines on the diagnosis and treatment of aortic diseases: Document covering acute and chronic aortic diseases of the thoracic and abdominal aorta of the adult. The Task Force for the Diagnosis and Treatment of Aortic Diseases of the European Society of Cardiology (ESC). *Eur Heart J.* 2014 Nov 1;35(41):2873–926. doi: 10.1093/eurheartj/ehu281. Epub 2014 Aug 29. Erratum in: Eur Heart J. 2015 Nov 1;36(41):2779

Lower limb peripheral arterial disease: Evidence Update November 2014: A summary of selected new evidence relevant to NICE clinical guideline 147 'Lower limb peripheral arterial disease: diagnosis and management' (2012) [Internet]. London: National Institute for Health and Care Excellence (UK); 2014

Moll FL, Powell JT, Fraedrich G, Verzini F, Haulon S, Waltham M, van Herwaarden JA, Holt PJ, van Keulen JW, Rantner B, Schlösser FJ, Setacci F, Ricco JB; European Society for Vascular Surgery. Management of abdominal aortic aneurysms clinical practice guidelines of the European society for vascular surgery. *Eur J Vasc Endovasc Surg.* 2011 Jan;41 Suppl 1:S1–S58. doi: 10.1016/j.ejvs.2010.09.011

Ricotta JJ, Aburahma A, Ascher E, Eskandari M, Faries P, Lal BK; Society for Vascular Surgery. Updated Society for Vascular Surgery guidelines for management of extracranial carotid disease. *J Vasc Surg.* 2011 Sep;54(3):e1–31. doi: 10.1016/j.jvs.2011.07.031. Erratum in: J Vasc Surg. 2012 Mar;55(3):894.

8.4

Thromboembolic disease

Jay Suntharalingam and James Harper

TABLE OF CONTENTS

8.4.1 Deep and superficial venous thrombosis 743
  Definition 743
  Epidemiology 743
  Risk factors 743
  Pathophysiology 744
  Clinical presentation 744
  Diagnosis of DVT 744
  Treatment of DVT 744
8.4.2 Pulmonary embolism 748
  Epidemiology 748
  Pathophysiology 748
  Clinical presentation 748
  Diagnosis of PE 749
  Risk stratification 749
  Investigation for acute pulmonary embolism 750
  Treatment of PE 750
  Duration of treatment 754
  PE in pregnancy 754
8.4.3 Chronic thromboembolic pulmonary hypertension (CTEPH) 755
  Definition 755
  Epidemiology 755
  Pathology 755
  Clinical presentation 756
  Diagnosis 756
  Treatment 757

8.4.1 Deep and superficial venous thrombosis

Definition
- Deep veins of the lower extremity: iliac, femoral, popliteal, tibial, peroneal, soleal, and gastrocnemial veins.
- Proximal deep veins include iliac, femoral, and popliteal veins
- Superficial veins of the lower extremity: great saphenous vein, small saphenous vein, non-saphenous veins

Epidemiology
- Annual incidence of VTE 104–183 per 100,000 person years
- Annual incidence of DVT without PE 45–117 per 100,000 person years

Risk factors
- Inherited thrombophilia
  - Factor V Leiden mutation
  - Prothrombin gene mutation
  - Protein C and S deficiency
  - Antithrombin deficiency

- Acquired thrombophilia
    - Malignancy (lung, pancreas, colorectal, kidney, and prostate most common)
    - Antiphospholipid antibodies
    - Lupus anticoagulant
    - Surgery in previous 3 months
    - Immobility for more than 48 hours
    - Current hospitalization
    - Hospitalisation in previous 3 months
    - Infection in previous 3 months
    - Trauma
    - Pregnancy
    - Intravenous drug use
    - Drugs: oral contraceptive, HRT, tamoxifen, bevacizumab, glucocorticoids, testosterone
- Systemic disease
    - Renal: CKD, nephrotic syndrome, renal transplant
    - Liver disease
    - Haematological: heparin-induced thrombocytopenia, hyperviscosity syndromes (hypergammaglobulinaemia and hyperfibrinogenaemia), myeloproliferative disease
    - Gastrointestinal: inflammatory bowel disease

Pathophysiology

- Virchow's triad—endothelial injury, venous stasis, and hypercoagulability predispose to thrombus formation
- Platelet aggregation, activation of the clotting cascade with subsequent fibrin clot formation

Clinical presentation

- Pain, swelling, and erythema of affected extremity
- Examination findings:
    - Difference in calf or thigh diameter
    - Dilated superficial veins
    - Tenderness along course of vein
    - Compartment syndrome with arterial compromise and venous gangrene can be seen with large proximal DVT
- The above signs and symptoms are all non-specific for making a diagnosis of DVT

Diagnosis of DVT

- If DVT is suspected use a 2-level Wells score for DVT (Table 8.4.1)
- DVT likely: 2 points or more
- DVT unlikely: 1 point or less
- Diagnosis is made by compression or duplex venous ultrasound

Treatment of DVT

Treatment of proximal DVT

- Initial treatment with either:
    - High-dose apixaban (10 mg BD for 7 days) or rivaroxaban (15 mg BD for 21 days)
    - Low molecular weight heparin (LMWH) for 5–10 days followed by either dabigatran 150 mg BD or edoxaban 60 mg OD.

Table 8.4.1 The Wells score for DVT.

Clinical feature	Points
Active cancer (treatment ongoing, within 6 months, or palliative)	1
Paralysis, paresis, or recent plaster immobilization of the lower extremities	1
Recently bedridden for 3 days or more or major surgery within 12 weeks requiring general or regional anaesthesia	1
Localized tenderness along the distribution of the deep venous system	1
Entire leg swollen	1
Calf swelling at least 3 cm larger than asymptomatic side	1
Pitting oedema confined to the symptomatic leg	1
Collateral superficial veins (non-varicose)	1
Previously documented DVT	1
An alternative diagnosis is at least as likely as DVT	−2

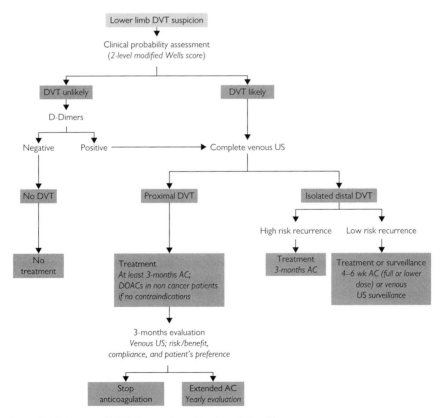

Figure 8.4.1 Proposed DVT diagnostic and treatment algorithm
AC = anticoagulation, DOAC = Direct oral anticoagulation
Mazzolai L, Aboyans V, Ageno W, et al. Diagnosis and management of acute deep vein thrombosis: a joint consensus document from the European Society of Cardiology working groups of aorta and peripheral vascular diseases and pulmonary circulation and right ventricular function. *Eur Heart J.* 2018 Dec 14;39(47):4208–4218. doi: 10.1093/eurheartj/ehx003 © European Society of Cardiology. With permission from Oxford University Press.

- LMWH followed by a vitamin K antagonist (VKA) to achieve INR 2–3. LMWH should be continued for 5 days or until the INR is greater than or equal to 2 for at least 24 hours, whichever is longer.
- Unfractionated heparin (UFH) for those with severe renal impairment (eGFR < 30 ml/min) or high bleeding risk
- Apixaban, rivaroxaban, and LMWH can be used as interim anticoagulation while awaiting leg vein ultrasound
- Subsequent treatment with either:
  - a direct oral anticoagulant (DOAC) (apixaban 5 mg BD, dabigatran 150 mg BD, edoxaban 60 mg OD or rivaroxaban 20 mg OD)
  - VKA to achieve INR 2–3
- In the absence of contraindications, a DOAC is recommended in preference to VKA in the absence of malignancy
- Dabigatran requires dose adjustment in the elderly. Edoxaban requires dose adjustment in renal impairment.
- DVT in association with malignancy can be treated with either LMWH or a DOAC
- Catheter directed thrombolytic therapy can be considered if the following are present:
  - Symptomatic iliofemoral DVT
  - Patients with good functional status and life expectancy > 1 year
  - Low bleeding risk
  - Duration of symptoms < 14 days

Treatment of distal DVT

- If severe symptoms and risk factors for extension of clot (positive D-dimer, extensive thrombus, thrombus close to proximal veins, DVT involving > 1 calf vein, bilateral distal DVTs, male sex, age > 50, no reversible provoking risk factor, active cancer, history of prior VTE inpatient status) are present, start anticoagulation as for proximal DVT.
- In the absence of severe symptoms and risk factors for clot extension, management options include a shorter duration of anticoagulation (4–6 weeks) or serial imaging of the leg veins at 1 and 2 weeks (or sooner if there is concern).
- Anticoagulation should be started if the thrombus extends but remains within the distal veins (grade 2C evidence) or if the thrombus extends into the proximal veins (grade 1B evidence).
- The same anticoagulants should be used as for proximal DVT.

Vena caval filters

- A temporary IVC filter can be inserted in patients with proximal DVT who cannot have anticoagulation. The filter should be removed when they become eligible for anticoagulation
- Caval filters can be considered for recurrent proximal DVT while on anticoagulation only after increasing target INR to 3–4 or switching to LMWH

Compression stockings

- Role of compression stockings to reduce the incidence of post thrombotic syndrome is uncertain but their use remains a reasonable option for controlling symptoms of acute proximal DVT

Duration of treatment

- Provoked proximal DVT (major transient risk factor for VTE present in the last 3 months, e.g. surgery, trauma, immobility, pregnancy, or puerperium or hormonal treatment).
  - Anticoagulation for 3 months

- Unprovoked proximal DVT
  - At least 3 months anticoagulation
  - Extended anticoagulation (no stop date) should be considered based upon the balance of bleeding risk and risk of VTE recurrence
  - Risk scores to help inform this decision include the Vienna prediction model, DASH score and HERDOO-2 score (Table 8.4.2).
  - Proximal DVT, obesity, old age, male sex, non blood group O, early post-thrombotic syndrome development, persistence of residual vein thrombosis at ultrasound, and high D-dimer values are all risk factors for DVT recurrence.
  - Patients taking extended anticoagulation should be re assessed annually, taking into account bleeding risk, risk of VTE recurrence, and patient preference.
  - The HAS-BLED score can be used to assess bleeding risk on anticoagulation (1 point scored for each of: hypertension, abnormal renal function, abnormal lover function, age ≥ 65, previous stroke, medication usage predisposing to bleeding, labile INR, alcohol use, and previous major bleeding or predisposition to bleeding). Consideration should be given to stopping anticoagulation if the HAS-BLED score is ≥ 4 and cannot be modified.
  - Low dose apixaban (2.5 mg BD) and rivaroxaban (10 mg OD) have been shown to be effective options as extended anticoagulation. Aspirin may be considered as extended treatment if anticoagulation is contraindicated.
- Distal DVT
  - If provoked and decision has been made to treat, then treatment should be for 3 months
  - If unprovoked, treatment for 3 months with assessment of risks and benefits of extended anticoagulation at that time
- Recurrent DVT
  - For second unprovoked DVT in those with low or moderate bleeding risk extended anticoagulation should be used
  - In those with high bleeding risk treat with 3 months anticoagulation

Table 8.4.2 Clinical prediction rules for assessing risk of VTE recurrence after first episode of unprovoked VTE.

Score	Vienna prediction model	DASH score	HERDOO-2
Parameters	D-dimer at 3 weeks and 3, 9, 15, and 24 months after stopping anticoagulation	Abnormal D-dimer 3–5 weeks after stopping anticoagulation	Abnormal D-dimer before stopping anticoagulation
	Male sex	Male sex	Post-thrombotic symptoms
	VTE location	Age < 50	Age ≥ 65
		VTE not associated with oestrogen-progesterone therapy in women	BMI ≥ 30
Comments	Nomograms available to calculate risk of VTE recurrence	Patients with score ≤ 1 have annual recurrence rate of 3.1%	Applies to women only. Patients with score ≤ 1 have annual recurrence rate of 1.3%

Mazzolai L, Aboyans V, Ageno W, et al. Diagnosis and management of acute deep vein thrombosis: a joint consensus document from the European Society of Cardiology working groups of aorta and peripheral vascular diseases and pulmonary circulation and right ventricular function. *Eur Heart J.* 2018 Dec 14;39(47):4208–4218. doi: 10.1093/eurheartj/ehx003 © European Society of Cardiology. With permission from Oxford University Press.

- Malignancy associated DVT
  - Anticoagulation for 3–6 months with review at this point to determine need for extended treatment

8.4.2 Pulmonary embolism

Epidemiology
- Major cause of morbidity, mortality, and hospitalisation
- Incidence of PE +/− DVT 29–78 per 100,000 person years
- 34% of VTE deaths present with sudden fatal PE

Pathophysiology
- Thrombus present within the pulmonary arterial tree. The thrombus most commonly arises from a coexistent DVT.
- PE causes both circulatory disturbances and abnormal gas exchange
- In acute PE there is a sudden increase in the pulmonary vascular resistance
- Compensatory mechanisms occur which aim to improve pulmonary arterial flow and maintain systemic BP:
  - Right ventricular (RV) pressure and volume increases leading to increased RV wall myocyte stretch. This initially increases RV output via the Frank Starling mechanism.
  - Neurohormonal activation with inotropic and chronotropic effects
  - Systemic vasoconstriction
- The unconditioned thin RV myocardium is unable to generate a mean pulmonary artery pressure (mPAP) > 40 mmHg
- In massive PE the increase in RV myocardial oxygen demand leads to RV ischaemia and decreased RV output
- The thin-walled RV is unable to generate the pulmonary pressure required to overcome pulmonary vascular resistance and becomes volume loaded.
- Bowing of the intraventricular septum occurs thus compromising LV filling in early diastole and further reduces cardiac output.
- RV coronary perfusion is compromised and worsening RV ischaemia results
- Thrombus within the pulmonary arterial tree causes ventilation perfusion mismatching and hypoxaemia. This further contributes to RV ischaemia and a decreasing cardiac output
- Ultimately systemic hypotension, cardiogenic shock, and death result from the failing right ventricle and compromised left ventricle.

Clinical presentation
- Dyspnoea
- Pleuritic chest pain represents pleural irritation secondary to pulmonary infarction—this tends to occur with more peripheral, low volume emboli and thus may not cause significant hypoxia.
- Anginal chest pain may be present reflecting RV ischaemia in large PE.
- Haemoptysis
- Syncope or pre-syncope due to haemodynamic disturbances in large PE
- Cough
- Fever
- Symptoms are non-specific and may be mild in otherwise healthy individuals even if large PE is present.

Diagnosis of PE
- Chest X-ray
    - May be normal—signs are all non-specific
    - Atelectasis
    - Pleural effusion—typically small and can be bilateral
    - Fleishner's sign: enlarged pulmonary artery
    - Westermark's sign: regional oligaemia
    - Hampton hump: peripheral wedge-shaped opacity due to lung infarction
- ECG
    - Non-specific changes
    - Sinus tachycardia or AF
    - RBBB and anterior T-wave inversion reflecting RV strain
    - $S_1Q_3T_3$ pattern is rare
- CT pulmonary angiography (CTPA) is the test of choice to confirm diagnosis
- Pulmonary embolism rule out criteria (PERC rule)
    - If clinical suspicion of PE is low, the PERC rule can be used to identify patients who do not need further investigation for PE
    - All of the following criteria must be met in order to identify patients who do not require further investigation: age < 50, heart rate < 100 beats/min, oxygen saturation > 94% on room air, no unilateral leg swelling, no haemoptysis, no recent trauma or surgery, no previous VTE, and no oral hormonal use.
- D-dimer testing
    - Age adjustment can be used, as for DVT.
    - Quantitative point-of-care tests can be used for those with a low pre-test probability of PE

Risk stratification
- PESI (PE severity index) and sPESI (simplified PESI) clinical risk scores predict mortality (Table 8.4.3).
    - PESI
        - Class I ≤ 65 points: very low 30 day mortality risk 0–1.6%
        - Class II 66–85 points: low mortality 1.7–3.5%
        - Class III 86–105 points: moderate mortality 3.2–7.1%
        - Class IV 106–125 points: high mortality 4–11.4%
        - Class V > 125 points: very high mortality 10–24.5%
    - sPESI
        - 0 points 30 day mortality risk 1%
        - ≥ 1 point 30 day mortality risk 10.9%
    - Indicators of RV dysfunction
        - Echo: RV dilatation, increased RV:LV diameter ratio, increased TR jet velocity, decreased TAPSE
        - CTPA: RV enlargement, straightening of the intraventricular septum, and reflux of contrast into IVC
        - Biomarkers of RV dysfunction and myocardial injury: BNP, NT-proBNP, and troponin
    - Shock or hypotension
        - Systolic BP < 90 mmHg for 15 minutes or more

Table 8.4.3 PESI and sPESI scores.

Clinical parameter	Original version	Simplified version
Age	Age in years	1 point if > 80
Male sex	+10	-
Cancer	+30	1 point
Chronic heart failure	+10	1 point
Chronic pulmonary disease	+10	
Pulse ≥ 110/min	+20	1 point
Systolic BP < 100 mmHg	+30	1 point
Respiratory rate > 30/min	+20	-
Temperature < 36°C	+20	-
Arterial oxygen saturation < 90%	+20	1 point
Altered mental status	+60	-

Konstantinides SV, Meyer G, Becattini C, et al; ESC Scientific Document Group. 2019 ESC Guidelines for the diagnosis and management of acute pulmonary embolism developed in collaboration with the European Respiratory Society (ERS). *Eur Heart J.* 2020 Jan 21;41(4):543–603. doi: 10.1093/eurheartj/ehz405. © European Society of Cardiology. With permission from Oxford University Press.

- Combined early mortality risk assessment
    - **High**: shock or hypotension present (systolic blood pressure < 90 mmHg or requirement for vasopressor to maintain blood pressure ≥ 90 mmHg or blood pressure drop ≥ 40 mmHg for longer than 15 minutes not caused by arrhythmia, hypovolaemia, or sepsis)
    - **Intermediate:**
        - **Intermediate-high**: PESI class III–IV or sPESI ≥1 or ≥1 Hestia criterion (Table 8.4.4) fulfilled OR/AND RV dysfunction on imaging AND positive biomarkers
        - **Intermediate-low**: PESI class III–IV or sPESI ≥1 or ≥ 1 Hestia criterion (Table 8.4.4) fulfilled OR/AND RV dysfunction on imaging AND negative biomarkers
    - **Low**: PESI class I or II or sPESI 0 or no Hestia criteria fulfilled. Assessment of RV dysfunction and biomarkers optional. If assessed both are negative

Investigation for acute pulmonary embolism

- Proposed diagnostic algorithm for patients with suspected high-risk PE, i.e. presenting with shock or hypotension—Figure 8.4.2
- Proposed diagnostic algorithm for patients with suspected pulmonary embolism without haemodynamic—Figure 8.4.3
- For investigation of intermediate and low risk PE, the 2-level Wells score for suspected PE can be utilized (Table 8.4.5)
    - PE likely if more than 4 points: CTPA to confirm diagnosis
    - PE unlikely if 4 points or less: D-dimer blood test can be done (CTPA if positive, consider alternative diagnosis if negative)

Treatment of PE

- High risk PE (with shock or hypotension)
    - Systemic thrombolytic treatment if bleeding risk not high
    - Alteplase, streptokinase, and urokinase are approved agents

Table 8.4.4 Hestia criteria. Absence of all risk factors indicates eligibility for outpatient management.

Is the patient haemodynamically unstable?	Yes/No
Is thrombolysis or embolectomy necessary?	Yes/No
Active bleeding or high risk of bleeding?	Yes/No
More than 24 hours of oxygen supply to maintain saturation > 90%?	Yes/No
Is PE diagnosed during anticoagulant treatment?	Yes/No
Severe pain needing intravenous pain medication for > 24 hours?	Yes/No
Medical or social reason to remain in hospital > 24 hours	Yes/No
Does the patient have creatinine clearance < 30 ml/min?	Yes/No
Does the patient have severe liver impairment (discretion of clinician)	Yes/No
Is the patient pregnant?	Yes/No
Does the patient have a documented history of heparin-induced thrombocytopenia?	Yes/No

Source data from Howard LSGE, Barden S, Condliffe R, et al. British Thoracic Society Guideline for the initial outpatient management of pulmonary embolism (PE). *Thorax.* 2018 Jul;73(Suppl 2):ii1–ii29. doi: 10.1136/thoraxjnl-2018-211539.

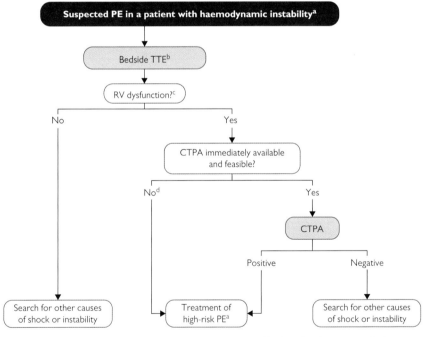

Figure 8.4.2 Diagnostic algorithm for patients with suspected high-risk pulmonary embolism presenting with haemodynamic instability. aSee text for definition of haemodynamic instability and high-risk PE. bAncillary bedside imaging tests may include TOE, which may detect emboli in the pulmonary artery and its main branches; and bilateral venous compression ultrasonography, which may confirm DVT and thus VTE. cIn the emergency situation of suspected high-risk PE, this refers mainly to a RV/LV diameter ratio >1.0. dIncludes the cases in which the patient's condition is so critical that it only allows bedside diagnostic tests. In such cases, echocardiographic findings of RV dysfunction confirm high-risk PE and emergency reperfusion therapy is recommended
Konstantinides SV, Meyer G, Becattini C, et al; ESC Scientific Document Group. 2019 ESC Guidelines for the diagnosis and management of acute pulmonary embolism developed in collaboration with the European Respiratory Society (ERS). *Eur Heart J.* 2020 Jan 21;41(4):543–603. doi: 10.1093/eurheartj/ehz405. © European Society of Cardiology. With permission from Oxford University Press.

8.4 Thromboembolic disease

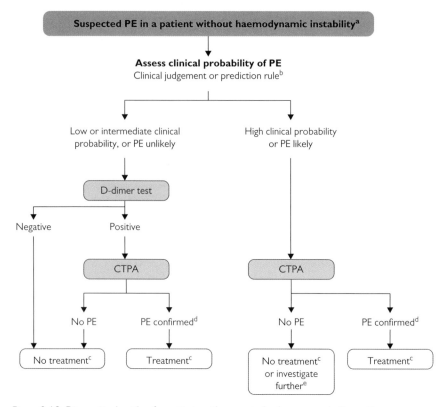

Figure 8.4.3 Diagnostic algorithm for patients with suspected pulmonary embolism without haemodynamic instability. [a]The proposed diagnostic strategy for pregnant women with suspected acute PE is discussed later in text. [b]Two alternative classification schemes may be used for clinical probability assessment, i.e. a three-level scheme (clinical probability defined as low, intermediate, or high) or a two-level scheme (PE unlikely or PE likely). When using a moderately sensitive assay, D-dimer measurement should be restricted to patients with low clinical probability or a PE-unlikely classification, while highly sensitive assays may also be used in patients with intermediate clinical probability of PE due to a higher sensitivity and negative predictive value. Note that plasma D-dimer measurement is of limited use in suspected PE occurring in hospitalised patients. [c]Treatment refers to anticoagulation treatment for PE. [d]CTPA is considered diagnostic of PE if it shows PE at the segmental or more proximal level. [e]In case of a negative CTPA in patients with high clinical probability, investigation by further imaging tests may be considered before withholding PE-specific treatment.

Konstantinides SV, Meyer G, Becattini C, et al; ESC Scientific Document Group. 2019 ESC Guidelines for the diagnosis and management of acute pulmonary embolism developed in collaboration with the European Respiratory Society (ERS). Eur Heart J. 2020 Jan 21;41(4):543–603. doi: 10.1093/eurheartj/ehz405. © European Society of Cardiology. With permission from Oxford University Press.

- Concomitant treatment with unfractionated heparin (UFH). UFH infusion should be stopped during administration of streptokinase or urokinase. UFH administration should be delayed if LMWH or fondaparinux has already been given.
- If high bleeding risk is present, systemic thrombolysis has failed or if shock is likely to cause death before systemic thrombolysis works, further options include:
  - Catheter-assisted thrombus removal
  - Catheter-directed thrombolysis
  - Surgical embolectomy

Table 8.4.5 2-level Wells score for suspected PE.

Clinical feature	Points
Clinical signs and symptoms of DVT (minimum of leg swelling and pain with palpation of the deep veins)	3
An alternative diagnosis is less likely than PE	3
Heart rate > 100 beats per minute	1.5
Immobilization for more than 3 days or surgery in the previous 4 weeks	1.5
Previous DVT/PE	1.5
Haemoptysis	1
Malignancy (on treatment, treated in the last 6 months, or palliative)	1

- Once stabilized ongoing oral anticoagulation as per intermediate and low-risk PE
- Intermediate and low-risk PE
  - Interim anticoagulation with LMWH, fondaparinux, rivaroxaban, apixaban, or UFH for those with severe renal impairment (eGFR < 30 ml/min) while awaiting results of diagnostic tests.
  - Subsequent treatment with a vitamin K antagonist or DOAC
  - Rivaroxaban, dabigatran, apixaban, or edoxaban are recommended DOACs
  - If a vitamin K antagonist is used, parenteral anticoagulation should be continued for 5 days or until the INR has been greater than or equal to 2 for at least 24 hours, whichever is longer. Target INR for treatment is 2–3.
  - Treatment with dabigatran 150 mg BD or edoxaban 60 mg OD should be preceded by 5–10 days of LMWH, UFH, or fondaparinux
  - Treatment with rivaroxaban (15 mg BD for 21 days followed by 20 mg OD) or apixaban (10 mg BD for 7 days followed by 5 mg BD) can be started directly or after 1–2 days of LMWH, UFH, or fondaparinux
  - A DOAC is recommended in preference to VKA in the absence of malignancy
  - PE in association with malignancy can be treated with a DOAC or LMWH. LMWH is preferred in patients with gastrointestinal cancer due to bleeding risk with DOACs.
  - Outpatient management of low risk PE:
    - Consider patients with confirmed PE who are classified as low risk (PESI class I or II or sPESI score of 0 or those who meet the Hestia criteria—Table 8.4.4) for outpatient management.
    - Patients assessed as low risk by PESI or sPESI should have a set of clinical and social exclusion criteria applied to confirm suitability for outpatient management.
    - Patients with suspected PE who are classified as low risk, may be treated with anticoagulation with subsequent outpatient imaging within 24 hours when same-day diagnostic imaging is not possible.
    - Where CT or echocardiography has identified RV dilatation in a patient who is otherwise suitable for outpatient management, negative cardiac biomarkers may be used to identify patients suitable for outpatient management
    - Patients with confirmed PE who are being treated as an outpatient should be offered either LMWH followed by dabigatran or edoxaban or a single-drug regime of either apixaban or rivaroxaban.
    - Patients with suspected PE who are being managed as an outpatient may be treated with LMWH, apixaban, or rivaroxaban pending diagnosis.

Duration of treatment
- Provoked PE
  - Major transient risk factor for VTE present in the last 3 months, e.g. surgery, trauma, immobility, pregnancy or puerperium, or hormonal treatment.
  - Anticoagulation for 3 months
- Unprovoked PE
  - At least 3 months anticoagulation
  - Extended anticoagulation (no stop date) for those with low or moderate bleeding risk.
  - Rivaroxaban 20 mg OD, dabigatran 150 mg BD or apixaban 5 mg BD should be considered as alternatives to VKA for patients needing extended anticoagulation
  - A reduced dose of rivaroxaban (10 mg OD) or apixaban (2.5 mg BD) can also be considered for extended anticoagulation after 6 months of full dose treatment.
  - Patients taking extended anticoagulation should be re assessed annually, taking into account bleeding risk, risk of VTE recurrence, and patient preference.
- Malignancy associated PE
  - Anticoagulation for 3–6 months with review at this point to determine need for extended treatment
- Recurrent PE
  - For second unprovoked PE in those with low or moderate bleeding risk extended anticoagulation should be used
- Subsegmental PE
  - If no proximal DVT is present and low clinical risk for VTE recurrence surveillance is recommended
  - Anticoagulate if high risk for VTE recurrence

PE in pregnancy
- PE in pregnancy is a leading cause of maternal mortality
- Breathlessness is a common phenomenon in pregnancy hence this symptom should be interpreted with caution
- Investigation
  - D-dimer use is not recommended in pregnancy
  - There is insufficient evidence to recommend the use of pre-test probability scoring (Wells score) in pregnancy
  - Baseline ECG and chest X-ray should be performed
  - In women with signs and symptoms of DVT, compression duplex ultrasound should be performed first. If this confirms DVT, treatment for VTE should start and no further investigation is required. If the duplex ultrasound is negative then further investigations to exclude PE should be performed
  - In the absence of signs and symptoms of DVT a V/Q scan or CTPA should be performed
    - When the chest X-ray is abnormal a CTPA should be performed in preference to V/Q
    - Women should be advised that compared to CTPA, V/Q carries an increased risk of childhood cancer (estimated increased risk of fatal childhood cancer to the age of 15 of 0.006% per mGy or a risk of 1 in 17,000 per mGy. Foetal radiation exposure with CTPA and V/Q is 0.1 and 0.5 mGy respectively).
    - CTPA carries an increased risk of breast cancer compared to V/Q (delivery of 10 mGy of radiation to the pregnant women's breast during CTPA is estimated to increase her lifetime risk of breast cancer by 13.6%. If the baseline lifetime risk of breast cancer is 0.1% then CTPA would increase this by 0.0136%)

- The ventilation component of a V/Q scan can often be omitted in pregnant women thus minimizing radiation risk to the foetus
- Treatment for suspected VTE should be started immediately while awaiting the results of definitive investigation for PE
- Treatment for VTE in pregnancy is low molecular weight heparin
  - LMWH does not cross the placenta
  - Warfarin and DOACs are contraindicated during pregnancy
  - LMWH dose should be based on the woman's booking or early pregnancy weight
  - There is insufficient evidence to guide whether a once daily dose or divided dose regime should be used and local protocols should be followed
  - Life-threatening high-risk PE should be treated with unfractionated heparin. A team of experienced clinicians including the on-call obstetrician should consider thrombolysis.
- Duration of treatment
  - Maintenance treatment should be with LMWH during pregnancy
  - Peak anti-Xa activity monitoring is recommended for women at extremes of weight (under 50 kg or over 90 kg) and in those with complicating factors such as renal impairment or recurrent VTE.
  - Treatment should continue for at least 6 weeks postnatally and until a total of 3 months of treatment has been given
  - Women should be given a choice of LMWH or oral anticoagulation postnatally
  - Postpartum warfarin should be avoided until at least the 5th day
  - Neither warfarin nor LMWH are contraindicated during breastfeeding.

8.4.3 Chronic thromboembolic pulmonary hypertension (CTEPH)

Definition
- Pulmonary hypertension caused by remodelling of pulmonary arterial system due to persisting pulmonary arterial thromboembolism.
- Classified as group 4 pulmonary hypertension

Epidemiology
- Estimated annual incidence of 5 per million
- Cumulative incidence of 0.1–9.1% within 2 years of a symptomatic PE
- CTEPH is thought to be underdiagnosed and thus prevalence may be higher

Pathology
- Occlusion of pulmonary arteries with thrombus is thought to be the trigger in CTEPH
- This thrombus persists and non-dissolution leads to formation of scar tissue with the development of fibrinous bands and webs within the pulmonary vasculature causing total or sub-total vascular occlusion.
- Pulmonary blood flow is subsequently diverted to non-occluded vessels, which exposes the endothelium to higher shear stresses.
- This leads to endothelial dysfunction and vascular remodelling, similar to that seen in PAH, further propagating the pulmonary hypertension.
- This explains the progressive nature of CTEPH even in the absence of recurrent thromboembolic events.

Clinical presentation
- 20–25% present with no history of documented prior thromboembolic event
- In those with antecedent thromboembolic event 'honeymoon' period between event and onset of symptoms can range from weeks to years
- Symptoms (e.g. exertional dyspnoea) may be non-specific or absent in early CTEPH.
- Symptoms indistinguishable from other forms of PH
- Signs and symptoms of right ventricular failure such as elevated JVP, peripheral oedema, loud pulmonary second heart sound, RV heave, syncope or pre-syncope and RV angina only manifest late in the disease when pulmonary hypertension is advanced.
- Left untreated the prognosis in CTEPH is very poor. Median survival is less than 2 years in patients with a mean PA pressure of greater than 30 mmHg at diagnosis.

Diagnosis
- CTEPH should be considered if breathlessness persists or new signs and symptoms of RV failure are present following an acute PE, having completed 3 months of anticoagulation. Patients with acute PE who are particularly at risk of CTEPH include those with
    - Unprovoked PEs
    - Initial large thrombus load
    - Longstanding symptoms prior to acute presentation
    - Elevated PASP (> 50 mmHg) during acute admission
- Due to the high prevalence of PE and relatively low risk of developing CTEPH routine screening for CTEPH in asymptomatic patients after an acute PE is not currently recommended. However selective screening for patients with risk factors may be appropriate.
- Risk factors for CTEPH
    - Splenectomy
    - Antiphospholipid antibody syndrome
    - Ventriculo-atrial shunt
    - Inflammatory bowel disease
    - Permanent central venous lines and pacemakers
    - Myeloproliferative disease
    - Chronic osteomyelitis
- CTEPH should also be considered as a diagnosis in anyone who presents with unexplained gradual onset breathlessness with no history of an antecedent thromboembolic event.
- Echo findings in CTEPH are similar to those seen in other forms of pre-capillary PH.
- A definitive diagnosis of CTEPH is made by right heart catheterization in combination with imaging to support the presence of chronic pulmonary arterial thrombus and vascular remodelling.
- Imaging
    - V/Q is the most sensitive and specific modality for the detection of chronic thromboembolic disease—a normal VQ scan essentially rules out CTEPH (Figure 8.4.4)
    - Direct signs of chronic thromboembolic disease on CTPA include organized pulmonary emboli, partial defects, or complete occlusion of pulmonary arteries as well as the formation of bands and webs within the pulmonary vasculature. Indirect signs include a mosaic perfusion pattern of the lung parenchyma and the presence of dilated bronchial arteries.
    - CTPA also has good sensitivity and specificity in expert hands. Additional information regarding the lung parenchyma is also obtained by CTPA. However, CTEPH should not be excluded on the basis of CTPA alone.
    - Magnetic resonance angiography may add additional useful information when used in conjunction with CTPA or V/Q if interventional treatment is being contemplated.

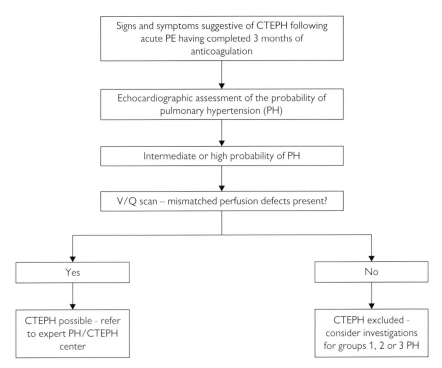

Figure 8.4.4 Investigation of suspected CTEPH. Reproduced from 2015 ESC/ERS Guidelines for the diagnosis and management of pulmonary hypertension

Galiè N, Humbert M, Vachiery JL, et al; ESC Scientific Document Group. 2015 ESC/ERS Guidelines for the diagnosis and treatment of pulmonary hypertension: The Joint Task Force for the Diagnosis and Treatment of Pulmonary Hypertension of the European Society of Cardiology (ESC) and the European Respiratory Society (ERS): Endorsed by: Association for European Paediatric and Congenital Cardiology (AEPC), International Society for Heart and Lung Transplantation (ISHLT). *Eur Heart J.* 2016 Jan 1;37(1):67–119. doi: 10.1093/eurheartj/ehv317. © European Society of Cardiology. With permission from Oxford University Press.

- Selective pulmonary angiography delineates the vascular anatomy accurately in order to assess operative feasibility.
- Right heart catheterization—findings in CTEPH are identical to those in PAH.

Treatment

- Surgical
  - Pulmonary endarterectomy (PEA) is the treatment of choice for CTEPH and can be curative. All patients with suspected CTEPH should be discussed at an MDT at an experienced PEA centre to determine operability.
  - Bilateral endarterectomy is performed under circulatory arrest and deep hypothermia.
  - Thrombi in the main, lobar, and segmental arteries can be accessed.
  - In hospital mortality of 2.2% in the most experienced centres
  - 5-year survival of 92.5%. Freedom from disease specific death at 5 and 10 years post PEA is 84% and 82% respectively.
  - Majority of patients experience significant improvement in symptoms and normalisation of pulmonary haemodynamics. All patients remain on lifelong anticoagulation following surgery.
  - Residual or recurrent pulmonary hypertension (mPAP ≥ 25 mmHg after leaving intensive care) is the most important cause of morbidity and mortality after PEA.

- Interventional
  - Balloon dilatation is increasingly being used for patients with inoperable CTEPH or with persistent disease post-PEA surgery.
- Medical
  - Optimum medical treatment includes lifelong anticoagulation with vitamin K antagonists, LMWH, or DOAC, diuretics for RV failure and oxygen for hypoxaemia.
  - Riociguat, a guanylate cyclase stimulator, is licensed for use in inoperable CTEPH or persistent/recurrent PH after PEA.
  - Riociguat has been shown to improve 6-minute walk distance, pulmonary vascular resistance, functional class and reduce levels of NT pro BNP in this group.
  - Off label use of drugs used in the treatment of pulmonary arterial hypertension (group 1 PH), e.g. endothelin receptor antagonists, phosphodiesterase type 5 inhibitors, and prostacyclin analogues may be used in inoperable CTEPH by expert centres.
  - Patients who progress despite optimal medical therapy should be considered for lung transplantation.

Further reading

Galiè N, Humbert M, Vachiery JL, Gibbs S, Lang I, Torbicki A, Simonneau G, Peacock A, Vonk Noordegraaf A, Beghetti M, Ghofrani A, Gomez Sanchez MA, Hansmann G, Klepetko W, Lancellotti P, Matucci M, McDonagh T, Pierard LA, Trindade PT, Zompatori M, Hoeper M. 2015 ESC/ERS Guidelines for the diagnosis and treatment of pulmonary hypertension. *Rev Esp Cardiol (Engl Ed)*. 2016 Feb;69(2):177. doi: 10.1016/j.rec.2016.01.002

Hoeper MM, Madani MM, Nakanishi N, Meyer B, Cebotari S, Rubin LJ. Chronic thromboembolic pulmonary hypertension. *Lancet Respir Med*. 2014 Jul;2(7):573–82. doi: 10.1016/S2213-2600(14)70089-X. Epub 2014 Jun 2

Howard LSGE, Barden S, Condliffe R, Connolly V, Davies CWH, Donaldson J, Everett B, Free C, Horner D, Hunter L, Kaler J, Nelson-Piercy C, O-Dowd E, Patel R, Preston W, Sheares K, Campbell T. British Thoracic Society Guideline for the initial outpatient management of pulmonary embolism (PE). *Thorax*. 2018 Jul;73(Suppl 2):ii1–ii29. doi: 10.1136/thoraxjnl-2018-211539. Epub 2018 Jun 13

Konstantinides SV, Meyer G, Becattini C, Bueno H, Geersing GJ, Harjola VP, Huisman MV, Humbert M, Jennings CS, Jiménez D, Kucher N, Lang IM, Lankeit M, Lorusso R, Mazzolai L, Meneveau N, Ní Áinle F, Prandoni P, Pruszczyk P, Righini M, Torbicki A, Van Belle E, Zamorano JL; ESC Scientific Document Group. 2019 ESC Guidelines for the diagnosis and management of acute pulmonary embolism developed in collaboration with the European Respiratory Society (ERS). *Eur Heart J*. 2020 Jan 21;41(4):543–603. doi: 10.1093/eurheartj/ehz405

Mazzolai L, Aboyans V, Ageno W, Agnelli G, Alatri A, Bauersachs R, Brekelmans MPA, Büller HR, Elias A, Farge D, Konstantinides S, Palareti G, Prandoni P, Righini M, Torbicki A, Vlachopoulos C, Brodmann M. Diagnosis and management of acute deep vein thrombosis: a joint consensus document from the European Society of Cardiology working groups of aorta and peripheral vascular diseases and pulmonary circulation and right ventricular function. *Eur Heart J*. 2018 Dec 14;39(47):4208–18. doi: 10.1093/eurheartj/ehx003

Thromboembolic disease in Pregnancy and the Puerperium: Acute Management. Green-top Guideline No. 37b. April 2015. Royal College of Obstetricians & Gynaecologists. https://www.rcog.org.uk/guidance/browse-all-guidance/green-top-guidelines/thrombosis-and-embolism-during-pregnancy-and-the-puerperium-acute-management-green-top-guideline-no-37b/

Venous thromboembolic diseases: diagnosis, management and thrombophilia testing. London: National Institute for Health and Care Excellence (UK); 2020. NICE Guideline. https://www.nice.org.uk/guidance/ng158

8.5

Pulmonary hypertension

Gerry Coghlan, Hossam Fayed, and Ruta Virsinskaite

TABLE OF CONTENTS

- 8.5.1 Overview and definitions 759
- 8.5.2 Haemodynamic classification 760
- 8.5.3 Clinical classification 760
- 8.5.4 Epidemiology and genetics 760
  - Epidemiology 760
  - Genetics 761
- 8.5.5 Pathophysiology of PH 762
- 8.5.6 Diagnosis 762
  - Symptoms 763
  - Signs 763
  - Investigations 764
- 8.5.7 Risk assessment in PAH 767
- 8.5.8 Treatment of pulmonary arterial hypertension 767
  - Non-pharmacologic 767
  - Specific pharmacologic therapy for PAH 768
  - Combination therapy 771
  - Adjunctive therapy 771
  - Surgical and interventional options 771
- 8.5.9 Specific types of pulmonary hypertension 772
  - Pulmonary hypertension due to left heart disease (PH-LHD or Group 2) 772
  - Pulmonary hypertension due to lung disease and/or hypoxia (PH-LD or Group 3) 773
  - Chronic thromboembolic pulmonary hypertension (CTEPH or Group 4) 773

8.5.1 Overview and definitions

- Pulmonary hypertension (PH) is a pathophysiological disorder that may involve multiple clinical conditions and may be associated with a variety of cardiovascular and respiratory diseases.
- Right heart catheterization (RHC) is the gold standard for diagnosing and classifying PH.
- Recent change in the definition and subtyping of PH has been presented at the ESC/ERS guidelines in 2022. The definition of PH is a mean pulmonary arterial pressure (mPAP) > 20 mmHg at rest as assessed by right heart catheterization (RHC), and precapillary PH is an mPAP > 20 mmHg with a pulmonary vascular resistance (PVR) of > 2 Wood's units (WU) and a pulmonary artery wedge pressure (PAWP) ≤ 15mmHg.
- The ESC/ERS guidelines 2022 has further expanded the definition of PH by including exercise PH as an increase in mPAP by greater than 3mmHg per litre increase in cardiac output, accepting that there is uncertainty about the reliability of this measure in people aged 60 years old and above.
- Pulmonary Arterial Hypertension (PAH) is the term used to describe patients with precapillary PH due to vasculopathy of the precapillary pulmonary arterioles. PAH is also referred to as Group 1 (see section 8.5.3) but is not synonymous to precapillary PH (see section 8.5.2).
- The recognition of PAH patients is vital as they can benefit from targeted specific therapy with vasodilators.

8.5.2 Haemodynamic classification

PH is classified according to the haemodynamic data obtained from cardiac catheterization as follows:

- Precapillary PH:
    - mean pulmonary artery pressure (mPAP) > 20 mmHg and pulmonary artery wedge pressure (PAWP) ≤ 15 mmHg and a pulmonary vascular resistance (PVR) > 2 WU.
    - Precapillary PH is not synonymous with PAH, other causes of precapillary PH include advanced lung disease, chronic thromboembolic PH or PH with unclear and/or multifactorial mechanisms (e.g. haematological disorders and chronic renal failure).
- Postcapillary PH:
    - mPAP > 20 mmHg and PAWP > 15 mmHg. This is typically caused by left heart disease but may also be seen with unclear and/or multifactorial mechanisms.

8.5.3 Clinical classification

Clinical diseases recognized to underlie PH are grouped into five distinct groups according to shared features (see Table 8.5.1).

8.5.4 Epidemiology and genetics

Epidemiology

- In the UK, the prevalence of PAH is estimated at around 100 cases per million with a female:male ratio of 1.8.
- In Europe, PAH prevalence is in the range of 15 – 60 subjects per million population and incidence is about 5–10 cases per million per year.
- In Europe and the US 5% of PH is due to PAH (Group 1).
- The most common cause of PH is left heart disease (Group 2). It is estimated 80% of all PH is due to left heart disease. Commonly in association with heart failure with preserved ejection fraction (HFpEF) but PH occurs in all forms left heart failure and left sided valve disease.
- Lung disease (Group 3) is the next most common group (around 10%).
- Worldwide the most common cause of PAH is thought to be schistosomiasis, in parts of the world without endemic schistosomiasis about half is due to idiopathic PAH and 10% are hereditary (HPAH).
- Idiopathic PAH most commonly presents in younger individuals (classically women in their thirties, however the mean age at diagnosis has been rising as more diagnostic efforts are made and is now closer to 60 years of age).
- Scleroderma associated PAH (SSc-PAH) is the most common form of connective tissue disease associated PAH (CTD-PAH) with a mean age of about 63 at presentation. Patients with SSc are thought to have lifetime risk of about 10-15% to develop PAH.

Table 8.5.1 Clinical classification of pulmonary hypertension according to the 2022 ESC/ERS Guidelines for the diagnosis and treatment of pulmonary hypertension.

Group 1 Pulmonary arterial hypertension (PAH)
1.1 Idiopathic
    1.1.1 Non-responders at vasoreactivity testing
    1.1.2 Acute responders at vasoreactivity testing
1.2 Heritable
1.3 Associated with drugs and toxins
1.4 Associated with:
    1.4.1 Connective tissue disease
    1.4.2 HIV infection
    1.4.3 Portal hypertension
    1.4.4 Congenital heart disease
    1.4.5 Schistosomiasis
1.5 PAH with features of venous/capillary (PVOD/PCH) involvement
1.6 Persistent PH of the newborn

Group 2 PH associated with left heart disease
2.1 Heart failure:
    2.1.1 with preserved ejection fraction
    2.1.2 with reduced or mildly reduced ejection fraction
2.2 Valvular heart disease
2.3 Congenital/acquired cardiovascular conditions leading to postcapillary PH

Group 3 PH associated with lung diseases and/or hypoxia
3.1 Obstructive lung disease or emphysema
3.2 Restrictive lung disease
3.3 Lung disease with mixed restrictive/obstructive pattern
3.4 Hypoventilation syndromes
3.5 Hypoxia without lung disease (e.g. high altitude)
3.6 Developmental lung disorders

Group 4 PH associated with pulmonary artery obstructions
4.1 Chronic thrombo-embolic PH
4.2 Other pulmonary artery obstructions

Group 5 PH with unclear and/or multifactorial mechanisms
5.1 Haematological disorders
5.2 Systemic disorders
5.3 Metabolic disorders
5.4 Chronic renal failure with or without haemodialysis
5.5 Pulmonary tumour thrombotic microangiopathy
5.6 Fibrosing mediastinitis

Humbert M, Kovacs G, Hoeper MM, et al; ESC/ERS Scientific Document Group. 2022 ESC/ERS Guidelines for the diagnosis and treatment of pulmonary hypertension. *Eur Heart J*. 2022 Oct 11;43(38):3618–3731. doi: 10.1093/eurheartj/ehac237. © European Society of Cardiology. With permission from Oxford University Press.

Genetics

- Mutations in PAH genes have been identified in familial PAH, IPAH, PVOD/PCH, and anorexigen-associated PAH.
- Heterozygous BMPR2 account for approximately 75% of familial PAH.
- It is estimated that about 25–30% of patients diagnosed with idiopathic pulmonary arterial hypertension have an underlying Mendelian genetic cause for their condition.
- Among other genes that also play a role in IPAH and/or HPAH are ALK1, 5HTT, ENG, SMAD9, CAV1 and KCNK3.

- In familial PVOD/PCH genome sequencing demonstrated mutations in EIF2AK4.

8.5.5 Pathophysiology of PH

- Ohm's law states that pressure = flow × resistance. Therefore, mPAP = (mean RV output × PVR) + PAWP.
- Increased pulmonary venous pressure (causing raised PAWP) occurs with left heart failure (with or without reduced systolic function) and mitral/aortic valve disease.
- Long-standing elevated pulmonary venous pressure may lead to secondary elevation of PVR (due to increased pulmonary vascular tone and vascular remodeling).
- In patients with pulmonary veno-occlusive disease (PVOD) pulmonary capillary pressure is raised due to narrowing of the pulmonary veins leading to pulmonary oedema. However, wedge pressure is not increased as there is no flow during balloon occlusion of the pulmonary vasculature and hence no resistance to pressure transmission from the left atrium.
- Increased flow due to congenital heart defects with left-to-right shunts (e.g. ASD), anaemia, liver cirrhosis, AV malformations or fistulas is usually accommodated by pulmonary vasodilation, but can ultimately lead to endothelial damage and increased PVR, this is especially likely where high flow is associated with high pressure (VSD or PDA) or exposure to endothelial toxins (portal shunts).
- In PAH increased PVR develops due to proliferative vasculopathy of the small pulmonary arteries and arterioles, characterized by vasoconstriction, cell proliferation, and microthrombosis.
- Pathologic changes affect all three layers of the vessel wall (intima, media, and adventitia) and is similar in all different types of PAH.
    - Initially medial hypertrophy and intimal hyperplasia dominates, then collagenous replacement of the intimal layer.
    - In advanced disease characteristic 'plexiform lesions' glomeruloid like complex vascular formations may develop, these are believed to be due to dysregulated neoangiogenesis.
    - Many vascular mediator pathways play a role including increased endothelin, decreased nitric oxide and prostacyclin levels which are targets for PAH specific therapy.
- Other causes of increased PVR include reduced cross-sectional area of the vascular bed (e.g. pulmonary emboli and interstitial lung disease) or hypoxia induced vasoconstriction.
- The ability of the RV to adapt to long-standing increased afterload plays an important role in the natural history of PH which ultimately leads to RV failure. Ventricular interdependency also plays a role in PH as both ventricles have the septum in common with common myocardial fibres and enclosed in the same pericardium.
- High right-sided pressures combined with reduced left-sided filling pressures causes diastolic leftward motion of the septum and ventricular dyssynchrony.
- In patients with very elevated right-sided pressures, the septum functionally acts as part of the hypertrophied right ventricle, resulting in systolic septal flattening and even bowing toward the left ventricle. Coupled with a reduction of cardiac output in advanced disease, this leads to underfilling of the left heart and a degree of 'disuse atrophy'.

8.5.6 Diagnosis

- PH diagnosis work up usually begins following clinical suspicion and suggestive echocardiographic features. The purpose of the diagnostic workup when PH is suspected is to confirm the presence of PH and then to classify according to aetiological, functional, and haemodynamic parameters (Figure 8.5.1).
- The diagnosis of PAH or CTEPH should be established in specialist centres before consideration of specific targeted therapies.

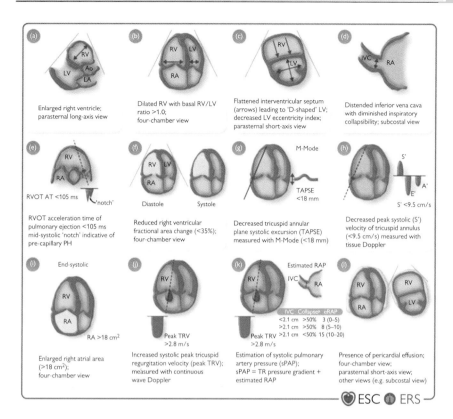

Figure 8.5.1 Transthoracic echocardiographic parameters in the assessment of pulmonary hypertension.
Humbert M, Kovacs G, Hoeper MM, et al; ESC/ERS Scientific Document Group. 2022 ESC/ERS Guidelines for the diagnosis and treatment of pulmonary hypertension. *Eur Heart J.* 2022 Oct 11;43(38):3618–3731. doi: 10.1093/eurheartj/ehac237. © European Society of Cardiology. With permission from Oxford University Press.

Symptoms

- Progressive effort-related breathlessness, lethargy, and in more advanced cases syncope or pre-syncope on exertion (from reduced cardiac output) and angina (due to RV ischaemia – demand/perfusion mismatch).
- As right ventricular failure advances ankle oedema, abdominal swelling due to hepatomegaly and ascites followed by cachexia develop.
- As these symptoms are not specific, the diagnosis of PH is often delayed or missed.
- PAH should be considered as soon as more common causes (like left heart and lung disease) are ruled out. This is even more important in patients with risk factors to develop PAH as family history, connective tissue disease (especially scleroderma), HIV, portal hypertension, or history of drug or toxin intake that is known to cause pulmonary hypertension.
- Less common symptoms include: cough, haemoptysis (from the bronchial vessels), hoarseness of voice (pressure on the recurrent laryngeal nerve).

Signs

- General physical signs generally only appear later in the course of the disease and include:

- Raised venous pressures and hepatomegaly (can be pulsatile) with tricuspid regurgitation.
- Peripheral oedema and ascites due to right ventricular failure.
- Cold peripheries due to reduced cardiac output in advanced pulmonary hypertension.
- Chest examination may reveal a parasternal heave, a loud P2, and in advanced cases a right ventricular gallop.
- Tricuspid regurgitation is common but only rarely causes a murmur (in patients with very high pulmonary pressures and modest regurgitation) and possibly a diastolic murmur of pulmonary regurgitation.
- Lung auscultation is usually clear unless if there is underlying lung disease or congestion due to heart failure or PVOD/PCH (crepitations).
- Pleural effusions may be present in advanced PH.
- Findings related to the underlying cause include e.g. signs of lung or left heart disease, cyanosis, clubbing (cyanotic heart disease, liver disease, interstitial lung disease, or PVOD), sclerodactly, telangiectasia, or digital ulceration (scleroderma).

Investigations

- ECG
  - Can be normal or may show P pulmonale, right axis deviation, RV strain, RV hypertrophy, or right bundle branch block.
  - PH may cause prolongation of QTc.
  - PH predisposes to atrial arrhythmias (atrial fibrillation suggests left heart disease while atrial flutter is more frequently observed in PAH).
  - In patients with PAH the development of atrial arrhythmias is a treatable cause of acute decompensation.
- CXR
  - Is abnormal in many patients with heart or lung disease irrespective of the presence of PH.
  - In PAH the CXR is abnormal in 90% of cases by the time of the diagnosis, though the abnormalities are subtle until disease is advanced.
  - Common features are dilatation of the main pulmonary artery and pruning of peripheral blood vessels (usually only identified on retrospective review after the diagnosis has been made).
  - At later stages an increased cardiothoracic ratio (RA and RV enlargement) can be seen.
  - Also, changes related to the cause can be seen (e.g. lung disease or pulmonary congestion due to left heart failure).
- Echocardiography
  - It is important to understand that whilst tricuspid regurgitation (TR) peak velocity (TV) strongly correlate with pulmonary systolic pressure, it often underestimates (especially if trivial or in severe TR) or overestimates PA systolic pressure and lacks reproducibility. However, a TV of > 3.4m/s is almost never observed in the absence of PH.
  - The TV should not be considered in isolation when assessing the likelihood of, or severity of PH. Additional variables related to RV morphology and function, such as RV/LV basal diameter/area ratio >1.0, flattening of the interventricular septum, TAPSE/sPAP ratio <0.55 mm/mmHg, RVOT acceleration time <105 ms and/or mid-systolic notching of the pulmonary systolic velocity envelope, early diastolic pulmonary regurgitation velocity >2.2 m/s, PA diameter >25 mm and/or > aortic root, IVC diameter >21 mm, with decreased inspiratory collapse, RA area >18 cm^2, are used to define the echocardiographic probability of PH (see Figure 8.5.1).

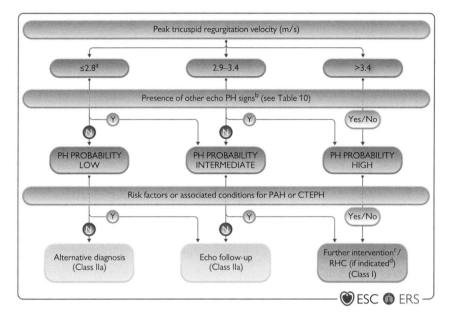

Figure 8.5.2 Echocardiographic probability of pulmonary hypertension and recommendations for further assessment.
Humbert M, Kovacs G, Hoeper MM, et al; ESC/ERS Scientific Document Group. 2022 ESC/ERS Guidelines for the diagnosis and treatment of pulmonary hypertension. *Eur Heart J.* 2022 Oct 11;43(38):3618–3731. doi: 10.1093/eurheartj/ehac237. © European Society of Cardiology. With permission from Oxford University Press.

- Echocardiographic probability of pulmonary hypertension and recommendations for further assessment are shown in Figure 8.5.2.
- Echocardiographers should report right ventricle size and basal RV-LV ratio, RV longitudinal function (TAPSE, S') and fractional area change, right atrial area (RA > 18 cm^2 has independent predictive value in the identification of PAH), septal curvature (systolic septal flattening suggests mPAP > 35mmHg irrespective of TV), RV outflow tract acceleration time, inspiratory collapsibility of inferior vena cava, presence of pericardial effusion.
- Echo is also very useful for looking for left heart-related causes of PH (e.g. left ventricular systolic and diastolic dysfunction, mitral and aortic valve heart disease, or congenital heart disease).
• CMR
    - Allows accurate and reproducible assessment of the RV (volumes, mass, morphology, and function).
    - Assessment of the haemodynamics (stroke volume, cardiac output, and reduced pulmonary distensibilty).
    - MR pulmonary angiography can support the assessment of CTEPH as obstructions in larger vessels can be demonstrated.
• Lung function tests
    - Are important for diagnosis of any underlying lung disease (Group 3).
    - Mildly abnormal spirometry and a slight reduction in DLCO is common in PAH.
    - A very low DLCO (< 45%) is uncommon in PAH, and should prompt consideration of PVOD/PCH, scleroderma, or emphysema/small airways disease.

- Sleep studies are useful if sleep apnoea or hypoventilation syndromes are suspected.
- High resolution CT
  - Allows quantification of the extent of lung fibrosis and emphysema, as well as identifying bronchial wall thickening, airway obstruction and 'mosaicism' or variations in xray density of the lung seen in CTEPH, small airways disease and also in advanced PAH.
  - Central to the diagnosis of PVOD.
- V/Q scans
  - Should be done in patients with PH to rule out CTEPH.
  - VQ scans have a greater sensitivity than CTPA for the exclusion of chronic thromboembolic disease except in expert centres, however there is a false positive rate, so where VQ scans suggest CTEPH, formal review of CTPA or pulmonary angiography is necessary to establish the diagnosis.
- Blood tests
  - Should include full blood count, renal profile, electrolytes, liver profile, clotting screening, and thyroid function tests.
  - BNP/NT-proBNP is particularly important in diagnosis and follow-up and is an important independent prognostic factor.
  - Autoimmune screening is necessary to rule out connective tissue disease-related PH.
  - Thrombophilia screen may be considered in the setting of CTEPH. HIV should be tested in all PAH patients.
  - Genetic testing recommended by specialist expert centres to patients with IPAH, familial PAH, and hereditary haemorrhagic telangiectasia (BMPR2, ACVRL1, and ENG). If these are negative then rarer mutations can also be considered (KCNK3, CAV1, etc.).
- Functional assessment: 6-minute walking distance (6MWD)
  - Widely used test that provides useful data on trends in functional capacity.
  - It has been validated in risk assessment of PAH patients.
  - Cardiopulmonary exercise test (CPET) is a more specific tool that can be useful in the initial workup of challenging cases and has also a role in risk assessment.
- Right heart catheterization
  - RHC is the gold standard for diagnosing and classifying PH.
  - The ESC/ERS 2022 guidelines stresses that this is carried out in expert specialist centers to ensure high quality data is recorded with a very low procedure related morbidity and mortality.
  - The minimum data set includes:
    - Documentation of the standardized zero reference point.
    - Right atrial mean pressure (mRAP).
    - Right ventricular systolic and end diastolic pressures (RVSP & RVEDP).
    - Pulmonary artery pressure (PA—systolic, diastolic, and mean).
    - Pulmonary arterial wedge pressure (PAWP).
    - Cardiac output (CO), cardiac index (CI), and PVR should be calculated using thermodilution and/or direct Fick's methods.
    - Indirect Fick should not be used at this lacks accuracy and reproducibility.
    - Oxygen saturations run (SVC, IVC, and PA oximetry) are required to rule out shunts (left to right shunts are more likely if the PA saturation is > 75%).
    - All pressure measurements, including PAWP, should be performed at end expiration (without breath-holding manoeuvre).
  - Calculated data includes:

- Transpulmonary gradient (TPG) is mean PAP − PAWP, (normally < 12 mmHg).
- Pulmonary Vascular Resistance (PVR) = TPG/CO.
- Vasoreactivity testing inhaled nitric oxide, inhaled iloprost, or i/v epoprostenol is recommended in patients with I/H/DPAH to detect those who can be treated with high doses of a CCB.
- Fluid challenge (500ml over 5 minutes) or left heart catheterisation (LHC) should be considered to measure LVEDP (if the PAWP > 12mmHg or there is a suspicion of left heart involvement).
- Pulmonary angiogram can also be done for detailed assessment of thromboembolic disease.

8.5.7 Risk assessment in PAH

- Comprehensive prognostic evaluation and risk assessment is recommended at diagnosis in the current ESC/ERS guidelines for pulmonary hypertension.
- The proposed multiparameter approach includes:
  - clinical (clinical signs of heart failure (HF), progression of symptoms, syncope, WHO functional class)
  - functional (6MWD or cardiopulmonary exercise test)
  - biomarkers (BNP or NT-proBNP)
  - imaging (right atrial area, TAPSE/sPAP, pericardial effusion, RVEF, SVI, RVESVI)
  - haemodynamics (RAP, CI, SVI and SvO2 (see Table 8.5.2).
- At diagnosis three strata are identified low, intermediate and high risk associated with a predicted one-year mortality of <5%, 5-20% and >20%, respectively.
- For follow up assessment a four-strata model is recommended (see Table 8.5.3). The main advantage of this model over the three-strata model is better discrimination within the intermediate-risk group (as high–intermediate group was associated with worse survival), which helps guide therapeutic decision-making and was included in the updated treatment algorithm.
- Another well-validated risk assessment method is the REVEAL 2.0 risk score which uses similar variables with slightly different cut-offs, but also includes others that are associated with adverse outcome. It provides accurate prediction when one key variable (WHO-FC, 6MWD, or BNP/NT-proBNP) is unavailable, but is no longer accurate when two of these variables are missing.
- Several studies have identified WHO-FC, 6MWD, and BNP/ NT-proBNP as the strongest prognostic predictors.

8.5.8 Treatment of pulmonary arterial hypertension

Non-pharmacologic

- PH is usually a chronic debilitating disease and patients need substantial support along their disease journey.
- This includes psycho-social support that can be supervised through specialist centres and patient support groups.
- Advice should be given for day-to-day life activities and specific advice regarding specific situations like pregnancy, travel, and surgery.
- It has been shown that improvement in functional capacity can be attained with supervised physical rehabilitation.

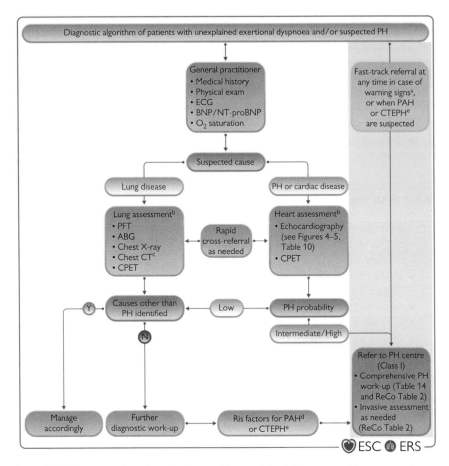

Figure 8.5.3 Diagnostic algorithm of patients with unexplained dyspnoea and/or suspected pulmonary hypertension.
Humbert M, Kovacs G, Hoeper MM, et al; ESC/ERS Scientific Document Group. 2022 ESC/ERS Guidelines for the diagnosis and treatment of pulmonary hypertension. Eur Heart J. 2022 Oct 11;43(38):3618–3731. doi: 10.1093/eurheartj/ehac237. © European Society of Cardiology. With permission from Oxford University Press.

- Advice against becoming pregnant, individual counselling and shared decision making are recommended. Pregnancy is associated with high mortality and therefore effective contraception should be provided (avoiding estrogenic agents).
    - There are reports of favourable pregnancy outcomes in women with PH, including, but not limited to, women with IPAH who respond to CCB therapy. But it remains associated with unforeseeable risks and may accelerate PH progression.
- For air travel supplemental O2 is recommended for patients using oxygen or whose arterial blood oxygen pressure is <8 kPa (60 mmHg). Similarly, these patients should be advised not to go to high altitude areas (>1500-2000 m) without supplemental oxygen.

Specific pharmacologic therapy for PAH

According to the revised haemodynamic definition, PAH may be diagnosed in patients with mPAP >20 mmHg and PVR >2 WU. Yet, the efficacy of drugs approved for PAH has only been demonstrated in patients with mPAP ≥25mmHg and PVR >3 WU.

Table 8.5.2 Comprehensive risk assessment in pulmonary arterial hypertension (three-strata model).

Determinants of prognosis (estimated 1-year mortality)	Low risk (<5%)	Intermediate risk (5–20%)	High risk (>20%)
Clinical observations and modifiable variables			
Signs of right HF	Absent	Absent	Present
Progression of symptoms and clinical manifestations	No	Slow	Rapid
Syncope	No	Occasional syncope	Repeated syncope
WHO-FC	I, II	III	IV
6MWD	>440 m	165–440 m	<165 m
CPET	Peak VO_2 >15 mL/min/kg (>65% pred.) VE/VCO_2 slope <36	Peak VO_2 >11–15 mL/min/kg (35–65% pred.) VE/VCO_2 slope 36–44	Peak VO_2 <11 mL/min/kg (<35% pred.) VE/VCO_2 slope >44
Biomarkers: BNP or NT-proBNP	BNP <50 ng/L NT-proBNP <300 ng/L	BNP 50–800 ng/L NT-proBNP 300–1100 ng/L	BNP >800 ng/L NT-proBNP >1100 ng/L
Echocardiography	RA area <18 cm² TAPSE/sPAP >0.32 mm/mmHg No pericardial effusion	RA area <18–26 cm² TAPSE/sPAP 0.19–0.32 mm/mmHg Minimal pericardial effusion	RA area >26 cm² TAPSE/sPAP <0.19 mm/mmHg Moderate or large pericardial effusion
cMRI	RVEF >54% SVI >40 mL/m² RVESVI <42 mLm/m²	RVEF 37–54% SVI 26–40 mL/m² RVESVI 42–54 mLm/m²	RVEF <37% SVI <26 mL/m² RVESVI >54 mLm/m²
Haemodynamics	RAP <8 mmHg CI ≥2.5 L/min/m² SVI >38 mL/m² SvO_2 >65%	RAP 8–14 mmHg CI 2.0–2.4 L/min/m² SVI 31–38 mL/m² SvO_2 60–65%	RAP >14 mmHg CI <2.0 L/min/m² SVI <31 mL/m² SvO_2 <60%

Humbert M, Kovacs G, Hoeper MM, et al; ESC/ERS Scientific Document Group. 2022 ESC/ERS Guidelines for the diagnosis and treatment of pulmonary hypertension. *Eur Heart J.* 2022 Oct 11;43(38):3618–3731. doi: 10.1093/eurheartj/ehac237. © European Society of Cardiology. With permission from Oxford University Press..

Table 8.5.3 Variables used to calculate the simplified four-strata risk-assessment tool.

Determinants of prognosis	Low risk	Intermediate–low risk	Intermediate–high risk	Hight risk
Points assigned	1	2	3	4
WHO-FC	I or II	–	III	IV
6MWD, m	>440	320–440	165–319	<165
BNP or NT-proBNP, ng/L	<50 <300	50–199 300–649	200–800 650–1100	>800 >1100

Humbert M, Kovacs G, Hoeper MM, et al; ESC/ERS Scientific Document Group. 2022 ESC/ERS Guidelines for the diagnosis and treatment of pulmonary hypertension. *Eur Heart J.* 2022 Oct 11;43(38):3618–3731. doi: 10.1093/eurheartj/ehac237. © European Society of Cardiology. With

- **Calcium channel blockers (CCB)**
    - Nifedepine, amlodipine, or diltiazem: can be used only in patients who were responsive to vasodilator testing on RHC and where efficacy is confirmed (close follow-up with complete reassessment after 3–4 months of therapy (including RHC) is recommended).
    - Efficacy is usually achieved in high doses (e.g. diltiazem 720 mg/d) and limitations include hypotension and peripheral oedema.
    - CCBs are not recommended in patients without a vasoreactivity study or non-responders, unless prescribed for other indications (e.g. Raynaud's phenomenon).
- **Phosphodiesterase type 5 inhibitors (PDE5i)**
    - Sildenafil or tadalafil: have been originally approved for erectile dysfunction. They act through enhancing the NO/cGMP pathway by inhibiting cGMP degradation.
    - These agents cause significant pulmonary vasodilatation and have modest antiproliferative effects *in vitro*.
    - They have shown improvement in functional and exercise capacity as well as time to clinical worsening.
- **Guanyl cyclase stimulator**
    - Riociguat: act on the same NO/cGMP pathway as PDE5i but through directly enhancing cGMP production.
    - It has been shown to have similar favourable effects.
    - To avoid profound hypotension, it is contraindicated in combination with PDE5is.
- **Endothelin receptor antagonists (ERA)**
    - Bosentan, ambrisentan, and macitentan: endothelin-1 causes vasoconstriction and mitogenic effects by acting on two receptors (A and B).
    - Bosentan (a dual receptor inhibitor) was first to be used of this class and has shown improvements in exercise capacity, functional class, haemodynamics, echo variables, and time to clinical worsening.
    - Monthly liver function monitoring is important as it has shown to cause dose dependent elevated transaminases in 10% of patients.
    - The newer ERA (ambrisentan and macitentan do not affect the bile transporter, so have not been associated with liver toxicity).
    - Ambrisentan acts only receptor A and has shown similar favourable outcomes and in combination with PDE5 inhibitors reduces disease progression.
    - Macitentan has also shown significant reduction in morbidity and mortality, alone or in combination with PDE5i.
- **Prostacyclin analogues**
    - Powerful vasodilators and are well known to have some cytoprotective and antiproliferative effects.
    - Parenteral agents (epoprostenol, treprostinil, and iloprost) have been used to treat PAH for decades and have proven efficacy.
    - Chronic ambulatory parenteral administration is complex as the patient needs to manage their infusion pump and have a permanent tunnelled catheter exposing the patient to the risk of sepsis.
    - Parenteral epoprostenol is a synthetic prostacyclin that has very short life (3–5 minutes), treatment is consistently associated with a significant reduction in mortality (IPAH) and improvement in symptoms, exercise capacity, and haemodynamics in IPAH and CTD associated PAH. Once established on high-dose therapy, interruption of the infusion can be very dangerous leading to rebound of PH that can be fatal.

- Iloprost, treprostinil can also be administered by inhalation with variable degree of evidence.
- Selexipag: is an oral selective prostacyclin IP receptor agonist that has demonstrated reduction in composite morbidity and mortality in randomized clinical trials of PAH patients. Treprostinil can also be delivered orally.

Combination therapy
- According to the 2022 ESC/ESR guidelines initial dual-combination therapy with an ERA and a PDE5i is recommended for newly diagnosed idiopathic, heritable, drug-associated, and connective tissue disease-associated pulmonary arterial hypertension (IPAH/HPAH/DPAH and PAH-CTD) patients without cardiopulmonary comorbidities, who present at low or intermediate risk. Initial monotherapy should be considered for patients, who are diagnosed with cardiopulmonary comorbidities.
- Patients, who present at high risk of death, initial combination therapy with a PDE5i, an ERA, and i/v or s/c prostacyclin analogues (PCA) should be considered.
- Adapted from the 2022 ESC/ERS Guidelines, pulmonary arterial hypertension initial treatment algorithm for patients with idiopathic, heritable, drug-associated, and connective tissue disease-associated pulmonary arterial hypertension in Figure 8.5.4.

Adjunctive therapy
- Management of right heart failure (e.g. diuretics and fluid restriction, digoxin for heart rate control and etc).
- Management of atrial arrhythmias, ideally re-establishing sinus rhythm, as these are a relatively common cause of significant deterioration.
- Management of anaemia and iron status.
- There are conflicting data from registries in respect of oral anticoagulation in IPAH, HPAH, and PAH due to anorexigens; on balance anticoagulation is not recommended in PAH but remains pivotal in the management of CTEPH.

Surgical and interventional options
- Pulmonary endarterectomy (PEA) is the treatment of choice in CTEPH with very good success rate leading to symptoms resolution and haemodynamic normalization.
- Balloon pulmonary angioplasty (BPA) can be considered in CTEPH patients who surgery is not suitable, and data are rapidly accumulating demonstrating the BPA is associated with a low adverse event rate and equivalent haemodynamic efficacy as PEA surgery.
- Balloon atrial septostomy:
  - Is a palliative procedure for functional class IV and RV failure resistant to treatment or severe syncopal symptoms.
  - It can be used as a bridging procedure to transplantation. This is however rarely used in adult patients where effective medical therapies are available.
  - The risks associated with atrial septostomy are not insignificant and increase rapidly as the right ventricle fails.
- Transplantation (either heart and lung or bilateral lungs transplantation) remains an important treatment option for patients with PAH refractory to optimised medical therapy and referral to a transplant center should be considered early. The survival rate has been reported previously at about 50% and more recently this seems to have improved to about 75% at 5 years.

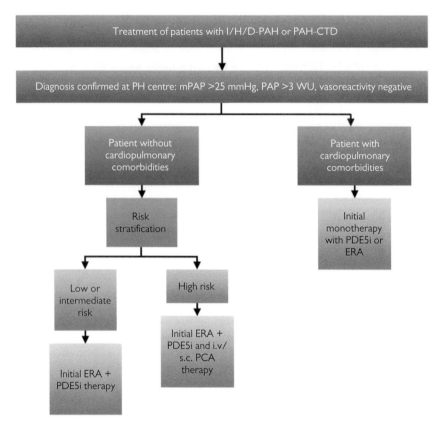

Figure 8.5.4 Pulmonary arterial hypertension initial treatment algorithm for patients with idiopathic, heritable, drug-associated, and connective tissue disease-associated pulmonary arterial hypertension.
Humbert M, Kovacs G, Hoeper MM, et al; ESC/ERS Scientific Document Group. 2022 ESC/ERS Guidelines for the diagnosis and treatment of pulmonary hypertension. *Eur Heart J.* 2022 Oct 11;43(38):3618–3731. doi: 10.1093/eurheartj/ehac237. © European Society of Cardiology. With permission from Oxford University Press.

8.5.9 Specific types of pulmonary hypertension

Pulmonary hypertension due to left heart disease (PH-LHD or Group 2)

- PH-LHD develops because the passively transmitted left-sided filling pressures.
- Chronically elevated left atrial pressure leads to elevated pulmonary vascular resistance in around one-third patients due to decreased NO availability, increased endothelin expression, desensitization to natriuretic peptide.
- A pulmonary vascular resistance exceeding 2 WU with an elevated PAWP (> 15 mmHg) is defined as 'combined pre and post capillary PH' (CpcPH).
- Based on recent data, a PVR >5 WU may indicate a severe precapillary component, the presence of which may prompt PH physicians to consider the use of PAH therapies in selected patients, despite the absence of supportive RCT evidence.

- The cornerstone of treatment of PH-LHD is the management of the underlying condition and optimizing fluid status.
- Non-specific vasodilators such as hydralazine and nitrates have been suggested with limited evidence.
- There is no consistent evidence base supporting the use PAH specific therapies in any form of PH-LHD.

Pulmonary hypertension due to lung disease and/or hypoxia (PH-LD or Group 3)

- Mild PH is relatively common with severe chronic obstructive pulmonary disease (COPD) or interstitial lung disease (ILD) but severe PH can also occur.
- Severe PH is seen commonly in patients with combined pulmonary fibrosis and emphysema (CPEF).
- PH causes significant deterioration of symptoms and is also associated with higher mortality when present in the setting of lung disease.
- Long-term oxygen therapy (LTOT) is recommended for patients with chronic hypoxaemia.
- It has been shown that LTOT slows the progression of PH associated with COPD but its role is less understood with ILD.
- Calcium channel blockers and vasodilators should not be used in Group 3 patients.
- Recent data shows that inhaled treprostinil is of symptomatic and morbidity benefit in ILD associated precapillary PH.
- As with Group 3 PH, treatment with PAH therapies may be considered if the PVR is substantially elevated (PVR >5WU).

Chronic thromboembolic pulmonary hypertension (CTEPH or Group 4)

- CTEPH has been previously been reported in up to 9.1% within the first 2 years after a symptomatic pulmonary embolism (PE), more recent data shows it is much more uncommon (<1%) and often there is evidence of chronicity on reviewing the 'acute' scans.
- Whilst CTEPH is very uncommon after an acute PE—residual breathless is not.
- PE guidelines recommend evaluation for CTEPH only in those remaining symptomatic after 3 months of anticoagulation.
- Where pulmonary thromboembolism is first identified during diagnostic work-up of breathless patients 3 months of anticoagulation is necessary before a diagnosis of CTEPH can be made.
- PH in this setting is not only a consequence of PA obstruction by organized fibrotic clots but can also be related to the associated microvasculopathy.
- Pulmonary endarterectomy is the treatment of choice in CTEPH with very good success rate leading to symptoms resolution and haemodynamic normalization but has an estimated 4.7% mortality risk though lower in high-volume centres.
- Long-term anticoagulation is indicated and riociguat has been shown to improve 6MWD and haemodynamics. Balloon pulmonary angioplasty has a role in non-operable patients and those with residual disease post surgery.

8.6

Adult congenital heart disease

Ali Khavandi, Graham Stuart and Victoria North

TABLE OF CONTENTS

8.6.1 Anatomical concepts in congenital heart disease 775
  Sequential segmental approach 775
  Distinguishing the morphological RV from the morphological LV 777
  Basic foetal and transitional circulation 777
8.6.2 Physiological concepts in congenital heart disease 778
  Pulmonary blood flow 778
  Cyanosis 780
  Flow-related development of cardiac chambers and vessels 782
8.6.3 General principles for use of diagnostic tests in patients with ACHD 782
8.6.4 Principles of intervention in ACHD 783
  Deterioration in functional status 783
  Heart failure 783
  Arrhythmia 783
  Infective endocarditis 783
8.6.5 Atrial septal defects and patent foramen ovale 784
8.6.6 Ventricular septal defects 786
8.6.7 Atrioventricular septal defects 788
8.6.8 Anomalous pulmonary venous drainage 789
8.6.9 Coarctation of the aorta 792
8.6.10 Coronary artery anomalies 794
8.6.11 Sinus of Valsalva aneurysms 795
8.6.12 Patent ductus arteriosus 796
8.6.13 Bicuspid aortic valve 796
8.6.14 Ebstein's anomaly 796
8.6.15 Transposition of the great arteries 797
8.6.16 Congenitally corrected transposition of the great arteries (ccTGA) 800
8.6.17 Tetralogy of Fallot 802
8.6.18 Functionally single ventricle and the Fontan circulation 804
8.6.19 Truncus arteriosus 806
8.6.20 Other considerations in adult congenital heart disease 807
  Infective endocarditis prevention 807
  Exercise prescription 807
  Genetic syndromes in ACHD 807

See Chapter 8.7 for pregnancy and adult congenital heart disease

8.6.1 Anatomical concepts in congenital heart disease

Sequential segmental approach

Describes anatomy based on the cardiac components and connections:

- Atria (via AV valve)
- Ventricles
- Great arteries

Atria

- Start at the atria (the morphological left and right atria are distinguished by the appendage, i.e. the 'left' atrium is not always on the left side; see Figure 8.6.1)

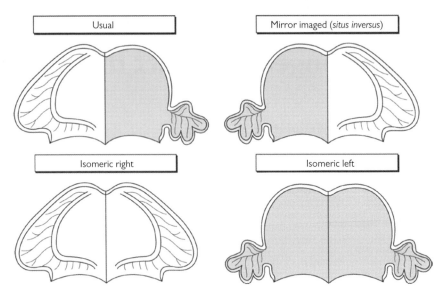

Figure 8.6.1 Right atrial appendage is broad and resembles 'Snoopy's nose'. The left atrial appendage is long and finger-like

Deanfield, John E., et al, 'Congenital Heart Disease in Children and Adults', in A. John Camm, Thomas F. Lüscher, and Patrick W. Serruys (eds), The ESC Textbook of Cardiovascular Medicine, 2 edn, The European Society of Cardiology (Oxford, 2009; online edn, Oxford Academic, 1 Aug. 2009), https://doi.org/10.1093/med/9780199566990.003.010

- The atrial location usually reflects the thoracic and abdominal visceral structures, e.g. the morphological left atrium is associated with the left bronchus (left lung) and the stomach and spleen (isomerism is more complex)
- Atrial arrangement can be described as:
  - *Usual*—LA on left, RA on right, also called **situs solitus**
  - *Mirror image*—RA on left, LA on right, also called **situs inversus**
  - *Right atrial isomerism*
    - More common in males
    - Unoperated survival to adulthood is rare
    - Asplenic with severe cyanotic heart disease lesions (e.g. single ventricle physiology)
  - *Left atrial isomerism*
    - More common in females
    - Polysplenia with absent sinus node and less severe spectrum of congenital cardiac lesions
    - Interrupted IVC—does not connect to right atrium (RA)—Azygos vein (Azygos continuity) drains from IVC into SVC
    - Note: embryologically the spleen is the only organ that is left sided from inception, and the IVC drains to the RA only, which explains the above findings

> **TIP**
>
> Isomerism = abnormal developmental symmetry in which morphologic structures that normally develop on one side are found on both sides of the body

Atrial → ventricular connections (AV)

Connections can be **concordant** (e.g. left atrium connects to left ventricle) or **discordant** (e.g. left atrium connects to right ventricle)

Distinguishing the morphological RV from the morphological LV

The morphological 'right' ventricle is not always on the right side, e.g. in congenitally corrected transposition of the great arteries the morphological LV is on the right and morphological RV is on the left

RV morphology:
- Increased trabeculations
- Moderator band
- More apically inserted tricuspid valve with *cordal attachment of the septal leaflet to the septum* (AV valve always follows the ventricle)—'offset of AV valve' on echo
- Discontinuity between AV valve and arterial valve

LV morphology:
- Muscular wall is smoother
- mitral valve (MV) has a higher insertion (mitral valve follows LV)
- Aorto-mitral continuity

Ventricular → great artery connections (VA)

Great arteries can be:

- *Concordant* e.g. LV to aorta
- *Discordant* e.g. LV to pulmonary artery
- *Double outlet*—usually RV to both great arteries
- Common trunk

For example, transposition of the great arteries (TGA) (see section on TGA):

- AV concordance with VA discordance
- Aorta arises from RV and aortic root is anterior to right pulmonary artery
- PA arises from LV

Other important anatomical terms:

- *Dextrocardia:* heart on the right side of thorax (apex points to the right)
- *Mesocardia:* heart centrally located with apex in midline
- *Levocardia:* heart on the left side of thorax (apex points to the left)
- *Levocardia with situs inversus:* heart on the left with a leftward pointing apex but mirror image of atria with thoracic and visceral structures

Basic foetal and transitional circulation

See Figure 8.6.2

- Oxygenated blood drains from the umbilical vein via the **ductus venosus** to the IVC and then RA
- Foetal pulmonary vascular resistance is high so blood bypasses the lungs via the **foramen ovale** (FO) and **ductus arteriosus** (DA) into the systemic circulation
- Transitional circulation develops when the newborn inflates lungs for the first time, pulmonary vascular resistance falls, flow increases, and LA pressure increases—FO closes
- DA flow reverses and it closes
- Results in **parallel pulmonary and systemic circulations**

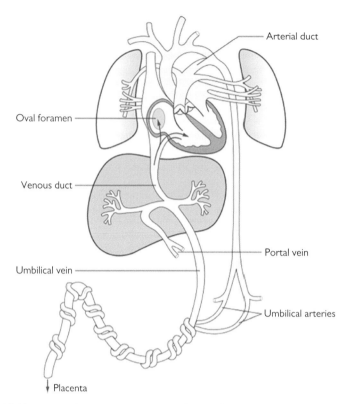

Figure 8.6.2 Venous circulation returning to the right heart bypasses the lungs via the oval fossa and arterial duct into the systemic arterial circulation

Deanfield, John E., et al, 'Congenital Heart Disease in Children and Adults', in A. John Camm, Thomas F. Lüscher, and Patrick W. Serruys (eds), The ESC Textbook of Cardiovascular Medicine, 2 edn, The European Society of Cardiology (Oxford, 2009; online edn, Oxford Academic, 1 Aug. 2009), https://doi.org/10.1093/med/9780199566990.003.010

8.6.2 Physiological concepts in congenital heart disease

Pulmonary blood flow

- Low pulmonary blood flow results in hypoxia
- High pulmonary blood flow results in pulmonary oedema and adverse vascular remodelling
- The muscular pulmonary arterial tree changes in the newborn over the first few months and becomes elastic and compliant
- If the lungs are exposed to high pressure and flow (e.g. via a left-to-right shunt) then this change does not occur and progressive irreversible adverse remodelling and pulmonary hypertension develop (Eisenmenger Syndrome, see Box 8.6.1)

If the flow is too high, an intervention is required to limit the flow:

- For example, surgical banding of the PA protects the distal vascular bed from high pressure whilst allowing adequate oxygenation
- Band is removed at definitive surgery (may develop PA stenosis at site of band)

If the flow is too little, an intervention is required to increase the flow:

- Low flow due to a pulmonary valve obstruction is treatable by valvotomy/valvuloplasty
- Otherwise a surgical shunt (arterial blood from aorta/subclavian redirected to PA) is used

BOX 8.6.1 EISENMENGER SYNDROME

- Occurs when a systemic to pulmonary shunt causes pulmonary arterial hypertension, which results in a reversal of the shunt direction (now from pulmonary to systemic) and therefore causing central cyanosis
- Symptoms: shortness of breath, cyanosis, fatigue, syncope, haemoptysis
- Negative prognostic factors: clinical evidence of right heart failure, decreasing exercise tolerance
- Treatment: targeted therapy for pulmonary arterial hypertension may be used with the input of a specialist centre

KEY CONCEPT
Protect the lungs from high pressures and flow to prevent irreversible adverse remodelling

Systemic arterial to pulmonary artery shunts (to increase pulmonary flow)
See Figure 8.6.3

Classical Blalock–Taussig (BT) shunt:
Usually right side via posterior thoracotomy
No longer used—subclavian is ligated and redirected to PA

Modified BT shunt (posterior thoracotomy):
Gortex tube between subclavian and PA

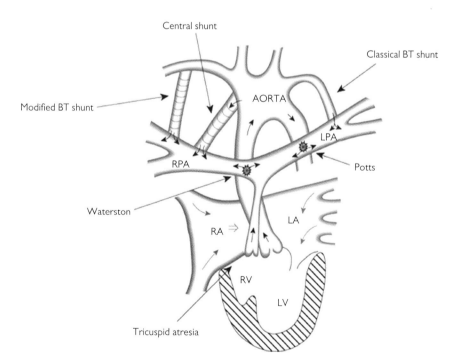

Figure 8.6.3 Blalock-Taussig shunt

Thorne, Sara, and Paul Clift (eds), ' Influence of pulmonary blood flow on management and outcome', in Sara Thorne, and Paul Clift (eds), Adult Congenital Heart Disease, 1 edn, Oxford Specialist Handbooks (Oxford, 2009), https://doi.org/10.1093/med/9780199228188.003.0005.

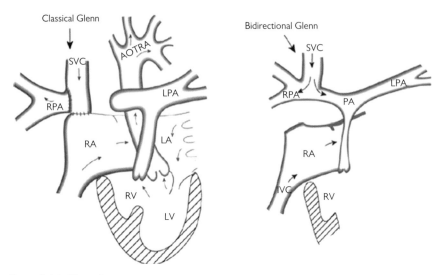

Figure 8.6.4 Glenn shunt
Thorne, Sara, and Paul Clift (eds), 'Influence of pulmonary blood flow on management and outcome', in Sara Thorne, and Paul Clift (eds), Adult Congenital Heart Disease, 1 edn, Oxford Specialist Handbooks (Oxford, 2009), https://doi.org/10.1093/med/9780199228188.003.0005.

Other shunts:
    Waterston: direct communication between ascending aorta and RPA
    Potts: direct communication between descending aorta and LPA
    Central: Gortex between brachiocephalic/aorta and PA

Systemic venous to pulmonary artery shunts

- After 6 months, infant pulmonary vascular resistance falls—systemic venous to pulmonary artery shunts become possible
- **Glenn shunt** (cavopulmonary shunt)—SVC to PA anastomosis (Figure 8.6.4): Classical Glenn—SVC anastomosis to RPA; RPA disconnected from main pulmonary artery (MPA)

Bidirectional Glenn—SVC anastomosis to RPA (RPA remains connected to MPA)
- If the IVC is also redirected to the PA then this constitutes a FONTAN circulation (discussed later)
- In childhood, SVC return is 75%—Glenn provides adequate flow
- In adults, SVC return is 25%—Glenn inadequate on its own
- Glenn shunts are associated with the development of pulmonary AV malformations (can contribute to right-to-left shunt, causing additional cyanosis or pulmonary haemorrhage)

Cyanosis

- Remember to consider if the pulmonary blood flow is high or low
- A cyanosed congenital patient has a right-to-left shunt (deoxygenated blood into systemic circulation)
- The combination of pulmonary blood flow (and size of right-to-left shunt) dictate the degree of cyanosis (systemic oxygenation):
  - **Low pulmonary flow**: greater cyanosis but lungs protected (blue but not breathless)
  - **High pulmonary flow**: less cyanosis but pulmonary congestion and damage to pulmonary vasculature (pink but breathless)

- In cyanosed congenital patients 'balancing' the pulmonary flow is essential, e.g. enough flow to achieve adequate systemic saturation whilst protecting the lungs
- In obligatory right-to-left shunt with 'balanced' pulmonary blood flow, systemic saturations will be around 85%
- Higher values suggest excess pulmonary blood flow and lower values inadequate flow

> **KEY CONCEPT**
>
> The degree of cyanosis reflects the balance between pulmonary blood flow and right-to-left shunt

Aetiology in congenital heart disease

Mixing of oxygenated and deoxygenated blood:
- Right-to-left shunt
- Bidirectional mixing via a univentricular heart or at great artery level
- Discordant VA connections (uncorrected TGA)—parallel circulations—shunt required to be compatible with life

Inadequate pulmonary blood flow:
- Obstructed or underdeveloped pulmonary vasculature
- Pulmonary hypertension (cyanosis always associated with a right-to-left shunt)

Important consequences of cyanosis

- Chronic cyanosis results in adaptive mechanisms to attempt to increase oxygen delivery to tissues, including erythrocytosis. These include:

Haematological:
- Polycythaemia, which can cause hyperviscosity and haemostatic abnormalities:
    - Venesection is not indicated unless there are clear clinical symptoms of hyperviscosity
    - When appropriate, venesection should be performed via exchange transfusion with saline replacement of volume
    - Care to avoid excess volume loss, which can lead to circulatory collapse and worsening iron deficiency
- Thrombocytopenia with impaired platelet function
- Iron deficiency, exacerbated by venesection
- Hyperuricaemia
- High levels of unconjugated bilirubin
- Coagulopathy: dysfunctional low platelets and clotting impairment. **INR falsely elevated** due to increased ratio of blood tube anticoagulant to plasma (high haematocrit)—discuss with lab when sending samples

Neurological:
- Stroke—usually secondary to paradoxical embolus (not due to hyperviscosity)
- Cerebral abscess—risk related to arterial saturation. **Should be suspected if cyanotic patient has neurological deterioration, odd headache, unexplained sepsis**
- Mental development is not significantly affected

Renal:
- Renal impairment
- Avoid nephrotoxic drugs

Other:
- Gout (urate excess) and pigment gallstones
- Acne
- Clubbing/scoliosis
- Haemoptysis—secondary to collaterals or pulmonary hypertension (PHT)—may be catastrophic and requires emergency investigation (CT) and preparation for aggressive resuscitation
- Avoid vasodilators as worsen cyanosis; beta-blockers acutely to reduce hypertension if required

Flow-related development of cardiac chambers and vessels
- Cardiac and arterial structures develop relative to the amount of blood flow
- If there is an interruption to blood flow then the structure will remain rudimentary/atretic
- If there is increased flow the structure will dilate and enlarge
- Illustrations of the concept:
    - Tricuspid atresia—no blood flow to RV—RV remains small and rudimentary
    - Aortic stenosis and large ventricular septal defect (VSD)—coarctation often present, with hypoplastic ascending aorta due to reduced aortic flow
    - Volume-loaded cardiac chambers or arteries enlarge (note: PAs remodel/hypertrophy in response to high degrees of flow)

8.6.3 General principles for use of diagnostic tests in patients with ACHD

- In general, the approach to diagnostic tests should be similar to that of any cardiac patient. Given the need for lifelong follow up for many ACHD patients, comparison of serial tests over time can be useful to determine the appropriate point for re-intervention, if required

Blood tests
- BNP/nT-pro BNP (trend over time more important than actual value)

Exercise testing
- Cardio Pulmonary Exercise Test (CPET)—using bike or treadmill—is a very useful functional test. 6-minute walk test (6MWT) is useful in the clinic setting, and is used particularly in the setting of pulmonary hypertension

Echo
- TTE is used routinely in the diagnosis and follow-up of ACHD patients
- TOE is used to answer specific questions such as looking for evidence of infective endocarditis, or providing detailed assessment of an ASD (often required to assess suitability for device closure)

CT
- Useful for assessing great vessels and coronary arteries
- Also often used when planning transcatheter valve implantation
- Be mindful of the young age of many ACHD patients and the need to reduce radiation exposure if possible

MRI
- Used to quantify ventricular volumes, shunts, pulmonary and systemic flows

Diagnostic cardiac catheterization
- Used to diagnose pulmonary hypertension, to assess shunts and pressure gradients, and to assess pressures within Fontan circulation
- Also has a role in identification of collateral vessels

8.6.4 Principles of intervention in ACHD

- All ACHD patients may come to require either medical treatment, catheter intervention, or redo surgery at some point in their lives
- Decisions regarding timing of intervention or redo surgery are usually taken by a multi-professional team in conjunction with the patient, with input from Cardiologists, Cardiac Surgeons, Radiologists, Clinical Nurse Specialists, Anaesthetists, and Clinical Psychologists
- Broadly speaking, the main reasons for medical/surgical or catheter intervention are:

Deterioration in functional status
- Requires assessment and treatment of any underlying reversible cause

Heart failure
- Requires assessment as above
- Conventional heart failure therapy if biventricular circulation and systemic LV
- Evidence for systemic RV/univentricular circulation is much more limited, and therefore needs expert management
- If no feasible targets for intervention, consideration of heart transplant (some ACHD patients may require heart/lung or heart/liver) or moving towards a palliative and supportive care approach

Arrhythmia
- Atrial and ventricular arrhythmia seen (depending on underlying pathology)
- Maintenance of sinus rhythm is the aim and referral to centre with expertise in arrhythmia and ACHD usually required:
    - Catheter ablation is recommended over long term medical therapy in patients with mild congenital heart disease and SVT
    - Should be considered in patients with moderate/severe congenital heart disease (in expert centre)
- Device implantation:
    - ICD for secondary prevention or for primary prevention in patients with biventricular circulation and systemic LV follows usual guidelines
    - Additionally, should be considered in Tetralogy of Fallot patients with multiple risk factors for VT
    - Evidence limited in patients with systemic RV or single ventricle

Infective endocarditis
- Managed as per local guidelines and early specialist centre input recommended
- See Chapter 3.7 for a summary of infective endocarditis management

8.6.5 Atrial septal defects and patent foramen ovale

The atrial septum is made-up of layers: **primum septum** (LA side) and **secundum septum** (RA side) with an overlapping flap in the region of the **fossa ovalis** (Figure 8.6.5).

Patent foramen ovale (PFO)

- Present in 25–30% of general population
- Clinical presentations:
  - Cryptogenic stroke in patients at low cardiovascular risk (paradoxical venous embolus)
  - Diving decompression illness (DCI, shunting of nitrogen bubbles)
  - Association with migraine (particularly with visual aura)
  - *Platypnoea-orthodeoxia syndrome* (dyspnoea and desaturation when moving from recumbent to standing or sitting position). Occurs due to transient right to left shunting in the upright position, and requires a PFO/ASD plus a functional component (e.g. pericardial effusion, emphysema, dilated aorta) causing deformation of the IAS on change of position
- Transthoracic echo (TTE) is usually normal unless the shunt is large (colour flow across septum) but PFO should be suspected if there is a significantly aneurysmal septum

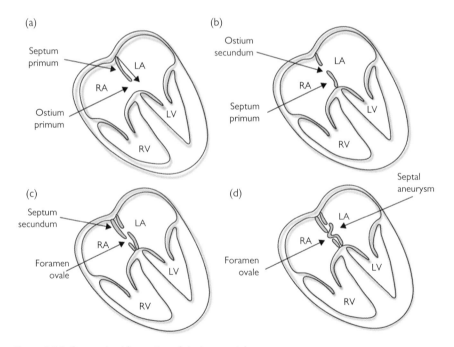

Figure 8.6.5 Summarised formation of the intra-atrial septum

A - first the septum primum comes down. If it does not complete then an ostium primum defect is created (defect involves atrial component of atrioventricular septum)

B - a hole develops in the middle of the primum septum = ostium secundum

C - a second muscular septum (septum secundum) forms on the RA side covering the hole. A large oval hole forms at the bottom = fossa ovalis. If the ositum secundum is not covered a ostium secundum ASD is created

D - at birth, increasing pressure in the LA pushes the two laminar septa together. In 25–30% the septa do not fuse and there is a flap or tunnel between the septa called a patent foramen ovale. If the septa are large and mobile a septal aneurysm results, which is almost always associated with PFO and confers an increased risk of paradoxical embolus stroke (compared to PFO on its own)

- PFO does not result in anatomical haemodynamic change, e.g. right volume load
- Investigation of choice: microbubble contrast transthoracic echo. Good technique requires repeated injection with high-quality Valsalva release (bubbles should cross on release of Valsalva manoeuvre) and sniff/cough manoeuvres
- Transcatheter closure indications:
  - Stroke without identifiable cardiovascular risk factors *and* no indication for long-term anticoagulation (e.g. intrinsic hypercoagulability) *and* no suspicion of left cardiac embolic focus (e.g. AF)
  - Patient with DCI who wishes to continue diving
  - Possibly migraine sufferers (controversial and subject of current research)
  - Platypnoea-orthodeoxia syndrome

Atrial septal defects

See Figure 8.6.6
Atrial septal defects are categorized into:

- Secundum (most common; 60%)
- Sinus venosus (difficult to detect on TTE and requires transoesophageal echocardiogram (TOE) assessment ('bicaval' 90° TOE view)
  - Superior (overriding SVC, defect at junction of vein into both atria; 15%)
  - Superior sinus venosus defects associated with partial anomalous pulmonary venous drainage—this represents an additional left-to-right shunt; most commonly right upper PV to RA or SVC
  - Inferior (rare)
- Coronary sinus (rare)
- Partial atrioventricular septal defects (20%, see section 8.6.5)
  - Sometimes referred to as 'primum ASD'
  - These defects are usually associated with an abnormality of the left AV valve and are *not* related to the primum septum
  - Due to a deficiency in the atrial component of the atrioventricular septum

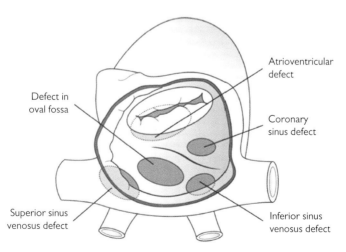

Figure 8.6.6 ASD locations
A. John Camm, Thomas F. Lüscher, and Patrick W. Serruys (eds), The ESC Textbook of Cardiovascular Medicine, 2 edn, The European Society of Cardiology (Oxford, 2009; online edn, Oxford Academic, 1 Aug. 2009), https://doi.org/10.1093/med/9780199566990

Atrial septal defect physiology

Chronic left-to-right shunting causes right heart volume overload and increased pulmonary arterial flow (with ageing, LA pressure increases—reduced LV compliance—and so the left-to-right shunt increases)

- Increased flow across PV and tricuspid valve (TV) can cause a murmur (signs can be confused with PS). Fixed split S2 classical
- Symptoms in childhood can be recurrent chest infections, failure to thrive, exercise intolerance
- Adults usually present in third or fourth decade with breathlessness and palpitations (or incidental; e.g. investigation of chest pain)
- Right heart volume loading causes right heart dilatation
- Right and left sided atrial arrhythmias are common
- Increased pulmonary flow can result in increased pulmonary vascular resistance (PVR) and PHT (late)
- Paradoxical embolus possible
- Endocarditis rare (low risk) with isolated secundum ASD
- ECG = right axis + incomplete RBBB (except primum or AVSD = left axis and RVH)
- One third of cases associated with genetic syndrome, e.g. Down's, Holt–Oram
- The association of first-degree heart block with a secundum ASD is suggestive of the familial (autosomal dominant) form and the family should be offered screening

Closure indications

1. ASD with 'haemodynamic consequences'—right heart dilatation
2. Symptoms—breathlessness or arrhythmia (may improve afterwards)
3. Protection of pulmonary vasculature (remodelling and progressive PHT)
4. Paradoxical embolus
    - Secundum defects (without other surgical lesions, e.g. anomalous PV drainage) up to 40 mm; anatomy usually suitable for transcatheter closure (Amplatzer device most common)
    - All other defects are currently only amenable to surgical intervention
    - In ASDs with established pulmonary hypertension caution is required—the ASD may act as a 'blow-off' valve to limit pulmonary pressure loading—closure may cause decompensation. Should still be possible with pressures < two-thirds systemic, shunt > 1.5:1 and demonstrated reversibility of PVR

> **LEARNING POINT**
>
> Partial atrioventricular septal defects and inferior sinus venosus defects cannot be closed using current technology by the transcatheter route

8.6.6 Ventricular septal defects

Ventricular septal defects (VSDs) are the second most common form of congenital heart disease after bicuspid aortic valve

The ventricular septum is composed of:

- Muscular septum—subdivided into
    - Inlet
    - Trabecular
    - Outlet
- Membranous septum—small area lying just below aortic valve

VSDs are classified according to their location within the septum and borders as viewed from the RV (Figure 8.6.7), e.g. muscular VSDs are bordered entirely by myocardium whereas perimembranous

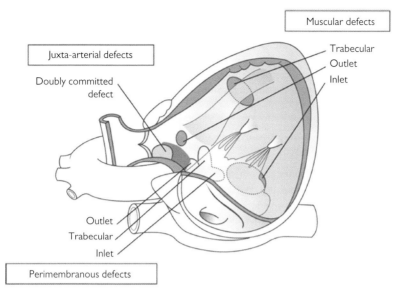

Figure 8.6.7 VSD locations
A. John Camm, Thomas F. Lüscher, and Patrick W. Serruys (eds), The ESC Textbook of Cardiovascular Medicine, 2 edn, The European Society of Cardiology (Oxford, 2009; online edn, Oxford Academic, 1 Aug. 2009), https://doi.org/10.1093/med/9780199566990

VSDs are bordered in part by the fibrous continuity of the AV valves and doubly committed VSDs border the fibrous continuity of the semi-lunar valves.

Restrictive ventricular septal defects

- Significant pressure gradient across defect from higher pressure left-to-right ventricle (high-velocity jet on echo)
- Shunt small (Qp/Qs < 1.5/1.0)
- No haemodynamic consequence
- Spontaneous closure in childhood common
- Asymptomatic (high-pitched murmur)
- Not always benign—restrictive perimembranous (including subarterial) VSD jet can 'suck' aortic valve leaflets via Venturi effect into the defect and the turbulence can cause leaflet damage/thickening:
    - Usually right coronary cusp of AV with signs of prolapse and progressive AR (requires close follow-up and is an indication for closure of VSD before irreversible valve damage results)
- A small perimembranous VSD may close while developing significant muscular right ventricular outflow tract obstruction
- Risk of endocarditis is not related to the size of defect

> **LEARNING POINT**
>
> A VSD-type murmur that recurs in a patient whose VSD was thought to have closed may represent the development of right ventricular outflow tract obstruction

Unrestricted ventricular septal defects

- The spectrum of clinical effect is dependent on the size of shunt and pulmonary versus systemic vascular resistance
- The haemodynamic burden and volume loading is on the **left ventricle—LV dilatation and failure, not RV dilatation, as RV is in systole during shunting**

- Pressure load affects the pulmonary vascular bed (and subsequently the RV)—increased flow/volume leads to increased PA pressure
- Moderate shunts lead to left heart dilatation and failure with atrial arrhythmias
- Large shunts lead to irreversible pulmonary vascular change and systemic pulmonary pressures unless pulmonary bed protected by pulmonary stenosis. End result is **Eisenmenger syndrome (right-to-left shunting, cyanosis)**

Management

The key indications for intervention are:

- Symptoms
- Progressive haemodynamic consequences of the shunt:
  - LV dilatation or increasing PA/RV pressures (usually when Qp:Qs > 2:1)
- Repair should be undertaken prior to irreversible pulmonary vascular change. In established PHT, repair may still be considered if there is evidence of pulmonary pressure reversibility associated with a moderate shunt
- Previous endocarditis and signs of AV valve prolapse/progressive regurgitation (in perimembranous defects) are other indications to prevent recurrence or valve damage

Intervention

- Generally surgical repair
- In perimembranous lesions—conducting tissues are vulnerable
- RBBB is common post-operatively and complete heart block (CHB) is possible
- Low threshold for permanent pacemaker (PPM) if there are persistent rhythm disturbances as there is a risk of late sudden death
- Transcatheter closure of muscular defects is possible in selected cases (requires no associated lesions and amenable anatomy)
- Perimembranous defects are also technically possible but rarely performed due to the higher incidence of unpredictable conduction problems (which can lead to late SCD)
- The aortic valve is also vulnerable and so highly specialist assessment is required

8.6.7 Atrioventricular septal defects

Consist of a defect of the AV septum with associated defect of the AV valve(s). There is a common AV junction (no offset on echo) and common AV ring.
Note: in AVSD the correct terminology is **left** and **right AV** valve as the valve anatomy is no longer 'mitral' or 'tricuspid'.

Common AV ring means that the aorta is displaced from its normal position between the two AV rings—LVOT is displaced anterosuperiorly and is elongated ('goose-neck') and narrowed—predisposes to obstruction.

Spectrum of anatomy (see Figures 8.6.8 and 8.6.9):

1. **Partial:** primum ASD + 'cleft' left AV valve but intact ventricular septum
2. **Intermediate:** primum ASD + restrictive VSD + separate but abnormal AV valves
3. **Complete:** continuous primum ASD and non-restrictive VSD + common AV valve (5 leaflets)
- **No AV offset on four-chamber echo = hallmark feature**
- 50% = trisomy 21 (Down's syndrome) but most partial AVSD do not have Down's syndrome (> 90%) and most complete AVSD do have Down's syndrome (> 75%)

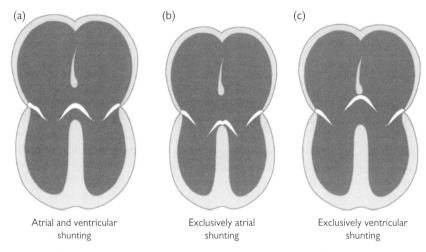

(a) Atrial and ventricular shunting (b) Exclusively atrial shunting (c) Exclusively ventricular shunting

Figure 8.6.8 Spectrum of anatomy and physiological consequences in AVSD relates to whether defect is ASD or VDS predominant and degree of left AV valve regurgitation
Source data from Craig B. Atrioventricular septal defect: from fetus to adult. *Heart.* 2006 Dec;92(12):1879–85. doi: 10.1136/hrt.2006.093344

- Physiology relates to whether the anatomy is ASD- or VSD-predominant and the degree of AV valve regurgitation, which is universal—partial/intermediate defects behave as large ASD physiology + left AV valve regurgitation
- Patients with trisomy 21 may present with established PHT (appear to have a propensity to developing PHT early possibly due to other intrinsic lung problems)
- ECG: first-degree AV block/higher degrees of AV block (defect affects the AV node)—heart block also a reasonably frequent post-surgical finding in this group
- All require surgical correction (unless established severe *irreversible* PHT)
- Long-term outcome is related to recurrence of left AV valve regurgitation (during initial repair, 'cleft' is sutured to create bi-leaflet left AV valve)
- Patients with operated AVSD who present with arrhythmia should have haemodynamic assessment, as the arrhythmia may be a manifestation of a structural lesion

8.6.8 Anomalous pulmonary venous drainage

Partial anomalous pulmonary venous drainage (PAPVD)

- *Definition*: at least one pulmonary vein drains to the right atrium (directly or indirectly via SVC or IVC)
- Most commonly right PVs to SVC or RA; left PVs less common—usually drain to coronary sinus or left brachiocephalic vein
- *Physiology*: As for ASD—left-to-right shunt; symptoms, signs, and indications for intervention the same as ASDs
- Associated with sinus venosus ASD—suspect partial anomalous pulmonary venous drainage (*PAPVD*) in **superior sinus venosus ASD** (commonly RUPV to SVC or RA)
- If there is only a single anomalous vein patients are usually asymptomatic (but this may be associated with other congenital lesions)

Scimitar syndrome

- Type of PAPVD
- Right PV to IVC ('scimitar vein')

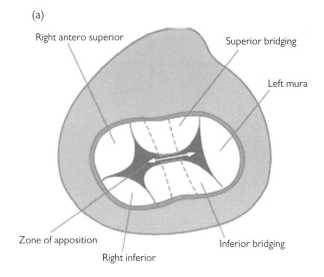
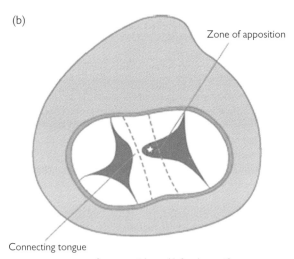

Figure 8.6.9 Anatomy of atrial septal defects: (a) Complete AVSD with common AV valve and (b) partial AVSD with 'cleft' mitral valve; Note the common AV ring and resultant anterior displacement of aorta

Source data from Craig B. Atrioventricular septal defect: from fetus to adult. *Heart*. 2006 Dec;92(12):1879–85. doi: 10.1136/hrt.2006.093344

- Anomalous systemic arterial supply to right lung (usually from descending aorta)
- Right lung hypoplasia and sequestration

Characteristic chest X-ray

Often diagnosed incidentally by radiologists (see Figure 8.6.10)

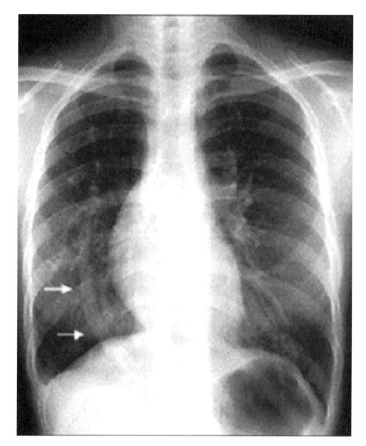

Figure 8.6.10 Scimitar syndrome. Arrows show 'scimitar' (curved middle-Eastern sword) vein and rightward displacement of the mediastinum.

Reproduced from Ashida K, Itoh A, Naruko T, et al. Familial scimitar syndrome: three-dimensional visualization of anomalous pulmonary vein in young sisters. *Circulation*. 2001 Jun 26;103(25):E126–7. doi: 10.1161/hc2501.092742 with permission from Wolters Kluwer.

Clinical presentation

- ASD physiology of left-to-right shunt (right heart volume loading/consequences of increased pulmonary flow):
    - Breathlessness or palpitations (secondary arrhythmias)
    - Frequent chest infections with possible haemoptysis due to lung sequestration
    - Incidental—murmur/CXR
- Indications for surgical intervention similar to ASD/PAPVD (right heart/PA consequences/symptoms/lung problems)
- 25% of patients have associated lesions that may require correction—ASD, VSD, patent ductus arteriosus (PDA), coarctation, tetralogy of Fallot (ToF)
- Intervention rarely required in adulthood

Total anomalous pulmonary venous drainage (TAPVD)

PVs join a confluence behind the LA—confluence drains into the right heart via the systemic venous circulation or atrium (see Figure 8.6.11):

1. Supracardiac: drains to brachiocephalic vein, azygos vein, SVC
2. Cardiac: drains to coronary sinus

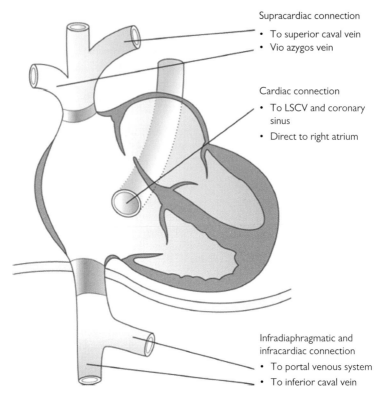

Figure 8.6.11 Total anomalous pulmonary venous drainage—entire pulmonary venous drainage is re-directed to a confluence, which in turn drains into a right sided/venous structure

Deanfield, John E., et al, 'Congenital Heart Disease in Children and Adults', in A. John Camm, Thomas F. Lüscher, and Patrick W. Serruys (eds), The ESC Textbook of Cardiovascular Medicine, 2 edn, The European Society of Cardiology (Oxford, 2009; online edn, Oxford Academic, 1 Aug. 2009), https://doi.org/10.1093/med/9780199566990.003.010

3. Infradiaphragmatic: to IVC; almost always with pulmonary venous obstruction (strongest predictor of poor outcome)
- TAPVD is always associated with ASD as all systemic and pulmonary venous return drains to the RA (obligatory right-to-left shunt, i.e. requires right-to-left shunt for life)
- ASD physiology of left-to-right shunt: right heart volume load and elevated pulmonary flow (leads to congestion and increased PVR)
- Requires early repair (no role for balloon septostomy)
    - Communication created between confluence and LA
    - ASD closed
    - Anomalous vein to systemic circulation ligated
    - Long-term outcomes excellent, and can be managed in primary care/general cardiology clinics

8.6.9 Coarctation of the aorta

Narrowing of the distal aortic arch usually at or beyond the site of the arterial duct, just distal to left subclavian (see Figure 8.6.12)

Spectrum of severity varies from mild to interruption of aorta or hypoplasia of the arch (collateral supply from arch to descending aorta)

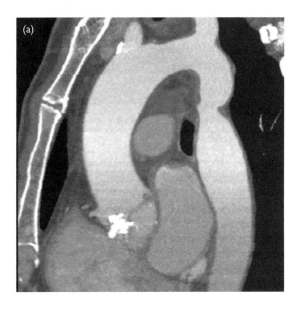

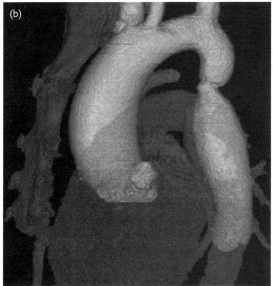

Figure 8.6.12 (a) CT image of aortic coarctation and (b) 3D reconstruction

Associated with:

- Bicuspid aortic valve (80%)
- Berry aneurysms of circle of Willis
- Turner's syndrome
- Multiple left heart obstructive lesions (Shone's syndrome: parachute MV, subvalvular and valvular AS and coarctation)

Presentation:

- Adults: uncontrolled hypertension or incidental finding
- Claudication, cerebral haemorrhage, and heart failure are less common presentations

Indications for intervention:

- Uncontrolled hypertension with evidence of significant anatomical obstruction or significant gradient (> 30 mmHg)

Surgical repair of coarctation:

1. End-to-end anastomosis
2. Subclavian flap repair: left subclavian artery used to augment aorta (left arm pulse diminished)
3. Dacron patch aortoplasty: now abandoned due to **risk of late aneurysm formation**

Transcatheter intervention:

- Transcatheter balloon angioplasty and stenting is an option for management of coarctation, and is frequently considered as an alternative to surgery, particularly in adults presenting with coarctation

Follow-up:

- Re-coarctation at the site of previous surgical repair is not uncommon; lifelong follow-up is required after surgery or transcatheter intervention as although relief of obstruction can reduce BP there is an inherent predisposition to hypertension and associated complications
- Measure BP in the right arm
- Ambulatory BP is commonly utilized to demonstrate hypertension
- Aggressive BP treatment, with ACE inhibitors/ARBs (caution in females of reproductive age) and BBs as the preferred agents
- Serial cross-sectional imaging is essential to assess the repair/stent—recoarctation, aneurysm formation, and stent fracture are all possible
    - **MRI** is the usual modality in native or surgical repair due to the avoidance of radiation and provision of physiological data. Baseline scans should look for cerebral berry aneurysm. However, MRI cannot identify stent structure/fracture and luminal data is limited due to stent interference
    - **Low dose localized CT**: higher resolution and useful in patients with stent follow-up
    - **Echo**: suprasternal aortic arch view. Align continuous wave with colour flow in descending aorta. Look for increased velocity and diastolic tail (Figure 8.6.13)

8.6.10 Coronary artery anomalies

- Incidence around 1%
- Range from minor with no clinical significance to those of major clinical importance
- Anomaly can be of:
    - Origin (i.e. not originating from sinus of Valsalva, or originating from wrong coronary sinus)—e.g. from Aorta or pulmonary artery, or e.g. right coronary artery from left coronary sinus
    - Anatomical course
    - Final communication (e.g. fistulous communication to ventricular cavity)
- Clinical importance depends on the ability of the anomaly to cause myocardial ischaemia, with the following being particularly important
    - Interarterial course (passing between the aorta and pulmonary trunk)—can become compressed—often during exercise when PA dilates

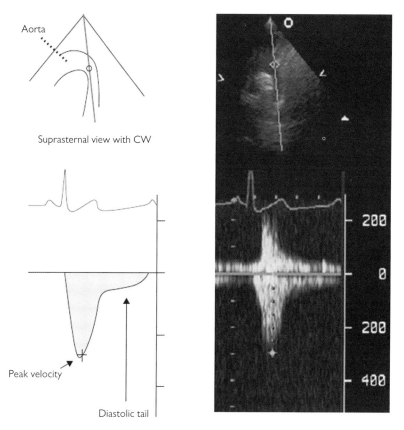

Figure 8.6.13 Echo assessment of coarctation. Suprasternal view and continuous wave Doppler trace demonstrating increased velocity with diastolic tail
Reproduced with permission from the *Oxford Specialist Handbook of Echocardiography*, eds. Paul Leeson, Andrew Mitchell and Harald Becher, copyright 2007 Oxford University Press

- Intramural course (coronary artery travels for some distance in the wall of the aorta)
- Origin from pulmonary trunk (e.g. left coronary artery from pulmonary artery—ALCAPA) which results in coronary steal—severity depends on development of collaterals

8.6.11 Sinus of Valsalva aneurysms

- Dilatation of one of the aortic sinuses
- Right coronary sinus most common site (75%)
- VSDs commonly associated
- Ruptured aneurysms can present acutely with chest pain and breathlessness (misdiagnosed as pulmonary embolus (PE) with loud continuous murmur or haemodynamic collapse and cardiac arrest/sudden death)
- Presentation depends on the site of rupture/receiving chamber and associated compromise of the coronary ostium
- Requires emergency intervention—most commonly surgery but transcatheter closure feasible and successful in expert hands

8.6.12 Patent ductus arteriosus

The foetal connection between proximal left pulmonary artery to descending aorta (just distal to left subclavian); foetal circulation bypasses lungs (see *Basic foetal circulation* in Figure 8.6.2)

Adult presentation

1. Incidental echo finding: very small, no murmur
2. Small: long ejection/continuous murmur radiating to back, no haemodynamic consequences, endocarditis risk
3. Moderate: continuous murmur, haemodynamic change (left-to-right shunt), increased pulmonary flow (risk of PHT) and left heart volume loading (left sided dilatation), collapsing pulses
4. Large—Eisenmenger physiology with pulmonary hypertension, differential cyanosis (lower body sats < right arm), toe clubbing
   - Associated with aortic coarctation
   - Transcatheter closure is the treatment of choice for children and adults
   - Incidental (silent) PDAs do not need closure (unless associated with an episode of previous endocarditis)
   - Small PDAs can be closed to protect against endocarditis
   - Haemodynamic PDAs should be closed unless severe irreversible PHT (act as 'blow-off' valve to limit pulmonary pressures)

8.6.13 Bicuspid aortic valve

- Most common congenital heart lesion—4.6 per 1000 live births
- 1.5× more prevalent in males
- Present in large proportion of cases of coarctation
- Majority spontaneous, although can be inherited
- May have associated aortopathy, e.g. dilated ascending aorta
- Anatomy:
  - Fusion/non-separation of two cusps—most common pattern is fusion of left and right coronary cusps
- Clinical presentation:
  - AS or AR
- Indications for intervention
  - As per usual indications for surgery for aortic valve disease (see Chapter 3.1)
  - Consider balloon valvuloplasty for younger patients with non-calcified valve
  - Consider 'Ross procedure' for younger patients requiring surgery, particularly when desire to avoid anti-coagulation, i.e. female of child-bearing age (aortic valve is replaced with the patient's own pulmonary valve, and a pulmonary allograft (cadaveric valve) is then used to replace the pulmonary valve, which should last longer than a tissue valve in place of the aortic valve where flow rate is higher)

8.6.14 Ebstein's anomaly

Failure of delamination of the TV leaflets. Results in (Figure 8.6.14):

1. Apical displacement of septal and posterolateral leaflets below the AV rings into the RV
2. 'Atrialization' of RV = smaller functional RV (large RA)

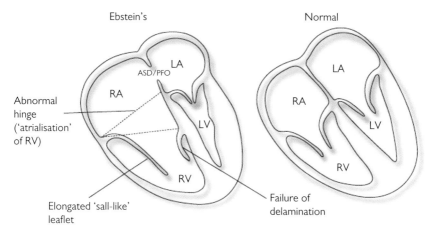

Figure 8.6.14 Ebstein's anomaly - elongated anterior leaflet and apical displacement of septal leaflet

3. TV dysfunction
4. Atrial shunt (PFO or ASD) in 50%
5. Accessory pathways in 25% (increased risk arrhythmias), often multiple

- Majority of cases sporadic (association with maternal lithium in first trimester may be false)
- There is a spectrum of Ebstein's malformation. Severity of the lesion dictates the natural history
- Adult presentation:
  - Consequences of TV/RV dysfunction or arrhythmia or complications related to a shunt (ASD/PFO; cyanosis, paradoxical embolus)
  - Echo diagnosis: hallmark is apical displacement of septal leaflet (+/− post leaflet) > 20 mm + elongated sail-like anterior leaflet
  - Elevated JVP is a late sign due to the large compliant RA

Intervention

- TV repair/replacement is indicated if there is significant TR with haemodynamic consequences (aim to intervene before significant right heart deterioration) *or* symptoms
- In addition to TVR the atrium can be 'plicated' to reduce the size, associated shunts closed, and arrhythmia surgery performed
- For high-risk patients, i.e. those with significant established right heart dysfunction, a bidirectional Glenn may be indicated to reduce RV preload
- Symptoms can be difficult to assess; regular objective functional testing is helpful (e.g. exercise testing)

8.6.15 Transposition of the great arteries

See Figure 8.6.15

- AV concordance with VA discordance (see segmental sequential approach)
- Aorta arises from RV and aortic root is anterior to right pulmonary artery (RPA)
- PA arises from LV

Systemic and pulmonary circulations are in parallel rather than in series:

- **Systemic circulation** (deoxygenated blood is re-circulated): SVC and IVC venous return to RA via tricuspid valve to RV, to aorta, to peripheral circulation, and back to SVC and IVC
- **Pulmonary circulation** (oxygenated blood re-circulated): PVs to LA via mitral valve, to LV, to PA, to lungs, and back to LA

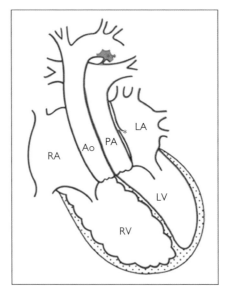

Figure 8.6.15 Transposition of the great arteries

Thorne, Sara, and Sarah Bowater (eds), Adult Congenital Heart Disease, 2 edn, Oxford Specialist Handbooks in Cardiology (Oxford, 2017; online edn, Oxford Academic, 1 Aug. 2017), https://doi.org/10.1093/med/9780198759959.001.0001

- CXR: narrow cardiac 'pedicle' representing the great arteries' parallel arrangement (normalized with arterial switch operation) compared to the normal crossing great arteries
- In the absence of a septal defect, the only way the two circulations can mix is via foetal shunts (foramen ovale and PDA). Otherwise the circulation is incompatible with life
- At birth, the PDA can be maintained via prostaglandin and/or the intra-atrial communication via percutaneous balloon septostomy

Atrial switch: Mustard or Senning operation

See Figure 8.6.16

- Intra-atrial baffles are used to re-route systemic and pulmonary circulation; systemic venous blood is redirected to the LV (pulmonary circuit pump) and oxygenated pulmonary venous return to the RV (systemic pump)
- The atrial switch has been superseded by the **arterial switch** (anatomical repair) since the late 1980s

TERMINOLOGY/NOMENCLATURE (POST-ATRIAL SWITCH)

Right sided atrium = pulmonary venous atrium
Left sided atrium = systemic venous atrium
Left ventricle = subpulmonary ventricle
Right ventricle = systemic ventricle

Definitions:

- Mustard operation uses prosthetic baffles (Dacron) or pericardium
- Senning operation uses baffles made of intrinsic atrial wall material
- Baffle is a saddle-shaped structure to redirect blood

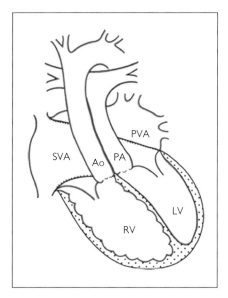

Figure 8.6.16 Atrial switch. Ao, aorta; LA, left atrium; LV, left ventricle; PA, pulmonary artery; RA, right atrium; RV, right ventricle; VC, valved conduit; PVA, pulmonary venous atrium; SVA, systemic venous atrium

Thorne, Sara, and Sarah Bowater (eds), Adult Congenital Heart Disease, 2 edn, Oxford Specialist Handbooks in Cardiology (Oxford, 2017; online edn, Oxford Academic, 1 Aug. 2017), https://doi.org/10.1093/med/9780198759959.001.0001

Long-term problems:

1. Venous pathway (SVC/IVC) stenosis/baffle leak; if this results in a right-to-left shunt will cause cyanosis
2. Atrial arrhythmias inevitable (focus is atrial surgical scar) and can cause circulatory collapse; **needs prompt DCCV**
3. Junctional rhythm common (AV node damage; PPM is indicated for symptomatic bradycardia or tachycardias secondary to the bradycardia; no proven prognostic benefit)
4. Eventual RV (systemic ventricle) or AV valve failure (not designed for systemic pressures). Options are transplant or consideration of arterial switch operation.

Arterial switch (anatomical repair)

- Aorta reconnected to LV and PA reconnected to RV
- Issues with distortion of the great arteries/valves:
    - Neo-aortic regurgitation/root dilatation
    - Supravalvular PS/RVOT obstruction
    - Coronary ostial stenosis

Rastelli operation

In TGA with a VSD and PS (see Figure 8.6.17):

- Parallel circulation blood mixed across VSD
- Excessive pulmonary blood flow prevented by stenosis (otherwise leads to increased PVR and PHT, i.e. Eisenmenger's)
- 'Balanced' cyanotic circulation that may allow survival

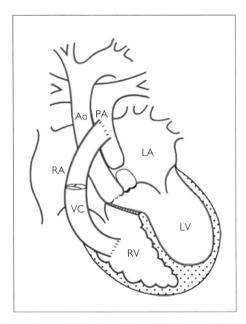

Figure 8.6.17 Rastelli operation in TGA with a VSD and PS. Ao, aorta; LA, left atrium; LV, left ventricle; PA, pulmonary artery; RA, right atrium; RV, right ventricle; VC, valved conduit; PVA, pulmonary venous atrium; SVA systemic venous atrium

Thorne, Sara, and Sarah Bowater (eds), Adult Congenital Heart Disease, 2 edn, Oxford Specialist Handbooks in Cardiology (Oxford, 2017; online edn, Oxford Academic, 1 Aug. 2017), https://doi.org/10.1093/med/9780198759959.001.0001

In a Rastelli procedure, VSD is closed to in such a way to commit the aorta to the LV (across non-functional RVOT) and the RV is directed to the PA via a valved conduit. The PA is ligated.

- Issues:
    - Conduit stenosis
    - Subaortic obstruction as a result of VSD patch
    - Residual VSD (shunt and endocarditis risk)

8.6.16 Congenitally corrected transposition of the great arteries (ccTGA)

In ccTGA there is AV and VA discordance, e.g. the ventricles are inverted (Figure 8.6.18).

- Associated lesions in the majority of cases:
    - VSD present in 75%
    - PS present in 75%
    - Left AV valve (tricuspid) abnormalities (Ebsteinoid)
- CXR: abnormally straight left heart border
- AV block is a very common complication (may be the presenting complaint); 2%/year incidence of CHB
- The problem with ccTGA is that the systemic circulation is supported by the RV and TV, which are not designed for this purpose. The circulations are in series and mix normally
- If there are no associated lesions the patient may be asymptomatic until early adulthood or middle age

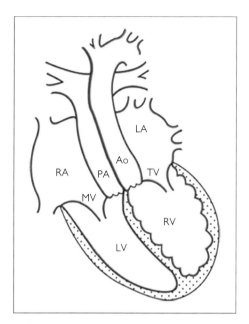

Figure 8.6.18 Isolated ccTGA. Ao, aorta; LA, left atrium; LV, left ventricle; PA, pulmonary artery; MV, mitral valve; RA, right atrium; RV, right ventricle; TV, tricuspid valve
Thorne, Sara, and Sarah Bowater (eds), Adult Congenital Heart Disease, 2 edn, Oxford Specialist Handbooks in Cardiology (Oxford, 2017; online edn, Oxford Academic, 1 Aug. 2017), https://doi.org/10.1093/med/9780198759959.001.0001

Adult presentation
- Progressive systemic ventricular (right ventricular) failure and/or left AV valve failure
- Heart block/arrhythmias

Management
- If asymptomatic and incidental it is reasonable to simply monitor the RV/TV (left AV valve) and treat with a PPM if CHB develops
- If significant TR develops early surgical intervention is indicated before the RV starts to fail
- **Anatomical surgical repair** or 'double switch' operation—Senning/Mustard and arterial switch, the LV becoming the systemic ventricle (LV may need to be 'retrained' with PA band)—considered if there is severe TR and RV dysfunction

As documented at the start of this section, 75% of patients with ccTGA have associated VSDs and PS. In the case of ccTGA with VSD and PS the presentation is paediatric:

- Heart failure if the VSD is large (high pulmonary flow and LV volume loading)
- Cyanosis if RVOT obstruction severe (low pulmonary flow but PAs protected)

Management: 'Classic repair'
- VSD patch closure
- LV redirected to the PA with a valved conduit
- TVR if significant valve problems

i.e. the RV remains the systemic ventricle with associated future problems

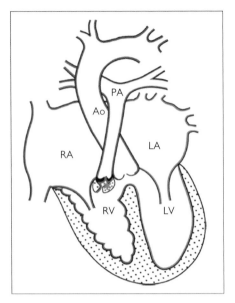

Figure 8.6.19 Tetralogy of Fallot. *deviation of outlet septum; Ao, aorta; LA, left atrium; LV, left ventricle; PA, pulmonary artery; RA, right atrium; RV, right ventricle

Thorne, Sara, and Sarah Bowater (eds), Adult Congenital Heart Disease, 2 edn, Oxford Specialist Handbooks in Cardiology (Oxford, 2017; online edn, Oxford Academic, 1 Aug. 2017), https://doi.org/10.1093/med/9780198759959.001.0001

8.6.17 Tetralogy of Fallot

See Figure 8.6.19. This is a combination of:

1. RVOT obstruction—valvular and infundibular pulmonary stenosis
2. VSD
3. Overriding aorta
4. RVH secondary to pulmonary stenosis

- Should be considered as a primary problem of the outlet (subarterial) ventricular septal formation and migration (anterocephalad deviation), with subsequent RVOT obstruction and overriding aorta
- 15% have a deletion of chromosome 22q11 (see Box 8.6.2)

Presentation

Depends on the degree of RVOT obstruction i.e. the 'balance' of systemic and pulmonary circulations:

- **Mild obstruction**—high pulmonary blood flow—cardiac failure and minimal cyanosis
- **Significant obstruction**—right-to-left shunt and cyanosis (majority)

Surgical management

- Palliative procedures to increase pulmonary blood flow—e.g. BT shunt—may be used if associated lesions complicate initial total repair
- Total repair (preferred treatment in infancy):
  - VSD closed with a patch
  - RVOT obstruction relieved by resection of infundibular muscle or transannular patch (literally cutting across the PV annulus and RVOT; almost always results in PR especially with associated dysplastic valves)

> **BOX 8.6.2 DIGEORGE SYNDROME (CATCH 22, 22Q11 SYNDROME)**
>
> Due to a deletion of chromosome 22 (22q11)
>
> C—cardiac defects (15% of ToF, interrupted aortic arch, truncus arteriosus)
>
> A—abnormal facies (microagnathia, short philtrum, low-set ears)
>
> T—thymic hypoplasia
>
> C—cleft palate
>
> H—hypocalcaemia
>
> 22—chromosome 22
>
> Behavioural and psychiatric disorders
>
> Inherited in an autosomal dominant manner and is highly variable
>
> Affected subjects have a 50% risk of passing the defect to offspring (e.g. if you have ToF with Catch 22 the implication is that there is a 50% of passing a congenital condition rather than 6% in isolated ToF); however, most cases sporadic
>
> FISH test for 22q11 should be offered to all patients with ToF considering pregnancy
>
> - 90% of patients have a *de novo* variant with 10% inherited from a parent who may or may not have already been diagnosed with the condition and can sometimes have very subtle clinical features only

- With successful repair, survival approaches that of the general population
- Long-term pulmonary regurgitation is inevitable after transannular patch—essentially the RVOT/pulmonary valve annulus has been longitudinally cut open and the often dysplastic pulmonary valve will not coapt as the RVOT grows/enlarges (the converse is residual stenosis)
- The development of severe PR leads to RV dilatation and dysfunction—indication for intervention (increasingly transcatheter or 'injectable' off-pump surgical valves)
- ECG shows RBBB (right bundle runs in the floor of the VSD and is often damaged during surgery)
- Non-sustained VT is common but is not in itself an indicator of SCD risk
- Antiarrhythmics are not indicated if asymptomatic
- The VT is normally of RVOT origin (surgical scar from infundibulectomy or VSD patch)
- Development of major arrhythmias (AF/flutter and sustained VT) normally reflect haemodynamic deterioration (PR, RV dilatation), and therefore haemodynamic assessment and correction of the lesion can correct the arrhythmia (with the option of surgical/catheter ablation)
- CXR—'coeur en sabot' or boot-shaped heart (classical)
- Aortic root dilatation and aortic regurgitation are recognised: can be due to damage to the aortic valve during VSD repair or intrinsic aortopathy (cystic medial necrosis type; root > 55 mm is surgical indication)

> **KEY CONCEPT**
>
> Change in QRS duration reflects RV size and is related to the risk of SCD and VT.
>
> QRS > 180 ms is a highly sensitive marker for SCD and VT in previous ToF repair (SCD accounts for one-third of late deaths)

Pulmonary atresia with VSD

- Is part of the ToF spectrum but instead of pulmonary stenosis there is an interruption (atresia) of the pulmonary outflow
- Associated with 22q11 micro-deletion

- Lack of PA flow results in different degrees of pulmonary vascular underdevelopment (cardiac structures develop relative to degree of blood flow)
- No blood passes directly from the right heart into the pulmonary tree (flow via VSD)
- Blood is redirected from systemic circulation back into PAs from either a large PDA or multiple systemic-to-pulmonary-artery collaterals—major aortopulmonary collateral arteries (MAPCAs)—usually from the descending aorta

8.6.18 Functionally single ventricle and the Fontan circulation

Functionally single ventricle

Complex **congenital heart disease** with a functionally single ventricle *and* a biventricular surgical repair not possible

Dominant ventricle can be morphologically right or left with an associated rudimentary ventricle. Common examples:

- **Tricuspid atresia** (no right AV connection = no blood flow = poor RV development = rudimentary RV); mixing via ASD
- **Pulmonary atresia** with intact ventricular septum (minimal flow into RV and so poor development = rudimentary RV)
- **Mitral atresia** (as per tricuspid atresia but for left)
- **Double inlet ventricle:**
    - Both AV valves connected to a single dominant ventricle
    - Main ventricle connected to a rudimentary chamber via 'VSD'
    - One great artery arises from main chamber and one from the rudimentary chamber
    - Left ventricle dominant in majority of cases
    - VA discordance (TGA type) common (aorta arises from rudimentary right ventricle)
    - Pulmonary obstruction protects the lungs from systemic pressures in 50%
- **Hypoplastic left heart syndrome**—varying hypoplasia of the LV, aorta and left-sided valves results in complex univentricular anatomy
    - Systemic and pulmonary blood is mixed in the dominant morphological right ventricle resulting in cyanosis
    - The degree of cyanosis and neonatal presentation depends on pulmonary blood flow (PA protected by PS or a restrictive 'VSD'—rare to have a balanced circulation)
    - **High pulmonary flow** = congestive heart failure and pulmonary vascular remodelling (mild cyanosis)—requires PA banding to protect lungs
    - **Low pulmonary blood flow** = severe cyanosis and circulatory collapse (requires emergency systemic-pulmonary shunt)

> **LEARNING POINT**
>
> There are now more adults than children with complex congenital heart disease, which reflects the success of paediatric cardiac surgery over the last 50 years

Fontan surgery

- A **palliative procedure** when a two ventricle repair is not possible (Figure 8.6.20)
- There are a number of modifications but in simple terms the systemic venous blood from the IVC and SVC is redirected (bypassing right heart) directly to PAs
- Functionally single ventricle to support the systemic circulation
- End result is a palliative procedure, e.g. limited life expectancy but improved symptoms and functionality

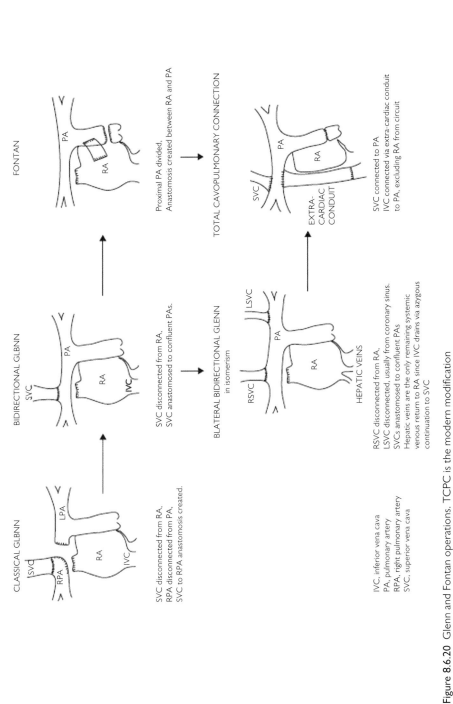

Figure 8.6.20 Glenn and Fontan operations. TCPC is the modern modification

Reproduced with permission from Thorne, S. A., 'Congenital heart disease in the adult', in David A. Warrell, Timothy M. Cox, and John D. Firth (eds), Oxford Textbook of Medicine, 5 edn, Oxford Textbooks (Oxford, 2010), https://doi.org/10.1093/med/9780199204854.003.1612_update_002. With permission from Oxford University Press

- Is usually a staged approach. There are many historical technical variations:
    - Originally an **atrio-pulmonary connection (e.g. RA connected to PA);** leads to massive RA dilatation and risk of arrhythmias. RA can behave as a swirling reservoir wasting passive blood flow energy, with risk of thrombus formation
    - Modern modification is the **total cavopulmonary connection (TCPC)**—SVC blood redirected via a Glenn shunt. IVC blood redirected via a lateral tunnel (within the RA) or an extracardiac conduit. The result is efficient laminar blood flow without RA loading. Note: as the SVC is usually disconnected from the RA the usual pacing lead route is not available

Stage 1:

- Correct pulmonary blood flow (PA band if high flow vs systemic-arterial shunt if low flow)

Stage 2:

- Glenn operation—cavopulmonary shunt—SVC connected to PAs
- SVC flow accounts for 70% venous return in infant
- Only possible when PVR low (3–4 months of age)

Stage 3:

- Complete Fontan: modern approach TCPC (stages 2 and 3 may be combined)
- TCPC can be 'fenestrated'. This will result in a right-to-left shunt with mild desaturation. Acts as a 'blow-off valve' for high venous pressures

> **KEY CONCEPT**
>
> By bypassing the RA (which acts as a reservoir with swirling blood) efficient laminar blood flow is redirected to the PAs
>
> **Flow is passive**—dependent on low pulmonary vascular resistance, good hydration/systemic venous pressure, and effective pulmonary venous atrium and systemic ventricular diastolic parameters (to 'suck' blood through the lungs)—therefore dehydration and arrhythmia can cause rapid life-threatening decompensation

Possible complications of Fontan circulation

- Atrial arrhythmias—common due to atrial surgical scarring. Potentially life-threatening due to slowing of passive flow—**acute arrhythmia in a Fontan patient is a medical emergency and requires immediate rhythm control (chemical or electrical)**
- Paradoxical embolus—use intravenous line filters to reduce risk if patient requires IV therapy
- The single systemic ventricle and AV valve may develop progressive dysfunction and eventual heart failure
- Any obstruction in the Fontan pathway or pulmonary circulation will obstruct passive flow
- At risk of thrombo-embolism and PE—all Fontan patients are anticoagulated
- Chronic venous hypertension leads to hepatic dysfunction and *protein-losing enteropathy* (5-year survival after diagnosis is 50%—test for low serum albumin but high stool alpha 1-antitrypsin in a 24-h collection)
- Progressive cyanosis (sats < 90%) suggests right-to-left shunt (opening up of venous collateral/pulmonary AVMs or shunting through Fontan fenestration); patients without a Fontan fenestration should have sats > 94%

8.6.19 Truncus arteriosus

- Single great arterial trunk arises from the ventricle (always associated with large VSD for mixing)
- PAs come off ascending aorta

- 'Truncal' valve dysplastic—the degree of valve dysfunction dictates prognosis
- One third have DiGeorge's syndrome
- Early corrective surgery is required before irreversible PHT develops (PAs subject to systemic pressures)

8.6.20 Other considerations in adult congenital heart disease

Infective endocarditis prevention
- Discrepancy exists between guidelines from ESC and NICE regarding endocarditis prophylaxis
- According to ESC, the following congenital heart disease patients are considered high risk of endocarditis and should receive antibiotic prophylaxis prior to dental procedures which require manipulation of the gingival or periapical region of teeth, or where the oral mucosa will be perforated:
    - Cyanotic ACHD, without repair, or where there is a residual defect, shunt, or conduit
    - ACHD after repair with prosthetic material (percutaneous or surgical) for 6 months after the procedure or until the material is judged to be endothelialized
    - Patients with a prosthetic valve or prosthetic material used for a valve repair
    - Patients with previous infective endocarditis
- Patients with ACHD should be counselled carefully regarding the risks of tattoos and piercings

Exercise prescription
- Exercise is recognized to be an important adjunct to medical care of the ACHD patient
- Indeed, sports and exercise should be discussed at every patient encounter and formal guidelines are available to help with this

Considerations for ACHD patients undergoing non-cardiac surgery or experiencing intercurrent, non-cardiac illness:
- Potential for cardiac condition to be destabilized by anaesthesia for planned surgery, or by acute non-cardiac illness
- Patient should be managed with guidance from the ACHD team who know the patient, and with an MDT approach including surgeon and anaesthetist
- Consideration should be given to:
    - Most appropriate location for surgery?
    - Need for anaesthetist with specific cardiac or ACHD expertise?
    - Most appropriate ward for patient to go to post-operatively? (e.g. general ITU, cardiac ITU, period of time on CCU after recovery)

Genetic syndromes in ACHD
Down syndrome
- Down syndrome is the most common chromosomal disorder with a birth incidence of about 1 in 1000 and is increasingly prevalent with advancing maternal age
- It is due to the presence of an extra, third copy of chromosome 21 (trisomy 21)
- Congenital heart disease is common, particularly AVSDs or VSDs
- Other common features include, characteristic facial features, short stature, learning difficulties, single palmar crease, sandal gap, hypotonia, and increased risk of leukaemia and dementia
- Testing is usually performed by QF-PCR if there are clinical features in a neonate

Noonan syndrome

- Noonan syndrome (NS) is an autosomal dominant condition cause by a variant in the RAS-MAPK pathway with a high incidence of CVD
- 1 in 1000–2500 births are affected
- Half are due to variants in the *PTPN11* gene where pulmonary stenosis is a frequent feature
- In contrast, those with a *RAF1* variant are more likely to have HCM
- It is usually a clinical diagnosis made by observing the typical features, but these may be subtle or absent
- Finding a pathogenic variant is extremely helpful in confirming a suspected clinical diagnosis
- Clinical features and cardiac defects are presented in Table 8.6.1 and Figure 8.6.21
- Abnormal ECGs are often seen, even in the absence of structural cardiac disease, and abnormalities include left axis deviation, small precordial R waves and features of HCM

Turner syndrome

- Turner syndrome affects about 1 in 2000 female births and is usually due to the presence of a single X sex chromosome
- There is commonly some degree of mosaicism, with each cell line having a slightly different karyotype, for example 46,XX/45,X0 mosaicism

Table 8.6.1 Summary of key genetic syndromes and their cardiac manifestations.

Genetic abnormality	Name of syndrome	Clinical features	Cardiac manifestations
Trisomy 21	Down syndrome	Characteristic facies Short stature Hypotonia Learning disability Early onset dementia	AVSD VSD ASD PDA ToF
45X0	Turner syndrome	Short stature Webbed neck Cubitus valgus Skeletal anomalies Renal anomalies Early ovarian failure	BAV Aortopathy CoA HLHS
22q.11 deletion	DiGeorge syndrome	Cardiac abnormality Abnormal facies Thymic anomalies Cleft palate Hypocalcaemia (CATCH 22)	ToF Truncus arteriosus VSD Aortic abnormalities
7q11.23 deletion	Williams syndrome	Dysmorphic facies 'Social personality' Short stature Endocrine abnormalities	Aortic stenosis (supra-valvar) Branch pulmonary artery stenosis Aortic abnormalities
Various	Noonan syndrome	Short stature Widely spaced eyes Pectus deformity Bleeding disorders	Pulmonary stenosis ASD ToF AVSD

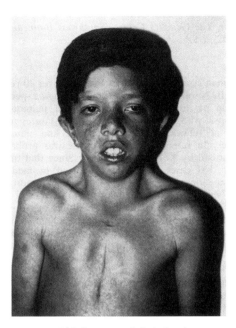

Figure 8.6.21 The phenotype is variable but generally includes short stature, facial dysmorphism, (hypertelorism with epicanthic folds, ptosis and low-set posteriorly rotated ears), unusual chest shape and cardiac defects
Reproduced from 'Noonan syndrome', J. E. Allanson, *J. Med. Genet.* 24(1), 9–13, copyright 1987 with permission from BMJ Publishing Group Ltd

- It is characterised by short stature, whilst other features include broad chest, lymphoedema, webbed neck, low-set ears, low hairline, gonadal dysfunction, thyroid abnormalities, increased risk of diabetes and autoimmune disease; learning difficulties are usually mild
- 30–50% have congenital heart disease: left-sided outflow tract abnormalities are common, including aortic coarctation, BAV, aortic valve stenosis, and rarely hypoplastic left heart. Aortic root dilatation is common, and the risk of dissection is known to be fivefold higher than the general population. In adult life premature cardiovascular disease is common
- MRI may identify vascular anomalies beyond the heart that would be missed by echo
- Genetic testing with karyotype analysis should be considered in females with these congenital heart diseases and in other girls and women with suggestive clinical features
- Karyotyping will usually identify individuals with at least 10% mosaicism

Williams syndrome

- Characterised by a typical facial appearance (see Figure 8.6.22), short stature, hypercalcaemia and other endocrine abnormalities, learning difficulties, hearing loss, and GI abnormalities
- Birth incidence is about 1 in 10,000 and most cases are *de novo*
- Younger children typically have a broad forehead, periorbital fullness, flat nasal bridge, full cheeks and lips, a pointed chin, and wide mouth; older children and adults share some of these features but become coarser over time
- It is caused by deletion of a specific region of chromosome 7. This deletion includes the elastin gene (ELN), variants in which can also cause the same range of cardiac defects but without the non-cardiac William's features

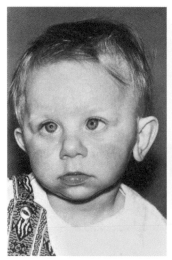 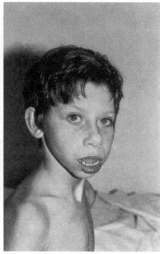

Figure 8.6.22 Appearance in Williams syndrome- same patient. (A) at 14 months and (B) at 17 years
Reproduced from 'Williams-Beuren Syndrome: phenotypic variability and deletions of chromosomes 7, 11, and 22 in a series of 52 patients', C. A. Joyce, B. Zorich, S. J. Pike, *J. Med. Genet.* 33, 986–992, Copyright 1996, with permission from BMJ Publishing Group Ltd

- Supra-valvular aortic stenosis is the most common cardiac defect which occurs in 50–75% of patients and may be associated with coronary artery abnormalities such as ostial stenosis or arterial dilatation
- Arterial narrowing at other sites, valve abnormalities and septal defects also occur
- FISH testing can confirm Williams syndrome by detecting a 7q11.23 deletion

Heart–hand syndromes

- This term is used to refer to a group of disorders where limb abnormalities are associated with cardiac defects
- One of the most commonly seen in clinical practice is Holt–Oram syndrome. This combines septal defects, usually atrial and/or AV node disease with abnormalities of the forearm and hand (ranging from subtle unilateral thumb hypoplasia to phocomelia)
- Usually due to dominant mutations in the *TBX5* gene and can be inherited from a very mildly affected parent

Further reading

Baumgartner H, Bonhoeffer P, De Groot NM, de Haan F, Deanfield JE, Galie N, Gatzoulis MA, Gohlke-Baerwolf C, Kaemmerer H, Kilner P, Meijboom F, Mulder BJ, Oechslin E, Oliver JM, Serraf A, Szatmari A, Thaulow E, Vouhe PR, Walma E; Task Force on the Management of Grown-up Congenital Heart Disease of the European Society of Cardiology (ESC); Association for European Paediatric Cardiology (AEPC); ESC Committee for Practice Guidelines (CPG). ESC Guidelines for the management of grown-up congenital heart disease (new version 2010). *Eur Heart J*. 2010 Dec;31(23):2915–57. doi: 10.1093/eurheartj/ehq249. Epub 2010 Aug 27. PMID: 20801927

Baumgartner H, De Backer J, Babu-Narayan SV, Budts W, Chessa M, Diller G-P, Lung B, Kluin J, Lang IM, Meijboom F, Moons P, Mulder BJM, Oechslin E, Roos-Hesselink JW, Schwerzmann M, Sondergaard L, Zeppenfeld K; ESC Scientific Document Group. 2020 ESC Guidelines for the management of adult congenital heart disease: The Task Force for the management of adult congenital heart disease of the European Society of Cardiology (ESC). Endorsed by: Association for European Paediatric and Congenital Cardiology (AEPC), International Society for Adult Congenital Heart Disease (ISACHD). *Eur Heart J.* 2021 Feb;42(6):563–645. https://doi.org/10.1093/eurheartj/ehaa554

Budts W, Pieles GE, Roos-Hesselink JW, Sanz de la Garza M, D'Ascenzi F, Giannakoulas G, Müller J, Oberhoffer R, Ehringer-Schetitska D, Herceg-Cavrak V, Gabriel H, Corrado D, van Buuren F, Niebauer J, Börjesson M, Caselli S, Fritsch P, Pelliccia A, Heidbuchel H, Sharma S, Stuart AG, Papadakis M. Recommendations for participation in competitive sport in adolescent and adult athletes with Congenital Heart Disease (CHD): position statement of the Sports Cardiology & Exercise Section of the European Association of Preventive Cardiology (EAPC), the European Society of Cardiology (ESC) Working Group on Adult Congenital Heart Disease and the Sports Cardiology, Physical Activity and Prevention Working Group of the Association for European Paediatric and Congenital Cardiology (AEPC). *Eur Heart J.* 2020 Nov 14;41(43):4191–9. doi: 10.1093/eurheartj/ehaa501. PMID: 32845299.

Pierpont ME, Brueckner M, Chung WK, Garg V, Lacro RV, McGuire AL, Mital S, Priest JR, Pu WT, Roberts A, Ware SM, Gelb BD, Russell MW; American Heart Association Council on Cardiovascular Disease in the Young; Council on Cardiovascular and Stroke Nursing; and Council on Genomic and Precision Medicine. Genetic Basis for Congenital Heart Disease: Revisited: A Scientific Statement From the American Heart Association. *Circulation.* 2018 Nov 20;138(21):e653–e711. doi: 10.1161/CIR.0000000000000606. Erratum in: Circulation. 2018 Nov 20;138(21):e713. PMID: 30571578; PMCID: PMC6555769

Pelliccia A, Sharma S, Gati S, Bäck M, Börjesson M, Caselli S, Collet JP, Corrado D, Drezner JA, Halle M, Hansen D, Heidbuchel H, Myers J, Niebauer J, Papadakis M, Piepoli MF, Prescott E, Roos-Hesselink JW, Graham Stuart A, Taylor RS, Thompson PD, Tiberi M, Vanhees L, Wilhelm M; ESC Scientific Document Group. 2020 ESC Guidelines on sports cardiology and exercise in patients with cardiovascular disease. *Eur Heart J.* 2021 Jan 1;42(1):17–96. doi: 10.1093/eurheartj/ehaa605. PMID: 32860412.

Villa ADM, Sammut E, Nair A, Rajani R, Bonamini R, Chiribiri A. Coronary artery anomalies overview: The normal and the abnormal. *World Journal of Radiology.* 2016; 8 (6): 537–55. doi:10.4329/wjr.v8.i6.537. PMID 27358682.

8.7

Cardiovascular disease in pregnancy

Stephanie Curtis and Yasmin Ismail

TABLE OF CONTENTS

8.7.1 Overview and epidemiology 813
8.7.2 Cardiovascular adaptations during pregnancy 814
    Plasma volume and cardiac output 814
    Heart rate 815
    Vascular resistance 815
    Haemostasis 815
    Delivery and post-partum period 815
8.7.3 Cardiac assessment 815
    History 815
    Examination 816
    Cardiac investigations in pregnancy 816
8.7.4 Maternal risk assessment in cardiac disease 817
8.7.5 General principles of pregnancy care for the cardiac patient 818
    Where to deliver 818
    Mode of delivery 818
    Third-stage management 819
    Regional analgesia/anaesthesia 819
    General anaesthesia 819
8.7.6 Specific cardiac conditions 819
    Valvular heart disease 819
    Management 821
    Congenital heart disease 823
    Acquired heart disease 827
8.7.7 Pharmacological treatment in pregnancy 833
8.7.8 Contraception 834

8.7.1 Overview and epidemiology

- Maternal disease complicates 1–4% of all pregnancies but this number is increasing.

View large Download slide

- Congenital heart disease occurs in 0.8% live births and 97% of these patients now reach adulthood due to improvements in paediatrics, surgery and intensive care.
- In developed countries, congenital heart disease and cardiomyopathies account for most of the cases seen. In developing countries cases are mainly rheumatic heart disease, though this is also increasing in developed countries due to immigration.
- Arrhythmia is the most common acquired problem atrial fibrillation is becoming more common with ageing mothers.
- Myocardial infarction (MI) in pregnancy is most commonly due to atheromatous disease. Less often it can be caused by spontaneous coronary artery dissection (SCAD).
- Coronary disease is seen most often in older women with traditional cardiovascular risk factors, such as smoking, hypertension, and diabetes.
- Cardiac death in pregnancy is rare. Morbidity is much more common.
- The Centre for Maternal and Child Enquiries produced a triennial report of maternal deaths, now succeeded by MBRRACE-UK (Mothers and Babies: Reducing Risk through Audits and Confidential Enquiries across the UK). The most recent report, published in October 2023 and examining deaths between 2019 and 2021, identified cardiac disease as the leading cause of maternal death after COVID-19s). The report identified markedly increased risks in women or minor ethnic groups

(an almost four-fold increase in deaths in black women and almost two-fold in Asian women) and those living in economic deprivation. More than half of deaths were in obese or overweight women and most cardiac deaths were in women not previously known to have heart disease.
- Historically the main causes of death have been: peripartum cardiomyopathy, myocardial infarction, aortic dissection, and pulmonary hypertension.
- Recently sudden adult death syndrome (SADS) has been identified as a rising cause of death, often in obese mothers.

8.7.2 Cardiovascular adaptations during pregnancy

- Characterized by significant haemodynamic changes to allow the foetus to receive adequate blood supply for development and protect the mother from blood loss at delivery.
- Hormonally mediated upregulation of nitric oxide synthesis and increases in prostaglandins and atrial natriuretic peptide seen.
- See Figure 8.7.1 for a list of physiologic changes during pregnancy.

Plasma volume and cardiac output

- Stimulation of the renin–angiotensin system results in an increase in plasma volume, which begins from six weeks' gestation, reaching a peak at 32–34 weeks, where it plateaus.
- Results in a relative anaemia, in spite of an increase in red cell mass.
- Returns to pre-pregnancy levels by 6–8 weeks post partum.
- Cardiac output increases by 40% by around 25 weeks due to increased stroke volume and heart rate. Patients who decompensate from an increase in preload and heart rate tend to present at around 18–22 weeks.

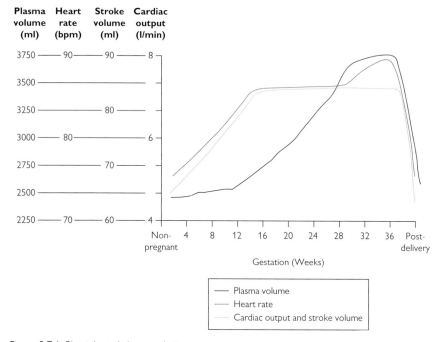

Figure 8.7.1 Physiological changes during pregnancy.
Reproduced from Thorne SA. Pregnancy in heart disease. Heart. 2004 Apr;90(4):450–6. doi: 10.1136/hrt.2003.027888 with permission from BMJ Group

- Blood pressure falls to lowest level in the mid second trimester then rises gradually towards term.
- In the supine position, IVC compression results in decreased venous return and can result in significant systemic hypotension. Pregnant women should be nursed in the left lateral decubitus position to avoid this.
- Serum colloid osmotic pressure decreases resulting in physiological oedema of extremities; pulmonary oedema may occur more readily.
- Pregnancy may therefore place a significant additional burden on an already compromised cardiovascular system or unmask a pre-existing but undiagnosed cardiac abnormality.

Heart rate

- Heart rate increases by 10–20 beats per minute (bpm) from around 6 weeks' gestation, reaching a peak at 36 weeks.
- Supraventricular tachyarrhythmias are commonly seen in pregnancy due to increased circulating catecholamines, increased sensitivity to catecholamines, and increased atrial wall stretch secondary to an increase in circulating plasma volume.

Vascular resistance

- Systemic vascular resistance (SVR) and pulmonary vascular resistance both decrease; the placenta is a low-resistance organ.
- Peripheral arterial vasodilatation seen in pregnancy causes aldosterone-mediated retention of sodium and water.

Haemostasis

- Pregnancy induces a state of hypercoagulability to minimize increased haemorrhage post partum. Women with atrial arrhythmias, surgical venous pathways, dilated cardiomyopathy, mechanical valves, and post-Fontan surgery are therefore at risk of thromboembolic events.
- Red cell mass increases but haematocrit decreases due to increase in plasma volume.
- Decreased tissue plasminogen activator (tPa); increased clotting factors.

Delivery and post-partum period

- Dramatic changes in haemodynamics during delivery and immediate post-partum period.
- Each uterine contraction causes an increase in venous return.
- Cardiac output increases by up to 25% during contractions in early labour, 50% during second stage, and 80% immediately post partum due to autotransfusion from contracted uterus and relief of caval compression.
- Sympathetic stimulation caused by pain and anxiety also augments heart rate, cardiac output, and blood pressure.
- Cardiac output and SVR mostly return to normal by two weeks post partum, and completely by 12–24 weeks' post partum.
- Clotting changes take six weeks to return to normal.

8.7.3 Cardiac assessment

History

- The following are normal in pregnancy: dyspnoea, fatigue, reduced exercise tolerance, palpitations, fainting, dizziness, and hyperventilation.

- Syncope or the development or progression of dyspnoea may be abnormal.
- Orthopnoea, exertional chest pain, and paroxysmal dyspnoea are not normal.
- Condition-specific issues need to be addressed, e.g. anti-coagulation in prosthetic valves.
- Drug history needs to be assessed for safety profile for mother and baby.

Examination
- Elevated jugular venous pressure, right ventricular heave, collapsing pulse, and ankle oedema are common.
- More than 90% of patients will have a 2/6 ejection systolic murmur, heard loudest at the left sternal edge, due to increased cardiac output. Soft continuous murmurs heard over the breasts also common due to increased blood flow to the breasts (mammary soufflés) and can be obliterated by pressure with the stethoscope.
- Diastolic murmurs in pregnancy are abnormal.
- 80% have an S3. S1 is often loud with an exaggerated split S2.

Cardiac investigations in pregnancy
- ECG: the following may be seen:
    - Sinus tachycardia in third trimester (exclude thyroid problems and pulmonary embolus). Resolves by two weeks post partum.
    - R wave can be increased V1 and V2.
    - Apex beat seen to shift to the left in normal pregnancy in third trimester, so may see a slight leftward axis shift (small Q wave in lead III).
    - Inferolateral ST depression/T wave inversion.
    - Isolated ventricular and supraventricular ectopics.
    - T wave inversion in III. P may be inverted in III.
    - First- and second-degree atrioventricular block.
- Echocardiography is a safe and non-invasive test that allows serial surveillance. In a normal pregnancy:
    - All four chamber sizes increase, but not beyond normal limits.
    - Transvalvular velocities increase and mild atrioventricular valve regurgitation also common due to increased cardiac output and mild annular dilatation.
    - Reducing velocities in left-sided obstructive valve disease may indicate left ventricular decompensation.
- CXR: avoid if possible, especially in early pregnancy. Pelvic shield recommended. In normal pregnancies, cardiac silhouette may be larger, lung markings more prominent, and small pleural effusions present.
- MRI: few indications. Gadolinium is contraindicated.
- CT: mainly used to diagnose pulmonary emboli. Avoid if possible and use techniques to minimize radiation dose otherwise. Iodine contrast can cause neonatal hypothyroidism, thus the infant must be screened at birth.
- Exercise ECG/cardiopulmonary exercise testing: unhelpful in pregnancy as heart rate and cardiac output already increased by the pregnancy itself. Useful as part of pre-pregnancy assessment of women contemplating pregnancy as risk stratification.
- Ambulatory ECG: useful investigation to identify the cause of palpitations.
- For any investigation involving radiation, risk to the foetus needs to be carefully weighed up against benefit for the mother. If the mother is unwell, the appropriate investigation for her health should be done, shielding the foetus where possible.

8.7.4 Maternal risk assessment in cardiac disease

Cardiac conditions can be thought of as low or high risk. The modified World Health Organization Category, described in the 2018 ESC guidelines for Cardiovascular Diseases in Pregnancy, can be used to help risk stratify women (see broad risk categories, Box 8.7.1). Patients at highest risk of cardiac events are those with:

- Left-sided valvular obstructive lesions.

BOX 8.7.1 RISK STRATIFICATION FOR HEART DISEASE IN PREGNANCY

Risk	Congenital Heart Disease and Cardiomyopathy	Valve Disease and Aortopathy	Ischaemic Heart Disease and Arrhythmia
mWHO I Very low	Small PDA, VSD Repaired ASD/VSD/PDA	Mild PS/PR Mild MR	
mWHO II Low	Unoperated ASD Good Fallot repair Repaired coarctation	Mild MS, AS Moderate PS/PR Moderate MR, AR	Revascularized IHD with no ongoing ischaemia and good LV function SVT
mWHO II–III Intermediate	Fallot with severe PR AVSD TGA, atrial switch, good systemic right ventricle Mild systemic ventricular impairment HCM	Moderate AS BAV Aorta < 45 mm	VT
mWHO III High	Good Fontan Unrepaired cyanotic heart disease Moderate systemic ventricular dysfunction Previous PPCM with normal LV	Moderate MS Severe asymptomatic AS Mechanical valve All Marfan 45–50 mm BAV 20–25 mm/m^2 TS	IHD not fully revascularized with no ongoing ischaemia and good LV function
mWHO IV Extremely high Pregnancy not advised	PH Severe (re) coarctation Fontan with complication TGA, atrial switch, impaired systemic right ventricle Severe systemic ventricular dysfunction Previous PPCM with residual LV impairment	Severe MS Severe symptomatic AS Operated Marfan > 45 mm Marfan > 50 mm BAV > 25 mm/m^2 TS	IHD with ongoing ischaemia Previous coronary dissection

AS—aortic stenosis, ASD—atrial septal defect, AVSD—atrioventricular septal defect, BAV—bicuspid aortic valve, HCM—hypertrophic cardiomyopathy, IHD—ischaemic heart disease, LV—left ventricular, MR—mitral regurgitation, MS—mitral stenosis, PDA—patient ductus arteriosus, PPCM—peripartum cardiomyopathy, PH—pulmonary hypertension, PR—pulmonary regurgitation, PS—pulmonary stenosis, SVT—supraventricular tachycardia, TGA—transposition of the great arteries, TS—Turner Syndrome, VSD—ventricular septal defect, VT—ventricular tachycardia, WHO—World Health Organization.

- Reduced systemic ventricular function.
- Inherited aortopathy.
- Cyanotic heart disease.
- Mechanical valves.
- Pulmonary hypertension (risk of death high; avoid pregnancy).
- Previous cardiac events.
- Severe pulmonary regurgitation and reduced subpulmonary ventricular dysfunction.

8.7.5 General principles of pregnancy care for the cardiac patient

Guidelines from European Society of Cardiology, the Royal College of Obstetricians and MBRRACE-UK describe ideal model of care:

- Individualized care is key.
- Cases must be reviewed in a multi-disciplinary team (MDT) meeting.
- Maternal Medicine Networks are responsible for ensuring that all women with pre-existing medical problems get timely specialist care and advice before, during and after pregnancy.
- Have a birth plan in the paper notes/electronic patient record and on labour ward.
- Care should be in a joint cardiac/obstetric clinic.
- Balance the mother's need with those of the foetus. If in doubt, treat the mother.
- Do not overmedicalize birth if not necessary.
- Allow for mother's input into birth plan.
- Those looking after patients should undergo formal training.
- Formalize pre-pregnancy counselling.

In addition:

- All patients with heart disease planning assisted conception should have cardiological assessment and optimization of treatment.
- Risks of assisted conception include multiple birth and the consequent haemodynamic stress of this, as well as the risk of ovarian hyperstimulation syndrome. Assisted conception is not safe in some cases.
- Pregnancy is an opportunity for refined genetic diagnosis and cascade family screening for women affected by inherited cardiac conditions.

Where to deliver

- Low-risk and some moderate-risk cases may be able to be delivered in local hospital, depending on available expertise.
- Otherwise delivery should be in a tertiary centre with consultant obstetric, cardiology, and anaesthetic cover.
- Wherever delivery planned, need to ensure that the resources for a safe delivery are in place including appropriately trained staff, equipment, and environment.

Mode of delivery

- Generally determined by obstetric indications.
- Generally a vaginal delivery with good analgesia is optimal.
- May need to limit active pushing to limit haemodynamic stress.

- Caesarean section results in more dramatic and sudden haemodynamic shifts and is therefore not usually recommended for cardiac reasons. Reserved for those with a high risk of aortic dissection if the risk of requiring cardiac surgery is high, those in whom warfarin has been taken in the previous three weeks, or if the mother is acutely unwell and rapid delivery is required. Needed if gestation too early for successful induction of labour.
- Induction of labour may be required for geographical or practical reasons.
- High-risk patients can be delivered with a carefully titrated combined spinal epidural and passive second stage, with ventouse or lift-out forceps if pushing is not advised for cardiac reasons (ventouse requires some pushing).

Third-stage management
- Complex fluid shifts occur as the placenta is delivered and the uterus contracts.
- High-risk patients are at greatest risk of cardiac events in the first 24–48 hours post partum and require high-dependency care. Aortic dissection risk persists for up to a week post partum.
- Drugs given routinely to prevent post-partum haemorrhage have significant haemodynamic side effects.
- Ergometrine should be avoided in most cases as it results in prolonged hypertension due to peripheral vasoconstriction. Also risk of coronary vasospasm.
- Low-dose infusion of syntocinon is recommended, rather than a bolus, which can cause profound hypotension and bradycardia.
- Misoprostol is usually safe.
- Senior input required if post-partum haemorrhage severe, as benefits of ergometrine may outweigh risks.

Regional analgesia/anaesthesia
- Good choice for effective pain relief.
- Used in most Caesarean sections but contraindicated if patient is fully anti-coagulated.

General anaesthesia
- Rarely indicated.
- Risks include failed intubation, aspiration, haemodynamic instability, and with induction/ maintenance of anaesthetic.
- General anaesthesia can result in death in patients with pulmonary hypertension.
- Risk of systemic air embolus if the patient has right-to-left shunting.
- Risk of neonatal respiratory depression and impaired bonding with baby.

8.7.6 Specific cardiac conditions

Valvular heart disease
Left-sided valvular heart disease in pregnancy
- Left-sided obstructive valve lesions are a significant risk factor for maternal morbidity and mortality. As plasma volume and heart rate increase and systemic vascular resistance decreases the effective obstruction increases.
- The foetus is at risk of death, growth restriction, low birth weight, and premature labour can occur.
- Left-sided regurgitant lesions, in contrast, are generally better tolerated in pregnancy due to the decrease in systemic vascular resistance.

Stenotic lesions
Mitral stenosis (MS)
- Usually rheumatic, increasingly common in high income countries due to increased immigration.
- Often presents for the first time in pregnancy.
- Moderate to severe stenosis poorly tolerated in pregnancy. Increased functional obstruction due to the increased preload and tachycardia of pregnancy. Resultant raised left atrial pressure and reduced cardiac output.
- Mild MS well tolerated.
- Pulmonary oedema occurs in a third of women with a pre-pregnancy valve area of ≤ 1.5 cm^2 and in half of those with an area ≤ 1.0 cm^2.
- Maternal risk also increased if symptomatic, estimated systolic pulmonary artery pressure > 30 mmHg on echo, and older age.
- Foetus at risk of intrauterine growth restriction (IUGR), prematurity, and death.

Clinical assessment:

- Presents with breathlessness, pulmonary oedema, or paroxysmal nocturnal dyspnoea, typically towards the end of the second trimester.
- May precipitate atrial fibrillation, which causes further decompensation and risk of thromboembolism.

Investigations:

- Mitral valve area (MVA) is a more reliable parameter in assessing MS severity in pregnancy than the pressure gradient across the valve, which is preload dependent.
- Assess valve morphology, area, peak and mean gradient, left atrial pressure (by E/E'), pulmonary artery pressure, and suitability for balloon mitral valvuloplasty (BMV).

Treatment:

- Options to reduce heart rate and optimize cardiac output include oxygen, bed rest, beta blockers, digoxin, and diuretics.
- Consider prophylactic low molecular weight heparin (LMWH) if the left atrium is large, even if in sinus rhythm due to the increased risk of left atrial thrombus formation.
- If in atrial fibrillation, full anticoagulation prophylaxis with LMWH needed. Aim to restore sinus rhythm if new onset. DC cardioversion is safe. Consider transoesophageal echo to assess thrombus in left atrial appendage.
- Balloon valvuloplasty should be considered, even if there is mitral regurgitation, to relieve pulmonary oedema and allow progress of pregnancy. 95% success rate with little risk to the mother or the baby. Should be performed in centre with established experience.

Delivery:

- Preterm delivery is likely with resultant low birth weight baby unless stenosis is mild.
- If mild, should be able to have a normal delivery.
- If moderate to severe, vaginal delivery with epidural analgesia is recommended, with careful balance of preload and afterload and the use of invasive monitoring.
- If maternal situation critical and foetus viable, stabilize on intensive care unit, deliver, and then treat mitral stenosis by BMV or surgery.
- Patients should be carefully monitored post partum with the use of diuretics to avoid pulmonary oedema.

Aortic stenosis (AS)
- Almost always due to bicuspid aortic valve disease in this age group.
- Mild and moderate stenosis well tolerated. Severe stenosis associated with increased maternal and foetal risk.
- Heart failure occurs in 1 in 4 women who have symptoms prior to pregnancy.
- Foetal risks include prematurity, IUGR and low birth weight; occurs in 20–25% with moderate and severe AS. Foetal loss in < 5%.

Management
- Monitor pressure gradient on echo. As with MS, severity can be overestimated if echo pressure gradient only used; increases throughout pregnancy due to increased cardiac output. Calculate area of valve and other echo parameters.
- In a patient who is asymptomatic and has isolated aortic stenosis, if good LV function with pre-pregnancy mean gradient < 50 mmHg/peak gradient < 80 mmHg, AVA > 1.5 cm^2, normal exercise capacity, and a normal exercise-tolerance test, pregnancy is likely to be well-tolerated.
- If becomes symptomatic admit for bed rest and consider delivery if foetus viable. Consider beta blockade and balloon valvotomy if still symptomatic in spite of this and foetus not yet viable.
- Signs of decompensation include worsening dyspnoea and/or tachycardia. May see decreasing pressure gradient on echo as a reflection of struggling left ventricle.
- Consider termination if adverse features present and severe aortic stenosis.

Delivery:
- If well at term should be able to have a normal delivery with epidural, and semi-passive second stage, depending on severity.
- In severe AS with adverse features premature delivery by Caesarean section should be expected with careful fluid balance and arterial line.
- If the mother deteriorates, interventions include balloon valvotomy (usually a bridging/palliative procedure with a risk of severe aortic regurgitation), or valve replacement can be considered with delivery of the foetus first if viable.
- Vaginal delivery with slow incremental low dose combined spinal epidural analgesia and careful fluid balance recommended to avoid rapid fluid shifts associated with Caesarean section.
- May need invasive monitoring depending on the severity of lesion.

Regurgitant lesions
Mitral regurgitation (MR)
- Usually well tolerated, even if severe, as long as left ventricular function is good
- If decompensating with heart failure, aim to treat medically with bed rest, nitrates, and hydralazine, *not* angiotensin converting enzyme (ACE) inhibitors, and deliver early if foetus viable.
- Caution with pre-pregnancy valve repair in case mechanical prosthesis required. Pregnancy with severe MR is lower risk than one with a mechanical mitral valve replacement.

Aortic regurgitation
- As with mitral regurgitation, aim to manage medically.

Prosthetic valves
- Significant risk to both mother and baby.
- Crucial to consider future pregnancies when selecting type of prosthetic valve in a woman of child-bearing age. Patient needs to be counselled regarding risks and benefits of each valve type with respect to pregnancy and anti-coagulation issues.

Bioprosthetic valves
- Low risk in pregnancy.
- Less thrombogenic than mechanical valves.
- Warfarin can be avoided, which significantly reduces maternal and foetal risk.
- Degenerate more rapidly in young patients, requiring re-operation, usually within 10 years. Pregnancy itself is not thought to cause degeneration.
- Mitral prostheses degenerate more rapidly than aortic.

Mechanical valves
- Problematic in pregnancy due to need for warfarin, which crosses the placenta.
- Hypercoagulable state of pregnancy increases risk of valve thrombosis and thromboembolism as well as risks of bleeding from warfarin.
- For the baby, risk of miscarriage, foetal loss, haemorrhage, foetal embyropathy and other risks (see below).
- Risks increased with older types of valve and those in mitral position.

Management of anticoagulation for prosthetic valves in pregnancy
- Difficult.
- Heparins, as a substitute for warfarin, do not cross the placenta and so are safe for the baby. However risk of valve thrombosis high, which can cause death

Unfractionated heparin
- Superseded by LMWH due to the risk of valve thrombosis, heparin-induced thrombocytopenia (HIT), and osteoporosis.
- Need to do periodic anti-factor Xa assay to guide therapy. APTT response to heparin often decreased due to decreased Factor VIII and fibrinogen.
- May need a three times daily regime or even an i.v. infusion to achieve this.

Low molecular weight heparin
- Does not cross the placenta.
- Lower incidence of HIT.
- Longer half-life thus harder to reverse effect.
- Multiple reports of valve thromboses in literature, resulting in maternal stroke and death despite careful monitoring and adequate anti-Xa levels.
- Need meticulous anti-factor Xa monitoring with at least weekly trough and peak levels. Aspirin 150 mg daily is usually added.
- Careful management around labour. Induction often required to facilitate this.

Warfarin
Causes four separate problems in the foetus:

- Warfarin embryopathy. Caused by exposure to warfarin between weeks 6 and 12 of gestation. Characterized by skeletal abnormalities and low birth weight. Risk related to the dose of warfarin taken.
- Central nervous system effects: spasticity and optic atrophy. Risk throughout pregnancy.
- Foetal haemorrhage.
- Foetal loss.

Options for anticoagulation

The following options must be discussed with the potential parents by an experienced multidisciplinary team, preferably pre-pregnancy. It is important that the mother and her partner are made aware of the risks of each option for the mother and the foetus. The woman is at most risk around the time of changing therapies.

- Warfarin throughout: most risk to foetus, least risk to mother (safest option for mother).
- LMWH–warfarin sandwich: i.e. LMWH for weeks 6 to 12, when the risk of embryopathy is high, warfarin from week 12–36, LMWH prior to and peri-delivery. Some risk to mother and foetus.
- LMWH throughout: least risk to foetus, most risk to mother.
- Aspirin: 150 mg aspirin may be used as an adjunct in second and third trimester but there is no consensus for this.

Note:

1. It takes three weeks to clear warfarin from the foetal liver so vaginal delivery is not safe. If the mother has taken warfarin within two weeks of onset of labour, Caesarean section must be performed.
2. Regional anaesthesia cannot be used if the mother is on warfarin.
3. Direct oral anticoagulants (DOACS) cross the placenta and are contraindicated in pregnancy. They are also contraindicated for use in patients with mechanical valves.

Congenital heart disease

General principles:

- All patients with congenital heart disease require pre-pregnancy risk assessment and counselling.
- Foetal echocardiography should be offered.
- At the first visit, the anatomy and physiology of the heart should be assessed.
- In complex congenital heart disease, prematurity and low birth weight infants are common.
- Infant mortality is higher than normal due to prematurity and recurrence of cardiac defects (recurrence 4–10% depending on lesion, compared to 1% in general population unless single gene defect).

Atrial septal defect (ASD)/ventricular septal defect/patent arterial duct

Unrepaired:

- Low risk if shunt small and pulmonary artery pressure normal.
- If large ASD, increase in cardiac output and atrial stretch may precipitate an atrial arrhythmia or ventricular dysfunction.
- For atrial septal defects care should be taken to reduce the risk of paradoxical thromboembolism, e.g. by using compression stockings post-partum and i.v. line filters. Consider LMWH if immobile.

Repaired:
- Low risk if no residual lesions, pulmonary artery pressure and ventricular function normal.

Repaired Tetralogy of Fallot

- Unrepaired Tetralogy of Fallot rare.
- Low risk if good functional capacity and good right ventricular function, even if severe pulmonary regurgitation.

- If severe pulmonary regurgitation and pulmonary valve replacement is indicated, this is best done pre-pregnancy.
- Need regular reviews during pregnancy with assessment of right ventricular function and cardiac rhythm. Risks include the development of arrhythmias and worsening ventricular function.
- Vaginal delivery usually recommended.

Ebstein's anomaly
- Rare.
- Can present with right heart failure due to significant tricuspid regurgitation, right ventricular dysfunction, atrial arrhythmias, and cyanosis (most have an inter-atrial shunt).
- Usually well tolerated and normal delivery can be expected if right ventricle is a reasonable size with good function and fully saturated.
- If cyanosed, increased risks to foetus (see below).
- Monitor during pregnancy for cyanosis, right heart failure, and arrhythmias.
- Left heart can be involved, most often mitral valve anomalies and cardiomyopathy with hypertrabeculation.

Cyanotic congenital heart disease
- Cardiac events relate to underlying lesion.
- Clotting factors and platelet function are impaired, so increased risk of haemorrhage and thromboembolic disease.
- Right-to-left shunting increases with decreased systemic vascular resistance so increased risk of paradoxical embolism and desaturation.
- Increased foetal loss (overall approximately 50%) and prematurity. Very high risk of foetal loss if oxygen saturation < 90%.
- Consider bed rest with oxygen, though saturations may not increase much as deoxygenated blood is bypassing lungs.
- Usually low birth weight and premature, so delivery by Caesarean section typical for foetal reasons.
- Meticulous haemostasis is required, with good hydration, avoiding vasodilatation, and using i.v. line filters.

Repaired univentricular hearts (Fontan)
- Risk of pregnancy considered at least moderate, but variable. Heart failure, thromboembolic events, haemorrhage, and arrhythmias can occur.
- Risk is lower if asymptomatic, good exercise tolerance, no previous thromboembolic event or arrhythmia, no cyanosis, good ventricular function, and minimal atrioventricular valve regurgitation.
- Biggest risk is to foetus. Foetal and neonatal complications occur in 75%: intrauterine growth restriction (which can be severe), miscarriage, prematurity, and small for gestational age.
- Fontan circulation dependent on good venous return and low pulmonary artery pressure so avoid dehydration, supine position, and venous thrombosis. All patients with a Fontan circulation should already be on warfarin so convert to LMWH as soon as possible.
- Careful and frequent monitoring of mother and foetus is required throughout pregnancy, with expectation of preterm delivery.
- Aim for a vaginal delivery with epidural, semi-passive second stage and assisted delivery.

Pulmonary stenosis
- Usually treated in childhood in UK.
- Aim to treat pre-pregnancy if severe.
- Pregnancy normally well tolerated if right ventricular function preserved, even if pulmonary stenosis severe.
- If severe may present with right heart failure, tricuspid regurgitation, or arrhythmias. If so, consider balloon valvuloplasty.
- Aim for vaginal delivery aiming to keep pre-load high and replace fluid losses promptly.

Pulmonary arterial hypertension
- Variety of causes, including Eisenmenger syndrome
- 30–50% maternal mortality in pregnancy, with foetal loss rate also of same magnitude. Due to:
    - Decrease in systemic vascular resistance resulting in an increase in the right-to-left shunting in Eisenmenger syndrome, decreased pulmonary flow, and progression to low output cardiac failure.
    - Failure of the right ventricle to cope with the additional haemodynamic strain and also presumed hormonal effects on pulmonary vasculature and vascular tone.
    - Death due to pulmonary hypertensive crises or heart failure; higher risk with higher pulmonary arterial pressure.
- If woman wishes to proceed with pregnancy, she should be managed in a centre with expertise in managing pulmonary hypertension and heart disease in pregnancy.
- Mortality risk may be 20% if carefully managed in an experienced centre.
- Management includes oxygen therapy, bed rest, prophylaxis against thromboembolism, diuretics, and pulmonary vasodilators. Endothelin receptor antagonists are contraindicated.
- Most deaths occur in the first few days post partum. Intensive care is required for at least a week with aggressive diuresis in first 72 hours. Deterioration may be sudden.

Coarctation of the aorta
- Usually has been repaired surgically or by stent.
- Biggest risk is hypertension, affecting 25–30%.
- Close monitoring of blood pressure crucial; BP should be measured in right arm as may be underestimated on the left
- Beta blockers are used as first line treatment to reduce blood pressure and risk of aortic dissection. Nifedipine and methyldopa can also be used safely.

Native coarctation
- Unrepaired lesions predispose the mother to the risk of severe systemic hypertension, heart failure, stroke, and aortic dissection. Placental and thus foetal blood flow is also compromised due to lower body hypoperfusion. Collateral vessels are variably present. Significant risk of intra-uterine growth retardation and foetal death.
- Treatment options are limited and termination of pregnancy should be strongly considered.
- Trans-catheter stenting is usually the treatment of choice in the non-pregnant state but carries a high risk of rupture or dissection during pregnancy and for 6 months afterwards due the changes in the vascular media.
- Surgical repair is associated with significant morbidity in the adult and cardiopulmonary bypass carries a high risk of foetal death.
- Medical therapy with anti-hypertensives can be considered if there is good collateral flow on CMR scanning. Monitor with regular growth scanning of the foetus.

Repaired coarctation
- Relatively common, though associated lesions also common and must be evaluated in own right (for example, bicuspid aortic valve and ascending aortopathy).
- CT or MRI 1–2 years prior to pregnancy should be available to ensure no aneurysm at repair site (high risk of rupture with pregnancy). If not, needs to be done in pregnancy.
- Blood pressure must be carefully controlled to avoid aortic wall stress. Management more aggressive than in normal pregnancy.
- Vaginal delivery with regional analgesia recommended. Consider limited pushing. Consider Caesarean section if aneurysm present.
- Risk of hypertension exists, even if no re-coarctation.

Bicuspid aortic valve
- See aortic stenosis and regurgitation.
- Associated ascending aortopathy common and confers increased risk of dissection and further dilatation (higher risk if coexisting coarctation).
- Treat as for aortopathies (see below).

Turner syndrome (TS)
- XO results in infertility so pregnancy occurs as a result of assisted reproductive techniques. Mosaics may spontaneously become pregnant.
- Patients commonly have bicuspid aortic valve, aortopathy, coarctation, and hypertension.
- Risk increases if heart disease or hypertension but TS itself is an independent risk factor for aortic dissection and risk higher than other patients with bicuspid aortopathy and coarctation.
- Up to 2% risk of death in pregnancy.
- Aortic measurements need to be corrected for smaller body surface area.
- Treat as Marfan with passive delivery in surgical centre.
- Caesarean section often considered due to body habitus.

Aortopathies
- Compliance of the aorta increases in pregnancy.
- Oestrogen inhibits collagen and elastin deposition in aortic media, increasing the risk of dissection. Haemodynamic changes and drugs given peri-partum also increase risk.
- Most aortic dissections occur in women with connective tissue diseases but pregnancy also increases the risk of aortic dissection in normal women.
- Aortic dissection accounts for 15% of maternal deaths; not decreasing.
- Slight Type A preponderance.
- Foetal mortality high; worse for type B.
- Risk of dissection is highest in third trimester or immediately post partum.

Marfan's syndrome
- Maternal complications in pregnancy include progressive aortic dilatation and dissection, aortic regurgitation, worsening mitral regurgitation due to mitral valve prolapse, early pregnancy loss, premature rupture of membranes, pelvic instability and back pain, post-partum haemorrhage, and poor wound healing.
- Risk dissection 3-4%, highest if aortic root dilated, recent rapid growth, family history of dissection, previous dissection/surgery, and hypertension.
- Most common in third trimester and post partum.
- Type B dissection is unpredictable.

- Foetal risk relates to maternal outcome if dissection and beta blockade during pregnancy, which results in IUGR.

Management in pregnancy:

- Pre-pregnancy counselling at specialist unit crucial. Pre-pregnancy root replacement should be considered if root > 45 mm.
- Meticulous blood pressure control and 4-weekly aortic root imaging by echo.
- Beta blockers are recommended for all patients, though evidence is limited. Monthly growth scans of foetus are required to check for IUGR.
- If patient dissects:
    - Surgical emergency; proceed to urgent surgery and deliver foetus by caesarean section if viable.
    - Meticulous blood pressure control critical; use beta blockers and hydralazine.
    - If the aorta dilates during pregnancy delivery should be expedited and aortic surgery considered.

Delivery:

- Aim for elective combined spinal-epidural with passive second stage if aorta less than 45 mm. If > 45 mm, Caesarean section with cardiac surgeon on stand-by.
- Dissection most common peripartum or in early post-partum period for up to a week.
- Consider recurrence in foetus.

Loeys–Dietz syndrome

- Dissection may occur without dilatation.
- Manage as for high-risk aortopathy with strict blood pressure control, frequent imaging and elective Caesarean section, with cardiothoracic surgeon on stand-by.

Vascular type (type IV) Ehlers–Danlos syndrome

- Rare; associated with vasculopathy, increased risk of large artery rupture, peri-/post-partum haemorrhage, and organ rupture, including uterus.
- Treat as high-risk aortopathy with elective Caesarean section, with cardiothoracic surgeon on stand-by.

Acquired heart disease
Maternal cardiac arrhythmias

General principles of arrhythmia management:

- Arrhythmias very common in pregnancy due to physiological changes.
- Most are benign.
- 60% of pregnant women have supraventricular or ventricular extrasystoles on Holter monitoring.
- Risk factors include congenital heart disease (especially if surgically repaired), any pre-existing acquired cardiac disease, or cardiac failure.
- Give reassurance for benign or self-limiting arrhythmias and avoid drugs if possible, especially in the first trimester.
- Treat only if arrhythmia is sustained, particularly troublesome, or is causing haemodynamic compromise to mother.
- If patient is haemodynamically stable, aim to manage tachyarrhythmias medically due to the associated risks of sedation/anaesthetic required for a DC cardioversion.

Use of anti-arrhythmic drugs in pregnancy:

- Flecainide, lignocaine, digoxin, adenosine, and cardio-selective beta blockers thought to be relatively safe, although limited data from human studies.
- Amiodarone may be teratogenic and is associated with foetal hypothyroidism, IUGR, and pre-term birth and thus its use is not recommended.
- Calcium channel blockers thought to be relatively safe but verapamil reported to cause foetal bradycardia, heart block, and hypotension.

Direct current cardioversion/defibrillation:

- Can be safely used at any stage of pregnancy if drugs ineffective.
- Recommend foetal heart scan post procedure with involvement of obstetric team.
- Patient should be intubated, because of increased risk of aspiration in pregnancy, and positioned in left lateral decubitus position.

Pacemakers/ICDs:

- Permanent pacemaker insertion is recommended for women presenting with symptomatic sinus node disease or non-transient second degree Mobitz type II/third-degree block in pregnancy, ideally after the first trimester.
- Pelvic shielding should be used to protect the foetus from radiation.
- No increased risks associated with pacemakers or implantable defibrillators per se implanted prior to pregnancy. Risks relate to underlying reason for needing device.
- Lower pacing rate of pacemakers needs to be increased in those implanted for sinus node disease to mirror the increased chronotropic state of pregnancy.
- Women who have devices will need special precautions such as the avoidance of unipolar diathermy and access to programming. Surgically implanted abdominal systems may have generator and/or leads close to the uterus.

Labour, delivery, and lactation:

- Normal vaginal delivery recommended.
- Intravenous adenosine useful for paroxysmal supraventricular arrhythmias in labour due to its short half-life. Intravenous esmolol also useful.
- All antiarrhythmics are excreted in breast milk although levels are generally low; amiodarone is an exception and should be avoided.
- Experience limited for many drugs, thus use with caution.

Inappropriate sinus tachycardia

- Heart rate persistently above 100 bpm.
- Usually resolves within 4 weeks post partum.
- Can occur at any time in pregnancy.
- May recur with subsequent pregnancies.
- Responds to beta blockers.

Supraventricular tachycardia (SVT)

- Common
- Known SVT has a high risk of recurrence in pregnancy; consider catheter ablation pre-pregnancy.
- In sustained SVT, vagal manoeuvres should be tried first. Intravenous adenosine safe and effective. Flecainide can be used if adenosine fails.

- Cardio-selective beta blockers and verapamil are useful in preventing paroxysmal SVT. Flecainde is best when there is pre-excitation.

Atrial flutter
- Haemodynamically unstable: DC cardioversion.
- Can rate control with beta blockers and digoxin.
- If haemodynamically stable, consider flecainide/propafenone combined with a small dose of a beta blocker to restore sinus rhythm.
- Need for continuing medication and anticoagulation will depend on whether further episodes develop.

Atrial fibrillation
- Rare in normal heart in pregnancy.
- Associated with increased morbidity and mortality in pregnancy due to haemodynamic effects in those with pre-existing heart disease and the increased risk of thromboembolism, especially in third trimester.
- If haemodynamically unstable: DC cardioversion.
- Aim to cardiovert pharmacologically; consider flecainide/propafenone in combination with a beta blocker.
- LMWH should be used for anticoagulation and continued for 4 weeks after sinus rhythm has been achieved.

Ventricular arrhythmias
- VT can occur in structurally normal hearts but is more commonly associated with underlying cardiac disease.
- In symptomatic VT, urgent therapy needed to preserve maternal circulatory status and protect foetus: DC cardioversion.
- Consider beta blockers, flecainide, and verapamil if haemodynamically stable and consult an electrophysiologist
- Inherited arrhythmia cases should be discussed between the electrophysiology, obstetric an anaesthetic teams. Women with long QT syndrome and catecholaminergic VT (CPVT) should be prescribed beta blockers throughout pregnancy and post partum. Long QT is associated with poorer fetal outcomes.
- A list of drugs to avoid in long QT and Brugada syndrome should be available in the mother's notes and she should have a consultation with an anaesthetist.

Bradyarrhythmias
- Usually seen in the context of repaired congenital heart disease.
- Transient first- and second-degree atrioventricular block can be seen in normal hearts during pregnancy.
- Complete heart block should always be taken seriously and pacing considered.
- In repaired congenital heart disease patients with sinus node dysfunction, second- or third-degree heart block, pacemaker insertion prior to pregnancy should be considered. If this has not been done, the patient needs to be carefully monitored for bradyarrhythmias.

Myocardial infarction (MI) and ischaemic heart disease
- Risk is increased threefold by pregnancy, but still rare (occurring in 3–8 per 100,000 pregnancies).
- 75% are ST elevation MIs (STEMIs).
- 24% present with severely impaired left ventricular function. Cardiogrnic shock and ventricular arrythmias are common.

- MI historically due to spontaneous coronary artery dissection (SCAD), though atheromatous disease increasing secondary to increasing obesity, smoking, and diabetes in mothers, as well as older mothers.
- Less common causes are thrombosis and coronary artery spasm.
- Mortality disproportionately high as multi-vessel dissection can occur and heart failure common. Maternal mortality 7%, foetal mortality 5%, mainly due to death of mother.
- Two-thirds of cases involve the anterior wall.
- Most occur in third trimester and post partum (75% of coronary dissections occur post partum).
- 75% occur in women over 30 years old.

Management:

- In STEMI emergency coronary angiography and percutaneous coronary intervention (PCI) as per usual protocols. If in doubt, treat the mother.
- In non-STEMI, consider conservative management due to high risk of iatrogenic coronary dissection by catheter. Seek senior advice from obstetric cardiologist, interventionist, and obstetrician.
- Minimise radiation by using an abdominal shield and radial approach with shortened fluoroscopy times.
- Avoid thrombolysis due to the risk of dissection being the cause. Thrombolytics do not cross the placenta but can cause subplacental bleeding.

Drug management:

- Aspirin and beta-blockers are safe and should be used.
- GPIIb/IIIa inhibitors and $P2Y_{12}$ inhibitors (e.g. clopidogrel) can be used in pregnancy if benefits outweigh risks. Limited data available. Heparin safe.
- Caution with i.v. nitrates (systemic hypotension and placental hypoperfusion)
- ACE inhibitors, spironolactone, and statins are contraindicated. Loop diuretics can be used with caution.
- $P2Y_{12}$ inhibitors preclude the use of regional anaesthesia for delivery. If possible, strategies should be pursued which avoid this but saving the life of the mother is paramount and decisions made in the cardiac catheterization laboratory should be based on this premise.

Delivery:

- Delivery should be delayed until 2–3 weeks post MI if possible.
- Best mode of delivery is vaginal with elective regional anaesthesia and passive second stage.
- Future pregnancy risk determined by left ventricular function, though should be avoided post SCAD. SCAD recurrence rate is approximately 10%.
- The risks to the baby of using drugs post partum for secondary prevention must be weighed up against the benefits of breast-feeding to both mother and child.

Stable coronary artery disease:

- Good prognosis if normal exercise tolerance prior to conception with no residual ischaemia.
- Low-dose aspirin should be continued after the first trimester.
- Statins, $P2Y_{12}$ inhibitors, and ACE inhibitors should be stopped.
- The development of angina may not indicate unstable coronary disease but rather a demand/supply mismatch in the myocardium due to flow-restricting lesions. Therefore, if the patient develops angina and the foetus is viable, delivery should be expedited. If not, symptom control with anti-anginals should be attempted.

- Angina at rest, with or without a troponin rise, should be treated by PCI. Close communication between cardiologists with experience of heart disease in pregnancy and obstetricians is crucial.
- Vaginal delivery best, as for myocardial infarction.

Cardiopulmonary bypass in pregnancy
- Only consider if no other options/mother's life at risk.
- Risk for mother not increased.
- Foetal risk of death 20% due to tissue pulsatility of bypass, hypothermia, and foetal bradycardia. Consider delivery if viable.
- Perform with full maternal and foetal monitoring, use normothermia, limit cross clamp and bypass time if possible.
- Best done in 2nd trimester (13–28 weeks).

Hypertension
- The commonest cardiovascular problem in pregnancy, affects 5–10% of all pregnancies.
- Important cause of maternal and foetal morbidity and mortality.
- Hypertension in pregnancy can be classified in to four subtypes:
    - Pre-existing or chronic hypertension
    - Gestational hypertension
    - Pre-eclampsia (occurs in 30% women with pre-existing hypertension)
    - Pre-eclampsia superimposed on chronic hypertension or gestational hypertension
- Generally managed by obstetricians, even if eclampsia. Cardiologists may get involved if there is cardiac decompensation, which is rare.

Management of hypertension in pregnancy:

- Severe hypertension (≥ 160/110 mmHg) in pregnancy requires admission and urgent treatment. Systolic blood pressure ≥ 160 mmHg should be treated. The threshold for treatment should be lower than this in some cases.
- Aim is to allow time for foetal maturation and a planned, safe delivery, often induced.
- Safe drugs for non-severe hypertension are labetalol, nifedipine and methyldopa.
- First-line agents for severe hypertension are intravenous labetalol and hydralazine.
- Oral nifedipine if no parenteral treatment.
- In pre-eclampsia, complete resolution of hypertension and associated features usually seen by 6 weeks' post partum but there is a risk of chronic hypertension long term.
- Post-partum hypertension can also occur.

Cardiomyopathies
- Most important are peripartum, dilated, and hypertrophic cardiomyopathy.
- Peripartum cardiomyopathy (PPCM) defined as an idiopathic cardiomyopathy presenting with heart failure secondary to left ventricular systolic dysfunction towards the end of pregnancy or in the months following delivery, where no other cause of heart failure is found where the ejection fraction is < 45% on echocardiography.
- Incidence approximately 1 in 1–4,000 pregnancies, with considerable geographical variation (e.g. 1 in 300 in Haiti).
- Risk factors include primigravidae, multiple pregnancy, hypertension (pre-existing, pre-eclampsia, or gestational hypertension), obesity, smoking, diabetes, multiparity, maternal age > 30 years, and Black race. Genetic predisposition likely.

- Usually presents with symptoms and signs of heart failure, but may present with arrhythmia or systemic emboli (5-9%) due to the formation of intracardiac thrombus. Cardiogenic shock occurs in a minority.
- Aetiology unknown, although recent interest in prolactin playing a casual role.
- Mortality rate is high but varies, depending on healthcare system, 7-20% in high income countries.
- Predictors of poor outcome include poor functional class, ejection fraction less than 30% and LVEDD > 6.0 cm at the time of diagnosis, as well as poor right ventricular function, the presence of LV thrombus and Black race.
- Left ventricle returns to normal in 50–80% by 6 months and may continue to recover for up to 2 years.
- Women should be advised against pregnancy if the left ventricle does not return to normal. Foetal risks: stillbirth, miscarriage, and preterm delivery.
- Risk in subsequent pregnancy strongly depends on recovery of left ventricle: if normalizes (EF>50%), 20% risk of deteriorating LV function, but severe deterioration rare and rate of subsequent recovery high. If does not recover, risk of further deterioration 50% with higher morbidity and mortality.

Management:

- Confirm diagnosis by echocardiogram and exclude other causes of heart failure.
- Manage with standard heart failure care but liaise with obstetricians/anaesthetists closely.
- ACE inhibitors if post-partum (enalapril is safe in breast-feeding).
- Delivery usually needs to be expedited. Ventricular function may deteriorate with continued pregnancy.
- Thromboembolic prophylaxis crucial due to high risk of embolic stroke. Consider full anticoagulation with low molecular weight heparin if EF<30-35%.
- Referral to transplant centre may need to be considered. Ventricular assist devices may be needed as a bridge to recovery.
- Bromocriptine has recently been shown to improve outcome in small trials but precludes breast-feeding and may increase clot risk.

Dilated cardiomyopathy (DCM)

- Often occult until the left ventricle has to deal with the volume load of pregnancy. May be difficult to differentiate from PPCM if occurs late in pregnancy.
- Typically presents at 17 to 20 weeks.
- Manage similarly to peripartum cardiomyopathy.
- Adverse risk factors: NYHA class ≥ III, EF <40%. Poor prognosis if EF < 20%, mitral regurgitation, right ventricular dysfunction, atrial fibrillation, and hypotension.

Hypertrophic cardiomyopathy

- Usually well tolerated in pregnancy if no symptoms pre-pregnancy and no severe left ventricular outflow tract (LVOT) obstruction.
- If symptomatic pre-pregnancy, consider beta blockers, septal myomectomy, and ICD implantation if high risk of sudden cardiac death.
- Avoid vasodilators that can worsen LVOT obstruction.
- Manage VT as in the normal heart.

- Atrial arrhythmias, worsening dyspnoea, and pulmonary oedema may occur (usually if history of these or large fluid boluses given at the time of delivery in the presence of diastolic dysfunction). A combination of loop diuretics and beta blockers is often effective.
- Caution with regional anaesthesia if obstruction. Avoid hypotension and rapid fluid shifts.

Maternal infective endocarditis (IE)
- Rare, involve obstetric cardiology and heart valve team urgently.
- Principles of treatment as for non-pregnant.

Prophylaxis and prevention of IE during pregnancy:

- Professional consensus-based guidelines rather than based on robust scientific data.
- Antibiotic prophylaxis no longer indicated for childbirth.
- If infection occurs, e.g. chorioamnionitis, prompt treatment with antibiotics is recommended.
- Prior to pregnancy ensure women at risk understand risks of endocarditis, how to prevent it, its clinical presentation, and need for early assessment.

8.7.7 Pharmacological treatment in pregnancy

- Evidence for drug treatment and safety in pregnancy based on case reports, observational studies, and clinical consensus, not from randomized clinical trials.
- Therefore, need to check every drug for safety profile and pharmacokinetics before use in pregnancy and lactation.
- Drugs may have unpredictable effects in pregnancy due to changes in gastric motility and drug absorption, changes in the volume of distribution and protein binding, increased renal blood flow as well as transfer of the drug transplacentally, which depends on the lipo/hydrosolubility of the drug, its molecular weight, and the pH of maternal and fetal fluids.
- Generally use drugs with a long safety record, at the lowest doses and for the shortest duration.
- See Table 8.7.1 for safety profile of drugs that are used in pregnancy.

Table 8.7.1 Safety profile of cardiac drugs commonly used in pregnancy.

Generally safe	Unsafe/inadequate data	Affect baby but used
Adenosine	Amiodarone	Beta blockers
Flecainide	ACE inhibitors	Sotalol
Furosemide	Angiotensin receptor antagonists	Lidocaine
Digoxin	Spironolactone	
Hydralazine	Thiazides	
Nitrates	Warfarin	
Aspirin	Statins	
GPIIb/IIIa inhibitors and $P2Y_{12}$ inhibitors	DOACs	
Nifedipine	Ivabradine	
Verapamil	SGLT2 inhibitors	

8.7.8 Contraception

- Contraception needs to be discussed in all women with known heart disease at each consultation and in those with congenital heart disease from puberty.
- Progesterones including the progesterone-based morning after pill are safe for all cardiac conditions.
- Need to consider efficacy of agent, thrombotic risk, drug interactions, infective risks, and risk of bleeding/vagal stimulation with insertion of intra-uterine devices.
- Sterilization should not be recommended as the most failsafe means of contraception. Hormonal contraceptives, such as Implanon/Nexplanon and the Mirena coil, are more effective and do not involve a surgical procedure with its attendant risks.
- Advice regarding termination of pregnancy should be sought for all women with heart disease from a cardiologist with expertise. Different methods of termination involve different risks and these need to be considered in the light of the original heart condition. Discussion between cardiologist, gynaecologist, and anaesthetist is recommended.

Further reading

Drenthen W, Boersma E, Balci A, Moons P, Roos-Hesselink JW, Mulder BJ, Vliegen HW, van Dijk AP, Voors AA, Yap SC, van Veldhuisen DJ, Pieper PG; ZAHARA Investigators. Predictors of pregnancy complications in women with congenital heart disease. *Eur Heart J*. 2010 Sep;31(17):2124–32. doi: 10.1093/eurheartj/ehq200. Epub 2010 Jun 28

Mandalenakis Z, Giang KW, Eriksson P, Liden H, Synnergren M, Wåhlander H, Fedchenko M, Rosengren A, Dellborg M. Survival in Children With Congenital Heart Disease: Have We Reached a Peak at 97%? *J Am Heart Assoc*. 2020 Nov 17;9(22):e017704. doi: 10.1161/JAHA.120.017704. Epub 2020 Nov 6. PMID: 33153356; PMCID: PMC7763707.

Presbitero P, Boccuzzi GG, Groot CJ, Roos-Hesselink JW. Pregnancy and heart disease. In Camm AJ, Lüscher TF, Serruys PW (eds). *The European Society of Cardiology Textbook of Cardiovascular Medicine*, 2nd edn. Oxford: Oxford University Press, 2009.

Regitz-Zagrosek V, Roos-Hesselink JW, Bauersachs J, Blomström-Lundqvist C, Cífková R, De Bonis M, Iung B, Johnson MR, Kintscher U, Kranke P, Lang IM, Morais J, Pieper PG, Presbitero P, Price S, Rosano GMC, Seeland U, Simoncini T, Swan L, Warnes CA; ESC Scientific Document Group. 2018 ESC Guidelines for the management of cardiovascular diseases during pregnancy. *Eur Heart J*. 2018 Sep 7;39(34):3165–241. doi: 10.1093/eurheartj/ehy340

Roos-Hesselink JW, Mark R. Johnson MR. *Pregnancy and Congenital Heart Disease (Congenital Heart Disease in Adolescents and Adults)*. Springer, 2019.

Silversides CK, Grewal J, Mason J, Sermer M, Kiess M, Rychel V, Wald RM, Colman JM, Siu SC. Pregnancy Outcomes in Women With Heart Disease: The CARPREG II Study. *J Am Coll Cardiol*. 2018 May 29;71(21):2419–30. doi: 10.1016/j.jacc.2018.02.076. PMID: 29793631.

Steer PJ, Gatzoulis MA (eds). *Heart Disease and Pregnancy*. Cambridge: Cambridge University Press, 2016.

Stout KK, Daniels CJ, Aboulhosn JA, Bozkurt B, Broberg CS, Colman JM, Crumb SR, Dearani JA, Fuller S, Gurvitz M, Khairy P, Landzberg MJ, Saidi A, Valente AM, Van Hare GF. 2018 AHA/ACC Guideline for the Management of Adults With Congenital Heart Disease: A Report of the American College of Cardiology/American Heart Association Task Force on Clinical Practice Guidelines. *J Am Coll Cardiol*. 2019 Apr 2;73(12):e81–e192. doi: 10.1016/j.jacc.2018.08.1029. Epub 2018 Aug 16. Erratum in: J Am Coll Cardiol. 2019 May 14;73(18):2361-2362. PMID: 30121239.

CHAPTER 9

CARDIOLOGICAL CONSULTATION

9.1

The patient undergoing non-cardiac surgery

James Rosengarten, Hiten Patel, and Thomas White

TABLE OF CONTENTS

9.1.1 Why is assessment important? 837
9.1.2 Physiological response to surgery 837
9.1.3 Risk assessment 838
  Surgery-related risk 838
  Type of surgery 838
  Patient-related risk 838
  Patients with cardiac symptoms and signs 839
9.1.4 Pre-operative assessment tools 839
  Risk scoring 840
  Frailty 841
  Functional capacity 841
  Investigations prior to NCS 841
  ECG and biomarkers 841
  Coronary angiography 842
9.1.5 Risk reduction strategies 842
  Lifestyle and CV risk factors 842
  Pharmacotherapy 842
  Antithrombotic agents 844
  Peri-operative thromboprophylaxis 846
  Patient blood management 847
9.1.6 Specific conditions 847
  Coronary artery disease 847
  Heart failure 848
  Valvular heart disease 848
  Arrhythmias 849
  Adult congenital heart disease 850
  Pericardial disease 851
  Pulmonary disease and pulmonary arterial hypertension 851
  Arterial hypertension 851
  Peripheral artery disease 851
  Cerebrovascular disease 852
  Renal disease 852
  Obesity 852
  Diabetes 852
  Cancer 852
  Coronavirus disease 2019 852
9.1.7 Peri-operative monitoring and anaesthesia 853
9.1.8 Peri-operative cardiovascular complications 853
  Peri-operative myocardial infarction/injury 853
  Venous thromboembolism 854
  Atrial fibrillation 854
  Peri-operative stroke 854

9.1.1 Why is assessment important?

- Globally it is estimated around 5% (300 million) of the world's population undergo non-cardiac surgery (NCS) annually.
- An increasing proportion of patients undergoing NCS have underlying cardiac pathology or cardiovascular risk factors. In a cohort of 40,000 patients aged ≥45 years undergoing inpatient NCS 1 of 7 experienced a major cardiac or cerebrovascular complication at 30 days.

9.1.2 Physiological response to surgery

- Surgery can evoke a series of neuro-hormonal and endocrine responses, known as a stress response.
- Tissue injury causes activation of the sympathetic nervous system leading to increased release of catecholamines amongst other stress hormones. The resulting tachycardia and hypertension can increase myocardial oxygen demand.

- Where there is already a reduced supply of blood to meet the metabolic demands of tissues, e.g. Ischaemic Heart Disease (IHD), a mismatch in the supply to demand ratio of coronary blood flow can lead to or precipitate myocardial infarction or arrhythmia.
- Surgery can lead to a hypercoagulable state by causing alterations in the balance between pro-thrombotic and fibrinolytic factors. Higher levels of fibrinogen together with other coagulation factors contribute to increased platelet activation and aggregation, which in turn lead to increased coronary thrombogenicity.
- Fluid shifts both physiological and iatrogenic can significantly increase the risk of surgery particularly when cardiac function is impaired. Release of stress hormones can lead to increased salt and water retention and fluid resuscitation to combat blood loss can exacerbate heart failure.

9.1.3 Risk assessment

Cardiovascular morbidity and mortality are determined by surgery-related and patient-related risks. These risks can be estimated through various risk scores and reduced by accurate pre-operative evaluation and proper selection of type and timing of the surgical procedure.

Surgery-related risk

- Surgical factors influencing decision-making in cardiac patients include urgency of surgery, degree of invasiveness, and duration. Physiological factors include changes in core temperature, fluid loss, and fluid shift.
- The need for further evaluation is dependent on the risk category of surgery, symptoms, and underlying clinical status. The risk–benefit balance of surgery must be considered as well as the urgency (see Table 9.1.1).

Type of surgery
Vascular surgery

- Generally, carries the highest risk of cardiac complications. Studies have shown taking adequate perioperative measures to address cardiac risk can reduce overall risk of surgery.
- Endovascular or video-assisted procedures should be considered for patients with high CV risk undergoing vascular or pulmonary surgery (ESC Class IIa).

Open vs laparoscopic or thoracoscopic procedures

- Laparoscopic surgery is associated with less tissue trauma, pain, and better post-operative pulmonary function when compared to open procedures.
- However, complications can arise secondary to gas insuflation required to perform these procedures. Raised intrabdominal pressures can result in reduced venous return. Pneumoperitoneum and the Trendelenburg position results in increased mean arterial pressure and systemic vascular resistance. All the above factors can contribute to impaired cardiac function.
- Therefore, CV risk is not necessarily reduced in patients undergoing laparoscopic surgery.

Patient-related risk

- Patient-related risk is determined by the patient's age, the presence or absence of CV risk factors or established CV disease and comorbidities.
- An accurate history and examination are important to obtain these details and assess if patients have any active cardiac symptoms and signs.

Table 9.1.1 Surgical risk estimate according to type of surgery or intervention

Low surgical risk (<1%)	Intermediate surgical risk (1–5%)	High surgical risk (>5%)
• Breast • Dental • Endocrine: thyroid • Eye • Gynaecology: minor • Orthopaedic: minor (meniscectomy) • Reconstructive • Superficial surgery • Urological: minor (transurethral resection of the prostate) • VATS minor lung resection	• Carotid asymptomatic (CEA or CAS) • Carotid symptomatic (CEA) • Endovascular aortic aneurysm repair • Head and neck surgery • Intraperitoneal: splenectomy, hiatal hernia repair, cholecystectomy • Intra-thoracic: non-major • Neurological or orthopaedic: major (hip and spine surgery) • Peripheral arterial angioplasty • Renal transplant • Urological or gynaecological: major	• Adrenal resection • Aortic and major vascular surgery • Carotid symptomatic (CAS) • Duodenal-pancreatic surgery • Liver resection, bile duct surgery • Oesophagectomy • Open lower limb revascularization or amputation or thromboembolectomy • Repair of perforate bowel • Pneumonectomy (VATS or open surgery) • Pulmonary or liver transplant • Repair of perforated bowel • Total cystectomy

CAS—carotid artery stenting; CEA—carotid endarterectomy; VATS—video-assisted thoracic surgery
Surgical risk estimate is a broad approximation of 30-day risk of cardiovascular death and myocardial infarction that takes into account only the specific surgical intervention, without considering the patient's comorbidities.
Adapted from data in Glance et al., Muller et al., Bendixen et al., and Falcoz et al.
Halvorsen S, Mehilli J, Cassese S, et al; ESC Scientific Document Group. 2022 ESC Guidelines on cardiovascular assessment and management of patients undergoing non-cardiac surgery. *Eur Heart J*. 2022 Oct 14;43(39):3826–3924. doi: 10.1093/eurheartj/ehac270. Erratum in: *Eur Heart J*. 2023 Nov 7;44(42):4421. © European Society of Cardiology. With permission from Oxford University Press.

- Standard laboratory tests should be measured in all patients undergoing intermediate to high-risk surgery. Some patients will require an ECG, biomarkers, assessment of functional capacity, and other investigations (see Figure 9.1.1)
- In patients with a family history of genetic cardiomyopathy, it is recommended to perform an ECG and TTE before NCS, regardless of age and symptoms.

Patients with cardiac symptoms and signs

- In patients with a newly detected murmur and symptoms or signs of CVD, a transthoracic echocardiogram (TTE) is recommended before NCS. A TTE is also recommended before high-risk NCS if the murmur is felt to be clinically significant, regardless of symptoms. (ESC Class I).
- In patients with chest pain or other symptoms suggestive of undetected CAD, further diagnostic work-up is recommended prior to elective NCS.
- In patients with dyspnoea and/or peripheral oedema, an ECG and an NTproBNP/BNP test is indicated before NCS. A TTE is recommended if NTproBNP levels are elevated.

9.1.4 Pre-operative assessment tools

In patients without unstable cardiac features, the assessment of risk factors can guide the need for further diagnostic testing and peri-operative management.

- Evidence suggests that in low or intermediate risk patients, non-invasive assessment does not alter outcome, provided optimal medical therapy is achieved.
- Testing should not be performed unless the results would affect perioperative management.

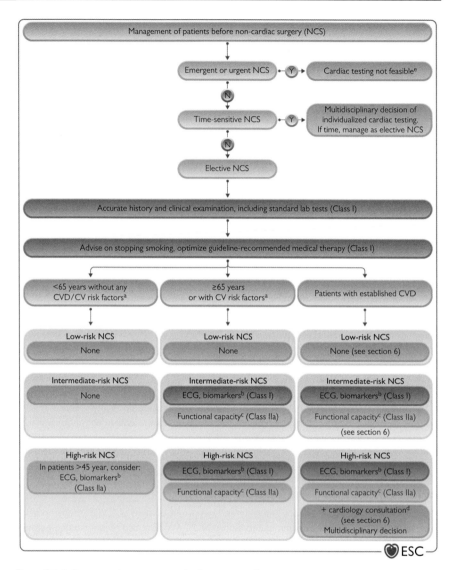

Figure 9.1.1 Pre-operative assessment before non-cardiac surgery.
[a]CV risk factors: hypertension, smoking, dyslipidaemia, diabetes, family history of CVD.
[b]Biomarkers: hs-cTn T/I (Class I) and/ or BNP/NT-proBNP (Class IIa). If pathological, consult a cardiologist.
[c]Functional capacity based on Duke Activity Status Index (DASI) or the ability to climb two flights of stairs (4 METs).
[d]For diagnostic and therapeutic efforts to be considered.
[e]Close follow-up after intervention and subsequent management of heart disease are advised.
Halvorsen S, Mehilli J, Cassese S, et al; ESC Scientific Document Group. 2022 ESC Guidelines on cardiovascular assessment and management of patients undergoing non-cardiac surgery. *Eur Heart J.* 2022 Oct 14;43(39):3826-3924. doi: 10.1093/eurheartj/ehac270. Erratum in: Eur Heart J. 2023 Nov 7;44(42):4421. © European Society of Cardiology. With permission from Oxford University Press..

Risk scoring

- Several risk indices have been in use over the last 30 years. Risk scores integrate patient-related and surgery-related risk factors, none of them include biomarkers.

- Previous ESC guidelines recommended utilizing the Lee's Revised Cardiac Risk Index or NSQIP risk scores. The most recent ESC guidelines 2022 recommend that selection criteria for further pre-operative testing should be based on clinical criteria and not based on a specific score.
- The American College of Surgeons (ACS) National Surgical Quality Improvement Programme (NSQIP) risk calculator is a comprehensive, externally validated risk calculator comprising 21 factors (20 patient factors plus the procedure). It is a predictive modelling tool derived from a database of >200,000 patients. It provides an estimate of the absolute 30-day probability of serious complications and complications compared with the average patient. The calculator is available online: https://riskcalculator.facs.org

Frailty

- Patients ≥70 years scheduled to undergo intermediate or high-risk NCS should be considered for frailty screening
- Frailty screening is an excellent predictor of unfavourable health outcomes in the older population. A simple approach is offered by the Clinical Frailty Scale. The Frailty Index and Frail Phenotype are the most recommended validated screening tools

Functional capacity

- Functional testing can help determine a patient's functional capacity or reserve in a more formal manner. It is measured in metabolic equivalents. One MET = metabolic demand at rest, 4 METs = climbing 2 flights of stairs, 10 METs = strenuous sport. The inability to climb 2 flights of stairs or run a short distance (<4 METs) indicates poor functional capacity and is associated with an increased incidence of post-operative cardiac events.
- The Duke Activity Status Index (DASI) (https://www.mdcalc.com/duke-activity-status-index-dasi#evidence) has a more precise estimation of cardiac risk than subjectively assessed functional capacity.

Investigations prior to NCS

Certain patients benefit from further investigations prior to NCS. The following recommendations are derived from the 2022 ESC Guidelines on cardiovascular assessment and management of patients undergoing non-cardiac surgery.

ECG and biomarkers

In patients undergoing intermediate or high risk NCS, who have known CVD or CV risk factors (including age ≥ 65 years), or symptoms or signs suggestive of CVD:

- A pre-operative 12-lead ECG is recommended (ESC Class IC)
- Measurement of high sensitivity troponin is recommended before surgery, at 24 hours and 48 hours afterwards (ESC Class IB)
- Measurement of NTproBNP or BNP should be considered (ESC Class IIa)

ECG and biomarkers should be considered in patients ≥45 years undergoing high-risk NCS
Transthoracic Echocardiography (TTE)

- TTE is recommended in patients with poor functional capacity and/or high NT-proBNP ((≥ 125 pg/mL) /BNP (≥ 35 pg/mL) or if murmurs are detected before high-risk NCS, to undertake risk reduction strategies (ESC Class I).
- TTE should be considered in patients with suspected new CVD or unexplained signs or symptoms before high-risk NCS (ESC Class IIa).

Stress imaging

- Stress imaging is recommended before high-risk elective NCS in patients with poor functional capacity[1] and high likelihood of CAD[2] or high clinical risk[3] (ESC Class IB).
- Stress imaging should be considered before high-risk NCS in asymptomatic patients with poor functional capacity[c] and previous PCI or CABG.

1. Physical capacity based on Duke Activity Status Index (DASI) or inability to climb 2 flights of stairs.
2. Pre-test probability.15% based on age, sex, and nature of symptoms, or two or more risk factors for CVD (dyslipidaemia, diabetes, hypertension, smoking, family history of CVD), or resting ECG changes (Q wave or ST-segment/T wave changes), or LV dysfunction suggestive of CAD.
3. One or more clinical risk factor according to the Revised Cardiac Risk Index (ischaemic heart disease, cerebrovascular disease, history of congestive heart failure, serum creatinine level 0.2 mg/dL, diabetes requiring insulin therapy).

Coronary angiography

- It is recommended to use the same indications for invasive coronary angiography and revascularization pre-operatively as in the non-surgical setting (ESC Class IC).
- CCTA should be considered to rule out CAD in patients with suspected CCS or biomarker-negative NSTE-ACS in case of low to intermediate clinical likelihood of CAD, or in patients unsuitable for non-invasive functional testing undergoing non-urgent, intermediate, and high-risk NCS (ESC Class IIa).

9.1.5 Risk reduction strategies

Lifestyle and CV risk factors

- It is important, where possible, to control CV risk factors prior to NCS including hypertension, dyslipidaemia, and diabetes (ESC Class IB).
- Smoking is associated with a higher rate of complications at 30 days and cessation is well documented in RCTs to improve outcomes, particularly when greater than 4 weeks prior to NCS (ESC Class IB).
- Pre-operative exercise programmes do not have large RCT backing but have been shown in smaller studies to reduce complications and so may be considered for patients requiring major or complex surgery. It is not recommended to attempt weight reduction in obese patients immediately prior to surgery.

Pharmacotherapy
Beta blockers

- Decrease myocardial oxygen consumption by reducing heart rate and contractility, as well as increasing diastolic filling time and helping prevent tachyarrhythmias.
- The POISE trial evaluated the effects of beta blockers in high-risk patients undergoing surgery and was associated with a reduction in the primary composite end point (cardiovascular death, non-fatal MI, or non-fatal cardiac arrest). However, there was an increase in overall mortality by up to 33% driven by hypotension and bradycardia.
- ESC guidelines suggest Class 1 indication for the continuation of beta blockers if already on it, especially for the treatment of angina and arrhythmia. Increased mortality and risk of AF has been reported in studies where they are withdrawn pre-operatively.
- There is a Class IIb indication for its initiation in patients undergoing high-risk surgery and with known CAD, myocardial ischaemia, or with two or more clinical risk factors (IHD,

cerebrovascular disease, renal insufficiency, diabetes). Atenolol or bisoprolol should be considered the first-choice agents.
- Routine initiation of beta blocker therapy peri-operatively is not recommended (ESC Class III).

Amiodarone

- It is unclear if there is net clinical benefit for the use of preventative amiodarone. A meta-analysis has shown a reduction in post-operative AF but there is the inevitable risk of non-cardiac side effects.

Statins

- The use of statins in patients at high risk of or with known CVD is well established. It is known to reduce cholesterol with additional plaque stabilizing properties through pleotropic effects thereby potentially preventing plaque rupture.
- Routine peri-operative initiation of statins is not recommended but continuation is recommended. If however a statin is already indicated for a patient, statin therapy should be considered peri-operatively, particularly for those undergoing high-risk surgery

Renin-angiotensin-aldosterone system (RAAS) inhibitors

- Peri-operative continuation of RAAS inhibitors appears to increase the risk of intra-operative hypotension and the need for vasopressors and inotropes with an associated risk of end-organ damage including kidney injury, myocardial infarction, and stroke. A converse increase in post-operative hypertension has been seen in trial patients for whom they were discontinued.
- In patients with stable HF, peri-operative continuation of RAAS inhibitors may be considered (ESC Class IIb) but in patients without heart failure, withholding them on the day of NCS should be considered (ESC Class IIa).
- If an RAAS inhibitor is withheld, it should be restarted as soon as possible to avoid inadvertent treatment cessation.
- There is no current data on the peri-operative use of angiotensin receptor neprilysin inhibitors (ARNI) but hypotension would be considered a risk.

Calcium channel blockers

- It is recommended to continue treatment with calcium channel blockers during the peri-operative period whilst omitting the dose on the day of surgery, particularly in those with vasospastic angina.
- There is conflicting data on the peri-operative initiation of calcium channel blockers with some a meta-analysis of 11 randomized trials including 1007 patients showing treatment significantly reduced episodes of myocardial ischaemia and supraventricular tachycardia but neither end point of mortality or MI reached statistical significance alone. Another case-control study with 1000 patients undergoing aortic aneurysm surgery suggested dihydropyridine use increased peri-operative mortality.

Diuretics

- Transient discontinuation of diuretic therapy to treat hypertension should be considered on the day of NCS (ESC Class IIa).
- Diuretic dose adjustments in heart failure should occur well in advance of NCS and careful attention should be paid to the patient's volume status and electrolytes in the peri-operative period.

Sodium-glucose co-transporter-2 (SGLT-2) inhibitors

- There is well-established benefit from the use of SGLT-2 inhibitors in patients with type 2 diabetes mellitus and also for patients with heart failure and chronic kidney disease.
- Several case reports have shown that euglycaemic diabetic ketoacidosis (a recognized but rare risk of SGLT-2 inhibitors) may occur after NCS in patients on such medication.
- ESC guidance suggests considering interrupting SGLT-2 use for at least 3 days prior to intermediate and high-risk surgery.

Antithrombotic agents

Antiplatelets

- The risk of ischaemic events in patients taking aspirin for primary prevention is low and so aspirin should be stopped prior to NCS with consideration of permanent discontinuation in low and moderate risk atherosclerotic cardiovascular disease risk patients and/or those with a high bleeding risk.
- In high bleeding risk procedures (such as spinal surgery or certain neurosurgical/ophthalmological operations) and where the bleeding risk is thought to outweigh the potential CV benefits, aspirin should be discontinued for at least 7 days prior to NCS (ESC Class IC).
- The POISE 2 trial did not show any significant difference in patients taking aspirin compared with placebo in rates of death or MI. However, bleeding rates were significantly elevated. There was, however, benefit seen in a post-hoc analysis of patients who had undergone previous PCI.
- ESC gives a Class IB recommendation for continuing aspirin in patients with previous PCI, if bleeding risk allows.
- For patients on clopidogrel monotherapy for chronic coronary syndromes, it should be interrupted in patients with high bleeding risk. For those on clopidogrel monotherapy after de-escalation following PCI/ACS or due to a recent stroke, peripheral arterial disease, or aspirin intolerance, decision-making will need to be individualized after an interdisciplinary evaluation, balancing the bleeding and ischaemic risk. Management may include continuing on $P2Y_{12}$ inhibitor monotherapy, bridging with aspirin or short interruption.
- If interruption of $P2Y_{12}$ inhibitor is required, ESC recommends withholding ticagrelor for 3–5 days, clopidogrel for 5 days and prasugrel for 7 days prior to NCS (ESC Class IB).
- If antiplatelet therapy has been interrupted it is recommended to resume as soon as possible, post operatively; ideally within 48 hours.

Dual antiplatelet therapy

- Those that are on dual therapy following stent insertion should remain on it for the prescribed duration and where possible surgery should be delayed until the recommended treatment period has passed.
- For patients with an ongoing indication for dual anti-platelet therapy undergoing non-cardiac surgery, discussion between surgeon, anaesthetist, and cardiologist is recommended to determine the risks of thrombotic complications vs bleeding.
- ESC recommends delaying elective NCS until 6 months after elective PCI and 12 months after ACS (ESC Class 1A), delaying time-sensitive NCS until a minimum of 1 month DAPT post-elective PCI (Class IC) or consider at least 3 months of DAPT for high-risk patients (STEMI or high-risk NSTE-ACS) prior to time-sensitive NCS (Class IIa).

Oral anticoagulants (OAC)

- Management of oral anticoagulation therapy depends on both surgery- and patient-related factors and the specific agent in use. Surgical factors include the bleeding risk, urgency, and the

9.1.5 Risk reduction strategies

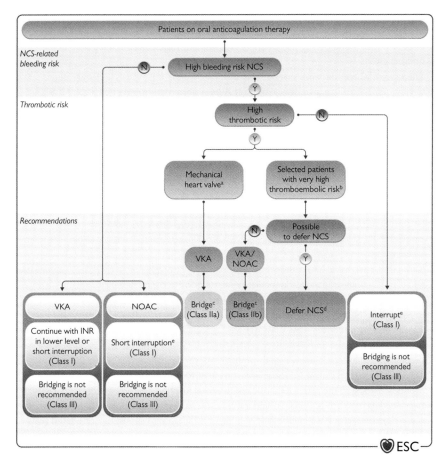

Figure 9.1.2 Recommendations for management of oral anticoagulation therapy in patients undergoing non-cardiac surgery.
[a] mechanical bileaflet AVR plus one other thromboembolic risk factor, older generation mechanical AVR or mechanical tricuspid or mitral valve replacement.
[b] recent stroke <3 months, high risk of VTE recurrence, left ventricular apex thrombus, AF with very high stroke risk.
[c] with unfractionated or low molecular weight heparin.
[d] For example >3 months after stroke/VTE.
[e] for further details on NOAC management during NCS see the ESC 2022 guidelines.
Reproduced from 2022 ESC Guidelines on cardiovascular assessment and management of patients undergoing non-cardiac surgery.

feasibility of mechanical compression of possible bleeding sites. Patient factors include age, thrombotic risk, prior bleeding history, medical comorbidities including renal insufficiency and concomitant medication. See Figure 9.1.2 for a summary of ESC guidance.

- Maintenance of therapeutic INRs in patients on vitamin K antagonists (VKA) with mechanical heart valves is essential. Minor surgical procedures and low bleeding risk procedures can be performed without VKA interruption with INR control at the lower end of the therapeutic range.
- Procedures with higher bleeding risks and requiring INR ≤ 1.5 require VKA interruption and bridging with heparin should be considered.

- There is concern regarding higher bleeding rates on heparin bridging. The recent PERI-OP trial comparing bridging versus placebo with either a mechanical heart valve, atrial fibrillation, or atrial flutter found no significant benefit in preventing major thromboembolism in the bridging group.
- Therefore ESC recommends that patients with mechanical heart valves and low risk of thromboembolism (e.g. mechanical bileaflet AVR in sinus rhythm) may not require bridging for their OAC interruption. Other patients at higher thromboembolic risk (e.g. mechanical bileaflet AVR plus one other thromboembolic risk factor (AF, previous thromboembolism, severe left ventricular dysfunction, hypercoagulable state), older generation mechanical AVR or mechanical tricuspid or mitral valve replacement) should be considered for bridging with heparin (ESC Class IIa).
- When a VKA is used for AF or VTE, the BRIDGE trial showed that 3–5 days of warfarin interruption without bridging was superior to heparin bridging (comparable arterial and venous thromboembolism but significantly lower incidence of major bleeding). Bridging therapy may be considered in patients with a high thrombotic risk (e.g. CHA_2DS_2-VASc score > 6, recent cardioembolic stroke < 3 months, or high risk of VTE recurrence), whilst weighing the relative bleeding risk.
- If required, reversal of VKAs should be with vitamin K or prothrombin complex concentrates and plasma administration (for immediate reversal prior to major surgery).
- In minor bleeding risk procedures uninterrupted OAC therapy is recommended (Class IB). In patients on NOACs, procedures should be carried out at trough levels if possible (usually 12–24 hr after last dose) (ESC Class IC).
- When interruption of an NOAC is required peri-operatively, bridging with heparin is not recommended except in a few high thrombotic risk circumstances (ESC Class III).
- Guidance should be sought for the specific timing of NOAC interruption for different agents according to the procedural risk and the renal function. For procedures with a very high bleeding risk such as spinal or epidural anaesthesia, interruption for up to 5 half-lives (i.e. 3 days for factor Xa inhibitors and 4–5 days for dabigatran) should be considered (ESC Class IIa).
- If reversal of a NOAC is required for unplanned and emergency procedures, use of specific reversal agents (idarucizumab to reverse dabigatran (ESC Class IIa) and andexanet alpha to reverse factor Xa inhibitors, off label) or, if these are unavailable, prothrombin complex concentrate (PCC) or activated PCC should be considered (ESC Class IIa).
- When patients are taking dual antithrombotic therapy with an OAC and an antiplatelet for instance for patients with AF and recent PCI, elective surgery should be postponed until the antiplatelet can be safely stopped (e.g. 6 months after elective PCI and 12 months after ACS). Management of the OAC should then be as above.

Peri-operative thromboprophylaxis

- A recent meta-analysis has challenged the traditional view linking peri-operative VTE to mortality and suggested it may be more of a marker of mortality rather than a causal factor.
- Decisions regarding thromboprophylaxis should be based on the individual patient and surgery specific factors (ESC Class IA).
- ESC recommends that for non-orthopaedic surgery, those patients at low VTE risk should receive mechanical rather than pharmacological VTE prophylaxis.
- If pharmacological thromboprophylaxis is required, the type of NCS, duration of immobilization and other patient factors should be considered when selecting the drug (LMWH, NOAC, or fondaparinux) and duration.

- In orthopaedic surgery, patients with low bleeding risk should be considered for peri-operative thromboprophylaxis of up to 14 or 35 days for total knee or hip arthroplasty, respectively (Class IIa), and NOACs at thromboprophylactic doses may be considered as alternatives to LMWH in these patients (ESC Class IIb).
- In most other cases it is recommended that thromboprophylaxis is continued until the patient is fully mobile or until discharge.

Patient blood management
Pre-operative anaemia
- Studies have shown that in patients undergoing major surgery, even mild anaemia significantly increased morbidity and mortality across all groups with associated increased length of hospital stay and need for intensive care.
- Furthermore, in a study of nearly 4500 cardiac surgical patients, pre-operative anaemia and intra-operative transfusion were both shown to independently decrease survival.
- It is recommended that haemoglobin is measured pre-operatively in patients awaiting intermediate and high-risk NCS and that anaemia is treated in advance of NCS to reduce the need for blood product transfusion (ESC Class IA).

Peri-operative blood loss
- Laboratory blood testing can cause a degree of blood loss enough to cause or aggravate hospital-acquired anaemia and so the volume of blood drawn should be minimized where possible by considering reduced frequency testing, using paediatric tubes or closed loop arterial sampling systems.
- Minimising intra-operative blood loss involves pre-operative considerations such as appropriate interruption of antithrombotic agents and intra-operative approaches such as advanced anaesthetic and surgical techniques with meticulous haemostasis including minimally invasive techniques, judicious diathermy use, physician awareness of blood loss, and the use of topical haemostatic agents.
- For procedures where blood loss is expected to exceed 500 ml, the ESC recommends the use of washed cell salvage (ESC Class IA) to minimize the need for allogenic red blood cell transfusion.
- For NCS where major bleeding is encountered, administration of tranexamic acid should be immediately considered (ESC Class IIa).

9.1.6 Specific conditions

Coronary artery disease
Acute Coronary Syndrome (ACS)
- In patients awaiting NCS who present with ACS, management should follow standard ACS guidance. In these circumstances it would be reasonable to consider only treating the culprit lesion, the use of newer generation drug-eluting stents, and reviewing the timing and peri-operative management of planned NCS should be considered. If safe to do so, NCS should be postponed for at least 3 months (ESC Class IA).
- In the rare cases of ACS and a concurrent life-threatening condition requiring urgent NCS, the treatment of the ACS and the surgical priorities should be discussed by a multidisciplinary team on an individualized basis (ESC Class IIa).

Chronic Coronary Syndrome (CCS)
- Routine myocardial revascularisation is not recommended prior to low to intermediate risk NCS.
- Revascularisation may be considered prior to high-risk non-cardiac surgery depending on the amount of ischaemic myocardium, refractory symptoms and coronary angiography findings, e.g. left main disease (ESC Class IIb).

Heart failure
- Heart failure (HF) is a known risk for post-operative mortality in NCS and features in several post-operative risk calculators. Furthermore, undergoing NCS also increases the risk of acutely decompensated HF in the post-operative period.
- The risk associated with HF depends on whether the LV systolic function is preserved or not, the presence or absence of haemodynamic compensation, and on the degree of symptoms.
- If HF is suspected or known in a patient awaiting high-risk NCS evaluation of LV function with an echo (< 6 months pre-op) and measurement of NT-proBNB/BNP levels is recommended (ESC Class IB).
- HF patients awaiting NCS should be optimally medically managed according to HF guidelines. Peri-operative regular assessment of volume status and signs of organ perfusion is recommended.
- Patients with hypertrophic cardiomyopathy with LV outflow obstruction (HCM) should have an echo pre-operatively to assess the extent of the hypertrophy, obstruction, and diastolic dysfunction. To maintain stroke volume and avoid precipitating increased outflow tract obstruction, it is important to avoid dehydration and prolonged fasting, vasodilating anaesthetic agents, tachycardia, and AF. Medications to treat obstruction should be continued.

Valvular heart disease
- Valvular heart disease (VHD) has a highly variable impact on the risk of peri-operative CV complications depending on its nature (particularly obstructive valve disease, e.g. severe aortic or mitral stenosis) and severity and the nature of the NCS.
- Clinical and echocardiographic assessment is recommended prior to intermediate or high-risk NCS in all patients with known or suspected VHD and in those for whom mild to moderate VHD was diagnosed more than 1 year ago (ESC Class I).

Aortic Stenosis (AS)
- The risk relating to AS depends on the severity, presence of coexisting CV disease, and the presence of symptoms with severe symptomatic AS being a significant risk factor for post-operative MI, heart failure, and mortality.
- In patients with symptomatic severe AS, intervention is recommended prior to intermediate or high-risk NCS (Class I). The choice between surgical aortic valve replacement (SAVR) and transcatheter aortic valve implantation (TAVI) should follow the recognized guidance regarding the management of aortic stenosis. For patients requiring time-sensitive NCS however, TAVI is a reasonable option.
- If definitive AS intervention is not possible or safe, balloon aortic valvuloplasty (BAV) may be considered prior to NCS as a bridge to more definitive intervention (ESC Class IIb).
- It is considered safe for asymptomatic patients to undergo low- and intermediate-risk procedures providing they are not associated with large volume shifts.
- Asymptomatic severe AS patients awaiting high-risk elective NCS should be considered for intervention after a Heart Team discussion (ESC Class IIa).

Aortic regurgitation (AR)
- NCS can be performed without additional risk in patients with mild to moderate AR.
- Patients with severe AR should be managed according to the recognized guidelines and for those requiring intervention, this should occur before intermediate or high-risk elective NCS (ESC Class IC).

Mitral stenosis (MS)
- The ESC recommends intervention (percutaneous mitral commissurotomy (PMC) or surgery) in patients with moderate to severe rheumatic MS when symptomatic or systolic pulmonary artery pressure (SPAP) > 50 mmHg prior to elective intermediate or high-risk NCS (ESC Class I).
- If asymptomatic and SPAP < 50 mmHg, moderate to severe MS patients can proceed with NCS with relatively low risk of complications.
- Heart rate and rhythm control and fluid balance management is critical in minimizing the risks for these patients in the peri-operative period.

Mitral regurgitation (MR)
- Patients with symptomatic severe primary MR or asymptomatic severe primary MR with LV systolic dysfunction (LVESD ≥ 40 mm and/or LVEF ≤ 60%) should be considered for valve intervention prior to intermediate or high-risk NCS (ESC Class IIa).
- Those with symptomatic severe secondary MR despite guideline directed medical therapy (including device therapy) should be considered for valve intervention prior to NCS (ESC Class IIa).

Prosthetic valves
- These patients can undergo NCS provided there is no evidence of valve dysfunction, albeit with sometimes problematic management of peri-operative anticoagulation.

Arrhythmias
- Unless life-threatening, tachyarrhythmias should not defer surgery. General measures to prevent them and reduce their risk should be taken including minimizing electrolyte and acid-base imbalance, myocardial ischaemia (including that caused by large blood loss and anaemia), and large volume shifts. Where possible, continue appropriate heart failure medications and antiarrhythmia drugs.

Supraventricular tachycardia (SVT)
- The management of peri-operative SVTs is as otherwise recommended in guidelines. They often respond to vagal manoeuvres but pharmacotherapy with adenosine, beta blockers, or calcium channel blockers, or rarely, prompt cardioversion, may sometimes be required.
- Ablation should be considered in symptomatic patients with recurrent or persistent treatment-resistant SVT prior to high-risk, non-urgent NCS (ESC Class IIa).

Atrial fibrillation/flutter
- Management of AF in the peri-operative period largely follows standard practice with an emphasis on treating causal factors (including but not limited to fluid shifts, anaemia, myocardial ischaemia, and infection). Digoxin may be ineffective in high adrenergic peri-operative conditions.
- In patients undergoing NCS who develop AF with haemodynamic instability, emergency electric cardioversion is recommended (ESC Class I) whilst amiodarone may be considered for acute rate control in this group (Class IIb).

Ventricular arrhythmias

- Premature ventricular contractions (PVCs) and non-sustained VT (NSVT) are common and historically thought of as benign, although recent studies suggest they may be associated with adverse outcomes, especially if frequent (>10–20% burden). For patients undergoing urgent NCS, they do not require treatment unless frequent and symptomatic.
- If treatment is required, beta blockers or, if not tolerated, amiodarone should be considered and, if awaiting elective NCS, further diagnostics are necessary, especially if frequent, symptomatic or in those with a family history of sudden cardiac death (SCD).
- Peri-operative VT or VF should prompt thorough investigation to exclude severe ventricular dysfunction, coronary artery disease requiring urgent revascularization, and other potential causes of arrhythmia including primary electrical disease such as long-QT and Brugada syndrome.
- Patients with VF or haemodynamically compromising VT should receive prompt defibrillation and cardioversion, respectively, and if recurrent, in the setting of ischaemia, may be effectively treated with beta blockers and amiodarone and consideration of revascularization.
- When patients have symptomatic monomorphic sustained VT associated with myocardial scar, despite medical therapy, ablation is recommended before elective NCS (ESC Class IB).

Bradyarrhythmias

- If pacing indications are met, NCS should ideally be deferred, and a permanent system should be implanted (Class IIa). Temporary pacing should be limited to those requiring urgent NCS and in whom the bradyarrhythmia is haemodynamically compromising despite chronotropic drugs or is leading to ventricular tachyarrhythmia.
- The equipment and expertise to perform emergency transcutaneous pacing should be available for patients with bifascicular block undergoing NCS or, alternatively, a permanent system may be considered.

Cardiac implantable electronic devices (CIEDs)

- All CIEDs should have had a check within 12 months (or 6 months for ICDs) prior to NCS.
- CIED check-up and reprogramming prior to NCS should be considered for patients with CRT or ICD devices, those that are pacing dependent, and those undergoing procedures with a high risk of electromagnetic interference (EMI), e.g. unipolar electrosurgery above umbilical area (ESC Class IIa).
- For patients with ICDs, if NCS has an anticipated risk of EMI, deactivation of the antitachycardia function with a magnet is recommended (leaving bradycardia pacing functions intact).
- EMI to the CIED should be avoided or minimized by the use of bipolar electrocautery, short bursts, use > 15 cm away from the device, and using the lowest possible energy. If using unipolar electrocoagulation, manufacturer's recommendations should be reviewed but in general the indifferent return electrode should be placed as far from the CIED as possible and ensure the surgical site is between the CIED and the return electrode.

Adult congenital heart disease

- Given the variability and complexity of patients with adult congenital heart disease (ACHD), a consultation with an ACHD specialist is recommended prior to intermediate or high-risk surgery (ESC Class IC).
- Intermediate and high-risk NCS is also recommended to be performed in a centre with experience in ACHD care (ESC Class IC).
- Patients with residual haemodynamic abnormality despite correction of their CHD would be considered at intermediate risk during NCS whilst those with uncorrected cyanotic heart

disease, pulmonary hypertension, complex CHD, ventricular dysfunction requiring medication, and those awaiting a heart transplant would be considered at severe risk.

Pericardial disease

- The treatment of pericardial disease should follow the recognized guidelines and acute pericardial disease such as pericarditis is a clear indication to postpone elective NCS. In the case of time-sensitive or urgent NCS however, care must be taken in terms of drug interactions and pharmacokinetics, for instance interactions between colchicine and central nervous system depressants.
- In patients with small or moderate pericardial effusion and constrictive pericarditis, careful attention must be paid to optimizing pre-load to the heart, including the use of pre-operative IV fluids, minimizing medications that reduce pre-load, and by minimizing, where possible, positive pressure ventilation.

Pulmonary disease and pulmonary arterial hypertension

- In patients with chronic obstructive pulmonary disease (COPD) undergoing NCS, the main aims are to optimize pulmonary function pre-operatively and minimize respiratory complications post-operatively. There is benefit from smoking cessation > 2 months prior to surgery.
- Obesity Hypoventilation Syndrome (OHS) is associated with increased peri-operative mortality alongside its association with angina pectoris, pulmonary hypertension, and cor pulmonale. Patients at risk of OHS should have the relevant investigations pre-operatively and, if indicated, positive airway pressure therapy should be initiated pre-operatively.
- Pulmonary arterial hypertension (PAH) is well recognized to be associated with increased morbidity and mortality in patients undergoing NCS, mostly associated with the right ventricle's haemodynamic response to acute increases in afterload.
- Meticulous planning is required prior to NCS in patients with PAH, often including pre-operative echocardiography and right heart catheterization. Planning should involve the expert multidisciplinary team and care should occur in a centre experienced in PAH.
- Patients with PAH should be medically optimized according to guidelines prior to NCS and it is recommended that chronic PAH therapy is continued in the peri-operative period (ESC Class IC). When right HF progresses post-operatively, diuretic optimization and, if necessary, IV prostacyclin analogues should be considered (Class IC).

Arterial hypertension

- It is recommended to screen for CV risk factors and hypertension-mediated end organ damage pre-operatively in newly diagnosed hypertensive patients awaiting high-risk NCS (ESC Class IC).
- It is usually not required to postpone NCS for patients with grade 1 or 2 hypertension but for those with systolic BP ≥ 180 mmHg and/or diastolic BP ≥ 110 mmHg deferring all but emergency NCS is advisable. One large observation study showed a 69% increase in 90-day post-operative mortality in patients with untreated hypertension 1 month prior to surgery.
- Large fluctuations in peri-operative blood pressure (particularly hypotension) should be avoided (ESC Class IA).

Peripheral artery disease

- Patients awaiting elective vascular NCS for peripheral artery disease (PAD) or abdominal aortic aneurysm (AAA) that have poor functional capacity or significant CV risk factors or symptoms should be referred for cardiac investigation and optimization prior to surgery (ESC Class IC).

Cerebrovascular disease

- Patents who are suspected to have had a transient ischaemic attack (TIA) or stroke in the preceding 6 months should receive a neurological consultation and appropriate neurovascular and brain imaging (ESC Class IC).
- The management of carotid artery stenosis should follow the same guidelines as in non-surgical settings (ESC Class IIa).

Renal disease

- Renal disease is associated with several cardiac conditions and is consistently shown to increase the risk of post-operative CV events including MI, stroke, and the progression of HF in patients undergoing NCS.
- Patients with cardiac comorbidities are more prone to developing acute kidney injury (AKI) after major NCS.
- For patients requiring peri-operative contrast-enhanced radiography, the risk of contrast induced AKI should be minimized by considering the use of balanced hydration with i.v. isotonic fluids and carefully selecting the type and volume of contrast media used (ESC Class IIa).
- Patients with risk factors for renal disease undergoing intermediate or high-risk NCS should have pre-operative renal function blood screening (Class IC) and a cystatin C measurement assay should be considered if available to confirm the diagnosis of chronic kidney disease (ESC Class IIa).

Obesity

- It is recommended to assess cardiorespiratory fitness rather than focusing on BMI measurements as a marker for peri-operative CV risk in patients with obesity, particularly for those undergoing intermediate and high-risk NCS (ESC Class IB).

Diabetes

- It is recognized that not only will patients with diabetes undergoing NCS be more likely to have coronary artery disease (CAD) than non-diabetic patients but that they also have a higher risk of silent ischaemia due to altered cardiac neural pathways. Diabetes is also a clear risk factor for cerebrovascular events and is associated with post-operative heart failure and wound infections.
- Patients with diabetes awaiting NCS should have had an HbA1c test done within 3 months. If this is ≥ 8.5% (69 ≥ mmol/mol), elective NCS should be postponed if safe and practical (ESC Class IB).
- Pre-operative cardiac assessment is recommended for diabetic patients with suspected or known CAD and for those with autonomic neuropathy, retinopathy, or renal disease awaiting intermediate or high-risk NCS (ESC Class IC).

Cancer

- The possibility of CV risk in patients with cancer undergoing NCS must be considered particularly given the specific risks posed by certain cancer treatments such as the HF risk of anthracyclines, trastuzumab cardiotoxicity, and the local cardiac effects of radiation in terms of fibrosis, CAD, and valvular heart disease.
- Cancer patients are also at higher risk of AF and thrombosis.

Coronavirus disease 2019

- Caused by the severe acute respiratory syndrome coronavirus 2 (SARS-CoV-2), coronavirus disease 2019 (COVID-19) appears in recent literature to be associated with an increased

risk of post-operative VTE and mortality. There is also the possible risk of myocardial injury associated with the infection.
- Generally, elective NCS should be postponed until patients have completely recovered from COVID-19 although some studies have reported greater risk of post-operative complications and mortality up to 7–8 weeks post COVID-19 diagnosis. These studies did not include high vaccine-prevalent populations.

9.1.7 Peri-operative monitoring and anaesthesia

- Most anaesthetic agents counter the physiological effects of surgery by reducing sympathetic activity. This can lead to changes in vascular tone leading to vasodilatation and in turn decreased blood pressure. There is a consensus that significant hypotension peri-operatively is associated with organ injury such as myocardial injury, stroke, and AKI.
- Significant fluctuations in BP should be avoided. The ESC recommends goal-directed haemodynamic therapy in patients undergoing high-risk NCS (Class IA) and to avoid intra-operative MAP decreases of > 20% from baseline or < 60–70 mmHg for ≥ 10 mins (ESC Class IB).
- Intra-operative tachycardia has previously been considered to be a risk for adverse outcomes, but this remains a subject of controversy. It seems sensible though to consider it at least as a marker of haemodynamic impairment.
- Post-operative pain should be avoided (ESC Class IB).
- General vs local anaesthesia can vary in the degree of stress response initiated. Careful choice must be considered between different strategies as less invasive anaesthetic techniques can lead to lower mortality in intermediate to higher risk non-cardiac surgery.
- In terms of the choice of anaesthetic agent, there is a suggestion that volatile anaesthetic agents offer better cardioprotective properties than i.v. agents with some data showing lower post-operative troponin release although there was no impact on clinical outcomes.

9.1.8 Peri-operative cardiovascular complications

- Post-operative STEMI, NSTE-ACS, acute HF, tachyarrhythmias, and venous thromboembolism should be treated as per guidelines in the non-surgical setting (ESC Class IC) although the use of antithrombotic agents immediately post-operatively would need careful consideration.

Peri-operative myocardial infarction/injury

- Peri-operative myocardial infarction/injury (PMI) is acute myocyte injury (with a post-operative high sensitivity troponin I/T release) with or without symptoms and with or without ECG changes. It is the most common CV complication of NCS and is associated with approximately 10% 30-day mortality risk.
- PMI is complicated by the fact that it is largely asymptomatic in approximately 90% of patients and therefore is regularly missed. Furthermore, post-operative pain, nausea, surgical wounds and drains may impede the early detection of acute CV complications such as PMI, Takotsubo cardiomyopathy, tachyarrhythmias, and acute HF.
- High awareness and surveillance (involving pre- and post-operative troponin measurements) for PMI in high-risk patients (known CAD, PAD, insulin-dependent DM, or cardiac symptoms) is recommended (ESC Class IB).

- The work-up for PMI should involve identification of the underlying cause and echocardiography is usually important and helps in the identification of conditions such as Takotsubo cardiomyopathy.

Venous thromboembolism

- In cases of post-operative PE, anticoagulation (preferably LMWH or fondaparinux) should be initiated as soon as possible (ESC Class IC). Rescue thrombolytic therapy is recommended when indicated, according to bleeding risk but surgical embolectomy or percutaneous catheter-directed treatment should be considered for patients with haemodynamic deterioration on anticoagulation treatment, especially if high bleeding risk.

Atrial fibrillation

- Post-operative AF is common and episodes are often self-terminating and some are asymptomatic. Nonetheless the risk of AF recurrence in the following 5 years is increased four- to five-fold and is a risk factor for stroke, MI, and death.
- Routine use of beta blockers for the prevention of post-operative AF in patients undergoing NCS is not recommended (ESC Class III).
- An RCT showed no net clinical advantage of rhythm vs rate control strategies for patients with post-operative AF and so decisions regarding management of stable patients after NCS should be based on symptoms and shared, informed decision-making.
- The available evidence suggests that post-operative AF after NCS conferred a similar long-term thromboembolic risk as non-surgical AF and so long-term OAC treatment should be considered in these patients as soon as is safe to, based on their individual stroke risk (ESC Class IIa).

Peri-operative stroke

- To minimize the risk of peri-operative stroke, anti-thrombotic agents should be continued whenever safe to do so during the peri-operative period and any drug interruptions should be as short as possible.
- Post-operative stroke should be acted on immediately with CT brain and angiogram and neurological/stroke/neurosurgical consultation with the aim of restoration of blood flow as soon as possible in acute thrombotic occlusion.

Further reading

Duceppe E, Parlow J, MacDonald P, Lyons K, McMullen M, Srinathan S, Graham M, Tandon V, Styles K, Bessissow A, Sessler DI, Bryson G, Devereaux PJ. Canadian Cardiovascular Society Guidelines on perioperative cardiac risk assessment and management for patients who undergo noncardiac surgery. Can J Cardiol. 2017 Jan;33(1):17–32. doi: 10.1016/j.cjca.2016.09.008. Epub 2016 Oct 4. Erratum in: Can J Cardiol. 2017 Dec;33(12):1735

Fleisher LA, Fleischmann KE, Auerbach AD, Barnason SA, Beckman JA, Bozkurt B, Davila-Roman VG, Gerhard-Herman MD, Holly TA, Kane GC, Marine JE, Nelson MT, Spencer CC, Thompson A, Ting HH, Uretsky BF, Wijeysundera DN; American College of Cardiology; American Heart Association. 2014 ACC/AHA guideline on perioperative cardiovascular evaluation and management of patients undergoing noncardiac surgery: a report of the American College of Cardiology/American Heart Association Task Force on practice guidelines. J Am Coll Cardiol. 2014 Dec 9;64(22):e77–137. doi: 10.1016/j.jacc.2014.07.944. Epub 2014 Aug 1

Glance LG, Lustik SJ, Hannan EL, Osler TM, Mukamel DB, Qian F, Dick AW. The Surgical Mortality Probability Model: derivation and validation of a simple risk prediction rule for noncardiac surgery. Ann Surg. 2012 Apr;255(4):696–702. doi: 10.1097/SLA.0b013e31824b45af

Halvorsen S, Mehilli J, Cassese S, Hall TS, Abdelhamid M, Barbato E, De Hert S, de Laval I, Geisler T, Hinterbuchner L, Ibanez B, Lenarczyk R, Mansmann UR, McGreavy P, Mueller C, Muneretto C, Niessner A, Potpara TS, Ristić A, Sade LE, Schirmer H, Schüpke S, Sillesen H, Skulstad H, Torracca L, Tutarel O, Van Der Meer P, Wojakowski W, Zacharowski K; ESC Scientific Document Group, Knuuti J, Kristensen SD, Aboyans V, Ahrens I, Antoniou S, Asteggiano R, Atar D, Baumbach A, Baumgartner H, Böhm M, Borger MA, Bueno H, Čelutkienė J, Chieffo A, Cikes M, Darius H, Delgado V, Devereaux PJ, Duncker D, Falk V, Fauchier L, Habib G, Hasdai D, Huber K, Iung B, Jaarsma T, Konradi A, Koskinas KC, Kotecha D, Landmesser U, Lewis BS, Linhart A, Løchen ML, Maeng M, Manzo-Silberman S, Mindham R, Neubeck L, Nielsen JC, Petersen SE, Prescott E, Rakisheva A, Saraste A, Sibbing D, Siller-Matula J, Sitges M, Stankovic I, Storey RF, Ten Berg J, Thielmann M, Touyz RM. 2022 ESC Guidelines on cardiovascular assessment and management of patients undergoing non-cardiac surgery. Eur Heart J. 2022 Oct 14;43(39):3826–924. doi: 10.1093/eurheartj/ehac270. PMID: 36017553.

Lee TH, Marcantonio ER, Mangione CM, Thomas EJ, Polanczyk CA, Cook EF, Sugarbaker DJ, Donaldson MC, Poss R, Ho KK, Ludwig LE, Pedan A, Goldman L. Derivation and prospective validation of a simple index for prediction of cardiac risk of major noncardiac surgery. Circulation. 1999 Sep 7;100(10):1043–9. doi: 10.1161/01.cir.100.10.1043

POISE Study Group, Devereaux PJ, Yang H, Yusuf S, Guyatt G, Leslie K, Villar JC, Xavier D, Chrolavicius S, Greenspan L, Pogue J, Pais P, Liu L, Xu S, Málaga G, Avezum A, Chan M, Montori VM, Jacka M, Choi P. Effects of extended-release metoprolol succinate in patients undergoing non-cardiac surgery (POISE trial): a randomised controlled trial. Lancet. 2008 May 31;371(9627):1839–47. doi: 10.1016/S0140-6736(08)60601-7. Epub 2008 May 12.

9.2

The patient with neurological symptoms

James Choulerton, Helen Sims, Oliver Watkinson, and Laura Pannell

TABLE OF CONTENTS

9.2.1 Stroke 857
Epidemiology 857
Ischaemic stroke classification 857
Aetiology of ischaemic stroke 858
Haemorrhagic stroke 861

9.2.2 Non-ischaemic neurological presentations 862
Transient loss of consciousness (TLOC) and syncope 862
Dizziness 862
9.2.3 Neuromuscular diseases with cardiac involvement 863

9.2.1 Stroke

Epidemiology
- Stroke is the second most common single cause of death in Europe, accounting for 405,000 deaths (9%) in men and 583,000 (13%) deaths in women each year
- Stroke is estimated to cost the EU economy €45 billion a year: around one-fifth of the overall cost of CVD
- More than half of all stroke survivors are left with disability and are dependent on others for everyday activities

Ischaemic stroke classification
Total Anterior Circulation Stroke (TACS)
- Large cortical stroke in the middle/anterior cerebral artery territory
  - Symptoms:
    - Unilateral weakness (and/or sensory deficit) of face/arm/leg
    AND
    - Homonymous hemianopia
    AND
    - Higher cerebral dysfunction (aphasia, visuospatial awareness)

Partial Anterior Circulation Stroke (PACS)
- Cortical stroke in the middle/anterior cerebral artery territory
- Symptoms:
  - TWO of the deficits in TACS

Lacunar Syndrome (LACS)
- Small subcortical stroke as a result of small vessel disease
- Symptoms:
    - No evidence of higher cerebral dysfunction, and one of:
        - Unilateral weakness (and/or sensory deficit) of face and arm, arm and leg, or all three
        - Pure sensory stroke
        - Ataxic hemiparesis

Posterior Circulation Stroke (POCS) (including brainstem)
- Stroke in posterior cerebral, basilar, vertebral, or cerebellar artery territories
- Affects the occipital lobes, cerebellum, or brainstem
    - Symptoms include one of:
        - Cerebellar or brainstem syndromes
            - Vertigo, nystagmus, dysdiadochokinesia, ataxia, slurred speech, tremor, diplopia, isolated cranial nerve palsies
        - Isolated homonymous hemianopia

Aetiology of ischaemic stroke
Cardiac embolism
- 15–30% of ischaemic strokes are secondary to cardiac embolism.
- Outcomes are worse than atherothrombotic strokes with 50% mortality at 3 years
- A CT or MRI brain demonstrating bilateral/multiple infarcts/multi-territory infarcts increase the index of suspicion of a cardioembolic cause of the stroke
- Standard trans-thoracic echocardiogram first-line investigation for all patients where this is suspected

Atrial fibrillation
- A major cause of ischaemic stroke (around a quarter of cases), the risk of stroke is increased fivefold in un-anticoagulated patients with AF—due to left atrial appendage thrombus formation
- *Investigation*
    - ECG
    - Ambulatory monitors
    - Implantable loop recorders (ILR)

N.B. more prolonged periods of monitoring have been shown to increase detection of AF (trials include Crystal AF for ILRs and Embrace AF for 30 day ambulatory ECG monitoring significantly improves the detection of AF by > 5×)

- *Management*
    - Patients with non-disabling stroke or TIA should be anticoagulated as soon as bleeding has been excluded
    - For larger ischaemic strokes anti-coagulate at day 7–14 depending on size as risk of haemorrhagic transformation is high acutely
        - High-dose antiplatelets used in the initial period prior to anticoagulation
    - Anticoagulation should be with either a DOAC or warfarin
        - DOACs are often preferred due to ease of prescribing and administration
        - Consider warfarin in patients unable to take DOACs or with specific indications such as metallic valves or moderate to severe mitral stenosis (excluded from trials)

- For patients unable to have anticoagulation
  - Antiplatelets are no longer recommended as an alternative for stroke prevention
  - Surgical ligation/resection or insertion of a left atrial appendage occlusion device (e.g. Watchman device) may be considered for those with contraindications to anticoagulation

Cardiac wall and chamber abnormalities

- Cardiomyopathies, e.g. DCM due to LV dysfunction, LVNC (left ventricular non-compaction)—mural thrombi form in deep intertrabecular recesses in the hypertrabeculated ventricle
- Recent/previous MI, resulting in LV aneurysm or LV thrombus formation overlying hypokinetic or akinetic myocardium; most commonly anterior infarct/apical myocardium.
- Atrial myxomas, papillary fibroelastomas and other tumours
  - Surgical resection should be discussed
- Septal defects and patent foramen ovale with paradoxical embolism

Patent Foramen Ovale (PFO)

- Present in about 25% of normal individuals; mostly asymptomatic
- Higher prevalence in those with stroke especially in younger patients with cryptogenic stroke (up to 40% quoted)
- PFO may act as a portal for paradoxical embolism into the arterial circulation causing stroke
- Suspect if stroke occurs in younger patients especially after a valsalva manoeuvre
- May however be incidental to stroke presentation
- *Investigation*
  - Bubble echocardiogram
  - Trans-oesophageal echocardiogram
  - Transcranial Doppler: detects microbubbles in mid-cerebral artery following i.v. injection of agitated saline to demonstrate right to left shunt
- *Management*
  - Meta-analyses have not shown a clear statistically significant difference between anticoagulation and antiplatelet therapy
  - Anticoagulation is not recommended unless there is another recognized indication, e.g. AF, DVT
  - Evidence conflicting with regard to benefit of closure—Cochrane meta-analysis found no significant benefit for the intervention and an increased risk of new-onset AF
  - Recent long-term follow-up of RESPECT trial indicates benefit of closure
  - Restricted commissioning in some areas limits availability for patients

Valve disorders

- Rheumatic mitral and aortic valve disease—significant mitral stenosis increases risk of left atrial thrombus formation
- Prosthetic valves
- Bacterial endocarditis with vegetation, which can be treated by surgical resection

Cardiac thrombus

- Left ventricular thrombus can create emboli leading to stroke, but is an uncommon cause
- *Investigation*
  - Echocardiogram: often only done in young patients (age < 55 years) or in those with abnormal ECG or cardiac murmurs

- Contrast echocardiography: improves visualization of the LV apex to assess for a thrombus or to differentiate thrombus from artefact/false tendons/trabeculations
- Management
  - Anticoagulation (usually for 6 months) to prevent embolic stroke either with DOAC or warfarin

Large and small vessel atherosclerosis
Aortic embolism
- Aortic atheroma is associated with systemic embolization resulting in stroke/peripheral embolism, e.g. limb/renal/mesenteric ischaemia
- Other complications include aortic dissection, pseudoaneurysm/aneurysm formation, and aortic rupture
- Atheroma formation is related to risk factors (discussed below): increasing age, smoking, hypercholesterolaemia, hypertension, and diabetes mellitus
- Factors which increase the risk of embolization:
  - Superimposed mobile thrombi
  - Plaques > 4 mm in depth
  - Complex ulcerated plaques
  - Non-calcified plaques
  - Cholesterol embolization from invasive procedures, e.g. during cardiac catheterization, cardiopulmonary bypass, intra-aortic balloon pump insertion
- Investigations
  - Allow diagnosis and characterization of plaques including evaluation of high-risk features mentioned above
  - CT/MR aortogram or transoesophageal echocardiography
- Treatment
  - The optimal therapeutic approach in patients remains unclear but include:
    - Statin therapy—may reduce plaque size and/or stabilize plaques reducing risk of embolization
    - Anticoagulation—reports suggest possible resolution of thrombi following treatment with warfarin

Diabetes
- An independent risk factor for stroke
- Hyperglycaemia has been shown to increase the size of ischaemic stroke and worsen clinical outcome
- Diabetic patients should have blood glucose levels tightly controlled in the hyperacute period as hyperglycaemia can further injure the ischaemic brain by creating anaerobic metabolism and lactic acidosis—sliding scales can be used
- Close working with diabetic specialists in order to optimize glucose control is important in order to reduce both micro- and macro-vascular disease (see Chapter 7.5)

Cholesterol
- Lipid modification is important in both primary and secondary prevention of stroke
- Large-scale evidence from randomized trials shows that each 1 mmol/L reduction in LDL cholesterol with statin therapy produces a proportional reduction of about 25% in the rate of major vascular events (including stroke) during each year that it continues to be taken
- PCSK9 inhibitors are a new option for controlling LDL cholesterol in those who do not tolerate statins—they specifically target receptors on the liver surface, which clear LDL cholesterol from the blood, increasing them in number (see Chapter 7.4)

Hypertension
- Elevated blood pressure is a major risk factor for stroke
- A 10 mmHg reduction in systolic BP is associated with a reduction in risk of stroke of approximately one-third
- There is no existing evidence to acutely lower blood pressure in acute ischaemic stroke. Acute blood pressure lowering may threaten the ischaemic penumbra thereby worsening the insult to the area of damaged brain
- However most stroke physicians would cautiously lower extremely high blood pressure (e.g. > 200 mmHg) as such pressures can increase haemorrhagic transformation risk
- Once extent of carotid disease is known, and after the first 24 hours, aim for improved control of hypertension
- Long-term blood pressure should be controlled aiming for BP < 130/80
- Blood pressure management is discussed in more detail in Chapter 7.3

Carotid atherosclerosis
- Narrowing of the carotid arteries through atherosclerosis or thrombosis causes turbulent blood flow, which can result in plaque/thrombus rupture and emboli causing stroke
- Patients presenting with symptoms of anterior circulation cerebral ischaemia who are considered suitable for surgical intervention should have urgent carotid imaging performed
- Patients with stable (non-disabling) neurological symptoms after stroke or TIA with symptomatic ipsilateral carotid stenosis of 50–99% should be referred for carotid endarterectomy as soon as possible (within 7 days); those with less than 50% stenosis should receive medical therapy alone
- CT angiogram or MR angiography is often needed to obtain more detailed information about the characteristics of the occlusion or stenosis
- All patients should receive optimal medical treatment: adequate blood pressure control, cholesterol lowering, antiplatelets, smoking cessation, etc.
- Completely occluded carotid arteries do not need surgical intervention as they are no longer at risk of causing emboli and stroke
- Patients who are unsuitable for endarterectomy, e.g. re-stenosis after endarterectomy, radiotherapy-associated carotid stenosis, should be considered for carotid stenting
    - Compared to endarterectomy, carotid stenting is associated with an increased risk of peri-procedural stroke (4.8% vs 3.5%)

Rarer causes
- Include: arterial dissection, vasculitis, antiphospholipid syndrome, hypercoagulability due to malignancy

Haemorrhagic stroke
Aetiology
- Haemorrhagic stroke is much less common than ischaemic stroke, making up only around 15% of stroke cases
- Most common cause is hypertension
- Other causes include:
    - Cerebral amyloid angiopathy: an abnormal build-up of amyloid proteins within the lining of blood vessels in the brain, resulting in weakened and friable walls which are more likely to rupture and bleed
    - Aneurysms
    - Ruptured arterio-venous malformations (AVMs)

- Use of anticoagulants or multiple antiplatelet medications
- Bleed into tumour (primary or metastases)
- Venous infarction (due to cerebral venous sinus thrombosis)

Diagnosis
- Certain examination findings such as decreased GCS, headache, vomiting, and seizure raise likelihood that stroke is haemorrhagic rather than ischaemic
- The initial investigation of choice is plain CT brain
- CTA or MRA can help diagnose aneurysms/AVMs
- Delayed (interval) MRI head is helpful in looking for underlying pathology, e.g. cerebral amyloid angiopathy (advanced small vessel ischaemia for age and lobar micro-haemorrhages) and underlying cerebral tumours

Medical treatment
- The mainstay of treatment in haemorrhagic stroke is control of BP and cessation of medications that increase bleeding
  - Patients presenting < 6 hours from symptom onset should have their BP tightly controlled at < 140/80 mmHg for at least the first 7 days, which may require labetalol or nitrate infusions
  - In the long-term BP should be controlled as for ischaemic stroke
- Any patient on anticoagulation requires reversal of these agents (unless absolutely required, e.g. metallic mitral valves), requiring urgent discussion with a Haematologist
  - Vitamin K and prothrombin complex concentrate for warfarin
  - Follow local protocols (and discuss with haematology) for DOAC reversal
  - Dabigatran is the only DOAC with a specific reversal agent (idarucizumab)
- In selected cases, antiplatelets or anticoagulants can be restarted at a later stage if indications exist, but ideally these patients should be enrolled in a relevant clinical trial
- Physiotherapy, occupational therapy, and speech and language therapy is as important in haemorrhagic as in ischaemic stroke, and is often the core component of treatment after the first 24 hours

Working with neurosurgery
- The role of neurosurgery in acute intracranial haemorrhage is relatively small. Patients with posterior fossa bleeds as well as those with hydrocephalus may be candidates for intervention as well as some lobar haemorrhages
- Neurosurgery or neuroradiological intervention may be appropriate for some underlying causes of bleeding such as solitary tumours, aneurysms, and AVMs

9.2.2 Non-ischaemic neurological presentations

Transient loss of consciousness (TLOC) and syncope
- May be due to syncopal or non-syncopal causes

See Chapter 4.2 for more detail

Dizziness
- Dizziness is a non-specific term used by patients. It can refer to:
  - Vertigo
    - Central causes, e.g. stroke and peripheral causes, e.g. BPPV, labyrinthitis

- Presyncope
    - Causes as for syncope
- Disequilibrium
    - Refers to a sense of imbalance that occurs primarily when walking. Can be due to peripheral neuropathy, musculoskeletal disorders that interfere with gait, vestibular and cerebellar disorders
- Non-specific dizziness
    - Often hard for patients to describe. Can be due to psychiatric disorders including anxiety and depression, fibromyalgia, hyperventilation, and hypoglycaemia

9.2.3 Neuromuscular diseases with cardiac involvement

- Neuromuscular disorders encompass a range of diseases in which pathologies of the peripheral nervous system or neuromuscular junctions lead to an impairment in the control and function of voluntary muscles
- Cardiac complications have been reported in nearly all neuromuscular disorders (listed below), but are particularly common and serious in Duchenne and Becker muscular dystrophies:
    - Muscular dystrophies (e.g. Duchenne, Becker, limb-girdle, Emery–Dreifuss)
    - Friedreich's ataxia
    - Myotonic dystrophy
    - Mitochondrial diseases (e.g. Barth syndrome)
    - Myofibrillar myopathies
- Problems can include conduction defects including heart block and heart muscle dysfunction—dilated cardiomyopathy is a leading cause of death among these patients

Duchenne muscular dystrophy (DMD)
- The most common muscular dystrophy, with an incidence of 30 per 100,000 live male births
- Predominantly X-linked recessive genetic disorder (males are affected, females are typically carriers) with one-third of cases due to spontaneous mutations
- Caused by mutation in the sarcolemmal protein dystrophin
- Results in progressive degeneration of skeletal muscles and serum CK is significantly elevated
- Males present with delayed motor milestones, abnormal gait, and calf pseudo-hypertrophy
- Cardiac manifestations include:
    - Dilated cardiomyopathy with progressive left ventricular dysfunction, though some may develop hypertrabeculation or non-compaction
    - Conduction defects leading to heart block
    - Malignant arrhythmias
- Cardiomyopathy is caused by cardiomyocyte hypertrophy, atrophy, and left ventricular wall fibrosis
- Death occurs in the patient's 20s due to cardiomyopathy or respiratory muscle weakness
- Cardiac investigations include:
    - ECG: 90% patients have an abnormal baseline ECG including sinus tachycardia, AF or flutter, premature ventricular complexes, tall R-waves, increased RS in V1, or deep Q-waves in left precordial leads
    - Echocardiography: LV dilation and dysfunction; should be considered routinely every 2 years up to the age of 10 and annually thereafter
    - CMR: demonstrates transmural myocardial fibrosis on late gadolinium enhancement (LGE) and helps assess LV function in patients with suboptimal echocardiographic images
    - Holter monitoring: for supraventricular and ventricular arrhythmias

- Treatments:
  - Non-curative but aim to slow the progression of LV dysfunction
  - ACEi, beta blockers, eplerenone
  - Corticosteroids (e.g. prednisolone slows the rate of progression)
  - Early trials of gene therapy have shown minimal to no improvement
  - Implantation of an ICD may be considered in patients with Duchenne or Becker muscular dystrophy and significant LGE on CMR (*Class IIb C*)

Becker muscular dystrophy

- Like DMD is an X-linked recessive disorder with mutation in the dystrophin gene
- Less common than DMD (3 per 100,000 live male births)
- Better prognosis than DMD and patients survive to age 40–50
- Cardiac involvement is independent of skeletal muscle severity
- Becker patients often have dystrophin variants that have partially functional proteins. In-frame variants have less effect on protein function
- Males with Becker muscular dystrophy develop a later onset myopathy and ambulatory problems. DCM is a significant cause of morbidity and the main cause of mortality
- Female carriers of dystrophin variants can sometimes display evidence of left ventricular dilatation and/or DCM, although typically it has a fairly indolent course
- ACE inhibitors and beta blockers have shown some benefit in Becker, reducing decline in LV function even in asymptomatic patients
- In both Duchenne and Becker muscular dystrophies, cardiac evaluation should be undertaken annually, including an ECG (*Class I*)
- All isolated males with DCM, or those with a family history consistent with X-linked inheritance, should be assessed for evidence of generalized skeletal myopathy and have their serum CK measured
- In female carriers, cardiac evaluation including echocardiography is recommended every 5 years from the age of 16 or from diagnosis
- As above, implantation of an ICD may be considered in patients with Duchenne or Becker muscular dystrophy and significant LGE on CMR (*Class IIb C*)

Other rarer muscular dystrophies

- May also develop cardiomyopathy
- Limb-girdle muscle dystrophy, characterized by weakness and wasting of proximal muscle groups of the shoulder and pelvic girdles
- Emery–Dreifuss muscular dystrophy:
  - Usually inherited in a dominant or X-linked manner
  - Characterized by weakness, muscle atrophy, and joint contractures
  - CK is often moderately elevated but may be normal
  - Cardiac involvement includes conduction defects, various arrhythmias, HCM, or DCM
- In patients with limb–girdle type 1B or Emery–Dreifuss muscular dystrophies and an indication for pacing, ICD implantation should be considered

Friedreich's ataxia

- Autosomal recessive disease with genetic defect in the mitochondrial protein frataxin due to trinucleotide GAA triplet repeat expansion
- Life expectancy is 40–50 years old

- Symptoms include:
    - Cerebellar symptoms (nystagmus, truncal ataxia)
    - Limb muscle weakness
    - Impaired sensation
    - Visual and auditory impairment
    - Diabetes mellitus
    - Dysarthria
- The most common cardiac manifestation is left ventricular hypertrophy (concentric or asymmetrical) and less commonly dilated cardiomyopathy; in the case of asymmetric LVH, outflow tract obstruction is uncommon
- Clinical phenotype and severity is highly variable
- The loss of contractile proteins and impaired mitochondrial function leads to the development of myocardial fibrosis and consequently LVH and conduction disease
- Symptoms include dyspnoea and palpitations
- Death is due to heart failure and arrhythmia (heart block, atrial or ventricular arrhythmias)
- *Investigations*
    - ECG: most common abnormality (85% patients) is t-wave repolarization abnormalities in inferior and lateral leads
    - Transthoracic echocardiography: assess LVH and LV function
    - CMR: demonstrates myocardial fibrosis
    - N.B. both routine echo and ECG monitoring should be conducted as co-morbidities, e.g. reduced mobility, may mask symptoms and progression of heart failure can occur rapidly before death
- *Treatment*
    - Beta-blockade may be harmful due to the loss of contractile proteins in Friedreich's ataxia
    - Pacemaker insertion for conduction abnormalities (e.g. AV block)
    - Pharmacological therapies have shown mixed results with no definitive treatment, which included the antioxidant Idebenone
    - Gene therapy has shown promise in mouse models of Friedreich's ataxia

Myotonic dystrophy (MD)

- Autosomal dominant trinucleotide repeat expansion disorder
- Onset in early adulthood
- The classic form MDI has an earlier onset, more trinucleotide repeats, and more severe symptoms than MDII
- Symptoms include muscle weakness, myotonia, and cataracts
- Cardiac manifestation is in the form of conduction disease and malignant arrhythmia with a high risk of sudden cardiac death due to cardiac fibrosis and fatty infiltration affecting all levels of the cardiac conducting system, providing a substrate for ectopic activity and re-entrant arrhythmias
- *Investigations*
    - 12-lead ECG/Holter monitoring to assess for conduction disease and ventricular/supraventricular arrhythmias
    - EP study can be used to identify patients with infrahisian disease who are at high risk of progression to complete AV block and benefit from prophylactic pacemaker insertion, particularly in those:

- With a sudden increase in PR interval or QRS duration
- With a PR interval ≥240ms or QRS duration ≥120ms
- >40 years old and have supraventricular arrhythmias or with significant LGE on CMR
    - EP study is also recommended for patients with syncope or palpitations suggestive of ventricular arrhythmia
- *Treatment*
    - Pacemaker implantation for conduction disease
    - Secondary prevention ICD implantation should be recommended for sustained ventricular tachyarrhythmias or aborted cardiac arrest
    - A primary prevention ICD may be considered if:
        - Pacing indication and additional risk factors such as CTG expansion, family history of sudden cardiac death, ECG conduction abnormalities (PR prolongation, LBBB, atrial arrhythmias), non-sustained VT, or LV dysfunction
        - Normal AV conduction and syncope highly suspicious for ventricular arrhythmia
        - Sustained VT induced during EP study if life expectancy >1 year

Mitochondrial diseases

- Heterogenous group of disorders, most frequently affect tissues with a high energy requirement, including the brain, eyes, endocrine organs, and skeletal muscle, along with the heart
- Examples include: mitochondrial encephalopathy with lactic acidosis and stroke-like episodes (MELAS), myoclonic epilepsy with ragged red fibres (MERRF), and Barth syndrome
- Abnormalities of mitochondria have been found to be associated with a wide range of cardiac phenotypes, including HCM, DCM, and conduction defects/arrhythmias
- Mitochondrial function is dependent on the DNA in the mitochondrial genome (mtDNA) which exists within the mitochondria and also nuclear genes, contained within the cellular nuclei
- Outside certain distinct disorders, genetic testing is complicated and should be undertaken with specialist clinical genetics input

Barth syndrome features:

- X-linked
- Neutropenia
- Disease is secondary to genetic mutations in proteins in the mitochondrial respiratory chain involved in ATP production
- *Investigations*
    - Skeletal muscle biopsy/cardiac biopsy
    - Genetics
- Cardiac involvement includes:
    - Hypertrophic
    - DCM
    - LVNC cardiomyopathy
- Develop heart failure and ventricular arrhythmias

Myofibrillar myopathies

- Mutations in sarcomeric proteins, e.g. BAG3, desmin, filamin c
- Predominantly autosomal dominant inheritance
- Proximal and distal muscle weakness

- Cardiac involvement:
  - Dilated or hypertrophic cardiomyopathy
  - Bradyarrhythmia requiring pacing
  - Malignant arrhythmia requiring ICD insertion
- Diagnosed by EMG, nerve conduction studies, muscle biopsy, genetic testing

Further reading

2022 ESC Guidelines for the management of patients with ventricular arrhythmias and the prevention of sudden cardiac death: Developed by the task force for the management of patients with ventricular arrhythmias and the prevention of sudden cardiac death of the European Society of Cardiology (ESC) Endorsed by the Association for European Paediatric and Congenital Cardiology (AEPC). *Eur Heart J*. 2022:ehac262. https://doi.org/10.1093/eurheartj/ehac262

Dellefave LM, McNally EM. Cardiomyopathy in neuromuscular disorders. *Prog Pediatr Cardiol*. 2007;24(1):35–46. doi: 10.1016/j.ppedcard.2007.08.005

Gladstone DJ, Spring M, Dorian P, Panzov V, Thorpe KE, Hall J, Vaid H, O'Donnell M, Laupacis A, Côté R, Sharma M, Blakely JA, Shuaib A, Hachinski V, Coutts SB, Sahlas DJ, Teal P, Yip S, Spence JD, Buck B, Verreault S, Casaubon LK, Penn A, Selchen D, Jin A, Howse D, Mehdiratta M, Boyle K, Aviv R, Kapral MK, Mamdani M; EMBRACE Investigators and Coordinators. Atrial fibrillation in patients with cryptogenic stroke. *N Engl J Med*. 2014 Jun 26;370(26):2467–77. doi: 10.1056/NEJMoa1311376. PMID: 24963566.

Kent DM, Dahabreh IJ, Ruthazer R, Furlan AJ, Weimar C, Serena J, Meier B, Mattle HP, Di Angelantonio E, Paciaroni M, Schuchlenz H, Homma S, Lutz JS, Thaler DE. Anticoagulant vs. antiplatelet therapy in patients with cryptogenic stroke and patent foramen ovale: an individual participant data meta-analysis. *Eur Heart J*. 2015 Sep 14;36(35):2381–9. doi: 10.1093/eurheartj/ehv252. Epub 2015 Jul 3. PMID: 26141397; PMCID: PMC4568404.

Li J, Liu J, Liu M, Zhang S, Hao Z, Zhang J, Zhang C. Closure versus medical therapy for preventing recurrent stroke in patients with patent foramen ovale and a history of cryptogenic stroke or transient ischemic attack. *Cochrane Database Syst Rev*. 2015 Sep 8;2015(9):CD009938. doi: 10.1002/14651858.CD009938.pub2. PMID: 26346232; PMCID: PMC7389291.

Mesa D, Franco M, Suárez de Lezo J, Muñoz J, Rus C, Delgado M, Ruiz M, Pan M, Romo E, Vallés F, Viñals M, Bescansa E. Prevalencia de foramen oval permeable en pacientes jóvenes con accidente isquémico cerebral de causa desconocida [Prevalence of patent foramen ovale in young patients with cerebral ischemic accident of unknown origin]. *Rev Esp Cardiol*. 2003 Jul;56(7):662–8. Spanish. doi: 10.1016/s0300-8932(03)76936-x. PMID: 12855148.

9.3

The patient with chronic kidney disease

Diana Vassallo and Dimitrios Poulikakos

TABLE OF CONTENTS

9.3.1 The patient with chronic kidney disease 869
9.3.2 Coronary artery disease and myocardial infarction 870
9.3.3 Congestive cardiac failure 877
9.3.4 Sudden cardiac death 879
9.3.5 Stroke 880
9.3.6 Atrial fibrillation 881
9.3.7 Peripheral arterial disease 882

9.3.1 The patient with chronic kidney disease

Introduction

- Patients with any stage of chronic kidney disease (CKD), as outlined in Table 9.3.1 are at an increased risk of cardiovascular (CV) morbidity and mortality and they usually have poorer outcomes compared to patients without CKD
- Besides shared conventional risk factors, reduced estimated glomerular filtration rate (eGFR) and proteinuria are both independent predictors of CV morbidity and mortality
- Patients with eGFR < 60 ml/min are more likely to die of CV disease than to progress to end-stage kidney disease (ESKD)
  - According to the US renal database up to around 40% of prevalent dialysis patients die due to underlying cardiac disease

Table 9.3.1 Stages of chronic kidney disease (CKD) by estimated glomerular filtration (eGFR) cutoffs; *CKD stages 1 and 2 fulfil the criteria for CKD only in the presence of evidence of kidney damage (urinary or radiological abnormalities).

CKD stage	Definition
Stage 1*	Normal function, ≥ 90 ml/min/1.73 m²
Stage 2*	Mildly decreased 60–89 ml/min/1.73 m²
Stage 3a	Mildly to moderately decreased, 45–59 ml/min/1.73 m²
Stage 3b	Moderately to severely decreased, 30–44 ml/min/1.73 m²
Stage 4	Severely decreased, 15–29 ml/min/1.73 m²
Stage 5	End-stage kidney disease (ESKD), < 15 ml/min/1.73 m²
Stage 5D	Dialysis-dependent CKD stage 5, including haemodialysis and peritoneal dialysis

- Dialysis patients are 20× more likely to die a CV death compared to the general population
- Despite the high burden of occlusive coronary artery disease (CAD) in patients with CKD, only 15% of cardiac deaths are directly due to acute myocardial infarction (AMI); indeed up to 60% of cardiac deaths in patients with CKD and ESKD are caused by sudden cardiac death, which accounts for 25% of overall mortality
- CKD significantly impacts on the pharmacokinetics and excretion of multiple cardiac drugs and so baseline and surveillance of renal function is crucial in cardiac patients
- Patients with CKD and ESKD have a high prevalence of left ventricular hypertrophy (LVH) and this probably underlies the heightened risk for cardiac arrhythmias
  - Potential causes for LVH in these patients (found in 75% of dialysis patients) include hypertension, anaemia, vascular calcification, vascular non-compliance, and volume overload
  - LVH contributes to diastolic dysfunction and indeed, while 85–90% of ESKD patients have preserved left ventricular systolic function on echocardiograms, up to 40% of incident ESKD patients present with circulatory congestion due to heart failure with preserved ejection fraction within the first year

9.3.2 Coronary artery disease and myocardial infarction

Epidemiology and pathophysiology

- The incidence and severity of obstructive CAD increases as eGFR declines; more than 50% of unselected ESKD patients demonstrate CAD on angiography
- In CKD, CAD characteristically shows a pattern of diffuse multi-vessel involvement with coronary calcification
- In patients with CAD, coexisting CKD confers a worse prognosis; CKD is considered an independent CV disease risk factor and a CAD equivalent for all-cause mortality
- Proteinuria or albuminuria is also an independent marker of adverse CV events in patients with CKD, and is independent of eGFR (microalbuminuria: ≥ 30–300 mg/g; macroalbuminuria: > 300 mg/g). It is a surrogate marker of the endothelial and microvascular damage that accompanies CKD and it also reflects the duration of hypertension and poor glycaemic control in diabetics
- In early CKD (stages 2 or 3), traditional CV risk factors are the major contributors to CV mortality
  - With worsening CKD, risk factors related to CKD drive the increased CV morbidity and mortality in these patients (Figure 9.3.1)
  - As a result, risk calculation tools based on traditional risk factors such as the Framingham risk score do not accurately predict coronary events in CKD
  - In advanced CKD, traditional risk factors such as hypercholesterolaemia, obesity, and blood pressure demonstrated a U-shaped association with mortality; reasons for this 'confounded epidemiology' are not completely clear

Diagnosis

- Routine investigations for CAD in CKD patients can be challenging to perform and interpret
- The classic triad of ischaemic symptoms, elevated cardiac biomarkers, and typical ECG changes is frequently absent in CKD patients; these patients are more likely to present with silent ischaemia, with symptoms of heart failure due to systolic or diastolic dysfunction, or with syncope

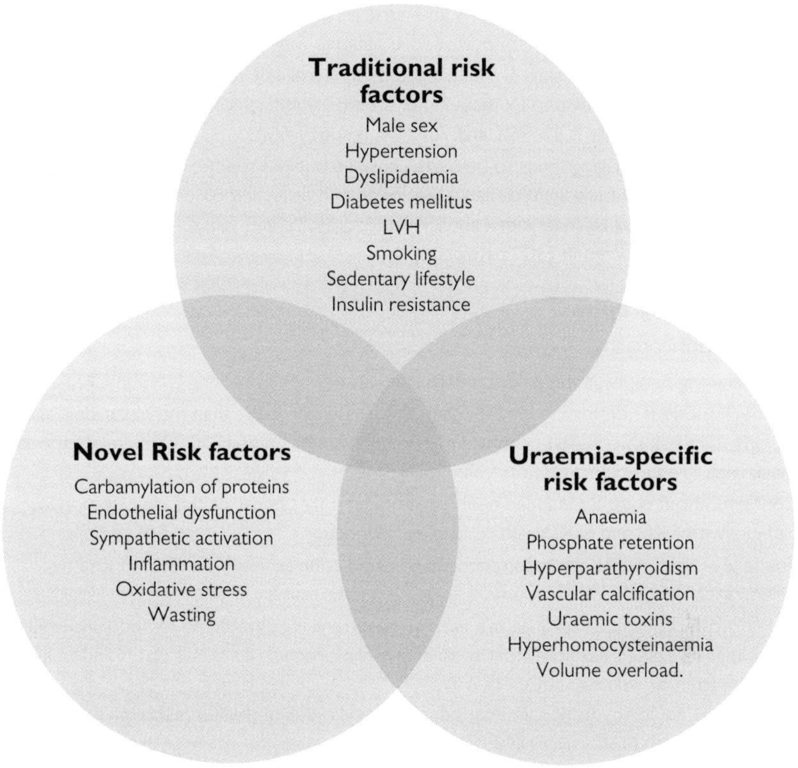

Traditional risk factors
Male sex
Hypertension
Dyslipidaemia
Diabetes mellitus
LVH
Smoking
Sedentary lifestyle
Insulin resistance

Novel Risk factors
Carbamylation of proteins
Endothelial dysfunction
Sympathetic activation
Inflammation
Oxidative stress
Wasting

Uraemia-specific risk factors
Anaemia
Phosphate retention
Hyperparathyroidism
Vascular calcification
Uraemic toxins
Hyperhomocysteinaemia
Volume overload.

Figure 9.3.1 Risk factors for cardiovascular disease in patients with chronic kidney disease

Electrocardiography (ECG) and echocardiography
- Kidney Disease Outcomes Quality Initiative (KDOQI) Guidelines recommend a baseline ECG at dialysis initiation and at annual intervals
- Dialysis patients not in sinus rhythm are 89% more likely to die and 164% more likely to suffer a stroke
- CKD patients with increased QRS and QT intervals have increased risk of adverse outcomes
- ECG interpretation can be difficult in CKD as LVH with a strain pattern can mask diagnostic ST depression
- KDOQI Guidelines recommend routine echocardiography in all dialysis patients after they achieve 'dry weight' targets 1–3 months after dialysis initiation and at 3-year intervals thereafter
- CKD patients with a left ventricular ejection fraction < 40% should be evaluated for CAD, except in paediatric or young adults with non-diabetic renal disease as these patients are at low risk for CAD

Stress tests
- The role of exercise ECG is limited in patients with advanced CKD due to often limited exercise capacity and the lack of specificity of the ST-segment abnormalities that are frequently noted on the ECG

- Pharmacologic stress echocardiography and nuclear perfusion techniques are operator dependent and results may be compromised in patients with LVH
- Stress echocardiography results are influenced by the small left ventricular (LV) cavity size found in patients with elevated LV mass index; sensitivity and specificity for pharmacological stress echocardiography is 69–95% and 76–94%, respectively
- Nuclear perfusion imaging tends to be more sensitive but less specific than stress echocardiography but the limited spatial resolution and disturbed coronary flow reserve that characterize elevated LV mass index and LVH affect results, and sensitivities and specificities < 80% have been reported in CKD patients

Coronary angiography
Contrast nephropathy
- Coronary angiography is the gold standard investigation for evaluating CAD in CKD and ESKD
- Although modern non-ionic contrast agents are less nephrotoxic than the older ionic agents, there is still a risk of contrast nephropathy in patients with an eGFR < 30 ml/min, especially in those with a reduced intravascular volume
- Concerns about contrast-induced nephropathy may limit the use of this investigation in patients with CKD and ESKD with residual renal function
- The following strategies are recommended to avoid contrast nephropathy induced by cardiological examinations:
    a. Perform echocardiography before elective coronary angiography to exclude unsuspected valvular disease or cardiomyopathy, to assess pre-procedure volume status and to assess left ventricular volume status
    b. Ensure adequate hydration and consider N-acetyl cysteine (NAC) (although the evidence of benefit with NAC is very limited)
    c. Minimize contrast dose if possible
    d. Avoid nephrotoxic medications
    e. Monitor renal function on a daily basis and optimize fluid balance
- Non-invasive coronary computed tomography (CT) angiography is again limited by contrast agent injection and also the high prevalence of coronary calcification in CKD patients (which limits quality of coronary assessment via CT)
- Non-invasive gadolinium-based magnetic resonance imaging in not recommended in patients with severe CKD (eGFR < 30 ml/min/1.73 m^2) due to concerns about nephrogenic systemic fibrosis

Biomarkers
- Cardiac Troponins (cTnT, cTnI):
    - In most CKD patients elevations in cardiac troponin should not be considered benign due to decreased clearance
    - Chronically elevated levels signify cardiac dysfunction probably indicating myocardial apoptosis or small vessel disease but do not necessarily reflect acute true myocardial necrosis
    - Trends in biomarker levels over time are better predictors of myocardial necrosis than single values
- Plasma brain natriuretic peptides (BNP and NT-proBNP):
    - These biomarkers reflect cardiac filling pressures and both predict decompensated heart failure
    - NT-proBNP is primarily cleared by the kidneys therefore may increase with declining eGFR

- However, both BNP and NT-pro-BNP are associated with abnormal echocardiographic findings and increased risk of CV events
- High-sensitivity C-reactive protein (CRP):
  - Inflammatory marker that is independently associated with adverse CV events

Risk prevention

- The role of medical therapy in CAD prevention in patients with CKD is unclear and the reason is twofold:
  - Patients with advanced CKD have been excluded from most clinical trials testing CVD therapies hence there is little evidence for the benefit of routine preventative strategies in these patients
  - Non-traditional risk factors also contribute proportionally more than traditional atherosclerotic disease towards the development of adverse cardiac events in patients with CKD
- The ISCHAEMIA-CKD trial has shown that among patients with advanced kidney disease and moderate to severe stress-induced ischaemia, an initial invasive strategy consisting of coronary angiography and revascularization (if appropriate) in addition to medical therapy did not reduce the risk of death or non-fatal MI
- The rationale for risk factor modification is the same as in the general population:
- *Lifestyle modifications* including smoking cessation, exercise, dietary salt reduction, and weight loss to optimal targets
- *Optimal blood pressure control* in non-dialysis CKD: use of Renin-Angiotensin System (RAS) inhibition together with SGLT2 inhibitors improve renal and cardiovascular outcomes:
  - CKD without proteinuria target BP is < 140/90 mmHg
  - CKD with proteinuria (urine albumin excretion ≥30 mg/g) target BP is < 130/80 mmHg and use of RAS inhibition and SGLT2 inhibitors is advised.

  Renin-Angiotensin System (RAS) Inhibition:
  - RAS inhibition with ACEi or ARB is recommended in diabetic and non-diabetic adults with CKD and urine albumin excretion ≥30 mg/g
  - RAS inhibition leads to generalized arterial vasodilatation resulting in lower systemic BP and reduced intra-glomerular pressure conferring a degree of renoprotection and reduced adrenal secretion of aldosterone. They may also have a beneficial effect on cardiac remodelling
  - Clinically significant hyperkalaemia and reductions in GFR can occur in patients receiving ACEi or ARB, particularly in patients with CKD, those who have renal-artery stenosis or reduced intravascular volume, or when these agents are used together with non-steroidal anti-inflammatory agents (NSAIDs), cyclo-oxygenase (COX)-2 inhibitors, or potassium-sparing diuretics
  - Reducing the dose or holding off on using ACEi or ARB until recovery is sensible in patients who develop inter-current illnesses that lead to dehydration as a result of diarrhoea, vomiting, or high fever
  - In view of the higher risk of side effects of RAS inhibition in CKD patients, the use of ACEi or ARB may not have the same risk-to-benefit ratio in CKD patients as in non-CKD populations; as described below, the development of novel oral potassium binders may allow continuation of renin-angiotensin blockade in patients with CKD
  - Combination of ACE and ARB to prevent progression of CKD is not recommended
  - Although optimal diabetes and blood pressure control can slow CKD progression in patients with pre-dialysis CKD, there is no evidence that attainment of specific BP goals or strict glycaemic control in ESKD patients on dialysis improves outcomes.

SGLT-2 Inhibitors:
- Large placebo-controlled randomised clinical outcome trials (CREDENCE, DAPA-CKD) have shown that SGLT2 inhibitors reduce progression of albuminuric CKD in both diabetic and non-diabetic patients.
- This is thought to occur through modulation of tubuloglomerular feedback, increased delivery of sodium to the macula densa and enhancement of glomerular afferent arteriolar vasoconstriction
- This leads to a reduction in intraglomerular pressure, leading to an acute reversible dip in kidney function (this is not generally an indication to stop treatment), reducing albuminuria and slowing rate of decline of renal function.
- It is advised to withhold SGLT2 inhibitors during periods of prolonged fasting, surgery or critical illness, due to risk of euglycaemic ketoacidosis in these circumstances. Once an SGLT2 inhibitor is started, it is reasonable to continue even if eGFR falls below 20 ml/min/1.73 m² unless it is not tolerated or renal replacement therapy is started.

- *Optimal blood pressure control* in dialysis patients:
  - In dialysis patients, a U-shaped association between pre-dialysis BP and outcomes has been reported (pre dialysis systolic BP < 110 or > 150 mmHg associated with higher mortality)
  - Consider pharmacokinetics and dialysability when prescribing anti-hypertensives in CKD
  - Examples of non-dialysable anti-hypertensives: ARBs, calcium channel blockers, α-blockers, carvedilol, labetalol, fosinopril
  - Examples of dialyzable anti-hypertensives: ACEi (apart from fosinopril), atenolol, metoprolol, bisoprolol
  - Non-pharmacological strategies to optimize blood pressure in dialysis patients
    1. Increased ultrafiltration
    2. Longer dialysis
    3. More than 3 dialysis treatments per week

- *Optimal diabetes control:*
  - Diabetic patients with CKD secondary to diabetic nephropathy have the highest risk of CVEs as both DM and CKD are strong CV risk factors. Besides being the earliest hallmark of diabetic nephropathy, microalbuminuria also predicts adverse CV and renal outcomes and management strategies focus on reducing progression to macroalbuminuria and overt diabetic nephropathy
  - *Glycaemic monitoring and targets in CKD*: HbA1c monitoring may not be as accurate among patients with ESKD as in the general population due to reduced red blood cell lifespan, blood transfusion, erythropoietin administration. An HbA1c target of around 48 mmol/mol has been recommended in CKD patients. Lower targets have been associated with adverse outcomes and patients with ESKD on dialysis are at an increased risk of hypoglycaemia. Individualized therapy is essential among patients with advanced CKD or on dialysis,
  - Pharmacological therapy:
    - *Metformin* is the first-line anti-diabetic agent but should not be used if the eGFR is < 30 ml/min/1.73 m² due to increased risk of lactic acidosis
    - SGLT2 inhibitors together with Metformin are now considered first-line agents in patients with diabetes and CKD. In addition, recent evidence has led to a paradigm shift in the clinical indication for SGLT2 inhibitors, with a shift in focus from hyperglycaemia control to management of cardiorenal risk in patients with CKD and CVD.

- SGLT2 inhibitors mediate their anti-hyperglycaemic effect by blocking the sodium-glucose high-capacity low-affinity transporter located mainly in the early proximal tubule, leading to glycosuria. This leads to increased sodium delivery to the macula densa, natriuresis and modulation of intraglomerular haemodynamics that results in improvement in microalbuminuria.
- SGLT2 inhibition as an adjunctive therapy to RAS blockade has been shown to decrease the risk of both CKD progression and heart failure or cardiovascular death in patients with CKD (eGFR ≥20 ml/min/1.73 m^2 and urinary albumin-to-creatinine ratio ≥250 mg/g) and with or without type 2 diabetes.
- GLP-1 receptor agonists have proven cardiovascular benefits in patients with Type 2 diabetes and CKD and are the recommended second-line agents in patients not attaining glycaemic goals despite SGLT2 inhibitors and metformin.
- Another addition to the therapeutic armamentarium for diabetic CKD are non-steroidal mineralocorticoid receptor antagonists (MRA) such as Finerenone. Two large clinical trials (FIDELIO-CKD and FIGARO-CKD) showed significant reductions in both the composite kidney outcomes and cardiovascular outcomes. These agents are recommended for patients with Type 2 diabetes, an eGFR ≥ 25ml/min/1.73 m^2, normal serum potassium concentration (<5 mmol/L) and albuminuria ≥30 mg/g despite maximum tolerated doses of RAS inhibitor. They can be used in conjunction with an SGLT2 inhibitor. In view of the risk of hyperkalaemia, serum potassium levels need to be monitored regularly after the initiation of a nonsteroidal MRA, with dose reduction or addition of a novel potassium binder if serum potassium rises >5.5mmol/L.
- *Insulin*—Patients who fail therapy with oral agents are treated with insulin. In CKD, the starting dose of insulin may need to be lower than would normally be prescribed

- *Aspirin*—Daily prophylactic aspirin in patients with CKD and ESKD may reduce CV risk but is associated with a higher incidence of bleeding; therefore aspirin is only indicated for secondary prevention of CVD in CKD
- *Statins*—Statin therapy may be of benefit in patients with moderate CKD but studies have not shown benefit in patients on haemodialysis
  - The KDIGO guidance suggests that patients aged ≥ 50 years who are non-dialysis dependent with eGFR < 60 ml/min/1.73 m^2 should be considered at sufficiently high risk for a CV event to warrant treatment with statin without the requirement for applying any formal risk calculation in individual patients
  - In patients with CKD aged 18–49 years who are not treated with chronic dialysis or kidney transplantation, statin treatment is recommended in patients with one or more of the following:
    - Known CAD (myocardial infarction or coronary revascularization)
    - DM
    - Prior ischemic stroke
    - Estimated 10-year incidence of coronary death or non-fatal MI > 10%
  - Although it is recommended that patients should continue treatment with statins when they are established on dialysis, statin treatment should not be initiated in dialysis patients for primary prevention
  - Prescription of statins in individuals with CKD should be based on doses that have shown benefit and safety profile in randomized trials in CKD patients (Table 9.3.2)
  - All statins may not be available in all countries, and lower doses than those used in major trials may be appropriate in Asian countries

Table 9.3.2 Recommended doses (mg/d) of statins in adults with CKD.

Statin	CKD Stage 1–2	CKD Stage 3a–5 including patients on dialysis or with a kidney transplant
Losuvastatin	GP	nd
Fluvastatin	GP	80
Atorvastatin	GP	20
Rosuvastatin	GP	10
Simvastatin/Ezetimibe	GP	20/10
Pravastatin	GP	40
Simvastatin	GP	40
Pitavastatin	GP	2

Abbreviations: eGFR—estimated glomerular filtration rate; GP—general population; nd—not done/studied.
From KDIGO clinical practice guideline for lipid management in CKD; Data based on ALERT, 4D, AURORA, SHARP (see further reading)

- Note that rosuvastatin 40 mg daily is not recommended for use in CKD 1–2 non-transplant patients as it may increase the risk of adverse renal events
- Cyclosporin inhibits the metabolism of certain statins resulting in higher blood levels
• Correction of anaemia to individualized targets using iron supplementation and erythropoiesis-stimulating agents
    - Complete correction of anaemia to normal targets have been associated with worse CV outcomes than in patients treated to lower targets

Treatment
• There is a paucity of randomized data on treatment of acute MI in CKD patients but standard acute coronary syndrome (ACS) management consisting of aspirin, clopidogrel, beta blockers, and renin-angiotensin blockade is still recommended in CKD patients
• The following points need to be taken in to account for management of ACS in CKD patients:
    - Aspirin and clopidogrel may carry a greater bleeding risk on CKD than in the general population, as platelet function is deranged in uraemia; they should not be administered if the bleeding risk is high
    - Glycoprotein IIb/IIIa inhibitors (eptifibatide) require dose reduction
    - Low molecular weight heparins require dose adjustment if eGFR < 30 ml/min
    - Non-renally cleared antithrombotic agents such as abciximab and unfractionated heparin may be preferable to renally-cleared agents such as enoxaparin in dialysis patients
    - Optimize fluid status—consider dialysis or diuresis in overloaded patients. However intermittent haemodialysis in the context of ongoing ACS is not recommended and continuous renal replacement therapy may be preferable if required
    - Maintain haemoglobin above 10 g/dl. In patients with fluid overload or hyperkalaemia, and in patients on haemodialysis, blood transfusions are delivered on dialysis
    - In acute ST-elevation MI, primary PCI should be the treatment of choice irrespective of CKD status

- Thrombolysis is not contraindicated in CKD or ESKD patients; thrombolysis is only contraindicated in the context of a recent renal biopsy, line insertion or uraemic pericarditis—in these situations PCI should be considered
- Beta blockers may need dose reduction; statins, calcium channel blockers and nitrates can be administered as usual
- While in the general population, early angiography is recommended in patients with non-ST elevation ACS, there is little evidence in advanced CKD and dialysis patients
- There are no trials evaluating the role of coronary revascularization (either CABG or PCI) in patients with advanced CKD and stable angina; there is a suggestion that the revascularization rate post-CABG is lower compared to post-PCI
- The incidence of operative mortality after CABG is 9–12.2% for ESKD patients on dialysis and three- to sevenfold higher in advanced CKD patients compared to non-CKD patients while PCI carries the risk of contrast-induced nephropathy. Retrospective studies suggest long-term survival may be better with CABG vs PCI; further studies are required

9.3.3 Congestive cardiac failure

Epidemiology and pathophysiology
- The prevalence of congestive heart failure (CHF) increases with declining eGFR
- CHF is the main CV condition in CKD patients; mortality is higher for diastolic than for systolic CHF
- The main mechanisms that lead to development of cardiomyopathy and LV failure in CKD are:
    - Pressure overload—Due to chronic hypertension and vascular non-compliance
    - Volume overload—Due to fluid overload
    - CKD-associated non-haemodynamic factors that induce changes in myocardium:
        - RAS activation
        - Oxidative stress
        - Inflammation
        - Stimulation of pro-hypertrophic and pro-fibrogenic factors (cardiotrophin-1, transforming growth factor-beta, fibroblast growth factor-23, chronic sympathetic over-activation)

Diastolic dysfunction
- CKD progression is associated with worsening LVH and diastolic dysfunction; impaired diastolic dysfunction may occur early in CKD and may precede LVH.
- It results from an imbalance between collagen synthesis and degradation.
- This leads to LV stiffness, increased LV filling pressures and abnormal diastolic filling, leading to diastolic dysfunction and failure (heart failure with preserved ejection fraction, HFpEF).

Systolic dysfunction
- In the absence of ischaemic heart disease or severe haemodynamic stress, CKD patients usually have normal or hyperdynamic resting LV systolic function.
- Haemodialysis patients suffer repeated haemodynamic instability and together with underlying microvascular dysfunction, this leads to myocardial ischaemia, 'myocardial stunning' and LV systolic dysfunction (heart failure with reduced ejection fraction, HFrEF).

Diagnosis
- The clinical presentation of CHF in CKD (exercise intolerance, oedema, shortness of breath) can be difficult to distinguish from volume overload
- Echocardiography
  - Key investigation that can identify LVH, diastolic and systolic dysfunction, and assess CV prognosis
  - Guidelines recommend echocardiograms for all ESKD patients 1–3 months after initiation of renal replacement therapy (RRT) and in subsequent 3-year intervals, irrespective of symptoms
- B-type natriuretic peptides (BNP and NT-proBNP)
  - Role in diagnosis and management of CHF is unclear as levels are influenced by both kidney function and CHF severity
- Troponins (cTNI and cTNT)
  - Strong predictors of all-cause mortality in ESKD, though their clinical significance in less advanced CKD is less clear
  - cTNT has been approved for risk stratification in ESKD
- Novel biomarkers
  - The role of novel biomarkers (such as tumour necrosis-α, haematocrit, interleukin-6, pre-albumin, and CRP) is unclear as the association with cardiac disease may be a reflection of chronic illness, inflammation, and malnutrition rather than causality
  - Levels of novel biomarkers such as neutrophil gelatinase-association lipocalin, kidney-injury molecule-1, and galectin-3 can also be dependent on GFR

Prevention and treatment
- CKD patients are underrepresented in randomized controlled trials in CHF
- Lifestyle advice:
  - Dietary salt restriction
  - Fluid restriction
  - Smoking cessation
  - Weight reduction
  - Optimization of diabetic control
- Cardioprotective medication:
  - Diuretic treatment may need to be more intensive due to excessive retention of salt and water
  - Aldosterone antagonists should be used with caution as they may precipitate hyperkalaemia, especially when used in combination with RAS inhibition
  - Registry data has shown that RAS blockade is associated with reduced mortality in patients with HFrEF and reduced renal function however close monitoring is required for patients with eGFR < 30 ml/min/1.73 m^2 as described above. It is unclear whether patients with HFpEF and CKD derive the same mortality benefit
  - Hyperkalaemia frequently limits or precludes the use of RAS blockade or aldosterone antagonists in patients with CHF and CKD. The development of novel oral potassium binders reduces the risk of hyperkalaemia in patients with CKD on RAS blockade or aldosterone antagonists, consequently allowing continuation and/or optimization of this cardioprotective therapy
  - The angiotensin receptor neprilysin inhibitor LCZ696 can have a haemodynamic effect in preserving GFR, with one study reporting smaller eGFR decline in patients with HFpEF on LCZ696 versus valsartan after 36 weeks of treatment. However, urinary

- albumin-to-creatinine ratios showed increases with LCZ696 versus valsartan, highlighting the need for monitoring
  - Beta blockers such as bisoprolol and carvedilol may improve survival in CKD patients with CHF
  - SGLT-2 inhibitors are the latest therapeutic pillars in the heart failure regimen. They should be initiated in those with stable symptomatic CHF (irrespective of ejection fraction) and in those with a uACR of ≥250 mg/g, excluding people with polycystic kidney disease or on immunological therapy for renal disease.
- Anaemia correction:
  - Haemoglobin levels > 10 g/dl can reduce LVH in CKD patients but total correction does not improve cardiac remodelling or CV outcomes further
  - Eryrthropoiesis-stimulating agents with or without IV iron may improve exercise tolerance but are not associated with any survival benefit
- Mitigating vascular calcification:
  - Optimal control of calcium, phosphate, PTH, and vitamin D levels is recommended; the impact on CV end-points in CKD is unclear
- Haemodialysis considerations:
  - Adequate ultrafiltration volumes—more frequent or longer dialysis sessions may be required
  - Use of lower dialysate sodium concentrations coupled to dietary sodium restriction
  - High-flow arteriovenous fistulae may precipitate high cardiac output failure

9.3.4 Sudden cardiac death

Epidemiology and pathophysiology

- Sudden cardiac death (SCD) accounts for 25% of dialysis patients' deaths, with an annual incidence rate of 5.5%
- SCD risk increases with decreasing GFR independent of cardiac or other comorbidities
- Haemodialysis confers an additional risk and the SCD risk is thought to double when ESKD patients start dialysis
- Unlike the general population, CAD and CHF are not the usual predisposing factors for SCD in CKD, hence current risk stratification tools may be inadequate in these patients
- Potential SCD risk factors in CKD/ESKD include LVH, fluid and electrolyte shifts on haemodialysis and vascular calcification
- Epidemiological studies suggest that the most common times for SCD to occur are towards the end of the long 72-hour weekend interval between dialysis sessions and in the 12 hours immediately after haemodialysis
- Haemodialysis is associated with arrhythmias and dynamic ECG changes
- While in the general population SCD is usually due to sustained VT and VF, the primary arrhythmic event in ESKD patients is unclear
- Factors such as pulmonary artery pressure and mitral regurgitation have been found to be independently associated with SCD in CKD patients, suggesting that the underlying pathophysiology of SCD in this group of patients is likely to be different to that of the general population

Prevention

- ECG and echo features:
  - The high prevalence of LVH in ESKD and dialysis patients limits its utility in SCD risk stratification

- LV dysfunction and ejection fraction ≤ 35% identifies a subgroup of patients at higher risk of SCD due to arrhythmia
- Biomarkers:
  - cTNT is associated with all-cause mortality and SCD
  - Other biomarkers associated with SCD in ESKD (markers of inflammation such as CRP and interleukin-6 or nutrition such as albumin and pre-dialysis serum creatinine) are non-specific and have not been validated
- Haemodialysis considerations:
  - Alteration to the dialysis prescription can influence the risk of SCD
  - Risk of intradialytic SCD is associated with use of low-potassium and calcium dialysate, large volume ultrafiltration, and pre-dialysis hyperkalaemia and hypokalaemia

Recommendations

- Avoidance of rapid fluid and electrolyte shifts and low-potassium dialysate in haemodialysis and ensure patient compliance with dietary K+ restriction to avoid hyperkalaemia
  - It is unclear whether other changes to the haemodialysis prescription such as frequency, time on dialysis, and blood flow rates can prevent SCD
- Beta blockers have been shown to improve survival and decrease SCD risk in ESKD patients with dilated cardiomyopathy
- Empirical administration of antiarrhythmic medication is unlikely to be of benefit
- Digoxin may be associated with increased mortality in ESKD patients and should be prescribed with caution and careful monitoring of K+ and digoxin level
- Implanted cardioverter-defibrillator devices are less effective in advanced CKD and have not been studied adequately in dialysis patients. Many dialysis patients experience SCD despite not fulfilling current criteria for implantation, making appropriate allocation of defibrillators uncertain

9.3.5 Stroke

Epidemiology and pathophysiology
- CKD Stage 3–4 is an independent risk factor for both ischaemic and haemorrhagic stroke (relative risk 1.4)
- The relative risk of stroke in dialysis-dependent ESKD patients is around 5–10 times that of an age-matched general population with an overall stroke rate of approximately 4% per year
- In dialysis-dependent ESKD patients, 87% of strokes were ischaemic
- Independent predictors of higher risk are age and diabetes, while African-American race has been associated with lower risk
- Around one-third of strokes occur during or shortly after haemodialysis treatment
- Stroke mortality in CKD 5 patients was around 5%, three times higher than that in patients with less advanced CKD

Prevention of non-cardioembolic ischaemic stroke:

- Blood pressure control
- Antiplatelet agents
- Statins
- Carotid endarterectomy if there is ipsilateral high-grade carotid stenosis, although the risk of peri-operative complications appears higher in CKD patients

Treatment:
- IV thrombolysis with tissue plasminogen activator administered < 4.5 hours of symptom onset is safe in with CKD stages 3–4 patients (risk of intracranial haemorrhage not increased)
- The safety of IV thrombolysis has not been defined in patients on haemodialysis with acute ischaemic stroke
- Heparin is administered during haemodialysis and recent heparin use with prolonged activated partial thromboplastin time is generally considered a contraindication to IV tissue plasminogen activator

9.3.6 Atrial fibrillation

Epidemiology and pathophysiology
- Most common cardiac arrhythmia in CKD patients with a prevalence of 15–20%

Role of anti-coagulation in mild to moderate CKD (CrCl > 30 ml/min):
- Randomized controlled trials have shown that new anti-coagulant agents (NOAC) are non-inferior to warfarin in patients with Cockcroft–Gault estimated creatinine clearance (CrCl) 30–50 ml/min and show a superior safety profile, with a 50% reduction in the risk of intracranial haemorrhage
- The dose of NOACs needs to be adjusted according to the eGFR (Table 9.3.3), and careful monitoring is required to detect decline in renal function and adjust dose accordingly. Recommended minimum frequency of renal function testing in months is calculated by dividing CrCl by 10

Role of anticoagulation in non-dialysis advanced CKD (CrCl 15–30 ml/min)
- There is no randomized controlled data about the efficacy of NOACs or vitamin K antagonists for stroke prevention in AF in more advanced CKD (CrCl 15– 29 ml/min)
- In the ARISTOTLE trial apixaban was associated with less bleeding events than warfarin for CrCl 25–30 ml/min
- Rivaroxaban, apixaban, and edoxaban (but not dabigatran) are approved in Europe for the use in these patients with dose adjustment in patients with CrCl 15–29 ml/min

Role of anti-coagulation in CrCl < 15 ml/min and in dialysis patients:
- The role of anticoagulation with warfarin in dialysis-dependent ESKD patients is unclear, due to an increased risk of anti-coagulant associated bleeding, vascular calcification, calciphylaxis, and labile international normalized ration (INR)
- A meta-analysis showed that oral anticoagulant agents (either warfarin or NOAC) were not associated with a reduced risk of thromboembolism in patients with AF on long-term dialysis, while a recent study exploring the role of apixaban as stroke prophylaxis in haemodialysis patients with AF showed similar bleeding rates to warfarin
- Hence routine anticoagulation in CKD 5D patients with AF is not recommended. There is a need for a multidisciplinary team and individualized approach to support decisions regarding starting oral anticoagulation in patients with AF and ESKD on dialysis, together with regular re-assessment of risk and benefits

Table 9.3.3 Dose adjustment for NOACs as evaluated in PHASE III trials.

	Dabigatran	Rivaroxaban	Apixaban	Edoxaban
Study	RE-LY	ROCKET-AF	ARISTOTLE	ENGAGE AF-TIMI
Drug renal clearance	80%	35%	25%	50%
Dose	150 mg or 110 mg bd	20 mg od	5 mg bd	60 mg or 30 mg od
Exclusion criteria for CKD	CrCL < 30 ml/min	CrCL< 30 ml/min	Serum creatinine > 2.5 mg/dl or CrCL< 25 ml/min	CrCL < 30 ml/min
Dose adjustment with CKD	None	15 mg once daily if CrCl < 30–49 ml/min	2.5 mg bd if serum creatinine ≥ 1.5 mg/dl (133 µmol/L) plus age ≥ 80 years or weight ≤ 60 kg	30 mg or 15 mg od if CrCl < 50 ml/min
Percentage of patients with CKD	20% with CrCl 30–49 ml/min	21% with CrCl 30–49 ml/min	15% with CrCl 30-50 ml/dl	19% with CrCl <50 ml/min
Reduction of stroke and systemic embolism	No interaction with CKD status	No interaction with CKD status	No interaction with CKD status	NA
Reduction in major haemorrhages compared to warfarin	Reduction in major haemorrhage with dabigatran was greater in patients with eGFR > 80 ml/min with either dose	Major haemorrhage similar	Reduction in major haemorrhage with apixiban	NA

CrCl—Creatinine Clearance; NA—not available.
Source data from Kirchhof P, Benussi S, Kotecha D, et al; ESC Scientific Document Group. 2016 ESC Guidelines for the management of atrial fibrillation developed in collaboration with EACTS. *Eur Heart J.* 2016 Oct 7;37(38):2893–2962. doi: 10.1093/eurheartj/ehw210. Epub 2016 Aug 27. PMID: 27567408.

9.3.7 Peripheral arterial disease

Epidemiology and pathology

- Patients aged > 40 years with eGFR < 60 ml/min/1.73 m² have a prevalence of peripheral arterial disease (PAD) of around 24%; the prevalence in dialysis-dependent ESKD patients can be as high as 48%
- Traditional risk factors for PAD such as diabetes, hypertension, increasing age, and dyslipidaemia account for the high prevalence of PAD in these patients
- In addition, 'renal-specific' factors such as dialysis vintage, dialysis adequacy, hyperphosphataemia, inflammation, hypoalbuminaemia, and low parathyroid hormone, also predispose to PAD
- CKD is an independent risk factor for PAD events

Diagnosis

- Screening is recommended for dialysis-dependent ESKD patients at the time of dialysis initiation however the diagnostic modality and optimal therapies for PAD in CKD are unclear
- CKD patients have a great prevalence of calcified vessels and the ankle-brachial index is an inadequate diagnostic tool. Alternative methods include toe-brachial index and pulse volume monitoring but data about these methods in CKD patients is limited

Prevention

- There is a lack of evidence-base for medical therapies for PAD in CKD patients but prevention is essential for reducing PAD-associated morbidity such as amputation
- Smoking cessation is of paramount importance
- Optimal diabetic control and adequate foot care
- Antiplatelets have not been specifically studied in the context of PAD and CKD, but may reduce CV events; careful monitoring is required as CKD patients have an increased risk of bleeding due to uraemia and heparin use on dialysis. There is evolving evidence regarding the role of low dose NOAC therapy (see Chapter 8.3)
- There is no data about the role of statins, renin-angiotensin blockade, and exercise therapy in prevention of PAD in CKD patients

Treatment

- In critical limb ischaemia, revascularization, or amputation is often required
- Percutaneous methods are preferred in CKD but outcomes are worse with higher rates of repeat percutaneous angioplasty, surgical revascularization, limb loss, and death
- Surgical revascularization is associated with high peri-operative mortality, prolonged hospitalization, and limb loss in dialysis patients

Further reading

Cheung AK, Chang TI, Cushman WC, Furth SL, Ix JH, Pecoits-Filho R, Perkovic V, Sarnak MJ, Tobe SW, Tomson CRV, Cheung M, Wheeler DC, Winkelmayer WC, Mann JFE; Conference Participants. Blood pressure in chronic kidney disease: conclusions from a Kidney Disease: Improving Global Outcomes (KDIGO) Controversies Conference. *Kidney Int.* 2019 May;95(5):1027–36. doi: 10.1016/j.kint.2018.12.025. PMID: 31010478

Heerspink HJL, Stefánsson BV, Correa-Rotter R, Chertow GM, Greene T, Hou FF, Mann JFE, McMurray J, Lindberg M, Rossing P, Sjöström CD, Toto RD, Langkilde AM, Wheeler DC; DAPA-CKD Trial Committees and Investigators. Dapagliflozin in patients with chronic kidney disease. *N Engl J Med.* 2020;383:1436–46.

House AA, Wanner C, Sarnak MJ, Piña IL, McIntyre CW, Komenda P, Kasiske BL, Deswal A, deFilippi CR, Cleland JGF, Anker SD, Herzog CA, Cheung M, Wheeler DC, Winkelmayer WC, McCullough PA; Conference Participants. Heart failure in chronic kidney disease: conclusions from a Kidney Disease: Improving Global Outcomes (KDIGO) Controversies Conference. *Kidney Int.* 2019 Jun;95(6):1304–17. doi: 10.1016/j.kint.2019.02.022. Epub 2019 Apr 30. PMID: 31053387

Sarafidis P, Ferro CJ, Morales E, Ortiz A, Malyszko J, Hojs R, Khazim K, Ekart R, Valdivielso J, Fouque D, London GM, Massy Z, Ruggenenti P, Porrini E, Wiecek A, Zoccali C, Mallamaci F, Hornum M. SGLT-2 inhibitors and GLP-1 receptor agonists for nephroprotection and cardioprotection in patients with diabetes mellitus and chronic kidney disease. A consensus statement by the EURECA-m and the DIABESITY working groups of the ERA-EDTA. *Nephrol Dial Transplant.*

2019 Feb 1;34(2):208–30. doi: 10.1093/ndt/gfy407. Erratum in: Nephrol Dial Transplant. 2020 Aug 1;35(8):1452. Wiecek, Andrej [corrected to Wiecek, Andrzej]. Erratum in: Nephrol Dial Transplant. 2020 Oct 1;35(10):1825. PMID: 30753708

Stevens PE, Levin A; Kidney Disease: Improving Global Outcomes Chronic Kidney Disease Guideline Development Work Group Members. Evaluation and management of chronic kidney disease: synopsis of the kidney disease: improving global outcomes 2012 clinical practice guideline. *Ann Intern Med*. 2013 Jun 4;158(11):825–30. doi: 10.7326/0003-4819-158-11-201306040-00007. PMID: 23732715

Wanner C, Tonelli M; Kidney Disease: Improving Global Outcomes Lipid Guideline Development Work Group Members. KDIGO Clinical Practice Guideline for Lipid Management in CKD: summary of recommendation statements and clinical approach to the patient. *Kidney Int*. 2014 Jun;85(6):1303–9. doi: 10.1038/ki.2014.31. Epub 2014 Feb 19. PMID: 24552851

Wanner C, Herzog CA, Turakhia MP; Conference Steering Committee. Chronic kidney disease and arrhythmias: highlights from a Kidney Disease: Improving Global Outcomes (KDIGO) Controversies Conference. *Kidney Int*. 2018 Aug;94(2):231–4. doi: 10.1016/j.kint.2018.05.005. Epub 2018 Jun 21. PMID: 29935952.

9.4

The patient with pulmonary disease

Patrick Murphy and Georgios Kaltsakas

TABLE OF CONTENTS

9.4.1 Chronic obstructive pulmonary disease (COPD) 885
    Epidemiology and prognosis 885
    Pathogenesis 886
    Clinical features 886
    Evaluation 887
    Diagnosis 887
    Severity assessment 887
    COPD exacerbation 888
    Cardiovascular implications of COPD 888
    Arrhythmia treatment considerations in COPD 890
    Respiratory treatment and arrhythmias 890
9.4.2 Obstructive sleep apnoea 891
    Definition 891
    Epidemiology 891
    Risk factors 891
    Clinical manifestations 891
    Diagnosis 892
    Treatment 892
    Pathophysiology of CV-associated disease 893
    Cardiovascular implications 893
9.4.3 Obesity hypoventilation syndrome 896
    Epidemiology 896
    Clinical features 896
    Pathogenesis 897
    Diagnosis 897
    Treatment 897
    Cardiovascular complications and prognosis 897
9.4.4 Central sleep apnoea 898
    Epidemiology 898
    Clinical manifestations 898
    Diagnosis 899
    Pathophysiology 899
    Treatment 899
    Central sleep apnoea in heart failure 899

9.4.1 Chronic obstructive pulmonary disease (COPD)

Epidemiology and prognosis

Prevalence in Europe:

- COPD is common; estimated prevalence 5–10% in the adult population, with an increasing prevalence with increasing age
- Despite high prevalence, it is considered to be under-diagnosed
- More common in men than in women, relating to previous trends in smoking habits
- Despite knowledge of harm, smoking rates in Europe remain between 20–40% of the adult population contributing to future morbidity due to COPD

Mortality:

- Overall, the COPD mortality rate for men and women in Europe, age-standardized to the European population, is approximately 18 per 100,000 inhabitants per year
- Despite significant respiratory morbidity, CVD and lung cancer remain the commonest causes of death in mild to moderate COPD

Pathogenesis

- Cigarette smoke or other noxious particles (biomass smoke) cause an inflammatory response within the lungs
- Some patients are susceptible to an altered inflammatory response leading to lung damage and COPD
- Disruption in normal repair and defensive mechanisms within the lung leads to damage to respiratory structures and a spectrum of clinical phenotypes (chronic bronchitis and emphysema)
- The abnormal inflammatory response is not confined to the lung with evidence of systemic inflammation and extra-pulmonary tissue injury
- The principal respiratory effect of these pathological changes is airflow limitation and gas trapping
- Chronic hypoxic vasoconstriction of the small pulmonary arteries leads to intimal hyperplasia and smooth muscle hypertrophy/hyperplasia of the pulmonary vasculature, leading to pulmonary hypertension

Clinical features

Smoking history:
- Most important risk factor for COPD
- Estimate use with 'pack years' smoked (packs of cigarettes per day multiplied by the number of years)—amount and duration of smoking contribute to disease severity
- A diagnosis of COPD is very unlikely in the presence of a pack-year history of < 10 pack years without a genetic or environmental factor
- Biomass fuel use is an important cause of COPD in patients from developing nations

Symptoms:
- Three cardinal symptoms of COPD:
  - Dyspnoea—exertional dyspnoea is the commonest presenting symptom
  - Chronic cough
  - Sputum production
- Less common symptoms:
  - Wheezing
  - Chest tightness
  - Weight gain or weight loss
  - Activity limitation
  - Depression and anxiety
  - Fatigue
  - Sleep disruption

COPD is a risk factor for:
- CVD, osteoporosis, metabolic syndrome, cognitive dysfunction, respiratory infections, anxiety and depression, DM, and lung cancer

Physical examination:
- Examination may be normal, or prolonged expiration or wheeze may be identified on forced exhalation at mild disease
- Due to hyperinflation: increased resonance to percussion, decreased breath sounds, distant heart sounds, increased anteroposterior diameter of the chest and a depressed diaphragm with limited movement, Hoover's Sign (intercostal retraction)
- Wheeze or crackles at lung bases

- Expiration through pursed lips
- Cyanosis

Evaluation

Spirometry:
- Measures forced expiratory volume in 1st second of expiration (FEV$_1$) and total forced expiratory volume (forced vital capacity; FVC)
- Required for diagnosis of COPD
- Assesses severity of airflow obstruction, which is itself defined by FEV1/FVC < 0.70
- Allows monitoring of disease progression

Pulse oximetry:
- Provides non-invasive assessment for hypoxaemia

Imaging:
- Not required for diagnosis of COPD
- Initial imaging should be a chest radiograph, which can be used for exclusion of other differential diagnoses: pneumonia, pneumothorax, heart failure, bullae, bronchiectasis, interstitial lung disease, thromboembolic disease, malignancy
- Further imaging such as CT or ventilation-perfusion scans are only required in specific clinical situations, e.g. assessment for specialist intervention such as lung volume reduction (surgical or bronchoscopic)

Diagnosis

- Spirometry is needed to make the diagnosis in the clinical context of symptoms and risk factors
- COPD should be considered in any patient with dyspnoea, chronic cough, and/or chronic sputum production with exposure to a risk factor (smoking or biomass fuel)
- A post-bronchodilator FEV$_1$/FVC < 0.70 confirms the presence of persistent airflow obstruction providing evidence of the diagnosis of COPD in patients with appropriate symptoms and significant exposure factors

Severity assessment

- The global initiative on obstructive lung disease (GOLD) therapeutic strategy suggests using a combination of the following to assess disease severity and guide therapy:
    - An individual's symptoms
    - History of exacerbations
    - Hospitalizations due to exacerbations
    - Severity of airflow obstruction, as measured by FEV$_1$
- Symptom burden can be assessed using commonly available scoring systems, e.g. COPD assessment tool (CAT) and the modified Medical Research Council dyspnoea score (mMRC-D)
- Post-bronchodilation spirometry and number of COPD exacerbations are also used to assess the future risk (Figure 9.4.1)

    Group A: Low risk, fewer symptoms: 0–1 exacerbation per year and no hospitalization for exacerbation; and CAT score < 10 or mMRC grade 0–1
    Group B: Low risk, more symptoms: 0–1 exacerbation per year and no hospitalization for exacerbation; and CAT score ≥ 10 or mMRC grade ≥ 2
    Group C: High risk, fewer symptoms: ≥ 2 exacerbations per year or ≥ 1 hospitalization for exacerbation; and CAT score < 10 or mMRC grade 0–1

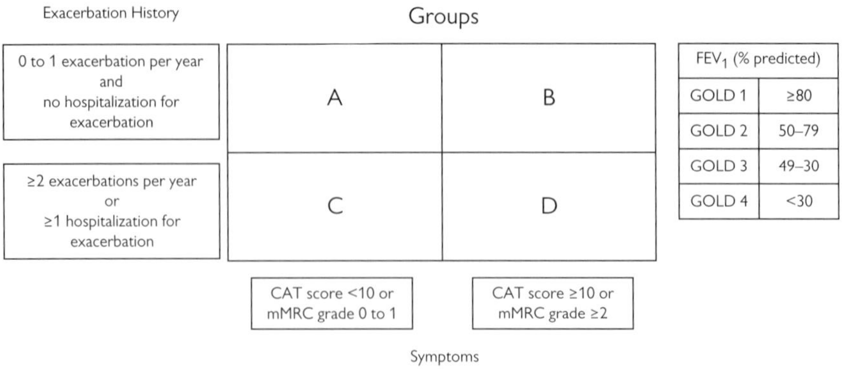

Exacerbation History	Groups		FEV$_1$ (% predicted)	
0 to 1 exacerbation per year and no hospitalization for exacerbation	A	B	GOLD 1	≥80
			GOLD 2	50–79
≥2 exacerbations per year or ≥1 hospitalization for exacerbation	C	D	GOLD 3	49–30
			GOLD 4	<30
	CAT score <10 or mMRC grade 0 to 1	CAT score ≥10 or mMRC grade ≥2		
	Symptoms			

Figure 9.4.1 COPD severity assessment

Group D: High risk, more symptoms: ≥ 2 exacerbations per year or ≥ 1 hospitalization for exacerbation; and CAT score ≥ 10 or mMRC grade ≥ 2

COPD exacerbation

- COPD exacerbations are an acute worsening of respiratory symptoms leading to the need for escalation of medical therapy
- Exacerbations of COPD negatively impact health status, rates of hospitalisation and readmission, and disease progression
- COPD exacerbations are complex events associated with increased airway inflammation, increased mucus production, and marked gas trapping
- These changes contribute to increased dyspnoea, increased sputum purulence and volume, and increased cough and wheeze
- The majority of exacerbations have an infective precipitant
- Due to the lack of a diagnostic test exacerbations are effectively a diagnosis of exclusion and therefore must be differentiated from common comorbidities in COPD such as ACS, pulmonary embolism, worsening of CCF, and pneumonia
- Acute exacerbations of COPD are categorized as:
  - Mild: treated with short-acting bronchodilators only
  - Moderate: treated with short-acting bronchodilators plus antibiotics and/or corticosteroids
  - Severe: requiring hospitalizations or assessment and treatment in the emergency department

Cardiovascular implications of COPD

The interrelationship between respiratory and CV system can be summarized in two types of association:

- Pathologies sharing similar risk factors such as cigarette smoking
- Dysfunction of the heart from primary lung disease such as secondary pulmonary hypertension

Coronary artery disease (CAD) and atherosclerosis

- There is a strong correlation between impaired lung function (FEV$_1$) and CV morbidity and mortality

- COPD and CAD share common risk factors, such as exposure to cigarette smoke and older age
- Higher risk of death by MI has been documented in patients with airflow limitation, and this is independent of age, sex, and smoking history
- Furthermore, for mild COPD, CVD is a more common cause of death than respiratory failure
- The prevalence of hypertension is also increased in COPD
- Patients with COPD and a recent severe exacerbation are at increased risk of an acute MI
- Low-grade systemic inflammation in COPD and atherosclerotic CVD might be the factor driving both diseases
- Although the strength of the associations and the mechanisms responsible have not been entirely elucidated, evidence suggest that patients with COPD should be screened for the presence of concomitant atherosclerosis and just as importantly, patients evaluated for the presence of atherosclerotic heart disease should be investigated for the concomitant presence of airflow obstruction

Heart failure (HF)

- The prevalence of impaired left ventricular (LV) function in COPD is largely unknown and clinically poorly defined due to the overlap in symptoms and signs
- Assessment of B-type natriuretic peptide or N-terminal pro-brain natriuretic peptide (NT-proBNP) can discriminate HF in COPD patients and may be useful to distinguish acute COPD exacerbations from decompensated HF
- LV dysfunction contributes to poor physical activity
- In patients with emphysema the cardiac size is decreased and the volume of the intra-thoracic blood is decreased due to hyperinflation; following lung volume reduction surgery, there is an increase in intra-thoracic blood volume and improvement in LV function, which is related to the changes in the intra-thoracic pressures

Pulmonary arterial hypertension

- Pulmonary arterial hypertension (PAH) at rest is uncommon in patients with mild to moderate COPD
- 1–3% of patients with COPD present with severe PAH that is disproportionate to the degree of airway obstruction
- 50% of patients with very severe COPD have moderate to severe PAH

Pathogenesis:

- Hypoxia:
    - Chronic hypoxia likely plays a role in the pathogenesis of PH in COPD by inducing vascular remodelling
    - In exercise, hypoxic vasoconstriction may become increasingly significant due to decreased mixed venous partial pressure of oxygen
- Vascular remodelling:
    - Intimal and medial structural thickening have been described in the small pulmonary arteries
    - Pulmonary artery endothelial dysfunction has also been described

Cardiac function at rest

- The majority of patients with milder COPD have normal right heart function at rest
- In some, but not all patients, there is a development of right ventricular dysfunction as the disease progresses in severity (more airflow limitation)

Cardiac function during exercise
- In the absence of overt primary CVD (such as valvular or IHD) the normal increase in cardiac output during exercise in COPD is impeded by two major physiological mechanisms:
  - Heart compression due to exercise-induced lung dynamic hyperinflation
  - Intra-thoracic hypovolemia secondary to decreased venous return resulting from persistent expiratory abdominal muscle recruitment
- Diminution of the degree of exercise-induced dynamic hyperinflation improves central haemodynamic responses in hyperinflated COPD patients

Cardiac arrhythmias
- COPD increases the risk of cardiac arrhythmias, which is higher during an acute exacerbation or thoracic surgery
- Risk factors for development of arrhythmias in COPD:
  - Hypoxaemia
  - Acidosis
  - Reduced FEV_1
- Multifocal atrial tachycardia (MAT):
  - Common in COPD
  - Frequently noted during acute exacerbations of COPD
  - Patients with COPD and MAT have a high mortality rate

Arrhythmia treatment considerations in COPD
- The general approach to treating arrhythmias in COPD is similar to that used in the general population
- SVTs (commonly AF and MAT) may persist for a long period of time and cause hypotension, systemic embolization, HF, and anxiety and may lengthen the post-operative hospitalization period

Respiratory treatment and arrhythmias
- β2-Agonists:
  - The relationship between β-agonist use and CV complications is controversial
  - Among subjects taking long-acting β2-agonists an increased incidence of tachycardia and hypokalaemia has been found
  - CV-related adverse events were not associated with salmeterol (a long-acting β2-agonist) in TORCH (TOwards a Revolution in COPD Health) study, in which more than 6000 patients with COPD were randomised to salmeterol alone, fluticasone alone, combination salmeterol–fluticasone, or placebo
- Corticosteroids:
  - A relationship has been reported between high-dose corticosteroid and development of AF
  - No increased arrhythmogenicity of inhaled corticosteroids has been shown
- Theophylline:
  - Can predispose to tachyarrhythmias even in the absence of elevated serum drug levels

Therapeutic implications
- Historically there have been concerns that beta blockers may provoke bronchospasm in COPD
- However, the use of cardio-selective beta blockers (e.g. atenolol and metoprolol), are safe and should not be routinely withheld in patients with COPD; this must be contrasted with the approach in patients with asthma when caution should be used

- Systemic and selective vasodilators are not routinely recommended for the treatment of PAH in COPD as they might inhibit hypoxic pulmonary vasoconstriction and induce further worsening of gas exchange. The vasodilators may improve the cardiac output, but the long-term effect on outcomes remains to be established
- Diuretics can be used to treat peripheral oedema in patients with cor pulmonale due to COPD. However, caution should be used, because increased RV afterload needs higher filling pressures to maintain the cardiac output and excessive use of loop diuretics can lead to a metabolic alkalosis
- Although there is heterogeneity in reported results, meta-analyses suggest that COPD is an adverse risk factor for major adverse cardiac events and mortality following PCI

9.4.2 Obstructive sleep apnoea

- Obstructive sleep apnoea/hypopnoea syndrome (OSAHS) is characterized by recurrent episodes of partial or complete upper airway collapse during sleep, resulting in reduction or cessation of airflow with ongoing respiratory effort
- An apnoea or hypopnoea must be associated with either an arousal from sleep or an oxygen desaturation

Definition

- An obstructive apnoea or hypopnea is an event that lasts for ≥ 10 s and is characterised by an absence (apnoea) or a decrease from baseline (hypopnea) in the amplitude of a valid measure of breathing during sleep that either reaches > 50% with an oxygen desaturation of 3% or an arousal (alternatively a 30% reduction with 4% desaturation)
- Events are scored per hour of sleep and expressed as an apnoea-hypopnoea index (AHI)
- OSA syndrome requires the presence of OSA and symptoms of daytime sleepiness or sleep disruption

Epidemiology

- The prevalence of OSA (defined by an AHI of > 5 events/h) is 24% in men and 9% in women
- The prevalence of OSA *syndrome* (AHI > 5/hr **and** symptoms of daytime sleepiness or sleep disruption) is 4% in males and 2% in females
- Prevalence of OSA is increasing in line with increasing rates of obesity in the general population

Risk factors
- Obesity
- Older age
- Male gender
- Genetic predisposition (shape of upper airway and jaw)
- Smoking
- Sedative drugs

Clinical manifestations
- Snoring
- Excessive daytime sleepiness due to the sleep disruption
- Witnessed apnoea
- Choking or gasping during sleep

- Recurrent awakenings from sleep
- Unrefreshing sleep
- Daytime fatigue
- Impaired concentration

Diagnosis

- The diagnosis of OSA is suspected from clinical features and is confirmed by a sleep study
- Sleepiness is often evaluated using the Epworth sleepiness scale, which assesses the global level of sleepiness and is independent of short-term variations in sleepiness
- It is important to appreciate that this is not a screening tool for OSA but an assessment of daytime somnolence from any cause
- Screening tests for OSA include STOP-BANG (see Box 9.4.1) which is well validated in many populations including the pre-operative population
- The gold standard for OSA diagnosis is overnight full polysomnography (PSG)
- Limited respiratory sleep studies, simple oximetry or other home sleep apnoea tests are validated for diagnosis of OSA in many countries where access to full PSG may be limited or reserved for more complex parasomnias

Treatment

- Gold standard treatment is with continuous positive airway pressure (CPAP); although long term compliance rates are poor at ~50%
- Other treatment options include:
  - Conservative: weight loss, sleep hygiene, positional sleep training
  - Mandibular advancement devices
- CPAP mechanisms of action on cardiovascular system:
  - Redistributing excess lung water to extra-thoracic compartments:
    a. Treats acute cardiogenic pulmonary oedema
    b. Reduces stimulation of pulmonary vagal irritant receptors and thus reduces the ventilation
    c. Increases lung compliance and as an effect unloads the inspiratory muscles
  - Significantly reduces LV afterload by lowering the transmural pressure in patients with compromised cardiac function and, thus, can augment cardiac output. The failing heart is insensitive to changes in preload

BOX 9.4.1 STOP-BANG

Snoring

Tiredness

Observed to stop breathing

Elevated or treated blood **P**ressure

Body mass index > 35 kg/m^2

Age > 50 years

Neck size > 43 cm (male) or 41 cm (female)

Gender (male)

0–2 = low risk of OSA; 3–4 = intermediate risk; > 4 = high risk

- Attenuates the sympathetic nervous activity and increases cardiac vagal modulation of the heart with improved blood pressure regulation
- Blood pressure can also be reduced with CPAP when compared with placebo, especially in patients using CPAP for ≥ 3.5 h/night and in those with > 20 desaturations of ≥4% per hour

Pathophysiology of CV-associated disease

- The negative intrathoracic pressure generated during breathing through obstructed airways contributes with two mechanisms:
  a. Increases LV transmural pressure and LV afterload
  b. Draws more blood into the thorax and increases RV preload
- Cardiac contractility and diastolic relaxation is impaired due to intermittent hypoxia
- Reduced endothelium-dependent vasodilation and decreased nitric oxide
- Increased sympathetic vasoconstrictor activity and inflammation
- Increased platelet activation

Cardiovascular implications

- OSA is associated with increased CV morbidity and mortality, being a significant risk factor for CVD
- While the effect of CPAP therapy on CV events has been explored in many studies, none has unequivocally shown benefits in the reduction in CV mortality, acute MI, and stroke
- CV risk appears more associated with OSA occurring during rapid eye movement (REM) sleep

OSA and hypertension:

- 50% of OSA patients are hypertensive
- Around 30% of hypertensive patients also have OSA, which is frequently undiagnosed
- Those patients with an attenuated nocturnal BP decline (non-dippers) may be more likely to have coexisting OSA
- Prevalence of hypertension in patients with OSA is increased, compared to controls, which remains significant after controlling for potential confounding factors such as age and obesity
- OSA is an independent risk factor for the development of essential hypertension as it can precede and predict the onset of hypertension
- It has been identified that there is a relationship between the severity of OSA and the likelihood of hypertension—AHI and 24-hour BP are related independent of confounding factors such as age, sex, BMI, and antihypertensive medications
- OSA is more strongly related to diastolic and/or combined hypertension, than to isolated systolic hypertension
- The association between OSA and hypertension is particularly prominent in patients with resistant hypertension (> 70% of patients with resistant hypertension have OSA)
  - Hypertension is considered resistant when BP remains above goal (≥ 140/90 mmHg) despite lifestyle modification and administration of three antihypertensive agents of different classes including a diuretic
- Effects of OSA on hypertension may be especially evident in middle-aged compared with older subjects
- The effect of OSA treatment on hypertension:
  - Positive airway pressure therapy for OSA reduces systemic BP, regardless of whether the patients are hypertensive at baseline
  - Effective CPAP treatment for OSA markedly and acutely decreases BP and sympathetic activation during sleep

- Mean systolic BP drop 2.6 mmHg
- Clinically relevant (reduction of 1–2 mmHg is associated with a reduction in major CV events and HF)
- Appears to be less than antihypertensive medication; when combining the two treatments the effect is greater
  - The presence of uncontrolled hypertension at baseline is an important predictor of reduction in BP with CPAP therapy, independent of OSA severity
  - The BP reduction achieved by CPAP therapy is less in patients without excessive daytime sleepiness than in patients with sleepiness and is related to the sleep apnoea severity
  - The use of conservative management (exercise and weight loss programmes) can be more effective on BP control than CPAP therapy in patients with OSA but without significant symptoms

Coronary artery disease (CAD)

- An increased risk for CV events related to CAD, independent of other shared risk factors has been noted in OSA, and OSA is a risk factor for worse outcomes in patients with established CAD
- OSA is related with multiple vascular risk factors and vascular disease markers:
  - Hypertension
  - Decreased high density lipoproteins
  - Increased C-reactive protein
  - Increased homocysteine
  - Diabetes mellitus
  - Coronary artery calcification
  - Increased troponin-I has been related to increasing severity of OSA and nocturnal hypoxia
- Clinical characteristics:
  - Higher incidence of fatal and non-fatal CV events (MI/ACS, stroke) for untreated, severe OSA than untreated patients with mild–moderate OSA, simple snorers, and healthy participants, even after adjustment for confounding variables
  - OSA may exacerbate pre-existing CAD
  - Although OSA is associated with significant CV risk, patients with OSA have smaller territorial MIs than matched controls, and it has been hypothesized that this is due to ischaemic preconditioning achieved in sleep-related desaturations
- Impact of CPAP:
  - Treatment with CPAP in OSA may reduce the incidence of CAD
  - Treatment of patients with symptomatic OSA (with CPAP) has been associated with a reduction of the likelihood of a MI, stroke, or ACS requiring a revascularization procedure compared with no treatment

Atrial fibrillation

- There is an increased prevalence of AF in patients with OSA, compared with controls or the general population (approximately ×3)
- The prevalence of OSA in patients with AF is high (30% to 80%)
- Characteristics of OSA promoting atrial arrhythmogenesis:
  - Autonomic dysfunction
  - Hypoxia
  - Hypercapnia (recovery phase)

- Increased negative intrathoracic pressures leading to increased juxtacardiac and transmural pressures affecting the thin-walled atria
- Clinical characteristics:
  - Increasing severity of sleep-disordered breathing associated with increasing prevalence of AF
  - OSA may be a modifiable risk factor for recurrent AF after cardioversion or ablation
- Effect of CPAP therapy
  - Limited data suggest that treatment of OSA reduces the risk of recurrent AF

Other arrhythmias and sudden death
- OSA is associated with nocturnal cardiac arrhythmias
- The bradycardia-tachycardia phenomenon may be observed with respiratory events (apnoea and hypopnoea). It is unknown whether or not the relationship is causal, but there may be a temporal relationship, with arrhythmias occurring more frequently after a respiratory event
- Higher prevalence of:
  - Nocturnal AF
  - Non-sustained VT (NSVT)
  - Complex ventricular ectopy (NSVT, bigeminy, trigeminy, and quadrigeminy)
- Patients with OSA appear to have a nocturnal (midnight to 6 a.m.) predilection to sudden death, with an approximately 3× increased risk, compared with the general population and those without OSA
- Nadir oxygen saturation is a predictor of sudden cardiac death
- Effect of CPAP therapy:
  - Preliminary data support a role for CPAP in reducing risk of cardiac arrhythmia and sudden death
  - Discontinuation of CPAP may increase the rate of sudden death

Heart failure (HF)
- OSA may be underdiagnosed in HF patients since typical symptoms of HF, such as nocturnal dyspnoea and nocturia related to diuretics, may be attributed to HF when they actually are signs and symptoms of OSA
- OSA is diagnosed in 11–37% of patients with HF resulting from systolic dysfunction who are referred for polysomnography and in 50% of HF patients with preserved systolic function
- Excessive daytime sleepiness appears less common in patients with OSA and HF
- Three months of CPAP has been reported to attenuate abnormalities in diastolic function, suggesting a potential aetiological role of OSA in diastolic HF
- The pathophysiology of sleep-disordered breathing and HF involves a variety of mechanisms
  - The most direct mechanism by which long-standing OSA might induce LV systolic dysfunction is by raising BP
  - Furthermore, it has been noted that LVH is more closely linked to hypertension during sleep than during wakefulness
  - Therefore, a high nocturnal BP in hypertensive patients with OSA may place them at risk in the long term for LVH and failure
  - OSA, which increase LV transmural pressures in response to increasingly negative intrathoracic pressure, results in reduction of LV preload and increased afterload
  - Nocturnal oxygen desaturation is an independent predictor of impaired diastolic function
  - In patients with HF, the coexistence of OSA may be related to higher sympathetic nerve activity and higher systolic BP during wakefulness, despite more intense antihypertensive therapy

- Cytokines, catecholamines, endothelin, and other growth factors produced in OSA may contribute to LVH independently of hypertension

Pulmonary arterial hypertension (PAH)
- Prevalence of PAH is approximately 20% in patients with moderate to severe OSA
- The degree of PAH is typically mild if no other lung disease coexist, but survival rates are lower among patients with PAH
- Characterized by reduced functional capacity and quality of life
- Risk factors for PAH are:
    - Co-morbid lung disease
    - Daytime hypoxaemia
    - Increasing apnoea hypopnoea index (AHI)
    - Co-morbid obesity hypoventilation syndrome
- Effect of treatment with CPAP:
    - Nasal CPAP can reduce PA systolic pressure and pulmonary vascular resistance in patients with OSA over a period of three to four months
    - The reduction of arterial systolic pressure is greater among patients who have OSA plus pulmonary hypertension than OSA alone

9.4.3 Obesity hypoventilation syndrome

- OHS ('Pickwickian syndrome') is a breathing disorder that affects obese individuals
- It is defined as the presence of awake alveolar hypoventilation which cannot be attributed to other conditions in patients with obesity and demonstrable sleep-disordered breathing

Epidemiology
- Not all obese people develop OHS but the prevalence increases with increasing BMI
- The prevalence of obesity hypoventilation syndrome in the general population remains unknown but is estimated at ~0.6%

Clinical features
- Risk factors in obese people:
    - Fifth and sixth decades of life
    - Severe obesity (BMI > 50 kg/m^2), where prevalence may be as high as 50%
    - Central obesity
    - Obesity attributed to an excess of food intake in relation to the energy expenditure requirements of the organism
    - Restrictive ventilatory defect in lung function
    - Reduced inspiratory muscle function
    - Severe OSA (AHI > 60 events per hour)
    - Male gender is NOT a risk factor (in contrast to OSA)
- Clinical presentation of OHS reflects the manifestations of:
    - Obesity
    - OSA (90% of OHS patients also have OSA which is often severe); in 10% the sleep-deprivation symptoms are also apparent, but without witnessed apnoea during sleep
    - OHS-related complications (e.g. pulmonary hypertension)

Pathogenesis
- One of the more interesting aspects of the interaction of respiratory function and obesity is that only some morbidly obese patients develop awake hypoventilation—a complex interaction between the following factors is likely to be involved in the pathogenesis of OHS:
    - Upper airway obstruction
    - Sleep-disordered breathing
    - Altered respiratory mechanics
    - Impaired ventilatory control

Diagnosis
- Diagnosis of daytime hypoventilation in an obese patient in the absence of other causes of alveolar hypoventilation:
    - Obesity (BMI > 30 kg·m^{-2})
    - Awake hypoventilation (PaCO$_2$ > 45 mmHg)
    - No alternative cause of hypoventilation
    - Evidence of sleep disordered breathing (OSA or isolated nocturnal hypoventilation)
- Sleep studies should be performed to characterize the type of underlying sleep-disordered breathing

Treatment
- First-line therapy is the combination of non-invasive ventilation (NIV) or CPAP and supervised and controlled weight loss
- A multidisciplinary approach utilizing experts in obesity, sleep, and ventilation is highly recommended
- CPAP is the usual mode chosen for OHS plus OSA, whereas BiPAP in the spontaneous timed mode is used for obesity hypoventilation plus sleep-related hypoventilation and in those that CPAP failed to control the hypoventilation
- For patients not complaint with NIV/CPAP, second-line therapeutic options are tracheostomy and bariatric surgery—these therapies are associated with high risk of adverse effects

Cardiovascular complications and prognosis
- Morbidity and mortality in OHS patients without treatment is high
- In addition to morbidity and mortality related to respiratory complications, patients with OHS also exhibit greater CV and metabolic morbidities compared with those with OSA or simple severe obesity
- Rates of systemic hypertension, HF, insulin resistance, cor pulmonale, and angina are higher among patients with OHS compared with those with eucapnic obesity
- Mild to moderate pulmonary hypertension is noted in up to two-thirds of OHS patients
- The impact of therapy, particularly non-invasive positive airway pressure on CV complications and mortality is uncertain and appears to be limited
- Even when sleep-disordered breathing is treated with positive airway pressure therapy, mortality in those with severe OHS remains substantially worse than individuals with OSA alone
- Presence of significant awake hypoxaemia at diagnosis and during NIV therapy has been associated with a poor prognosis
- The main cause of death is generally from CVD, and hospitalization rates and ICU admissions are higher in OHS compared with eucapnic obese individuals

9.4.4 Central sleep apnoea

- Transient loss of neural output to the respiratory muscles causing cessation or reduction of ventilation for a period ≥ 10 s (in adults) defines central sleep apnoea/hypopnoea
- Recurrent central apnoeas are the hallmark feature of CSA, and they are usually due to hyperventilation, but can be caused by hypoventilation
- Cheyne–Stokes respiration (CSR) is a periodic pattern of waxing and waning hyperventilation followed by periods of apnoea
- In contrast to OSA, there is an absence of respiratory effort in CSA

Epidemiology

- CSA is common, although less prevalent in the general population than OSA and its actual prevalence is unknown
- Less than 5% of patients referred to a sleep laboratory reveal predominant CSA—however, in certain conditions, including HF, neuromuscular disorders, opioid use, and high altitude, the prevalence of CSA is high
- Idiopathic CSA, by definition, is not associated with any comorbid condition
- Risk factors for CSA are provided below in Box 9.4.2

Clinical manifestations

- Patients with CSA typically present with:
    a. Symptoms of disrupted sleep:
        - Excessive daytime sleepiness
        - Poor subjective sleep quality
        - Insomnia
        - Inattention
        - Poor concentration
        - Fatigue
        - Poor exercise tolerance
    b. Symptoms and signs due to the recurrent central apnoeas:
        - Paroxysmal nocturnal dyspnoea
        - Morning headaches

BOX 9.4.2 RICK FACTORS FOR CENTRAL SLEEP APNOEA

- Male gender
- Older age (> 60 years)
- Congestive heart failure
- Hypocapnia
- Atrial fibrillation
- Stroke
- Chronically use of opioids, including methadone maintenance therapy
- During initiation of CPAP therapy in certain patients with OSA
- CSR observed during the day
- Pulmonary hypertension
- Neuromuscular disease
- Acromegaly
- Renal failure
- Low cervical tetraplegia
- Primary mitochondrial diseases

- Nocturnal angina.
- Episodic oxyhaemoglobin desaturation
- Pauses in breathing
- Nocturnal arrhythmias

Diagnosis
- Requires overnight sleep study (full polysomnography or limited respiratory polygraphy)

Pathophysiology
- The source of CSR is regarded to be the increased pulmonary venous pressure due to left HF, as pulmonary congestion stimulates stretch receptors that sensitise the peripheral chemoreceptors to carbon dioxide through vagal afferents
- $PaCO_2$ is then driven below the apnoeic threshold attributed to the increased ventilatory sensitivity to carbon dioxide
- Additionally, hypoxia that follows apnoea/hypopnea contributes to an enhanced post-apnoeic hyperventilation

Treatment
- CSA-specific therapies are indicated for patients with significant symptoms and signs such as excessive daytime sleepiness or severe episodic oxyhaemoglobin desaturation during sleep
- For patients with CSA associated with symptomatic HF with reduced systolic function (LVEF < 50%), a trial of CPAP may be beneficial, but adaptive servo-ventilation (ASV) should not be used in these patients due to possible increase in CV deaths
- CPAP, bi-level ventilation, and oxygen have limited evidence of benefit in CSA

Central sleep apnoea in heart failure
- Although OSA has been identified as a possible independent risk factor for the development of heart and vascular disease, CSA more often is a consequence of such CV illness
- Among patients with moderate to severe HF (LVEF ≤ 55%) the prevalence of sleep apnoea (both obstructive and central) is very high irrespective of the clinical suspicion
- CSR/CSA in HF patients is associated with poor prognosis, and mortality is increased even after controlling for the severity of HF, age, sex, and other potential confounders, particularly in patients presenting with daytime CSR during physical activity
- Therapy in HF:
    - Optimized medical therapy of HF is the first step
    - Cardiac resynchronization and heart transplantation may also alleviate CSR/CSA
    - CPAP may also be required, if medical therapy alone is ineffective
    - CPAP increases the intrathoracic pressure, which reduces both afterload and preload by decreasing transmural ventricular pressure and venous return so that cardiac function improves in patients with increased filling pressures. Additionally, CPAP stabilizes CSR by raising the end-expiratory lung volume
    - Nocturnal CPAP has been shown to improve nocturnal CSR/CSA, oxygen saturation, LVEF, sympathetic nervous system activity, and 6-min walking distance. Furthermore, there are data showing a survival benefit in a subgroup of patients in whom CPAP sufficiently suppressed CSR/CSA
    - There are contradictory data regarding the use of supplemental nocturnal oxygen: a reduction in CSR/CSA, along with improvements in physical performance or quality of life in some studies, whilst others failed to reproduce these benefits

Further reading

Bradley TD, Floras JS. Obstructive sleep apnoea and its cardiovascular consequences. *Lancet*. 2009 Jan 3;373(9657):82–93. doi: 10.1016/S0140-6736(08)61622-0. Epub 2008 Dec 26

Falk JA, Kadiev S, Criner GJ, Scharf SM, Minai OA, Diaz P. Cardiac disease in chronic obstructive pulmonary disease. *Proc Am Thorac Soc*. 2008 May 1;5(4):543–8. doi: 10.1513/pats.200708-142ET

Han MK, McLaughlin VV, Criner GJ, Martinez FJ. Pulmonary diseases and the heart. *Circulation*. 2007 Dec 18;116(25):2992–3005. doi: 10.1161/CIRCULATIONAHA.106.685206

Parish JM, Shepard JW Jr. Cardiovascular effects of sleep disorders. *Chest*. 1990 May;97(5):1220–6. doi: 10.1378/chest.97.5.1220

Somers VK, White DP, Amin R, Abraham WT, Costa F, Culebras A, Daniels S, Floras JS, Hunt CE, Olson LJ, Pickering TG, Russell R, Woo M, Young T; American Heart Association Council for High Blood Pressure Research Professional Education Committee, Council on Clinical Cardiology; American Heart Association Stroke Council; American Heart Association Council on Cardiovascular Nursing; American College of Cardiology Foundation. Sleep apnea and cardiovascular disease: an American Heart Association/American College Of Cardiology Foundation Scientific Statement from the American Heart Association Council for High Blood Pressure Research Professional Education Committee, Council on Clinical Cardiology, Stroke Council, and Council On Cardiovascular Nursing. In collaboration with the National Heart, Lung, and Blood Institute National Center on Sleep Disorders Research (National Institutes of Health). *Circulation*. 2008 Sep 2;118(10):1080–111. doi: 10.1161/CIRCULATIONAHA.107.189375

9.5

The patient with rheumatic disorders

John D. Pauling and Lesley-Anne Bissell

TABLE OF CONTENTS

9.5.1 The patient with rheumatic disorders 901
9.5.2 Rheumatoid arthritis 902
9.5.3 Spondyloarthopathies 905
9.5.4 Systemic lupus erythematosus 907
9.5.5 Antiphospholipid syndrome 909
9.5.6 Primary Sjögren's syndrome 911
9.5.7 Myositis spectrum disorders 912
9.5.8 Systemic sclerosis 914
9.5.9 Primary systemic vasculitis 916
9.5.10 Cardiac disease in miscellaneous rheumatic disorders 919

9.5.1 The patient with rheumatic disorders

- Rheumatic disorders include a diverse range of conditions associated with musculoskeletal impairment and include:
    - The inflammatory arthritides
    - Systemic vasculitides
    - Autoimmune connective tissue diseases (e.g. Systemic Lupus Erythematosus (SLE))
    - Crystal arthritides
    - Primary disorders of bone (e.g. Paget's)
    - Inherited disorders of the connective tissue (e.g. Marfan's)
- Cardiac involvement in the rheumatic diseases is diverse and can affect all the tissues of the heart, leading to a diverse range of symptoms and clinical signs
- Autopsy and multi-modality imaging studies suggest a very high prevalence of cardiac involvement across the spectrum of rheumatic diseases, though symptomatic cardiac disease remains generally uncommon
- Recent attention has focused on increased CV risk secondary to accelerated atherosclerosis which occurs within many of the rheumatic diseases—both inflammatory disease processes
- Clinical presentation of cardiac involvement mirrors that of idiopathic disease, making it essential that cardiologists are alert to the clinical features that might indicate the presence of an underlying rheumatic disease
- Management of cardiac disease in rheumatic disease can be challenging due to disease-associated co-morbidities complicating both the clinical picture and considerations concerning management

Features that should alert cardiologists to the possible presence of rheumatic disease

Clinical

- Clinical evidence of autoimmunity in the form of autoantibody generation and organ-specific autoimmunity (e.g. arthritis, skin rashes, myositis, etc.)
- Vasculopathy often manifesting as Raynaud's phenomenon but also affecting other vascular beds such as the lungs (pulmonary arterial hypertension) or kidneys (e.g. the scleroderma renal crisis)
- Aberrant tissue remodelling such as fibrosis of the skin, lungs, or gastrointestinal tract
- Constitutional symptoms of ill health such as fatigue, fever, weight loss, and generalized malaise
- Extra-articular manifestations of inflammatory arthritis, e.g. interstitial lung disease (ILD), scleritis, uveitis, rheumatoid nodules
- Extra-articular features of crystal arthritis, e.g. gouty tophi
- Phenotypic features that might indicate the presence of a collagen vascular disorder (e.g. arachnodactyly and high-arched palate in Marfan's disease)

Laboratory

- Presence of autoantibodies targeting ubiquitously expressed nuclear or cytoplasmic cell constituents, e.g. anti-DNA autoantibodies in SLE or anti-synthetase antibodies in myositis-spectrum disorders
- Raised inflammatory markers within the autoimmune rheumatic diseases, e.g. elevated plasma viscosity (PV), erythrocyte sedimentation rate (ESR), and C-reactive protein (CRP)
- Leukopenia common in autoimmune rheumatic diseases, e.g. SLE
- Laboratory features of immune complex disease, e.g. hypocomplementaemia
- The identification of genetic polymorphisms can be used to confirm inherited disorders of bone and connective tissue

Systemic inflammation in atherosclerosis

- CRP has been found in atherosclerotic lesions in histological studies
- CRP can induce adhesion molecule expression on endothelial cells, reduce endothelial nitric oxide synthase, augment monocyte migration into the atherosclerotic lesion, and mediate monocyte's uptake of LDL-C
- Higher levels of interleukin-6 (IL-6) have been associated with development of CVD, and interruption of IL-6 signalling has been associated with reduced IHD
- Positron emission tomography (PET) imaging using 18F-fluorodeoxyglucose (FDG) has illustrated inflammatory lesions within arterial wall plaques, correlating with CV risk factors and inflammatory markers
- CRP can predict future CV events; odd ratios (OR) 1.5–3 for CRP in the highest tertile vs lowest, and it is independently associated with CVD mortality
- Lower CRP is associated with better CV outcomes; as seen in statin trials
- CRP and ESR associated with arterial stiffness, endothelial dysfunction, and fibrosis
- However, evidence is inconsistent as to the benefit of adding CRP in to CV risk models

9.5.2 Rheumatoid arthritis

Summary

- Rheumatoid arthritis (RA) is characterized by a symmetrical, sometimes erosive, inflammatory polyarthritis

- Prevalence approximately 1% with a female predominance
- An accelerated risk of CVD secondary to atherosclerosis is observed in those with RA, comparable to those with DM, and thought secondary to the presence of traditional CV risk factors and systemic inflammation associated with RA
- Treatment guidelines recommend the multiplication of CV risk scores by 1.5 to reflect this increased risk, along with the management of traditional CV risk factors and minimizing RA disease activity

Cardiovascular involvement in RA
Epidemiology
- Patients with RA have an accelerated risk of CVD and MI secondary to atherosclerosis comparable to those with diabetes
- Data suggest the risk is reducing in those recently diagnosed with RA with the advent of earlier recognition and aggressive treatment of RA
- Patients with RA have an increased risk of HF after adjustment for IHD and CV risk factors suggesting an alternative pathophysiology other than that of atherosclerosis
- Pericardial effusions (in up to 30%) and pericarditis (2%) have been reported
- Valvular nodules can occur (usually on mitral or aortic valve) or valvular insufficiency or thickening/stenosis (tricuspid, aortic, and mitral)
- Myocarditis and conduction defects are rare

Pathophysiology
- Accelerated atherosclerosis is the key driver of CV morbidity in RA, driven by both traditional CV risk factors and systemic inflammation
- Synovitis is the result of a complex auto-immune process involving both innate and cell-mediated immunity, with the activation of both T and B cells, macrophages, fibroblasts, endothelial cells, and the release of cytokines which are thought to also initiate and augment atherosclerosis
- Evidence for endothelial dysfunction in RA; increase in markers of endothelial activation which are increased in IHD and predict CV events in the general population, in addition to reduced flow mediated dilatation (FMD)
- Increase in mediators of atherosclerotic plaque destabilization in RA, and those released following plaque rupture associated with CV events and mortality in the IHD population
- Arterial stiffness greater in RA; by similar degree to those with DM
- Ultrasound-measured carotid intimal media thickness (CIMT) greater in RA, and associated with future CV events in RA
- Autopsy studies in patients with RA and CVD reveal less severe coronary artery lesions but more evidence of vulnerable plaques, with more inflammatory change
- Autopsy studies in RA have revealed microvasculitis and microthrombosis without macroscopic evidence for MI in those with perfusions defects on dipyridamole Thallium-201 (T1) scintigraphy, associating with inflammatory markers

Disease phenotype most at risk
CV risk factors
- Hypertension in up to 57%; not clear if this is greater compared to general population, but has predicted CV events in RA
- Hypertension can be exacerbated by use of corticosteroids and NSAIDs
- Smoking increase CV risk, and is also an independent risk factor for developing RA, predicting severe disease, and poor treatment response

- Dyslipidaemia in up to 30% with abnormalities seen up to 10 years before diagnosis. Individual lipid measures (e.g. total cholesterol) can be influenced by systemic inflammation (levels dropping with increasing CRP), described as the 'lipid paradox'

Disease-specific factors

- Combining traditional CV risk factors with RA disease-specific factors has yielded strong prediction for future CV events

RA disease-specific factors associated with CVD:

- RA duration is an independent determinant of arterial stiffness, and associated with reduced diastolic dysfunction
- RA activity; reported commonly as DAS-28 (composite score of tender and swollen joints, physician visual assessment score, and an inflammatory marker, e.g. CRP), is associated with multiple cardiac complications including fibrosis
- Subcutaneous nodules
- Erosions
- Physical inactivity

Medication

- No evidence to be stricter with NSAID treatment compared to those without RA, current practice is to minimize their use, especially in those at higher risk of CVD
- Corticosteroids associated with increased risk of CV events (relative risk (RR) ~1.5), possibly through exacerbation or induction of hypertension, increasing risk of DM and obesity or affecting lipid metabolism (European League Against Rheumatism (EULAR) advocates the use of ≤ 7.5 mg/day of prednisolone to minimize CV risk)
- Leflunomide and ciclosporin (disease-modifying anti-rheumatic drugs, DMARDs) can exacerbate or induce hypertension
- Tocilizumab (IL-6 receptor inhibitor) can increase lipids, however changes do not translate into increased risk of CVD in RA
- Recent data suggest Janus Kinase (JAK) inhibitors, in comparison to Tumour Necrosis Factor (TNF) inhibitors, are associated with an increased risk of CV events in older patients with RA with an existing CV risk

Laboratory investigations

- N-terminal pro-brain natriuretic peptide (NT-proBNP) is raised in RA and an independent predictor of mortality in established RA
- RF and ACPA positivity

Echocardiography

- Systolic impairment and diastolic dysfunction in early and established RA
- Often a higher LV mass index
- May detect higher mean systolic pulmonary artery pressure secondary to either generalized diastolic heart dysfunction or pulmonary abnormalities
- Mitral valve thickening or insufficiency seen in 5–35%, and aortic valve lesions in 5–14%
- Asymptomatic pericardial effusions in up to one-third
- Stress-echocardiography may reveal areas of ischaemia with normal angiography; thought secondary to microvascular disease

Imaging
- Angiography studies determined greater burden of coronary plaque in RA with greater multi-vessel disease after adjustment for CV risk factors
- Dipyridamole Thallium-201 (T1) scintigraphy studies demonstrated perfusion abnormalities associated with inflammatory markers
- Cardiac magnetic resonance (CMR) has utility in the assessment of CVD in RA. In contrast to echocardiography data, reduced LV mass index is reported, myocardial oedema on T2-weighted images, focal fibrosis with late gadolinium enhancement (transmural and sub-endocardial in up to one-third) and diffuse fibrosis with increased extracellular volume (ECV)

Management

Screening
- Calculate patient's 10-year CV risk score using nationally recommended models at least once every 5 years in line with ESC guidance, repeating more frequently if patient is at intermediate/high CV risk or if there have been substantial changes in RA therapy
- Multiply CV risk score by 1.5 if RA not already incorporated into the risk model (e.g. in QRISK2)
- Consider carotid ultrasound to detect asymptomatic atherosclerotic plaques to improve risk evaluation
- If symptomatic, assess as per general population

Prevention
- Patient education is key: greater risk of CVD in RA, smoking cessation, healthy diet
- Advise regular exercise: lowers CRP levels, reduces body fat, and improves vascular function in RA with no data to support any adverse effects

Treatment
- Treatment of modifiable CV risk factors and established CVD should not differ in RA from general population
- Pericardial disease generally asymptomatic and does not usually require intervention

N.B. Synthetic and biological DMARDs have been associated with a reduction of CV events and mortality in RA

9.5.3 Spondyloarthropathies

Summary
- Spondyloarthropathy (SpA) encompasses a spectrum of inflammatory disorders that can affect peripheral and axial joints, along with disease at the enthesis and extra-articular sites:
    - Ankylosing spondylitis (AS)
    - Psoriatic arthritis (PsA)
    - Inflammatory bowel disease (IBD)-related arthritis
    - Reactive arthritis
- Effects an estimated 0.5–2% of the population
- CV manifestations in SpA depend on the disease, but include accelerated atherosclerotic CV disease (similar to that seen in RA), conduction defects and valvular insufficiency

Cardiovascular involvement in SpA
Epidemiology
- Accelerated risk of atherosclerotic disease and MI seen in SpA, though less data reported in comparison to RA
- AS strong independent predictor of CABG at young age
- Relative risk (RR) for CV mortality in AS reported as 1.6–1.9, but difficult to determine if this risk is independent of CV risk factors
- Little data in IBD-related SpA, but increased risk of CVD seen in general IBD population; risk greater in women and young patients (< 40 years)
- Aortic root involvement seen in up to 60% of AS: aortitis, aortic root dilatation, and aortic valve insufficiency, thickening, or valve nodules
- Aortic insufficiency associated with increasing age, AS disease duration (~10% after 10 years), HLA-B27 and peripheral joint involvement
- Aortic prolapse ~4% of AS patients, mitral regurgitation is rare
- Conduction defects seen in 3–33% of AS patients. Associated with HLA-B27, can occur during flare and improve with NSAIDs
- Cardiomyopathy with diastolic/systolic dysfunction recognized in AS
- Myocarditis rare

CV risk factors
- Increased prevalence of traditional CV risk factors in PsA and AS (e.g. type 2 DM, hyperlipidaemia, hypertension, raised BMI)
- Increased prevalence of metabolic syndrome in AS and PsA

Pathophysiology
- Chronic inflammation thought to drive accelerated atherosclerosis
- Evidence for endothelial dysfunction and increased arterial stiffness in AS and PsA
- Aortic root involvement occurs due to sclerosing inflammatory process of aortic root and aortic valve cusps
- Autopsy studies show thickened and shortened aortic valve, fibrosis of aortic wall and above sinuses of Valsalva, extending below base of aortic valve. Inflammation and fibrosis of the interventricular septum may affect the AV node and can extend to mitral valve and interventricular septum
- Thickening of ventricular septum ('sub-aortic bump') in up to 30% of AS patients

Laboratory investigations
- HLA-B27 (associated with aortic insufficiency and conduction defects)
- Cardiac enzymes including troponin I may indicate myocarditis or recent MI
- NT-proBNP

Imaging
- In AS, echocardiography can demonstrate increased aortic root diameter at sinus of Valsalva, ascending aorta, valve thickening or regurgitation, and impaired function
    - Recent studies suggest reducing prevalence related to advancements in treatment
- CMR helpful in diagnosis of IHD and detection of myocarditis

Management
Screening and prevention
- EULAR CV recommendations (discussed in 9.5.1) apply to AS and PsA

Treatment
- Treat modifiable CV risk factors and established CVD as per general population
- Acitretin (used in treatment of psoriasis) can increase lipids, but has not been shown to increase CV risk
- Aortic valve disease and conduction defects (can improve with NSAIDS) should be managed as per the general population; valve replacement is rarely required (permanent pacemakers rarely required)

9.5.4 Systemic lupus erythematosus

Summary
- SLE is one of the commonest autoimmune CTDs (affects ~ 1 in 1000 people)
- Female predominance (9:1) and symptoms often present in the 3rd or 4th decades
- Dysregulated inflammation (sometimes driven by immune complex deposition) is the pathological hallmark of the disease
- As a heterogeneous, multisystem disease potentially involving most tissues within the body, this can sometimes lead to delays in diagnosis
- Mucocutaneous and musculoskeletal involvement are the commonest disease manifestations
- Other pathological features of CTD can be present such as vasculopathy (Raynaud's, pulmonary hypertension (PH)) and aberrant tissue remodelling (e.g. ILD)

Cardiac involvement in SLE
- All the tissues of the heart can be affected in SLE, and sensitive methods for cardiac involvement identify abnormalities in > 50% of patients
- Symptomatic cardiac involvement is less common
- The presence of cardiac involvement often reflects poorly controlled active disease
- Accelerated atherosclerosis and increased incidence of CVD is an important and modifiable cardiac manifestation

Epidemiology
- Pericardial disease often a presenting feature (or a feature of recent relapse)
    - Symptomatic pericarditis is common but pericardial tamponade, constrictive pericarditis, or purulent pericarditis are rare
    - Pericardial disease is evident on echocardiography in up to half of patients with SLE and often associated with disease activity elsewhere
- Atypical verrucous endocarditis (also termed Libman–Sacks endocarditis) valve disease (typically aortic or mitral valves) is evident in 40–50% using TTE, 50–60% using TOE, and up to 75% on autopsy studies
    - May be more common in conjunction with positive antiphospholipid antibodies
    - Usually asymptomatic (and can resolve spontaneously) but complications can occur including regurgitant disease, infective endocarditis, and embolic disease
- Myocarditis and myocardial fibrosis less common in SLE since widespread use of DMARDs (7–10%). Positive anti-Ro antibodies might be a risk factor for myocardial involvement
- CAD occurs in ~10% of patients and the RR is 4–8× more common in SLE than healthy controls making accelerated atherosclerosis
- Focal arteritis might account for minor coronary artery involvement
    - Coronary ischaemia in younger patients with active disease and shorter disease duration should raise suspicion regarding possible coronary arteritis

- Older patients/more stable disease at greater risk of accelerated atherosclerotic disease
- Rhythm and conduction disturbances are often asymptomatic but can result in palpitations and fatigue
    - Arrhythmias can be the result of primary myocardial involvement, antimalarial drug use, electrolyte disturbance, or thyroid disease

Pathophysiology

- Acute and chronic pericardial disease can occur in SLE
- Deposition of C3 and immunoglobulins can be identified in acute pericardial disease
- Verrucous endocarditis consists of fibrin clumps, focal necrosis, and lymphocytic infiltrates during acute phase, and replaced with vascularized fibrous tissue (+/− calcification) in established disease
- CAD can be caused by atherosclerotic disease or focal arteritis
- The enhanced CV risk associated with SLE is consistent with the underlying procoagulant, proinflammatory, and atherosclerotic lipid profile typically present
- Risk factors for atherosclerotic disease include cumulative exposure to glucocorticoids, cumulative disease activity, accrued damage, and conventional CV risk factors (which themselves might be augmented by disease process, e.g. atherogenic lipid profiles)
- Immune complex and complement deposition within the vessel walls and perivascular myocardium can be identified in SLE-associated myocarditis

Laboratory investigations

- Raised inflammatory markers
- Low C3 levels
- Raised anti-DNA binding levels
- Elevated cardiac enzymes
- Elevated LDL-C and total cholesterol

Electrocardiography

- ECG abnormalities consistent with valve disease, pericarditis, myocardial ischaemia, and arrhythmias are similar to idiopathic variants
- Sinus tachycardia is commonest ECG abnormality (caused by anaemia, fever, or primary myocardial involvement)
- Conduction disturbance including AV and BBB can be seen in SLE (either due to parenchymal cardiac involvement or antimalarial drug therapy)
- Neonatal lupus secondary to placental transfer of anti-Ro antibodies to the neonate can result in congenital heart block in approximately 2% of births from mothers with SLE carrying anti-Ro antibodies (the rate increasing if previous pregnancies affected)

Echocardiography

- LV diastolic dysfunction is present in up to half of patients and E/E' ratios are higher in SLE than healthy controls (particularly with advancing disease duration)
- Systolic septal motion velocity is lower in SLE compared with healthy controls
- Segmental wall abnormalities may indicate primary myocardial involvement in SLE

Imaging

- Large pericardial effusions may be evident on CXR
- Myocarditis and myocardial fibrosis can be identified using cardiac MRI
- Cardiac scintigraphy can be used to identify perfusion defects

Treatment

- Myocarditis:
    - Should be managed aggressively (high-dose short-term corticosteroids, cyclophosphamide and maintenance DMARD therapy)
- Pericarditis:
    - NSAIDs or short course of corticosteroids (e.g. prednisolone 30 mg daily for 1 week) often effective for acute pericarditis
    - DMARDs (e.g. methotrexate, mycophenolate, or azathioprine) should be considered for chronic or recurrent pericardial disease
    - Pericardiocentesis, pericardial window or pericardial stripping rarely needed
- Valve disease:
    - Does not necessarily warrant management if asymptomatic, resolution of valve lesions have been noted with immunosuppressive therapy
    - Anticoagulation might be considered for cases of embolic disease of valvular lesions in the presence of positive antiphospholipid antibodies
    - Valve replacement sometimes required for incompetent valves (mechanical valves preferable to porcine valves in SLE)
- Conventional CV factors should be treated aggressively to modify future CV risk
- Hydroxychloroquine has favourable effects on lipid profiles that would be expected to reduce the CV risk of SLE
- Symptomatic cardiac dysrhythmias should be managed accordingly with anti-arrhythmic therapy and/or pacemaker insertion (rarely required in SLE)

9.5.5 Antiphospholipid syndrome

Summary

- Antiphospholipid syndrome (APS) is an autoimmune condition characterized by a hypercoagulable state resulting in thrombotic complications ranging from recurrent pregnancy loss, venous thromboembolic disease, and arterial thrombosis that can affect the coronary and cerebral circulation
- Prevalence is ~450 per million
- It is one of the few autoimmune rheumatic diseases (ARD) where autoantibodies (anticardiolipin antibodies, lupus anticoagulant, and/or anti-beta$_2$-glycoprotein I) may directly contribute to disease pathogenesis and hypercoagulability
- The condition can be primary or secondary to:
    - Other ARD (notably SLE)
    - Infections
    - Malignancy
    - Drug-induced APS

Cardiac involvement in APS

Epidemiology

- Relatively rare (~25% of cases) but can be life-threatening and leading cause of mortality
- Cardiac involvement includes:
    - Valve disease (~14%)
    - Primary cardiomyopathy (~3%)
    - CAD (~8%)
- RV strain can occur secondary to PAH (~2%)

Pathophysiology

- Valve pathology is the commonest symptomatic cardiac manifestation of APS:
    - Mitral valve most frequently affected, followed by aortic valve, typically regurgitant
    - Libman–Sacks endocardial lesions are present in 10% of patients with SLE and APS, most commonly on the ventricular surface of the mitral valve
- Progressive diastolic dysfunction can occur independent of ischaemic or valve disease
- Microvascular thrombosis and endomyocardial fibrosis may contribute to pathogenesis
- Intracardiac thrombosis is rare but can result in pulmonary or systemic embolic disease
- PH can occur secondary to chronic pulmonary thromboembolic disease, primary pulmonary vascular remodelling, or mitral valve disease, and may be more common in SLE-APS
- MI occurs in ~5.5% of patients and there is a 2.7% rate of coronary by-pass re-thrombosis
- Coronary vasospasm (Prinzmetal's angina) can result in significant ischaemic events in absence of coronary thrombosis

Physical examination

- The presence of livedo reticularis (lace-like blanching erythematous changes often present on the thighs or shins) should alert clinicians to the possible presence of APS

Laboratory investigations

- Anticardiolipin antibodies, lupus anticoagulant, and anti-beta$_2$-glycoprotein I

Coronary angiography

- The absence of atherosclerotic lesions elsewhere within the coronary circulation may suggest the presence of a pro-coagulable state/embolic event following an MI

Echocardiography

- Should be considered in all patients as part of initial assessment of APS, particularly in the presence of any potentially cardiac symptoms
- Valve disease present in 30–40% of APS using TTE, rising to 82% using TOE
    - Defined as thickening (> 3 mm) or irregular nodules on atrial face of mitral valve or vascular face of aortic valve
- LV thrombus present in ~2%

Imaging

- Myocardial perfusion abnormalities present in ~30% of cases using nuclear imaging
- Cardiac CT can be used to differentiate pseudotumours from intracardiac thrombus
- CT pulmonary angiography can exclude pulmonary embolic disease
- Cardiac MRI is increasingly valuable for identifying sub-endocardial perfusion defects, myocardial fibrosis, and LV thrombus in APS

Treatment

- Valvular disease often persistent or progressive despite anticoagulation
- Most patients remain asymptomatic but valve replacement may be required
- Immunosuppression (e.g. cyclophosphamide, i.v. immunoglobulin, rituximab, or plasma exchange) can transiently reduce APL antibodies and should be considered during life-threatening manifestations, e.g. multi-organ involvement in Catastrophic APS (CAPS)
- Primary prevention with low-dose aspirin now has a role in patients with APL antibodies
- Traditional CV risk factors should be modified aggressively and potential pro-coagulable medications such as the oral contraceptive pill avoided

- Anticoagulation with warfarin (target INR 3.0) should be instituted for definite APS following arterial or venous thrombosis

9.5.6 Primary Sjögren's syndrome

Summary
- Primary Sjögren's syndrome (pSS) is a systemic autoimmune disorder characterized by lymphocytic infiltration of exocrine glands
- Predominantly affects females, with an age of onset usually between 40 and 60 years
- Common with other associated autoimmune rheumatic diseases, dysregulated inflammation often occurs within other organs and can be accompanied with vasculopathy and aberrant tissue remodelling
- The term secondary Sjögren's is used to describe sicca symptoms occurring in the context of other rheumatic diseases such as RA, SLE, or SSc

Cardiovascular involvement in pSS
Epidemiology
- Mortality is higher in pSS and CVD is leading cause of death, but no clear evidence to support a higher rate of CV events in pSS
- Pericardial effusions are common, but usually mild and asymptomatic
- Symptomatic pericarditis is rare, so it is important to exclude the occurrence of another autoimmune disease (e.g. SLE)
- Asymptomatic diastolic dysfunction (up to 50%)
- Autonomic dysfunction reported
- Case reports of atrioventricular and intraventricular conduction defects
- Myocarditis is very rare
- Smoking less common due to exacerbation of xerostomia symptoms

Pathophysiology
- Very little data investigating pathophysiology of cardiac disease in pSS
- Autopsy case report revealed atherosclerosis and lymphocyte infiltration in the bundle of His in case of sudden death

Echocardiography
- Can demonstrate mild mitral (up to 30%), tricuspid (up to 10%), and aortic regurgitation (up to 23%)
- Pericardial effusions (up to 33%)
- Left ventricular diastolic dysfunction (50%)
- PH (up to 22%)

Cardiovascular MRI
- Could help determine cardiac function and exclude myocarditis

Management
- Pericardial disease is generally asymptomatic and does not usually require intervention
- Manage valve and conduction disease as per the general population
- Case reports describe improvement of conduction defects with corticosteroid

9.5.7 Myositis spectrum disorders

Summary
- Myositis spectrum disease (MSD) includes:
  - Polymyositis (PM)
  - Dermatomyositis (Dm)
  - Cancer associated myositis (CAM)
  - Necrotizing autoimmune myositis (NAM)
  - Sporadic inclusion body myositis (IBM)
- PM and Dm are the principle and most widely investigated forms autoimmune rheumatic disease-related MSDs for cardiac disease
- Clinically overt cardiac involvement in MSD is rare (~6%), however the prevalence of subclinical cardiac disease is high and CVD disproportionately contributes to disease-related mortality (10–20% of deaths)
- Greater recognition of the burden of cardiac disease in MSD and improved methods of detection are hoped to lead to earlier identification and treatment of CVD in MSD

Cardiac involvement in MSD
Epidemiology
- Cardiac involvement appears to be more common in PM than Dm
- Prevalence of cardiac involvement varies from 9 to 72% depending on patient selection and investigative approach (higher prevalence in autopsy studies)
- Subclinical cardiac involvement in MSD in up to 70% of patients
- Cardiac symptoms not necessarily related to activity of skeletal muscle disease and can occur late in the disease course
- Symptomatic pericarditis in ~10%

Pathophysiology
- Autopsy studies have identified endomysial (PM) and perivascular (Dm) mononuclear cell inflammatory infiltrates, fibre degeneration and necrosis of cardiac myocytes, and aberrant tissue remodelling with myocardial fibrosis and regenerating muscle fibres
  - Involvement of myocardium and conduction tissue
- Microangiopathy may contribute to myocardial ischaemia (particularly in Dm), and associated Raynaud's phenomenon may be a risk factor for Prinzmetal's angina and secondary myocardial ischaemia
- Conventional CV risk factors (hypertension and diabetes) may be higher in MSD compared with the background population, increasing the risk of IHD
- ~6% prevalence of MI with a 16-fold increased death rate from MI compared with the general population

Laboratory investigations
- Troponin I more reliable biomarker of myocarditis (elevated CK-MB and Troponin T are released by regenerating skeletal muscle in MSD without cardiac involvement)
- NT-proBNP may be elevated and useful to monitor HF
- Endomyocardial biopsy is seldom necessary to diagnose cardiac involvement in MSD following the emergence of non-invasive imaging techniques

Electrocardiography

- ECG should be performed annually in asymptomatic patients and 24-hour Holter monitoring for symptoms consistent with conduction defects (e.g. pre-syncope)
- ECG and Holter abnormalities in 25–85% (e.g. frequent atrial or ventricular premature beats, atrial tachycardia, VT, AF, conduction disturbance, abnormal Q-waves, and non-specific ST/T-wave abnormalities)
    - Commonest are non-specific ST/T-wave changes and conduction defects
    - Higher prevalence of LVH and rhythm/conduction disturbances in PM vs Dm
    - Complete heart block rare but can be fatal

Echocardiography

- Abnormalities reported in up to 62%
- LV diastolic dysfunction common and increases with disease duration
- Left atrial or ventricular enlargement and LVH present in up to 15% with MSD
- Mitral valve prolapse is the commonest valve abnormality
- Small pericardial effusions are not uncommon (up to two-thirds) but usually asymptomatic
- Features of PAH can occur in patients with severe LVSD or severe ILD

Imaging

- Technetium99m-pyrophosphate (99mTc-PYP) scintigraphy may facilitate early detection of cardiac involvement and abnormal uptake has been reported in up to 57% of patients
- 99mTc-PYP scintigraphy has identified regional wall motion abnormalities (with preserved LVEF) in 15% of MSD patients and is associated with a poor prognosis
- CMR can help differentiate myocardial ischaemia from myocarditis/fibrosis (due to sparing of sub-endocardial layer on delayed enhancement) and primary myocardial inflammation appears more common in PM compared to Dm

Treatment

- Modify traditional CV risk factors and treat HF and conduction defects in accordance with existing recommendations
    - Evidence for the role of immunosuppressive therapy for HF and/or conduction disturbances is contradictory
- Pericardial disease generally asymptomatic and rarely require intervention
- Beta blockers might exacerbate Raynaud's symptoms but are not contraindicated
- Myocarditis should be managed aggressively with immunosuppressive therapy to prevent irreversible myocardial damage:
    - Controlled trials are needed to facilitate an evidence-based management
    - An appropriate treatment regime might include high-dose corticosteroids and cyclophosphamide as 'induction' treatment followed by maintenance therapy with conventional steroid-sparing agents (e.g. mycophenolate mofetil)
- B-cell-depleting therapies (such as rituximab) are likely to be more widely used to manage severe organ-specific manifestations (such as cardiac involvement) in the future
- Intravenous immunoglobulin (IVIG) may have beneficial effects but its use might be limited by volume of treatment administered
- High-dose calcium channel blockers might have a role in suspected Prinzmetal's angina in patients with MSD (particularly in association with Raynaud's phenomenon)

9.5.8 Systemic sclerosis

Summary
- Systemic sclerosis (SSc) or Scleroderma is a chronic systemic autoimmune disease characterized by inflammation, vasculopathy and fibrosis
- Usually presents between the ages of 30 to 50 years, and predominantly affects women
- CVD can present as a result of atherosclerosis or as a direct result of the disease process, termed SSc-cardiomyopathy or primary myocardial disease
- Although evidence is limited, those with poor prognostic features of SSc are most at risk of SSc-cardiomyopathy and may justify more intensive monitoring for SSc-cardiomyopathy and its complications

Cardiac involvement in SSc
Epidemiology
- 20–30% of deaths in SSc are secondary to CV causes
- Associated with poor prognosis (hazard ratio of 2:3 for death in SSc)
- Prevalence varies from 7% to 39% depending of definition of cardiac disease
- Manifestations vary from palpitations, arrhythmias, diastolic dysfunction, HF, myocarditis, MI, and sudden death (~6%)
- More common in diffuse cutaneous SSc (23–32% vs 12–23% in limited cutaneous)
- Other features associated with SSc-cardiomyopathy include:
    - Male gender
    - Antibody positivity (especially anti-topoisomerase, anti-Ku, anti-Histone, anti-RNA polymerase, and anti-U3-RNP antibodies)
    - Rapid skin thickness progression
    - Age of onset > 65 years
    - Presence of: tendon friction rubs, digital ulcers, lung involvement, myositis
- Risk of atherosclerotic-related CVD does appear to be accelerated in SSc although relatively understudied
- Valve thickening and prolapse has been seen
- Modified Medsger Severity Scale for cardiac involvement grades cardiac involvement from 0–4 (0 = no involvement, 4 = end-stage)

Pathophysiology
Myocardial fibrosis
- Cardinal feature of SSc-cardiomyopathy and can affect endocardium, myocardium, and pericardium, explaining the varied clinical presentations
- CMR studies demonstrate sparing of the sub-endocardium, an area usually affected in atherosclerotic heart disease
- Data suggest this may be preceded by micro-perfusion abnormalities
- Perfusion abnormalities can be independent of atherosclerotic heart disease and present in association with digital ulcers

Myocarditis
- Cellular inflammatory change on endomyocardial biopsies
- Described in association with peripheral myositis
- Can lead to secondary fibrosis with resolution of initial inflammatory process

Atherosclerotic-related CVD
- Endothelial dysfunction with microvascular fibro-proliferation (both hallmarks of the disease pathogenesis) may be accountable, inflammation plays much smaller role
- Invasive angiography studies have confirmed a reduced coronary reserve in patients with SSc, and evidence of calcific disease using CT angiography
- Autopsy findings have also included pericarditis, nodular abnormalities of valve tissue, and sterile vegetation

Clinical factors
- Features suggesting active SSc, e.g. progressive skin tightening or worsening ILD, would support a low threshold for investigation for SSc-cardiomyopathy

Laboratory investigations
- Raised CRP reflects active SSc
- Creatine kinase (CK) and troponin I raised in myositis, though CK may be raised if concomitant peripheral myositis
- NT-proBNP: raised in context of heart failure, PAH (now recommended in risk stratification of PAH), and also SSc-cardiomyopathy

Electrophysiology
- Abnormalities in up to half, most common being supraventricular and ventricular ectopics or conduction defects
- Late ventricular potentials are prevalent in SSc
- 24-hour ECG studies suggest more abnormalities in dcSSc

Echocardiography
- Routine tool used as a screen for PAH
- Standardized Scleroderma Doppler echocardiography protocol recommended, and tissue Doppler may be the preferred method if available
- Most common abnormalities include pericardial effusions (~18%) and diastolic dysfunction (up to 63%), independently associating with disease duration
- No echocardiography evidence for impaired LV systolic function in SSc

Cardiac MRI
- Recent studies confirm the presence of subclinical diastolic dysfunction, with normal LV systolic function, and myocardial oedema in ~12%
- Late gadolinium enhancement indicating focal fibrosis seen in up to two-thirds:
    - Usually in basal and mid-cavity LV segments
    - In all layers of myocardium, with sparing of the sub-endocardium suggesting alternative pathology to atherosclerosis
    - Associated with disease duration and poor prognostic markers
- Diffuse fibrosis is increased in SSc and a poor prognostic marker
- Perfusion defects reported in up to 79%, but can be difficult to identify atherosclerotic-related disease

Screening
- Regular clinical review
- Annual lipid profile and HbA1c monitoring

- Routine screening with CK, troponin I and NT-proBNP not yet validated for SSc-cardiomyopathy (consider annually or more frequently if symptoms)
- Annual ECG (repeating more frequently if symptoms suggest)
- Annual echocardiography (more frequently if symptoms/disease evolves)
- Stress perfusion testing as done in general population if IHD suspected
- Triggers for CMR (in the absence of other pathologies):
  - Regional wall motion abnormality on echocardiography
  - Troponin/NT-proBNP rise
  - Right/left ventricle dysfunction
  - Significant pericardial effusion
- EP studies should be considered as in standard practice

Treatment

- Modify traditional CV risk factors in accordance with existing recommendations
- Decision to treat with immunosuppression should be made with rheumatology input
- No robust evidence for the treatment of SSc-cardiomyopathy with immunosuppression
- Corticosteroid (< 15 mg/day) +/− pulse cyclophosphamide may be considered if myocarditis or other features of active SSc cardiomyopathy are evident
- Indications for cyclophosphamide include myocarditis, moderate–severe LV dysfunction (not secondary to IHD) and life-threatening cardiac arrhythmias
- Use steroids with caution due to association with SSc renal crisis
- Arrhythmias, conduction defects, heart failure, and IHD should otherwise be managed according to standard practice, e.g. pacemaker insertion for complete heart block
- Beta blockers might exacerbate Raynaud's symptoms but are not contraindicated

9.5.9 Primary systemic vasculitis

Summary

- Primary systemic vasculitides (PSV) is an umbrella term used to describe a broad range of rheumatic diseases in which the vessel wall is a key inflammatory target
- Unsurprisingly, CVD is common within this group of related disorders and a major cause of disease-associated morbidity and mortality
- PSV is typically classified according to affected vessel size with specific diseases falling under the auspices of:
  - Large (e.g. Giant Cell Arteritis (GCA), Takayasu's Arteritis (TAK))
  - Medium (e.g. Kawasaki's disease (KD), polyarteritis nodosa (PAN))
  - Small (e.g. ANCA-associated systemic vasculitis (AAV) and Henoch–Schönlein purpura (HSP))
- The small-vessel AAV include:
  - Granulomatosis with polyangiitis (GPA, formerly Wegener's granulomatosis)
  - Microscopic polyangiitis (MPA)
  - Eosinophilic granulomatosis with polyangiitis (EGPA, formerly Churg–Straus)
- Some diseases are associated with mixed vessel involvement (e.g. Behcet's disease)
- The annual incidence of PSV is ~50 patients/million but the exact prevalence is impacted by a number of factors including ethnicity, age, gender, and environmental factors

- Improved treatment of potentially life-threatening organ manifestations of PSV has resulted in longer survival and greater recognition of the long-term CV risk associated with cumulative glucocorticoid exposure

Cardiac involvement in PSV
Pathophysiology
- Endothelial activation and damage is the pathological hallmark of PSV and caused by a diverse range of pathological mechanisms (differing according to disease)
- Immune complex-mediated activation of the complement cascade occurs in PAN, SLE, and cryoglobulinaemia
- ANCA-associated vasculitis is associated with aberrant neutrophil–endothelial interaction
- Long-standing vessel wall inflammation, endothelial dysfunction, altered carotid baroreceptor sensitivity, disturbed lipid metabolism, and atherogenic fibrinolytic profiles are all putative mechanisms linking accelerated atherosclerosis with PSV
- Increased arterial stiffness and subclinical atherosclerosis has even been identified in children with KD

Cardiovascular involvement in large vessel vasculitis
- Aortic involvement in TAK often results in stenosis but aneurysmal dilation can occur
- Functional aortic regurgitation can follow ascending aorta aneurysm in GCA or TAK (likelihood increases if antiphospholipid antibodies present)
- PH identified in 15% of TAK patients
- CAD is common in TAK and includes stenosis or occlusion at the coronary ostia, diffuse or focal coronary arteritis, and coronary aneurysm formation
- TAK associated with metabolic syndrome (dyslipidaemia, diabetes mellitus) which might further increase future CV risk
- Hypertension (~85%) and CCF (~40%) common in TAK (hypertension usually caused by renovascular involvement)
- Cardiac involvement in GCA rare
- Aortic involvement in GCA can result in aortic aneurysm or dissection (sometimes preceding the disease)
- The RR of coronary heart disease is increased in GCA (often as a long-term sequelae)
- Statin use might reduce risk of developing GCA

Cardiovascular involvement in medium vessel vasculitis
- KD is commonest cause of acquired heart disease in children in the UK and is associated with coronary arterial aneurysms (20–40% of untreated patients)
- 50% of coronary aneurysmal lesions (usually smaller 3–4 mm) regress within 5 years, but giant coronary artery aneurysms (> 8 mm) unlikely to resolve and can result in stenosis, thrombosis, MI, and death
- Subclinical myocardial involvement can be identified on speckle-tracing 2-dimensional echocardiography and CMR
- ECG abnormalities reported in ~four-fifths of children with KD
- Autopsy study of PAN identified sub-epicardial coronary arteritis, perivascular fibrosis, and pericardial involvement. Clinically overt cardiac involvement rare but associated with poorer prognosis and increased mortality when present

Cardiovascular involvement in small vessel vasculitis
- Cardiac involvement most common in EGPA (~66% of adults and ~44% of children)
- Approximately 25% of patients with EGPA have symptomatic cardiac disease and is a poor prognostic factor (including if subclinical)
- EGPA associated with pericardial disease, cardiomyopathy, endomyocardial fibrosis, microangiopathy causing ischaemic events (often with normal coronary angiography), valvular insufficiency (mitral most commonly), and arrhythmias
- Clinically relevant cardiac involvement in GPA occurs in ~3.3% of patients and can include pericarditis, cardiomyopathy and conduction defects, though subclinical involvement in ~three-fifths
- Primary cardiac involvement (identified using multimodality screening) or cardiac symptoms at presentation in GPA and EGPA associated with increased mortality
- CCF occurs in ~15–20% of patients with MPA and pericardial disease in ~10%
- CAD, valve disease and endocardial involvement are all rare in GPA and MPA
- Hypertension present in ~one-third of cases of MPA with CCF affecting one-fifth of patients
- Hypertension (and pre-eclampsia) can occur many years after resolution of kidney involvement in HSP and may predispose to accelerated atherosclerosis

Cardiovascular involvement in variable-vessel vasculitis
- Behcet's disease can affects vessels of various sizes and the scope of CV involvement is broad: pericardial disease, cardiomyopathy, IHD, conduction disturbance, valvular disease, accelerated atherosclerosis, and intra-cardiac masses/thrombus

Investigation of cardiovascular involvement in PSV
- Patients with large vessel vasculitis (particularly in the presence of hypertension) should be monitored for aortic aneurysm disease
- Investigation of symptomatic cardiac disease, e.g. angina, pre-syncope, HF, PH, should follow standard approaches

Cardiovascular risk modification secondary to immunosuppressive therapy
- DMARDS (e.g. methotrexate or azathioprine) and biologic agents (e.g. rituximab and anti-TNFi) have generally favourable effects on HDL-C metabolism, atherosclerotic plaque formation, and long-term CV event risk
- In contrast, glucocorticoid increased CV risk due to its effects on lipid metabolism and hypertension, with a daily dose of 10 mg or greater increasing the risk of MI

Management
- Traditional CV risk factors should be managed aggressively in all patients
- Induction therapy for PSV typically includes short-term high-dose glucocorticoids (although steroid light approaches are gaining popularity), used alongside cytotoxic agents (e.g. cyclophosphamide) if organ-threatening manifestations present
- Low-dose aspirin is recommended in GCA and may reduce CV events
- Early intervention with immunosuppressive therapy modifies coronary aneurysm formation in KD
- Surgical intervention is sometimes necessary (e.g. renovascular or incompetent aortic valves in TAK)
- Cardiac transplantation has been associated with good outcomes in EGPA

9.5.10 Cardiac disease in miscellaneous rheumatic disorders

Summary
- In addition to the major rheumatic diseases discussed, cardiac involvement can occur in a number of the rarer rheumatic diseases, though there are a number of other multisystem diseases (e.g. sarcoid) associated with both rheumatic and cardiac manifestations that are beyond the scope of this chapter

Paget's disease of bone
- Paget's disease is a condition of disorganized bone turnover
- It results in one (monostotic) or multiple (polyostotic) areas of localized bone changes characterized by expansion of the bone cortex resulting in deformity (e.g. bowing of the femur), fracture and neurovascular compression

Cardiac issues
- Dysregulated bone turnover results in the production of highly vascular new bone that can result in high-output HF
- Electrolyte abnormalities (e.g. hypercalcaemia) can result in cardiac dysrhythmias
- The clinical features and management of high-output congestive cardiac failure are synonymous with idiopathic disease

Collagen vascular disorders
- The collagen vascular disorders are a diverse group of inherited conditions affecting the structure and function of connective tissue
- Clinical features include joint hypermobility/subluxation/dislocation, skin hypermobility, bleeding diathesis, dysmorphia (e.g. arachnodactyly in Marfan's disease), bone fracture, and organ-specific complications of connective tissue insufficiency e.g. ocular lens dislocation
- Marfan's syndrome (MS) is an autosomal dominant disorder involving mutations to the fibrillin gene affecting approximately 1 in 3000 people
- Ehlers–Danlos syndrome (EDS) is a group of related disease involving collagen production and/or function affecting approximately 1 in 5000 people

Cardiac issues
- Prolapse of the mitral or aortic valves occurs in both MS and EDS
- There is an increased incidence bacterial endocarditis affecting regurgitant valves and increased risk of dehiscence of valve prostheses
- Aortic root dilation (may result in aortic dissection) is the most serious cardiac manifestation of MS and EDS
    - Patients with suspected MS and EDS should have baseline TTE to measure the aortic root with periodic screening thereafter
    - CT or MRI is required to fully assess the aortic root and ascending aorta
- EDS is also associated with arterial rupture (particularly in the more serious type IV EDS, which has a reduced median life expectancy in the 5th decade)
- 60% of patients with type IV EDS experience a vascular complication by the age of 40 years and procedure-associated morbidity is high due to haemorrhage, graft failure, thrombosis, and aneurysms
- Postural orthostatic tachycardia syndrome (POTS) and other conduction abnormalities can occur in EDS

Relapsing polychondritis
- Relapsing polychondritis (RP) is a rare (prevalence ~5 per million) autoimmune condition characterized by inflammation of cartilaginous tissues within the ears, nose, respiratory tract, eyes, and joints
- Often occurs in conjunction with other autoimmune or haematological disorders

Cardiac issues
- Cardiac valve disease occurs in ~10% of patients with RP, mostly affecting mitral or aortic valves, and periodic TTE is recommended
- Can also experience: pericarditis, conduction disturbance, coronary artery disease

Crystal arthritides
- Includes gout (monosodium urate crystal deposition) and CPPD (calcium pyrophosphate dehydrate crystal deposition)
- Serum urate can be normal in acute attacks of gout, and synovial aspirates do not always demonstrate crystals

Cardiac issues
- Gout is associated with increased risk of atherosclerotic CVD
- Hyperuricaemia is associated with obesity, hypertension, increased lipids (particularly triglycerides), and atherosclerotic CVD
- No clear evidence to support lowering serum urate in the treatment of hypertension or CVD

Rheumatic fever
- Clinical manifestations include fever, arthritis, carditis, chorea, and cutaneous disease such as erythema nodosum
- Laboratory investigations typically reveal high inflammatory markers and a positive anti-streptolysin-O titre (ASOT)
- Prompt treatment of streptococcal pharyngitis with penicillin has resulted in a sharp decline in incidence in developed nations

Cardiac issues
- The major cardiac feature is valvulitis, typically affecting the mitral (most often) or aortic valve. Right-sided or isolated aortic valve disease is rare
- Globally, non-suppurative autoimmune valvular damage secondary to streptococcal infection is the major cause of CV morbidity in adolescence, accounting for approximately 1.4 million deaths annually
- Pericardial effusions can occur but are often asymptomatic
- Myocarditis can occur with perivascular infiltrates that can contribute to cardiac failure but does not result in overt myocardial necrosis
- Episodes can resolve without sequelae but recurrent or prolonged episodes result in rheumatic heart disease (RHD) in approximately 60% of cases
    - Clinically relevant mitral valve regurgitation is the commonest feature of RHD
- Managed primarily with antibiotics to eradicate the offending streptococcal infection and NSAIDS/corticosteroids to control active inflammation
- Secondary prophylaxis with antibiotics (e.g. penicillin V 250 mg twice daily) is used to prevent further attacks

- Management of RHD sometimes requires valve replacement or percutaneous mitral balloon commissurotomy (for less severe mitral stenosis with favourable valve morphology) to manage symptomatic valve compromise

Further reading

Agca R, Heslinga SC, Rollefstad S, Heslinga M, McInnes IB, Peters MJ, Kvien TK, Dougados M, Radner H, Atzeni F, Primdahl J, Södergren A, Wallberg Jonsson S, van Rompay J, Zabalan C, Pedersen TR, Jacobsson L, de Vlam K, Gonzalez-Gay MA, Semb AG, Kitas GD, Smulders YM, Szekanecz Z, Sattar N, Symmons DP, Nurmohamed MT. EULAR recommendations for cardiovascular disease risk management in patients with rheumatoid arthritis and other forms of inflammatory joint disorders: 2015/2016 update. *Ann Rheum Dis*. 2017 Jan;76(1):17–28. doi: 10.1136/annrheumdis-2016-209775. Epub 2016 Oct 3

Bissell LA, Anderson M, Burgess M, Chakravarty K, Coghlan G, Dumitru RB, Graham L, Ong V, Pauling JD, Plein S, Schlosshan D, Woolfson P, Buch MH. Consensus best practice pathway of the UK Systemic Sclerosis Study group: management of cardiac disease in systemic sclerosis. *Rheumatology (Oxford)*. 2017 Jun 1;56(6):912–21. doi: 10.1093/rheumatology/kew488

Doria A, Iaccarino L, Sarzi-Puttini P, Atzeni F, Turriel M, Petri M. Cardiac involvement in systemic lupus erythematosus. *Lupus*. 2005;14(9):683–6. doi: 10.1191/0961203305lu2200oa

Misra DP, Shenoy SN. Cardiac involvement in primary systemic vasculitis and potential drug therapies to reduce cardiovascular risk. *Rheumatol Int*. 2017 Jan;37(1):151–67. doi: 10.1007/s00296-016-3435-1. Epub 2016 Feb 17

O'Sullivan M, Bruce IN, Symmons DP. Cardiovascular risk and its modification in patients with connective tissue diseases. *Best Pract Res Clin Rheumatol*. 2016 Feb;30(1):81–94. doi: 10.1016/j.berh.2016.03.003. Epub 2016 May 26

Woldu B, Bloomfield GS. Rheumatic heart disease in the twenty-first century. *Curr Cardiol Rep*. 2016 Oct;18(10):96. doi: 10.1007/s11886-016-0773-2

9.6

The patient with erectile dysfunction

Greg Shaw, Piotr Pawel Swiniarski, and David Ralph

TABLE OF CONTENTS
9.6.1 The patient with erectile dysfunction 923
9.6.2 Epidemiology 923
9.6.3 Aetiology and- pathophysiology 923
9.6.4 Natural history 924
9.6.5 Symptoms 924
9.6.6 Examination and investigation 924
9.6.7 Management 925
9.6.8 Follow-up 927

9.6.1 The patient with erectile dysfunction

- Erectile dysfunction (ED) is defined as the persistent inability to attain and maintain an erection sufficient to permit satisfactory sexual intercourse
- It should be regarded as a potential warning sign for CVD, and its diagnosis can improve the sensitivity of screening for asymptomatic CVD in men with DM
- ED significantly increases the risk of CVD, CAD and stroke, which all cause mortality, and the increase is probably independent of conventional CV risk factors
- The risks of CVD and death increase steadily with the severity of ED
- ED shares both unmodifiable and modifiable common risk factors with CVD (e.g. obesity, DM, dyslipidaemia, metabolic syndrome, lack of exercise, and smoking)

9.6.2 Epidemiology

- There is a high prevalence and incidence of ED worldwide, affecting up to 50% of men aged 40–70 years
- The overall prevalence in men aged 40–70 years in the Massachusetts Male Aging Study (MMAS) was 52%; the severity was: mild in 17.2%, moderate in 25.2%, severe in 9.6%
- ED has an age-related increase from 2.3% to 53.4% among men 30–80 years old, as well as age-related increase in disease severity
- One in four patients seeking help for the first time for ED is younger than 40 years
- Almost 50% of presenting patients have severe ED

9.6.3 Aetiology and pathophysiology

- Erection is a neurovascular phenomenon under psychological control, and either or both can cause ED

- Vasculogenic (70%)
    - CVD (hypertension, CAD, peripheral vasculopathy, etc.)
    - DM
    - Hyperlipidaemia
    - Smoking
- Neurogenic
    - Central (e.g. degenerative disorders, spinal cord trauma/disease, stroke)
    - Peripheral
        - Neuropathy: DM, CKD, polyneuropathy
        - Iatrogenic: Major pelvic surgery or localized radiotherapy
- Anatomical (e.g. hypo-/epi-spadias, micropenis, Peyronie's disease, penile cancer, phimosis)
- Hormonal (e.g. hypogonadism, hyperprolactinaemia, endocrine disorders)
- Drug-induced (e.g. antihypertensives, antidepressants, antipsychotics, antiandrogens, recreational drugs)
- Psychogenic (e.g. generalized or situational)
- Traumatic (e.g. penile or pelvic fracture)

9.6.4 Natural history

- With organic causes, ED usually starts as mild or moderate; however if the risk factors are not managed it will progress to severe disease
- In traumatic, post-operative cases ED has an acute onset and is usually severe
- In psychogenic cases, ED has an acute and intermittent course depending on specific trigger factors however, morning erections are always preserved

9.6.5 Symptoms

- Difficulty/inability to attain or maintain an erection
- Decrease in penile rigidity and failure of penetration
- Lack of spontaneous night and/or morning erections (in organic and post-traumatic ED)

9.6.6 Examination and investigation

- Basic work-up to identify common causes of ED, reversible risk factors, and psychosocial status
    - Onset, course, and duration of ED
    - Medical and surgical history
    - Sexual history:
        - Sexual orientation
        - Relationship issues with partner
        - Previous traumatic sexual experience
        - Frequency of intercourse
        - Enquire about libido, quality of erection, ability to penetrate partner, ejaculation, orgasm, and morning erections
    - Physical examination (secondary sexual characters, penile and scrotal examination)
    - Laboratory testing (FBC, lipid profile, testosterone, prolactin, fasting glucose)

Table 9.6.1 Cardiac risk stratification in ED.

Low-risk category	Intermediate-risk category	High-risk category
Asymptomatic, < 3 risk factors for CAD (excluding sex)	≥ 3 risk factors for CAD (excluding sex)	High-risk arrhythmias
Mild, stable angina (evaluated and/or being treated)	Moderate, stable angina	Unstable or refractory angina
Uncomplicated previous MI	Recent MI (> 2, < 6 weeks)	Recent MI (< 2 weeks)
LVD/CHF (NYHA class I or II)	LVD/CHF (NYHA class III)	LVD/CHF (NYHA class IV)
Post-successful coronary revascularization	Non-cardiac sequelae of atherosclerotic disease (e.g. stroke, peripheral vascular disease)	Hypertrophic obstructive and other cardiomyopathies
Controlled hypertension		Uncontrolled hypertension
Mild valvular disease		Moderate-to-severe valvular disease

CAD—coronary artery disease; CHF—congestive heart failure; LVD—left ventricular dysfunction; MI—myocardial infarction; NYHA—New York Heart Association

- Extended evaluation
    - Nocturnal penile tumescence and rigidity test
    - Intracavernous injection test
    - Colour Duplex Doppler ultrasound of the penis (Vmax < 25 cm/s = arteriogenic ED)
    - Cavernosometry and cavernosography for selected cases showing signs of veno-occlusive dysfunction on penile duplex
    - Internal pudendal arteriography for selected cases showing signs of reduced penile blood flow on penile duplex
    - Neurological studies (e.g. bulbocavernosus reflex latency, nerve conduction studies) for selected cases
    - Endocrinological evaluation
    - Psychiatric assessment
    - Penile abnormalities requiring surgical correction
- Cardiac risk stratification (based on 2nd and 3rd Princeton Consensus)—Table 9.6.1 and Figure 9.6.1
    - Low risk—initiate or resume sexual activity or treatment for sexual dysfunction
    - Intermediate risk—CV assessment and re-stratification
    - High risk—sexual activity deferred until stabilization of cardiac condition

9.6.7 Management

- Identification of all the risk factors and possible causes of ED
- Modifying reversible risk factors and treatment in curable causes
- Lifestyle management: e.g. smoking, recreational drug use, diet, and exercise
- Patient and partner education and psychosexual counselling for selected cases
- Lifestyle modification and pharmacotherapy for CV risk factors may improve sexual function in men with ED

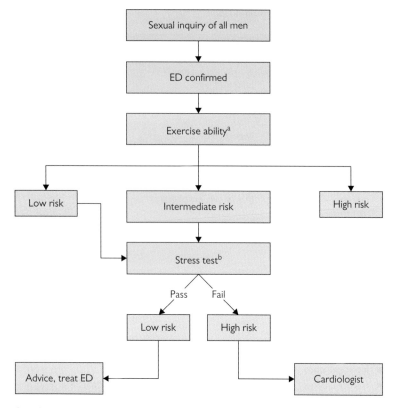

[a] Sexual activity is equivalent to walking 1 mile on the flat in 20 min or briskly climbing two fights of stairs in 10 s.
[b] Sexual activity is equivalent to 4 min of the Bruce treadmill protocol.

Figure 9.6.1 EAU Guidelines treatment algorithm for determining level of sexual activity according to cardiac risk in ED (based on 3rd Princeton Consensus)
Reproduced from Hatzimouratidis K, Amar E, Eardley I, et al; European Association of Urology. Guidelines on male sexual dysfunction: erectile dysfunction and premature ejaculation. *Eur Urol.* 2010 May;57(5):804–14. doi: 10.1016/j.eururo.2010.02.020 with permission from Elsevier.

First-line treatment—medical management
- PDE5i:
    - Sildenafil (Viagra)
    - Tadalafil (Cialis)
    - Vardenafil (Levitra/Staxyn)
    - Avanafil (Stendra/Spedra)
- Side effects of PDE5Is
    - Headache
    - Flushing
    - Rhinitis
    - Altered (blurred) vision
    - Palpitations
    - Dyspepsia

- Myalgia
    - Priapism
- Safety issues for PDE5 inhibitors
    - All PDE5Is are contraindicated in:
        - patients who have suffered from an MI, stroke, or life-threatening arrhythmia within the last 6 months
        - patients with resting hypotension (blood pressure < 90/50 mmHg) or hypertension (blood pressure > 170/100 mmHg)
        - patients with unstable angina, angina with sexual intercourse, or HF categorized as NYHA grade IV
    - Nitrates are *absolutely contraindicated* with PDE5 inhibitors
    - Co-administration of PDE5Is with antihypertensive agents (ACEi, ARB, calcium blocker, beta blocker, and diuretic) may result in small additive decreases in BP
    - All PDE5Is show some interaction with alpha blockers, which under some conditions may result in orthostatic hypotension
    - Dosage adjustment with interfering medication

Second-line treatment

- Vacuum-erection devices (VED)
- Low-intensity extracorporeal shockwave therapy (LI-SWT)
- Alprostadil
    - intracavernosal injections (Caverject™, Edex/Viridal™)
    - intraurethral pellet (MUSE™)
- Other intracavernosal injections (papaverine, phentolamine, Invicorp)
- Possible side effects include: priapism, bruises/swelling of penis, urethral injury, pain in penis/urethra/testicles, dizziness, rash, penile discharge, haematuria
- Priapism is an andrological emergency, and if prolonged (> 4 hours) erection occurs this requires emergency treatment

Third-line treatment—surgical management

- Penile (corpora cavernosa) implants

Future therapy

- Stem cell therapy
- Gene therapy
- Platelet-rich plasma therapy

9.6.8 Follow-up

- Assess response to treatment
- Consider combination therapy if needed, e.g. daily tadalafil + on-demand sildenafil/daily tadalafil + on-demand ICI/daily tadalfil + shockwave therapy
- Assess treatment compliance and side effects
- Ask about patient's and partner satisfaction

Further reading

Gandaglia G, Briganti A, Jackson G, Kloner RA, Montorsi F, Montorsi P, Vlachopoulos C. A systematic review of the association between erectile dysfunction and cardiovascular disease. *Eur Urol.* 2014 May;65(5):968–78. doi: 10.1016/j.eururo.2013.08.023. Epub 2013 Aug 23. PMID: 24011423

Gupta BP, Murad MH, Clifton MM, Prokop L, Nehra A, Kopecky SL. The effect of lifestyle modification and cardiovascular risk factor reduction on erectile dysfunction: a systematic review and meta-analysis. *Arch Intern Med.* 2011 Nov 14;171(20):1797–803. doi: 10.1001/archinternmed.2011.440. Epub 2011 Sep 12. PMID: 21911624

Nehra A, Jackson G, Miner M, Billups KL, Burnett AL, Buvat J, Carson CC, Cunningham GR, Ganz P, Goldstein I, Guay AT, Hackett G, Kloner RA, Kostis J, Montorsi P, Ramsey M, Rosen R, Sadovsky R, Seftel AD, Shabsigh R, Vlachopoulos C, Wu FC. The Princeton III Consensus recommendations for the management of erectile dysfunction and cardiovascular disease. *Mayo Clin Proc.* 2012 Aug;87(8):766–78. doi: 10.1016/j.mayocp.2012.06.015. PMID: 22862865; PMCID: PMC3498391

CHAPTER 10

GENETICS AND CLINICAL PHARMACOLOGY

10.1

Genetics

Victoria McKay and Stewart Brown

TABLE OF CONTENTS

10.1.1 Introduction 931
10.1.2 Mendelian inheritance 932
    Autosomal dominant inheritance 932
    Autosomal recessive inheritance 933
    X-linked recessive inheritance 933
10.1.3 Non-Mendelian inheritance 935

Mitochondrial inheritance 935
Multifactorial/polygenic inheritance 936
Mosaicism 936
Chromosomes 936
10.1.4 Chromosomal and genetic testing 937

10.1.1 Introduction

- Genetics in cardiology is an evolving field
- There is a significant overlap between inherited conditions
- The main roles of genetics within cardiology are:
    - To confirm diagnosis
    - To allow screening and preventative treatment in at-risk family members
    - Prediction of phenotype; e.g. *LMNA* variants confer a high risk of sudden cardiac death (SCD)
    - Commence genotype-specific treatments e.g. sodium channel blockers in Long QT Syndrome 3
- A gene is a sequence of nucleotides that codes for a specific product. This may be instructions on how to build a certain protein like a cardiac sodium channel (SCN5A) but genes can also have other functions, e.g. regulation of other genes
- Different versions of the same gene exist which are called alleles. Each person usually has two alleles per gene; one from each parent
- To have a single disease-causing allele (and one non-disease allele) is termed a heterozygote
- To have two identical disease-causing alleles is termed a homozygote
- The terms variants and mutations are used interchangeably: the term 'variant' will be used throughout this chapter as it is the preferred term in the genetic literature at present
- Monogenic diseases are usually caused when a person is a heterozygote or a homozygote for disease-causing variants

10.1.2 Mendelian inheritance

- Mendelian inheritance is a set of genetic principles for monogenic diseases
- All of the genes, excluding those on the sex chromosomes and the mitochondrial genes, are termed autosomal
- Autosomal genes usually occur in pairs (one from each parent)
- Inheritance can be autosomal or X-linked
- Mitochondrial inheritance does not follow Mendelian segregation patterns

Autosomal dominant inheritance

- Dominant inheritance patterns occur when the presence of a single variant in one of a pair of autosomal genes, known as the **genotype**, causes a specific set of clinical features, known as the **phenotype**.
- Variants can either be inherited from a parent or occur *de novo* (a spontaneous new variant).
- The offspring of an individual with an autosomal dominant condition has a 50:50 chance of inheriting the disease, irrespective of gender (see Figure 10.1.1).
- **Penetrance** is the proportion of people with a specific genotype who manifest the phenotype.
- For some dominant conditions, the presence of a disease variant may not always lead to the phenotype; this is termed **incomplete penetrance**.
- Some conditions show **variable expression**, meaning different signs and symptoms can occur in a population with the same genetic condition, with some more severely affected than others.

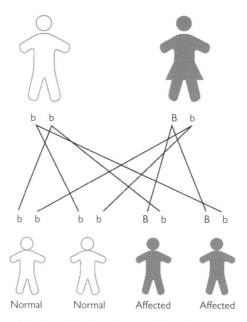

Figure 10.1.1 Autosomal dominant inheritance from an affected parent

Reproduced from Discern Genetics, available at www.discern-genetics.org. Copyright University of Oxford 2005, with permission from the University of Oxford

Autosomal recessive inheritance

- If the presence of a variant in both copies of an autosomal gene is required to cause a condition it is termed autosomal recessive.
- Usually, each parent has one allele with the variant and one allele without and is termed a **carrier**.
- There is a one in four chance of having an affected child, irrespective of gender, if both parents are carriers (see Figure 10.1.2).
- As a general rule:
    - Carriers of recessive conditions do not display features of the condition
    - A person with variants in both copies of an autosomal recessive gene will be affected by the condition, although there are rare exceptions such as the low penetrance in hereditary haemochromatosis

X-linked recessive inheritance

- Apart from a small number of genes present on both the X and Y chromosomes (the pseudo-autosomal region) most of the genes on the X chromosome are present in two copies in females and one copy in males.
- Most X-linked conditions are carried by females but only affect males (**X-linked recessive inheritance**) (Figure 10.1.3).
- X-linked recessive inheritance should be suspected when there is mother-to-son transmission.
- All daughters of an affected father will be carriers for that condition and all sons will be unaffected (see Figure 10.1.4).
- Rarely, females may be affected by these conditions, most commonly where there is also an abnormality or absence of the other X chromosome, i.e. Turner syndrome.

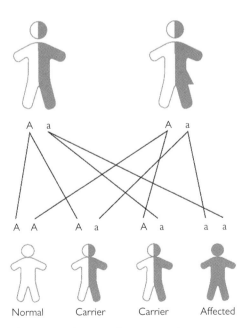

Figure 10.1.2 Autosomal recessive inheritance from two carrier parents

Reproduced from Discern Genetics, available at www.discern-genetics.org. Copyright University of Oxford 2005, with permission from the University of Oxford

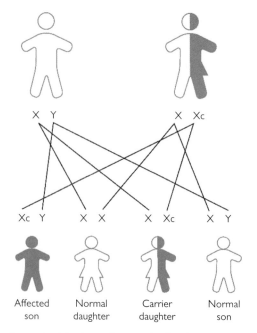

Figure 10.1.3 X-linked recessive inheritance from carrier female
Reproduced from Discern Genetics, available at www.discern-genetics.org. Copyright University of Oxford 2005

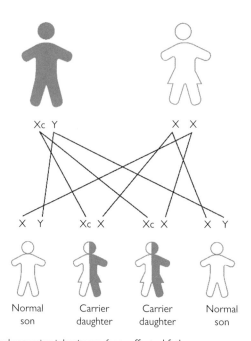

Figure 10.1.4 X-linked recessive inheritance from affected father
Reproduced from Discern Genetics, available at www.discern-genetics.org. Copyright University of Oxford 2005

- Some X-linked conditions can give rise to the condition in females: **X-linked dominant inheritance**.

10.1.3 Non-Mendelian inheritance

Mitochondrial inheritance

- Disorders of the mitochondria are an uncommon but important cause of cardiac disease, most commonly cardiomyopathy and/or conduction disease, either as an isolated finding or as a part of multi-system disease.
- Mitochondria have their own DNA, although the majority of genes essential for mitochondrial function are in the nuclear genome (these usually cause mitochondrial disease in an autosomal recessive pattern).
- Mitochondria are only passed to the resulting embryo from the ovum and not the sperm (see Figure 10.1.5).
- All children of a mother with a mitochondrial variant will inherit it, whereas no children of a father with a mitochondrial variant will inherit it.
- There are tens to hundreds of mitochondria in each cell and frequently only a proportion of the mitochondria in a cell will have a particular variant. This level can vary in different cells, tissues, and organs, affecting the phenotype and known as **heteroplasmy**.
- A threshold level of the variant must be surpassed to give rise to clinical features, this level being variable depending on the particular variant, organ, and condition involved.

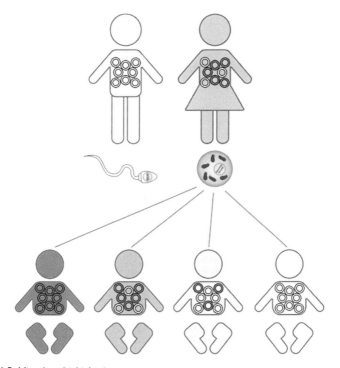

Figure 10.1.5 Mitochondrial inheritance
Reproduced with kind permission of Clinical Tools Inc.

Multifactorial/polygenic inheritance
- This refers to the majority of medical disorders, where multiple genes and environmental factors interact to give rise to the condition.
- The importance of the genetic component varies between conditions, and even between individuals with the same disorder.
- The role of a single individual genetic factor is likely to be very small but together these factors have a cumulative effect. This either then leads to the condition itself or increases the risk of a disease.

Mosaicism
- When a new DNA mutation occurs after several cell divisions of a fertilised egg, not all the cells in the body will be affected.
- This variant will then only be seen in a proportion of cells of the body, known as **mosaicism**.
- In general, those with a mosaic variant will have a milder clinical phenotype than those with the equivalent non-mosaic variant.

Chromosomes
- 22 autosomal chromosomes are inherited, one from each parent, as well a sex chromosome from each parent, giving rise to a complete set of 23 pairs.
- The sex chromosomes are XX in females (see Figure 10.1.7) and XY in males.
- Each chromosome has two arms joined by a centromere, the short arm (termed p) and the long arm (termed q).
- Genetic material is organized within the cell nucleus as chromosomes.
- Chromosomes incorporate DNA and structural proteins (e.g. histones).

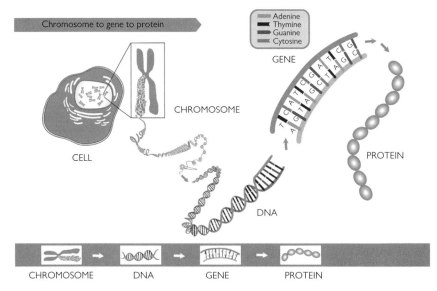

Figure 10.1.6 Representation of the organization of genetic material and translation of genes into proteins

Illustration from *Genetic Counseling Aids* 5th Edition. Copyright Greenwood Genetic Center 2007. Reproduced with kind permission from Greenwood Genetic Centre

10.1.4 Chromosomal and genetic testing

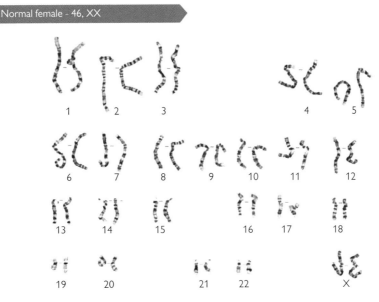

Figure 10.1.7 Normal female karyotype
Illustration from *Genetic Counseling Aids* 5th Edition. Copyright Greenwood Genetic Center 2007. Reproduced with kind permission from Greenwood Genetic Centre

- Structural proteins facilitate efficient packaging of DNA and assist in the regulation of gene transcription (the copying of DNA into RNA) and replication (see Figure 10.1.6).
- The complement of chromosomes is referred to as the karyotype.

10.1.4 Chromosomal and genetic testing

Chromosomal testing
- Testing of chromosomes in cardiology is most frequently performed in congenital heart disease but may also be appropriate with other cardiac disease, particularly in the presence of other physical or developmental problems.
- Array comparative genomic hybridisation (array CGH or microarray), allows analysis at a much higher resolution, permitting detection of copy-number variants across the whole chromosomal complement, and detecting both recurrent abnormalities (such as 22q11.2 microdeletion) as well as novel regions of chromosome imbalance or copy-number variants.
- More specific chromosome tests may sometimes be appropriate, e.g. fluorescent *in-situ* hybridization (FISH) testing for specific disorders of chromosomal copy-number variants, such as 22q11.2 microdeletion.
- If chromosome analysis is being considered, discussing with or referring to clinical genetics may be appropriate.

Genetic testing
Background
- Identifying the patient's genotype can support diagnosis, inform prognosis and risk of certain clinical events, facilitate genotype-specific treatment and pre-implantation genetic testing, and identify at-risk family members.

- Next-generation sequencing refers to the highly efficient methods by which large volumes of DNA are tested for variants against a reference sequence.
- DNA from a patient is denatured and exposed to probes, strands of DNA complementary to those of interest to the clinician. These segments of double-stranded DNA are labelled and read by the sequencer.
- This information then undergoes bio-informatic quality control before the results are made available.
- A selection of variants in known disease-causing genes can be tested for using this technology, known as **gene panel testing**.
- Sequencing beyond gene panels may be used in paediatrics, rare disease, and as a research tool (to find new variants), e.g. **whole exome sequencing** (WES) and **whole genome sequencing** (WGS).
- The protein-coding DNA sequences are found in the exons which make up about 1% of the total DNA in an individual's genome. Collectively, all of the exons are known as the exome. Most pathogenic variants are found in exons.
- WES can be useful when gene panel testing is negative but there remains a strong suspicion of familial disease.
- WGS tests all of the introns and exons (coding and non-coding DNA) and needs a greater amount of computing power to assess (generates > 100× more data than WES).
- In cases of suspected sudden cardiac death and a normal post mortem, a molecular autopsy may be helpful to inform cascade screening in at-risk family members.
- DNA from the spleen of the affected individual can be tested for variants associated with conditions causing sudden cardiac death, such as channelopathy and cardiomyopathy variants.

Interpreting a laboratory genetic test result
- An EDTA blood sample is sent to a regional genomics laboratory hub; specific tests may only be available in a small number of centres in the country.
- Reports should be interpreted in collaboration between laboratory scientists, specialist cardiologists, and clinical geneticists.
- Not all genetic variants cause disease. Benign variation exists between individuals and accounts for the differences seen between individuals like eye colour, blood type, etc. These variants are highly prevalent in the population and are known as **polymorphisms**.
- A variant may be present in a known disease-causing gene but not all variants will cause disease. This is because some variants (polymorphisms) do not negatively affect gene function.
- Variants are categorised depending on the likely pathogenicity (Table 10.1.1). Pathogenicity is determined by variant type (e.g. missense), variant databases, literature review, frequency in the general population, and *in silico* analysis using software tools. Pathogenic variants are deemed to be causative of the disease in question.
    - Missense variants are defined as those where the nucleotide change leads to the substitution of one amino acid for a different amino acid.
- **Variants of unknown significance** (VUS) are variants found in known disease-causing genes but currently lack evidence to meet the pathogenicity criteria. They are not a positive result and must be treated with caution. They are not suitable for cascade screening. As new evidence arises, some VUS may be re-classified as benign and some as pathogenic, whilst others may not accrue any new evidence and remain a VUS.
- Where a pathogenic variant is identified the clinical diagnosis is confirmed and family genetic screening is possible.

Table 10.1.1 American College of Medical Genetics classification system of variants.

Class	Pathogenicity	Description
1	Pathogenic	• This variant directly contributes to the development of disease • Some pathogenic variants may not be fully penetrant • In the case of recessive or X-linked conditions, a single pathogenic variant may not be sufficient to cause disease on its own • Additional evidence is not expected to alter the classification of this variant
2	Likely pathogenic	• There is a high likelihood (greater than 90% certainty) that this variant is disease-causing • Additional evidence is expected to confirm this assertion of pathogenicity, but there is a small chance that new evidence may demonstrate that this variant does not have clinical significance
3	Uncertain significance	• There is not enough information at this time to support a more definitive classification of this variant
4	Likely benign	• This variant is not expected to have a major effect on disease; however, the scientific evidence is currently insufficient to prove this conclusively • Additional evidence is expected to confirm this assertion, but we cannot fully rule out the possibility that new evidence may demonstrate that this variant can contribute to disease
5	Benign	• This variant does not cause disease

- In the setting of a diagnostic test it is rare that absence of a variant will change the clinical diagnosis.
- In a predictive test for an at-risk but unaffected relative, the absence of a variant is usually sufficient to reassure the patient they are not at increased risk. In this scenario, ongoing clinical screening is usually not required.
- Information about individual genes, variants and their role in disease can be found at https://www.omim.org/ and https://www.ncbi.nlm.nih.gov/clinvar/.

Genetic counselling

- Genetic counselling is the process of helping people understand and adapt to the medical, psychological, and familial implications of the genetic contributions to disease.
- All patients who have or are at-risk of an inherited heart disease should have genetic counselling.
- Key points to communicate about a potentially inherited heart conditions include:
    - The genetic origin (and certainty of this)
    - The likely mode of inheritance
    - The probability of other family members and children being affected
    - The clinical features of the disorder and its natural history
    - Particular advice regarding pregnancy
    - The role and benefits of cardiac screening for the family
    - The availability and role of genetic testing
    - Information regarding appropriate patient associations and sources of reliable and understandable medical information.

Family testing

- **Predictive genetic testing**, often referred to as **cascade screening**, offers a DNA blood test to identify whether an at-risk relative carries the same pathogenic variant detected in the first person tested in a family, who is known as the **proband**.
- Genetic testing of first-degree relatives of an affected individual is frequently indicated as an initial step in inherited heart diseases where dominant inheritance is likely. Immediate testing of more distant relatives is less commonly indicated.
- The main aim of cascade screening is to identify those who would benefit from clinical investigations, treatment, health and lifestyle advice, or discussion of reproductive options, and/or to clarify whether other family members may be affected.
- The availability of a predictive genetic test, i.e. a test for a disorder that a patient may develop in the future but does not currently have signs or symptoms of, can help clarify some of these issues.
- Only class 4 and class 5 pathogenic variants should be used in cascade screening.

Drawing a pedigree

- Information on pedigree drawing, along with many other useful educational resources, can be found at the National Genetics Education and Development Centre website (see Further reading).
- In brief, when drawing a pedigree (see Figure 10.1.8):
  - Males are drawn as a square and females as a circle
  - It is easiest to start with the youngest generation and work back up generations on both sides
  - The proband is marked with an arrow, often to the bottom left
  - Those affected by the condition are shaded in, and a key should be drawn
  - Where someone is deceased a line through the symbol is used
  - Siblings are traditionally drawn from eldest on the left to youngest on the right, and in couples the male is on the left and female on the right.

Genetic testing in cardiomyopathy

- Mendelian pattern of inheritance is common, predominantly autosomal dominant.
- Inheritance pattern can sometimes be determined from the pedigree.
- Genetic testing in cardiomyopathies has many potential issues:
  - A proportion of genes are unrecognised and some of those recognised may not be available as a clinical test
  - **Genetic heterogeneity**, i.e. variants in several different genes, can all give the same phenotype
  - Most cardiomyopathies are clinically variable despite there being the same underlying cause: **variable expressivity**
  - A proportion of those with a pathogenic genetic variant do not display clinical features: **incomplete penetrance**. This is more common in younger individuals as features may develop over time, known as **age-related penetrance**
  - Incomplete penetrance makes it difficult to remove individuals from ongoing cardiac screening on the basis of one normal clinical assessment.
- Family clinical surveillance is often instituted following the diagnosis of cardiomyopathy, unless an acquired cause is demonstrated.
- Continued follow up through adulthood is often advised. The age to which this is continued will usually be based on clinical judgement and patient wishes. Current recommendations are

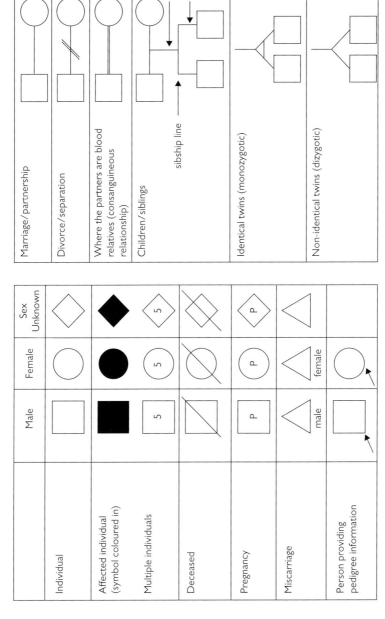

Figure 10.1.8 Examples of commonly used pedigree symbols and relationship lines

Reproduced with permission of the National Genetics Education and Development Centre (http://www.geneticseducation.nhs.uk/), from 'Taking and Drawing a Family History', Copyright 2008 NHS National Genetics Education and Development Centre

every 3–5 years when there is no known familial variant, with those who do have an identified familial variant being seen more frequently.
- The age to commence clinical screening is also uncertain. Starting between 8 and 12 years old may be appropriate for most cardiomyopathies.

Further reading

Genomics England Panel App: https://panelapp.genomicsengland.co.uk/

HEE resources for drawing a family pedigree: https://www.genomicseducation.hee.nhs.uk/wp-content/uploads/2019/05/Family-history-worksheet-blank.pdf

Kumar D, Elliott P. *Principles and Practice of Clinical Cardiovascular Genetics.* Oxford: Oxford University Press, 2010.

National NHS E Genomics Test Directory: https://www.england.nhs.uk/publication/national-genomic-test-directories/

10.2

Clinical pharmacology

Christopher N. Floyd and Alexander Carpenter

TABLE OF CONTENTS

10.2.1 Pharmacokinetics 943
10.2.2 Pharmacogenetics 945
10.2.3 Cardiovascular side effects of non-cardiovascular drugs 945
  QT prolongation 946
  Left ventricular impairment 946
  Bradycardia 946
  Metabolic syndrome and accelerated atherosclerosis 946

10.2.1 Pharmacokinetics

- Pharmacokinetics (PK) describes the passage of a drug and its metabolites through the body as a function of time
- Broadly it can be thought of as 'what the body does to a drug', and contrasts with pharmacodynamics (PD) which describes 'what the drug does to the body'
- There are four PK processes which must be considered and are abbreviated to the acronym ADME:
  - **Absorption**—how the drug enters the body (e.g. from the gastrointestinal tract, intravenous, or transdermal)
  - **Distribution**—how the drug moves between compartments (e.g. from plasma into tissues)
  - **Metabolism**—how the drug is changed to a different molecule (e.g. hepatic metabolism)
  - **Excretion**—how the drug is removed from the body (e.g. biliary or renal excretion)
  (The term 'elimination' is also used to combine metabolism and excretion)
- Commonly, PK is described in terms of the plasma concentration-time curve as phlebotomy provides an easy method of measuring drug concentrations compared to tissue biopsy or cerebrospinal fluid sampling
- However, it is important to note that a drug will only work if/when it reaches its target, which is clinically evident when administering:
  - Rapidly acting intravenous drugs, which usually take a few minutes to demonstrate effect (e.g. IV flecainide), vs
  - Oral drugs, which generally take much longer as absorption from the gastrointestinal tract is not instantaneous
- The plasma concentration-time curve introduces a number of important descriptive PK parameters (illustrated in Figure 10.2.1):
  - The maximum plasma concentration (C_{max})
  - Time to maximum plasma concentration (t_{max})
  - Half-life ($t_{1/2}$)
  - Total drug exposure (area under curve; AUC)

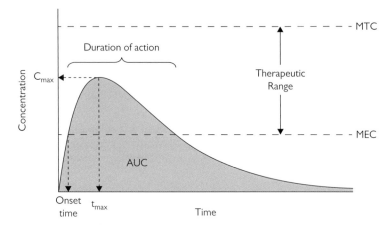

Figure 10.2.1 Plasma-concentration-time-curve showing a typical profile following administration of an oral medication; Cmax, maximum concentration; tmax, time to Cmax; AUC, area under the curve; MEC, minimum effective concentration; MTC, maximum tolerated concentration

Reproduced from Mehrotra N, Gupta M, Kovar A, Meibohm B. The role of pharmacokinetics and pharmacodynamics in phosphodiesterase-5 inhibitor therapy. *Int J Impot Res.* 2007 May-Jun;19(3):253–64. doi: 10.1038/sj.ijir.3901522 with permission from Springer Nature.

- However, the descriptive PK parameters do not provide any insight on how the body is handling a drug, but rather the *outcome* of ADME processes. We therefore need to consider three conceptual parameters:
    - **Clearance (CL)**—the ability of the body to eliminate (a combination of metabolism and excretion) a drug from the systemic circulation (expressed as volume/time)
    - **Bioavailability (F)**—the proportion of an administered dose that reaches the systemic circulation (expressed as a percentage)
    - **Volume of distribution (V)**—the theoretical volume that would be necessary to contain the total amount of an administered drug at the same concentration that it is in plasma (expressed as a volume)
- The relevance of both descriptive and conceptual PK parameters to clinicians is that they determine dosing regimens in both health and disease:
    - *The half-life* (time taken by plasma concentration to fall by 50%) determines how quickly a drug will reach steady state (~4–5 $t_{1/2}$), washout when stopped (~4–5 $t_{1/2}$), and the dosing interval required to maintain steady-state with acceptable fluctuations in plasma concentrations. As it is derived from the relationship between V and CL ($t_{1/2}$~V/CL), conditions which affect either parameter will alter $t_{1/2}$. For example, renal failure will reduce CL for a renally excreted drug and correspondingly increase $t_{1/2}$
    - *The bioavailability* determines how dosing differs between different routes (e.g. intravenous versus oral). Bioavailability of oral drugs is invariably less than intravenous due to both variable absorption and first-pass metabolism
    - *Drug toxicity* is often determined by C_{max} (e.g. ototoxicity with intravenous furosemide or postural hypotension with doxazocin) and so rate of absorption might need to be modified (e.g. furosemide infusions or modified-release doxazocin)
- Changes in PK parameters (both acute and chronic) will have a greater effect on drugs with a narrow therapeutic range (alternatively called therapeutic index or therapeutic window) between which they achieve their desirable pharmacological effect (minimum effective concentration; MEC)

and unacceptable toxicity (maximum tolerated concentration; MTC). Examples of cardiovascular drugs with a narrow therapeutic range include digoxin, flecainide, and warfarin
- It should be noted that the most common reason for therapeutic failure is medication non-adherence

N.B. Strategies to address this can be found in the 2009 NICE guidelines, 'Medicines adherence: involving patients in decisions about prescribed medicines and supporting adherence'

10.2.2 Pharmacogenetics

- Pharmacogenetics is the study of how an individual's genes affect their response to a drug, dealing with both inherited and acquired genetic variation, and spans both PK and PD
- The term 'pharmacogenomics' is often used interchangeably with 'pharmacogenetics', but the former encompasses the effects of multiple genes on drugs response (e.g. a genome-wide association approach) compared to the latter which focuses on single drug–gene interaction
- The potential for genes to vary drug response (usually through single nucleotide polymorphisms; SNPs) is unlimited, but there are common variants which are relevant to cardiovascular medicine. Table 10.2.1 provides some examples
- Clopidogrel is a pro-drug which requires two cytochrome-mediated steps to generate its active metabolite. Cytochrome 2C19 (CYP2C19) makes a substantial contribution to both of these steps and so loss-of-function mutations (either hetero- or homozygous) impairs the generation of active metabolite
    - Of note, omeprazole is a moderate inhibitor of CYP2C19 which is why co-administration with clopidogrel may be avoided
- Warfarin inhibits vitamin K epoxide reductase (encoded by VKORC1 gene) and has a narrow therapeutic window. Individuals with a common VKORC1 SNP produce lower levels of the enzyme and so require reduced warfarin dose to achieve the same level of anticoagulation. Warfarin is a racemix and S-warfarin is the more potent enantiomer. It is metabolized by CYP2C9 and so loss-of-function mutations therefore increase warfarin concentrations and risk of bleeding
- The SLCO1B1 enzyme (encoded by the SLCO1B1 gene) is a hepatic drug transporter which clears simvastatin from the blood. Loss-of-function SNPs increase plasma concentration and increase the risk of myopathy
- Despite ever increasing understanding of the interaction between genetics and drug response, no genetic testing is currently standard of care in cardiovascular pharmacotherapy

10.2.3 Cardiovascular side effects of non-cardiovascular drugs

- The list of non-cardiovascular medications with cardiovascular side effects is exhaustive, and several key ones have been highlighted below

Table 10.2.1 List of common drug–gene interactions.

Drug	Genes
Clopidogrel	CYP2C19
Warfarin	CYP2C9, VKORC1
Simvastatin	SLCO1B1

QT prolongation
- The most common cause of drug-induced QT prolongation (also referred to acquired long QT syndrome; aLQTS) is blockade of the hERG K⁺ channel—(encoded by the 'human Ether-à-go-go-Related Gene', also known as KCNH2)
- QT prolongation increases the risk of Torsades de Pointes (TdP)
- Nowadays, drugs undergo testing for hERG inhibition during drug development
- Blockade of hERG and potential for drug-induced QT prolongation is much more likely if multiple potentially QT-prolonging medications are used concurrently
- Electrolyte abnormalities (particularly K^+, Mg^{2+}, and Ca^{2+}) are likely to exacerbate aLQTS and the risk of TdP, as are overdoses of QT-prolonging medication
- Individuals with congenital LQTS are, of course, at much higher risk
- Potent hERG inhibitors can be found in many different classes of drugs; http://www.crediblemeds.org contains a useful list stratified by risk (see also chapter 4.1)
- Management usually involves careful monitoring of heart rhythm and corrected QT interval, withdrawal of offending drugs if possible, stabilization of electrolytes and management of arrhythmia if it occurs
- Although patients starting one or more potentially QT-prolonging medications should be considered for ECG screening pre-initiation, there is no consensus on this, or subsequent ECG monitoring

Left ventricular impairment
- Multiple drugs, in particular chemotherapeutic agents, can cause LVSD, and this can occur via various mechanisms (see Chapter 5.5 for further details)

Bradycardia
- It is rare for a non-cardiovascular drug to cause clinically important bradycardia at usual doses
- Medications that can include:
    - The peripherally acting acetylcholinesterase inhibitor neostigmine can result in increased vagal tone and bradycardia
    - Clonidine can produce striking bradycardia, thought to be via vagus nerve stimulation
    - Cholinesterase inhibitors such as donepezil, used in the treatment of dementia

Metabolic syndrome and accelerated atherosclerosis
- Antipsychotic medications, such as chlorpromazine, promote weight gain and subsequently the development of metabolic syndrome
- Premature coronary atherosclerosis related to antiretroviral drugs is a recognized problem

Further reading
Mehrotra N, Gupta M, Kovar A, Meibohm B. The role of pharmacokinetics and pharmacodynamics in phosphodiesterase-5 inhibitor therapy. *Int J Impot Res.* 2007 May-Jun;19(3):253–64. doi: 10.1038/sj.ijir.3901522. Epub 2006 Sep 21. PMID: 16988721

Raj SR, Stein CM, Saavedra PJ, Roden DM. Cardiovascular effects of noncardiovascular drugs. *Circulation.* 2009 Sep 22;120(12):1123–32. doi: 10.1161/CIRCULATIONAHA.107.728576. PMID: 19770411; PMCID: PMC2773827

Index

For the benefit of digital users, indexed terms that span two pages (e.g., 52–53) may, on occasion, appear on only one of those pages.
Tables, figures, and boxes are indicated by t, f, and b following the page number

abciximab, ACS 132
abdominal aortic aneurysm see aortic aneurysms
Academic Research Consortium for High Bleeding Risk 133t
accessory pathways (APs)
  ablation 366
  definition 344–49
ACE inhibitors 636
  abdominal aortic aneurysm 706
  ACM 478
  ACS 138
  angina 163
  aortic regurgitation 202
  atrial fibrillation 357
  cancer 528
  diabetes 670
  heart failure 433–45, 435t, 473
  hypertension 636–38, 794
  peripartum CM 492
  pregnancy contraindication 639, 830, 833t
  RCTs 437t
  renal artery stenosis contraindicated 741
  restrictive CM 483
  SCD prevention 575
acetylcholinesterase inhibitor, bradycardia 946
acetylsalicylic acid see aspirin
ACHD patients undergoing non-cardiac surgery 807
acute aortic syndromes 708–17
  ESC recommendations 710t
  high-risk clinical features 710t, 711f
  management 714t
  Stanford classification 711f
acute cardiovascular care
  acute kidney injury 553–55
  analgesia 558–59
  assessment of 540t, 554–55
  deteriorating patient 541
  discharge from intensive care 565
  fluid management 549
  gastrointestinal issues 562–64
  haematological issues 559–62
  haemodynamics 546–49
  hypertension 552
  hypotension 549–51
  infective issues 564–65
  inotropes 549–51, 550t
  medical/surgical 539–40
  neurological issues 555–58
  pacing 552–53
  palliation, and end-of-life care 566
  renal issues 553–55
  stroke 557–58
  time course 542t
  vasoactive medications 549–51
  vasopressors 549, 551t
  see also ICU; ventilation
acute chest pain, emergency echocardiography, 63t
acute coronary syndrome (ACS)
  atherosclerotic plaque rupture 123–24
  bradyarrhythmias, with haemodynamic compromise 142
  chronic kidney disease 143
  co-morbidities 142–44
  default antithrombotic therapy regimens 132f
  diagnostic coronary angiography and revascularization 139–40
  diagnostic criteria 126–27
  diagnostic techniques 127–29
  early and late complications and their management 140–42
  frailty 144
  free wall/papillary muscle rupture 141
  heart failure and cardiogenic shock 142–43
  high-sensitivity cardiac troponin (hs-cTN) 127–28
  multivessel disease 139–40
  non-atherosclerotic causes 124–26
  non-cardiac surgery 847
  non-invasive imaging 128–29
  older person 144
  pathophysiology 123–24
  pharmacotherapy 130–38
  risk scores 127

acute coronary syndrome
      (ACS) (cont.)
   selective invasive
         strategy 139
   timing of invasive
         approach 139
   ventricular septal
         rupture 141
acute dyspnoea, emergency
      echocardiography,
      63t
acute heart failure 456–58
acute kidney injury 553–55
   AKIN classification 555t
   indications for renal
         replacement 554–55
   management 554
   renal replacement
         mechanisms 554–55
   RIFLE criteria 554t
adenosine
   nuclear cardiology 110
   termination of supraventricular
         tachycardia 372
adenovirus 489b
ADME mnemonic 943
adult congenital heart disease
      (ACHD) 775
   diagnostic tests 782–83
   heart failure 783
   non-cardiac surgery 850–51
   pregnancy and 823–27
   principles of intervention in
         ACHD 783
   see also atrial septal defects;
         circulation; patent
         foramen ovale; shunts
advanced life support 568,
      568f
aerobic capacity 611–12
after-load, definition 547–48
Agatston score 100, 103
airport metal detectors,
         pacemakers 333, 409
albuminuria 635, 636f
alcohol 624
alcoholic cardiomyopathy 491
alkaptonuria 204
Allen's test 168
ambulatory blood pressure
      monitoring
      (ABPM) 631
amiodarone 338–39
   non-cardiac surgery 843
amyloid heart disease 481–82
   investigations 482, 482t

management 483
prognosis 483–84
amyloidosis, CMR 78
anabolic steroids 598
anaemia
   ACS 143
   multi-valvular disease 241
   non-cardiac surgery 847
anaerobic threshold 610–11
analgesia
   acute cardiovascular
         care 558–59
   simple analgesics 558
anaphylaxis, contrast-related 183
Andersen-Tawil syndrome
      (LQT7) 385
Anderson–Fabry disease 78, 485
   cardiovascular presentation
         485–87
aneurysmal dilatation 101
angina
   microvascular 162–63
   refractory 163
   rheumatic valve disease 205
   variant 124–25
   vasospastic/Prinzmetal 124,
         163
   without obstructive disease,
         epicardial coronary
         arteries 162–63
angina (in absence of coronary
      artery disease) 200
angina pectoris 152
angina pectoris Canadian
      Cardiovascular
      Society (CCS) 154b
   clinical assessment 153–56
angiosarcoma 523
angiotensin receptor blockers
      (ARBs) 138, 636,
      701
ankylosing spondylitis 200, 905
anomalous coronary arteries,
      SCD 596–97
anomalous pulmonary venous
      drainage 789–92
anomalous systemic vein
      connections 88
anthracycline 530b
anti-ischaemic drugs 159
antiarrhythmic drugs
   classes 1-4 336–39
   pharmacology 336–40
   triggered activity 336
   Vaughan–Williams
         classification 336t

antibiotic prophylaxis 564
antibiotics
   outpatient parenteral
         antibiotic therapy
         (OPAT) 262–63
   Staphylococcus species 261
anticoagulants 135–36
   direct acting oral
         (DOACs) 561–62
   factor Xa inhibitors 136
   heparin 135
   long-term oral anticoagulants
         136–37
   new anticoagulant
         agents 881, 882t
anticoagulation 561
   cancer patients 532–33
   non-cardiac surgery 844–46,
         845f
   for prosthetic valves,
         pregnancy, 822–23
antiphospholipid
      syndrome 909–11
antiplatelet therapy 561, 624
   ACS, pre-treatment and
         duration 132–33
   agents, ACS 130–32
   and CABG 135
   dual (DAPT) 132f
   long-term oral anticoagulants
         136–37
   non-cardiac surgery 135,
         844
   risk criteria for extended
         treatment
         with a second
         antithrombotic
         agent 134t
   shortened and extended 134
   single (SAPT) 136–37, 136f
antithrombotics
   non-cardiac surgery 844–46
   single antiplatelet therapy
         (SAPT) 136–37,
         136f
   triple antithrombotic therapy
         (TAT) 136–37
aorta
   atheromatous disease 720
   branches, CMR 87
   coarctation 102
   dimensions, normal
         values, 63t
   genetic diseases 717–19
   imaging modalities 695t,
         695–97

European Society
of Cardiology
recommendations
696t
normal 693
pathology 693–95
thrombotic or cholesterol
emboli 720
traumatic rupture
aetiology 723
endovascular repair 724
pathogenesis 723
wall stress
investigations 694f,
695–97
Laplace law 694, 694f
aortic aneurysms
abdominal aortic
aneurysms 705–8
aetiology 697–98
contained rupture 717
dissection, and aortic
coarctation before/
after repair 87
endovascular repair 703–4
ESC recommendation
2014, threshold
intervention 701–3
risk factors 697–98
surgical/endovascular
management 701
thoracic 698
thoracoabdominal aneurysms
(TAA) 704
variables 700t
aortic annulus
ECG gated CT 101
normal values, 63t
aortic atheromatous
disease 720
aortic coarctation 57, 102, 633,
792–94
pregnancy, 825–26
aortic disease
atheroma, thrombotic
or cholesterol
emboli 720
pathophysiology 200
peripheral signs 201
aortic dissection
endovascular therapy 715
intramural haematoma 716
penetrating aortic ulcer 716
SCD 598
aortic embolism 860
aortic pseudoaneurysm, 716–17

aortic regurgitation
acute severe 200
aetiology 199–200
aortic valve replacement
dysfunction,
assessment 104
assessment of severity by
echo, 47–49
cardiac auscultation 201
chronic severe 200
echo 47–49
echo parameters for assessing
severity 202t
grading of severity by
echo, 50t
indications for surgery 203
non-cardiac surgery 849
precordial palpation 201
sport and 607
see also multi-valvular disease
aortic root anatomy,
normal 169
aortic root dilatation, sport
and 608–9
aortic root surgery 203
aortic size index 700
aortic stenosis 37, 189
aetiology
congenitally abnormal
valve 203
subvalvular 204
supravalvular 203
valvular 203–4
assessment of severity by
echocardiography, 38t
asymptomatic patients 204
examination
cardiac auscultation 205
cardiac
catheterization 207
cardiac CT 207
carotid pulse 205
CMR 207
echo 206–7
low-flow, low-
gradient, 37–38
haemodynamic
parameters, 37
follow-up 210
interventions 207–8
ACC/AHA 2020 guideline
recommendations
208–9
ESC guideline 2021
recommendation
208

medical management 207
non-cardiac surgery 848
pathophysiology
calcific 'degenerative' 203
fibrosis on LGE imaging 81
rheumatic valve
disease 203
pregnancy, 821
sport and 607
symptoms 205
see also multi-valvular disease
aortic valve area 189
aortic valve disease,
anatomy 199
aortic valve replacement
dysfunction,
assessment 103–4
aortic valve stenosis 103
calcium scoring and stenosis
assessment 99–100,
103
aortic variants, CMR 88
aortitis 719–20
aortopathies, pregnancy, 826
apolipoprotein B
atherogenesis risk
screening 621
cardiovascular risk 647
ARNIs, angiotensin receptor
and neprilysin
inhibitors 435t, 437t,
439–40
arrhythmias
ACS 142
adult congenital heart disease
(ACHD) 783
with cancer therapies 531
definitions 299–300
detection and ICD
programming
393–98
non-cardiac surgery
849–50
pregnancy, 829
arrhythmogenic
cardiomyopathy
recommendations for
competition 601–2
SCD 597
arrhythmogenic RV
cardiomyopathy
(ARVC) 298–99,
450, 474, 475–79
clinical presentation 476
CMR 77
diagnostic features 477b

arrhythmogenic RV
            cardiomyopathy
            (ARVC) (cont.)
    diagnostic testing 476
        ambulatory
            monitoring 476
        electrocardiography 476
        endomyocardial
            biopsy 476
        genetic testing 476
    differential diagnosis 476–78
    echo major/minor 2DE
            criteria, 35–36
    epsilon wave (major
            criterion) 592t
    genetic testing 476
    key facts 577–78
    management 478–79, 478t
    physiology vs pathology 600
    prognosis and outcome 479
    RVOT VT 381
    SCD risk 577–79
    ventricular tachycardias 299
arterial hypertension 629–32
arterial switch 799
aspirin
    ACS 130
    bleeding and 875
    post surgery 561
    in primary prevention 624
asymmetrical septal
            hypertrophy, 34
atherogenic dyslipidaemia 625,
            670, 671f
atherosclerosis
    coronary angiography 153
    coronary fat attenuation
            index 100
    coronary physiology 151
    large/small-vessel 860–61
    pathogenesis 147–49, 148f
    plaque erosion 124
    plaque rupture 123–24
    risk factors 149–51
    systemic inflammation 902
atherosclerotic cardiovascular
            disease, SGLT2
            inhibitors 673
athlete's heart 589–94
    electrical changes 589–91
atrial conduction 275
atrial fibrillation
    ACS 142
    associated morbidity and
            mortality 356
    beta blockers 361

catheter ablation 364–65
classification 355–56
Cox Maze III 'cut and sew'
            procedure 365
definition 355
diagnostic
            assessment 358–59
epidemiology 356, 881
European Heart Rhythm
            Association AF
            symptom scale 358t
familial 367
management 359–66
new anti-coagulant
            agents 881, 882t
pacemaker and AV node
            ablation 365
pathophysiology 357, 881
pharmacological
            cardioversion 363
post-operative 367
pre-disposing
            conditions 357–58
pregnancy 366–67, 829
recommendations for
            competition 603–4
rhythm control 362
risk factor modification 361
summary 367–68
ventricular rate
            control 361–62
atrial fibrillation/flutter, non-
            cardiac surgery 849
atrial flutter
    atypical atrial flutter 371–72
    correlation with other atrial
            arrhythmias 370
    ECG characteristics 370
    pregnancy, 829
    summary 373–74
    treatment 371
    see also atrial fibrillation
atrial septal defect 785
    closure 786
    echo, 55–56
    physiology 786
    pregnancy and 823
atrial septum, structure 784
atrial situs solitus or inversus,
            CMR 86
atrial switch: Mustard or Senning
            operation 798–99
atrial tachycardia 372–73
    electrophysiology study
            (EPS) 373
atrio-pulmonary

            connection 806
atrioventricular
            arrangements 86
atrioventricular (AV) block
    bradycardia, indications
            for permanent
            pacing 321b
    first degree 289
    pacing 321
    second degree 290
    third degree 291
atrioventricular (AV)
            conduction
            disease 319–20
atrioventricular conduction
            324
atrioventricular node
            ablation 365
atrioventricular node 275
atrioventricular septal
            defects 788–89
atropine, nuclear
            cardiology 110
Austin Flint murmur 201
automated external
            defibrillators 567
AV node re-entry tachycardia
            (AVNRT)
    accessory pathways 342–49
    ECG features 343
    EPS features 351–53
    management 343–44
    pathophysiology 342–43
AV re-entrant tachycardia
            (AVRT)
    acute management 348
    asymptomatic pre-excited
            ECG 349
    definition, 344
    ECG features 346–47
    long-term management 348
    management 348
    pathophysiology 340–41
    pathophysiology 345–46
    risk stratification 349
AVID study, ICD vs
            antiarrhythmic
            drugs 391

Barth syndrome 866
basic life support 567–68
Beck triad 509
beta blockers 637
    ACS 137
    atrial fibrillation 361

CCS 160
non-cardiac surgery 842–43
see also antiarrhythmic drugs, Class II
bicuspid aortic valve 796
pregnancy, 826
bile acid sequestrants 653–54
biomarkers
  brain natriuretic peptides (BNP) 872
  cardiac troponins 872
  chronic kidney disease 872–73
  high-sensitivity cardiac troponin (hs-cTN) 127–28
  natriuretic peptides, 422–23, 422b
bioprosthetic valves, pregnancy, 822
bleeding
  Academic Research Consortium for High Bleeding Risk 133t
  ICU 559–60
  major/minor criteria for high risk 133t
  management 559–60
  prevention 559
  risk factors 559
blood glucose, management 563–64
blood pressure
  ABPM 631
  Australian National Blood Pressure Study (ANBP2) 637
  definitions of hypertension grade 630t
  home monitoring 631–32
  measurement 630–32
blood pressure, cholesterol and smoking, combined risk assessment 620t, 621
Blood Pressure Lowering Treatment Trialists Collaboration (BPLTT) is a meta-analysis 636–37
blood products 560
Body Mass Index (BMI) 622
body size, scaling, echo 24–27
Borrelia burgdorferi, tick-borne Lyme disease 491
bradyarrhythmias

guideline management 569–70
  with haemodynamic compromise 142
bradycardia
  acetylcholinesterase inhibitor, 946
  atrioventricular (AV) conduction disease 319–20
  bundle branch block (BBB) 320, 946
  classification and indications for pacing 317–20
  history and evaluation 323
  indications for permanent pacing 321b
  investigation 323
  sinoatrial (SA) node disease 318–19
  treatment 323–24
brain injury, post cardiac arrest 556
brain natriuretic peptides (BNP) 872
Brugada syndrome 337, 386–88
  ECG patterns 292
  genetics 387–88
  ICD implantation 580, 604
  management, 387
  risk of SCD 579–80
  SCD 598
  Shanghai Score System for diagnosis 386t, 387f
bundle branch block
  bi-and tri-fascicular block 320
  pacing 321
  bradycardia, indications for permanent pacing 321b
bundle of His 275
  infra-His conduction 275
  see also left bundle branch block (LBBB); right bundle branch block (RBBB)
Butler-Leggett ECG voltage, RVH criteria 282t
bypass graft disease 100
BYPASS-CTCA trial 100

C-reactive protein (CRP) 873
cadmium-zinc-telluride (CZT) gamma cameras, MPS 109
calcific degenerative

  disease 204
  multi-valvular disease 233
calcium channel antagonists 160
calcium channel blockers 636, 770
  non-cardiac surgery 843
calcium scoring
  ESC/EACST 2021 guidelines 103
  and stenosis assessment 99–100, 103
cancer
  ACS 143
  lifetime risk 108
  non-cardiac surgery 852
  see also cardiac masses and tumours; cardio-oncology
cancer treatment
  cardiac side effects 527–30, 528b
  chemotherapy 529t
cancer-associated myositis 912
cangrelor, ACS 131
cannabis 598
cardiac amyloidosis 78
cardiac arrest
  assessment of survivors 581–82
  automated external defibrillators 567
  emergency echocardiography, 63t
cardiac arrhythmias
  driving regulations 314t
  pregnancy, 827–29
cardiac auscultation 201, 205
cardiac axis
  calculation from limb leads 277f
  estimation 277, 277t
  left and right axis deviation 278t
cardiac catheterization
  2021 ESC/EACTS guidelines 201
  aortic stenosis 207
  diagnostic 783
  invasive coronary angiography 169–74
  laboratory equipment 166
  normal aortic root anatomy 169
  radiation protection 165–66

cardiac catheterization (cont.)
  restrictive
    cardiomyopathy 480
  vascular access 166–68,
    167f, 167t
cardiac chambers, anatomy,
  size, function, 27–32
cardiac CT
  acquisition 91–98
  acquisition mode and image
    interrogation 95–97
  3D volume rendering/
    cinematic
    rendering, 97
  multiplanar reconstruction
    (MPR) 96–97
  patient selection and
    preparation 97–98
  spiral CT 96
  step and shoot/axial
    acquisition 95
  ECG synchronization 93–94
    prospective ECG
      gating 94
    retrospective ECG
      gating 93
  intravenous contrast
    timing 92
  spatial resolution 92
  temporal resolution 92
  test bolus technique 92
cardiac cycle
  electrical vectors 275–77
  stages by surface ECG 276t
cardiac drugs, pregnancy, 833t
cardiac implantable electronic
  devices (CIEDs), non-
  cardiac surgery 850
cardiac ion channel
  dysfunction 292–94,
  383
  long QT syndrome 383–85
  VT and 382
cardiac lymphoma, 524
cardiac magnetic resonance
  (CMR)
  artefacts, motion
    artefacts 66
  artefacts 66–67
  blood flow
    assessment 71–72
  comprehensive 86
  contrast agents, 69
  dobutamine stress
    imaging 71
  examination, overview 69

methodology 69–72
  cardiac anatomy 69
  cardiac function 69–70
  stress imaging 70–71
  tissue characterization 70
MR angiography 72
physics 65–66
safety and
  contraindications 68
safety terminology and
  labelling for medical
  devices and
  implants 68t
specific heart diseases 73–79
cardiac masses and
  tumours 82–85, 104
  arrhythmia 518
  assessment of 82
  benign tumours 518–23
  clinical features 517–18
  CMR 518
  diagnosis 518
  echo 54–55, 55t, 518
  gated computed
    tomography 518
  metastases 524–25
  obstruction 517
  see also cancer;
    cardio-oncology
cardiac MRI 129
  ESC/EACTS guidelines
    (2021) 202
cardiac output (CO)
  calculation, 59
  echo grading, 58
  Fick 188
  thermodilution method 188
cardiac rehabilitation 679
  access to 680–81
  audit and evaluation of
    programmes
    688–89
  core components 681–82
  defined 679
  dietary advice and weight
    management 686–87
  early activity after cardiac
    surgery 684
  education 685–86
  exertion scales 685t
  long-term rehabilitation
    management 688
  'mets' for specific
    activities 684b
  physical activity and
    exercise 682–85

psychological status and
  quality of life 687
structure of programmes
  680
tailored CR programmes
  683–85
types of intervention 682
cardiac resynchronization
  therapy (CRT)
  CRT-D and CRT-P 409
  HFrEF 409–12
  at implant 410
  conduction system
    pacing 412–14
  ESC indications by evidence
    level 411b
  NICE guidelines 410t
  non-response 411–12
  practical device considerations
    414–15
  trials of CRT in heart
    failure 410
cardiac surgery, management
  post-surgery
  541–42
cardiac syncope 305
cardiac tamponade see
  tamponade
cardiac thrombus, stroke
  risk 859–60
cardiac trauma 104–5
cardio-oncology 527
  ideal service 535
  imaging 533–34
  multidisciplinary team (MDT)
    approach 535
cardiomyopathies
  classification of phenotypes
    461, 462f
  CMR 75–79
  markers of increased risk of
    SCD 601–2
  pregnancy, 831–32
  Takotsubo 126
    CMR, 79
  VT and 382
  see also arrhythmogenic
    RV —; dilated —;
    hypertrophic —;
    non-dilated LV —;
    restrictive —
cardioprotection, RCT
  data 534–35
cardiopulmonary bypass
  hypothermia 541–42
  in pregnancy 831

cardiopulmonary exercise testing (CPET), sport and 609–16
cardiotoxicity
  BSE/ BCOS echocardiographic definitions 534t
  defined 79
  late effects 535
cardiotropic viruses 489b
cardiovascular care see acute cardiovascular care
cardiovascular disease
  evaluation of patients 615–16
  see also cardiovascular risk
cardiovascular risk 617–18
  additional risk screening options 621
  age groups 626–27
  apolipoprotein B 647
  assessment tools 618–21, 619t, 620f
  cigarette smoking, BP, cholesterol 621–22
  HDL 646–47
  LDL 646
  NICE Guidelines 630
  other factors 621–22
  risk profile management 622–25
  triglycerides 647
CARE-HF trial 410
carotid artery disease 734–37
carotid artery stenting (CAS) 736
carotid atherosclerosis 861
carotid pulse, palpation 205
CARTO® (Biosense Webster) 353f, 353
catecholaminergic polymorphic VT (CPVT) 388–89, 574
  competitive sports not recommended 604
  risk of SCD 580–81, 598
  SCD 598
catheter ablation
  paroxysmal and persistent AF 364–65
  pulmonary vein isolation (PVI) 364
cavo-tricuspid isthmus (CTI) 369f
central sleep apnoea 898–99
central venous catheter associated complications, cancer patients 532–33

cerebrovascular disease, non-cardiac surgery 852
cervical arteries, diseases, CT 105–6
Chagas disease 490–91
channelopathies 292
chemotherapy 529t
  cardiac side effects 527–30
chemotherapy-related cardiotoxicity 79
chest pain
  differential diagnosis 154, 155t
  non-cardiac 154–56, 155t
chest radiograph 201
chest trauma, emergency echocardiography, 63t
chlorpromazine 946
cholesterol
  BP, and smoking, combined risk assessment 620t, 621
  lipid modification in prevention of stroke 860
  risk assessment 621
cholesterol synthesis inhibitors 656
chronic coronary syndromes
  clinical assessment 153–56
  clinical likelihood of coronary artery disease 156
  diagnostic management 156–59
  management 159–61
  pharmacological management 159–61
  prognosis 152–53
  risk stratification 152–53
  see also atherosclerosis
chronic kidney disease
  acute coronary syndrome (ACS) 143
  biomarkers 872–73
  coronary angiography 872–77
  coronary artery disease and myocardial infarction 870–77
  diagnosis 870–71
  dialysis patients 874
  electrocardiography and echocardiography 871
  glomerular filtration rate (eGFR) 869t

GLP-1 receptor agonists 875
glycaemic monitoring and targets 874
insulin 875
ISCHAEMIA-CKD trial 873
KDOQI Guidelines 871
metformin, increased risk of lactic acidosis 874
mineralocorticoid receptor antagonists (MRA) 875
risk assessment 620, 622
risk factors 871f
stages 869t
statins 875, 876t
stress tests 871–77
see also renal disease
chronic obstructive pulmonary disease (COPD) 885
  arrhythmias 890–91
  cardiac function at rest 889
  cardiovascular implications 888–90
  clinical features 886–87
  diagnosis 887
  epidemiology and prognosis 885
  evaluation 887
  exacerbations 888
  heart failure 889
  pathogenesis 886
  risk of comorbid disease 886
chronic thromboembolic pulmonary hypertension (CTEPH) 755–58, 773
  clinical presentation 756
  diagnosis 756–57
  epidemiology 755
  medical treatment 758
  surgical treatment 757–58
chronic total occlusions (CTO) 103
Churg–Strauss syndrome 79
chylomicrons 645–46
cigarette smoking 124
  BP, cholesterol, combined risk assessment 620t, 621
  cessation 623
circulation
  basic foetal and transitional circulation 8.6S9, 778f
  Blalock–Taussig shunt, classical vs modified 779

circulation (*cont.*)
  flow-related development of cardiac chambers and vessels 782
  parallel pulmonary and systemic circulations 8.6S9
  systemic arterial to pulmonary artery shunts (to increase pulmonary flow 762, 779–80
clinical pharmacology 943–46
clopidogrel 561, 945
  ACS 130–31
  CAD 134
coarctation of aorta 57, 102, 633, 792–94
  pregnancy, 825–26
cocaine, SCD 598
cognitive dysfunction, post-op (POCD) 557
colchicine, Cardiovascular Outcomes Trial (COLCOT), 138
collagen vascular disorders 919
commotio cordis, SCD 598
compartment syndrome 183
COMPASS-PAD trial 730
computed tomography electrocardiogram-gated (ECG-gated CT), 91
  multidetector (MDCT) 91
computed tomography coronary angiography (CTCA) 91, 129
conducting system of heart *see* electrical activity of heart
conduction disturbances
  atrioventricular conduction, 275, 324
  electrophysiology study (EPS), 286–92, 324
  sinus node dysfunction 324
congenital heart disease
  in adult 775
  aetiology 781
  anatomical concepts 775–77
  atria
    -situs inversus 775–76
    -ventricular connections 776
  CMR 85–86
  CT imaging 105
  ECG gated CT to document cardiac venous anatomy 102
  echo 55–57
  LV/RV
    anatomical terms 777
    great artery connections 777
    morphological RV vs morphological LV 777
  physiological concepts 778
  pulmonary blood flow 778–80
  pregnancy, 823–27
congenitally corrected transposition of great arteries (ccTGA) 800–1
congestive cardiac failure
  diagnosis 878
  epidemiology and pathophysiology 877–79
  prevention and treatment 878–79
Conn's disease 633
constrictive pericardial disease 510–15
  aetiology 512–14
  diagnosis 512
constrictive pericarditis
  causes 192, 193*t*
  diagnostic approach 513*t*, 514*f*
  echo 53–54
  management 515
  physical signs 512*t*
contraception, advice in pregnancy, 834
contrast agents
  echo 14*t*
  left heart, 15*t*
contrast echocardiography, 12–14
contrast nephropathy, coronary angiography 872–77
Corbi or Farbe's disease 486*t*
Cornell ECG voltage, LVH criteria 280*t*
coronary anatomy, invasive coronary angiography 169–74
coronary angiography
  atherosclerosis 153

cardiac output (CO) 188
catheter selection and views 174–77, 175*f*–77*f*
chronic kidney disease 872–77
complications 182–85, 182*t*
contrast nephropathy 872–77
contrast-related complications 183–84
coronary complications 184–85
coronary perforation/rupture 184
in-stent restenosis 185
indications 179
invasive functional assessment and intracoronary imaging 179–82
in non-cardiac surgery 842
and PCI, complications 182–85
radiation protection 165–66
right heart catheterization and cardiac haemodynamics 185–92, 185*t*, 186*f*
stent embolization 184
stent thrombosis 185
coronary arteries
  arising from pulmonary artery 174
  arising from wrong sinus 170, 171*f*–73*f*
  common native vessel variations 170
  CT coronary angiography (CTCA), 91
  end-systole 94
  non-cardiac surgery 847–48
  normal course and nomenclature 170
  single 173, 173*f*
  sport and 605*t*
coronary artery
  anomalies 100–1, 170–74, 794–95
  risk of SCD 579
coronary artery bypass grafting (CABG) 140
  antiplatelet therapy 135
  screening 730
coronary artery calcium score (CACS)
  Agatson units 621
  Agatston score 100

coronary artery disease
(CAD) 98–100
  antiplatelet therapy, risk
    criteria for extended
    treatment 134t
  assessment of,
    likelihood 156, 157f
  chronic coronary
    syndromes 156
  and chronic kidney
    disease 870–77
  chronic total occlusions
    (CTO) 103
  computed tomography
    coronary angiography
    (CTCA) 129
  coronary blood flow 151
  hybrid imaging 117–18
  key facts 574–76
  leading cause of SCD 574
  myocardial complications 101
  myocardial complications,
    interventional
    guidance 101–2
  myocardial perfusion
    scintigraphy
    (MPS) 108–16
  pre-test probability 156,
    157t, 158f
  spontaneous coronary
    artery dissection
    (SCAD) 125
  standardized reporting
    nomenclature 98–99
  stratifying patients 99
  testing (ESC Guidelines
    2019) 156
  testing in patients with
    established
    chronic coronary
    syndromes 158t
  testing (UK NICE Guidelines
    2016), 158–59
  see also acute coronary
    syndrome (ACS)
coronary artery dissection,
  SCD 597
coronary artery embolism
  (CE) 126
coronary blood flow 151
coronary bypass grafts,
  saphenous vein
  (SVG) 170
coronary fat attenuation
  index 100
CRISP CT study 100

coronary ostia 169, 169f
coronary revascularization
  161–62
  PCI vs CABG 161–62
coronary sinus defect,
  echo 56
coronary stents 100
coronavirus disease 2019,
  non-cardiac
  surgery 852–53
Cox Maze III 'cut and sew'
  procedure 365
Coxsackie virus 489b
CPET data, interpretation
  613–15
crystal arthritides 920
CT fractional flow reserve
  (CTFFR) 99
CT scanner, photon-counting
  CT scanner 100
CTCA
  calcium scoring and stenosis
    assessment 99–100
  chronic coronary syndrome
    setting 103
  coronary anomalies 100–1
  CT fractional flow reserve
    (CTFFR) 99
CULPRIT-SHOCK trial,
  ACS, 142
Cushings syndrome 633
cyanosis 780–82
  consequences 781–82
cyanotic congenital heart
  disease, pregnancy
  and 824
cystic tumour of the AV
  node 523
cytotoxic agents
  cardiac assessment prior to
    initiation 533
  cardiac side effects 529t
  echo, anthracyclines
    and/or
    trastuzumab 534
  monitoring 533–35

deep venous thrombosis
  743–48
  clinical prediction rules
    assessing risk of
    recurrence 747t
  epidemiology 743
  pathophysiology 744
  treatment 8.4F1

unprovoked proximal
  DVT 747
Wells score 745t, 745f
defibrillation 568–69
DEFINITE trial, ICD 392
delirium 555–56
DeMusset sign 201
dermatomyositis 912
dextrocardia 777
diabetes
  ACS and 143
  actions and effects of anti-
    diabetes drugs 674t
  acute coronary
    syndromes 677
  atherogenic dyslipidaemia
    670, 671f
  atherothrombotic risk 670,
    671f
  blood pressure control 673
  CAD and 143
  cardiomyopathy 671
  classification,
    pathophysiology and
    diagnosis 665–67
  complications 668–71
  definition 665
  diabetic nephropathy
    669–70
  diabetic neuropathy 670
  diabetic retinopathy 668–69
  drugs 7.5T1
  epidemiology 668
  foot disease 730
  GLP-1 receptor agonists 875
  glucose control,
    ICU 563–64
  glycaemic control 672–73
  heart failure 677
  lifestyle 676–77
  macrovascular
    complications 670–71
  management of
    dyslipidaemia 673
  microvascular
    complications 668–70
  non-cardiac surgery 852
  optimal control 874
  platelet stabilization
    673–76
  prevention and management
    of cardiovascular
    disease 671–77
  risk assessment 620
  risk of stroke 860
diastolic murmur 201

diathermy 331–32
diet
  lipid goals 647–49
  trans fats 648
DiGeorge syndrome 803b
digoxin 296, 340
dilated CM 471–74
  cardiac MRI 473
  cardiopulmonary exercise testing 472
  clinical course and prognosis 472
  CMR 76–77
  echo 473
  echo techniques, 33–36
  electrocardiography 472
  endomyocardial biopsy 473
  management 473
  physiology vs pathology 600
  recommendations for competition 602
  risk assessment, screening and prognosis 473–74
  SCD 597
dipyridamole, nuclear cardiology 110
direct acting oral anticoagulants (DOACs) 561–62
diuretics, non-cardiac surgery 843
diuretics (thiazide-like) 637
dizziness 862–63
dobutamine, nuclear cardiology 110
dobutamine stress CMR imaging 71
  contraindications 71
Doppler-based strain analysis, 12
Down syndrome 807, 808t
DPD scintigraphy 118
Dressler's syndrome 505
  ACS 142
driving regulations
  pacemakers 414–15
  transient loss of consciousness (TLOC) 314
drugs
  bioavailability 944
  causes of QT prolongation 295b
  clearance 944
  comparison trials 637

therapeutic index 944–45
toxicity 944
volume of distribution 944
drug–gene interactions 945t
ductus arteriosus, patent 57, 796
Duplex ultrasound 734
Duroziez sign 201
dyslipidaemias 643–46
  classifying 658–62
  secondary causes 662, 662t

early repolarisation syndrome 389–90
Early Warning Scores (EWS), deteriorating patient 541
Ebstein's anomaly 796–97
  pregnancy, 796–97
echocardiography, transthoracic, non-cardiac surgery 841
echocardiography techniques 3–16
  2D-mode, 4–5
  3D-mode, 7–9
  deformation imaging, 12
  Doppler (blood flow, tissue), 9–11
  echo/stress modalities, 14
  emergency, 63t, 64
  global LV and RV systolic and diastolic function, 16–24
  M-mode, 3–4
  non-invasive haemodynamics 58–59
  primary and secondary cardiomyopathies, 33–36
  stress meta-analysis 116
  stress-echo modalities, 14
  transoesophageal 15–16
  complications post surgery 562
  transthoracic 128
Ehlers–Danlos syndrome 200
  pregnancy, 827
eicosapentaenoic acid (EPA) 655
Eisenmenger syndrome 779b
ejection systolic murmur 201
electrical activity of heart 273–75, 276f

anatomy and physiology of conducting system 274
cardiac ion channel dysfunction 292–94
cellular and molecular mechanisms 273
chamber hypertrophy 278–82
common artefacts and lead reversal ECGs 278
common causes of signal artefact 278b
conduction disturbances 286–92
early repolarization (ER) 294
ECG voltage criteria for left ventricular hypertrophy 280t
exercise ECG testing 301–2
ischaemia and infarction 282f, 283–86
long-term ambulatory ECG 300–1
mnemonic for ECG evidence of lead mal-position 279t
palpitations 300–2
phases 0–4 273
pre-excitation 292
repolarization disturbances 294–96
REVERSE mnemonic for ECG evidence of lead mal-position 279t
sinus node 274–75
ST-elevation myocardial infarction 283f
electro-anatomic mapping, 3D EAM 353–54
electrocardiogram 201
  cardiac pathology 278–99
  ECG gated CT, aortic annulus 101
  electrical vectors throughout cardiac cycle 275–77
  suspected ACS 127
Emery–Dreifuss muscular dystrophy 864
end-diastolic (EDV) and end-systolic (ESV) LV volumes 16
  echo parameters, 18t
endocarditis see infective endocarditis

Index

endomyocardial biopsy
　graft failure 80
　myocarditis 80
endomyocardial inflammation, eosinophilic myocarditis 79
endothelin receptor antagonists (ERA) 770
EnSite Array, non-contact mapping (St Jude Medical) 354
EnSite NavX® (St Jude Medical) 353–54
enteral feeding 563
Enterococcus species, antibiotics 261
eosinophilic myocarditis 79
eptifibatide, ACS 132
erectile dysfunction 923–27
　cardiac risk stratification 925t
　epidemiology 923
　first-line treatment, medical management 926–27
　second-line treatment, 927
ESC 2018
　hypertension, treatment targets 634
　hypertension-mediated organ damage (HMOD) 632, 634
escape rhythm failure, Stokes–Adams attacks 292
Europe, SCORE model 630
EUROscore, CCS 162
event prevention drugs, CCS 161
exercise ECG, CCS 153
exercise intolerance, cardiovascular vs pulmonary aetiology 613
exercise physiology 588
exercise stress test 202–3, 202f, 311–12
exertion scales 685t
extra-cranial carotid artery disease 734–37

18F-fluorodeoxyglucose (FDG), positron emission tomography 117
18F-flupiridaz, positron emission tomography 117
Fabry disease 204

Fallot tetralogy 802–4
familial combined hyperlipidaemia (FCH) 660
familial hypercholesterolaemia 204, 659–60
　Simon Broome Register diagnostic criteria 660t
familial primary hypoalphalipoproteinemia 661–62
fascicular block, left anterior/posterior 323f
fat intake/diet, goals 647–49
fetal circulation 778f
fibrates, mechanism of action 652–53
fibrinolytic therapy 137
　contraindicated absolutely 137
fibroma 82–85, 521–22
fibrosarcoma 524
fluid management 549
　acute cardiovascular care 549
fluoropyrimidines 530
fluoroscopy, radiation protection 165–66
foetal circulation 778f
fondaparinux, factor Xa inhibitor 136
Fontan surgery 804–6, 805f
　pregnancy, 824
Food and Drug Administration (FDA), MR safety terminology and labelling for medical devices and implants 68t
fractional flow reserve (FFR) CT 99
　definition 180
　post PCI FFR and subsequent events rates and FFR 181t
Framingham Heart Study 618, 619t
Fredrickson classification system, lipid profile abnormalities 658t
Friedreich's ataxia 864–65
functionally single ventricle and the Fontan circulation 804–6

gadolinium, late gadolinium enhancement (LGE) 75, 79
gadolinium-based compounds CMR 69
gastrointestinal issues, acute cardiovascular care 562–64
genetic counselling, 939
genetic syndromes in ACHD 807–10, 808t
genetics
　autosomal dominant inheritance 932
　cardiology 931
　chromosomal testing 937
　chromosomes 936–37
　dominant inheritance 932
　drawing a pedigree 940
　family testing 940
　genotype testing 937–38
　heteroplasmy 935
　laboratory genetic test result 938–39
　Mendelian inheritance 932–35
　mitochondrial inheritance 935
　mosaicism 936
　multifactorial/polygenic inheritance 936
　non-Mendelian inheritance 935–37
　recessive inheritance 933
　whole genome sequencing 938
　X-linked recessive inheritance 933–35
global LV and RV systolic and diastolic function, 16–24
glomerular filtration rate, chronic kidney disease 869t
glucose control, ICU 563–64
glycogen storage disease (GSD) 486t
　investigations 429
　management 487–88
glycoprotein IIb/IIIa inhibitors, ACS 132
glycosphingolipids 485
　deposition 78
Gorlin formula 189
GRACE (Global Registry of Acute Coronary Events) Score 127

graft failure, endomyocardial biopsy 80
great vessel diseases, CT imaging, 105
guanyl cyclase stimulator 770
Gubner ECG voltage, LVH criteria 280*t*

haemachromatosis 486*t*
haemangioma 82–85, 521–22
haematological issues, acute cardiovascular care 559–62
haemodynamic instability, emergency echocardiography, 63*t*
haemodynamics, acute cardiovascular care 546–49
haemoglobin degradation products 73
haemopericardium 105
Hakki formula 189
hazard ratios, lipids and CAD 648*f*
HDL
  primary disorders 661
  secondary disorders 661
heart
  blunt trauma, management 725
  penetrating trauma
    aetiology 724
    investigations 724–25
    management 725
    prognosis 725
heart failure
  2009 INTERMACS classification 452*t*
  adult congenital heart disease (ACHD) 783
  aetiology 426–29
  anaemia and iron deficiency 455
  arrhythmia, pacing and device therapy 445–48
  causes of cardiomyopathy 427*t*
  classification 421–24
  CMR 75
  co-morbidities and multidisciplinary care in HF 454–55
  definitions 419
  diagnosis of HFpEF 423–24
  diastolic function 423–24
  endomyocardial biopsy 431
  epidemiology and prognosis 420–21
  ESC categories 421*t*
  evaluation of patients 615
  grading
    ACC/AHA vs NYHA classification 425*t*
    Weber-Janicki classification 426*t*
  grading of HF severity 424
  H2 FPEFF score (2018) and HFA-PEFF Score (2019) 423
  HFmrEF 445
  HFpEF 423–24
  imaging 432
  indications for CRT 447*t*
  inter-atrial shunt devices 450
  intervention for secondary mitral regurgitation/HFrEF 449–50
  investigations 429–33
    99mTc-DPD scintigraphy 431
    blood laboratory testing 430–31
    ECG abnormalities 430*t*
    exercise testing 431
  key CRT studies 448
  key randomized controlled trials 437*t*
  long-term follow-up and monitoring 455
  mechanical circulatory support (MCS) 450–53
  medical management 433–45
  multidisciplinary team management recommendations 455
  natriuretic peptides (NPs), 422–23, 422*b*
  non-cardiac surgery 848
  palliative care 458–59
  pathophysiology 428–29
  pharmacology
    ARBs 441
    ARNIs 439–40
    beta blockers 438–39
    digoxin 444–45
    diuretics 442
  hydralazine and isosorbide dinitrate (H-ISDN) 442–43
    little/no benefit therapies 445
    mineralocorticoid receptor antagonists 439
    SGCSs 444
    SGLT2 inhibitors 440–41
  pharmacology for use in HFrEF 433
    dosage 435*t*
    RAAS and NP system 438*f*
    with reduced ejection fraction *see* cardiac resynchronization therapy
  rheumatic valve disease 205
  SGLT-2 inhibitors 433, 434, 435*t*
  signs and symptoms 420*t*
  symptoms 200
  Weber classification for grading severity 615*t*
  see also acute heart failure; congestive cardiac failure
Heart Failure Survival Score (HFSS) 616
Heart Team, CCS 162
heart transplantation 453
  contraindications 454*t*, 496
  indications 496
  patient factors 454*t*
  selection for 615–16
hemitruncus arteriosus, 86
His bundle 275
His bundle pacing, CRT 412
HIV cardiomyopathy 490
homocysteine, defective methionine metabolism 151
HOPE trial, ramipril 138
hybrid imaging 117–18
hypercalcaemia 295
hypercholesterolaemia, familial 204, 659–60
hyperglycaemia 563–64
hyperkalaemia 294
  and reductions in GFR 873
hyperparathyroidism 204
hypertension 552, 629–32
  acute cardiovascular care 552

Index 959

age groups 638
anti-hypertensive
    treatment 634, 635f
    single pill combination
        (SPC) 634–38, 635f
anti-hypertensives vs
    placebo 636–37
diabetes 638–39
grade definitions 630t
hypertensive emergencies
    641t
malignant
    hypertension 640–41
multi-valvular disease 241
non-cardiac surgery 851
pregnancy 639, 831
renal disease 639
resistant 639–40
secondary causes 633
specific considerations 635
sport and 605–6, 607t
stroke 639
stroke risk 861
summary of evidence 638
treatment targets (ESC
    2018) 634
when to treat 634, 635f
see also arterial hypertension
hypertension-mediated
    organ damage
    (HMOD) 633–34
hypertrabeculation/non-
    compaction,
    LV 494–95
hypertriglyceridaemia,
    causes 662t
hypertrophic CM 462–71
    abnormalities of mitral valve
        apparatus 463–64
    aborted 576
    cardiac MRI 466–67
    clinical presentation 464
    CMR 75–76
        late gadolinium
            enhancement
            (LGE) 75
    diagnosis 464–67
    diastolic dysfunction 464
    differential diagnosis, 35t
    ECG guidelines to
        diagnosis 466b
    echo guidelines to
        diagnosis 465b
    echo techniques, 33–34
    electrocardiography 465
    genetic testing 465

genetics 463
key to diagnosis 462
LGE pattern 75
management 468
    alcohol septal
        ablation 469
    atrial tachyarrhythmias
        469
    dual chamber pacing 469
    heart failure 469
    LVOT obstruction 468–69
    primary/secondary
        prevention 471f
    SCD 470
    ventricular septal
        myectomy 468–69
microvascular ischaemia, 464
myocardial fibrosis 463
    CMR 76
    extracellular volume (ECV)
        fraction CMR 76
    pathophysiology 463–64
physiology vs
    pathology 599–600
prognosis and
    outcome 467–68
recommendations for
    competition 601–2
risk factors for SCD 467b
SCD 597
screening 467
T1 mapping 76
hypocalcaemia 295
hypokalaemia 294
hypomagnesaemia 295
hypotension 549–51
hypothermia 296
    temperature management
        and warming 541–42

[123]iodine-metaiodobenyzl-
    guanidine
    (mIBG), sympathetic
    innervation
    imaging 118
ICU
    communication, palliation,
        and end-of-life
        care 566
    oxygenation and ventilatory
        support 542–43
    respiratory failure in acute
        care 542
    temperature management
        and warming 541–42

thromboprophylaxis 560–61
time course 542t
see also acute cardiovascular
    care
imaging, cardio-oncology
    533–34
immune checkpoint
    inhibitors 528
implantable cardioverter
    defibrillator 313–14,
    391
anti-tachycardia pacing
    (ATP) 399
arrhythmia detection 396
box plots 402
complications and
    deactivation 403–4
defibrillation safety margin
    (DSM) 393
defibrillation threshold
    (DFT) 393–94
device interrogation and
    follow-up 402–3
device therapy 398–99
ESC guidelines 392
essential features of all
    ICDs 391
NICE guidelines (UK) 393,
    394b
and pacemakers,
    competitive sports
    recommended 604
primary prevention
    trials 392
programming 396–97
secondary prevention
    trials 391–92
shock vectors 394
subcutaneous ICDs 399–402
SVT discriminators 398
troubleshooting 404–7
wearable ICDs 402
inborn errors of
    metabolism 486t
incidental findings, CMR 89
inclusion body myositis 912
infective endocarditis 103–4,
    200
adult congenital heart disease
    (ACHD) 783
affecting cardiac implantable
    electronic devices
    (CDRIE) 264–65
antibiotic prophylaxis 267
antibiotic treatment 260–62
classification, high risk 268t

infective endocarditis (cont.)
  classification and terminology 250
  complications 258–59
  computed tomography 257
  definition 249
  diagnosis 252–59
    ESC algorithm 255, 255f
    ESC criteria 252b
  echocardiography 51–52, 256–57
  epidemiology 249–50
  ESC IE new guidelines 268–69
  magnetic resonance imaging 257
  microbiological diagnosis 257–58
  microbiology 251
  multi-valvular disease 233
  multidisciplinary management 265–67, 266f
  non-antibiotic prevention 268–69
  non-bacterial thrombotic endocarditis (NBTE) 265
  nuclear imaging 257
  pathophysiology 251–52
  pregnancy, 833
  prevention 807–10
  prognosis 259–60
  surgical treatment 263–64
infective issues, acute cardiovascular care 564–65
inferior vena cava (IVC), size and respiratory changes, 60
infiltrative myocardial disease, CMR 77
inflammatory bowel disease (IBD)-related arthritis 905
inflammatory cardiomyopathy 461, 490f
  viruses 489b
inotropes 549–51
instantaneous wave free ratio (iFR)
  compared to FFR 181
  definition 179
insulin therapy, blood glucose management 541–42
intensive care unit (ICU) see acute cardiovascular care

intramyocardial haemorrhage (IMH), 73
intravascular ultrasound (IVUS) 181
  myocardial revascularization 181
intraventricular conduction 324
intraventricular conduction delay 288
Ionising Radiation (Medical Exposure) Regulations 165
Irbesartan Diabetic Nephropathy Trial (IDNT) 636
iron overload cardiomyopathy, CMR 78
ischaemia, pregnancy, 829–31
ischaemia and infarction 282f, 283–86
ISCHAEMIA-CKD trial 873
ischaemic heart disease
  CMR 73
  concealed 596–97
  evaluation of infarct size and myocardial viability 73
  SCD 596–97
  sport and 605
  see also myocardial ischaemia
ischaemic stroke
  classification 857–58
  see also stroke
ivabrodine, CCS 160

J-wave, or Osborne wave 296
Jervell–Lange–Nielsen syndrome 385
Joint British Societies recommendations on prevention of cardiovascular disease 630

Kussmaul's sign 193t, 509

lacunar syndrome 858
Laplace law, aorta wall stress 694
LDL
  cardiovascular risk 646
  primary disorders 659

LDL-C, intervention strategies 656–57, 657f
left anterior/posterior fascicular block 323f
left atrial ablation 365
left atrial appendage thrombus 102
left atrium
  echo 30–32
  normal values for LA linear and area measurements, 31t
left bundle branch area pacing (LBBAP) 413
left bundle branch block (LBBB)
  bi-and tri-fascicular block 285, 286–92, 287b, 288
  conduction disturbances 286–92
  hemi-fascicular block 287
  Sgarbossa criteria 127
left heart contrast agents, echo 15t
left ventricle
  anatomy, size, function, 27–28
  regional LV function: ischaemia, 23–24
  relative wall thickness and hypertrophy, 27f
  scoring to assess wall motion, 25t
  systolic and diastolic function, reference values, 18t
left ventricle filling pressure, echo grading, 58
left ventricle mass, scaling for body size, and hypertrophy, 24–27
left ventricle myocardial non-compaction, 36
left ventricle outflow tract
  elliptical vs circular, 59
  measurement, 59
  obstruction, 34
left ventricle systolic function, echo assessment of 18
left ventricular assist device (LVAD) 453
  complications 453
left ventricular dysfunction 547–48

left ventricular hypertrabeculation/
non-compaction
494–95
left ventricular
hypertrophy 201
concentric 78
ECG features 281
ECG voltage criteria 280f
multiple voltage criteria 280t
Romhilt–Estes Score, 281t
left ventricular impairment 946
left ventricular
non-compaction 79
physiology vs pathology 600
left ventriculography 177, 178f
leucocyte scintigraphy 118
levocardia 777
levocardia with situs
inversus, 777
Lewis ECG voltage, RVH
criteria 282t
lifestyle
body weight 650
cigarette smoking, BP,
cholesterol 620t
interventions to reduce
TC and LDL-C
levels 649t
physical activity 650
specific lifestyle changes 649t
target changes 635
lipid control, pharmacological
strategy 656–58
lipid goals, saturated fat
intake 647–49
lipid molecules and
metabolism 643–46
cholesterol/ esters 643
lipid profile abnormalities,
Fredrickson
classification system
7.4T2
lipid treatment goals 647–50
lipid-modifying therapy 625
lipids
hazard ratios, CAD 648f
LDL-C recommendations
650
triglycerides 650
lipoma 82–85
interatrial septum 520
lipoproteins
chylomicrons 645f, 645–46
HDL 645
LDL 645
lipoprotein(a) 151, 646

plasma lipoproteins and
apolipoproteins 644
triglycerides 643–44
VLDL 645–46
liver congestion and venous
flow, echo 60–64
Loeffler's endocarditis 79
Loeys–Dietz syndrome
aortic dissection 598
pregnancy, 827
long QT syndrome 383–85
genetics 385
LQTS score 292–94, 384t
management 385
risk of SCD 580
SCD 598
sports participation 604
sub-types 384–85
low density lipoprotein
(LDL) 204
Lown-Ganong-Levine
syndrome 350
lupus erythematosus 204
LV aneurysm, ACS 140
LV dysfunction, ACS 140
LV thrombus, ACS 140–41
Lyme disease 491
lymphoma, 82–85, 524

macro aggregated albumin
(MAA) 118–19
MADIT study, ICD 392
MADIT-CRT 410
Mahaim physiology 350
Marfan syndrome 693, 700
aortic disease 200, 203
pregnancy, 826–27
mesocardia 777
mesothelioma 82–85
metabolic cardiomyopathy
491–92
metabolic syndrome
and accelerated
atherosclerosis 946
CVD risk 625
definition 625
diagnosis 625t
first-line therapy 625
metformin, increased risk of
lactic acidosis 874
methionine, defective
methionine
metabolism 151
micronutrients, dietary
supplementation,

no evidence of CV
benefit 687
mineralocorticoid receptor
antagonists 439
minute ventilation/carbon
dioxide (VE/VCO2)
slope 612–13
mitochondrial diseases 866
mitochondrial encephalopathy
with lactic acidosis
and stroke-like
episodes 866
mitral regurgitation 104, 192
aetiology 211–12
assessment of MV
morphology, 41
assessment of
severity, 41–44
asymptomatic severe
primary 214–15
colour Doppler imaging, 41
examination
cardiac auscultation 213
precordial palpation 212
fibrosis on LGE imaging 81
functional 215
investigations
cardiac MRI 213
chest radiograph 213
electrocardiogram 213
grading severity of primary
MR, 44t
medical management 213,
216f
non-cardiac surgery 849
pathophysiology 212
pregnancy, 821
secondary (functional) 141,
212
severe secondary 215
TEER 215
sport and 608
surgical/percutaneous
management, ESC
guidelines 214–15,
214f
see also multi-valvular disease
mitral stenosis 38–40, 190–91,
191t, 693, 700
aetiology 215–16
assessment of severity, 41t
examination 217–18
investigations 218
medical management 219
pathophysiology 217
sport and 608

mitral stenosis (cont.)
    surgical management 219,
        220f
        Wilkins classification
            219t
    symptomatic rheumatic
        MS 219–21
    symptoms 217
    see also multi-valvular
        disease
mitral valve
    anatomy 211
    interventions 102
mixed valvular disease see
    multi-valvular
    disease
modified Rankin Scale 735t
molecular-targeted agents,
    cardiac side
    effects 529t
Morris index, defining LA
    enlargement by ECG
    criteria 279
MR angiography 72
MRI conditional pacemakers
    414
multi-detector computed
    tomography
    (MDCT) 91
    requirements 92
multi-valvular disease 235–41
    abnormal loading
        conditions 234
    aetiologies 233, 234
    chamber remodelling and
        annular dilation 234
    echocardiographic
        assessment 235
    impact of concomitant
        co-morbidities 241
    management and
        follow-up 242
    progressive valvular
        dysfunction (stenosis
        or regurgitation) 234
    symptoms of
        co-morbidities 241
muprocin 564
muscular dystrophy
    Becker 864
    cardiac manifestations
        493t
    cardiomyopathy 492
    Duchenne 863–64
Mustard or Senning operation,
    atrial switch 798–99

myocardial bridging 101
myocardial diseases
    inflammatory myocardial
        disease 488–91
    secondary 491–96
myocardial infarction
    and chronic kidney
        disease 870–77
    classification 130
    ECG changes in an
        ST-elevation MI 283
    fourth universal
        definition 129–30
    loss of R-wave and
        development
        of pathological
        Q-waves 284
myocardial thinning 101
pregnancy, 829–31
RV 284
ST-elevation ECG
    changes 283f
ST-elevation MI (STEMI)
    equivalents 283f, 284
myocardial infarction/
    injury, non-cardiac
    surgery 853–54
myocardial ischaemia 151–52
    oxygen supply/demand
        mismatch 152f
    quantified burden 114t, 114f,
        115f
    see also ischaemic heart
        disease
myocardial oedema 79
myocardial perfusion
    scintigraphy
    (MPS) 108–16
    cameras and isotopes 109–10
    clinical value 113–16
    image interpretation 113
    limitations 116
    reporting 116
    sensitivity and specificity 129
myocardial revascularization
    2018 ESC guidelines 167
    2018 recommendations,
        FFR or iFR first
        line 179
    intravascular ultrasound
        (IVUS) 181
myocardial stunning,
    hibernation, and
    viability 152
myocardial viability
    assessment 128, 129, 152

myocarditis 297–98
    cardiotropic viruses 489b
    CMR 77
    endomyocardial biopsy 80
    Lake Louise Consensus
        Criteria 80
    protozoal 490–91
    recommendations for
        competition 602
    SCD 597
myoclonic epilepsy with
    ragged red fibres
    (MERRF) 866
myofibrillar myopathies 866–67
myositis spectrum
    disorders 912–13
myotonic dystrophy 865–66
myxoma 82–85
    atrial 519

necrotizing autoimmune
    myositis 912
nephrogenic systemic fibrosis
    (NSF) 69
nerve blocks 558
neurological issues, acute
    cardiovascular
    care 555–58
neurological symptoms, see
    also dizziness; stroke;
    syncope
neuromuscular diseases
    with cardiac
    involvement 863–67
nicorandil, CCS 161
nitrates
    long-acting 159–60
    short-acting 159
non-cardiac surgery 837
    cardiac symptoms 839
    ECG and biomarkers
        841–42
    functional capacity or
        reserve 841
    myocardial infarction/
        injury 853–54
    open vs laparoscopic 838
    peri-operative monitoring
        and anaesthesia 853
    physiological response to 841
    pre-operative assessment
        839–42, 840f
    risk assessment 838–39
    risk reduction 842–47
    surgical risk estimate 839t

Index 963

non-cardiovascular drugs, side effects 945–46
non-dilated left ventricular CM 474–75
  clinical course and prognosis 474
  diagnostic testing 474–75
    ambulatory monitoring 474
    cardiac MRI 475
    electrocardiography 474–75
    endomyocardial biopsy 475
    genetic testing 474
  management 475
  risk assessment, screening and prognosis 475
Noonan syndrome 808, 808t
nuclear cardiology 107
  certification 108
  other nuclear cardiology investigations 118–19
  radiation protection 108
  SPECT 111
  see also myocardial perfusion scintigraphy (MPS); positron emission tomography (PET); radionuclide ventriculography (RNV)
nutrition 623–24

obesity
  Body Mass Index (BMI) 623
  multi-valvular disease 241
  non-cardiac surgery 852
obesity hypoventilation syndrome 896–97
  cardiovascular complications and prognosis 897
  epidemiology 896
  pathogenesis 897
  treatment 897
obstructive sleep apnoea
  arrhythmias and sudden death 895
  atrial fibrillation 891–96
  coronary artery disease (CAD) 894
  heart failure 895–96
  and hypertension 893–94
  pathophysiology of CV-associated disease 893

pulmonary arterial hypertension 896
ochronosis 204
Ohm's law 327
older person, ACS 144
omega-3 (n-3) fatty acids 655
omeprazole 945
opiates 558
optical coherence tomography (OCT) 182
orthostatic hypotension 306–7
  aetiology 307
  echo 311
  electrocardiography 311
  evaluation 307–9
  investigations 309–12
  lifestyle measures 312
  orthostatic challenges 310
  risk stratification 308–9
  subtypes 306–7
  see also syncope
oxygen uptake, VO2 max 588

P wave, P-pulmonale 280
P2Y12 inhibitors, ACS 130
pacemaker (P) cells 274
pacemaker syndrome 328
pacemaker-mediated tachycardia (PMT) 329
pacemakers
  competitive sports recommended 604
  failure to capture 330
  follow-up 333
  nomenclature 324
  oversensing 330
  permanent 324–28
  practical considerations 331–33
  sensing and sensitivity 327
  troubleshooting 329–33
  undersensing 331
pacing
  airport metal detectors 333
  complications of pacemaker implantation 327
  DAVID trial 328
  defibrillation 332
  failure 329–30
  ICU 552–53
  indications for permanent pacing 321b
  lead impedance 327

magnet mode 328
MRI 332
relationship between threshold, pulse duration, lead impedance, and energy 326
stimulation threshold 325–27
unipolar vs bipolar pacing 325
Paget's disease of bone 919
Paget's disease 204
pain see analgesia
pain, adjuvant medications 558
palliation, and end-of-life care 566
palpitations 300–2
  sudden onset and sudden offset 342
pannus, aortic valve replacement dysfunction, assessment 103–4
papillary fibroelastoma 520–21
papillary muscle rupture, ACS 141
paraganglioma 82–85
parenteral feeding 563
paroxysmal SVT with pre-excitation, recommendations for competition 603
paroxysmal SVT without pre-excitation, recommendations for competition 603
parvovirus B19 489b
patent ductus arteriosus, 57, 796
patent foramen ovale 784–85, 784f
patient assessment 632
  risk stratification 632t
penicillin allergy 260, 261
percutaneous coronary intervention (PCI)
  ACS patients 131, 132
  complications 182–85
  contrast-related anaphylaxis 183
  fractional flow reserve, post PCI FFR and subsequent events rates and FFR 181t
peri-arrest arrhythmias 569

peri-operative blood loss, non-cardiac surgery 847
pericardial anatomy 499
pericardial cyst, 54, 523
pericardial disease
 CMR 82
 CT 105
 echo signs 52–54
 elderly people 516
 non-cardiac surgery 851
 pregnancy and lactation 515–16
 rare causes 515
 see also constrictive pericardial disease
pericardial effusion 82, 297–98, 502
 assessment 508t
 cancer patients 532
 diagnostic evaluation 507–8
 management 508
pericardial masses and tumours 82–85, 515
 cardiac metastases 524–25
 malignant, 523–25
pericardial physiology 500–1
 ventricular interdependence 501
pericardiocentesis 511b
pericarditis 297–98
 ACS 142
 acute 502–7
 aetiology 504–5, 504f
 clinical diagnosis 502, 505f
  ECG 503t
  physical signs 503t
 management 506
 recommendations for competition 602
 recurrent and chronic 506–7
 systemic disease 505
 see also Dressler's syndrome
pericardium, congenital absence, 54
peripartum cardiomyopathy 492–94, 493b
peripheral arterial disease
 abdominal aortic aneurysm 737–39
 acute limb ischaemia 732–33, 733t
 assessment 728
 CABG screening 730
 carotid artery stenting (CAS) 736

carotid intervention prior to cardiac surgery 737
carotid stenosis, ACAS (1995) and ACST (2004, 2010)
 trials 735–36
classification of severity 729t
critical limb-threatening ischaemia 731–32
diagnosis 883
epidemiology 728, 882–83
extra-cranial carotid artery disease 734–37
imaging 728
 CT 105–6
intermittent claudication 730–31
medication 730
mesenteric artery disease 739–40
modified Rankin Scale 735t
non-cardiac surgery 851
pathophysiology 728, 882–83
prevention 883
renal artery stenosis 740–41
revascularization, 731
upper limb ischaemia 733–34
vertebral artery disease 737
permanent pacemakers 324–28
persistent junctional reciprocating tachycardia (PJRT) 350
phaeochromocytoma 633
pharmacogenetics 943–45
pharmacokinetics 943–45
phosphodiesterase type 5 inhibitors (PDE5i) 770
photon-counting CT scanner 100
plasma concentration-time curve 944f
plasminogen activators (TPA) 137
PLATO trial, ticagrelor 131
polygenic hypercholesterolaemia 661
polymyositis 912
Pompe's disease 486t
positron emission tomography (PET) 107, 117
 ACS 129

post-atrial switch: Mustard or Senning operation 798–99
post-operative cognitive dysfunction (POCD) 557
Potts shunt 780
prasugrel
 ACS 131
 CAD 134
pre-load, definition 547
precordial palpation 205
pregnancy
 adult congenital heart disease (ACHD) 823–27
 anaesthesia 819
 cardiac assessment 815–16
 cardiac conditions 819–33
 cardiovascular adaptations during 814–15, 814f
 care for the cardiac patient 818–19
 CVD 813–14
  epidemiology 813–14
 delivery
  and post-partum period 815
  third stage 819
  where, mode of 818
 heart disease, risk stratification 817b
 hypertension 639
 maternal risk assessment in cardiac disease 817–18
 pulmonary embolism 754–55
 termination of pregnancy 825
pregnancy and lactation 366–67, 515–16
premature ventricular contractions, recommendations for competition 603
primary Sjögren's syndrome 911
primary systemic vasculitis 916–18
Prinzmetal's angina 124, 163
pro-protein convertase subtilisin/kexin type 9 inhibitors 655
prostacyclin analogues 770
prosthetic valves 51, 243–48
 anticoagulation management 244t, 244–45

assessment 104
choice of prosthesis
    type 243
complications 245
complications of valvular
    heart disease 103
echo parameters (identifying
    aortic valve prosthesis
    malfunction), 52t
endocarditis 104
follow-up 248
haemodynamics of 245–48
haemolysis and paravalvular
    leak 246
management of mechanical
    prosthetic
    thrombosis 246f
morphological findings, 52
non-cardiac surgery 849
non-obstructive left-sided
    thrombus 246–48
obstructive left-sided
    thrombus 245
pregnancy, 821
prosthesis–patient
    mismatch 246–48
structural valve
    degeneration 248
thrombosis 245–48, 247f
types, 51t
protamine, heparinization 560
proteasome inhibitors 528
proton pump inhibitor
    (PPI), stress ulcer
    prophylaxis 563
protozoal myocarditis 490–91
pseudoaneurysm 183
pseudoxanthoma
    elasticum 200
psoriatic arthritis 905
psychogenic pseudo-syncope 307
pulmonary artery pressure
    (PAP)
    echo parameters, 61t
    grading probability of PH
        being present, 58
pulmonary atresia with
    VSD 803–4
pulmonary disease, non-cardiac
    surgery 851
pulmonary embolism
    clinical presentation 748
    diagnosis 749
    epidemiology 748
    with haemodynamic
        instability 751f

Hestia criteria 751t
imaging 119
pregnancy 754–55
risk stratification 749–50
treatment 750–53
Wells score 753f
without haemodynamic
    instability 752f
pulmonary haemodynamics,
    echo parameters, 61t
pulmonary hypertension 58,
    192, 759
clinical classification 760,
    761t
diagnosis 762–67
diagnostic algorithm
    of unexplained
    dyspnoea 768f
epidemiology and
    genetics 760–62
haemodynamic
    classification 760
investigations 764–67
    blood tests 766
    CMR 765
    echo signs, grading
        probability of PH
        being present, 58t
    echocardiographic
        assessment 763f, 765f
    lung function tests 765
    right heart
        catheterization 759,
        766
non-cardiac surgery 851
and normal left atrial
    pressures 192t
pathophysiology 762
pregnancy, 825
risk assessment 767, 769t
    variables calculation of
        simplified 4-strata
        assessment
        tool, 769t
specific types
    PH-LD 773
    PH-LHD 772–73
symptoms 763
treatment
    adjunctive therapy 767–71
    combination therapy 771
    specific pharmacologic
        therapy 768–71
    surgical and interventional
        options 771
    treatment algorithm 772f

pulmonary perfusion, and
    right-to-left
    shunting 118–19
pulmonary regurgitation
    aetiology 229
    assessment of
        severity, 50–51
    investigations 230
    see also multi-valvular
        disease
pulmonary stenosis
    aetiology 230
    investigations 231–32
    pathophysiology 38, 231
    pregnancy, 825
pulmonary vascular
    resistance 189
pulmonary vein isolation
    (PVI) 102
pulmonary veins, number and
    location, CMR 88
pulse oximetry
    plethysmography
    168
pulsus paradoxus 509

QResearch database 619t
QRS complex, cardiac
    axis 277f
QRS morphology, right
    ventricular
    hypertrophy 280
QT prolongation 946
    drug causes 295b, 946
    Torsades de Pointes 381
Quincke's pulse 201

[82]Rubidium, positron emission
    tomography 117
RAAS inhibitors 469, 843, 873
    non-cardiac surgery 843
radiation
    cardiac complications
        from 488t, 531
    inverse-square law of
        radiation 166
radiation protection
    nuclear cardiology 108
    strategies 166
radiolabelled leucocyte
    scintigraphy 118
radionuclide ventriculography
    (RNV) 107, 116–17
    equilibrium RNV, 116–17

Index

radiotherapy
  cardiac side effects 531
  see also radiation
randomized controlled trials
    (RCTs), key (ACE-I,
    BB, ARNI, If) 437t
ranolazine, CCS 160
RAS inhibitors 873
  albuminuria 635, 636f
Rastelli operation 799–800
reactive arthritis 905
red blood cell transfusion 560
reflex syncope (neurally
    mediated) 305–6
regadenoson, nuclear
    cardiology 110
relapsing polychondritis 920
renal disease
  non-cardiac surgery 852
  parenchymal disease 633
  see also chronic kidney
    disease
renal issues, ICU 553–55
renal vascular disease 633
respiratory failure 542
  in acute care 542
restrictive cardiomyopathy
    192, 479–85
  amyloid heart
    disease 481–82
  cardiac catheterization 480
  clinical presentation 479,
    480f
  diagnosis 483
    electrocardiography
      and ambulatory
      monitoring 479
  diagnostic testing, CMR 78,
    479
  endomyocardial
    biopsy 480
  genetic testing 480
  management 481
  prognosis and outcome 481
  secondary RCM 481
resuscitation
  drugs 571t
  ethics 572
  post resus care 570
revascularization
  aorto-iliac occlusive
    lesions 731
  femoro-popliteal occlusive
    lesions 731
  intravascular ultrasound
    (IVUS) 181

REVERSE, mnemonic for ECG
    evidence of lead
    mal-position 279t
REVERSE trial 410
rhabdomyoma 522
rhabdomyosarcoma 524
rheumatic disorders 901–2
  miscellaneous 919–21
rheumatic fever 920–21
rheumatic valve disease 204,
    233
  angina 205
  heart failure 205
rheumatoid arthritis 902–5
RIFLE criteria, acute kidney
    injury 554t
right atrium
  echocardiography 32
  enlargement, causes 279
  sulcus terminalis 274–75
right atrium pressure
  grading probability
    of PH being
    present, 58
  mean, 61t
right bundle branch block
    (RBBB)
  bi-and tri-fascicular
    block 285, 286–92,
    287b, 288
  conduction disturbances
    286–92
right heart catheterization 759,
    766
  cardiac haemodynamics
    185–92, 185t
right ventricle
  anatomy, size,
    function, 28–29
  normal values for the RV size
    parameters, 28t
right ventricle cardiomyopathy,
  arrhythmogenic,
  echo, 35–36
right ventricle systolic
    function 16–24
  normal values for
    echocardiographic
    parameters, 23t
right ventricle volumetric
    analysis, 29
right ventricular
    dysfunction 548–49
right ventricular hypertrophy
  Butler-Leggett ECG voltage
    criteria 282t

  criteria 282t
  ECG features 282
  QRS morphology, 280
right ventricular infarction 284
right-to-left shunting 118–19
rivaroxaban, CAD 134
Romano–Ward syndrome 385
Romhilt–Estes Score,
    left ventricular
    hypertrophy 281t

saphenous vein coronary
    bypass grafts
    (SVG) 170
sarcoid heart disease 483–84
  clinical presentation 484
  diagnosis 484, 484t
  management 484–85
sarcoidosis
  CMR 78
  LGE 78
sarcoma 82–85
  angiosarcoma 523
  fibrosarcoma 524
  rhabdomyosarcoma 524
sarcomeric protein
    mutations 463b
sarcomeric variants, HCM 573
Scimitar syndrome 789–91
SCORE, ESC Ten-year
    cardiovascular risk
    categories 631t
SCORE2 study 618, 619t, 621
sedentary behaviour and
    physical activity
  definitions 622
  guidelines 622
selective cholesterol absorption
    inhibitors 654–55
septal hypertrophy,
    asymmetric, 34
Sgarbossa's criteria, LBBB 285t
SGCSs, soluble guanylate
    cyclase receptor
    stimulators 444
SGLT-2 inhibitors
  atherosclerotic cardiovascular
    disease 673
  CKD 874
  heart failure syndromes 433,
    434, 435t
  ICD 392–93
  non-cardiac surgery 844
  VT 382
shock therapy 399

shock/haemodynamic
        instability, emergency
        echocardiography,
        63t
short QT syndrome
        (SQTS) 292, 389
    SCD 598
shunts 188f
    atrial and ventricular
        shunting 789f
    Glenn shunt 780
    inter-atrial shunt devices 450
    Potts shunt 780
    pulmonary (Qp) to systemic
        (Qs) blood flow 189
    right-to-left shunting 118–19
    systemic venous to
        pulmonary artery
        shunts 780
    Waterston shunt 780
signal artefact, common
        causes 278b
Simpson's algorithm, echo, 18t
single nucleotide
        polymorphisms 945
sinoatrial (SA) node
        disease 318–19
sinus node 274–75
sinus node disease 321b
sinus of Valsalva
    aneurysms 795
    normal values, 63t
sinus venosus defect, 56
situs solitus or inversus,
        CMR 86
Sjögren's syndrome,
        primary 911
SMILE trial, ramipril 138
Society of Thoracic Surgeons
        (STS) score,
        CCS 162
sodium channel blockers
        (Class I
        antiarrhythmics) 336
Sokolow-Lyon ECG voltage
    LVH criteria 280t
    RVH criteria 282t
sotalol 339
    Torsades de Pointes 363
speckle-tracking, deformation
        imaging, 12
spondylitis, ankylosing 200, 905
spondyloarthropathies 905–7
spontaneous coronary
        artery dissection
        (SCAD) 125

sports cardiology
    abnormal ECG findings in
        athletes 590t
    aortic root dilatation 608–9
    arrhythmogenic
        cardiomyopathy 600
    cardiomyopathies, markers
        of increased risk of
        SCD 601–2
    criteria for interpretation of
        athlete's ECG 591
    differentiating adaptation
        from
        cardiomyopathy
        599–600
    dilated cardiomyopathy
        600
    exercise physiology 588
    further investigations 592t
    heart, structural changes in
        athletes 594
    hypertrophic
        cardiomyopathy
        599–600
    International Consensus
        Standards for
        Electrocardiographic
        Interpretation in
        Athletes: Definition
        of ECG criteria 590t
    left ventricular mass
        index 594f
    left ventricular
        non-compaction 600
    recommendations 601–9
    SCD
        causes, all
            conditions 594–98
        primary prevention in
            athletes 599
        secondary prevention in
            athletes 599
Staphylococcus species, infective
        endocarditis 261
statin therapy
    ACS 137–38
    CAD 137
    chronic kidney disease 875,
        876t
    ESC recommendations
        653f
    intolerance to 656
    lipid-modifying therapy 625
    mechanism of action 650–
        51, 651f
    non-cardiac surgery 843

    side effects 652
STEMI
    posterior 284
    ST segment depression
        and T-wave
        inversion 286, 286f
    ST-elevation MI
        equivalents 284
stenotic lesions,
        pregnancy, 820–21
stent, carotid artery stenting
        (CAS) 736
stent patency 100
sternal wound infections 564
sternum, re-do
        sternotomy 100
Stokes–Adams attacks, escape
        rhythm failure 292
storage diseases 485–88
Streptococcus gallolyticus
        (formerly S. bovis)
        group 260–61
streptokinase, fibrinolytic
        therapy 137
stress
    exercise stress test 202–3,
        202f, 311–12
    image interpretation 113
    LVEF post stress 115
    nuclear cardiology 110
    protocols 110–11
    reconstructed SPECT
        images 112f
    stress echocardiography 129,
        153
    ACS 128–600
    meta-analysis 116
stress myocardial
        scintigraphy 153
stress tests, non-invasive 153
stress ulcer, prophylaxis,
        ICU 563
stroke
    acute cardiovascular
        care 557–58
    aetiology 858–61
    classification 857–58
    CT angiography of neck
        arteries/ circle of
        Willis 106
    diagnosis 862
    epidemiology 857, 880
    haemorrhagic stroke
        861–62
    medical treatment 862
    modified Rankin scale 735t

stroke (cont.)
  pathophysiology 880
  posterior circulation stroke 858
  prevention and management 558
  risk factors 557
  transient loss of consciousness and syncope 862
  treatment 881
stroke rate, CHA2 DS2-VASc score 360t
stroke volume
  calculation, 59
  echo grading, 58
Study on Cognition and Prognosis in the Elderly (SCOPE) 636
sudden arrhythmic death syndrome (SADS) 581
sudden cardiac death
  aborted 576
  aetiology 574
  in athletes 594–96
  autopsy and molecular autopsy 581
  definitions 573t
  epidemiology 573–74, 879–80
  pre-disposing conditions 574–81
  prevention 575
  recommendations 880
superficial venous thrombosis 743–48
supraventricular tachycardia
  classification and management 340–50
  pregnancy, 828–29
  termination 372
surgical site infection 564–65
surgical site infection reduction, skin preparation 564
sympathetic innervation imaging 118
syncope
  cardiac pacing 313
  driving regulations 314t
  electrophysiology study 312
  evaluation 307–9
  investigations 309–12
  pharmacological therapy 313
  physical counter-pressure manoeuvres 312

psychogenic pseudo-syncope 307
reflex, pacing 321
risk stratification 308–9
smartphone applications 312
treatment options 312–14
see also orthostatic hypotension
SYNTAX score, CCS 162
SYNTAX score II, CCS 162
systemic inflammation, in atherosclerosis 902
systemic lupus erythematosus 907–9
systemic and pulmonary vascular resistance 189
systemic sclerosis 914–16
systemic venous to pulmonary artery shunts 780

tachyarrhythmias
  automaticity 335
  electrophysiology study (EPS) 350–54
  mechanisms 335–36
  see also antiarrhythmic drugs
tachycardia
  classification and management 340–50
  guideline management 569
  invasive SVT management 350–54
  narrow complex, ECG diagnosis 340
  pathophysiology 345–46
  persistent junctional reciprocating tachycardia (PJRT) 350
  re-entrant (AVRT), pathophysiology 340–41
tachycardia-related cardiomyopathy 492
Takotsubo cardiomyopathy, CMR, 77, 79, 126, 495–96
tamponade 508–10, 551–52
  echo 53
  indications 509t, 510f
  investigations 509, 552
  management 552
Tc-99m macro aggregated albumin (MAA) 119
Tc-99m tetrofosmin study
  cameras and isotopes 109–10

image acquisition, reconstruction, and display 111
lifetime risk of cancer 108
stress protocols 110–11, 111f
Tei index, 19
temperature management and warming 541–42
teratoma 82–85
tetralogy of Fallot, pregnancy 802–4
TGFBR1 or TGFBR2 mutation (including Loeys–Dietz) 203
thallium-201 study
  cameras and isotopes 109–10
  image acquisition, reconstruction, and display 111
  lifetime risk of cancer 108
  stress protocols 110–11, 111f
thoracoabdominal aneurysms (TAA) 704
thrombocytopenia, ACS 144
thromboelastography (TEG) 559–60
thromboembolic disease
  chronic thromboembolic pulmonary hypertension (CTEPH) 755–57
  deep venous thrombosis 743–48
  pulmonary embolism 748–55
thromboprophylaxis 561
  cardiac surgery patients 560–61
  ICU 560–61
  non-cardiac surgery 846–47
thrombosis see deep venous thrombosis
thrombus, aortic valve replacement dysfunction, assessment 104
ticagrelor
  ACS 131
  CAD 134
tick-borne Lyme disease 491
tirofiban, ACS 132
tissue Doppler imaging (TDI-derived RIMP), 19
tissue plasminogen activators (recombinant TPA) 137
Torsades de Pointes 337, 363, 381

total anomalous pulmonary
    venous drainage
    (TAPVD) 791–92
total cavopulmonary connection
    (TCPC) 806
transcatheter aortic valve
    implantation
    (TAVI) 101–2
  permanent pacing 322
transient loss of consciousness
    (TLOC)
  classification and
    pathophysiology
    305–7
  driving regulations 314
  glossary 303, 304b
  prevalence 303
  see also syncope
transoesophageal
    echocardiography
    15–16
  complications post
    surgery 562
transplant cardiomyopathy,
    CMR 80
transposition of great
    arteries 86, 797–800
  congenitally corrected
    (ccTGA) 800–1
transthoracic echocardiography
    128
Traube's sign 201
trauma, aorta or heart 723–24
tricuspid annular plane
    systolic excursion
    (TAPSE), 19
tricuspid annulus, TDI, S-wave
    velocities, 19
tricuspid regurgitation
  aetiology 223–24
  assessment of
    severity, 45–46
  assessment of TV
    morphology, 45
  echo 45–46
  examination 224
  grading of severity, 48t
  pathophysiology 224
  surgical management (ESC
    guidelines 2021) 225,
    226f
tricuspid stenosis
  aetiology 225
  assessment of severity, 41t
  echo 40–41
  investigations 227

pathophysiology 225
  see also multi-valvular disease
triglycerides
  cardiovascular risk 647
  hypertriglyceridaemia 657–58
  metabolism
    disorders 661–62
trimetazidine, CCS 161
TRITON-TIMI 38,
    prasugrel 131
troponins
  biomarkers for chronic kidney
    disease 872–73
  high-sensitivity cardiac
    troponin
    (hs-cTN) 127–28
truncus arteriosus, 86, 806–7
Trypanosoma cruzi, protozoal
    myocarditis 490–91
Turner syndrome 808–9, 808t
  pregnancy, 826

upper limb ischaemia 733–34

vacuum-assisted closure
    (VAC) 565
valve assessments 189–92
valvular heart disease 80–81
  and endocarditis 103–4
  epidemiology
    developing world 197
    Western world 197
  fibrosis on LGE
    imaging 80–81
  pregnancy, 819–21
  SCD 598
  sport and 606–8
  stroke risk 859–60
  valvular morphology and
    function, 37–51
vascular disease
  CMR 87–88
  non-cardiac surgery 848–49
vascular endothelial growth
    factor (VEGF),
    signalling pathway
    inhibition 528
vasoactive medications 549–51
  acute cardiovascular
    care 549–51
vasopressors 549, 551t
Vaughan–Williams classification,
    antiarrhythmic
    drugs 336t

vena cava
  liver congestion and venous
    flow, 60–64
  respiratory changes, liver
    congestion and
    venous flow, 60–64
venous thromboembolism 561
  prophylaxis 561
ventilation, ICU
  extra-corporeal membrane
    oxygenation
    (ECMO) 543
  failed extubation 545–46
  following extubation 545–46
  high-flow nasal oxygen 543
  lung-protective
    ventilation 543–45
  mechanical ventilation 543
  non-invasive ventilation
    (NIV) 543
  prolonged ventilation 545
  rapid shallow breathing index
    (RSBI) 545
  spontaneous breathing
    trial 544–45
  ventilator settings 544
  weaning/assessing for
    extubation 544
ventilatory equivalents 611
ventricular arrhythmia
  diagnosis 375–77
  ECG characteristics 376, 376f
  morphology of ECG 379f
ventricular diastolic dysfunction,
    multi-valvular
    disease 241
ventricular function 103
ventricular
    interdependence 501
ventricular septal defect 57,
    786–88
  pregnancy and 823
  restrictive 787
ventricular septal rupture,
    ACS 141
ventricular tachycardia
  acute management of
    VT 378–80
  fascicular VT 381
  long-term management
    381–82
  management 378–82
  'normal heart' 381
  polymorphic VT 380
  right ventricular outflow tract
    (RVOT) VT 381

ventricular tachycardia (*cont.*)
  specific conditions that predispose to VT 382
ventriculography and/or aortography, automated injector system 166
viruses, inflammatory cardiomyopathies 489*b*

VO2, cardiac output at rest/peak exercise 612*f*, 612
VO2 max, aerobic capacity 611–12
VOYAGER PAD trial 730

warfarin 245, 359–60, 361, 367, 445, 553, 561, 945

water hammer or Corrigan pulse 201
Waterston shunt 780
Williams syndrome 808*t*, 810*f*
Wolff–Parkinson–White syndrome 344
  accessory pathways (AP), ablation and 366
  pre-excitation 292
  SCD 598